TEXTBOOK OF MEDICAL TREATMENT

TEXTBOOK
OF
MEDICAL TREATMENT

By Various Authors

EDITED BY

D. M. DUNLOP

B.A.(Oxon.), M.D., F.R.C.P.(Edin.)

Professor of Therapeutics and Clinical Medicine, University of Edinburgh
Physician, Royal Infirmary, Edinburgh

L. S. P. DAVIDSON

B.A.(Camb.), M.D., F.R.C.P.(Edin.), M.R.C.P.(Lond.)

Professor of Medicine and Clinical Medicine, University of Edinburgh
Physician, Royal Infirmary, Edinburgh
Formerly Regius Professor of Medicine, University of Aberdeen

J. W. McNEE

D.S.O., D.Sc., M.D.(Glas.), F.R.C.P.(Lond.)

Physician, H.M. the King in Scotland
Regius Professor of Practice of Medicine, University of Glasgow
Physician, Western Infirmary, Glasgow
Consulting Physician, University College Hospital, London

With a Foreword by

A. J. CLARK

B.A.(Camb.), M.D., D.P.H., F.R.C.P.(Lond.), F.R.S.

Professor of Materia Medica, University of Edinburgh

Reprint

EDINBURGH
E. & S. LIVINGSTONE
16 & 17 TEVIOT PLACE
1940

First Edition . . June 1939
Reprint . . February 1940

Made and Printed in Great Britain.

PREFACE

This book has been written for students and practitioners in the hope that it may fill the therapeutic gap left by the majority of textbooks on general medicine in which, owing to exigencies of space, the section devoted to treatment is often inadequate. In addition, the information given is not infrequently couched in such indefinite terms as to be of little value in helping the practitioner to determine whether a particular line of treatment is worthy of trial and, if so, how it can be put into practice. The following statements, for instance, are frequently made: "vaccines may be of value," "arsenic may be tried," "a well-balanced diet should be given," "the general health should receive attention." Further, it is not uncommon for many drugs and measures recommended by our forefathers to continue to be included in such works year after year in spite of the fact that some of them have been shown to be useless and others are known to be less efficacious than modern substitutes.

An attempt has therefore been made by the authors of this book to be extremely explicit in regard to the treatment recommended, in the hope that the directions given will suffice to enable a doctor without much previous experience to carry out the measures which have been described. As far as possible the indications, contraindications and dangers of each recommended method or drug are fully discussed.

Further, an attempt has been made to indicate why and when certain drugs and methods formerly widely used should no longer be employed for the particular purpose under discussion. From this it follows that the number of drugs advised are considerably fewer than in some books of therapeutics, but this we believe to be wise, for undue reliance on the "bottle of medicine" has tended in the past to obscure and diminish the importance of certain general measures of paramount importance which may be included under the heading "General Management of the Patient," *i.e.*, diet, rest, exercise, nursing, etc., which in the past have received too little attention in medical teaching and textbooks. In addition, the general problem of handling patients and relations under the various circumstances which continually confront the young doctor is dealt with. This entails a consideration of what information should or should not be given to the relatives and patient in certain circumstances, and general advice on where and when to send patients to sanatoria, spas or for a change of air and climate. Lastly, the good management of a case frequently requires a knowledge of common-sense psychological principles which are so important in the art of medicine.

It is well recognized that in some diseases where no specific therapy exists a variety of methods of treatment may be advocated by different authorities. In others, even though the general principles of treatment are unanimously approved, yet the details of their practical application may vary widely in different hands. For example, it would be generally admitted that a case of severe diabetes requires insulin, but opinion differs upon the type of insulin to be used, the details of its administration, and upon the quantity of carbohydrate to be allowed in the diet. No attempt has been made in this book to give a comprehensive description of all the possible methods of treatment which have been recognized to be of value. To do so would greatly increase the size of the book and would, in addition, defeat the object aimed at, namely, to present to the student and general practitioner the subject of medical therapeutics in a simple and rational form. Accordingly the authors have selected for description those methods which from their personal experience they have found to be most useful. When the procedures are of such a specialized nature as to be outside the scope of the general practitioner, only a brief outline is given.

The work is not a small handbook of treatment, nor yet a vast encyclopædia, since there are already a number of such books. Neither is it a textbook of pharmacology, since a large portion of the book deals not with drugs but with the "Management of the Case" in the widest sense of the term. It is not concerned with surgery, but includes sections on the treatment of venereal diseases, tropical medicine, some diseases peculiar to infants, common diseases of the skin, industrial diseases and the neuroses. There is, in addition, a section which describes in detail the technique of certain essential medical procedures—such as lumbar puncture, venesection, paracentesis, blood transfusion, oxygen therapy, etc.

It is a pleasure to acknowledge the help received from Mr T. H. Graham and Miss Margaret P. Russell, M.A.—Librarian and Assistant Librarian in the Royal College of Physicians,

Edinburgh—for their help in proof-reading and in the compilation of the index; to various editors and publishers who have given us permission to use certain plates and diagrams appearing in their journals, and in particular to Messrs Lippincott, of Philadelphia, the publishers of "Body Mechanics," and to Messrs Oliver & Boyd, publishers of the *Edinburgh Medical Journal*; and, lastly, to Mr McDonald Walker, of Messrs E. & S. Livingstone, who on all occasions has assisted us in every possible way.

D. M. DUNLOP.
L. S. P. DAVIDSON.
J. W. McNEE.

1939.

PREFACE TO THE REPRINT

THE hope entertained by the Editors that a book of this nature on rational therapeutics would prove to be of some service to medical practitioners and students has been realized by the fact that a large first edition of the work has been exhausted within seven months of publication. It has been felt that a completely new edition so soon after publication would be premature, and indeed its compilation would have been fraught with considerable difficulty owing to the dispersal on war service of many of the contributors. The opportunity has, however, been taken of bringing the present reprint up to date.

The whole book has been revised and certain errors of omission and commission corrected, to many of which our attention has been drawn by kindly critics. Owing to the rapid advance of sulphonamide chemotherapy these emendations have been particularly numerous and extensive in the sections devoted to Cerebrospinal Fever, Septicæmias, Venereal Diseases and Respiratory Diseases. Further, the growing importance of sex hormones in therapeutics has made it necessary to devote a separate section to this subject. For the sake of convenience in reprinting this has been added at the end of the book. Lastly, a serious omission has been rectified by the insertion of some pages on the treatment of alcoholism and drug addiction.

D. M. DUNLOP.
L. S. P. DAVIDSON.
J. W. McNEE.

1940.

CONTRIBUTORS

Infectious Diseases.	W. T. Benson, B.Sc., M.D., F.R.C.P.Ed., D.P.H., D.T.M.&H., late Assistant M.O.H., Edinburgh; late Medical Superintendent, Edinburgh City Hospital.
Septicæmia and Erysipelas.	W. R. Snodgrass, M.A., B.Sc., M.D., F.R.F.P.S.Glas., Physician, Southern General Hospital, and Assistant Physician, Western Infirmary, Glasgow. T. Anderson, M.B., Ch.B., M.R.C.P.Ed., Deputy Physician Superintendent, Ruchill Fever Hospital, Glasgow.
Tuberculosis.	D. M. Dunlop, B.A.Oxon., M.D., F.R.C.P.Ed., Professor of Therapeutics and Clinical Medicine, Edinburgh University. Bruce M. Dick, M.B., Ch.B., F.R.C.S.Ed., Lecturer in Tuberculosis and Clinical Surgery, Edinburgh University.
Common Diseases of the Skin.	G. H. Percival, Ph.D., M.D., D.P.H., F.R.C.P.Ed., Physician, Department of Diseases of Skin, Royal Infirmary, Edinburgh.
Venereal Diseases.	Robert Lees, M.D., F.R.C.P.Ed., Assistant Medical Officer, V.D. Department, Royal Infirmary, Edinburgh; Assistant, V.D. and Ante-Natal Department, Royal Maternity Hospital, Edinburgh.
Common Tropical Diseases and Helminthic Infections.	Lt.-Col. E. D. W. Greig, C.I.E., D.Sc., M.D., C.M., F.R.C.P.Ed., late Lecturer in Diseases of Tropical Climates, Edinburgh University.
Some Common Disorders in Infancy and Early Childhood.	G. B. Fleming, M.B.E., B.A., M.D.Camb., F.R.F.P.S.Glas., Professor of Medical Pædiatrics, Glasgow University. S. G. Graham, M.D., F.R.F.P.S.Glas., Lecturer on Medical Diseases of Infancy and Childhood, Glasgow University.

Industrial Diseases.	T. Ferguson, D.Sc., M.D., D.P.H., F.R.C.P.Ed.
Metabolic Diseases— Diabetes, Obesity.	Professor Dunlop. Ruth Pybus, Sister Dietitian, Royal Infirmary, Edinburgh.
Deficiency Diseases.	Noah Morris, D.Sc., M.D., D.P.H., F.R.F.P.S.Glas., M.R.C.P.Lond., Professor of Materia Medica and Therapeutics, Glasgow University.
Diseases of the Ductless Glands— Thyroid.	I. G. W. Hill, M.B., Ch.B., F.R.C.P.Ed., Assistant Physician, Royal Infirmary, Edinburgh.
Suprarenals, etc.	Professor Morris.
Diseases of the Blood, Spleen and Lymphatic Glands.	L. S. P. Davidson, B.A.Camb., M.D., F.R.C.P.Ed., M.R.C.P.Lond., Professor of Medicine, Edinburgh University. H. W. Fullerton, M.A., M.D.Aberd., Lecturer in Medicine, Aberdeen University.
Diseases of the Alimentary Canal.	J. W. McNee, D.S.O., D.Sc., M.D., F.R.C.P.Lond., Regius Professor of Practice of Medicine, Glasgow University. David Smith, M.D., F.R.F.P.S.Glas., Physician, Royal Infirmary, Glasgow.
Diseases of the Liver, Gall-bladder and Biliary Tract, Pancreas and Peritoneum.	Professor McNee.
Diseases of the Heart and Circulation.	A. Rae Gilchrist, M.D., F.R.C.P.Ed., M.R.C.P.Lond., Physician, Royal Infirmary, Edinburgh. I. G. W. Hill.
Diseases of the Blood Vessels of the Limbs.	J. R. Learmonth, Ch.M., F.R.C.S.Ed., Professor of Surgery, Edinburgh University. W. M. Arnott, B.Sc., M.D., F.R.C.P.Ed., Lecturer in Therapeutics, Edinburgh University.
Diseases of the Nose, Throat and Ear.	I. Simson Hall, M.B., Ch.B., F.R.C.P.Ed., F.R.C.S.Ed., Surgeon, Ear, Nose and Throat Department, Royal Infirmary, Edinburgh.

Diseases of the Respiratory System.	Professor Davidson. Ian Gordon, B.Sc., M.B., Ch.B.Aberd., M.R.C.P.Lond., Assistant Physician, Royal Infirmary, Aberdeen.
Renal Diseases.	J. D. S. Cameron, M.D., F.R.C.P.Ed., Assistant Physician, Royal Infirmary, Edinburgh. J. N. Cruickshank, M.C., D.Sc., M.D., F.R.F.P.S.Glas., F.R.C.P.Lond., Physician, Royal Infirmary, Glasgow.
Chronic Rheumatic Diseases and Diseases of Bone.	Professor Davidson. J. J. R. Duthie, M.B., Ch.B.Aberd., Assistant in Department of Medicine, Edinburgh University.
Diseases of the Nervous System.	W. Ritchie Russell, M.D., F.R.C.P.Ed., M.R.C.P.Lond., Assistant Physician, Royal Infirmary, Edinburgh; Lecturer in Neurology, Edinburgh University.
Psychotherapy in General Practice.	D. R. MacCalman, M.D.Glas., Lecturer in Psycho-pathology, Aberdeen University; Medical Officer in Charge of Department of Psychological Medicine, Royal Infirmary, Aberdeen.
Female Sex Endocrinology.	T. N. MacGregor, M.D., F.R.C.S.Ed., M.R.C.O.G., Junior Assistant Obstetrician and Gynæcologist, the Royal Infirmary, Edinburgh.
Technical Procedures and Oxygen Therapy.	Professor Learmonth. I. G. W. Hill.

CONTENTS

INFECTIOUS DISEASES

	PAGE
General Management	1
Anthrax	11
Cerebrospinal Fever	13
Chickenpox	18
Diphtheria	19
Bacillary Dysentery	25
Chronic Dysentery	29
Enteric Fever	30
Encephalitis Lethargica	37
Glandular Fever	38
Influenza	40
Measles	42
Mumps	47
Acute Poliomyelitis	49
Psittacosis	52
Rubella	53
Scarlet Fever	54
Smallpox	60
Tetanus	64
Typhus Fever	67
Whooping-cough	70
Serum Sickness	74

SEPTICÆMIA AND ERYSIPELAS

Septicæmia	78
Erysipelas	88

TUBERCULOSIS

Prevention	92
Pulmonary Tuberculosis	100
General Management	100
Tuberculin	116
Gold	119
Collapse Therapy	121
Symptomatic Treatment	130
Pleurisy with Effusion	136
Laryngeal Tuberculosis	138
Renal Tuberculosis	141
Tuberculosis of the Epididymis	143
Glandular Tuberculosis	143
Tuberculous Peritonitis	147
Tuberculosis of the Skin	148

COMMON DISEASES OF THE SKIN

Introduction	150
Bacterial Infections	162
Impetigo Contagiosa	162
Furunculosis	164
Sycosis	165
Parasitic Infections	167
Ringworm	167
Scabies	171
Pediculosis	172
Acne	173
Rosacea	175
Dermatitis	176
Due to External Causes	177
Due to Internal Causes	179
Dermatitis—*contd.*	
Varicose Dermatitis	181
Occupational Dermatitis	182
Pruritus	182
Urticaria	185
Drug Eruptions	186
Bullous Eruptions	186
Herpes Simplex	186
Herpes Zoster	187
Alopecia	187
Pityriasis Rosea	188
Lichen Planus	188
Psoriasis	189

VENEREAL DISEASES

	PAGE
Introduction	192
Gonorrhœa	193
Management of Male Case	198
Management of Female Case	201
Vulvovaginitis of Children	204
Infection of the Eye	205
Syphilis	206
Management of Early Syphilis	210
Management of Late Syphilis	212
Syphilis during Pregnancy	214
Syphilis—*contd.*	
Cardio-vascular Syphilis	214
Congenital Syphilis	215
Syphilis of the Central Nervous System	216
Chancroid	224
Lympho-granuloma Inguinale	225
Venereal Warts	225
Herpes Genitalis	225
Balanitis	226

COMMON TROPICAL DISEASES AND HELMINTHIC INFECTIONS

Introduction	227
Malaria and Blackwater Fever	228
African Trypanosomiasis	233
Leishmaniasis	235
Infectious Jaundice	238
Rat-bite Fever	239
Undulant Fever	240
Cholera	241
Amœbic Dysentery	244
Sprue	247
Leprosy	250
Yaws	252
Rabies	254
Tropical Neurasthenia	255
Helminthic Infections	256
Schistosomiasis	256
Cestodiasis	258
Filariasis	260
Ankylostomiasis	262
Enterobiasis	264
Ascariasis	264
Trichuris Trichiura	265

SOME COMMON DISORDERS IN INFANCY AND EARLY CHILDHOOD

Introduction	266
Nursing	266
Special Methods of Feeding	268
Special Methods of Giving Fluid	269
Neo-natal Conditions	271
Prematurity	271
Inanition Fever	273
Sepsis Neonatorum	273
Melæna Neonatorum	274
Hæmolytic Anæmia and Jaundice	274
Birth Injuries	275
Diseases of the Digestive System	278
Stomatitis	278
Vomiting	279
Constipation	282
Gastro-enteritis	283
Acute Ileocolitis	284
Diseases of the Digestive System—*contd.*	
Cœliac Disease	285
Milk Modifications	286
Diseases of the Respiratory System	287
Colds	287
Otitis Media	287
Bronchitis and Pneumonia	288
Empyema	290
Pulmonary Fibrosis and Bronchiectasis	290
Atelectasis	292
Diseases of the Nervous System	292
Convulsions	292
Mental Deficiency	295
Enuresis	296
Cyclical Vomiting	297
Pink Disease	299

INDUSTRIAL DISEASES

	PAGE		PAGE
Introduction	300	Poisonous Gases	310
Effects of High Temperatures	302	Industrial Dust Diseases	315
Work in Compressed Air	304	Industrial Dermatitis	317
Work with Pneumatic Drills	304	Industrial Cancer	319
Miners' Nystagmus	305	Injury from Radio-active Substances	320
Poisoning by Metals	306		

METABOLIC DISEASES

Diabetes Mellitus	323	Obesity—*contd.*	
Dietetic Treatment	323	Thyroid Treatment	396
Insulin Treatment	341	Management of Case	398
Diabetic Coma	351	Deficiency Diseases	401
Zinc Protamine Insulin	354	Introduction	401
Diabetes in Children	363	Vitamin A Deficiency	402
Diabetes and Pregnancy	372	Beri-beri	404
Complications of Diabetes	376	Pellagra	408
The Surgical Diabetic	382	Scurvy	410
Obesity	387	Rickets	413
Introduction	387	Teta	423
Dietetic Treatment	389		

DISEASES OF THE DUCTLESS GLANDS

The Thyroid	428	The Suprarenal Glands	450
Simple Goitre	428	Addison's Disease	450
Cretinism	430	Tumours of the Adrenals	453
Myxœdema	431	Diseases of the Gonads	454
Hyperthyroidism	432	Diseases of the Pituitary	456
The Parathyroid Glands	447	Diabetes Insipidus	456
Tetania Parathyropriva	447	Adenomata	457
Hyperparathyroidism	449	Pituitary Infantilism	458
		Simmond's Disease	459

DISEASES OF THE BLOOD, SPLEEN AND LYMPHATIC GLANDS

Introduction	460	Splenic Anæmia	497
Classification	461	Polycythæmia Vera	502
Anæmias due to Iron Deficiency	462	Enterogenous Cyanosis	506
Chronic Nutritional Hypochromic Anæmia	464	The Purpuras	507
Nutritional Hypochromic Anæmia of Infancy	473	Hæmophilia	518
Post-hæmorrhagic Anæmia	475	Agranulocytic Angina	521
Pernicious Anæmia and Other Macrocytic Anæmias	480	Diseases of the Reticulo-endothelial System	524
Hæmolytic Anæmias	488	The Leukæmias	524
Aplastic and Hypoplastic Anæmia	494	Aleukæmic Leukæmia	529
		Hodgkin's Disease	530

DISEASES OF THE ALIMENTARY CANAL

	PAGE
Diseases of the Œsophagus	532
Œsophagitis	532
Dysphagia	533
Peptic Ulcer of Œsophagus	535
Diseases of the Stomach	536
Gastritis	540
Peptic Ulcer	542
Cancer of the Stomach	561
Anorexia Nervosa	562
Common Functional Disorders	563
Uncommon Disorders	564
Diseases of the Intestines	565
Diarrhœa	567
Constipation	573
Regional Ileitis	584
Mucous Colitis	585
Ulcerative Colitis	587
Diverticulosis and Diverticulitis	591
Idiopathic Steatorrhœa	591
Intestinal Obstruction	593
Megacolon	594
Diets for Intestinal Diseases	595

DISEASES OF THE LIVER, GALL-BLADDER AND BILIARY TRACT, PANCREAS AND PERITONEUM

	PAGE
Diseases of the Liver	602
Jaundice	606
Acute Yellow Atrophy	609
Cirrhosis	610
Diseases of the Gall-bladder and Biliary Tract	614
Cholecystitis	616
Diseases of the Gall-bladder and Biliary Tract—*contd.*	
Gall-stones	619
Carcinoma of the Gall-bladder or Bile Ducts	622
Diseases of the Pancreas	623
Diseases of the Peritoneum	625

DISEASES OF THE HEART AND CIRCULATION

	PAGE
Introduction	627
The Heart and Circulation in Infections	633
Rheumatic Carditis	633
Non-Rheumatic Endocarditis	639
Pericarditis	640
Circulatory Failure in Acute Infections	643
Focal Sepsis in Relation to Heart Disease	644
Management of the Ambulant Cardiac Patient	645
Essential Hypertension	650
Cardiovascular Syphilis	654
The Senile Heart	658
Heart Disease in Relation to Pregnancy	660
Congenital Heart Disease	663
Heart Failure	665
Congestive Heart Failure	666
Anginal Heart Failure	692
Dyspnœic Heart Failure	699
Disorders of Rhythm	703
Auricular Fibrillation	703
Auricular Flutter	707
Paroxysmal Tachycardia	708
Heart-block	711
Extra-systoles	712
Surgery in the Treatment of Cardiac Disease	713
The Cardiac Neuroses	718
Acute Circulatory Failure	723
Simple Syncope	724
Cardiac Syncope	725
Collapse and Shock	727

DISEASES OF THE BLOOD VESSELS OF THE LIMBS

PAGE
Physiology 731
Classification 732
Sudden Obstruction of Larger Arteries 733
Gradual Obstruction of Arteries 734
Intermittent Obstruction of Arteries 740
Erythro-cyanosis . . . 741

DISEASES OF THE NOSE, THROAT AND EAR

The Nose 743
Physiology 743
Injuries 745
Rhinitis 749
Ozæna 750
Polypi 750
Nasal Allergy 751
Foreign Bodies 751
Sinusitis 752
The Pharynx 755
Tonsillitis 755
Pharyngitis 760
The Pharynx—*contd.*
Retropharyngeal Abscess . 761
Pharyngeal Neuroses . . 761
The Ear 762
Diseases of the External Ear 762
Affections of the Drum . 764
Acute Otitis Media . . 764
Chronic Otitis Media . . 768
Middle-ear Deafness . . 770
Deaf Aids 770
Laryngitis 771

DISEASES OF THE RESPIRATORY SYSTEM

Prevention 775
Acute Coryza 779
Acute Bronchitis and Broncho-pneumonia 782
Chronic Bronchitis and Emphysema 792
Lobar Pneumonia 795
Acute Empyema . . . 809
Spontaneous Pneumothorax . 810
Bronchiectasis . . . 812
Abscess and Gangrene of the Lung 818
Post-operative Pulmonary Complications . . . 820
Intrathoracic New Growths . 822
Asthma 823
Hay Fever 843
Paroxysmal Rhinorrhœa . 846

RENAL DISEASES

Nephritis 851
Introduction 851
Acute Nephritis 852
Nephrosis 858
Azotæmic Nephritis . . 861
Hydronephrosis 867
Infections of the Urinary Tract 869
Renal Calculus . . . 882
Phosphaturia 884
Oxaluria 885

CHRONIC RHEUMATIC DISEASES AND DISEASES OF BONE

Introduction 886
Classification 889
Prophylaxis 891
Rheumatoid Arthritis . . 894
Osteo-arthritis . . . 923
Chronic Menopausal Arthritis . 925

CHRONIC RHEUMATIC DISEASES AND DISEASES OF BONE—*contd.*

	PAGE
Spondylitis	927
Fibrositis	931
Surgery in Rheumatic Diseases	942
Physio-therapeutic Methods in Rheumatism	945
Gout	962
Diseases of Bone	966

DISEASES OF THE NERVOUS SYSTEM

Introduction	969
Disorders of Muscle	971
Dermatomyositis	971
Volkmann's Contracture	971
The Muscular Dystrophies	971
Cramps and Spasms	973
Disorders of Peripheral Nerves	974
Interstitial Neuritis	974
Traumatic Neuritis and Pressure on Nerves	977
Coccygodynia	978
Polyneuritis	978
Neurofibromatosis	980
Disorders of the Skull, Vertebræ and Meninges	980
Osteomyelitis	980
Meningitis	981
Tumours	982
Osteitis Deformans	983
Disorders of the Brain and Spinal Cord	983
Infections	983
Disseminated Sclerosis	983
Amyotrophic Lateral Sclerosis	985
Myelitis	986
Paraplegia	986
Subacute Combined Degeneration	988
Vascular Lesions of the Cord	989
Compression of the Cord	989
Syringomyelia	990
Spina Bifida	990
Disorders of the Brain and Spinal Cord—*contd.*	
Injury	990
Congenital Degenerative Disorders	991
Congenital Diplegia	991
Infantile Hemiplegia	992
Hereditary Ataxias	992
Disorders of the Extra-Pyramidal Motor System	992
Encephalitis Lethargica	992
Paralysis Agitans	994
Chorea	994
Disorders of the Cerebral Circulation	995
Hæmorrhage	995
Aneurysm	996
Thrombosis	996
Arteriosclerosis	997
Embolism	997
Venous Thrombosis	997
Disorders of Cranial Nerves	999
Hydrocephalus and Intracranial Tumour	1003
Injury to the Skull and Brain	1005
Disorders of Cerebral Function	1008
Epilepsy	1008
Migraine	1011
Narcolepsy and Cataplexy	1012
Spasmodic Torticollis	1012
Sleeplessness	1012
Remedial Exercises	1014

PSYCHOTHERAPY IN GENERAL PRACTICE

Introduction	1016
Parent-child Relationships	1021
Adjustment of the Sexual Instinct	1023
Attitude of the Patient to Disease	1027
Therapeutic Procedures	1033
Scope and Limitations of Psychotherapy	1042
Alcoholism	1046
Drug Addiction	1054

FEMALE SEX ENDOCRINOLOGY

	PAGE
Introduction	1056
Gonadotropic Hormones	1057
Ovarian Hormones	1058
Functional Uterine Bleeding	1061
Ovular Bleeding	1062
Amenorrhœa	1063
Minor Menstrual Disorders	1065
Recurrent Abortion	1065
The Menopause	1066
Post-menopausal Disturbances	1067
Dysmenorrhœa	1067

TECHNICAL PROCEDURES AND OXYGEN THERAPY

Subcutaneous Administration of Fluid	1070
Rectal Administration of Fluid	1070
Venipuncture	1071
Intravenous Infusion	1075
Blood Transfusion	1079
Intradermal Injection	1084
Hypodermic Injection	1085
Intramuscular Injection	1086
Paracentesis of the Abdomen	1087
Aspiration of the Pleural Cavity	1088
Lumbar Puncture	1090
Cisternal Puncture	1095
Epidural Injection	1096
Oxygen Therapy	1098

Conversion Table for Weights and Measures . . . 1107

Index 1109

FOREWORD

I HAVE felt for several years that a work of the character of a "Textbook of Medical Treatment" was needed and hence I welcome its appearance with particular pleasure.

The volume summarizes the remarkable therapeutic advances that have occurred during the present century and gives a systematic account of rational therapeutics. Modern therapeutics is a difficult subject, because, like all living and growing things, it cannot be described with rigid accuracy. This difficulty has hindered systematic treatment of the subject, and as a result the extent of its development has not been generally appreciated. A glance at the history of therapeutics during the past century suffices, however, to show the remarkable nature of the transformation that has occurred.

In the middle of last century, leaders of medicine noted regretfully that whilst basic medical sciences were developing rapidly, therapeutics remained an art rooted in the traditions of the past, which at the best were empirical traditions of a craft and in many cases were merely superstitions. The rapid advance of pathology and bacteriology during the second half of last century diverted attention from drug therapy during that era and resulted in the nihilist attitude that was dominant at the commencement of this century.

A study of the literature of that period, such for instance as the annual reviews of medical progress published by *The Lancet*, shows that all interest as regards curative therapy was directed towards sera and vaccines, and the likelihood of the development of curative drug therapy was scarcely recognized. For example, in 1908 the possibilities of a serum treatment for syphilis were considered of greater interest than the results reported from the use of atoxyl. Few recognized the future developments adumbrated by this latter discovery or by the commencement of substitution therapy that had been made with thyroid administration. Drugs such as anæsthetics, hypnotics, purgatives and disinfectants, etc., were recognized as useful and indeed indispensable agents, but drugs as a whole were regarded as placebos—or at best palliatives rather than as serious curative agents. Furthermore, the polypharmacy engendered by the love of elegant prescriptions tended to obscure the merits of valuable drugs such as digitalis, which like all active agents only produce their desired effect when given in adequate dosage.

The discovery of salvarsan by Ehrlich in 1910 inaugurated a new science since it provided dramatic proof of the successes that might be attained when chemical and pharmacological methods were combined in a systematic search for new therapeutic agents.

Since that date rapid progress has been made along two lines—namely, chemotherapy and autopharmacology. Chemotherapy first provided curative agents for the majority of the diseases produced by animal parasites and recently has made an advance of the first magnitude by discovering synthetic drugs capable of checking the invasion of the body by bacteria.

The development of endocrinology and the discoveries initiated by the work of Loewi have revealed a complete system of chemical control of the body functions. The fact that in several cases the production of these regulating agents is dependent on materials contained in the diet is linking up endocrinology with deficiency diseases. These advances promise in the future to provide interpretations and possible cures for many functional disorders.

These developments in chemotherapy and in autopharmacology have been accompanied by important advances in many other directions. For example, new anæsthetics, hypnotics, analgesics and analeptics are appearing in increasing numbers. In general it may be said that the efficiency of what may be termed palliative, as opposed to curative treatment, is showing a slow but steady advance.

The dominant feature in medical progress during the last quarter of a century has been the increasing part played by the organic chemist. Anæsthetics were the first synthetic organic drugs of major importance to be used in therapeutics and these were followed by the hypnotics, analgesics and disinfectants. One outstanding contribution during the present century has been the discovery of chemotherapeutic agents such as salvarsan, atebrin and the sulphonamide group. Equally important, and even more remarkable from the technical standpoint, has been the achievement of the organic chemists in analysing the mechanisms by which the functions of the body are controlled. The progress made in sex hormone therapy may serve as a typical example. Evidence for the existence of these substances has been known since the dawn of history, but their structure was only established a few years ago, yet already synthetic substitutes have been introduced and are gradually finding their place in practice.

These developments have brought therapeutics to a difficult stage in respect of drug therapy. The older drugs fall into two classes, namely, a minority which produce some definite effect, and the others which are administered from force of habit and tradition and to gratify in an innocuous manner the popular love for a bottle of medicine. The modern drugs fall into three classes—a small minority which represent important therapeutic advances, a large number which have actions similar but not clearly superior to those of established drugs, and finally a certain number which show no superiority over the ancient placebos. A special difficulty as regards modern drugs is that they appear in groups rather than as individuals, and their nomenclature usually gives no hint of their relationships.

This situation tends to produce in medical men two forms of reactions: some react positively to advertisement and try every new drug that appears and always believe that the latest is the best, others react negatively and disregard all innovations.

This volume provides a basis for the rational and critical judgment of modern therapeutic agents. A complete break has been made from the use of drugs as talismans of doubtful efficacy, which serve chiefly as placebos to physician and patient by convincing both that treatment is being given and received. Attention is centred on drugs which produce a recognizable effect and the nature of the desired effect is clearly indicated.

The common characteristic of all such drugs is that they are sharp-edged tools, the incorrect use of which is highly dangerous. Hence the detailed account of the exact manner in which these drugs should be used is extremely valuable.

The development of synthetic organic agents and of knowledge regarding the natural agents, the hormones and vitamins, have been the most spectacular change in therapeutics during the present century. Drug therapy is, however, only a part of therapeutics and a special feature of the volume is that it shows clearly the relationship of all the various forms of therapy. It is particularly interesting to note the importance of dietetics in the treatment of a wide variety of disorders. The same rational methods have been applied to those other branches of therapy as have been applied to drug therapy; only those procedures are mentioned which are capable of producing some definite effect, and full instructions regarding their mode of employment are provided. It is recognized, moreover, that a large proportion of a doctor's work is connected with functional disease: the adjustment of the individual in his particular social and environmental relationships constitutes an important factor in maintaining physical and mental health and in the prevention of disease. The importance of this aspect of therapeutics is fully recognized in this book.

Hence the volume provides a very practical account of the methods of rational therapeutics of which a large proportion have been evolved during this century.

A. J. CLARK.

INFECTIOUS DISEASES

GENERAL MANAGEMENT OF THE FEVERED PERSON

FEVER may be regarded as a reaction of the tissues to invasion by micro-organisms and their toxins. Whilst pyrexia, arising from a toxic interference with the function of the heat regulating centre, is a cardinal sign of fever, in some cases, and those the most toxic, the temperature may not be raised above normal. Wasting, due to increased catabolism; dry hot skin, acceleration of the pulse and respiration; coated tongue, anorexia, vomiting and constipation or diarrhœa; headache, restlessness, insomnia and delirium; and quantitative and qualitative changes in the urine are all symptoms of fever resulting from the action of bacterial toxins on the various organs and tissues of the body.

In certain diseases we can materially assist the tissues in their struggle against the infecting organism or its toxins by the injection of an appropriate antiserum, *e.g.*, diphtheria, scarlet fever, tetanus, etc. Unfortunately, in many of the acute infections, our therapeutic efforts are of necessity still limited to the application of certain broad physiological principles of treatment and the relief of distressing symptoms.

It may be some consolation, if not a source of professional satisfaction, to remember that most febrile cases tend to recover if placed in good hygienic surroundings and competently nursed.

The primary essentials in the treatment of the fevered person are (*a*) rest; (*b*) skilled nursing; (*c*) fresh air; (*d*) a suitable diet with copious intake of water; and (*e*) relief of symptoms.

Rest.—Confinement to bed is essential as long as the temperature remains elevated, and should be continued for a varying period in convalescence. A strictly recumbent position should be enforced in those diseases characterized by a marked toxic action on the cardio-vascular system, *e.g.*, diphtheria, enteric fever.

A single bed and firm mattress are preferable for nursing

purposes. In prolonged fevers a sponge rubber or air mattress adds greatly to the patient's comfort. The bedclothes should be light and varied in amount according to the temperature of the patient and of the sickroom. The general tendency towards excess of coverings must be guarded against.

Quietness in the sickroom and its environment is essential. Whilst it is preferable to select a sickroom with a sunny exposure, the writer would, during the acute stage of the more serious infections, be tempted to sacrifice sunshine for freedom from noise. Traffic in and out of a sickroom should be cut down to a minimum, and attendants should wear soft-soled shoes. Mental rest is of great importance. Measures should be taken to allay worry and anxiety. Business matters and domestic problems should be shelved until the patient is fit to cope with them. Visitors should be limited to near relatives, whose stay should be brief.

The ideal sickroom is a large, airy, bright, well-ventilated room opening on to a balcony and heated by an open coal fire. Proximity to a bathroom, which should if possible be reserved for the patient's use, is advantageous. An upper floor is usually quieter and more removed from household activities. The temperature of the sickroom should be kept around 55° F. except in the case of infants or the aged, when it may with advantage be raised to between 60° and 65° F.

The bed must be so placed that the patient is readily accessible from both sides, out of direct draught, and not directly facing a window or other source of bright light.

Furniture, hangings and carpets should be reduced to a minimum, and those retained of such a type as to permit of subsequent disinfection if considered necessary.

A prominent warning notice on the door of the sickroom will serve the same purpose as the time-honoured sheet moistened with disinfectant. The risk of aerial conveyance of infection from the sickroom is negligible.

Nursing.—The value of skilled nursing in fevers is generally recognized, but, unfortunately, the ideal of a fever-trained nurse for every infectious patient is as yet unattainable.

Broadly speaking, the notifiable infectious diseases should not be treated at home unless trained nurses can be provided. The non-notifiable infections, such as measles and whooping-cough, present a special problem. Young children suffering from these diseases require skilled nursing care, but, owing to lack of hospital accommodation, must of necessity be treated at home. When circumstances permit, at least one fever-trained nurse should always be obtained.

In most cases, providing the child is looked after by a sensible mother or near relative who can be relied upon to carry out conscientiously the detailed instructions given by the physician, progress will be satisfactory. If the attendant has not already suffered from the particular disease, the risk of contracting infection should be pointed out, and advice must be given as to how the risk of personal infection and the conveyance of infection to other members of the family may be minimized. Overalls, kept in the sickroom, should be provided for the use of the attendant and physician, and a bowl containing a solution of perchloride of mercury, lysol or dettol should be available for disinfection of the attendant's hands.

Whilst it is not within the scope of a book of this type to describe minute details of nursing technique, it may be advantageous to emphasize one or two points about which the practitioner may be called upon to instruct the unskilled attendant.

The skin should be kept clean by sponging with soap and warm water night and morning, especial care being paid to areas liable to soiling. These should be freely dusted with talcum powder. The body should be washed and dried limb by limb and the windows kept closed during the process.

In serious illness the position of the patient should be changed every four to six hours.

Food should be given at strictly regular intervals and should be removed from the sickroom between meals; food remains should be burnt. Cold water must be given without stint and be offered at frequent intervals. In young children the mouth should be gently cleansed after each meal by inserting the index finger enveloped in cotton-wool soaked in warm water or warm solution of bicarbonate of soda (30 gr. to 1 pint). In older children the teeth should be brushed and the mouth rinsed with warm water or mild antiseptic solution. The lips may be smeared with vaseline or boracic ointment.

Nasal discharge must be promptly removed on rags or paper handkerchiefs, and the nostrils gently cleaned with a cotton-wool swab soaked in warm normal saline or bicarbonate solution. Older children should be encouraged to clear the nose by gentle blowing. Vaseline or boracic ointment applied to the nostrils and upper lip will prevent crusting and excoriation.

The eyes may require regular cleansing as detailed in the section on the Treatment of Measles.

In young children the temperature should be taken by inserting the clinical thermometer into the rectum, groin or axilla, and not into the mouth.

All excreta should be removed from the sickroom and consigned to the closet as quickly as possible. Care must be taken to avoid contamination of water-closet seats. Specimens required for the physician's inspection should be placed in covered fly-proof receptacles. Articles soiled with excreta must be disinfected. Swabs used for wiping away discharges from the mouth, nose, ears, eyes and other organs must be burnt.

Food should be protected from flies, and measures taken to exterminate these pests.

Fresh Air.—Free ventilation of the sickroom is essential. Apart from the diminished concentration of bacteria in the atmosphere, the free movement of cool air has a very important tonic influence on the patient. The appetite and circulation improve, the patient is less restless and sleeps better. In equable weather treatment in the open air is the ideal, failing this the bed should be moved close to a widely opened window. The patient must be kept warm by extra hot bottles and blankets if necessary, and sheltered from strong winds and excessive sunlight. Caution must be exercised in exposing young infants and the aged to open-air conditions.

Diet.—The characteristic change in the metabolism of fever is the greatly increased destruction of the nitrogenous-containing tissues of the body. Instead of endeavouring to make good this loss by an increased nitrogenous intake it is a better policy to supply an abundance of "protein sparers" in the form of carbohydrates. Fever patients strongly dislike fatty foods. On theoretical grounds a high caloric intake is indicated, but in actual practice, owing to loss of appetite and actual distaste for food, this is impossible to attain during the height of the fever. Whilst the semi-starvation diet favoured by Hippocrates, who fed his fever patients on thin barley gruel and wine, may be appropriate in fever of a few days' duration, there can be no question that in more prolonged attacks the patient should be fed up to the limit of his digestive capacity. The absorption of light articles of diet is almost as perfect in the febrile person as in health.

In drawing up a diet it is essential that the likes and dislikes of the patient should be studied and no article for which the patient expresses a strong predilection withheld unless there is a good reason for doing so. Sudden changes in diet are better avoided.

When the febrile period does not exceed four or five days, the diet should be restricted to fluids and "feeding up" is to be deprecated. One and a half to three pints of milk daily usually form the basis of the diet. Not more than 5 to 6 oz. should be given at a feed. The milk may be boiled, diluted, citrated (2 gr. of sodium citrate to 1 oz.), peptonized, treated with lactic acid, or flavoured with tea or coffee according to circumstances. Whether administered hot or cold is a matter of taste. Glucose is a most valuable and easily assimilated food, which should be given freely in the form of sweetened lemon or orange juice drinks. From 5 to 10 oz. of glucose can readily be administered in the twenty-four hours. Cane sugar is not a satisfactory substitute. Albumen water, jellies, clear soups and custards may be given if desired. Because of their low nutritive value, high content of extractives, and relative cost, the various commercial beef-juice preparations have little to commend them.

Feeds should be given at two-hourly intervals during the day and every four hours during the night if the patient is awake.

The free intake of water favours the elimination of toxins, hence the patient should be encouraged to drink cold or hot water freely between feeds. Including glucose lemonade, the water intake should amount to at least 4 pints in the twenty-four hours, the greater the consumption of water the better.

Alcohol should not be administered as a routine except to alcoholics or elderly patients, to whom ½ oz. of whisky diluted with twice its volume of water may be given at two to four-hourly intervals.

When the febrile period exceeds one week the above diet will require to be supplemented on the lines described in the section on the Treatment of Enteric Fever.

Relief of Symptoms

Pyrexia.—A drug should only be prescribed when there are definite indications for its use, and should be administered in draught or powder form, not in tablets. Unless otherwise stated, the doses prescribed in this section are for administration to adult patients.

A raised body temperature is in itself not harmful, and, unless excessively high, does not call for active treatment. In mild cases of fever the following simple diaphoretic mixture may be administered every four hours :—

℞		
	Pot. Cit.	gr. xx
	Liq. Ammon. Acet. Dil. . . .	ʒii
	Syr. Aurantii	ʒi
	Aq. . . . . ad	℥ss

When the temperature exceeds 103° F., sponging the skin of the whole body with warm (98° F.), tepid (80° F.), or even cold water, according to the height of the pyrexia, is the correct treatment. The sponging may have to be repeated at two to four-hourly intervals as indications arise. Apart from its effect in reducing temperature, the application of tepid or cold water to the skin exerts an important reflex tonic effect on the nervous, respiratory and circulatory systems, and is very refreshing for the patient.

Hyperpyrexia (106° F. or over) can be controlled by the cold pack, rubbing the skin with ice or by the cold bath. The application of the cold pack consists of wrapping a sheet wrung out of cold or iced water around the patient. The cold-bath treatment is difficult to apply in general practice and, in fact, is rarely necessary. The patient should be immersed in water at 85° F., which is then gradually cooled by the addition of ice or cold water. During the application of any of these procedures, ice or cold water should be applied to the head, the condition of the patient carefully watched, and the treatment stopped when the temperature has fallen to 102° F.

Drugs such as pyramidon, phenacetin, aspirin, etc., should not be prescribed for the reduction of temperature.

Headache and Malaise.—A combination of aspirin and Dover's powder (7½ to 10 gr. of each) administered at intervals of six hours usually gives relief. Should headache persist, phenacetin, caffeine and antipyrin (3 gr. of each) may be prescribed in place of the above ; the powder to be repeated every two hours for three or four doses. Diminution of intra-cranial pressure by lumbar puncture affords immediate relief in infections of the central nervous system. In the most intractable cases a hypodermic injection of ¼ gr. of morphine will be necessary. When headache is severe a quiet environment and the exclusion of bright light add to the comfort of the patient. A prolonged hot bath is very soothing for general aches and pains.

Insomnia and Delirium.—Restlessness and inability to sleep are characteristic symptoms in febrile cases and should always be taken seriously. Nursing technique should first be reviewed and everything done to make the patient comfortable. Where sleeplessness is due to worry or anxiety, a hot toddy with 30 gr. of ammonium bromide is frequently successful. The relief of headache may cure the insomnia. If pain is keeping the patient awake, then either 15 gr. of Dover's powder or 15 minims of tincture of opium should be prescribed ; relief may only be obtained following the hypodermic injection of $\frac{1}{6}$ to $\frac{1}{4}$ gr. of morphine.

Where there is no definite cause for the insomnia beyond a feeling of general discomfort, the following mixture of chloral and bromide given well diluted is useful :—

℞		
℞	Chloral. Hydratis	gr. xx
	Pot. Brom.	gr. xxx
	Syr. Aurantii	ʒss
	Aq. . . . . ad	℥ss

Paraldehyde is another excellent and safe hypnotic; unfortunately it has a most unpleasant taste and odour. It may be administered well diluted with whisky or brandy and water.

℞		
℞	Paraldehydi	ʒii
	Ext. Glycyrrhiz Liq.	ʒii
	Syr.	℥i
	Aq. . . . . ad	℥ii

Paraldehyde may be administered by the rectum, 4 drachms in 4 oz. of starch mucilage.

Barbitone or soluble barbitone, in a dose of $7\frac{1}{2}$ gr., and soneryl, $1\frac{1}{2}$ gr., are excellent hypnotics.

Once a sleeping draught has been prescribed it is essential to see that the desired result is attained. This may necessitate repetition of half the initial dose at hourly intervals up to the limit of safety for the particular drug employed. Detailed written instructions regarding dosage should be given to the attendant.

Whilst mild delirium can usually be controlled by chloral and bromide, active delirium calls for the hypodermic injection of $\frac{1}{4}$ gr. of morphine with, in cases of maniacal excitement, the addition of $\frac{1}{100}$ gr. of hyoscine hydrobromide; the injection may be repeated after an interval of one hour.

Nausea and Vomiting.—Common initial symptoms in many febrile conditions, nausea and vomiting are rarely sufficiently severe or persistent to call for active treatment.

In the majority of cases the symptoms will rapidly subside following the administration of a purgative and restriction of food intake to 5 per cent. glucose lemonade and water. If nausea continues, fragments of ice may be sucked, and a powder consisting of sod. bicarb. and bismuth. oxycarb. (10 gr. of each) administered four-hourly, stirred in a little water.

Persistent vomiting should be treated by the intravenous infusion of 5 per cent. glucose saline. Where circumstances do not permit of this procedure, 5 per cent. glucose saline may be administered four-hourly by the rectum. A mustard plaster applied to the pit of the stomach and the hourly administration by mouth of 1 minim of tincture of iodine in a teaspoonful of water for eight doses are sometimes helpful procedures.

Constipation.—The bowels should be thoroughly cleared out during the early stages of the illness. Calomel in $\frac{1}{4}$-gr. doses every half hour for six doses, followed by a draught of $\frac{1}{2}$ to 1 oz. of magnesium sulphate six to eight hours later is an excellent prescription. In children, $\frac{1}{2}$ oz. of milk of magnesia is more readily taken than Epsom salts. Half an ounce of castor oil or double the dose of the patient's usual aperient may be prescribed. Drastic purgatives should be avoided thereafter.

During the course of the illness only the mildest aperients should be administered, such as liquid paraffin in 2-teaspoonful doses thrice daily or an occasional evening dose of 1 teaspoonful of liquorice powder.

In the more serious infections, following initial purgation, the bowels should be kept open by the administration of a soap and water enema every other day.

The reduction of milk in the diet with an increase of sugar, fat and broths will tend to soften the motions and correct constipation.

Disinfection

The aim of disinfection is to destroy the germs which are cast off from the patient in the various excretions. Objects with which the patient comes into contact are liable to be contaminated with pathogenic organisms, particularly clothing and utensils, and may remain a potential source of infection to others for a varying period of time.

The daily disinfection carried out in the sickroom is termed "current" disinfection. The disinfection of the sickroom after removal of the patient to hospital, or after recovery, is termed "terminal" disinfection. The more efficiently "current" disinfection is performed the less need will there be for an elaborate disinfecting ritual after recovery.

Current Disinfection.—Immediate disinfection and careful disposal of all infected material during the course of the illness are essential procedures in the nursing of a case of infectious disease. Whilst a conscientious fever-trained nurse can be relied upon to practice "current" disinfection, an untrained attendant, or even a general trained nurse, should receive detailed instructions regarding the disinfecting procedures appropriate to the particular disease.

The principal objects that require disinfection are (1) discharges from the body; (2) towels, handkerchiefs, bed-gowns and bedding; (3) cutlery, crockery, food remnants, etc.; (4) nursing utensils, clinical thermometer, toilet articles, etc.; and (5) the hands of those who come in contact with the infection.

Discharges from the Body.—The patient should be instructed to hold a piece of gauze or cloth over the mouth and nose whilst coughing or sneezing.

Nasal discharge and sputum should be received on a small piece of gauze, cloth, soft tissue paper or on a paper handkerchief. A bowl should be placed at the bedside for the reception of these soiled swabs, which should subsequently be burnt. When the sputum is considerable, an enamel or earthenware bowl or a flask containing a 5 per cent. solution of either carbolic acid or chlorinated lime should be provided. The contents of the flask should be mixed with sawdust and burnt and the container boiled.

Soiled dressings should, on removal, be placed in a suitable receptacle and subsequently burnt. The receptacle must be sterilized by boiling or scalding.

Fæces should be received into a receptacle containing either 5 per cent. carbolic acid, 2 per cent. cresol or lysol, or 5 per cent. chlorinated lime. Pour a liberal amount of the disinfectant over the stool and mix thoroughly with a small stick; the stick may either be burnt or dropped into the mixture. Allow the excretal matter to stand for two hours in a covered receptacle before the contents are either emptied down a drain or buried in the ground. The receptacle must be thoroughly cleaned and disinfected before it is used again.

If no chemical antiseptics are available, a bucket of boiling water poured over one stool and allowed to stand until cool is an effective disinfecting agent.

At least an equal volume of one of the above disinfectant solutions should be added to urine; the receptacle is then covered and allowed to stand for two hours, after which the urine may be emptied down a drain. Cleanse and disinfect the receptacle before it is used again.

Vomit should be treated in the same manner as fæces.

Towels, Bedding, Overalls, Fabrics, etc.—Towels, handkerchiefs, napkins, bed and body linen, provided they are not soiled with excreta, pus or blood, may be boiled. If soiled, they should be disinfected by soaking in either a 5 per cent. solution of carbolic acid or a 2 per cent. solution of lysol or cresol for twelve hours before being washed; blankets should be similarly treated. If soiled articles are boiled without preliminary soaking they will become permanently stained. Blankets must never be boiled. The householder should be warned that it is illegal to send infected clothing to a laundry.

Cutlery, Crockery, Food, etc.—Plates and cutlery should be set aside for the patient's use, and sterilized by boiling or scalding after each meal. Food remains should be burnt.

Nursing Utensils, etc.—Bed-pans, urinals, etc., should either be swilled out with boiling water or stored in one or other of the disinfecting solutions recommended above. The disinfecting solution must be washed off prior to use. Enema nozzles should be boiled. The clinical thermometer, toothbrush, nailbrush, etc., should be kept in either a 2 per cent. solution of dettol or a 2½ per cent. solution of carbolic acid.

Hands.—After thorough washing with warm running water and soap (a nailbrush should be used) the hands should be immersed for two minutes in either a 1 : 1,000 solution of perchloride of mercury or a 5 per cent. solution of dettol.

A bowl containing one or other of these solutions should be kept in the sickroom.

Nursing and Visiting Ritual.—At least two overalls should be hung just inside the sickroom door. On entering the sickroom the attendant rolls up her sleeves, puts on an overall, attends to the patient, removes the overall and then washes and disinfects her hands. The same ritual should be enforced for visitors, who should not, however, be permitted to approach within 1 yd. of the patient's bed.

The attendant may, if desired or considered advisable, be masked whilst nursing such diseases as diphtheria, scarlet fever, poliomyelitis, cerebrospinal fever, etc. A mask to be effective should consist of eight folds of fine meshed sterile gauze, and should be re-sterilized after use.

Terminal Disinfection

In the common infectious diseases less importance is now attached to the terminal disinfection of the sickroom. It is now realized that the patient is the real danger and that there is little risk of infection arising from contamination of the walls, floor or furnishings of the sickroom.

Viruses in particular appear to loose their infecting power very rapidly after leaving the human body.

The fumigation or spraying of wards between the reception of different infectious diseases was given up some years ago in the Edinburgh City Hospital. The confidence placed in the disinfecting power of a thorough domestic cleansing and airing has been justified.

Domestic Cleansing.—Provided current disinfection is conscientiously practised throughout the course of the illness, a thorough domestic cleansing is all the terminal disinfection that is required in the majority of the infectious diseases dealt with in this section. Bed and body linen should be treated in the manner already described. The mattress, outer garments, carpets, etc., should be exposed to fresh air and sunlight for a day or two ; carpets should be run over with a vacuum cleaner or well beaten. The room and furniture should be washed with soap and warm water. Following thorough ventilation for twenty-four hours, the room may be put in order for the next occupant.

Formalin Spray.—The elaborate disinfecting procedure necessary after the removal of a case of smallpox is carried out by the local Public Health Department and includes such measures as the steam disinfection of all bedding and clothing, the spraying of the room with formalin, 8 oz. to the gallon of water, followed by closure for six hours, and the stripping and washing down of walls.

In typhus fever special measures have to be taken to destroy lice.

The reader is referred to textbooks on Hygiene for details of these procedures.

ANTHRAX

Anthrax is a gastro-intestinal infection which affects horses, cattle, sheep and goats. The disease is conveyed to man through contact with infected animals or with skins and hides, wool, hair or bristles which are contaminated with secretions containing the spores of the anthrax bacillus. The disease is essentially an occupational risk, and in man is more or less confined to workers with animals or in wool, hair or hides. Infected shaving brushes have in the past been responsible for the conveyance of anthrax infection in several instances.

Infection usually enters through minute wounds or abrasions on the exposed skin, giving rise after an incubation period of about twenty-four to thirty-six hours to a cutaneous lesion, the " malignant pustule." Early diagnosis of the lesion, by enabling prompt treatment, greatly improves the prognosis. The spores are occasionally ingested or inhaled, giving rise to the gastro-intestinal or pulmonary forms of the disease, which are almost invariably fatal within three to four days.

Anthrax is not a notifiable disease, but information regarding cases occurring in factories and workshops must be forwarded to the Chief Inspector of Factories at the Home Office.

Preventive Treatment.—Various legal enactments dealing with the disposal of anthrax-infected animal carcases, the disinfection of infected cattle sheds, etc., the disinfection of wool and hair imported from Asia and Egypt, and the prohibition of importation of Japanese shaving brushes have played an important part in diminishing the incidence of the disease in this country.

Special preventive measures are enforced in factories, including the provision of exhaust ventilation, the wearing of overalls, the provision of ample washing accommodation, etc. Workers with skin lesions are excluded.

So far as the individual is concerned great care must be taken in handling infected material. Rubber gloves should be worn and are essential if there are any abrasions on the hands. Nurses or attendants must handle infective discharges from the " pustule " or the respiratory and intestinal tracts with great care. Contaminated dressings should be promptly burnt and discharges disinfected.

Individuals who have run a serious risk of infection should receive an intramuscular injection of 10 c.c. of Sclavo's anti-anthrax serum.

Curative Treatment.—*Serum Treatment.*—Early and repeated injections of Sclavo's anti-anthrax serum is the most effective treatment for the cutaneous form of the disease. An initial intravenous injection of 100 c.c. of serum should be followed by a daily intravenous or intramuscular dose of 60 c.c. until improvement ensues ; a total dose of from 300 to 600 c.c. of serum may be required. Large doses of serum must be administered when the lesion is on the face or neck, when there are marked signs of toxæmia or when the diagnosis has been delayed. Intensive serum treatment should be tried in cases of internal anthrax, 100 c.c. intravenously at eight-hour intervals (see p. 75).

Arsenical Compounds.—According to Pijper[1] (1926) and Gilbert[2] (1935), organic compounds of arsenic are very effective in the treatment of cutaneous anthrax. If serum is not available, 0·6 to 0·9 gm. of neosalvarsan should be administered intravenously and the injection repeated on the following day. In exceptionally severe cases a third injection may be given on the fourth day. One injection of salvarsan appears to be

[1] Pijper, A., *Lancet* (1926), **1**, 88.
[2] Gilbert, F. W., *Lancet* (1935), **2**, 1283.

sufficient to effect a cure in some cases. Eurich [1] (1933) usually combines salvarsan administration with intravenous serum injections.

Treatment of the Lesion.—Immobilization of the affected area either by sandbags or splints is essential. The lesion should be dressed with gauze soaked in eusol or 2 per cent. formalin. Hodgson [2] (1928), Brentnall [3] (1930) and Eurich (1933) report excellent results following purely medical treatment, and are opposed to excision of the local lesion. With this opinion the writer is disposed to agree.

General Management.—Owing to the ever-present risk of septicæmia it is wise to confine the patient to bed even if there is no fever.

When constitutional disturbance is present the case should be treated on the lines indicated for any acute febrile condition, and preferably in the open air.

Vomiting, diarrhœa, headache, delirium, convulsions and cardio-vascular failure, common symptoms in septicæmic attacks, require appropriate symptomatic treatment.

Attendants should wear rubber gloves whilst dressing the "pustule." In the internal form of the disease the respiratory, gastric and intestinal excretions contain anthrax bacilli and must be burnt or disinfected.

CEREBROSPINAL FEVER

Cerebrospinal fever is most commonly met with in children under five years of age ; epidemics also occur among older children and young adults. The causal organism, *N. meningitidis*, is spread by droplet infection mainly through the agency of carriers, direct spread from one patient to another being unusual. A high percentage of the urban population may carry the meningococcus in the nasopharynx during epidemic periods. A carrier commonly harbours the organism for two to three weeks, but the carrier state may be more persistent. Whilst a relatively small proportion of any community contracts the typical disease, abortive and atypical clinical infections are probably common. The most important factors favouring the spread of the meningococcus are overcrowding and bad ventilation. In a susceptible individual the organism is usually conveyed from the nasopharynx to the meninges by the blood stream. The incubation period varies from one

[1] Eurich, F. W., *Brit. Med. Jour.* (1933), **2**, 50.
[2] Hodgson, A. E., *Lancet* (1928), **2**, 594.
[3] Brentnall, C. G., *Lancet* (1930), **2**, 1174.

to seven days, but is commonly from three to five days. Cerebrospinal fever is a notifiable disease.

Preventive Treatment.—*Vaccine Prophylaxis.*—The published reports on the prophylactic value of inoculation with a multivalent meningococcal vaccine are conflicting.

Zrünek and Feierabend [1] (1931) employing a vaccine containing 4,000 million meningococci per c.c. found the method ineffective in the Czechoslovak army. On the other hand, promising results have been obtained by Pergher and Portois,[2] (1936), who vaccinated over 120,000 persons. These authors attribute their success to the employment of large doses of vaccine freshly prepared from local strains.

Owing to the feeble contagiosity of cerebrospinal fever, the method is not worth while in general practice.

General Measures.—On the occurrence of a case in a household or during epidemic prevalence the home conditions should be reviewed. Children should not be permitted to sleep in the same bed, overcrowding should be corrected where possible, and the necessity for free ventilation emphasized. Predisposing factors such as fatigue, chill, and catarrhal infections should be avoided. Children should not attend cinemas, theatres, parties or other assemblies, and those who have been in intimate contact with a clinical case must be kept away from school for three weeks from the date of their last contact. Adults who have recently been in close contact with a cerebrospinal fever patient may continue to attend business, but should so far as possible avoid contact with young children. The kissing of children must be forbidden and the potential danger attached to the common use of handkerchiefs pointed out.

In dormitories the minimum distance between the edges of adjacent beds should be 3 ft., and the occupants should lie alternately with head or feet next the wall.

In a closed community, or under other special circumstances, the isolation of meningococcal carriers may be advisable, but owing to the widespread prevalence of the meningococcus, this method of control is impracticable among the general population. In searching for carriers the upper end of the posterior pharyngeal wall should be swabbed and culture plates promptly inoculated. At least two reports of swabs taken at an interval of three days should indicate the absence of meningococci before the carrier state can reasonably be excluded.

[1] Zrünek, K., and Feierabend, B., *Trav. Inst. d'Hyg. Pub. Etat Tchécoslav.* (1931), **2**; abstr. *Med. Ann.* (1932), 92.

[2] Pergher, G., and Portois, F., *Ann. Soc. Belge de Méd. Trop.* (1936), **16**, 343; abstr. *Bull. Hyg.* (1937), **12**, 2, 109.

Contacts and known carriers should remain in the open air as much as possible, this being the most effective means of clearing up the carrier condition. The routine use of nasal douches and gargles is of very doubtful value either in lessening the risk of contracting the disease or in clearing up the carrier condition. The writer strongly deprecates the use of strong antiseptic solutions for this purpose. If desired, a 1 per cent. solution of chloramine T. may be sniffed from the palm of the hand into the nose and returned through the mouth, and also sprayed on to the pharyngeal wall morning and evening for a fortnight after exposure to infection.

It is wise to regard the occurrence of febrile or catarrhal symptoms, with or without headache, in known contacts, as evidence of an abortive attack of cerebrospinal fever. Such individuals should be promptly isolated and steps taken to confirm the diagnosis.

Curative Treatment.—*Serum.*—The treatment of meningococcal meningitis with serum may now be regarded as a thing of the past. Sulphonamide chemotherapy has taken the place of serum and its action against the meningococcus represents an outstanding therapeutic advance.

Sulphonamides.—Banks[1] (1939) reports a fatality rate of 1·4 per cent. in a series of 72 cases of cerebrospinal fever adequately treated with either sulphanilamide or sulphapyridine. Bryant and Fairman[2] (1939) and Somers[3] (1939), during an outbreak of meningococcal meningitis treated under field conditions in the Sudan, record recovery rates of 95 and 90 per cent. in two series of 189 and 143 respectively following sulphonamide therapy. These are remarkable results when one considers that over a long period of years the annual fatality rate for patients suffering from cerebrospinal fever in the Edinburgh City Hospital, in spite of intensive serum treatment, varied from 50 to 75 per cent.

Prompt administration and high dosage during the first three days of treatment, followed by a diminished dosage for four or five days thereafter, are the essentials of successful sulphonamide therapy.

The slightest clinical suspicion of acute meningitis is an indication for the immediate administration of either sulphapyridine or sulphanilamide. Confirmation of the diagnosis by lumbar puncture and bacteriological examination of the cerebrospinal fluid may be done at leisure. It may be noted

[1] Banks, S. H., *Lancet* (1939), **2**, 921.
[2] Bryant, J., and Fairman, H. D., *Lancet* (1939), **1**, 923.
[3] Somers, R. B. U., *Lancet* (1939), **1**, 921.

in passing that these drugs are also the most effective method of treatment for pneumococcal and streptococcal meningitis. According to Maegraith and Vollum [1] (1938) sulphapyridine (M. & B. 693) is the most effective bacteriostatic agent against *N. meningitidis*. This has been borne out by recent clinical experience where it has been found that a concentration of sulphapyridine as low as 1 to 2 mg. per 100 c.c. cerebrospinal fluid is curative, whereas in the case of sulphanilamide a concentration lower than 5 mg. per 100 c.c. cerebrospinal fluid appears to be therapeutically unsafe. The correct dosage of sulphapyridine has still to be worked out and may prove to be smaller than that suggested by Stanley Banks, as indicated in the following table :—

Dosage of Sulphapyridine or Sulphanilamide.		
Age in Years.	Daily Dosage in Grammes.	
	1st to 3rd Days.	4th to 8th Days.
Under 2	3·0	1·5
2 to 4	4·5	2·25
5 to 9	6·0	3·0
10 to 14	7·5	3·75
15 +	9·0	4·5

The tablets should be crushed, suspended in water, milk or fruit juices and administered at four-hourly intervals, the patient being aroused at night. To enable a high concentration of the drug in the cerebrospinal fluid to be rapidly attained, the first two doses should be double the succeeding doses, 1 to 3 gm. being given instead of $\frac{1}{2}$ to $1\frac{1}{2}$. In the vast majority of cases the drug can be administered orally ; in comatose patients administration can be effected by the nasal tube. Should a dose be vomited, it should be repeated when the patient is settled. In exceptional cases the soluble sodium salt of sulphapyridine may have to be injected intramuscularly. This salt is now put up in ampoules containing 1 gm. in 3 c.c. This injection may be repeated in four hours, but oral administration should be started as soon as possible.

Following oral or intramuscular administration, the concentration of sulphapyridine or sulphanilamide in the cerebrospinal fluid rises within a few hours to only slightly less than that of the blood. There is no advantage in the intrathecal injection of these drugs.

[1] Maegraith, B. G., and Vollum, R. L., *Brit. Med. Jour.* (1938), **2**, 985.

A marked amelioration of symptoms may be expected within forty-eight hours of commencing chemotherapy and within the same space of time the cerebrospinal fluid is usually sterile. Pressure symptoms are less prominent than in serum therapy and in the majority of cases lumbar puncture is only required for diagnostic purposes, though it may be repeated if severe headache persists. Owing to the rapid clearing of the cerebrospinal fluid with quick absorption of the meningeal exudate there appears to be a remarkable freedom from relapses and complications due to pressure and adhesions (hydrocephalus).

Chemotherapy appears to be equally effective in infections with groups I. and II. meningococci.

For details of the toxic effects that may arise during the administration of the sulphonamides, see p. 86.

General Management.—Absolute rest in bed, a quiet environment and skilled nursing are essential. The patient's eyes should be screened from bright light. The skin, mouth, nose and eyes require regular and careful cleansing. Discharges from the nose, mouth and eyes are potentially infective and should be burnt or otherwise disinfected. The bowels must be kept open by enemata or liquid paraffin. The fluid diet of the first few days may be rapidly supplemented by soft solids, and solid food may be given as soon as the temperature has settled. If coma or dysphagia be present, nasal feeding will be necessary.

Retention of urine is apt to occur and should be relieved by regular catheterization.

Headache is usually relieved by lumbar puncture and the withdrawal of cerebrospinal fluid, but may require appropriate drug treatment. A mixture of chloral and bromide usually allays excitement and delirium and enables the patient to sleep, but the hypodermic injection of morphine with or without hyoscine may be necessary.

Regular hot baths are very soothing.

Treatment of Complications.—Internal hydrocephalus is a serious complication, liable to arise in cases where chemotherapy has been delayed. Sulphonamides should be administered and pressure relieved by ventricular puncture. In infants the puncture is made through the lateral angle of the anterior fontanelle and is a simple procedure. In older children and adults trephining is required.

Chemotherapy is worth a trial in the treatment of arthritis and orchitis which, however, usually respond readily to simple measures. These new drugs may also prove helpful in the treatment of serious eye complications such as purulent iridochoroiditis.

Nothing can be done for deafness due to a lesion of the auditory nerve. There is evidence that this complication may arise in spite of sulphonamide treatment.

Convalescence.—Even in mild attacks it is wise to keep the patient in bed for at least ten days after the temperature has settled. The patient may be released from isolation as soon as he is fit. Examination of post-nasal swabs prior to discharge is unnecessary. Work should not be resumed for at least two months from the commencement of the illness, and after a severe attack three to six months' holiday is advisable.

CHICKENPOX

A virus disease of high infectivity, chickenpox is probably spread by droplet infection and by conveyance of material from the skin lesions either on the hands or clothes of a third person, or possibly by air. The incubation period is usually from thirteen to sixteen days. It is rarely less than eleven days or more than twenty days. There is good reason to believe that the disease is infective for at least twenty-four hours before the appearance of the rash. The duration of infectivity is uncertain, but for practical purposes may be regarded as persisting until the last primary crust has separated from the skin.

Chickenpox is not a notifiable disease, but should smallpox be prevalent in a particular area, chickenpox cases may have to be reported to the local Public Health Authority.

Preventive Treatment.—There is no effective specific method of prophylaxis against chickenpox.

Children who have not previously suffered from the disease should be kept away from school for twenty-one days from the date of last contact. Where the date of exposure is accurately known, quarantine need only be enforced from the tenth to the twenty-first days inclusive.

Susceptible adult contacts need not stay away from their employment unless it involves close contact with children, *e.g.*, school teachers, nurses, etc.

Children who have not previously suffered from chickenpox should not needlessly be exposed to a case of herpes zoster.

Curative Treatment.—*General Management.*—The treatment of chickenpox is on general lines, no specific method being available. Even in mild attacks it is wise to confine the patient to bed during the efflorescence of the eruption. When the rash is profuse, bed should be enforced until the lesions have crusted. If there is a tendency to scratch the pocks, the hands may be wrapped in lint or gauze, or the arms lightly splinted.

The skin must be kept scrupulously clean by a daily warm bath, either coloured claret with potassium permanganate or to which a handful of boracic crystals has been added. After gentle drying, the skin should be dusted freely with either a good talcum powder or with a powder consisting of equal parts of boric acid, zinc oxide and starch. If itching is intense, the application of either calamine lotion or $2\frac{1}{2}$ per cent. phenol in vaseline or olive oil will give relief.

A mild antiseptic mouth wash should be used after meals.

In severe eruptions the writer favours daily painting of the whole skin surface with a 1 per cent. solution of permanganate of potash.

The light diet of the febrile stage can rapidly be followed by a return to normal food.

Complications.—Whilst complications are rare, secondary infection of the skin lesions with *S. pyogenes*, staphylococci or even the diphtheria bacillus may lead to serious and even fatal results. Appropriate serum treatment combined with the administration of a sulphonamide compound in the streptococcal infections should supplement frequent antiseptic baths and dressings.

Convalescence.—Chickenpox is one of the mildest of the infective diseases, and no special measures are required during convalescence. Isolation should be continued until the last primary crust has separated from the skin. Work or school may be resumed a day or two after release from isolation.

DIPHTHERIA

Apart from case to case infection, diphtheria is frequently transmitted by faucial or nasal carriers of *C. diphtheriæ*. During epidemic prevalence from 1 to 3 per cent. of the urban population may at any given time be carriers of virulent diphtheria bacilli. The organism is conveyed either by droplet infection or by articles contaminated with secretions from the upper respiratory tract; the latter may remain contagious for some considerable time. Milk infected from a human source is an occasional source of infection. The incubation period of diphtheria is usually from two to four days, but may extend to seven days.

Diphtheria is a notifiable disease.

The importance of the early diagnosis of diphtheria cannot be too strongly emphasized. Careful examination of the fauces should be a routine procedure in every febrile case. Apart from the presence of "false membrane," marked faucial and palatal œdema, accompanied by an acute gross enlargement of the cervical glands, should, in a child, always be treated as diphtheria until proved otherwise.

Preventive Treatment. — *Schick Test.* — Susceptibility to diphtheria can be ascertained by the application of the Schick test—an intradermal injection into the left forearm of 0·2 c.c. of diluted diphtheria toxin. Individuals showing an area of erythema from 1 to 4 cm. in diameter around the site of injection two to four days after the application of the test are said to be Schick positive, an indication of susceptibility to the disease. No local reaction appears in those who are immune (Schick negative reactors). In individuals above nine years of age a precisely similar injection is made into the skin of the right forearm, but with toxin which has been previously inactivated by heat. This control test enables us to discriminate between local reactions arising from sensitization to the protein present in the test fluid and the true positive Schick reaction. Reliable Schick and control test material can be obtained commercially.

Among children in this country the proportion susceptible to diphtheria varies from 15 to 90 per cent. according to age and social environment ; the highest proportion of susceptibles is found in the pre-school age group and among the well-to-do.

Active Immunization.—Every child should be actively immunized against diphtheria as soon after its first birthday as possible. A preliminary Schick test may be omitted.

Various immunizing preparations, termed diphtheria prophylactics, are available commercially, of which the best are alum precipitated toxoid (A.P.T.), formol toxoid (F.T.) and toxoid-antitoxin floccules (T.A.F.). Two intramuscular injections of 0·2 and 0·5 c.c., respectively, of alum toxoid, administered at an interval of four weeks, will render at least 95 per cent. of children immune to diphtheria within six weeks of the final injection. The writer is not in favour of the single dose, or as it is frequently termed, the "one-shot" method of immunization (1 c.c. of alum toxoid), which, in his experience, cannot be relied upon to produce either an effective or lasting immunity.

Formol toxoid (F.T.) is an excellent immunizing agent. In the writer's opinion a course of three intramuscular injections of this preparation (F.T.), each of 1 c.c., administered at fourteen-day intervals, affords the highest and most lasting degree of protection against diphtheria.

Above nine years of age toxoid-antitoxin floccules (T.A.F.), owing to its freedom from unpleasant reactions, is the immunizing preparation of choice—the course to consist of three intramuscular injections, each of 1 c.c., at fourteen-day intervals.

The usual sites for injection are either into the deltoid muscle or immediately above and behind the elbow.

From four to eight weeks after completion of the immunizing course, evidence of satisfactory immunity should be obtained either by the application of the Schick test or by the estimation of the antitoxic content of the blood. The latter procedure is the more reliable but is not practicable in general practice.

Should susceptibility still persist, as indicated by a positive Schick reading, the immunizing course must be repeated and a re-test applied one month later.

Whilst absolute protection against diphtheria cannot be guaranteed in every successfully immunized individual, marked modification in the severity of a subsequent attack is to be expected. The duration of immunity varies, but in all except a small percentage of children lasts for some years. In addition to pre-school immunization, the writer advises the administration of a single intramuscular injection of either 0·5 c.c. alum toxoid, or 1 c.c. formol toxoid, when the child commences his school career. The immunizing injections do not, with rare exceptions, give rise to marked local or systemic disturbance in young children.

Passive Immunization.—Passive immunity against diphtheria can readily be attained by the intramuscular injection of 1,000 units of diphtheria antitoxic serum. Immunity develops within twenty-four hours of the injection and lasts for some two to three weeks.

General Measures.—Following the isolation of the suspected case and disinfection of all articles likely to be contaminated with the faucial or nasal secretions of the sick person, household or institutional contacts must be examined for evidence of a missed infection. Individuals with chronic nasal or aural discharge, or obviously unhealthy tonsils are isolated, and the nose and throat of every contact swabbed. Efficient swab taking is an unpleasant procedure for the individual, but the need for a thorough and careful technique must be emphasized if reliable bacteriological findings are to be obtained. It is a wise policy promptly to inject young children who have been in intimate contact with a case of severe diphtheria with 2,000 units of diphtheria antitoxin intramuscularly.

Schick negative contacts must not return to school or business until two consecutive negative reports for diphtheria bacilli, with an interval of forty-eight hours between the swabs, have been obtained from throat and nose.

Schick positive contacts must be kept under medical supervision for ten days from the date of last contact, and, if found to be carrying diphtheria bacilli, should be passively immunized.

Individuals reported as having morphological diphtheria bacilli in either throat or nose must be strictly isolated until the virulence of the organism is ascertained. If the organisms are non-virulent, the individual may resume his normal activities. If the organisms are virulent, strict isolation must be continued until the carrier condition clears up (see p. 25).

Curative Treatment.—The four essentials in the treatment of a case of diphtheria are: (1) early adequate serum administration; (2) absolute rest in bed for a varying period of time according to the severity of the disease; (3) skilled nursing; and (4) the free administration of glucose.

Antitoxic Serum.—An intramuscular injection of at least 4,000 units of diphtheria antitoxic serum should immediately be administered to any patient suspected to be suffering from diphtheria. *Bacteriological confirmation of the clinical diagnosis should follow and not precede the administration of antitoxin. When the clinical picture is typical of diphtheria, negative bacteriological findings should be ignored and adequate serum treatment immediately instituted.* There is considerable difference of opinion regarding the optimum dosage of antitoxin in the treatment of diphtheria. Broadly speaking, mild attacks should receive from 2,000 to 8,000 units intramuscularly; cases of moderate severity from 10,000 to 30,000 units intramuscularly; severe or toxic attacks from 50,000 to 100,000 units of antitoxin intravenously. When the diphtheritic infection is limited to the larynx, 10,000 units of antitoxin is usually sufficient, and in purely nasal diphtheria, unless toxæmia is severe, 4,000 to 8,000 units is adequate.

When treatment is delayed, or in the case of young children, relatively larger doses of antitoxin are required. Owing to the slow rate of absorption a therapeutic dose of serum should never be administered subcutaneously. The total dose of serum considered necessary for the treatment of the case should be administered in a single injection; the method of administering a series of relatively small doses at twelve-hour intervals is to be deprecated. The middle third of the outer side of the thigh is an excellent site for intramuscular injection.

In assessing dosage, extensive clinical experience is the only reliable guide, and if the practitioner be in doubt, an expert opinion should always be obtained.

Glucose.—Glucose lemonade should be freely administered to every diphtheritic patient. In severe infections the dose of serum may, with advantage, be diluted with 2 or more pints of 5 per cent. glucose saline and administered by continuous intravenous infusion. This should be followed by the daily intravenous injection of either 200 c.c. of a 25 per cent. solution of glucose, or 1 to 2 pints of a 10 per cent. solution (drip method), until the toxæmia lessens. The writer is satisfied that dextrose therapy provides the best means of combating cardio-vascular failure in severe diphtheria.

General Measures.—With the exception of the mildest attack a case of diphtheria should not be treated at home unless fever-trained night and day nurses can be provided. From the moment that diphtheria is suspected, the patient must be confined to bed in a strictly recumbent position. Owing to the risk of cardio-vascular complications, any attempt to sit up, reach over to a chair or bedside table, etc., must be strictly prohibited. The patient should not even feed himself. The period of recumbency varies from fourteen days in mild attacks to eight weeks or longer in severe cases, according to the condition of the cardio-vascular system and the incidence of paralysis.

Following the addition of a second and a third pillow at intervals of two clear days, the patient is permitted to sit up, and may leave his bed seven to ten days later. The rate of progress will vary according to the severity of the attack and the response of the cardio-vascular system to increased exertion. Care should be taken to curtail activity when the patient gets on to his feet.

A fluid diet with the addition of ice cream and jellies is the most suitable so long as the throat is inflamed. A glucose intake by mouth of from 3 to 5 oz. daily in the form of glucose lemonade is of definite therapeutic value. As the throat improves the diet may be increased and varied, but food must still be given in small amounts at two-hourly intervals and indigestible articles carefully excluded.

When grossly inflamed and foul or necrotic the throat should be douched two-hourly with either warm normal saline or bicarbonate solution, and small pieces of ice sucked. It is unwise, owing to resultant exhaustion, to persist with faucial treatment in a resistive child. In most cases of diphtheria local treatment is unnecessary. The mouth should be cleansed after each feed. Hot fomentations may be applied to the neck if the swollen cervical glands are painful.

Except in slight attacks, when mild aperients may be administered, the bowels should be opened by enemata every alternate day.

The possible development of ocular paresis requires to be

borne in mind and reading restricted to two hours daily ; the print must be large and the page well illuminated.

Complications.—The prevention of serious toxic damage to the heart and vessels by the early application of the measures detailed above is the fundamental principle in the treatment of diphtheria. Once well-marked signs of cardio-vascular weakness appear, little can be done to ward off death. The foot of the bed should be raised. Vomiting due to cardiac failure necessitates the replacement of oral feeding by the regular administration of rectal or intravenous glucose salines. The mouth may be moistened with sips of water or pieces of cracked ice. Epigastric pain, restlessness and anxiety are best relieved by repeated hypodermic injections of morphine : $\frac{1}{36}$ gr. for a child of two years, $\frac{1}{18}$ gr. at five years, and $\frac{1}{12}$ gr. for a child of ten years.

The writer is not impressed with the value of the various vasomotor or cardiac stimulants in the treatment of circulatory failure in diphtheria. One or other of the following drugs may, however, be administered if desired : adrenalin chloride solution (1 : 1,000) in subcutaneous doses of 5 minims every two hours ; camphor in oil, $1\frac{1}{2}$ gr. intramuscularly every four hours ; strychnine, $\frac{1}{48}$ gr. four-hourly ; caffein sodium benzoate, $1\frac{1}{2}$ gr. four-hourly. The doses indicated are suitable for a child five years of age.

Digitalis or strophanthus are definitely contraindicated. The routine administration of alcohol has nothing to commend it.

Apart from involvement of the pharyngeal and respiratory muscles no anxiety need be felt regarding the outcome of the post-diphtheritic palsies, since they tend to recover spontaneously within a few weeks. In palatal paresis the fluid part of the diet should be replaced by semisolids. In pharyngeal paralysis the foot of the bed should be raised 18 in., saliva and mucus aspirated at frequent intervals from the pharynx and food administered by the nasal tube. On the slightest indication of weakness of the intercostal or diaphragmatic muscles the patient must be treated in a mechanical respirator.

Late generalized muscular weakness improves with massage, hot and cold douching, graduated exercise, fresh air and good food.

Convalescence.—It is advisable to obtain two consecutive negative cultures at an interval of one week from both throat and nose before the patient is released from isolation. Even after a mild attack the patient should not resume school or work for at least a fortnight after release from isolation. The convalescent period may require to be prolonged to six months or even longer following toxic diphtheria. Strenuous exercise must be forbidden during convalescence. A change of air to the country or seaside and the administration of iron is very beneficial.

Carriers

The first essential in dealing with a persistent convalescent or contact carrier of morphological diphtheria bacilli is to ascertain whether the organisms present are virulent or non-virulent. Carriers of non-virulent bacilli are not dangerous to the community and need not be segregated.

The only effective method of ridding a faucial carrier of virulent diphtheria bacilli is by tonsillectomy. This procedure should not be undertaken hastily or without due consideration of the patient's physical condition. Antiseptic applications to the tonsils are useless. Persistent nasal or aural carriers should be examined by an aural surgeon. The carrier condition may clear up following appropriate radical measures directed at the underlying pathological condition.

Laryngeal Diphtheria

On the slightest suspicion that a child is suffering from a diphtheritic laryngitis the practitioner should immediately inject 8,000 units of antitoxin intramuscularly, and arrange for the prompt removal of the patient to hospital. The steam kettle, hot fomentations to the neck and the administration of 10 to 20 minims of paregoric every four hours are helpful in the early stages of the attack.

In hospital practice the diagnosis can be confirmed by endoscopy, and relief of respiratory distress attained either by aspiration, intubation or tracheotomy.

Laryngeal diphtheria calls for constant watchfulness, skilled care and highly specialized treatment. In an emergency the practitioner may be called upon to perform a tracheotomy. The reader is referred to surgical textbooks for the appropriate technique.

BACILLARY DYSENTERY

Shiga dysentery, the most fatal type of the disease, is common in the tropics, but, with the exception of occasional outbreaks in mental hospitals, is rarely met with in this country. According to Hurst and Knott[1] (1936) infections with Flexner and Sonne strains of *B. dysenteriæ* are more common in Great Britain than is generally realized. The incidence of the disease appears to be increasing. From

[1] Hurst, A. F., and Knott, F. A., *Lancet* (1936), 2, 1197.

investigations in the Glasgow area, Carter[1] (1937) found the disease most prevalent between July and November, and that two-thirds of the dysentery cases occurred in children under fifteen years of age. The infection is spread mainly by convalescent carriers and by unrecognized or atypical cases. Infection may be conveyed in the same manner as enteric fever. The incubation period is commonly two to three days, but may vary from one to seven days.

In every case of febrile diarrhœa with blood and mucus in the stools an attempt should be made to obtain bacteriological confirmation of dysenteric infection. In mild Sonne infections the stools are loose, but may not contain blood or obvious mucus, and the clinical picture may simulate food-poisoning. The stool specimen must be forwarded to the laboratory within twelve hours, or preferably less, of its passage.

In the writer's experience the ileocolitis, which is a fairly frequent complication of measles and whooping-cough during convalescence, particularly in hospital practice, is usually a dysenteric infection. Ward outbreaks of dysentery tend to spread with great rapidity in spite of strict measures of control. Bacillary dysentery is a notifiable disease.

Preventive Treatment.—*Vaccines.*—Conflicting reports have been published regarding the prophylactic value of vaccination against bacillary dysentery (Newman[2] (1929), Walker and Wats[3] (1930), and Johns and Chalk[4] (1933)). The results on the whole are not very encouraging.

General Measures.—As household infection commonly arises from a missed case or carrier, the practitioner, in addition to prompt isolation of the patient, should question other members of the family regarding recent attacks of diarrhœa and arrange for bacteriological examination of the stools where necessary.

Contacts should be kept away from school for one week from the date of last exposure to infection. Adults whose occupation entails the handling of milk or other foods, or contact with water supplies, should not be permitted to resume their duties until at least three stool examinations, spread over a period of one week, have proved negative for dysentery bacilli.

Those in attendance on the patient must practice the same precautions as in dealing with a case of enteric fever, and must on no account prepare or handle food which is to be consumed by other members of the family.

[1] Carter, H. S., *Jour. Path. Bact.* (1937), **45**, 447.
[2] Newman, R. E. U., *Jour. Roy. Army Med. Corps* (1929), **52**, 7.
[3] Walker, W., and Wats, R. C., *Jour. Roy. Army Med. Corps* (1930), **54**, 190.
[4] Johns, E. P., and Chalk, S. G., *Canad. Med. Ass. Jour.* (1933), **29**, 40.

Curative Treatment. — *Serum.* — The early intravenous administration of 100 c.c. of antidysentery serum (Shiga) is of undoubted value in the treatment of severe attacks of Shiga dysentery. The serum may, with advantage, be diluted with 2 to 3 pints of normal saline and administered by the drip method. The injection should be repeated daily until definite improvement ensues.

Whilst the writer has occasionally observed marked and rapid improvement follow the intravenous or intramuscular administration of daily doses of 50 c.c. polyvalent antidysentery serum (Flexner) in severe cases of Flexner dysentery, serum therapy is on the whole disappointing in this type of infection.

Bacteriophage.—Judging from the published reports and from limited personal experience the writer has still to be convinced of the value of bacteriophage in the treatment of bacillary dysentery.

General Management.—The patient must be confined to bed and kept warm from the first symptom of the disease. Except in the mildest attacks the bed-pan should be employed. When the call to stool is incessant the bed-pan is dispensed with and the motions received into tow which, when soiled, is collected and burnt. The attendants should wear rubber gloves. Specimens of stool must be collected daily for inspection by the practitioner.

There is considerable difference of opinion as to the most suitable diet in the treatment of dysentery. Providing the diet prescribed is nutritive, easily assimilable and with little residue, considerable latitude is permissible.

During the acute stage albumen water, arrowroot, jellies, thin gruels, chicken-tea and clear soups may be given in small amounts, slightly warmed, at two-hourly intervals. As the symptoms abate, milk and additional carbohydrates may be administered. The writer has employed an apple diet in Flexner and Sonne infections with satisfactory results. Ripe eating apples are skinned and cored, grated down, and the pulp, sweetened to taste with glucose, is administered two-hourly. Children take the pulp freely, and 2 to 3 lbs. of apples may be administered daily.

In subacute or chronic cases a fairly generous diet may be allowed. It should be low in residue and fat, but fairly high in protein. Carbohydrates should be given in a dextrinized form as crisp toast. An example of such a diet is given below.

Early Morning—

Juice of 1 orange with water.

Breakfast—

Baked apple or apple sauce, prune pulp or grape juice.
1 egg (poached, boiled or scrambled) or 2 strips of bacon (grilled), or small helping of white fish.
1 slice crisp toast buttered sparingly.
1 cup of weak tea, with sugar if desired.

10 *a.m.—*

Drink of acidophilus milk or buttermilk.

Lunch—

Small glass of tomato juice.
Small helping of chicken, white fish, sweetbreads or very tender meat *finely divided* (not fried).
1 slice crisp toast.
If desired, water biscuit with small piece of St. Ivel cream cheese.

Tea—

1 slice crisp toast with butter, or 2 water or tea biscuits.
Honey or jelly.
1 finger plain cake.
1 cup weak tea, with sugar if desired.

Dinner—

Milk soup (very little seasoning) ; marmite may be used for flavouring.
Vegetables may be used in soup, but it must be strained.
Average helping of meat (this should be finely divided, and may be cooked in any manner, except fried. Avoid much seasoning).
Average helping of potato (baked, mashed or diced).
Custard, curds, jelly or whip.
Weak coffee, with sugar if desired.

As the symptoms abate, milk, cream, butter, puréed fruit and, eventually, carefully sieved and puréed vegetables may be added very gradually to the diet.

An initial dose of ½ oz. of castor oil combined with 15 minims of tincture of opium, followed by the administration of 1 drachm of sodium sulphate every two hours for the first twenty-four hours, and thereafter every four hours until the stools become fæculent, is a routine method of treatment. The dehydration and loss of chlorides resulting from this treatment in severe cases can, with advantage, be counteracted by the continuous intravenous infusion of 3 or more pints of hypertonic saline (2 drachms of NaCl to 1 pint) daily ; this procedure also helps to ward off collapse.

Water, or $2\frac{1}{2}$ per cent. glucose lemonade, preferably with the chill removed, should be freely administered.

Griping and colicy pains are relieved by the application of the hot bag or hot fomentations or poultices to the abdomen.

A rectal irrigation of warm saline followed by the administration of either an enema containing 40 minims of tincture of opium in 1 to 2 oz. of starch mucilage, or a suppository containing $\frac{1}{4}$ gr. morphine, should be prescribed for the relief of tenesmus. If irrigations afford relief and are well borne, they may be repeated twice daily during the febrile period.

When the abdominal pain is severe, either tincture of opium in doses of 1 to 2 minims every two hours may be administered by mouth, or $\frac{1}{4}$ gr. morphine combined with $\frac{1}{100}$ gr. atropine sulphate injected twice or thrice in each twenty-four hours.

The mild Sonne and Flexner infections met with in this country usually run a course of three to four days and call for little medicinal treatment. Three doses, each of from 10 to 30 gr., of magnesium sulphate administered daily at 8, 9 and 10 A.M., is an alternative to the routine saline treatment. The administration of 30 gr. of bismuth carbonate, and either 1 minim of laudanum or 1 gr. of Dover's powder every two to four hours, is more effective in allaying pain and tenesmus. When large doses of bismuth are prescribed it is advisable to empty the bowel by a dose of castor oil or salts every third day.

CHRONIC DYSENTERY

The diet should be generous but carefully regulated on the lines already described. A small dose of a saline aperient should be administered daily. A course of autogenous or stock vaccine is sometimes followed by improvement. The initial subcutaneous dose should not exceed 1,000,000 bacilli, and subsequent injections may be administered bi-weekly with cautious increase in dosage.

Washing out the large bowel on alternate days either with warm saline, warm boric lotion, or with 2 pints of eusol diluted one and a half times with warm water, sometimes proves effective.

The injection into the lower bowel of 6 to 8 oz. of either protargol ($\frac{1}{2}$ to 1 per cent.), albargin (2 per cent.), nitrate of silver ($\frac{1}{2}$ gr. to the ounce of distilled water) or yatren 105 ($\frac{1}{2}$ per cent.), is worth a trial in obstinate cases.

As a last resort surgical measures may have to be considered.

Patients suffering from chronic dysentery must be warmly clad and should take precautions against chill. Bathing in cold water and the consumption of alcoholic drinks must be forbidden. A change of air or a sea voyage sometimes effects a rapid cure.

ENTERIC FEVER

Recent epidemics in Hawick, Croydon and Bournemouth indicate that, in spite of sanitary precautions, the risk of contamination of water and food supplies with the enteric group of organisms still persists. *B. typhosus* and *B. paratyphosus B.*, the organisms commonly met with in the British Isles, are excreted in the stools and urine during the course of the illness. Temporary and chronic carriers play a very important part in the dissemination of enteric fever. It is estimated that from 2 to 5 per cent. of all cases of enteric fever become permanent carriers. That the incidence of the chronic carrier state is four times higher in women than in men is unfortunate when we consider the possibilities of contamination of food in course of preparation. Whilst the fæcal carrier is more commonly encountered, the urinary carrier is potentially more dangerous. The organisms are discharged intermittently in both stools and urine, so that repeated bacteriological examinations are essential before the carrier state can be excluded. The results of recent studies by Felix[1] (1938) and Bhatnagar[2] (1938) indicate that the presence of Vi antibody in the serum is a certain serological sign of the presence of living typhoid bacilli in the body and that Vi agglutination should be employed in the routine detection of carriers.

Nurses may contract the disease in the course of their routine duties; such a sequence usually indicates insufficient cleansing of the hands. Commonly a case or carrier contaminates water or food. Milk and milk products, prepared meats, uncooked vegetables, fruit and shellfish are the usual vehicles of infection. Flies and infected dust have been proved to convey the disease.

The incubation period of enteric fever is usually from twelve to fourteen days, but may apparently vary from seven to twenty-one days.

The importance of blood culture as a diagnostic aid in obscure febrile conditions is perhaps insufficiently appreciated.

Preventive Treatment.—The control of enteric fever is essentially a problem for the local Sanitary Authority and embraces such factors as an efficient system of sewage disposal, a safe water and milk supply, the detection of carriers, the

[1] Felix, A., *Lancet* (1938), **2**, 738.
[2] Bhatnagar, S. S., *Brit. Med. Jour.* (1938), **2**, 1195.

purification of shellfish, the control of the house-fly and protection of food against contamination by rats and mice.

Early diagnosis of each case and a close liaison between practitioners and the local Public Health Department are important points in the control of epidemic spread.

The simultaneous appearance of a group of cases in a community with good sanitation indicates contamination of the water or milk supply or some food substance; the occurrence of one or two isolated cases of enteric fever suggests household infection from a carrier.

During epidemic prevalence drinking water and milk should be boiled and the consumption of milk products, raw green vegetables and shellfish forbidden until the vehicle of infection has been discovered. Flies should be destroyed.

The routine method of detecting carriers includes a careful medical history, application of the Widal test (O, H and Vi agglutinins) and at least three bacteriological examinations of both stools and urine.

Carriers should be promptly notified to the local Public Health Department, which will arrange for their isolation or supervision.

Adult contacts, whose occupation entails the handling of milk or food, and school children should be quarantined for three weeks from the date of last contact. In the case of the former, particular care should be taken to exclude the carrier condition prior to resuming work.

Vaccination.—T.A.B. vaccine usually contains 1,000 millions of *B. typhosum* and 750 millions each of *B. paratyphosum A* and *B* in each cubic centimetre. The initial dose in adults is 0·5 c.c. followed seven to ten days later by 1·0 c.c.; to children between three and ten years of age 0·25 and 0·5 c.c. may be administered. The injection is given subcutaneously below the clavicle, and as systemic disturbance is liable to follow, the individual should be confined to bed for twenty-four hours after each dose. Contraindications to inoculation are pulmonary tuberculosis, diabetes mellitus and chronic kidney or vascular disease. The vaccine should not be administered during late pregnancy or during the course of an acute infection.

A high degree of protection is attained within two weeks of the final injection, and after lasting for some months gradually lessens over a period of two or more years. Inoculation materially diminishes, but does not exclude, the risk of subsequent enteric infection.

Oral administration of vaccine has been extensively employed on the Continent, in Japan, and elsewhere. The course consists of three successive daily doses each of 50,000 million *B. typhosum* and 25,000 million *B. paratyphosum A* and 25,000 million *B. paratyphosum B* accompanied by a 3-gr. keratin-coated ox-bile tablet. The vaccine should be taken first thing in the morning on an empty stomach, followed two hours later by a light breakfast of tea and toast. A more effective immunity is produced by the subcutaneous injection of vaccine, and oral administration should not be resorted to except under special circumstances.

Topley [1] (1938), in discussing the rôle of active immunization in the control of enteric fever, expresses the following views: Individuals going abroad or to an area where enteric fever is epidemic should be inoculated. There is something to be said for the inoculation of contacts of isolated cases. On the other hand, inoculation of contacts during the height of a brief epidemic due to water or milk is inadvisable. The sanitary breakdown in such epidemics is usually rapidly discovered and rectified, thus removing the major source of infection. Wholesale inoculation in such circumstances would result in the injection of individuals actually incubating the disease, thus leading to "provocation typhoid" with sudden onset and severe course.

Passive Immunization.—The prophylactic value of antityphoid serum requires further investigation. Fenton and Hay [2] (1938) administered from 5 to 10 c.c. of antityphoid serum intramuscularly to thirty-one home contacts; none contracted typhoid fever. According to Felix [3] (1938) the prophylactic dose of antityphoid serum for an adult should amount to from 20 to 30 c.c. administered intramuscularly. Passive immunization should be confined to home or institutional contacts who have been exposed recently and intimately to typhoid infection.

Curative Treatment.—*Serum.*—Whilst statistically inconclusive, the reports so far published on the therapeutic value of the antityphoid serum prepared by Felix at the Lister Institute have been favourable (Felix [4] (1935), Cookson and Facey [5] (1937), M'Sweeney [6] (1937)). The writer has observed marked and rapid improvement following serum administration in a few cases of typhoid fever, but in many others no apparent beneficial effect has been noted.

The usual dose of typhoid serum is 30 c.c. administered intramuscularly on each of two or three successive days as early in the course of the illness as possible.

[1] Topley, W. W. C., *Lancet* (1938), **1,** 181.
[2] Fenton, J., and Hay, C. P., *Brit. Med. Jour.* (1938), **1,** 1090.
[3] Felix, A., *Brit. Med. Jour.* (1938), **1,** 1091.
[4] Felix, A., *Lancet* (1935), **1,** 799.
[5] Cookson, H., and Facey, R. V., *Brit. Med. Jour.* (1937), **1,** 1009.
[6] M'Sweeney, C. J., *Brit. Med. Jour.* (1937), **2,** 1118.

Vaccines, etc.—Typhoid vaccine and various forms of non-specific therapy have been extensively employed in the treatment of enteric fever. The intravenous injection of typhoid vaccine during the first week of the illness may abort the disease, but this method of treatment is not entirely devoid of risk and cannot be recommended.

Bacteriophage.—The published reports on the value of D'Herelle's bacteriophage in the treatment of typhoid fever are so conflicting that it may be reasonable to assume that the preparation is of doubtful value.

General Management.—A practitioner who undertakes the treatment of a case of enteric fever must not only satisfy himself that the home arrangements and resources are adequate, that two nurses experienced in the management of the disease are available, but also be prepared to visit his patient at least twice daily for a period of some three to four weeks. Hospital is the ideal place for treatment, and it is very important that the patient should be removed there at an early stage of the illness.

The patient must be kept strictly recumbent, but his position should be altered several times daily. Mental rest is essential, and visitors should be excluded. A four-hourly chart must be kept and arrangements made for the prompt notification of serious symptoms to the physician. Stools, urine and other discharges, wash water, soiled linen, nursing utensils, etc., require to be carefully disinfected, and the patient's crockery, cutlery, etc., must be boiled after use. Measures should be taken to rid the sickroom of flies. The nurse must on no account prepare or handle food which is to be consumed by other members of the household.

The mouth and skin require regular and careful cleansing, and precautions have to be taken to prevent the development of pressure sores.

Retention of urine is liable to occur and should receive appropriate treatment. Inspection of the stools, abdomen, lung bases and heart should form part of the physician's daily routine examination.

Diet.—Whilst Ker successfully treated many hundreds of cases of enteric fever with a diet limited to milk and beef tea, modern opinion favours a more liberal diet. It is very difficult to get a typhoid patient to take nourishment, but with the aid of a tactful nurse and careful attention to the patient's idiosyncrasies a daily intake of at least 2,000 calories may be attained. During the early days of the illness a fluid diet should be administered. Towards the end of the first week, in addition to 2 pints of milk daily, such readily digestible articles as lightly boiled eggs, custard, ice cream, junket, cream cheese, milk shapes, milk puddings, jellies, mashed potatoes with butter or gravy, prepared breakfast foods, stewed apples, plain chocolate, thin bread and butter, sponge cake, and minced chicken or beef may be administered. Not more than 5 oz. of milk should be administered at one time and each feed should be consumed within fifteen minutes.

Feeds should be given at two-hourly intervals, between 7 A.M. and 9 P.M., and twice during the night when the patient is awake.

Plain cold water or fresh orange, lemon or grape fruit drinks sweetened with lactose or glucose should be administered at least every half hour between feeds. A daily fluid intake, apart from meals, of at least 4 pints is desirable. An occasional cup of weak tea may be appreciated.

Constipation.—Apart from a dose of calomel followed by salts administered during the first week of the illness, purgatives should be avoided and constipation treated by the administration of a soap and water enema every other day. Liquid paraffin, however, may safely be prescribed.

Diarrhœa.—Severe and persistent diarrhœa necessitates restriction and modification of the diet. If curds are present in the stools, milk should be restricted in amount, diluted or peptonized; it may be necessary to replace milk by whey. The carbohydrate intake should be diminished, lactose substituted for glucose and soups excluded. Colonic lavage with warm water or saline once or twice daily followed by a starch and opium enema in the evening is a useful procedure. An occasional dose of 5 gr. of Dover's powder is often effective in lessening the frequency of the motions.

Meteorism.—On the first indication of increasing abdominal distension the diet must be restricted as for the treatment of diarrhœa. If meteorism becomes severe, food should be restricted to whey, albumen water and cold meat juice. A soft rubber catheter should be introduced some 12 in. into the rectum and left *in situ* for twenty minutes. This procedure may be repeated from time to time. Turpentine may be prescribed either by the mouth, 20 minims in a capsule every four hours, or by the rectum, $\frac{1}{2}$ oz. added to a 1-pint soap and water enema. In obstinate cases either 0·5 c.c. of pituitrin, $\frac{1}{50}$ gr. of physostigmine sulphate or 0·1 gm. of acetylcholine may be injected at four-hourly intervals.

Toxæmia.—In severe attacks of enteric fever toxæmia is profound, and by the third week nervous symptoms are prominent and circulatory failure is liable to occur.

Cold water should be freely administered by the mouth. The intravenous injection of from 4 to 8 pints of 5 per cent. glucose saline daily, by the drip method, is very beneficial.

Tepid or cold sponging every four hours is a valuable procedure. Immersing the patient in a bath at 85° F. four-hourly is a very effective but a difficult procedure to carry out in private practice. Delirium calls for appropriate drug treatment (chapter on Management), and cardio-vascular failure for the intravenous injection of 50 per cent. glucose saline. Cyanosis and dyspnœa are indications for the continuous administration of a mixture of oxygen and carbon dioxide by the nasal catheter.

Hæmorrhage and Perforation (see p. 475).—The practitioner must be on the outlook for these serious complications during the third week of the illness. A suitable blood donor should be on call. On the first appearance of blood in the stools or a sudden drop in temperature accompanied by a rising pulse rate, all food and water should be stopped and $\frac{1}{4}$ gr. of morphine plus $\frac{1}{100}$ gr. of atropine sulphate promptly injected. When the effect of the morphine begins to wear off, 5 gr. of Dover's powder may be administered every four hours until the bleeding stops. In severe or persistent hæmorrhage the motions should be received into tow, the foot of the bed raised on blocks, the lower limbs bandaged from below upwards, extra hot bottles inserted and blood transfusions administered. Preparations such as hæmoplastin 2 c.c. subcutaneously every four hours or coagulen-ciba 20 c.c. subcutaneously twice daily may be tried, but are no substitute for transfusion.

Nothing should be given by mouth, except water and fragments of ice to suck, until the hæmorrhage has ceased. Feeding may then be resumed by the hourly administration of dessert-spoonfuls of glucose lemonade, diluted milk, etc., the amount to be cautiously increased day by day until the intake is again adequate.

If the bowels have not moved, an olive oil enema may be given two days after the hæmorrhage has ceased.

Surgical asistance must be summoned immediately perforation is suspected. Morphine should be withheld until the diagnosis is confirmed and operation decided upon.

Phlebitis.—Thrombosis of the veins of the lower limbs is a common complication during convalescence. The affected limb is immobilized with pillows or sand-bags for four weeks, after which period gentle massage and passive movements may be started. The application of hot fomentations will help to relieve the early pain.

Other Complications.—The pain of cholecystitis can be ameliorated by the local application of hot fomentations and the hypodermic injection of morphine and atropine. Suppurative cholecystitis or perforation of the gall-bladder will necessitate surgical aid.

Suppurative bone lesions must be treated on surgical lines. Pus from a periosteal abscess may contain typhoid bacilli, and soiled dressings should be handled with care.

Convalescence.—It is advisable to confine the patient to bed for at least fourteen days after the temperature has returned to normal. Relapse is not uncommon. Three consecutive negative cultures for enteric organisms must be obtained at weekly or bi-weekly intervals from both stools and urine prior to the release of the patient from isolation. Pus from bone lesions or other sources will also require to be examined bacteriologically.

The duration of convalescence varies greatly according to the severity of the illness—ranging from one month in a mild attack of paratyphoid B fever to six months or even longer after a severe infection with *Bact. typhosum.*

Treatment of Carriers.—Enteric organisms continue to be excreted in the stools and/or urine for a variable period of time during convalescence. Ten to twenty grains of urotropine three times daily will clear up most urinary carriers. The urine must be acidified with 30 gr. of acid sodium phosphate thrice daily prior to the administration of urotropine, which should always be prescribed separately. Should the carrier condition persist in spite of three weeks treatment with urotropine, sulphanilamide or ammonium mandelate may be tried. Neither drug, vaccine nor dietetic treatment can be relied upon to cure the chronic intestinal carrier. It is impracticable to isolate the persistent convalescent carrier indefinitely and the practitioner, when faced with this difficulty, should apply to the local Medical Officer of Health for advice. An individual should not be classified as a chronic carrier until he has been excreting typhoid bacilli for one year. Prior to release from isolation, typhoid carriers must be given detailed written instructions regarding personal hygiene, and must undertake not to engage in any occupation entailing the handling of food. Members of the household to which the carrier returns should be inoculated against enteric fever.

Cholecystectomy will cure 75 per cent. of chronic intestinal carriers, and nephrectomy has proved successful in selected urinary carriers.

Where typhoid bacilli continue to be excreted in the pus

from a chronic bone lesion, appropriate surgical measures are usually effective in clearing up the condition.

ENCEPHALITIS LETHARGICA

The incidence of this serious disease of the central nervous system, which reached a peak in Great Britain in 1924, has, fortunately, diminished during recent years. The causal agent is thought to be a filterable virus which is probably disseminated by droplet infection and presumably gains entry through the upper respiratory passages. The infectivity is low, case to case infection being unusual, but there is reason to believe that mild and abortive attacks are not uncommon and along with carriers probably play the major part in the spread of the disease.

The duration of the incubation period is uncertain, but according to different observers may vary from one day to as long as three weeks.

Encephalitis lethargica is a notifiable disease.

Preventive Treatment.—As yet there are no specific or general measures available which can be relied upon to control the spread of encephalitis lethargica. The patient must be promptly isolated. Children should be excluded from school for three weeks from the date of last contact with the case. The nose and throat of contacts may be douched or sprayed with a 1 : 5,000 solution of permanganate of potash in normal saline morning and evening. During epidemic prevalence the same general preventive measures should be applied as recommended for the control of poliomyelitis and cerebrospinal fever (pp. 50, 14).

Curative Treatment.—The effective treatment of a case of encephalitis lethargica is limited to skilled nursing and the relief of symptoms.

General Management.—Confinement to bed is essential even in mild attacks. Isolation should be continued for three weeks from the onset of the illness. The fauces and nasopharynx should be sprayed and the mouth swabbed with a 1 : 1,000 solution of permanganate of potash in normal saline every four hours. If conjunctivitis be present the eyes should be cleansed with warm boric lotion thrice daily. Discharges from the mouth, nose and eyes must be carefully collected and either burnt or disinfected. Lethargic patients require to be fed at regular intervals on the lines laid down for the treatment of enteric fever. Feeding by the nasal tube may be necessary.

At least 4 pints of plain water or glucose lemonade should be administered daily.

Constipation is a feature of the disease which necessitates the regular use of laxatives or enemata. The condition of the bladder requires to be watched and retention promptly treated. Headache and general aches and pains may be relieved by the ice-bag and the administration of either a combination of aspirin with Dover's powder, 10 gr. of each, every six hours, or the hypodermic injection of morphine. Radiotherapy may be tried for the relief of severe and persistent neuralgic pains. If the cerebrospinal fluid is under pressure, repeated lumbar puncture is beneficial. Insomnia, restlessness and delirium are best treated by the prolonged hot bath, or hot pack, and the exhibition of chloral and bromide or other sedatives.

Even large doses of sedatives sometimes fail to relieve persistent hiccough, which may only be controlled by the inhalation of chloroform.

Convalescence.—Convalescence is usually slow and tedious. The patient should be in the open air as much as possible. Rigidity or residual paralysis improve following massage, passive and active movements and hydrotherapy.

After a varying period of apparent recovery various distressing sequelæ, such as Parkinsonism, and mental changes frequently appear, leading to chronic invalidism. For their treatment see p. 992.

ERYSIPELAS

For the treatment of erysipelas see p. 88.

GLANDULAR FEVER

Epidemics of this acute infectious disease of unknown ætiology have of recent years occurred in various schools and institutions, and sporadic cases are not uncommon among the general population. Whilst susceptibility to the disease appears to be almost universal, the degree of infectivity is not high. The writer has treated cases of glandular fever in a mixed ward with no ill results. The disease may perhaps be spread by droplet infection. The incubation period lies usually between five and fifteen days. Fever accompanied by acute enlargement of the lymph glands, particularly of the neck, is the form of the disease commonly met with in children. Febrile and anginose types occur in young adults. A mononuclear leucocytosis is characteristic of the disease. The sheep cell agglutination test described by Bunnell[1] (1933) has proved a valuable aid to diagnosis.

Glandular fever, or infective mononucleosis as it is sometimes called, is not a notifiable disease.

Preventive Treatment.—There is no specific method of prophylaxis against glandular fever.

Providing reasonable precautions are taken and the patient isolated, there is little chance of other members of the household becoming infected (Tidy,[2] 1934). Contact children should be kept under observation for a period of three weeks, dating from the last contact, but need not be kept away from school. In residential schools the isolation of contacts usually proves ineffectual in limiting the spread of the disease.

Curative Treatment.—There is no therapeutic measure yet available which will cut short the disease. The treatment of glandular fever is purely symptomatic.

General Management.—The patient should be confined to bed and kept there until the temperature has been normal for one week and the glandular swelling markedly diminished. The diet is limited to fluids and soft solids during the febrile stage of the illness, and water freely administered. Hot fomentations may be applied to the neck if the swollen glands are painful. The anginose type in adults simulates diphtheria, but the faucial exudate does not respond to treatment with diphtheria antitoxin. The throat should be sprayed with hydrogen peroxide diluted with two parts of warm water and subsequently douched with hot saline several times daily. The membrane may persist for many days.

The febrile type with high and prolonged pyrexia, lasting several weeks, requires to be treated on the same lines as a case of enteric fever.

Whilst little is known regarding infectivity, it is probably a wise precaution to disinfect the secretions from the upper respiratory tract.

Epistaxis, hæmaturia and conjunctivitis are occasional complications.

Convalescence.—Recrudescences are very liable to occur. Even after mild attacks anæmia and slight debility may persist for several months. A change of air is definitely beneficial, and Blaud's pill (45 gr. daily) or iron and ammonium citrate (90 gr. daily) should be prescribed.

[1] Bunnell, W. W., *Amer. Jour. Med. Sci.* (1933), **186**, 346.
[2] Tidy, H. L., *Lancet* (1934), **2**, 236.

INFLUENZA

That epidemic influenza is primarily a virus infection has been proved by the work of Smith, Andrewes and Laidlaw [1] (1933) (1935). The virus can be recovered from the nose and throat during the early stages of the illness. A highly infectious disease, influenza has as yet defied all attempts at control. The virus is usually transmitted by direct contact (droplet infection), but may also be conveyed by articles recently contaminated with nasal or buccal secretions. Infectivity probably persists throughout the febrile stage of the illness. The incubation period is approximately forty-eight hours.

An abrupt onset with marked constitutional disturbance is characteristic of epidemic influenza. In febrile catarrh, which is frequently confused with influenza, symptoms such as coryza, sore throat and cough usually precede the fever by several days.

Influenza is only notifiable when complicated by pneumonia.

Preventive Treatment.—Prophylactic inoculation with living or dead virus is still in the experimental stage, but Andrewes [2] (1937) is hopeful that an effective vaccine against influenza may yet be produced. By analogy with other virus infections the intramuscular injection of 5 c.c. of serum or 15 c.c. of whole blood from a convalescent might result in either complete temporary immunity or a modification in severity of the subsequent attack.

Free ventilation, avoidance of crowds, a healthy mode of life, and an adequate and balanced diet are measures which will lessen the risk of contracting influenza.

Whilst the wearing of masks has proved ineffective in preventing the spread of influenza among the general population, there is something to be said in favour of the efficient masking of those in attendance on influenza patients.

The routine employment of antiseptic gargles or sprays is, in the writer's opinion, of very dubious prophylactic value.

Vaccination against the secondary invading organisms associated with the serious complications of influenza has been extensively practised. A mixed vaccine containing 400 million *B. Pfeiffer*, 200 million pneumococci and 100 million streptococci in each cubic centimetre may be injected subcutaneously in doses of 0·1, 0·2, 0·4, 0·8, 1·2 and 1·5 c.c. every fourth day.

[1] Smith, W., Andrewes, C. H., and Laidlaw, P. P., *Lancet* (1933), **2**, 66; *Brit. Jour. Exp. Path.*, (1935), **16**, 291.

[2] Andrewes, C. H., *Brit. Med. Jour.* (1937), **2**, 513.

Curative Treatment.—*General Management.*—Immediately influenza is suspected the patient must be isolated and confined to bed in a freely ventilated room. There is no specific serum or drug treatment of proven value for influenza. In severe or complicated attacks, however, the intramuscular injection of convalescent human serum or whole blood in repeated doses of 50 c.c. may be worth a trial.

The diet should be restricted to warm fluids administered at two-hourly intervals during the day and four-hourly during the night if the patient is awake. Water flavoured with fresh orange, lemon or grape-fruit juice, and sweetened with glucose, must be given freely.

The bowels should be freely opened at the commencement of the illness, and thereafter regulated by mild aperients.

The mouth, nose, eyes and skin require regular and careful cleansing. Sponging the skin with warm or tepid water adds greatly to the patient's comfort and should be performed every four hours when the temperature exceeds 103° F.

Aspirin and Dover's powder, 10 gr. of each every six hours, is usually effective in alleviating the headache, insomnia and general discomfort. For the treatment of such symptoms as severe headache, persistent insomnia and nausea and vomiting the reader is referred to the section on General Management of the Fevered Person (see p. 6).

Cough is frequently troublesome and exhausting, and may be relieved by 1-drachm doses of syrup of codeine or a diamorphine linctus administered at intervals of four to six hours. The inhalation of steam impregnated with either tincture of benzoin or oil of eucalyptus three or four times daily is a useful procedure. When chest symptoms are prominent, expectoration will be aided by a simple expectorant mixture such as the following, administered three or four times daily :—

℞ Tinct. Ipecac. . . . . . . ♏x
Tinct. Opii camph. . . . . . ♏x
Syr. Prun. Serot. . . . . . ʒi
Aq. Chlorof. . . . . . ad ℥ss

The slightest degree of cyanosis is an indication for the continuous administration of oxygen, either by the oxygen tent or by the nasal catheter. Four-hourly or even two-hourly hypodermic administration of either adrenalin (5 to 10 minims), pituitrin ($\frac{1}{2}$ c.c.), strychnine ($\frac{1}{32}$ to $\frac{1}{16}$ gr.) or camphor (3 gr.) may be of some assistance in warding off cardio-vascular failure ; glucose should be injected intravenously.

Complications.—Every case of influenza is a potential case of broncho-pneumonia. Pleurisy, empyema, and œdema or emphysema of the lung may develop. Acute suppurative otitis media, paranasal sinus suppuration, myocarditis, nephritis and neuralgia are other common complications, for the treatment of which the reader is referred to the appropriate sections of this book.

Convalescence.—The importance of an adequate period of convalescence after influenza must be impressed upon the patient. Owing to the toxic effect of influenza on the myocardium it is advisable to keep even the mildest case in bed for at least three days after the temperature has settled. In more severe attacks this period should be extended to one to two weeks. The response of the heart to increased exertion must be carefully watched, and further rest enforced if this be unsatisfactory. Fresh air, sunlight, ample good food and exercise short of fatigue will hasten recovery. A change of surroundings is very beneficial, particularly to patients suffering from the characteristic mental depression or residual tracheitis. Cough due to tracheitis is sometimes very persistent, but is usually relieved to some extent by the administration of 1-drachm doses thrice daily of either elixir diamorphinæ et terpini cum apomorphina or syrup of codeine. Infected nasal sinuses may be the exciting factor and should receive appropriate treatment.

Before permitting the patient to resume work the practitioner should satisfy himself by a careful clinical examination, particularly of the cardio-vascular, respiratory and nervous systems, that recovery is complete.

MEASLES

Measles is one of the most important and most highly infectious diseases of childhood. Owing to the risk of a complicating broncho-pneumonia it is a particularly serious infection in children under three years of age. The causal agent, a filterable virus, is commonly spread by direct contact (droplet infection), particularly during the catarrhal stage of the illness, a stage at which measles is seldom diagnosed. Except for those who have previously suffered from the disease, susceptibility to measles appears to be practically universal. During an epidemic a small proportion of exposed susceptible children may, however, as the result of a process of latent immunization, either escape the disease entirely or suffer from it in a highly modified form. The incubation period is usually from nine to eleven days, but may vary from seven to fourteen days.

Measles should always be suspected when a child who has not previously suffered from the disease develops catarrhal symptoms accompanied by an evening temperature. The diagnostic importance of Koplik's spots is not even yet sufficiently appreciated. Prodromal rashes are of common occurrence.

In certain areas the first case of measles occurring in a household has to be notified to the Medical Officer of Health. Otherwise the disease is not notifiable.

Preventive Treatment.—*Passive Immunization.*—The intramuscular injection of an appropriate dose of one or other of the following preparations, namely: (1) human convalescent serum or whole blood; (2) the serum or whole blood of adults who have previously suffered from measles; or (3) immune globulin (human) can be relied upon to prevent or modify an attack of measles in an exposed susceptible child. As the supply of human convalescent serum, the most effective prophylactic preparation, is necessarily limited, its use should be reserved for the passive immunization of children under four years of age.

Certain progressive Sanitary Authorities have arranged for the collection and issue to practitioners of convalescent or adult measles serum. Immune globulin (human) is obtainable commercially.

Except in an ailing or weakly child, the aim should be to attenuate rather than to prevent an attack of measles. Such a procedure will enable the child to gain a lasting immunity.

The dose of the various prophylactic preparations suitable for a child under five years of age is set out in the following table. Owing to variations in the antibody content of human serum, complete protection cannot, however, always be relied upon to follow the administration of the dosage indicated.

Dosage of Measles Prophylactic Preparations

	Day of Exposure.	Convalescent.		Adult.		Immune Globulin.
		Serum.	Whole Blood.	Serum.	Whole Blood.	
Complete Protection.	First to Fourth.	5·0 c.c.	10 c.c.	20 c.c.	30 c.c.	4 c.c.
Attenuation .	First to Fourth.	2·5 c.c.	5 c.c.	10 c.c.	15 c.c.	2 c.c.
	Fifth to Eighth.	5·0 c.c.	10 c.c.	15 c.c.	20 c.c.	4 c.c.

Whilst immune globulin has the advantage of being readily obtained, mild systemic reactions not uncommonly follow its injection, and on rare occasions even severe and alarming collapse has been noted (Eason [1] (1938)).

Should the practitioner fail to obtain a supply of convalescent or adult serum, blood may be withdrawn from a vein of either parent into a sterile syringe and forthwith injected intramuscularly into the exposed child. No anti-coagulant is necessary. There is no risk of anaphylaxis. Needless to say, the parent must have suffered from measles at some previous date.

General Measures.—Contacts who have not previously suffered from measles are usually excluded from school for three weeks from the date of onset of the last case in the house. Forbes [2] (1936) is of the opinion that home contacts should continue to attend school, unless under exceptional circumstances, provided they are inspected daily by the school nursing staff, or by teachers trained to recognize the early symptoms of measles. This procedure, he maintains, would lead to early diagnosis and prompt isolation, and would ensure proper medical care and nursing from the onset of the attack. No restrictions need be applied to children who have previously suffered from measles. When measles is prevalent susceptible children should not attend parties, the cinema or other gatherings.

The view widely held among the public that, as a child will probably contract measles some time, the sooner it passes through an attack the better, cannot be too strongly condemned. Every precaution should be taken to prevent the exposure of young children to measles.

Curative Treatment.—*Serum.*—There is no specific of proven value in the treatment of measles. The intramuscular injection of human convalescent serum has not, in the writer's experience, been followed by any demonstrable clinical improvement.

General Management.—Immediately measles is suspected, the child must be isolated and confined to bed in a freely ventilated yet warm (60° to 65° F.) room. The real danger of measles lies in the complications arising from invasion with such organisms as *S. pyogenes*, the pneumococcus and Pfeiffer's bacillus. Whilst in some cases the patient may be harbouring these organisms in the upper respiratory tract prior to the onset of measles, in others infection arises through droplet spread from individuals in the patient's environment. Under

[1] Eason, G. A., *Brit. Med. Jour.* (1938), **1**, 488.
[2] Forbes, D., *Lancet* (1936), **2**, 457.

no circumstances should attendants or visitors suffering from acute or chronic catarrhal infection be allowed into the sickroom unless efficiently masked. The fewer visitors the patient sees the better.

Discharges from the mouth, nose and eyes should be collected on rags or paper handkerchiefs and promptly burned.

The bed should be placed so that the patient does not face the light. Excess of bedclothes is a common fault; a sheet and one or, at most, two layers of blanket is ample. The patient should wear a single cotton or flannel nightgown and be kept warm by hot-water bottles. The whole skin surface should be sponged with soap and warm water once daily. The bowels should be freely opened at the commencement of the illness by the administration of either castor oil or in older children a dose of salts. Milk of magnesia or other mild aperient may be administered as indications arise.

The mouth and nose must be gently cleansed at regular and frequent intervals. In very young children the mouth can be swabbed with cotton-wool soaked in warm saline or a solution of bicarbonate of soda (20 gr. to 1 pint). In older children the mouth should be rinsed with warm saline after each meal and the teeth cleansed. The throat may be sprayed with a warm solution of bicarbonate of soda. The lips may be smeared with vaseline or boric ointment.

Nasal discharge should frequently be removed, the anterior nares gently swabbed with warm bicarbonate solution, and along with the upper lip subsequently smeared with simple vaseline. Older children may be encouraged to clear the nose by gentle blowing.

The eyes should be irrigated with warm boric lotion (4 gr. to 1 oz.) at varying intervals, from twice daily to hourly, according to the severity of the conjunctivitis. Vaseline or boric ointment smeared on the edges of the lids after each treatment prevents adhesion. In the more severe infections one drop of 10 per cent. solution of argyrol in each eye thrice daily will hasten cure. Irrigation with a $\frac{1}{2}$ per cent. solution of zinc sulphate is more effective when the conjunctivitis tends to persist in a subacute form.

When the temperature reaches 104° F., an effort should be made to reduce it by tepid sponging at four-hourly intervals. This procedure is very valuable for the relief of restlessness and insomnia.

Inflammatory catarrh of the whole gastro-intestinal tract is present to some degree in every case of measles, hence the necessity for dietetic discretion. In a short infection like uncomplicated measles the intake of food can be left to the patient's inclination. In infants, milk, suitably diluted with water according to age, is given at the same intervals as prior to the onset of measles—every three to four hours. Between feeds drinks of water flavoured with orange or lemon juice and sweetened by the addition of from 2 to 5 per cent. of glucose should be offered, slightly warmed, every half hour. Should diarrhœa prove troublesome, the milk should be omitted for twenty-four hours and then resumed, previously citrated or peptonized. In older children, undiluted milk may be supplemented by thin gruels or milk puddings if desired. As soon as the temperature begins to fall the appetite tends to return, and a full diet may be administered when the temperature is again normal.

The irritating cough may be relieved by the inhalation of steam impregnated with Friar's balsam, and a nightly dose of either compound tincture of camphor or Dover's powder. A simple cough mixture may be prescribed if desired, but the writer has little faith in expectorants. When the child has difficulty in expelling abundant secretions, alternate hot and cold fomentations or hot mustard baths may prove beneficial by stimulating increased respiratory movements.

Complications.—Broncho-pneumonia is by far the most common of the serious complications of measles.

The treatment of broncho-pneumonia following measles in no way differs from the treatment of broncho-pneumonia in general. The great value of an abundance of fresh air or, preferably, treatment in the open air cannot be over-emphasized. Bronchitis is a frequent complication. For details of treatment of these conditions the reader is referred to the section on Respiratory Diseases (see p. 782).

A mild degree of laryngitis is a common early symptom in measles. The occurrence of severe dyspnœa during the stage of eruption or in early convalescence usually indicates a diphtheritic or coccal infection of the larynx, and should be regarded as an indication for the intramuscular injection of 16,000 units of anti-diphtheritic serum and the immediate removal of the patient to hospital. The diagnosis and subsequent treatment of the condition is on the lines described in the chapter on Diphtheria (see p. 19).

If the gastro-intestinal symptoms characteristic of the acute stage of measles continue into convalescence, or become more severe, then active treatment should be applied. Milk should be stopped, and 1 to 2 oz. of half-strength normal saline with the addition of 2½ per cent. glucose administered by mouth every hour for twenty-four hours. Whey, albumen water or lactic acid milk (2 drops of lactic acid (B.P.) to 1 oz. of skimmed cow's milk) with added sugar may then be cautiously administered, 2 oz. every three hours, and saline liberally supplied between feeds. If vomiting is troublesome, glucose saline must be administered rectally, subcutaneously, intraperitoneally or intravenously. Drugs do not appear to be of much value in this condition.

In hospital practice the condition is frequently due to a superimposed infection with dysentery bacilli.

The appearance of corneal ulceration calls for dilatation of the pupil, either by atropine drops or ointment ($\frac{1}{4}$ per cent.) and the use of 10 per cent. argyrol drops thrice daily.

Convalescence.—In an uncomplicated case the child may be allowed out of bed about the tenth to twelfth day from the onset of the disease, and out of isolation on the fourteenth day. Plenty of good wholesome food and exercise in the open air will hasten convalescence. A holiday at the seaside or country is very beneficial, particularly to cases with residual pulmonary catarrh. A course of ultra-violet ray treatment and the administration of cod-liver oil are useful measures during the winter months.

MUMPS

The infective agent in mumps is a filterable virus which is present in the saliva during the acute stage of the illness. The disease is commonly spread by direct contact (droplet infection), and possibly by articles recently contaminated with infective saliva. Infectivity probably persists from the onset of the first symptom until the swelling of the salivary glands has subsided. The incubation period varies from twelve to twenty-six days, but usually lies between seventeen and twenty-one days.

Whilst the parotid is the gland most frequently involved, it is well to remember that the submaxillary or sublingual salivary glands may be exclusively affected and that abortive attacks of mumps, owing to the lack of facial deformity, may readily be missed. The occurrence of a lymphocytosis is of some diagnostic value.

Mumps is not a notifiable disease.

Preventive Treatment.—*Specific Prophylaxis.*—The intramuscular injection of 10 c.c. of serum or 20 c.c. of whole blood from a mumps convalescent has been successfully employed as a prophylactic. It is doubtful if the method is worth while in such a habitually mild disease.

General Measures.—The patient must be promptly isolated. The quarantine period for mumps contacts is twenty-six days, but where the date of exposure is definitely known, an exposed child may safely attend school for the first ten days of this period. In actual practice, providing a contact is examined daily and isolated on the first suspicion of illness, exclusion of contacts from school in the case of a mild infection like mumps seems unnecessary. A child who has previously suffered from the disease may, for practical purposes, be regarded as immune and need undergo no restrictions. Adult contacts may continue their business activities.

Curative Treatment.—*General Management.*—There is no specific treatment for mumps.

The patient should be confined to bed as long as the parotid swelling persists. Owing to the risk of orchitis, a minimum period of ten days in bed is probably wise in the case of adolescent and adult males. Difficulty in opening the mouth and pain on mastication are indications for the restriction of the diet to fluids and soft solids.

Hot dry cotton-wool or hot fomentations applied to the swollen glands will help to relieve pain and local discomfort.

The mouth should be washed out with a 1 : 5,000 solution of permanganate of potash or other mild antiseptic preparation four times daily.

Following preliminary purgation, the bowels may be regulated by the administration of mild aperients.

Treatment of Complications.—Orchitis usually develops when the parotid swelling is at its height and may be expected in approximately 20 per cent. of males above the age of puberty. Surround the scrotum with hot dry cotton-wool and support the inflamed parts either by a pillow placed between the thighs or by a suspensory bandage. The bowels should be freely opened by the administration of $\frac{1}{2}$ to 1 oz. of magnesium sulphate.

Symptoms of gastric disturbance are usually due to pancreatitis. A hot bag or hot fomentations applied to the site of the pain, with limitation of food and the exclusion of fat from the diet, will give relief. If the pain be severe, $\frac{1}{4}$ gr. of morphine may be injected hypodermically.

Meningeal symptoms are liable to be met with in some epidemics, and, if severe, should be relieved by repeated lumbar puncture.

There is no effective treatment for acute labyrinthitis, which is fortunately a very rare complication.

Convalescence.—Convalescence is usually rapid. Isolation

of the patient should be continued for one week after the parotid swelling has subsided. The minimum isolation period is fourteen days. To diminish the risk of orchitis, adult patients should avoid erotic excitement, cycling or riding for at least one month after recovery.

ACUTE POLIOMYELITIS

The incidence of paralytic cases gives a very erroneous impression of the actual prevalence of acute poliomyelitis. The presence of neutralizing antibodies in the blood serum of from 50 to 60 per cent. of the adult population indicates that a large proportion of urban dwellers have suffered from an unrecognized or abortive attack of poliomyelitis. The disease is transmitted through the transfer of the secretions of the nose and throat from person to person by droplet infection, by fingers and the common use of articles recently contaminated with these secretions. The virus attaches itself to the olfactory hairs. Ascending by way of the olfactory nerves it invades the nerve cells with more or less extensive spread from brain to spinal cord.

Carriers and unrecognized or abortive cases play a very important part in the spread of this serious disease.

The duration of infectivity is unknown. The virus has been isolated from the nasopharynx during the third week of convalescence, and in one case as late as four months after the onset.

The incubation period appears to be from two to fourteen days, the average period being about ten days.

Acute poliomyelitis, including acute polioencephalitis, is a notifiable disease.

Preventive Treatment.—*Specific Prophylaxis.*—Human convalescent or adult serum has been extensively used as a prophylactic against poliomyelitis, but the results have been disappointing. If it be desired to give the method a trial, either 10 c.c. of human convalescent serum or 20 c.c. of whole blood from an adult may be injected intramuscularly.

Attempts to produce an active immunity against poliomyelitis by means of vaccines have not so far proved successful.

Nasal Spray.—Recent efforts have been directed at preventing the passage of the poliomyelitis virus along the olfactory nerves by spraying the nose with various coagulating solutions such as 1 per cent. zinc sulphate, or a combination of picric acid with sodium aluminium sulphate, 0·5 per cent. of each in normal saline.

Apart from the technical difficulties associated with this method of prophylaxis, an analysis of the results obtained with the zinc sulphate spray during the Toronto epidemic of 1937 indicates that the method is of no prophylactic value.

One must conclude with regret that as yet there is no effective specific method of control of poliomyelitis.

General Measures.—The probability that the virus of poliomyelitis may be more or less widely distributed among the contacts, even by the time the first clinical case is recognized, raises difficult problems in control.

On the occurrence of a case of poliomyelitis in a household the patient must be promptly and effectively isolated. Children who have been in contact with the patient are strictly quarantined and kept under medical surveillance for a period of three weeks from the date of last contact. Adult contacts may continue their occupation providing it does not entail mixing with children as in the case of nurses and school-teachers. They should, however, abstain from all social activities for three weeks from the date of last contact ; kissing or playing with young children must be strictly forbidden.

A contact who suffers from a febrile catarrh or other symptoms suggestive of an abortive attack of poliomyelitis should be strictly isolated until recovery ensues.

The importance of free ventilation cannot be too strongly emphasized. Contacts should spend as much time in the open air as possible. Children should not sleep together in the same bed. The common use of handkerchiefs must be discouraged.

The routine use of an antiseptic gargle and nasal douche or spray is of very doubtful prophylactic value. Warm normal saline may, if desired, be sniffed up the nostrils twice or thrice daily, and returned through the mouth.

The prevention of epidemic spread of poliomyelitis in residential schools and institutions is a problem for the local Medical Officer of Health. Adequate spacing of beds in dormitories and free ventilation are of paramount importance. The closure of infected residential schools is not to be recommended because of the risk of introducing the poliomyelitis virus into non-infected communities.

Whilst an epidemic prevails, young children should not be permitted to enter any house wherein there is a case of poliomyelitis, and all gatherings of children should be avoided. Closure of day schools may have to be considered.

Curative Treatment.—*Serum Treatment.*—Very divergent views have been expressed regarding the value of human convalescent serum in the treatment of acute poliomyelitis. The difficulty in diagnosing the disease in the pre-paralytic stage and variations in the antibody content of the serum employed are probably responsible for this unsatisfactory state of affairs, and much more work will have to be done before the value of the remedy can be accurately appraised. In a disease fraught with such serious possibilities it is perhaps wise, if serum be available, to give the patient the benefit of the doubt. Serum treatment is useless once paralysis has appeared, hence the importance of early diagnosis. During epidemic prevalence the occurrence of such symptoms as fever, vomiting, sweating, headache, stiffness of the neck and drowsiness with irritability should lead to immediate examination of the patient's cerebrospinal fluid; only if the changes characteristic of poliomyelitis are present in the fluid should serum be administered.

Opinions differ as to the best route of administration of the serum—whether intrathecal only, intravenous only or by both routes. The writer favours the intravenous injection of from 25 to 50 c.c. of serum; the dose to be repeated after an interval of twelve hours.

Practitioners desiring a supply of human convalescent poliomyelitis serum should apply to the local Public Health Department. The serum is not available commercially, and the supply from private sources is extremely limited.

General Management.—Pre-paralytic Stage.—Absolute rest, quiet surroundings, the minimum of handling and the relief of pain and insomnia are the essentials in the treatment of the pre-paralytic stage of acute poliomyelitis. If trained day and night nurses cannot be obtained, the patient should be transferred to hospital.

Isolation should be strictly enforced and visitors discouraged. Discharges from the nose and throat must be carefully collected on rags or paper handkerchiefs, which are promptly burnt. The urine and stools may be infective and require to be disinfected.

Hyperæsthesia and fear of pain on handling are usually prominent symptoms. The painful limb or muscles should be wrapped in hot dry cotton-wool and kept warm by extra hot bottles. When the weight of the bedclothes causes distress a cradle should be employed. Aspirin in doses of 2 to 10 gr. every four hours will help to relieve pain. Chloral and bromide should be prescribed for restlessness or insomnia. Otherwise the treatment of the case is on general lines.

Paralytic Stage.—When paralysis is evident, the extent of muscular involvement must be carefully assessed and the affected limbs kept in the appropriate position by means of sand-bags or light splints. Paralysed legs should be kept extended, adducted and rotated in with the feet kept at right angles to the legs; a small pillow should be inserted beneath the knees and the child kept flat. In the case of paralysis of the deltoid muscle the arm should be abducted to a right angle with the body. Involvement of the muscles of the back necessitates a strictly supine and straight position in bed until such time as a proper spinal support can be applied. In pharyngeal paralysis, the foot of the bed should be raised eighteen inches, secretions aspirated from the pharynx at regular intervals by a soft rubber catheter, and food administered by the nasal tube, supplemented if necessary by intravenous or rectal glucose salines. The mechanical respirator affords the only effective therapeutic measure in cases suffering from paralysis of the respiratory muscles.

Convalescence.—After the temperature has been normal for several days and all muscle tenderness has disappeared, plaster cases and splints should be applied under the guidance of an orthopædic surgeon, who should, in fact, be called upon to supervise the case from the onset of paralysis. Daily gentle massage and passive movements of the affected limbs may be supplemented by the local application of radiant heat. Treatment in the open air is of great value. After an isolation period of six weeks, arrangements should be made to secure continued orthopædic supervision and treatment, preferably by transfer of the patient to an orthopædic hospital.

PSITTACOSIS

Human infection with the virus of psittacosis arises through contact with diseased parrots, budgerigars or other members of the parrot family. The bird may show signs of illness. On the other hand, apparently healthy home-bred birds may carry the virus and prove to be a very real danger. The filterable virus is excreted in the bird's droppings, and the portal of infection in man is probably the respiratory tract. Human case to case infection has been suspected but not proven.

The duration of the incubation period is uncertain, but may be seven days or longer.

Psittacosis is not a notifiable disease.

An acute febrile illness with combined typhoidal and pneumonic symptoms occurring in a person who has to do with parrots, etc., is probably psittacosis. The diagnosis can be confirmed either by the isolation of the virus from the blood or sputum, or by the complement fixation test. An attempt should be made to demonstrate psittacosis virus in the suspected bird even though the latter may appear healthy.

Preventive Treatment.—Following the epidemic of psittacosis in this country in 1930, the immigration of birds of the parrot family was strictly controlled. Unfortunately, this policy has failed to banish the human disease. The simple and obvious method of prevention rests with the public, who, if they do not wish to run the risk of psittacosis should not keep these birds in their homes.

Actually the risk of contracting the disease from birds that have been in a household for many months or years is negligible, but newly acquired birds should be suspect.

Persons owning these pets should (1) avoid fondling and petting the birds; (2) protect food and water from fouling by the birds; and (3) keep the cage thoroughly clean. An ailing bird of little monetary value should be killed and burnt; if of value, it should be isolated and laboratory aid enlisted to arrive at a diagnosis. Extreme care must be taken in handling and disinfecting all articles with which the bird has come in contact.

Curative Treatment.—There is no effective specific treatment for psittacosis.

Treatment is purely symptomatic and the general management of the case is on the lines recommended for enteric fever and pneumonia.

Although isolation need not be enforced, it is probably wise to regard the patient as potentially infective. Sputum, urine and stools should be disinfected.

RUBELLA (Syn: German Measles)

Probably a virus infection, rubella is spread by direct contact and, possibly, by fomites. There is no information available regarding the conveyance of infection by carriers.

Infectivity appears to be limited to the prodromal and eruptive stages of the illness.

The incubation period is usually from fourteen to eighteen days, but may vary from twelve to twenty-one days.

Rubella is not a notifiable disease.

Preventive Treatment.—There is no specific method of prophylaxis against rubella.

Contact children who have not had the disease should be excluded from school for three weeks from the date of last exposure to the patient. When the date of exposure to infection is definitely known, absence from school may safely be curtailed to the period from the eleventh to the twenty-first day inclusive. If quarantine is not practised, school contacts must be inspected daily, and promptly isolated on the appearance of slight catarrh or swollen cervical glands. Apart from nurses, school-teachers, etc., adults who have been in contact with a case of rubella may continue their business activities.

Curative Treatment.—Treatment is purely symptomatic. The patient should remain in bed until the temperature has subsided and the rash faded. The illness is usually so mild that the patient can be kept on an ordinary diet and no special treatment is required.

Complications are rare.

An isolation period of one week from the appearance of the rash is ample.

SCARLET FEVER

That scarlet fever is an infection of the throat by certain strains of *S. hæmolyticus*, which produce a soluble toxin, was proved by the work of the Dicks. The rash and constitutional symptoms are due to absorption of the toxin. Mild cases of the disease are liable to be missed and are a frequent source of infection. Individuals immune to the toxin may suffer from a local faucial infection with the scarlet fever organism and yet show no rash. Such cases, along with carriers, play an important part in the spread of scarlet fever and render control of the disease practically impossible.

Infection is usually conveyed either by direct contact or by articles contaminated with oral or nasal secretions. Milk, infected from a human source, has been responsible for epidemic spread.

The duration of infectivity of a case of scarlet fever is uncertain and may extend to many weeks.

The incubation period is usually from two to four days, but may vary from one to seven days.

Scarlet fever is a notifiable disease. Notification is still restricted to cases showing the typical skin eruption.

Preventive Treatment.—*The Dick Test.*—Susceptibility to scarlet fever can be ascertained by the intradermal injection of 0·2 c.c. of diluted scarlet fever toxin (Dick test) which, if the person be susceptible, will produce within twelve hours an area of erythema 1 cm. or more in diameter. A control injection, with heated toxin, is unnecessary in children under ten years of age. Reliable Dick-test products can be obtained commercially. The technique is the same as for the Schick test in diphtheria.

Experience with the Dick test indicates that the majority of infants, especially during the first six months of life, are immune to scarlet fever, and that the susceptibility rate in children from one to nine years of age varies from 15 to 90 per cent., according to age and environment.

It is to be noted that a Dick negative reactor, although immune to clinical scarlet fever, may yet suffer from a tonsillo-pharyngitis due to infection with scarlatinal strains of streptococci.

Active Immunization.—At least 90 per cent. of Dick positive reactors can be rendered Dick negative by the subcutaneous injection at weekly intervals of 500, 2,000, 8,000, 25,000 and 50,000 skin-test doses of sterile scarlatinal toxin. A susceptibility test should be performed four weeks after completion of the course. The immunity so attained, which is purely antitoxic, will in the majority of individuals last for years, but cannot be relied upon to prevent upper respiratory tract infections with the scarlatinal streptococcus. A modified course of 500, 3,000, 12,000 and 30,000 skin-test doses of toxin, administered at weekly intervals, will in most cases produce a satisfactory but shorter lived immunity.

Unfortunately, the immunizing injections are liable to give rise to unpleasant but not serious reactions. Whilst active immunization is the most effective procedure in the prevention of epidemics of scarlet fever in residential schools and institutions, this method of prophylaxis is unsuitable for general application during the present mild phase of scarlet fever.

Where one member of a household has previously died from scarlet fever, or where there is a family history of undue susceptibility to the disease, the practitioner should attempt to immunize the remaining susceptible members of the family.

Passive Immunization.—Within a few hours of the intramuscular injection of 5 to 10 c.c. of a potent scarlet fever antitoxic serum the majority of susceptible individuals will have become immune to the disease. This passive immunity only lasts from ten to fourteen days. The infectivity of scarlet fever is so capricious that, as a general rule, there is little to recommend the passive immunization of susceptible contacts in the course of general practice. When an ailing or weakly child has been intimately exposed to infection ; when the type of disease is exceptionally severe ; or when the parents express a desire for prompt prophylactic measures, passive immunization may be employed.

Sulphanilamide.—The writer is not yet prepared to recommend the indiscriminate use of sulphanilamide and its derivatives, a potentially toxic group of drugs, as a prophylactic agent against scarlatinal infection.

General Measures.—The patient must be promptly and effectively isolated. Contact children should be excluded from school for one week after removal of the patient to hospital. When the patient is treated at home, the local Health Authority may insist on the remaining susceptible children of the household being kept away from school throughout the period of treatment. Where arrangements can be made for susceptible home contacts to live with adult relatives, loss of school time can be materially diminished.

A quarantine period of at least one week must be strictly enforced in the case of adult contacts whose occupation entails the handling of milk, or close contact with children. The throat and nose of such adult contacts should be bacteriologically examined, and any individual heavily infected with hæmolytic streptococci quarantined until either the strain is proved non-pathogenic or the carrier condition clears up.

If an epidemic of scarlet fever is to be stamped out in a residential school or institution it is essential to isolate cases of hæmolytic streptococcal tonsillo-pharyngitis and carriers of this organism, in addition to patients showing the classical erythema. Bacteriological assistance must be employed as a routine measure.

The practical problems presented by the application of these, the only really effective measures of control of "scarlet fever," to the general population have still to be solved.

Curative Treatment.—*Serum Treatment.*—The early administration of scarlet fever antitoxic serum rapidly alleviates the toxæmic symptoms, and thus renders the patient more comfortable. Serum treatment diminishes the incidence, but is no guarantee against the development of complications. The following recommendations for serum treatment are based on the writer's personal experience :—

1. Toxic and septic attacks or cases of simple scarlet fever with an evening temperature of 103° F. or above, should receive serum treatment.
2. Serum need not be administered to mild cases of scarlet fever unless the child was previously ailing, weakly or rheumatic.

3. Serum must be administered within seventy-two hours of the onset of the illness ; the earlier the better.
4. Intramuscular injection gives satisfactory results, and is the route of administration recommended for use in general practice. In severe attacks, however, intravenous injection is preferable.
5. From 10 to 30 c.c. of serum is adequate for the treatment of a case of simple scarlet fever. A toxic or severe attack may require from 60 to 120 c.c. of serum. The total dose should be given in one injection. The administration by the intravenous drip method, of serum diluted with 3 pints of 5 per cent. glucose saline, gives excellent results in toxic cases of scarlet fever.

Sulphanilamide.—The treatment of scarlet fever with sulphanilamide or its derivatives is still in the experimental stage. There is not yet sufficient evidence to justify the routine administration of these new drugs to cases of simple scarlet fever. On the other hand, in septic cases serum treatment may with advantage be supplemented by the oral administration of from 0·15 to 0·5 gm. of sulphanilamide four-hourly for five consecutive days and thrice daily thereafter for three days to children between one and five years of age.

General Management.—Where circumstances permit, there is much to be said in favour of the home treatment of simple scarlet fever. Toxic and septic attacks require hospital care. The services of a fever-trained nurse should, if possible, be obtained, but mild cases of scarlet fever can be safely entrusted to the care of a competent relative, providing nephritis or other serious complications do not arise. The nursing care is on the lines described in the chapter on General Management (see p. 1).

The administration of Dover's powder with aspirin will help to allay headache, insomnia and general discomfort.

In young children mild angina requires no local treatment. In older patients the throat may be sprayed with warm saline or warm ½ per cent. solution of bicarbonate of soda. A grossly inflamed, dirty or ulcerated throat should first be sprayed with hydrogen peroxide diluted with two parts of warm water, and then freely irrigated with hot normal saline solution to which ½ per cent. phenol may be added. The treatment may be repeated every two to four hours. Steam inhalations with or without the addition of Friar's balsam are sometimes appreciated, and sucking fragments of ice helps to relieve pain and diminish swelling.

Young children suffering from septic scarlet fever are very difficult to handle, and in such cases, even though the throat be grossly inflamed, it is wiser to limit local treatment to occasional spraying than to risk resultant exhaustion from more vigorous faucial cleansing.

The nose should be sprayed or gently swabbed every two to four hours with warm saline or warm bicarbonate of soda solution. Forcible irrigation is probably unwise because of the risk of conveyance of infective material into the Eustachian tube. The nostrils and upper lip should be smeared with boric ointment or vaseline to prevent crusting and excoriation.

Discharge from the mouth and nose must be carefully collected on rags or paper handkerchiefs and promptly burnt.

Hot fomentations applied to the swollen and painful cervical glands usually afford some relief.

The free application of boro-calamine lotion or sponging with a tepid solution of bicarbonate of soda (1 teaspoonful to 2 pints) will diminish the itching and burning of the skin arising from the rash.

As soon as the temperature falls, the fluid diet of the acute stage may be supplemented by soft solids, and as the appetite returns the patient may be given normal fare. The composition of the diet during early convalescence has no influence on the subsequent incidence of nephritis.

The urine should be tested for albumen daily up to the twenty-fourth day of disease, and every second day thereafter until the patient is released from isolation.

A daily inspection of the ear drums, especially in young children, facilitates the early diagnosis of otitis media and permits of treatment by paracentesis. It is well to remember that pain may not be complained of in this condition.

Complications.—Otitis media, nephritis, arthritis, adenitis and rhinitis are common complications for the treatment of which the reader is referred to appropriate sections of this book.

Toxic and Septic Attacks.—Toxic scarlet fever, fortunately of rare occurrence in recent years, is characterized by an abrupt onset, a temperature from 105° to 107° F., persistent vomiting, profuse diarrhœa, delirium and extreme prostration; the rash is frequently inconspicuous. The onset of such symptoms in a child who has been in recent contact with scarlet fever is an urgent indication for immediate intravenous serum-glucose-saline administration. The treatment of the case is otherwise purely symptomatic, special measures being taken to combat cardio-vascular failure.

The septic type of scarlet fever usually met with in young children is essentially a septicæmia. Apart from the injection of serum, plus the oral administration of sulphanilamide, the treatment is symptomatic. Particular emphasis is placed on the value of the open balcony. The grossly inflamed and painful throat and blocked nostrils may necessitate the rectal or intravenous administration of 5 per cent. glucose saline. Septic complications and broncho-pneumonia are of common occurrence.

Convalescence.—Providing the condition of the myocardium and the pulse is satisfactory, mild uncomplicated cases of scarlet fever may be allowed out of bed on the twelfth day of disease, and in suitable weather into the open air three days later. Patients suffering from severe or complicated attacks should be confined to bed for at least three weeks.

An isolation period of four weeks is ample for a clean case, but two weeks more should elapse before the individual returns to school or work. During this latter period the patient should sleep by himself, have crockery, cutlery, handkerchiefs, towels, etc., reserved for his own use, and remain out of doors as much as possible.

The writer has for some years past shortened the isolation period in selected adult cases of scarlet fever to from sixteen to twenty-one days. No ill results either to the individual or his associates have resulted from this procedure.

Carriers

The persistence of discharge from the nose, ears, glands or skin, or of an unhealthy condition of the tonsils is an indication for continued isolation until the pathological condition has been cured. Exercise in the open air, good food and the administration of cod-liver oil combined with simple local cleansing treatment will, given time, effect a cure in most patients. Rhinitis and otorrhœa are sometimes very intractable sequelæ (the nasal discharge in particular is highly infective), and should they continue into the eighth week of convalescence, either removal of infected tonsils and adenoids or investigation of the paranasal sinuses will have to be considered.

The persistence of *S. hæmolyticus* in the fauces or nose cannot be regarded as a reliable index of infectivity, and the routine bacteriological examination of scarlatinal convalescents is to be deprecated. Nevertheless, a rich growth of this organism from either the throat or nose of certain patients, *e.g.*, dairy workers, nurses, medical men, school-teachers, may reasonably be regarded as an indication for continued isolation until the carrier condition has ceased.

Tonsillectomy will rid most faucial carriers of *S. hæmolyticus.* Antiseptic applications to the fauces and pharynx are ineffective. The cure of a persistent nasal carrier is a very difficult problem, and the condition may defy even surgical measures.

SMALLPOX

Of recent years two distinct varieties of smallpox have been epidemic in this country—variola major and variola minor. Clinically the two types are very alike, but, whereas the fatality rate of major smallpox is around 15 per cent., that of minor smallpox rarely exceeds 0·2 per cent. The minor form is apparently due to a smallpox virus of low virulence which breeds true. Vaccination is equally protective against both forms of the disease.

Smallpox is usually spread by direct contact, but the virus may also be conveyed by infected clothing, letters or other articles, or on the clothing or hair of a third person, or by flies. A smallpox corpse is highly contagious.

The virus probably enters by the respiratory tract.

The incubation period is usually twelve days, but may vary from eight to sixteen days.

Infectivity probably persists from the onset of symptoms until all the crusts have separated from the skin.

Smallpox is a notifiable disease.

Preventive Treatment.—The control of smallpox is essentially a public health problem. The accurate diagnosis of the initial case or cases rests, however, with the practitioner, and herein lies a grave responsibility. Early diagnosis, followed by prompt isolation of the primary case, the immediate vaccination and continued supervision of all contacts, and thorough disinfection of the patient's house and its contents are the essentials of successful smallpox control.

The practitioner should not hesitate to obtain the opinion of an expert from the local Public Health Department on any case which he has the least reason to suspect might be smallpox. The initial case or cases in a smallpox epidemic are commonly misdiagnosed as chickenpox.

There can be no doubt as to the wisdom of promptly removing every case of variola major to hospital. Hospital isolation should be enforced during an epidemic of variola minor so long as accommodation is available. In the event of continued spread of the minor form, circumstances may justify or necessitate home treatment. These matters of policy are for the local Medical Officer of Health to decide.

Following the removal of the patient to hospital, every member of the family and every known contact should be immediately vaccinated. Children, unless recently successfully vaccinated, should be excluded from school for sixteen days from the date of last contact with the patient. Adult contacts who accept vaccination may continue their occupation, but should be examined morning and evening for a period of sixteen days. Adult contacts who do not accept vaccination should be strictly quarantined.

If a case of variola minor is treated at home, isolation of the patient should be strictly enforced and every member of the household vaccinated. Current disinfection must be conscientiously performed.

Vaccination.—In this highly effective method of prophylaxis against smallpox, introduced by Jenner in 1798, vaccinia, or cowpox, is inoculated into the human subject. Vaccinia may be regarded as a modified form of variola resulting from the passage of the smallpox virus through animals.

Whilst the vaccination of infants before the sixth month is compulsory in this country, exemption can readily be obtained on the grounds of conscientious objection to the procedure.

Primary vaccination should not be performed until the fourth month, and should be postponed if the child is debilitated, febrile, eczematous or has recently been exposed to infectious disease. Exposure to smallpox, however, justifies immediate vaccination. Fresh glycerinated calf lymph, which is issued in sealed capillary tubes, should be employed. The lymph should be stored in a cool dark cupboard or in a refrigerator. The contents of a tube once unsealed must not be kept for use on a future occasion. The lymph must be expelled from the tube by a rubber teat—such as that used on an infant's feeding-bottle ; the mouth must not be applied directly to the tube.

The usual site for vaccination is over the insertion of the left deltoid muscle, but for æsthetic and other reasons the inner and posterior aspect of the arm or the outer aspect of the thigh or leg may be chosen. The skin should be cleansed with soap and warm water, wiped with industrial methylated spirit or ether and allowed to dry. A drop of lymph is then expelled on to the cleansed area, and a single linear scratch $\frac{1}{4}$ in. long made through the lymph in the long axis of the limb with a sterile needle. The scratch should not draw blood. The arm must not be covered until the lymph has dried. If the patient tends to scratch the vaccination site, a dressing of sterile gauze or lint may be strapped on, but in most cases a dressing is unnecessary.

One capillary tube of lymph should suffice to vaccinate at least six people.

When the maximum degree of protection against smallpox is desirable, then the number of insertions may be increased up to four, situated at least 1 in. apart. Vaccination should be performed with the minimum of trauma to the tissues, and cross scarification avoided.

At least three attempts should be made with different varieties of lymph before an individual may be regarded as insusceptible to vaccination.

The duration of complete protection against smallpox afforded by primary vaccination is uncertain and probably variable. Following infantile vaccination by the single insertion technique, revaccination should be performed when the child is five years old, and again between the ages of fourteen and sixteen years.

In the event of exposure to smallpox, vaccination should immediately be performed unless there is reliable evidence of successful primary vaccination within the previous three years or successful revaccination within the previous five years.

Owing to the risk of vaccinal encephalitis, slight as it may be, primary vaccination should not be performed in school-children or in adolescents, unless they have been directly exposed to smallpox.

Successful vaccination within the first four days of the incubation period will in most cases prevent an attack of smallpox, and even if delayed to the seventh day may modify the severity of the attack.

Curative Treatment.—There is no specific treatment for smallpox. The constitutional disturbance of the prodromal stage is treated on the lines already laid down (p. 1). The diet at this stage is limited to fluids, and water must be administered freely.

During the papular and vesicular stages of the eruption the regular application of an antiseptic dusting powder (equal parts of boric acid, zinc oxide and starch) or boro-calamine lotion will help to allay the skin irritation. Along with the daily permanganate bath little else need be done in the treatment of variola minor. In this form of smallpox the rash often aborts, secondary fever is usually absent and the prognosis is uniformly good.

Iced boric compresses applied to the face and distal parts of the limbs, and frequently changed, will be found comforting in the confluent eruption of major smallpox. Prolonged warm baths, spraying with a 1 : 40 solution of phenol or smearing the skin with 3 per cent. carbolic vaseline are alternative methods of treatment. In children the arms may require to be splinted or the hands bandaged to prevent scratching. Chloral and bromide given internally may give some relief and facilitate sleep ; morphine aggravates skin irritation.

When the pocks begin to rupture the patient, if not too ill, should be immersed three times daily for half an hour each time in a bath at 98° F. ; either potassium permanganate may be added until the water has a claret tinge or a double handful of boric crystals.

The offensive smell associated with confluent cases of major smallpox can be masked to some extent by sprinkling eucalyptus oil on and around the bed.

The application of starch or linseed poultices spread thinly on lint will hasten the separation of the scabs, and subsequent tenderness of the skin can be alleviated by the application of sterile talcum powder or zinc oxide ointment.

Of the many applications recommended for the treatment of the rash the writer favours the daily painting of the skin with a 1 to 5 per cent. (according to skin sensitivity) aqueous solution of potassium permanganate as suggested by Balfour. The painting should be continued until the crusts have separated.

Owing to the presence of the eruption on the mucous membranes, the eyes, mouth, throat, nose and larynx require careful treatment. The eyes should be bathed with warm boric lotion at four-hourly intervals, and 1 drop of 10 per cent. argyrol inserted morning and evening if conjunctivitis be severe. Vaseline applied to the margins prevents gumming together of the lids. The mouth and throat must be cleansed at regular intervals ; either a 1 : 5,000 solution of permanganate of potash or peroxide of hydrogen diluted with two parts of water may be employed as a spray or mouth wash. Frequent inhalations of steam, impregnated with Friar's balsam or creosote, help to alleviate laryngeal and bronchial symptoms. Dysphagia may be lessened by sucking fragments of ice or by spraying the throat with a 4 per cent. solution of cocaine before each feed.

The fluid diet of the prodromal period requires to be supplemented by soft solids during the eruptive stage. Fresh fruit juice drinks sweetened with glucose must be administered freely throughout the illness.

Complications.—Boils and abscesses are of frequent occurrence, and should be treated on surgical principles. Severe laryngitis sometimes necessitates tracheotomy. Bronchopneumonia is a common and frequently fatal complication. Keratitis and panophthalmitis are liable to occur in severe cases, particularly if the eyes have not been carefully treated from the first.

Convalescence.—The patient should be kept in bed until the eruption has crusted. In variola minor and in mild attacks of major smallpox convalescence is usually rapid and the patient fit for discharge from hospital or isolation as soon as he is free from infection. School or business activities may be resumed from two to four weeks after release from isolation.

After severe attacks, several months may elapse before the patient is fit to resume his normal activities.

Isolation must be continued until the last crust has separated from the skin. This period varies from three weeks in mild cases to three months or longer in severe attacks. Detachment of the crusts can be hastened by warm baths and the application of linseed or starch poultices, olive oil or vaseline. The thick skin of the palms and soles may be softened by frequent soaking in hot water, and the buried crusts picked out with a sterile penknife as recommended by Ker.

A thorough soap and water bath and shampoo precedes the transfer of the patient to a non-infected room in which he puts on clean clothes.

TETANUS

The normal habitat of *Cl. tetani* is the intestinal tract of horses, cows and other herbivora. The bacilli are sometimes found in human fæces. Heavily manured soil is particularly liable to be contaminated with the highly resistant spores of the tetanus bacillus. Introduced through a punctured wound commonly made by a splinter or nail the bacilli, or spores, particularly in the presence of pyogenic infection, laceration of tissues and a foreign body, tend to multiply and produce the powerful toxin which acts on the nervous system.

Whilst the potential risk of tetanus following deep suppurating wounds is well recognized, the very real danger of infection following superficial septic abrasions in children or mild septic skin lesions in farm workers is not sufficiently appreciated. Imperfectly sterilized catgut has been responsible for the development of post-operative tetanus.

The length of the incubation period has a very important bearing on prognosis. When this period is less than seven days, recovery is unlikely. Should the spores lie latent in the tissues, the incubation period may be weeks or even months.

Early diagnosis is very important. Stiffness of the jaw, pain in the neck or back increased by manipulation and associated with the characteristic facial expression should lead to immediate specific treatment.

Tetanus is not a notifiable disease.

Preventive Treatment. — *Passive Immunization.* — If all accidental wounds were promptly and thoroughly cleansed and, in circumstances favourable to infection, tetanus antitoxin employed as a prophylactic, the disease would virtually disappear.

Where a wound is liable to be contaminated by dirt from manured soil, stables or farmyards, in lacerations by farm implements, in bites or wounds from horses, in gunshot wounds etc., in addition to early and thorough cleansing of the injury an intramuscular injection of from 1,500 to 3,000 units of tetanus antitoxin should be given promptly. If the risk of tetanus appears to be great, then the prophylactic dose may be repeated eight days later, and invariably if the wound has to be re-opened.

Active Immunization.—Tetanus toxin which is subjected for a prolonged period to the action of formalin and heat becomes converted into a harmless yet antigenically efficient toxoid.

Ramon [1] (1936) suggests the immunization of agricultural workers, gardeners and soldiers by a course of three injections of 1, 1·5 and 1·5 c.c. of tetanus toxoid at intervals of three weeks, to be followed one year later by a single injection of 2 c.c.

Brown [2] (1937) states that following the injection of two doses of alum toxoid at an interval of three months, the majority of individuals inoculated develop a complete and permanent immunity, and recommends the employment of combined immunization against typhoid and tetanus in the Army.

Active immunization against tetanus has recently been offered to all regular troops in the British Army. The course consists of two doses of 1 c.c. of formol toxoid with an interval of six weeks between the injections.

Curative Treatment.—The three essentials in the treatment of tetanus are (1) the early administration of antitoxic serum ;

[1] Ramon, G., *L'Echo méd. du Nord.* (1936), **5**, 873; abstr. *Bull. Hyg.* (1937), **12**, 64.

[2] Brown, H. H., *Brit. Med. Jour.* (1937), **1**, 494.

(2) thorough cleansing of the wound ; and (3) attempts to control the spasms.

Antitoxic Serum.—Whilst there is general agreement regarding the undoubted value of massive doses of antitoxic serum (from 200,000 to 800,000 units) in the treatment of tetanus, opinions differ as to the best route of administration. The intrathecal route has long held the field, but Cole [1] (1936), and other clinicians with an extensive experience of tetanus favour the intravenous injection of serum. A single early massive intravenous dose of 200,000 units of antitoxin, as recommended by Cole [2] (1936), appeals to the writer as sound practice. The combined method of administration of serum by intrathecal (lumbar or cisternal), intravenous and intramuscular injections is still the most popular.

Cleansing of Wound.—Owing to the possibility of increased toxic absorption it is a wise procedure to delay cleansing the wound until an hour or two after the intravenous administration of antitoxin.

Scabs and foreign bodies should be removed, penetrating wounds freely opened up and whitlows incised. Following the evacuation of all septic material and the removal of lacerated tissue, the wound should be syringed with hydrogen peroxide and dressed with light porous gauze. Dressings should be changed every four hours. Free drainage is essential, the wound being kept open and allowed to granulate from the bottom.

General or regional anæsthesia may be required, but local anæsthesia or cauterization of the wound are inadvisable.

Control of Spasms.—In mild cases without convulsions 30 gr. of bromide of potassium administered every six hours is all that is required. If the spasms are severe, the period of onset less than four days or the patient becoming exhausted, then avertin is the most efficacious drug to employ. From 0·07 to 0·1 gm. per kg. of body-weight should be administered by the rectum at intervals of six to eight hours. As the spasms diminish, the time interval between doses may gradually be increased. Apart from some respiratory difficulty and slight cyanosis, which is usually relieved by atropine hypodermically, and oxygen administration by the nasal catheter, no toxic effects have been observed.

Among the less reliable drugs that have been employed are chloral hydrate, from 15 to 30 gr. every three hours ; paraldehyde in doses of 2 to 6 drachms in 3 to 9 oz. of normal

[1] Cole, L., *Brit. Med. Jour.* (1936), **1**, 1191.
[2] Cole, L., *Brit. Med. Jour.* (1936), **1**, 1191.

saline by the rectum ; and morphine sulphate hypodermically up to 2 gr. daily.

Inhalations of nitrous oxide and oxygen, chloroform or ether, may be necessary in severe respiratory spasm until the avertin effect is obtained.

General Management.—The patient should lie on an air mattress or water-bed with the bedclothes supported by a cradle. Isolation is not essential. Trained day and night nurses are necessary. Noise must be excluded, the sickroom darkened and nursing duties performed quietly and preferably at times when the patient is deeply under sedatives.

A minimum daily food intake of 2,000 calories in an adult patient, whilst a highly important part of the treatment, is very difficult to attain. One of the main duties of the nurse is to feed the patient at hourly or even half-hourly intervals with milk, egg flip, thin gruels and glucose lemonade. To facilitate feeding, teeth may have to be extracted. Plain water or glucose saline should be given freely by the mouth or rectum. In severe cases feeding may have to be carried on through the nasal tube left in position or supplemented by the intravenous administration of 5 per cent. glucose saline by the drip method.

The bowels should be moved by enemata, and retention of urine watched for and relieved by catheterization.

TYPHUS FEVER

Apart from a few sporadic cases occurring from time to time, particularly in Ireland and such ports as Glasgow and Liverpool, typhus fever, once so prevalent, has disappeared from this country. Exanthematic or epidemic typhus, the type of disease still prevalent in Eastern Europe, is caused by intracellular infection with Rickettsia prowazeki bodies, and is transmitted from man to man by lice. The Rickettsia bodies are present in the blood vessels of the skin, brain, kidneys, etc., and have also been found in the intestinal epithelium of lice taken from cases of exanthematic typhus. Infection is conveyed either through the bite of an infected louse or through the louse excreta being scratched into the skin. There is good reason to believe that typhus fever cannot be conveyed by droplet infection or by human discharges.

The incubation period is usually from twelve to fourteen days, but may vary from five to twenty-one days.

Typhus fever is a notifiable disease.

Of recent years a group of typhus-like diseases have been

noted as occurring in various parts of the world—so-called endemic typhus. The group, in which ticks, mites and fleas are known vectors, includes among other diseases eruptive Mediterranean fever, Brill's disease in America, Australia and elsewhere, and tropical typhus.

Preventive Treatment.—*Active Immunization.*—Vaccines have been prepared from the intestine of infected lice or from the internal organs of infected guinea pigs and rats. Blanc [1] (1936) and Laigret [2] *et al* (1937) report favourable results in the control of typhus epidemics in Morocco, Tunis and Algeria following vaccination. Whilst the immediate efficacy of vaccination appears to be proved, the method does not appear to be entirely free from risk either to the individual or to the community.

Passive Immunization.—Nicolle [3] (1935) considers that the subcutaneous injection of 10 c.c. of human convalescent typhus serum, repeated at intervals of seven to twelve days, is the most effective specific prophylactic method against typhus fever. The serum should be obtained during the second week of convalescence. Whilst the protection conferred is transient, this method of prophylaxis is particularly valuable for those who have been bitten by lice whilst attending typhus patients.

General Measures.—The essential factor in limiting the spread of typhus fever is the prompt delousing of patients and contacts.

Doctors, attendants and nurses must wear one-piece overalls, caps, rubber gloves and boots whilst handling infested patients or contacts, and should bathe and change their clothing at the end of the day's work.

The patient's clothing should either be burnt or placed in a canvas bag and removed for disinfection by steam.

The hair of the head should be cut short with a machine clipper, and all body hair shaved. The hair clippings must be burned. This procedure is followed by a thorough scrubbing with soft soap and hot water. The patient is then dressed in clean hospital clothing or his own disinfected garments. When the hair of the head is not cut short the application of paraffin soaks followed by a shampoo with soft soap and subsequent thorough tooth combing will effectively kill or remove lice and nits.

[1] Blanc, G., *Bruxelles-méd.* (1936), **17**, 116.
[2] Laigret, J., Durand, R., and Belfort, J., *Bull. Office Internat. d'Hyg. Publique* (1937), **29**, 743-7.
[3] Nicolle, C., *Rev. d'Immunol.* (1935), **1**, 9.

All clothing and bedding must be removed for steam disinfection. Leather and rubber articles may be disinfected by immersing for ten minutes in a watery emulsion of 2 per cent. cresol with 5 per cent. soft soap.

Contacts are kept under daily observation for three weeks from the date of last exposure. Adults, following disinfestation, may be permitted to attend business, but children should be kept away from school throughout the quarantine period.

Curative Treatment.—*Serum Treatment.*—Favourable therapeutic results have been reported following the injection of convalescent human typhus serum or immune horse or ass's serum, but the value of these specific methods of treatment still awaits confirmation.

General Management.—Typhus fever is essentially a disease for hospital treatment, where, if possible, the patient should be nursed on the open balcony. Once the patient has been thoroughly freed from vermin there is apparently no risk of the spread of contagion to nurses or attendants.

Skilled nursing is essential.

The diet and management of the case is on the same lines as advised for the treatment of a severe case of enteric fever.

Pyrexia, headache, insomnia and delirium call for frequent tepid sponging and the exhibition of hypnotics.

The bladder should be percussed morning and evening, particularly in delirious patients, and retention of urine relieved by appropriate measures.

The myocardium suffers severely in typhus fever, and every precaution should be taken to conserve the patient's strength. Daily intravenous injections of 5 per cent. glucose saline by the drip method may advantageously be employed in toxic cases. Adrenalin, camphor in oil, coramine, etc., may be administered at two to four-hourly intervals in the attempt to combat cardio-vascular failure.

Complications.—Whilst complications are uncommon, laryngitis, bronchitis, broncho-pneumonia and myocarditis may give rise to anxiety during the acute stage of the illness. Thrombosis in the veins or arteries, particularly in the lower limbs, is a feature of some epidemics.

Convalescence.—Strength is usually rapidly regained, but the reaction of the cardio-vascular system to increased effort must be carefully watched. The patient may be permitted to sit up in bed one week after the temperature has settled, and may get up a few days later. The appetite returns early and the diet may be rapidly increased. Cod-liver oil and iron may be administered. As the patient may be regarded as non-infective from the time of delousing, he may be permitted to leave hospital when fully recovered, but should not resume work for at least another four weeks.

WHOOPING-COUGH OR PERTUSSIS

A particularly dangerous disease in infancy, whooping-cough is one of the most important infections of early childhood. The disease is highly infective, particularly during the catarrhal stage of the illness, the stage at which clinical diagnosis is very difficult. The causal organism, *H. pertussis*, is spread by direct contact, droplet infection and perhaps by fomites.

Abortive and unrecognized attacks are common, particularly in adults, and frequently prove an unsuspected source of contagion.

The incubation period varies from three to eighteen days.

Whooping-cough is not yet a notifiable disease.

The disease may be diagnosed during the catarrhal stage by making the patient cough on a plate of special media held about 5 in. in front of his mouth, the total period of exposure to amount to 10 to 15 seconds. After incubation the plate is examined for *H. pertussis*. The practitioner may be able to obtain diagnostic " cough plates " from the local Public Health Laboratory. The complement-fixation test is useful for the late diagnosis of atypical attacks of pertussis ; a positive reaction may be expected from the fourth to the eighth week of the disease.

A severe cough associated with a marked leucocytosis and a lymphocytosis of over 60 per cent. may safely be diagnosed as pertussis, but a normal leucocyte and differential count does not exclude the disease.

Preventive Treatment.—*Active Immunization.*—The experience of Madsen[1] (1933) (1937) and Sauer[2] (1937) indicates that the injection of a vaccine prepared from recently isolated hæmolytic strains of *H. pertussis* affords either complete or partial protection against whooping-cough. Whooping-cough vaccine containing 10,000 million organisms in each cubic centimetre can be obtained commercially. Modern practice favours a total prophylactic dose of at least 80,000 million bacilli administered in three subcutaneous injections of 2, 3 and 3 c.c. of the vaccine at weekly intervals. Systemic reactions to pertussis vaccine rarely occur and local reactions are usually mild.

[1] Madsen, Th., *Jour. Amer. Med. Ass.* (1933), **101**, 187; " The Control of Syphilis and Other Infectious Diseases " (Baltimore, 1937).

[2] Sauer, L. W., *Jour. Amer. Med. Ass.* (1937), **109**, 487.

Children should be immunized, preferably during the latter half of infancy, but when whooping-cough is epidemic this method may be employed in protecting children of pre-school and school age.

The duration of immunity is uncertain and apparently variable, but infantile immunization may at least lessen the risk of infection with *H. pertussis* during the early years of life.

Passive Immunization.—Debré [1] (1923), Bradford [2] (1935) and Meader [3] (1937) have reported satisfactory prophylactic results following the injection of the serum of convalescents or of the whole blood of those who have previously suffered from whooping-cough.

Failing convalescent serum (10 c.c.), which is practically unobtainable, the practitioner should inject 20 c.c. of parental blood intramuscularly into exposed susceptible children under four years of age, with a view to preventing or modifying the severity of the attack.

Until a reliable skin test for immunity is available it is wise, although not necessarily accurate, to assume that a child who has not previously suffered from whooping-cough is susceptible to the disease.

General Measures.—Every precaution should be taken to prevent the exposure of young children to whooping-cough.

During epidemic prevalence of the disease older children and adults suffering from a febrile catarrh should not be permitted to come into close contact with younger members of the household until a diagnosis of whooping-cough can be excluded.

Susceptible contacts require to be quarantined for three weeks, and, if attending the infant classes, must be kept at home during this period.

Adult contacts may continue their work, but must be promptly isolated on the first appearance of suspicious symptoms.

Curative Treatment.—*Specific Treatment.*—The treatment of whooping-cough with human convalescent serum or whole blood or with the serum of horses immunized against pertussis is still in the experimental stage; the favourable results so far reported require confirmation.

Vaccine treatment has in the writer's experience proved ineffective.

[1] Debré, R., *Bull. Acad. de Med.* (1923), 3 e. sér., **89,** 348.
[2] Bradford, W. L., *Amer. Jour. Dis. Child.* (1935), **50,** 919.
[3] Meader, F. M., *Amer. Jour. Dis. Child.* (1937), **53,** 760.

General Management.—As soon as whooping-cough is suspected the patient must be confined to bed. Free ventilation of the sickroom is essential, and if the weather be equable the patient may with advantage be nursed in the open air during the daytime. During the catarrhal stage the following simple expectorant mixture may be administered three or four times daily :—

℞	Tinct. Opii Camph	♏iv
	Tinct. Ipecac.	♏v
	Syr. Scillæ	♏x
	Aq.	ad. ʒii

Provided the attack is afebrile, uncomplicated and not unduly severe, the child, if over three years of age, may be allowed out of bed about the fourth day of the whoop. When the paroxysms exceed thirty in the twenty-four hours, when there is a previous history of respiratory disease, or in the case of young children, confinement to bed until convalescence is well established is a wise policy. During the paroxysmal stage the patient should spend most of the time in the open air, unless the weather be inclement. Mild exercise should be encouraged, and precautions taken to avoid contact with susceptible children.

In infants and young children a flannel binder firmly applied round the abdomen affords support during the strain of coughing.

Excitement should be avoided, and some trustworthy individual must be constantly in attendance to support and comfort the child during the paroxysms. A towel or suitable receptacle should be at hand to receive respiratory discharges and vomit. Discharges from the mouth and nose must be burnt or disinfected.

An occasional dose of syrup of figs or liquorice powder will keep the bowels in order.

The dietetic management of a severe case of whooping-cough presents a difficult problem. Food should be administered in small amounts about ten minutes after each paroxysm. In infants " feeding by the clock " may have to be adjusted to the necessities of the case. If vomiting and loss of weight continue, then the time between feeds should be shortened, and the bulk of each feed lessened. Milk may require to be either diluted, boiled and citrated, treated with lactic acid or peptonized, or replaced by glucose, whey, albumen water and raw meat juice. Mouth feeding can be supplemented or replaced if necessary by the rectal, intravenous or intraperitoneal administration of 5 per cent. glucose saline.

In older children no material alteration in diet is necessary. Milk, eggs, butter, fish, chicken, meat and vegetable soups are better than an excess of starchy and saccharine foods. Biscuits, rusks, oatcakes or similar dry crumbly foods, irritating to the pharynx, should be avoided.

Fresh orange or lemon juice drinks sweetened to taste with glucose should be administered freely.

In severe attacks, in spite of the painstaking endeavours of a tactful nurse, some degree of malnutrition must be expected.

There is no specific drug treatment for whooping-cough.

In a mild attack there is no need for medication, but the simple expectorant mixture recommended for the catarrhal stage may be continued throughout the illness if desired. The inhalation of steam impregnated with the compound tincture of benzoin or with eucalyptus oil is soothing.

When the paroxysms are frequent and severe, seriously interfering with sleep and the taking of food, a sedative or antispasmodic drug should be prescribed. One or other of the following preparations may be administered every four hours to a child one year old, until either improvement ensues or the child becomes drowsy: 2 gr. chloral hydrate with 2 gr. potassium bromide; $\frac{1}{2}$ gr. Dover's powder; or 10 minims of syrup of codein phosphate. One-sixth of a grain of phenobarbital administered at six-hourly intervals, or an evening dose of $\frac{1}{4}$ gr., is sometimes effective in lessening the severity of the paroxysms. This drug must be employed with caution and care taken to avoid cumulative poisoning. If belladonna is prescribed, it must be pushed to the physiological limit. Commence with 3 minims of the tincture of belladonna three times daily; providing no idiosyncrasy is present, promptly change to four-hourly administration with a daily increase of 1 drop per dose until dryness of the mouth or dilatation of the pupils is evident.

Conflicting reports have been published on the value of Roentgen rays in the treatment of whooping-cough. The verdict so far is not proven. In exceptional cases, however, where the paroxysmal stage is unduly prolonged, the application of X-rays to the interscapular space may, by diminishing the enlarged tracheo-bronchial glands, be followed by rapid improvement.

Whilst of value as a general tonic, ultra violet light has, in the writer's experience, no specific curative effect on the paroxysmal stage of whooping-cough.

Complications. — Broncho-pneumonia, convulsions and gastro-enteritis are serious complications and a frequent cause of death in young children. Epistaxis and other hæmorrhages, whilst of comparatively common occurrence, are not of serious import. Well-marked cardiac dilatation may occur in severe cases. Otitis media is not uncommon.

When a child under two years of age is suffering from pertussis, the parent should be warned of the possibility of convulsions, and instructed to treat the complication by the prompt administration of a hot mustard bath or pack with the application of cold water to the head.

A few whiffs of chloroform will usually terminate the convulsion. Morphine sulphate should then be administered hypodermically, $\frac{1}{24}$ gr. to a child one year old, and the sedative effect continued by rectal chloral, 5 gr. in 1 oz. of warm milk repeated as necessary. Lumbar puncture is a useful procedure when the convulsions are repeated.

Convalescence.—Fresh air and plenty of good wholesome food are the essential requirements in convalescence. Care must be taken to protect the child against catarrhal infection or chill. If circumstances permit, a change of air to the seaside or to the country will prove very beneficial, particularly to cases with a persisting catarrhal condition of the lungs. Cod-liver oil and iron may be prescribed.

A paroxysmal cough may persist for months in some cases, and only disappear after the removal of infected tonsils and adenoids.

The tendency of whooping-cough to rouse into activity any latent tuberculous process should be borne in mind.

The duration of infectivity in whooping-cough probably varies from case to case, but rarely exceeds four weeks. As a general rule, the patient should be isolated for four weeks from the commencement of the paroxysmal stage of the illness. After this period has elapsed, the child may, though still "whooping," safely mix with other children or even return to school if physically fit.

SERUM SICKNESS

Serum disease was the name applied by von Pirquet and Schick to the various clinical manifestations such as skin rashes, œdema, fever and arthritis following the injection of horse serum. The occurrence of this group of symptoms indicates that the individual is sensitized to the foreign protein in the serum.

The incidence of serum sickness following the use of therapeutic sera may vary from 10 to 70 per cent. according to the purity of the preparation employed, the age group injected and the volume of serum administered. Intravenous, intrathecal and intraperitoneal injections of serum are more liable to produce severe and rapid anaphylactic symptoms than intramuscular or subcutaneous injections.

As commonly met with, the symptoms do not appear until some eight to twelve days after the injection. But in individuals who are hypersensitive "immediate" or "accelerated" reactions may occur in which more or less severe symptoms appear within a few minutes to seven days after the administration of serum. Individuals liable to asthmatic or hay-fever-like attacks when in the proximity of horses must be regarded as highly serum-sensitive, as must also be, to a lesser degree, those who have received an injection of horse immune serum more than nine days previously.

Preventive Treatment.—Whilst the risk of severe anaphylactic shock and death following the administration of horse immune sera is infinitesimal, nevertheless, the indiscriminate use of serum for prophylactic and therapeutic purposes is to be deprecated. Before injecting serum, the practitioner should satisfy himself that this form of treatment is essential, and, in the case of prophylactic use, should bear in mind that as a result of the injection the individual will become sensitized to subsequent serum administration.

Before injecting serum, the practitioner should put the following questions to the patient :—

1. Do you sneeze, cough or develop asthmatic symptoms whilst in the proximity of horses ?
2. Do you suffer from asthma, hay fever, or attacks of nettle-rash (urticaria) ?
3. Have you received injections of serum on a previous occasion ? Did you suffer from serum sickness ?

If the answer to all these questions is in the negative, serum may be administered by any route with an easy mind. Serum sickness may follow the injection, but it will be of the "normal" type and without danger to life.

If the patient is a definite "horse asthmatic," immune horse serum should not be injected by any route. Endeavour to obtain an immune ox serum. If the history is in the least suggestive, then a skin test may be applied.

If the answer to either question (2) or question (3) is in the affirmative, serum may be administered by the subcutaneous or intramuscular route with comparative safety following desensitization, but particular care must be exercised when serum is injected intravenously.

Skin Test.—Within half an hour of the intracutaneous injection of 0·1 c.c. of a 1 : 50 dilution of sterile horse serum in sterile normal saline an urticarial wheal will appear in an individual sensitized to horse serum. If no wheal appears within one hour of the injection the test is negative. An equal volume of sterile normal saline should be injected in the same manner some 2 in. distant as a control.

Desensitization.—The following two methods of desensitization, whilst not invariably effective, are suitable for application by the practitioner, and may be relied upon to give reasonably satisfactory results.

Providing the serum is not going to be administered intravenously, a single subcutaneous desensitizing injection of 0·5 c.c. of the immune serum administered at least four hours before the therapeutic dose will usually prevent severe serum sickness.

Prior to intravenous administration, inject subcutaneously at hourly intervals 0·25, 0·5 and 1 c.c. of the immune serum followed after an interval of two hours by the intravenous injection of the remainder of the full therapeutic dose. The first few cubic centimetres of serum should be injected into the blood stream very slowly and the patient carefully watched for the development of untoward symptoms.

Curative Treatment.—Whenever serum is given intravenously, intrathecally or intraperitoneally, a syringe containing 15 minims of adrenalin chloride (1 : 1,000) should be ready for immediate use. If anaphylactic symptoms appear, the administration of serum must immediately be stopped and 10 to 15 minims of adrenalin promptly injected intramuscularly. If the dyspnœa is severe, adrenalin may be supplemented by $\frac{1}{100}$ gr. of atropine sulphate injected subcutaneously. The general treatment for shock should be applied.

In the usual type of serum sickness the patient suffers great discomfort from pruritis due to the urticarial rash. Ephedrine by mouth in doses of from $\frac{1}{6}$ to $\frac{1}{2}$ gr. every six hours according to age sometimes affords relief, but the writer has found the subcutaneous injection of 5 to 10 minims of adrenalin more effective in severe cases. If administered in the evening, adrenalin will enable the patient to get a few hours sleep.

The oral administration of either calcium lactate or calcium chloride, 20 gr. four-hourly, or the intramuscular or intravenous injection of calcium gluconate (10 c.c. of a 10 per cent. solution) at intervals of twelve hours have been recommended, but are of very doubtful utility.

A soothing application, such as calamine lotion with 1 per cent. phenol added, or menthol ointment (10 per cent. menthol in vaseline) should be applied to the affected skin.

Headache and pains in the muscles and joints are usually relieved by 5 gr. of aspirin administered every two hours. A mixture containing chloral hydrate and potassium bromide may be required for the relief of insomnia.

W. T. Benson.

SEPTICÆMIA AND ERYSIPELAS

SEPTICÆMIA

THE varied clinical manifestations of this condition have their common basis in the signs and symptoms due to an infection of the blood. Transient invasion by pathological organisms, however, may often occur without any signs or symptoms of disease. Thus blood cultures taken immediately after extraction of a tooth usually show a growth of streptococci, while four hours later no growth can be obtained. On the other hand, streptococci may be obtained from many local conditions of the body, a joint, a tonsil, a tooth abscess, without any infection of the blood.

The causes underlying the production of the clinical state of septicæmia are not fully understood, but undoubtedly they include two main factors :—

1. The infection of fixed tissues by micro-organisms and the spread therefrom to the main blood stream by veins or lymphatics. This probably takes place by septic thrombo-phlebitis of minute vessels in the infected area ;
2. The failure of the natural or acquired immunological properties of the blood, and of phagocytosis to overcome the entry of organisms into the blood stream.

These two factors underlie all our ideas concerning treatment and find expression in two therapeutic principles :—

1. Attempts to eradicate safely any focal sepsis ;
2. Attempts to overcome the blood infection by stimulating the natural defence mechanisms of the body (*a*) directly, (*b*) by phagocytosis, or (*c*) by chemotherapeutic efforts to lower the numbers of infecting organisms to a level at which the body can deal with the remainder.

A further factor to be considered is the virulence of the infecting organism. Septicæmia derived from a hæmolytic streptococcus acquired during the conduct of a post-mortem examination may lead to death within twenty-four hours, while a patient suffering from subacute bacterial endocarditis caused by the non-hæmolytic streptococcus viridans may linger for a year. The appreciation of the therapeutic principles involved therefore demands a consideration of the interaction of the two opposing sets of factors. On the one side is the infecting agent: its quantity and virulence; its powers of multiplication; its augmentation by supplies from a focal source; its liberation of toxins or bodies inimical to the host. On the other side are the natural defences of the body: its natural immunity; its immunizing power derived from acquired immunity at the source of focal infection; its powers of phagocytosis. The illness, therefore, may be very varied in its character, but several main types can be described in each of which the different therapeutic measures available may acquire different relative degrees of importance:—

1. The signs of infection are rapidly progressive. The patient goes from bad to worse, and death usually ensues within a week. A few cases suddenly and apparently spontaneously get better, but this is exceptional. Many cases of infection by a virulent strain of hæmolytic streptococcus are included in this group and immunological treatment seems of little avail. The chief hope would appear to be in the application of successful chemotherapeutic treatment.

2. The infection progresses by stages, and the duration of the illness is to be counted in weeks or months. A period of oscillating fever is succeeded, perhaps seven or ten days later, by a swing which reaches yet higher and lower levels and by increased prostration and graver signs of toxæmia. Recovery is relatively more common than in the first group and usually takes place by a corresponding series of stages of decreasing illness rather than by dramatic improvement. Many organisms may produce such a picture. As a rule, if the infecting agent be staphylococcus the outcome is fatal. Stimulation of the defence mechanisms of the body was of value in this type of septicæmia, but now, granted a suitable infective organism, the use of the sulphanilamide series of drugs gives additional help. The two methods of treatment are supplementary.

3. Sometimes a moderately severe illness of some ten to twenty-one days' duration ends in apparent recovery, but a recrudescence takes place about one week later. There may be several such relapses. Recovery is, on the whole, the rule, and such cases are rarely associated with cryptogenic septicæmia. They are rather the product of focal sepsis, and indicate the

importance of searching for and treating any local lesion. Failure is sometimes due to the production of a secondary focal abscess in some inaccessible organ of the body.

4. A short, sharp illness of a few days' duration ends, almost invariably, in recovery. The septicæmia of septic abortion is often an example of this type. In many instances there is barely time to make an accurate clinical diagnosis or to secure a positive blood culture before recovery takes place.

5. A terminal septicæmia may occur in cachectic states after a long debilitating illness. Little need be said of such conditions. They usually represent the final breakdown of the resistance of the body to infection rather than the vigorous attack of a pathogenic organism.

The first part of the management of a case of septicæmia lies, therefore, in an attempt to estimate the extent and severity of the infection, and the probable subsequent course of the disease. The scope of this article does not include the clinical description of septicæmia, nor the differential diagnosis, and at this stage the reader would do well to refresh his memory by recourse to a standard textbook of medicine. Certain points bearing more directly on the therapeutic outlook must be indicated briefly.

It is important that the correct diagnosis be reached as quickly as possible. Where septicæmia follows a medical lesion such as lobar pneumonia, or a definite surgical condition such as puerperal sepsis, there is little room for doubt, as also when the condition is secondary to a frank and obvious surgical wound. Much delay, however, may take place in those cases where the wound is trifling, or often indeed healed by the time advice is sought, and where the onset of symptoms and signs is gradual, and the incubation period reckoned in weeks. Blood cultures should be taken as soon as any suspicion of septicæmia is entertained, and should be repeated, if negative in result, on several occasions, choosing the time of a rigor or the gravescent stage of a febrile period at which to withdraw the blood. Cultures should never be omitted in frank cases of septicæmia, for it is of vital importance to obtain as quickly as possible all available bacteriological information concerning the type, the strain and, if possible, the quantity of the infecting organism. When a positive result has been obtained, cultures should be repeated at regular and appropriate times during the course of the illness. The bacteriologist must help the clinician throughout the progress of the disease—his information may vary and such variation may call for rapid changes in therapeutic measures.

Certain clinical points are of great importance in prognosis, such as the height and variations of the temperature, the rate and quality of the pulse, the colour and dryness of the tongue, the depth and duration of delirium. The spleen is frequently enlarged, but a variation in size seems difficult to correlate with clinical progress, though often an increase in splenic dullness immediately precedes a change for the worse. Increasing prostration is a bad sign, particularly if accompanied by a diminution in the severity of the variations of the temperature.

A daily and careful search should be made for signs of local infection, whether primary or secondary. The skin, the meninges, the heart, the sinuses, the throat, the ears and the pelvic organs all call for regular scrutiny. Frequent examination of the blood is necessary not only to detect the presence of progressive anæmia but more particularly to determine the response of the leucocytes to infection. In this connection it is well to remember that leucopenia is often seen in septicæmia caused by organisms of the coli-typhoid group.

The examination in detail of the therapeutic measures available may now be considered.

Treatment of any Focal Lesion.—All pyæmic cases are associated with septicæmia, but the converse is not necessarily true, and frequently evidence of abscess formation only appears during the later stages of illness. Such abscesses may be in any of the tissues or organs, and their localization depends to some extent upon whether infection is by systemic veins or lymphatics, by the portal system of drainage or through arterial blood. In any case the surgical treatment of all accessible collections of pus is similar to the treatment of a primary wound or focal sepsis. Complete excision of an infected area can only rarely be practised and free drainage of septic foci is the recognized practice, but care must be taken not to open up fresh channels of infection. Dressings should be such as to facilitate drainage, and probably in the early stages hot boracic lint foments are most generally useful. When drainage is established, often after incision, hot moist applications of hypertonic (5 per cent.) saline are advised.

Treatment designed to aid the Natural Defences of the Body.—*Blood Transfusion.*—The administration of whole blood from a suitable donor was the earliest method, but a series of experiments designed to increase the antibacterial efficacy of the donor's blood calls for brief review.

Sir Almroth Wright added a quantity of stock vaccine of the appropriate organism to the donor's defibrinated blood. This mixture was injected one hour later. The results obtained appeared to be due to protein shock rather than, as Wright suggested, to an elaboration of non-specific bactericidal substances from the leucocytes of the donor's blood.

Colebrook and Storer tested the phagocytic properties of the patient's blood. If these were reduced much below normal they employed a method of immuno-transfusion whereby the donor received a subcutaneous injection of 1,000 million stock staphylococcus vaccine, and his blood was utilized some hours later. Various workers employed citrated or defibrinated blood or direct methods of transfusion.

Many attempts have been made to induce a high state of immunity in the donor by giving him a series of injections of a vaccine prepared from the organism found in the patient's blood. Such preparation must take at least one week, and its clinical benefits are somewhat doubtful.

Non-specific immuno-transfusion may be more easily practised by giving the donor a preliminary protein shock by any of the recognized methods. The blood is used a few hours after the acute reaction has subsided.

Cadham utilizes serum taken from rabbits inoculated with vaccines made from the infecting organism. This is given frequently in small doses along with small quantities of serum from a human donor to make up deficiency of complement.

The value of these varied methods is not proven—they are difficult to apply except under hospital conditions, and the practitioner is strongly advised at present to rely upon simple transfusion.

Do not overload the patient with large quantities of blood. Give 200 to 300 c.c. of blood: give it within forty-eight hours of making a diagnosis: repeat such transfusion from time to time, more particularly if even transient benefit be noticed. Remember that in the early stages a blood transfusion is given to administer normal active serum and leucocytes; only in the later stages, when anæmia becomes marked, is it intended primarily to supply hæmoglobin and erythrocytes.

Injections of sodium nucleinate (1 to 5 c.c. of 5 per cent. solution) have been used to produce a leucocytosis. Though of theoretical value, the practical results are doubtful.

Sera and Vaccines.—The early administration of serum is often of benefit, especially when the infecting organism is a hæmolytic streptococcus or a meningococcus. It is, however, desirable to use an appropriate serum whenever the infecting organism can be determined. Serum should be given at the earliest possible moment, and repeated daily for about a week, or even at twelve-hourly intervals for the first day or two.

There are many reliable brands of the commoner sera, and the practitioner is advised not to carry out the instructions given by the manufacturer, but to administer large doses. The serum may be given directly by the intramuscular route or by the intravenous route when diluted with twice its volume of normal saline, and precaution must be taken against anaphylaxis. If the intracutaneous administration of one drop of the serum is not followed by a marked local erythema in fifteen minutes, anaphylaxis is improbable. In all cases, however, the patient should be asked if he has ever had serum administered before, and, if the answer be yes, special precaution in administration is necessary. Give one drop of serum intracutaneously, ten minutes later give 0·5 c.c. serum subcutaneously, and thereafter, unless very marked local reaction be noticed, the whole dose may be given very slowly. The subcutaneous injection of $\frac{1}{2}$ to 1 c.c. of $\frac{1}{1000}$ watery solution of adrenalin hydrochloride is of great value in dealing with immediate anaphylactic reactions.

Vaccines are of no value in acute septicæmia and probably of little value in the more chronic stages of infection.

Chemotherapy.—Numerous substances have been used in the past in the hope of exercising a selective antiseptic action on the infecting organism. Hexamine, chlorine preparations, methylene blue, gentian violet, brilliant green, neutral acriflavine, mercurochrome and neoarsphenamine have all been praised, and have all accomplished very little. Probably the best of these preparations is flavine, and the intravenous administration of from 80 to 120 c.c. of a 1 : 500 watery solution of neutral acriflavine has been of value. Such an injection should be repeated every second day if needed, and should not be dismissed as useless until four or five injections have been given. It has been found of benefit in staphylococcus infection.

In recent years, however, these drugs have been completely superseded by the sulphanilamide series of preparations.[1] The first experimental work was published in 1935 by Domagk. This concerned a reddish powder, an azo dye, sulphamido-chrysoidin, termed Prontosil "red." In 1936 Trefouël, Nitti and Bovet showed that a portion of this drug, para-amino-phenyl-sulphonamide, now commonly termed "sulphanilamide," was as potent in experimental infections as the parent substance.

[1] An azo dye contains the linkage $-N=N-$. Sulphonamide contains a benzene ring and has the formula

$$H_2NO_2S-\langle\bigcirc\rangle-NH_2.$$

Since then numerous compounds have been made using sulphanilamide as a component, and many of them have considerable human therapeutic activity. The search goes on, and laboratory interest is roused by a series of products in which the azo linkage of sulphonamide is replaced by a sulphone. Such sulphones are not yet of major clinical importance. In this article the sulphanilamide preparations to be considered will be sulphanilamide, Rubiazol (a French preparation, an azoic dye, carboxy-sulphamideo-chrysoidine), a sulphonamide linked to a pyridine ring, commonly called sulphapyridine (manufactured by Messrs May & Baker Ltd., under the trade name of Dagenan or M. & B. 693) and Uleron (a di-sulphanilamide, marketed by Messrs Bayer Products Ltd.).

Sulphanilamide, Rubiazol and sulphapyridine are active against infection caused by streptococci, particularly those of beta-hæmolytic strains, meningococci, *B. coli,* the bacillus of gas gangrene and *B. abortus.* Though all three are active against pneumococci and gonococci, sulphapyridine is undoubtedly the drug of election in such infections. Uleron has been recommended particularly for staphylococcal infections, but it is very doubtful if it is as efficacious in this respect as sulphanilamide or sulphapyridine. These drugs have little action in cases of infection by *Streptococcus viridans, H. influenzæ, B. typhosus* or in virus diseases.

The sulphonamide group of drugs act *in vivo* and only to a lesser extent *in vitro,* requiring the presence of human serum to achieve their best results. The mode of action is not understood, but on the whole they are considered at present to inhibit the growth of bacteria in the body by interfering with their metabolism, thus rendering the organisms more susceptible to natural defences. They act as well when given by the mouth as when given parenterally. The optimum dosage is not yet settled, nor indeed need it necessarily prove to be the same for all members of this group or for septicæmias caused by different organisms. Therapeutic benefit is only noticeable when the concentration of the drug reaches a certain level in the body and only continues when that concentration is maintained. Sulphanilamide is quickly excreted. Ninety-five per cent. of the drug is soon recoverable from the urine and little storage action is to be expected. It is suggested that the main action of the pyridine in sulphapyridine may be to delay excretion of sulphanilamide. It follows that to secure effective concentration in the blood an adequate dose must be given at regular periods and in the first stages of treatment these should not exceed four-hourly intervals. Sulphanilamide and sulphapyridine are sold in tablets of 0·5 gm. ($7\frac{1}{2}$ gr.), Rubiazol in tablets of 0·2 gm. (3 gr.), and it is suggested that a suitable dosage and mode of administration for an adult is to give two tablets crushed and taken with at least half a glass of water every four hours for the first three or four days. Such a dosage may be maintained for seven to ten days in the absence of toxic effects and thereafter two tablets thrice daily will probably be sufficient. Treatment should be continued if possible for at least seven days after apparent cure to diminish a tendency to relapse or recurrence. It has been shown that the liability to serious complications such as agranulocytosis is increased if the treatment is continued for periods longer than two weeks. Accordingly if it is decided to continue chemotherapy for a longer period the administration of the drug should be suspended for three or four days to allow complete elimination and to diminish the incidence of toxic symptoms. Treatment may then be recommenced if indicated, usually with a change of drug. The preliminary choice of the drug to be used depends upon the nature of the infection.

If the causal organism is unknown sulphapyridine should be employed because it is the most effective member of the sulphonamide group in pneumococcal and gonococcal infections and is at least equal, if not superior, in infections due to hæmolytic streptococci, meningococci, Friedländer's bacillus, bacillus of gas gangrene (*Clostridium welchii*), *B. abortus* and *B. coli*. Until recently Uleron (Bayer) in a dosage of not more than 4 gm. a day was recommended if the septicæmia was found to be of staphylococcal origin. Recent publications suggest that sulphapyridine may be equally effective, but the matter is still *sub judice*. Rubiazol is the least toxic of the sulphonamide drugs and should be tried when symptoms of toxicity are such as to suggest the inadvisability of continuing with sulphapyridine.

In a small proportion of cases the patient is unconscious or too ill to swallow. In such an event the drug must be given by nasal tube or by intramuscular injection. It is inadvisable to administer it by the intravenous route, and, in view of the rapid penetration of sulphanilamide into the cerebrospinal fluid, the intrathecal route is unnecessary. The preparations mentioned above can only be employed orally, and for injections one may use either Prontosil "soluble," a complicated but soluble derivative of Prontosil "red," the sodium salt of sulphapyridine, or Soluseptasine, a benzyl compound of sulphanilamide. The directions for administration given by the manufacturers with these products may be followed. As soon as the patient is able to swallow, the appropriate drug for oral use should be commenced.

The sulphonamide series must not be employed to the exclusion of other methods of treatment. So far clinical work shows definitely that better results are obtained if it is given in collaboration with other therapeutic agents.

Toxic symptoms are common. In many cases a degree of cyanosis appears. This is usually due to methæmoglobinæmia, and is not necessarily a reason for stopping the use of sulphonamide. Only a spectroscopic examination of the blood will settle finally the differential diagnosis between this and sulphæmoglobinæmia which necessitates the immediate stoppage of all sulphonamides. In general practice it is not easy to live up to this ideal and the practitioner is accordingly advised to adopt the following plan: (1) Administer methylene blue in pill form in a dosage of 2 gr. thrice daily. If the cyanosis is due to methæmoglobinæmia it will improve or disappear with this treatment. (2) Continue the use of the sulphonamide preparation when clinically advisable. (3) If cyanosis deepens, but no complaint is made, use Rubiazol in place of the sulphonamide previously employed. The dosage should be 0·2 or 0·4 gm. every four hours in the case of an adult. (4) Wherever cyanosis deepens and sickness, lassitude, shallow breathing and mental distress appear, stop the administration of all sulphonamide preparations. Sulphæmoglobinæmia often develops if the patient is taking sulphur in any form. This is more serious and death may ensue if the use of drugs of the sulphonamide series be continued. Medicines containing sulphur must therefore be avoided. Thus saline purgatives containing sulphates and liquorice powder are prohibited, as also is iron in the form of sulphate. Onions and eggs contain a fair proportion of sulphur, and their use should be restricted, although no harmful effect has been noticed following the taking of eggs in moderate quantity.

Drug fever, erythematous and morbilliform rashes, headache, giddiness, anorexia, nausea, vomiting and diarrhœa have all been noted as toxic effects. Their severity and the progress of the case must determine whether the drug is to be stopped or not. Rashes have been seen particularly on parts of the body exposed to bright sunlight, and this should be remembered.

A rarer, but more serious, complication is agranulocytosis marked by great diminution in the number of leucocytes. This must be watched for, and calls for immediate cessation of the drug and the administration of blood transfusions and iron.

Certain details in the management of the patient have been

found of value in the prevention of these toxic symptoms. Constipation and stasis of the bowel is a causal factor and must be prevented. Prior to treatment a soap and water enema should be given, and thereafter the bowel should be regulated to secure a daily evacuation with paraffin or any simple laxative not containing sulphur if paraffin proves inadequate, or enemata. Drugs which produce a watery stool should be avoided.

General Measures.—*Diet* should be light but ample. Fluid intake should be high and amount to at least 3,000 c.c. in the twenty-four hours for an adult. Glucose is valuable and the administration of 4 oz. a day is of benefit to the heart muscle. Additional quantities of vitamin A (cod-liver oil), vitamin B (marmite or yeast) and vitamin C (orange or lemon juice) should be given. Eggs, in moderate quantity, milk, soups and soft foods should make up a diet with a high calorific value giving a low residue, and should be administered in frequent small feeds. If the disease be chronic, little restriction should be placed on the patient's natural desires. Alcohol, approved by some, disapproved by others, is probably only of benefit in an emergency. Its food value is easily supplanted by glucose, its stimulant effect by aromatic spirit of ammonia. Champagne, iced and in small quantity, is probably the best variety to employ.

Drugs, other than specifics, should be kept to a minimum. Coramine, 1 ampoule injected either once daily or as frequently as two-hourly, is a definite cardiac stimulant. Its use in the treatment of acute circulatory failure is fully discussed on p. 729. Aromatic spirit of ammonia (30 to 60 minims) is a good diffusible stimulant, and strychnine ($\frac{1}{30}$ to $\frac{1}{10}$ gr.) may be given by injection. If pain be present do not hesitate to employ omnopon ($\frac{1}{3}$ to $\frac{1}{2}$ gr.) or morphia tartrate ($\frac{1}{6}$ to $\frac{1}{4}$ gr.) by injection. For sleeplessness any favourite hypnotic may be employed; there are no special indications. An enema or a glycerin suppository is preferable to laxatives by mouth other than paraffin, but here, too, any routine laxative treatment may be given, avoiding any preparation containing sulphur.

If anæmia develops, 30 gr. of iron and ammonium citrate should be given three times a day (avoid ferrous sulphate).

The practitioner must never regard the prognosis as hopeless in a case of septicæmia. If a septic focus can be adequately drained, if sulphanilamide can inhibit bacterial growth in the body and if immunity can be stimulated, the most dramatic results can be achieved. At present the therapeutic measures of first importance comprise blood transfusion, immune sera and the sulphanilamide series of drugs. Their relative values and methods of employment have only been indicated here in a routine manner, but the actual management of any given case of septicæmia calls for the highest grade of clinical observation and judgment, and the successful outcome not infrequently is a measure of the care of the doctor alike in the employment of the major methods of therapy and in the handling of the minor symptoms which may arise from day to day in the course of the illness.

Prophylaxis.—Many occasions arise where doubt exists as to whether or not an organism capable of producing septicæmia has been introduced into the body. Severe laceration at child-birth, the prick of a surgical needle, wounds inflicted by a dirty weapon or contamination by soil may be instanced. The advantage of the administration of anti-tetanic or anti-gas-gangrene serum is well known, and these should be given when the need is indicated. If streptococcal infection be suspected the immediate and repeated administration of concentrated anti-streptococcal serum, given with precautions against anaphylaxis, can do no harm, and this should be combined with either sulphapyridine or sulphanilamide by mouth.

Because of their limited time range of effective action these drugs should be employed in the dosage already indicated in order to maintain an effective concentration in the blood serum. They should be given for four or five days in absence of symptoms. Septicæmia is so fatal, and the proliferation of the streptococcus and the effect of its toxins so rapid, that it is surprising indeed that more attention is not given to the prophylactic side of this infection. For war wounds the use of anti-tetanic and anti-gangrene sera is routine, yet these diseases are relatively infrequent. For civilian wounds much more should be done to prevent streptococcal infection, but if a drug of the sulphonamide series be employed it must again be emphasized that the value of any one dose is of short range, and that repeated dosage is the only method of therapeutic value.

W. R. SNODGRASS.

ERYSIPELAS

Erysipelas is a notifiable disease : some local authorities do, in fact, arrange for the treatment of such cases in hospital. The infectivity is, however, slight, and, provided simple aseptic precautions are taken, there is no reason why the patient should not be treated at home.

The general measures to be adopted are similar to those applicable to any other acute infection. Careful nursing is important since the disease frequently attacks elderly patients, often as a complication of some other disease.

It is doubtful if any type of local treatment has a beneficial effect upon the dermatitis. The assessment of the value of any form of treatment in erysipelas is exceedingly difficult owing to the natural tendency of the disease towards spontaneous cure. Many so-called specific treatments have thus gained a reputation through the observation of their effects in small and uncontrolled series of cases. It is only when large numbers of patients have been treated that the inefficacy of certain methods can be proved. Thus the application of mild antiseptic ointments to the lesion has no value in limiting its spread, while painting the spreading margin with tincture of iodine or with collodion is equally ineffective. Local applications, however, do have a place in the treatment of certain cases owing to their value in relieving pain and œdema. Compresses of carbolic lotion 1 : 60 or 1 : 80, anhydrous magnesium sulphate (50 per cent.) in glycerin, or even simple hot fomentations may here be of great benefit, and they should always be used in cases of facial involvement where gross œdema is present. In certain cases, too, the desquamation which appears on the site of the lesion, especially when there has been much vesication, gives rise to discomfort. The application of the following salve gives great relief: oil of cloves, 1 per cent.; oil of eucalyptus, 5 per cent.; soft paraffin to 100.

Certain methods of treatment have been advised with a view to increasing the local or general resistance of the body. The exposure of the spreading margin of the lesion, and the skin immediately beyond it, to the rays of a mercury-vapour lamp is apparently often successful in promoting more rapid recovery. The lamp should be held from 1 to 2 ft. from the skin surface and a dose of one and a half to two "erythema doses" applied. It is important that all of the healthy skin surrounding the lesion be exposed to the rays.

As the disease is of streptococcal origin the administration of scarlet fever antitoxin has been advised. I have employed this serum both locally and intravenously and have failed to observe any beneficial effect on the toxæmia, pyrexia or the lesion itself.

The use of the sulphanilamide group of drugs, however, has so greatly hastened recovery that no other form of treatment is, as a rule, required. (For a more detailed reference to these drugs, reference should be made to the section which deals with the treatment of septicæmia.) Many favourable reports upon the value of these drugs in the treatment of erysipelas have been published. Proof of their undoubted effect has been furnished by Snodgrass and myself in a controlled series of over 500 consecutive cases reported to the Therapeutic Trials Committee of the Medical Research Council. Cure of the disease can be established in practically all cases within a period of three or four days. The best results are obtained with either the original red dye—sulphamido-chrysoidin or its derivative *p*-amino-benzene-sulphonamide, usually referred to as sulphanilamide. While many other derivatives of this group of drugs have now been advocated, the practitioner is advised, in the meantime, to make his choice between these two, which are of proved efficacy.

The following table shows the range of dosage which should be employed in different age-groups. Children tolerate the drug exceedingly well, and since the disease is often most severe in infancy, relatively large doses should therefore be employed.

Age Group.	Dosage in Grammes per Twenty-four Hours.	
	Sulphamido-chrysoidin.	Sulphanilamide.
Adults . . .	9 to 12	6 to 9
Five to ten years .	6 ,, 9	4·5 to 6
Under five years . .	3 ,, 6	3

In order to maintain an effective concentration of sulphanilamide in the blood, the drugs should be given by mouth at four-hourly intervals, and if a dose be omitted for any reason, that following should be doubled in amount. Preparations of the drugs may be obtained for parenteral administration (prontosil soluble (5 per cent.) or sulphanilamide (1 per cent.)). This method of administration shows no therapeutic advantage over the oral route, and its use should be reserved for critically ill patients first seen late in the disease where it is desired to obtain a high blood concentration in a short time.

If the drugs are used in the suggested doses the lesion will cease to spread within forty-eight hours, and in the majority of cases the temperature will regain normal in three or four days. Should the latter not occur, first the correctness of the diagnosis should be reviewed; secondly, the presence of some septic complication should be excluded; and thirdly, the question of fever, directly due to the drug, should be considered.

After the cessation of primary pyrexia, administration of the drugs should be continued for a further period of ten to fourteen days, a dose of 1 gm. three times daily being employed. When this is done, recurrence of the disease is unusual.

(*N.B.*—During the administration of these drugs certain rules should be rigidly applied. Reference should again be made to the section dealing with the treatment of Septicæmia (p. 86).)

Certain symptoms are commonly present which require attention. (The drugs which are suggested for their treatment have all been found effective and do not increase the tendency to toxic effects from sulphanilamide.) *Headache* is frequently complained of, but is usually relieved by acetyl-salicylic acid (5 to 15 gr.). *Insomnia*, when present, should be treated early because of its exhausting effect upon the patient and also because, if untreated, it may lead to the appearance of delirium. Syrup of chloral hydrate ($\frac{1}{2}$ to 2 drachms), Dover's powder (5 to 15 gr.), Battley's solution of opium (5 to 30 minims) or sulphonal (25 gr.) are all suitable. *Delirium* in the early stage is not uncommon. Morphine tartrate ($\frac{1}{4}$ gr.) and hyoscine hydrobromide ($\frac{1}{100}$ gr.) should be given and, if necessary, repeated. When a history of alcoholism is obtained it is advisable to continue moderate doses of whisky during the acute stage.

The incidence of complications is exceedingly low if treatment with sulphanilamide is begun early. Inflammation of the associated lymph glands is frequently present but will usually subside without any local treatment. Should the glands suppurate, simple hot fomentations are helpful. Incision should be delayed until complete coalescence has occurred and fluctuation is definitely present. Healing is then more rapid. Subcutaneous abscesses are not infrequent. Here, again, incision should not be made too early. The abscess frequently underlies the original erysipelatous lesion and healing is more rapid if its cure has first been established. Acute nephritis, usually of focal type and early in its appearance, rapidly subsides with cure of the local lesion. Since gross failure of renal secretion is rarely demonstrated, there is no contraindication to the use of sulphanilamide. Rarely does septicæmia or pyæmia develop. Its presence calls not only for an increase in the dose of sulphanilamide, but for the employment of all the additional methods of treatment which such a serious condition demands.

T. Anderson.

TUBERCULOSIS

THE PREVENTION OF TUBERCULOSIS

CAUSES of Decline in Tuberculosis Mortality.—It is well known that in the majority of Western European countries and in North America the mortality from tuberculosis has been declining for many years. In England and Scotland, for example, it has fallen during the last fifty years by about 75 per cent. Moderately reliable tuberculosis mortality statistics became available coincidently with Koch's discovery of the tubercle bacillus, which discovery set on foot the organized campaign against the disease. The decline in tuberculosis mortality thus became apparent at much the same time as the anti-tuberculosis measures were initiated, and since then the fall in the one has run parallel with the development of the other. It is natural enough, therefore, for many to ascribe this gratifying decline entirely to the great campaign which has been waged against tuberculosis. There is much evidence to suggest, however, that the mortality from tuberculosis had been declining for many years prior to the special measures taken to combat the disease. It has thus been suggested, with considerable evidence for the assumption, that we are at present at the end of a protracted epidemic of tuberculosis, and that the disease is subject to the same epidemic waves as measles, scarlet fever and diphtheria, with this difference, that whereas the epidemic waves of these more acute diseases are relatively short, that of tuberculosis may last a hundred years or more. This is according to expectation in a disease which may continue for the lifetime of an individual, in contrast to epidemic diseases of a more evanescent type. Further, it is probable that during the course of such an epidemic communities which have been exposed particularly to the infection have acquired a strong resistance to it, and that those individuals who are peculiarly susceptible to the tubercle bacillus have died at an early age leaving relatively few descendants who may have inherited their peculiar susceptibility. Lastly, the number of young people alive to-day is relatively less in proportion to the number of people over forty than was the case in the Victorian age, and it is well known that tuberculous disease, particularly where females are concerned, reaches its most lethal peak between the ages of twenty-five and thirty-five. Thus the decline in the mortality from tuberculosis may be due to the fact that the virulence of the infective agent is diminishing, and that there is a proportionately smaller number of susceptible persons on which the infection can produce its effects.

Whether or not we believe that these are potent factors in producing the fall in the mortality from tuberculosis, it should not lead to a fatalistic attitude in regard to the preventive aspects of the disease. There is no reason to believe that an epidemiological curve cannot be modified beneficially by human efforts. No one, for example, would suggest that the worst effects of epidemics of acute infectious diseases cannot be ameliorated by popular education, by social and public health measures and by the private efforts of medical practitioners. The same can be said of tuberculosis. The recognition of the fact that we may be unable complacently to congratulate ourselves that the *entire* fall in the mortality from tuberculosis has been due to anti-tuberculosis measures, does not justify the opposite attitude not infrequently adopted. It is unfair and unwise to make light of the great efforts which have been made to combat the disease, or to deny that these have been a potent contributory factor in lowering the mortality from tuberculosis. We have only to look, for example, to the increase in tuberculosis in Germany during the war of 1914-18, to its disproportionate incidence in certain trades, to its wide occurrence in districts smitten by poverty and unemployment, and to the virtual absence of glandular and bone and joint tuberculosis in countries with a clean milk supply, to be certain that epidemiology, immunity and natural selection are not the only factors in this great problem.

Infection.—The factors contributing to the spread and morbidity of tuberculosis are many, but the essential cause is contagion from a human or animal source. It therefore becomes of interest to inquire to what extent such infection can be avoided, and whether attempts to prevent infection should occupy an important place in anti-tuberculosis measures, and if so, to what extent. The answer to this question depends on whether adult exogenous infection occurs with significant frequency in civilized communities. Opinions differ on this matter, but it is an important one for the practitioner whose opinion may be sought by patients as to whether they are likely to infect their husbands, wives or adult friends, and by employers as to the danger to others of a tuberculous employee in their office or works. We believe that adult tuberculosis usually occurs as a late manifestation of an earlier disease. Just as general paralysis is a late visceral manifestation of syphilis, so it is exceptional for an adult to develop tuberculous disease as the result of an outside superinfection, provided he is protected by tubercle bacilli acquired in childhood and is tuberculin positive. It should be remembered that in older children and adults a positive tuberculin reaction is a desirable rather than an undesirable acquisition. When tuberculous disease does occur in an adult, therefore, it is usually due to the breakdown of his resistance to an infection which he already harbours and not to the fact that he has been reinfected from without.

Occasionally a high rate of tuberculous morbidity is witnessed among medical students and nurses as the result of professional contact with cases of open tuberculosis. Heimbeck has pointed out, however, that this excessive morbidity chiefly occurs among those few probationers and students who exhibit a negative tuberculin test on starting training, and who are thus, to some extent, comparable as regards susceptibility to tuberculosis to the Red Indian when first brought into contact with white men. All nurses and young adults about to be brought into close and continuous contact with cases of open tuberculosis should be tested with tuberculin, and those who are negative reactors should, if at all possible, be prevented from taking such a considerable risk.

Immunity in tuberculized adults to exogenous reinfection may occasionally disappear just as it occasionally disappears in the case of the common exanthemata. A doctor cannot, therefore, *guarantee* that an adult will not be reinfected, just as he cannot *guarantee* that an individual will not take measles twice, but he can say that the risk is extremely slight. No doubt, also, this adult immunity may be temporarily in abeyance as the result of one of the acute infectious fevers like measles, or during the puerperium, when a massive exogenous infection may cause tuberculous disease. Care should therefore be taken at such times that the patient is not nursed by, or brought into close contact with, cases of open tuberculosis in the household.

In the great majority of cases, however, it is as difficult to reinfect a previously tuberculized adult as Koch found it to reinfect a tuberculous guinea-pig. How else can one explain the fact that cases of tuberculous adenitis in sanatoriums are not superinfected by cases of open tuberculosis in the same ward; that insurance companies do not see fit to load the premiums of tuberculosis officers; and, above all, that there is no statistical evidence to suggest that the tuberculous husband infects his healthy consort with any frequency, or vice versa? We believe, therefore, that with the precautions noted above the practitioner can advise his patients that the risk of one adult infecting another in civilized communities is comparatively slight.

If it be true that a tuberculized adult is not usually susceptible to a secondary exogenous infection, the attempt to prevent infection in adults is not a matter of primary importance. Our efforts should rather be directed to the prevention of massive primary infection in the young child, who, like the savage, forms virgin soil for the tubercle bacillus. It is highly desirable that infection with tuberculosis should be delayed as long as possible, since the younger the child when the infection occurs the greater is the chance of a fatal issue. It would seem, from the results of tuberculin tests, that in this country the tuberculization of the community is, on the average, occurring at a later age than heretofore, and this is desirable.

In the absence of sufficient proof as to the efficacy or harmlessness of the B.C.G. vaccine, efforts to prevent massive infection in young children must continue to be directed along two main channels: their segregation from close contact with cases of open tuberculosis and the provision of a clean milk supply. These two measures, if effectively carried out, would go far in themselves to diminish mortality and morbidity from tuberculosis in childhood. They would probably go further: they would tend very considerably to reduce the incidence of pulmonary tuberculosis and other late visceral manifestations of the disease in adult life, since experience suggests that such manifestations occur very frequently in adults who were subjected to repeated massive infections in childhood.

The segregation of young children from close and continuous contact with open cases of tuberculosis in their family is often a matter of great difficulty. The chief ways in which the risk of infection from the human type of the bacillus in a child's home life can be prevented, or reduced to a minimum, are by the removal of an open case of tuberculosis among the parents or those living in the house to a residential tuberculosis institution, or by the removal of the child from the tuberculous home. The second method, or Grancher system, though practised to a considerable extent in France and to a limited extent in this country, seems an impossible and perhaps undesirable practice to be universally adopted. It is much more satisfactory to remove and treat the adult patient, who is the potential source of the infection. Unless patients are adequately informed of the risk of infecting their children, they will often refuse such segregation. When this is carefully and considerately explained to them, however, it is very rare for them to object, no matter how painful the separation may be.

With the limited number of beds at our disposal in tuberculosis institutions, however, it is not always possible to remove all infectious cases from risk of contact with their young children. Again, it is sometimes undesirable to continue to keep a patient in a sanatorium who may have recovered sufficiently to resume his occupation, but who may still have tubercle bacilli in his sputum. In such cases, if it is impossible to remove the young child to the home of a relative or to an institution, every effort should be made by the family doctor to ensure that the child is kept as far as possible from close contact with the tuberculous patient. In certain overcrowded houses this may present almost insuperable difficulties, and it is unfortunately not uncommon to find a case of open tuberculosis not only sleeping in the same room but even in the same bed as a young child. This is, of course, an administrative and social scandal, and disaster under such circumstances is almost inevitable. In cases where it is unfortunately found impossible to avoid having an open case of tuberculosis and a young child in the same house, it should usually be possible to arrange for the patient to have a separate sleeping room into which the child should never go, and to have separate utensils for eating and drinking and separate towels and bedclothes. All infected sputum should be ejected into a sputum flask or paper handkerchief, which latter should be promptly burned. Further, the patient should as far as possible avoid touching the child, who should never be taken on his knee and never on any account kissed. It should always be remembered that contact with a tuberculous patient, or the conveying of infected material to the mouth, are probably much more common causes of massive infection than "droplet infection," which receives such a prominent place in tuberculosis literature.

If the segregation of the young child from massive human infection is a matter of extreme difficulty, its segregation from massive infection from milk is eminently practicable. There is no doubt that tuberculosis due to the bovine bacillus is responsible for a considerable percentage of tuberculous morbidity among children, particularly in Scotland. Though the bovine type of disease is mostly to be found in glandular, lupoid, abdominal, bone and joint and meningeal lesions, yet it may on occasion cause any type of tuberculosis—not even excluding the pulmonary variety. Having regard to the great prevalence of tuberculosis among the dairy herds of this country, and to the absence of a comprehensive national plan for dealing with it, it is clear that if conditions are allowed to remain as they are, large numbers of children are doomed to die of bovine tuberculosis, or to become crippled by it. In several countries, notably America and New Zealand, bovine tuberculosis has been largely eradicated by ensuring a clean milk supply, but in this country large quantities of tuberculous milk are still consumed. It is common to hear the remark that a child is all the better for being immunized by a small dose of bovine bacilli. Unfortunately one cannot regulate the dose, and no one would be so bold as to suggest that it is good for a child to drink a teaspoonful of tuberculous pus in its milk.

Wherever possible certified or tuberculin-tested milk should be given to young children. Unfortunately it is often impossible to procure such milk, and even when procurable its expense makes it prohibitive to large sections of the community. Until, therefore, the ideal of a national clean milk supply is achieved, it seems only common sense that all milk given to young children should be pasteurized. It is true that this method is not an absolutely complete safeguard in preventing the occasional occurrence of tubercle bacilli in milk, and that in the process certain insignificant losses occur in respect of its vitamin and mineral content. No one, however, with any knowledge of the subject can believe that these drawbacks are at all comparable to the great risks children run by consuming unpasteurized milk from herds which have not been tuberculin tested.

Even pasteurized milk is, however, often unprocurable, especially in rural districts. In such cases milk for young children should be boiled, or dried milk should be used. When these expedients are resorted to, orange juice must also be given to make good the vitamin deficiency which might otherwise occur.

Such measures to prevent bovine tuberculous infection are not so necessary in the case of older children and adults whose tuberculin reactions have already become positive. Clean milk is, however, *ideal* for them also as tuberculosis is not the only disease conveyed through milk.

Resistance.—Having taken steps against the massive contamination of virgin soil by segregation and by the provision of a safe milk supply, the factors which conduce to tuberculous disease must be looked for, not so much among the seed as in the soil in which the seed is sown. That is, infection is almost certain to take place—ideally in small and infrequent doses—and thereafter all our efforts should be directed, not so much to the prevention of infection as to raising the resistance of the infected individual, particularly the young adult, against the infection becoming a disease.

Apart from the question of race and breeding, over which we have no control, the resistance of an individual to his tuberculous infection will depend very largely on certain environmental conditions ; housing, nutrition, habits and intercurrent infections.

One has only to glance at the innumerable statistics produced from all over the world to see that tuberculosis and overcrowding go hand in hand, though the relative importance of overcrowding will depend to some extent on the nature of the other adverse conditions present. Overcrowding is a factor which is capable of correction in the course of time, and the problem is being steadily tackled in this country. There is every reason to believe that the better housing of the future will cause a marked diminution in the incidence of the disease. Overcrowding is a national problem rather than one for the private medical practitioner, though he may on occasion assist to procure more suitable accommodation for the tuberculous families in his practice.

If, on the other hand, good environmental conditions as regards housing are only obtained at the expense of increased rents, and therefore in a reduction of the family's food-purchasing power, the advantages which accrue from good housing may be considerably outweighed by nutritional depreciation. There is indeed definite statistical foundation for the statement that under-nourishment is one of the most important factors in predisposing an individual towards tuberculous infection. Up till now the principles of good nutrition have been largely neglected in the medical curriculum. While every doctor can prescribe bottles of medicine, comparatively few can give sound advice as to how money can be expended most profitably on food. An educational campaign by family doctors on the subject of nutrition, particularly among girls and housewives, might be far more conducive to national physical fitness and the prevention of tuberculosis than the less prosaic campaign now being waged on the subject of playing fields. At the same time it must be confessed that it would tax the ingenuity of the most competent dietitian to provide entirely adequate diets in respect of first-class protein, vitamins and minerals on the income of many of our working-class families.

Early Diagnosis.—It is apparent that all preventive measures taken against tuberculosis cannot be expected to be entirely successful without the early diagnosis of the disease. When a case of tuberculosis occurs in a household it is the family doctor's duty, in conjunction with the district tuberculosis officer, to search for a possible focus of infection among the other members of the family. A child dying from tuberculous meningitis is frequently found to have a parent or grandparent supposed to be suffering from chronic bronchitis, whom more careful examination will show to be in reality suffering from chronic pulmonary tuberculosis. Further, all the other children and young adults in such a family should be carefully examined, preferably with the help of X-rays, to eliminate the possibility of early tuberculous disease, and any subsequent illness from which they may suffer must be regarded by the family doctor in the light of the family history.

In the past over-emphasis has been laid on gross physical signs in the chest in the diagnosis of tuberculosis, such as impairment of the percussion note and the presence of bronchial breathing and crepitations. These are frequently difficult to elicit or entirely absent in early pulmonary disease. On the other hand, too little importance is attached to the general signs of tuberculous toxæmia, common to all forms of the disease, which are often apparent to the patient's relatives and friends but overlooked by the doctor, obsessed by his hunt for crepitations in the lungs. Again, the significance of history-taking in the diagnosis of early tuberculosis is often insufficiently appreciated, and yet the vast majority of patients repeat with variations the same history with the regularity of a theme in a symphony. Early disease can usually only be *suspected* by the practitioner, and to clinch the diagnosis an appeal has often to be made to radiological and bacteriological examinations. These special services for the diagnosis of tuberculosis are available free of cost in all parts of this country and full use should be made of them.

Lastly, it should always be remembered that other diseases, such as measles, whooping cough, diabetes, silicosis and influenza, predispose towards tuberculosis. The prevention of such diseases and their correct treatment would assist indirectly in the prevention of tuberculosis, and suspicious symptoms occurring in the victims of such diseases should be regarded particularly seriously.

PULMONARY TUBERCULOSIS

GENERAL MANAGEMENT

In the following pages the general management of a case of pulmonary tuberculosis will be described. Pulmonary tuberculosis is only one of the local manifestations of the disease, and the general treatment of pulmonary tuberculosis applies no less to other forms of the disease.

When a patient develops pulmonary tuberculosis there is often a natural disinclination on the part of the family doctor to tell him exactly what is the matter with him. Euphemisms such as " a spot on the lung " or " a slight inflammation of the lung " are often used. This is undoubtedly a great mistake and often deludes the patient into a sense of false security, so that instead of putting himself immediately under strict treatment he compromises by going away for a holiday or by going to bed for a week or two. Valuable time in an early case is thereby lost. A patient has a right to know the true diagnosis of his condition, even if it causes considerable temporary distress.

The word tuberculosis has an unfortunate connotation. Patients think of it as an incurable and fatal disease, and feel that some sort of stigma is associated with it. It should be explained to them that tuberculosis, as we recognize it nowadays, is quite a different thing to the " consumption " of the Victorian era. The disease was then seldom recognized till it had reached an incurable stage. Even if it was diagnosed relatively early, the correct method of treatment was not known. The patient can be told that tuberculosis, far from being incurable, is a condition to which human beings are peculiarly resistant; that nearly all of us are infected by it, and that many of us without having been aware of the fact have indeed suffered from it slightly and have completely overcome it. Accordingly he must be made to realize that with wise management there is no reason at all why he should not make a complete recovery. Even moderately advanced cases should be encouraged in this way, for hope is a great therapeutic agent, and there are indeed few cases so severe when first seen that a hopeless prognosis can be given with any degree of certainty. At the same time the patient must be told that it is of the utmost importance for him to go under strict treatment at once, and that this will consist, among other things, in complete rest for an unspecified period. He will then almost certainly ask how long he will have to stop work. It is very unwise for the doctor to commit himself on this point, especially as he himself can only have a vague idea of the probable duration of the disease. Too often the patient is told that three months in a sanatorium will put him right. The patient makes his arrangements accordingly and may be seriously inconvenienced when it is found later that he will have to stay there for a considerably longer time. In addition, the physician in charge of the sanatorium may be put in a difficult position. On the other hand it is often injudicious to depress the patient at the beginning of treatment by the statement that he may have to be off work for a year or more. It is wiser, and more honest, therefore, to answer the patient's question by saying that it is quite impossible at the outset to say how long he will have to be under strict treatment, since this entirely depends upon how he reacts to it. He will have to reckon its duration, however, in terms of many months and not in terms of weeks. A young person may be encouraged by the suggestion that it is worth while spending some months in enforced inactivity to begin with in order to insure his health for the rest of his life.

Sanatorium Treatment.—The majority of patients with active tuberculosis should be advised that the first stage of treatment is best carried out in a sanatorium. This advice does not apply to elderly patients suffering from chronic fibroid disease, whose management presents a special problem of its own (see p. 115) or to patients so ill that the prospect of procuring arrest of their disease is very bad. Unless young children are present in the house it is wiser to treat such patients at home. For the average case of exudative tuberculosis in a young adult, however, a period of sanatorium treatment is invaluable. Quite apart from any active form of curative treatment, such as collapse therapy, the experience gained by the patient through the routine of sanatorium life is most useful in educating him in the implications of his disease and in methods for regulating his life in the future. Very few patients gain this knowledge if they are treated from the beginning in their own homes. It is often difficult to explain to a patient the benefits which he may expect to derive from going to a sanatorium. He is apt to say: "Surely if I have to do nothing except to lie in bed in the fresh air and to have good nourishing food, I can be cured at home just as well as in a sanatorium." The conditions at home are, of course, often quite unsuitable for rest in physiological surroundings. Even when they are apparently suitable it may be impossible to obtain mental as well as physical rest in the domestic atmosphere. All the circumstances of home life remind the patient of the active life which he formerly led and which he has had to abandon. In this connection it must be remembered that mental rest is only secondary in importance to physical rest. The doctor should try to persuade the patient to divorce himself entirely from his previous associations, to place himself confidently and unreservedly in the hands of others and to accept the situation in a placid and co-operative spirit. Once patients have made up their minds to do this they usually settle down into the sanatorium routine with relief. They then realize, perhaps for the first time, how ill they are and what an effort it had been to carry on their ordinary life. It is only with returning health that they once more begin to wish for a resumption of their normal activities.

Sanatorium treatment is available free of cost for all in this country. Many of these public institutions are admirably run, and the after-care by the tuberculosis authorities in conjunction with the family doctor is excellent. Unfortunately this is not invariably the case. In some districts there is a scarcity of sanatorium beds, necessitating tedious delay in admitting patients in urgent need of treatment, and causing premature discharge of others long before their disease has had a chance of becoming quiescent.

The financial difficulties of a family deprived of its bread-winner will also have to receive the practitioner's consideration. In this respect the help of the Care Committee attached to the local tuberculosis dispensary should be solicited.

Another problem may often arise among those well able to afford a private nursing home for an acute illness but quite unable to face the expenses (seven or eight guineas a week) of a private sanatorium for six months or a year. If the local public sanatorium is a good one, such patients should be strongly advised to go there for their treatment rather than to put themselves to unwarranted financial strain for the sake, perhaps, of a single room and the small additional comforts of a private sanatorium. Since the salary of such patients may be temporarily suspended and their earning capacity considerably reduced in the future, it is very important for them to conserve their finances in every way possible.

Climate.—There is a common idea among the well-to-do that tuberculosis spells institutional treatment abroad—particularly in Switzerland. This is a complete fallacy. Climate is of much less importance in the treatment of tuberculosis than the excellence of the physiological régime which is instituted, and there are several admirably run private sanatoria in this country. A patient may be cured of his disease in the centre of a large city just as well as in the middle of a pine forest, or on the slopes of a Swiss mountain. It is scandalous the way seriously ill patients are sometimes sent to die far away from their friends, relatives and home comforts. That they should be subjected to the fatigue of a long journey, and the indifferent nursing frequently encountered in a foreign institution because of the common illusion of the magical curative properties of the air and sunshine of some foreign health resort, is deeply to be deplored. No patient who is suffering severely from the toxæmia of tuberculosis should be sent abroad. On the other hand, in the case of a wealthy patient whose acute systemic intoxication has subsided under treatment, but whose further progress has become unduly slow, a change of scene to Switzerland may be beneficial. There is no doubt that high mountain air has certain tonic and hæmopoietic properties, and the sunshine and novel surroundings often have a stimulating psychological effect. This may be more than counterbalanced, however, if the nursing in the foreign institution is inadequate as it so often is. No patient should therefore be sent abroad who is not well enough to be out of bed for a part of the day, and able to attend to some extent to his own requirements.

Rest.—In tuberculosis the traditional therapeutic triad—fresh air, good food and rest—has stood the test of time, but the greatest of these is rest. To give insufficient rest is the commonest mistake in the treatment of the condition. Perhaps the surgeon now appreciates the importance of rest in the cure of tuberculosis of the bones and joints more fully than the physician in the cure of the pulmonary variety of the disease. In this respect the surgeon is helped by anatomical considerations which may favour the easier acceptance of a long period of rest by the patient. Further, it is comparatively easy to immobilise a tuberculous knee joint in a plaster case, but it is impossible to immobilize a lung completely which opens and shuts in the process of breathing some 30,000 times a day. It is true that this immobilization can be facilitated to a great extent by collapse therapy (see p. 121). Rest in bed, however, is of primary importance in ensuring that the respiratory movements should be sufficiently quiet and shallow to allow the formation of fibrous tissue to take place.

The factors which contribute to the inadequate prescription of rest so common in the treatment of tuberculosis have been enumerated by Roche[1] as follows :—

1. The doctor is often influenced by the teaching which

[1] H. Roche, *Brit. J. Tuberculosis* (1938), **32**, 89.

used to stress unduly the value of graduated labour and exercise of all kinds in the open air at an early stage in the disease. No doubt carefully graduated exercise and occupational therapy are most beneficial in the final stages of treatment, but they should not be started too soon.

2. The severe symptoms of tuberculous toxæmia often disappear under treatment long before the local lesion is sufficiently healed to make it permissible for exercise to be started. The patient therefore feels too well to lie in bed, and the doctor too often yields to his importunities to be permitted a little more latitude. Patience on the part of both doctor and patient is perhaps the most important of all qualities in the treatment of tuberculosis. No intelligent person, however, can be expected to exercise this quality to the necessary extent unless the reasons for long-continued rest are carefully explained to him. The cultivation of a co-operative spirit between the doctor and the patient, and the psychological ascendancy of the former over the latter, are essentials of successful treatment.

3. Public or individual economic difficulties may militate against prolonged rest : an inadequate number of institutional beds may conduce towards hurried treatment, owing to the length of the waiting list ; or private economic insecurity may unsettle a patient, so as greatly to curtail the desirable period of treatment.

4. Perhaps the most important cause of insufficient rest in the treatment of tuberculosis lies in the inadequate appreciation of the criteria on which the control of rest is based. There is no single method which will give this information. The control of the case must be determined by weighing the evidence derived from a number of sources, the most important of which are : Temperature, pulse-rate, weight, general symptoms, X-rays, blood sedimentation rate, the polymorph-lymphocyte-monocyte ratio. The extent of the tuberculous lesion itself is no criterion of the amount of rest which should be prescribed. A patient with a small circumscribed lesion may be seriously ill and in need of absolute rest, whereas extensive fibroid disease affecting both lungs may be no contraindication to a moderately active life.

Temperature.—A carefully kept record of the temperature taken night and morning is an essential in the treatment of all cases of active tuberculosis. Occasionally four-hourly recordings may be instructive. While the rectal temperature may be more accurate than the temperature taken in the mouth, its inconvenience makes the oral method preferable. Axillary skin temperatures are too inaccurate and should not be used. The thermometer should be kept in the closed mouth for at least three minutes, and no hot or cold foods or liquids should be taken immediately beforehand. It should be remembered that 98·4° is not a normal temperature for a patient who is confined to bed all day. In such cases the diurnal swing of the temperature should be below this level, and a chart which shows persistent readings along the so-called "normal" line usually indicates a mild degree of pyrexia. On the other hand, an occasional isolated reading up to 99° need not be regarded as of great significance provided all the other available data are satisfactory.

A high swinging temperature is an indication for complete rest in bed. When the pyrexia is only moderate and there are no other contraindications, the patient should be allowed up for washing and toilet purposes, as this greatly conduces to his mental and physical comfort. Apart from this, however, rest in bed throughout the twenty-four hours should be the rule for a patient with exudative tuberculosis until the temperature has entirely settled. A few cases of chronic fibroid tuberculosis with cavitation invariably have an evening temperature of 99° or even 100°. A certain amount of latitude in the matter of exercise should be allowed such patients whose management (see p. 115) is very different from that of the young adult with exudative tuberculosis. When the patient is allowed out of bed the temperature should be taken following exercise, and any instability of temperature at this time, especially a delay in returning to normal limits, will suggest caution.

While the temperature is a most valuable guide in determining how much rest or exercise should be prescribed, too much dependence should not be placed on it alone. Some cases of progressive disease who are not fit to be out of bed may be practically apyrexial; on the other hand, an occasional small rise of temperature may be of little significance if all the other signs are favourable.

The Pulse-rate.—As a general rule a resting pulse-rate of ninety per minute or over is an indication for the continuance of complete rest. A slow, steady pulse of good tension is a favourable sign. In most cases the temperature and pulse-rate rise and fall simultaneously, but in some the pulse remains elevated long after the temperature has become persistently normal or vice versa. In such cases the abnormal rather than the normal feature should be the controlling factor.

When exercise is started the pulse-test as used at Frimley is of value; the average resting pulse-rate is taken as being normal for the patient, who is then sent to take his prescribed amount of exercise; he lies down as soon as he returns and the pulse-rate is estimated immediately, and again in five minutes and half an hour. If a raised pulse-rate is due to mechanical cardiac embarrassment, such as may occur in pulmonary fibrosis or emphysema, the pulse-rate usually returns to normal in half an hour. If it is due to toxæmia, however, the tachycardia will be more persistent and will demand a reduction in the patient's activities.

Just as in the case of the temperature, the pulse-rate is simply a link, though a valuable one, in the chain of evidence which should govern the doctor's prescription of rest or exercise.

Radiography.—Good X-rays taken at regular intervals are more useful than the stethoscope in determining whether or not a patient is fit for exercise. The extension or limitation of the disease can be determined radiologically with considerable accuracy, and such findings furnish useful criteria for the prescription of further rest or increased activity for the patient.

The X-ray appearances, however, must be interpreted in light of the clinical picture. To make a prognosis from the X-ray picture alone is the worst possible practice. In this connection the use of X-rays is limited by the fact that it is not always possible to tell whether a shadow on the X-ray plate indicates active or healed disease. This is specially the case where many shadows are present. Further, foci of active disease may be concealed by the heart shadow, and the extent of their activity may not always be apparent even when lateral or oblique views are taken. Lastly, where a patient has a fibrous cavity in the lung, the radiological findings may not indicate whether or not a patient should be allowed to take exercise. This will depend on the presence and extent of toxæmic signs and symptoms.

The Blood Sedimentation Rate (for Technique see p. 959).—This test should never be omitted when any doubt exists as to whether a patient should be allowed out of bed or as to the amount of exercise he should be permitted to take. The test is so simple and easy to perform that there is no reason why it should not be widely used in general practice where it will be found to have numerous applications.

Generally speaking, it may be said that patients with healed tuberculous lesions, and otherwise in good health, have a normal sedimentation rate (below 6 Westergren); in quiescent cases, and in fibroid tuberculosis without toxæmic symptoms, the sedimentation rate will be slightly accelerated (6 to 14); and in progressive cases—particularly where the disease is exudative in type—it may vary from 14 to 100 depending upon the severity of the process. The test has thus the same significance in tuberculosis as fever, tachycardia and emaciation, but it is usually a more sensitive expression of the activity of the disease than any of them. Thus an increased rate of sedimentation may be noted long after the temperature, pulse-rate and nutrition have returned to normal, and may sound a warning note against the premature prescription of exercise, just as it does under similar circumstances in rheumatic fever.

Ideally, all patients with exudative disease who appear to have a reasonable hope of cure should be kept in bed till their blood sedimentation rate has fallen below 20, and preferably below 12. Thereafter, as long as the sedimentation rate, performed once a fortnight, keeps within normal limits, and provided the other prognostic data are satisfactory, the amount of exercise allowed can be steadily increased.

The Polymorph-Lymphocyte-Monocyte Ratio (Medlar count). —This test is complementary to the blood sedimentation rate, and is also of great service in the control of treatment of a tuberculous case. It would take too long to describe the details and rationale of the test here, and those unfamiliar with it are referred to the original papers on the subject. The practical objections to the test for routine use are that it demands some experience in differential blood counting, it is time-consuming and requires uniform interpretation by the same observer.

Weight.—In the average case the weekly weight of the patient is a useful guide to the progress of the disease, provided the various other factors enumerated above are taken into consideration. No patient should be allowed out of bed till the nutrition has become reasonably satisfactory, and a careful watch should be kept on the weight and on the muscular tone while exercise is being increased.

Symptoms.—The exacerbation of existing symptoms or the appearance of fresh ones such as dyspnœa, tiredness, increased cough or sputum, hæmoptysis, pleural pain or undue sweating requires an immediate re-assessment of the case and possibly a limitation of the patient's activities. The psychology of the patient must, however, be taken into account in assessing the significance of such symptoms.

In summary, then, a patient with exudative tuberculosis in whom there is a chance of obtaining arrest of the disease should be kept in bed till his temperature, pulse, nutrition, X-ray picture and blood tests are satisfactory. Thereafter exercise should be very gradually increased in proportion as the prognostic criteria noted above continue to be favourable. It is far better to make the mistake of increasing exercise too slowly than too quickly. It is exceedingly disappointing to a patient who has reached a certain stage in treatment to have to curtail his exercise or possibly to go back again to complete rest in bed. Finally, every effort should be made to induce the patient to cultivate some suitable hobby. There is nothing more conducive to morbid introspection than complete idleness.

Fresh Air.—Since the beginning of the century fresh air and tuberculosis have been spoken of in the same breath. In fact, they have been so linked together in people's minds that there has been a tendency to believe that open-air treatment is specifically beneficial for tuberculosis and for nothing else. This is entirely fallacious. There is nothing specific in the effect of open air on tuberculosis. The free exposure of a patient to fresh circulating air is of the greatest therapeutic value in raising his resistance towards any infection, particularly to respiratory infections. With a few exceptions all sick persons do better if they are nursed in the fresh air, provided conditions of heat and cold are not too rigorous, and provided shelter can be obtained against wind and rain. Old people, infants and patients suffering from a few diseases, such as acute nephritis, are exceptions to this rule. In many diseases, where various forms of specific treatment are employed, the use of fresh air as a therapeutic agent is often neglected. In tuberculosis, where treatment largely consists in raising the resistance of the individual through natural means, the importance of fresh air has been well recognized.

Rest in the fresh air produces remarkable changes which have to be seen to be believed. Night sweating can almost be guaranteed to disappear in the first few days of open-air treatment. Sleep becomes sounder and more refreshing, provided the patient is not allowed to become chilled through insufficient bedclothes. The appetite, which is usually poor in untreated tuberculosis, is rapidly regained and may indeed become unusually keen. The temperature abates much more rapidly in the real fresh air of a sanatorium than it does in the moderately fresh air of a ward in a general hospital. Cough and expectoration are diminished. Perhaps the most striking changes occur in the appearance of the patient, whose tissues regain tone and whose complexion improves. Shabby looking people begin to bloom and even to become beautiful. As the patient experiences the tonic influences of fresh air and notices the disappearance of his symptoms, his mental state often improves as much as his physical condition. Hope returns and with it a determination to get well.

The benefits provided by fresh air are due to its cutaneous or physical properties rather than to its respiratory or chemical qualities; that is, the effects depend on the tonic influences of circulating air on the skin rather than on the chemical composition of the air breathed. A stuffy atmosphere is not usually detrimental to health because of its chemical constitution—such as an excess of CO_2—but because its air is stagnant and laden with moisture and possibly with pathogenic organisms. Thus the therapeutic effects of fresh air can often be obtained almost as well in a room as outside, provided the room can be thoroughly ventilated; and town air may be as beneficial as country air, provided it circulates freely and does not have to reach the patient in a small back court or down a shaft in the middle of a tenement.

To nurse a patient outside in a comfortable shelter or verandah ensures for him real open-air treatment. Such conditions are usually obtainable without inconvenience in a sanatorium or a country house. As we have seen, however, it is not essential to live outside in order to get fresh air, and many a patient in the town is put to great inconvenience by attempting to do so. He is much better in his own comfortable bedroom, provided it can be well ventilated, than in a shed in his back yard. His bedroom must have its window or windows open top and bottom, however, and the bed should be drawn across the window or otherwise arranged so that the patient obtains the maximum of fresh air. Curtains, hangings and furniture should be reduced to a minimum in his room. Many persons consider that sufficient fresh air is obtained by opening their bedroom window a few inches, and the doctor will have to make it quite clear that more than this is required. Further, he may find it difficult to get suitable conditions owing to the fear that the patient, or the members of the family who attend him, will catch colds or chills. He will have to explain that infections of this nature are never caught from fresh air. With perseverance the patient will soon constitute himself the doctor's best ally in this respect, as he will quickly become used to fresh air and finally intolerant to a stuffy atmosphere.

Cold air is no drawback to treatment. Young patients can habituate themselves with benefit to most of the low temperatures encountered in this country, and can continue in open-air conditions throughout the winter. Indeed after a little training they soon find the atmosphere of the ordinary household extremely oppressive. A fetish is, however, sometimes made of "hardening" patients. The writer has seen snow-drifts forming in the corners of sanatorium wards, and has encountered institutions where any form of heating in the wards, even a coal fire, was forbidden. Such rigors are quite unnecessary and only succeed in making patients unhappy; indeed, when applied to elderly or cachectic patients, they can do much harm. Plenty of clothing is necessary for patients under a sanatorium regimen in cold weather, both for the person and for the bed. Such clothing should, however, be light rather than heavy. It is warmer and more beneficial to allow several light wraps rather than a single thick one. Shetland woollens are extremely suitable for this purpose, being warm and yet permitting the free circulation of air. In cold weather the hands of patients in bed should be protected by woollen gloves.

Heat, especially humid heat, should be avoided even more than cold. The bed, in hot weather, should be kept in the shade, and should be placed so as to get any breeze that may be present. Electric fans may be useful in such circumstances. The problem of excessive heat is not, however, a difficult one to cope with in this country.

While heliotherapy is undoubtedly of service in tuberculosis of the skin, glands, bones and joints, it has probably no value in pulmonary tuberculosis. Any benefit claimed from exposing the chests of patients with chronic pulmonary tuberculosis to sunshine is most likely due to the stimulus of fresh air on the skin or to psychological causes. In active exudative cases heliotherapy is definitely contraindicated and may have detrimental effects, comparable to an excessive dose of tuberculin. Such patients should therefore be guarded against direct exposure to strong sunshine in the summer time.

Patients frequently inquire whether smoking will interfere with the benefits of open-air treatment. Since fresh air, as we have seen, produces its effects through its action on the skin rather than through the lungs, it is improbable that smoking will be harmful from this point of view. It is our custom to allow patients with pulmonary tuberculosis to smoke in moderation, provided laryngitis or bronchitis is not a feature of the case and provided the cough is not obviously exacerbated by smoking as is occasionally the case. The inhaling of tobacco smoke should be avoided as much as possible.

Diet.—A large number of dietetic systems have been recommended from time to time as specifics in the treatment of tuberculosis. These range from the excessive or even forcible feeding of consumptives which was in vogue about the turn of the century to the Gerson-Sauerbruch diet introduced during recent years. Fishberg has said with truth that a good cook is more useful in the management of a tuberculous case than a detailed diet sheet. It is, indeed, unwise to lay down strict dietetic rules applicable to all cases of tuberculosis, since the individual's economic position, his likes and dislikes as regards food and the state of his digestion should all be taken into consideration in arranging his diet. None the less it may be helpful to consider certain broad general principles as regards dietetics in tuberculosis, though it is well to remember that in tuberculosis no dish is definitely contraindicated provided the digestion is good.

Since tuberculosis is a wasting disease, and many of the patients who suffer from it are in addition poor and under-nourished, it is plain that on the whole more food should be given to tuberculous than to ordinary people. On the other hand, the grossly excessive feeding which used to be so popular only succeeds in causing dyspepsia, and the patient should never be forced to take more food than he wishes. Three good meals a day are sufficient. In addition there is no objection to a small tea, and a glass of milk may be taken before going to sleep at night. Otherwise small feeds in between the principal meals should be discouraged as being detrimental to appetite and likely to cause dyspeptic symptoms.

As wasting of muscle is a common feature of exudative tuberculous disease, it is important to see that the diet contains an adequate amount of animal protein in the day, otherwise a negative nitrogen balance is apt to occur. There is no need, however, to stuff the patient with huge quantities of expensive protein food. The administration of 1·5 gm. of protein per kilogram of body-weight is amply sufficient to prevent a negative nitrogen balance in all cases of tuberculosis. This protein intake will be ensured provided the patient takes a good helping of meat and fish, an egg and a pint of milk in the course of the day.

It used to be a popular vogue to force quantities of raw eggs upon consumptives. While raw eggs are well tolerated by some patients, and form useful sources of protein and fat, yet they are ill-borne by others, and raw eggs have probably been responsible for a great deal of dyspepsia among tuberculous patients. Raw white of egg has an inhibitory effect on gastric secretion and opposes the tryptic activity of the pancreatic juice. As many tuberculous people have already deficient digestive secretions, the use of raw eggs may still further upset their digestive powers.

Tuberculous patients should have plenty of milk. At least 1 pint and preferably 2 pints should be taken daily. Many patients protest that they cannot take milk. This is in the great majority of cases a fad with no foundation, but, unfortunately, occasional cases of true milk intolerance do occur. In such patients the drinking of milk is invariably followed by abdominal discomfort, flatulence and sometimes diarrhœa.

Protein will not fatten a patient, and a diet containing plenty of fat has been recommended from the earliest times in the treatment of tuberculosis and is probably beneficial. It must be remembered, however, that many patients are intolerant to large amounts of fat, which may produce nausea and gastro-intestinal disturbances. It is useless to attempt to give fat in large amounts to such patients. Butter is probably the most easily assimilated form of fat and can usually be taken freely. Fat fish such as herring, salmon, fish roe, mackerel and sardines are also useful sources of fat which are generally well borne. Those who can tolerate fat easily can take in addition cream, fat bacon, ham and other fat meats. For generations cod-liver oil has been looked upon as a sheet-anchor in the treatment of tuberculosis. It is a rich source of fats and of vitamins A and D. Fat can, however, be given in much more palatable forms, and provided a good mixed diet is being taken there is no reason to believe that tuberculous people are peculiarly liable to vitamin A and D deficiency. The old theory that demineralization occurs in tuberculosis has never been proved, and there is no trustworthy evidence to show that the calcification of tuberculous lesions is accelerated by the administration of cod-liver oil. Cod-liver oil should be prescribed, especially in winter, to those indigent people who can tolerate it and whose diet may not be adequate in fats or vitamins. The pure oil should be taken in amounts varying from ½ to 1½ oz. a day. If patients dislike the pure oil, concentrates of vitamin A and D can be used (see p. 415).

The diet should contain plenty of fruit and green vegetables.

An excess of starchy carbohydrates should not be taken. If large quantities of white bread, cereals, pastries and sweets are eaten the patient may not have any appetite left for the more vital foodstuffs. Further, there is some evidence to suggest that an excess of carbohydrate food may further the spread of the exudative process in the lung.

Extra nourishment can be obtained for necessitous cases by application to the local tuberculosis authorities.

After-care.—When a patient's disease has become quiescent, or when he has become sufficiently well to be discharged from a sanatorium, he should none the less continue under medical supervision. The family doctor, in conjunction, perhaps, with the local Tuberculosis Authorities, should keep a close watch upon him. To begin with he should report for clinical examination at least once a month. Ideally, a blood sedimentation test should be performed at the time of the examination, and a radiological examination should be made every three or four months during the first year of convalescence. It will depend on the patient's temperament as to whether he should be asked to keep a chart of his temperature during this time. Such a record is useful in diagnosing at an early stage a possible recrudescence of the disease. On the other hand, the continual taking of the temperature may be a factor in inducing a hypochondriacal state in the patient. For the unduly optimistic type of patient continual warnings may be necessary. The well-known *spes phthisica*, however, is by no means universal, and many patients are morbidly introspective and anxious about themselves. These latter require much encouragement and reassurance from their doctor, who should make every effort to stop them from brooding on their disease. It is usually unwise to ask such patients to keep a temperature chart.

Provided a patient has been fit for a full amount of exercise for some months, and provided the various prognostic criteria enumerated above continue to be satisfactory, a return to work should not be unduly delayed. A patient kept idle for too long is apt to become introspective and neurotic or lazy and unemployable.

On first returning to work, the patient should be warned that he should spend the time in resting which others spend in recreation. Thus the ordinary division of the twenty-four hours into eight hours' work, eight hours' play and eight hours' rest should for him be divided, as far as possible, into eight hours' work and sixteen hours' rest. It may occasionally be wise to advise him to stay in bed entirely on Sunday.

Further, the patient must be warned against reverting to bad habits as regards inadequate fresh air. He should avoid as much as possible stuffy, crowded atmospheres, such as are often found in cinemas and theatres, and should take every precaution against contracting upper respiratory tract infections (see p. 775). A cold in the head should be treated seriously by him and he should go to bed till the worst of the infection is over.

Finally, every effort should be made to see that meals are ample and well cooked. The hurried consumption of small starchy meals at snack counters should be avoided as far as possible.

Employment.—The question will at once arise as to what sort of work he should undertake ; if at all possible he should return to his original employment. There are, of course, certain forms of employment involving great physical exertion, or work in dusty atmospheres and in extremes of heat and cold which are manifestly unsuitable for people who have suffered from tuberculosis. Likewise, where a woman's employment brings her into close contact with young children, as, for instance, in the case of a teacher in an infant school, or where the work involves contact with food, as in the case of a dairymaid, new employment will have to be sought.

Apart, however, from these obviously unsuitable vocations the patient should attempt to return to his or her original employment. Even when this is not entirely suitable from a tuberculosis point of view, it is much less strain for the patient to do the work to which he is accustomed than to attempt an entirely new occupation in strange surroundings for which he may be totally unsuited.

It should be remembered that it is more important for a tuberculous individual to obtain sedentary work rather than work in the open air, though light work in fresh air is the ideal. Too often a bank clerk is advised to become a chicken farmer, an occupation which may involve much physical exertion and for which he may have no aptitude.

Marriage.—The practitioner will sometimes be asked as to the advisability of one of his tuberculous patients marrying. Provided the healthy partner understands thoroughly the implications of marrying a person who has or has had tuberculosis, marriage may be beneficial in some respects to the patient. Thus a man may have a more restful and comfortable home with better-cooked meals than he had when a bachelor ; and a tuberculous woman, who has had to earn her own living previously, may obtain protection, security and possibly an easier life through matrimony than she had when single. On the other hand matrimony may increase a man's responsibilities necessitating harder work for him, and it may be the beginning of an anxious and strenuous life for a woman. It all depends on the circumstances of the case, and on the position and mentality of the persons concerned. These matters will have to be taken into consideration by the practitioner in coming to a difficult decision.

In any case, no tuberculous person should be allowed to marry unless the healthy partner is fully conversant with the tuberculous history. The risks of a possible breakdown in health and of the patient's physical capabilities should be explained fully to the fiancé, with whom the family doctor should have a private interview. No woman with tubercle bacilli in the sputum should be allowed to have a baby. Though pregnancy may be borne reasonably well, the disease tends to progress disastrously during the puerperium. Further, the risks which an infant runs under such circumstances of fatal infection from its mother are very great. So great, indeed, are the dangers of pregnancy to a woman with active pulmonary tuberculosis that therapeutic abortion may be considered if the pregnancy has not progressed beyond the third month. It is probably inadvisable for a woman to start a family for at least two years after her sputum has become negative, her symptoms in abeyance and the various prognostic tests satisfactory. Naturally these implications will have to be carefully explained to the woman's fiancé. There is no reason why two tuberculous people should not marry provided their circumstances are such as to make it possible for them to live an easier life married than single.

Chronic Fibroid Pulmonary Tuberculosis.—The management of a case of chronic fibroid tuberculosis provides a very different problem to that presented by a patient suffering from exudative disease. When the chronic disease is unilateral, the patient may often be saved from permanent invalidism by one or other of the methods of collapse therapy—particularly thoracoplasty (see p. 128). The feasibility of inducing collapse must, therefore, be seriously considered in all unilateral cases. Collapse therapy is impracticable, however, in advanced chronic disease affecting both lungs. In such cases all that can be done is to regulate the life of the patient so as to keep his activities as far as possible well within the bounds imposed by his limited capacity, to treat symptoms as they arise (see p. 130), and to attempt to prevent him from infecting other people by giving him advice as to personal hygiene and by keeping him from close contact with children (see p. 95).

In some cases a considerable degree of systemic intoxication may be present owing to the retention of secretions in fibroid cavities and in collapsed portions of lung. Where toxæmia is marked, the patient must be kept in bed, and the general measures adopted must approximate to those already mentioned. It is usually unnecessary and unwise to send such patients away from home to an institution. Far too many beds in sanatoriums are occupied by elderly patients suffering from chronic fibroid phthisis, sometimes to the exclusion of early and curable cases. Where, however, the home conditions are obviously unsuitable for proper nursing, or where young children are present in the house, it may be necessary to segregate the patient in a hospital for advanced cases. The principles as regards rest in bed, which have been recommended for curable cases, need not be applied so rigidly to patients with advanced chronic disease. They are often happier, and indeed better, if they are allowed to be up for a short time each day, usually in the morning when their temperature may be normal and when they feel at their best. Much can be done to make them more comfortable by careful treatment of their symptoms as they arise. Such treatment is fully described later (see p. 130).

When a patient first develops pulmonary tuberculosis, the chances of his dying within five years are very considerable. If he lives for five years, however, his chances of survival for a further period are proportionately greater. He has proved himself resistant to the disease, and even though it persists it usually becomes progressively less virulent and less toxic. Thus, the longer a patient survives, the less he tends to suffer from the systemic effects of tuberculous toxæmia, and the more from the effects of pulmonary fibrosis, complemental emphysema and right-sided cardiac embarrassment. Thus extensive fibroid disease, even when associated with gross cavitation, is not necessarily inconsistent with many years of active and useful life. Systemic intoxication is minimal and the patient frequently lives almost in symbiosis with his tubercle bacilli, suffering to a greater or less degree from cough and dyspnœa on exertion, but otherwise feeling comparatively well. Many of them are able to attend to their work and businesses, and should not be prevented from doing so. Their treatment should be very similar to that suggested for patients suffering from chronic bronchitis and emphysema (see p. 792).

TUBERCULIN TREATMENT

Under the influence of rest, fresh air and good food the great majority of patients suffering from pulmonary tuberculosis show some improvement; whereas, if they do not receive these benefits the majority get worse. We *know*, therefore, that these are useful methods of treatment in tuberculosis. The same cannot be said for other forms of treatment for, with the exception of collapse therapy, which is simply an extension of the principle of rest, none of them gives good results with any constancy. It is, indeed, exceedingly difficult to gauge the effect of any remedy in a disease which may last a lifetime, which is subject to natural fluctuations in severity and to the strongest tendency to spontaneous healing under an ordinary physiological regimen. Further, many patients suffering from tuberculosis are highly suggestible and will react favourably to any harmless drug, or even to distilled water if it is administered with impressive gravity especially by the hypodermic route. This favourable reaction will be magnified if the administrator himself believes firmly in the efficacy of the nostrum and is able to impart his faith in it to the patient. Hence, tuberculosis, like disseminated sclerosis, is a happy hunting-ground for the uncritical therapeutic enthusiast and for the quack.

Among serious workers opinion is unanimous that there is no specific remedy for tuberculosis comparable to quinine in malaria, arsenic in syphilis or antitoxic serum in diphtheria. Here, however, unanimity ends and controversy is particularly acute in regard to the efficacy of tuberculin treatment. More than fifty years after its introduction by Koch as a remedy for tuberculosis, one group of workers remain fanatical exponents of its excellence, while another, and larger group, as hotly proclaim its complete therapeutic worthlessness. We have seen many patients improve remarkably while receiving tuberculin, but the improvement could well have been ascribed to the regimen under which they were living at the time and to the fact that the disease might have been spontaneously healing without the help of tuberculin. Further, it is well to remember that tuberculin treatment is only indicated in cases without marked toxæmic symptoms, and especially in extra-pulmonary disease such as glandular or bone and joint tuberculosis. That is, it is supposed to be most efficacious in just those cases where the prognosis is most favourable. Again, there is no scientific proof that any experimental animal has ever been cured of tuberculosis by the use of tuberculin. Lastly, the advocates of tuberculin treatment are by no means unanimous as to dosage and the best method of its administration. Indeed, they are apt to be very contemptuous of any technique except their own. Some believe in large doses with the production of a general reaction, others in homeopathic doses producing no general reaction, while others take up an intermediate position. In addition, the subcutaneous, intradermal and percutaneous methods of administration each have their protagonists. Since tuberculin is exceedingly difficult to standardize, it is apparent that under the present circumstances wide variations occur in the amount administered, depending not only on the prescribed dosage but on the method of administration and the batch of tuberculin employed.

Tuberculin should never be used in the treatment of exudative tuberculosis with signs of systemic intoxication. In chronic cases without toxæmia large doses of tuberculin are dangerous and may cause an exacerbation of the disease. In such cases small doses given with due precautions are harmless, but in view of the considerations which have been enumerated, we are sceptical of their value. Tuberculin may, however, be of some service, and certainly often has a beneficial psychological effect. Further, all patients should be given some form of active therapy in addition to rest, fresh air and good food, and it is useful to have some treatment to give when a patient is reporting weekly for observation. Under such circumstances, tuberculin treatment may appeal particularly to intelligent patients who have some knowledge of the principles of immunity.

When tuberculin is used diagnostically, the intradermal or Mantoux test is the most successful. When used for therapeutic purposes, however, it is best given either subcutaneously or percutaneously by inunction in the form of tuberculin ointment. The latter is the method of choice when a child is the patient, as it is preferable to avoid using the hypodermic needle on children whenever possible. Tuberculin ointment should be prescribed thus :—

Koch's old tuberculin . .	10, 20, 30, 40, 50 per cent.
Lanolin	1 oz.

After washing the skin thoroughly with soap and water and then ether, in order to get rid of its natural fats, a small quantity of the ointment—about the size of a split pea—is rubbed in with the aid of a glass rod for four or five minutes. No dressing is necessary afterwards. The front of the chest is the most convenient site for the inunction. In a tuberculized patient a red rash appears at the site of the inunction within forty-eight hours and slowly fades during the succeeding days. The severity of the local reaction will determine the strength of the ointment which should be used. It is advisable to start with the 10 per cent. ointment and to work gradually upwards. The inunction should be repeated once a week, or twice a week in less sensitive children. This is a very safe method of administering tuberculin and practically never produces a general reaction.

For the treatment of adults, Koch's old tuberculin should

be suitably diluted and injected subcutaneously. The diluent employed is sterile water containing 0·8 per cent. sodium chloride and 0·5 per cent. phenol. Unless tuberculin is being used in large quantities in an institution, the dilutions are best made up by a chemist and procured from him in very small quantities at a time. Undiluted tuberculin keeps for a long time, but when diluted it rapidly loses its potency and should not be kept for longer than a month. The dilutions commonly employed for treatment are 1 : 100,000, 1 : 10,000, 1 : 1000, and very occasionally for patients who are extremely tolerant to the drug 1 : 500. 0·1 c.c. of 1 : 100,000 tuberculin is a safe dose to start with and is unlikely to cause any general reaction even in an extremely sensitive patient. Thereafter the dose should be increased by 0·1 c.c. at a time till a significant local, but not general, reaction is caused. The ideal local reaction is a slightly red, tender induration in the subcutaneous tissues. Once this is procured no further injections should be given until the reaction has entirely died down, and no increase in dosage need be made as long as a satisfactory reaction is produced. The drug can usually be given once every five or six days. It is probably unwise to increase the dose above 1 c.c. of the 1 : 1000 dilution, except in unusually tolerant patients, and even this dose should only be given if no local reaction occurs with the weaker dilutions. The needle should always be cleansed of all tuberculin adhering to it before making an injection ; otherwise an intra-dermal skin reaction may be caused. The temperature and pulse-rate should be taken night and morning following the injection, and any significant systemic reaction should be avoided.

GOLD TREATMENT

Many of the remarks which have been made about the efficacy of tuberculin apply equally to gold treatment in tuberculosis. There can be no doubt as to its dangers, but there is considerable dubiety as to its efficacy. It is generally agreed that gold is of no service in chronic fibroid cases and that it is contraindicated in cases with acute exudative disease with severe toxæmic symptoms. It is advocated in exudative or fibro-caseous cases where toxæmia is mild, or absent, and where the disease is slowly progressing. In some cases it certainly appears to cause the disappearance of tubercle bacilli from the sputum and to reduce its quantity.

If gold has a beneficial effect, its mode of action is not clear. Almost certainly it has no bactericidal effect on tubercle bacilli within the body, though very weak solutions of gold salts will inhibit their growth in culture. It is supposed to stimulate the defensive forces of the patient and to increase the tendency to fibrosis in tuberculous lesions.

The gold preparations which have been most extensively employed in tuberculosis are the double thiosulphate of gold and sodium (sanocrysin) which was first prepared by Moellgaard in 1923. It is obtained from the chemist as a crystalline powder in hermetically sealed ampoules. The crystals are readily soluble and should be given intravenously dissolved in 5 c.c. of sterile distilled water. It is wise to start with a small dose of 0·05 gm. in order to test for any idiosyncrasy to the drug. Thereafter weekly doses can be given in steadily increasing strengths. In a case which shows no unpleasant reactions to the drug, the scale should be climbed each week as follows: 0·05, 0·1, 0·25, 0·3, 0·4, 0·5 of a gramme. It is unwise to give a larger single dose than 0·5 gm., and the total amount given in one course of treatment should never exceed 5 gm.

When a preparation which is given intramuscularly is preferred to one given intravenously, solganol B. oleosum (Schering) can be used instead of sanocrysin. This oily suspension of solganol is sold in ampoules, and a course should consist of not less than 3 gm. and not more than 5 gm. An average scheme of dosage is appended, but it must be clearly understood that gold should never be given by rule-of-thumb methods, but must be administered with due regard to the reactions which may occur.

Dose 1 . .	0·01 gm. in 1·5 c.c. of oil—two doses in first week.	
Dose 1A . .	0·02 gm. in 1·5 c.c. of oil—two doses in second week.	
Dose 2 . .	0·05 gm. in 1·5 c.c. of oil—two doses in third week.	
Dose 3 . .	0·1 gm. in 2 c.c. of oil—one dose fourth, fifth and sixth weeks.	
Dose 4 . .	0·2 gm. in 2 c.c. of oil—one dose in each subsequent week until total dose has been given.	
Dose 5 . .	0·3 gm. in 3 c.c. of oil	Only to be employed where patient is very tolerant to the drug.
Dose 6 . .	0·4 gm. in 3 c.c. of oil	

The complications of gold treatment, which are numerous and dangerous, are fully discussed on p. 903. Whenever gold is being given the doctor should be constantly on the outlook for early manifestations of intolerance to the drug. The occurrence of stomatitis, glossitis, jaundice, leukopenia, erythema of the skin, hæmaturia or more than a faint trace of albumen in the urine should be a sign to stop the treatment permanently. Similarly, *severe* febrile reactions, vomiting and diarrhœa, or pains in the joints and limbs should be indications for the termination of treatment. *Slight* febrile, gastro-intestinal or arthritic reactions, however, need not necessarily be contra-indications to further treatment, though the next injection should be delayed until the reaction has entirely subsided and then a smaller dose than the one producing the reaction should be given. To patients who appear to have improved under gold therapy, and who have shown themselves tolerant to the drug, a further course of treatment may be given in six months' time.

Numerous other methods of treatment have been advocated from time to time in tuberculosis—creosote, arsenic, iodine, sodium morrhuate, vaccines, protein shock, calcium and parathyroid extract. They have all had their day and have been found wanting. Apart from preventive measures, the only great advance which has been made in the treatment of tuberculosis since the introduction of rest and the sanatorium régime has been collapse therapy.

COLLAPSE THERAPY

Many cases of pulmonary tuberculosis remain active or tend to progress in spite of strict sanatorium treatment. Failure to heal may be due, *inter alia*, to poor resistance, to the type of the disease, or to secondary mechanical factors, and each requires careful individual assessment. In the lungs, as in other structures, healing is favoured if sustained physiological rest can be secured, and for that purpose there are now available for selected subjects a choice of several measures known collectively as collapse therapy. Their value is now definitely established, and their use should not be withheld if the proper conditions for their application are present.

The specific effect of all forms of collapse therapy is the reduction of lung volume regionally or generally, with resulting diminution of tension (atmospheric and mechanical), so that reparative processes may not be inhibited or, if already present can proceed unhampered. The methods of established value are :—

1. Artificial pneumothorax.
2. Intrapleural (cautery) division of adhesions.
3. Phrenicectomy (crushing or evulsion of the phrenic nerve).
4. Extrapleural thoracoplasty (local or extensive resection of the ribs).
5. Extrapleural pneumothorax.

General Indications and Choice of Method.—The appropriate method of collapse and the time for its adoption depend on the special pathological conditions within the lung and pleura ; each case must be decided on its individual features. Haphazard interventions will be avoided if the operator has ascertained the full history of the case—clinical and radiographic. The simpler methods, such as artificial pneumothorax, are employed in early and progressive cases in which the lesion will be of the exudative or caseous type. The more drastic measures which involve rib resection are reserved for established fibrotic disease, especially when cavity formation predominates. Sometimes the methods are employed in combination, *e.g.*, artificial pneumothorax and phrenicectomy may be combined advantageously in certain circumstances.

Troublesome symptoms, such as persisting irritating cough and recurring hæmoptysis, irrespective of the type of disease, may be controlled by artificial pneumothorax or phrenicectomy, even though the prospect of cure of the underlying disease is unlikely.

In the selection of cases there are certain rules and limitations which apply broadly to all methods of collapse therapy. Early and exudative cases present an urgent problem in treatment, whereas the patient with chronic fibroid disease does not suffer by reasonable delay. The prospects of success are greatest when the disease is unilateral, although in special circumstances, to be defined later, limited disease in the healthier lung need not necessarily contraindicate such treatment. Active and extensive bilateral disease is an obvious barrier to treatment. The patient's age must be taken into consideration : the simpler methods may give very gratifying results in young subjects, even children, but thoracoplasty should be avoided before the age of seventeen years as scoliosis usually follows. When there is myocardial weakness, emphysema and bronchitis, collapse therapy aggravates dyspnœa and should not be attempted. In consequence, these methods have a rather more limited scope in subjects over the age of forty-five.

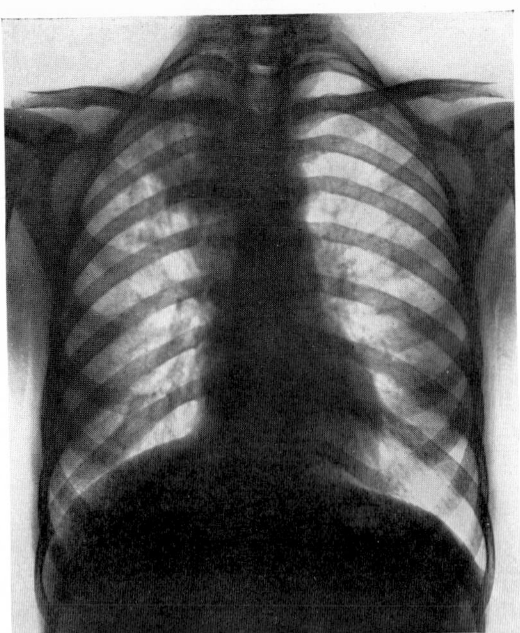

PLATE 1.—Moderately Early Right-sided Pulmonary Tuberculosis occurring in an Adolescent Female and affecting the Upper Lobe in which a small cavity has developed.

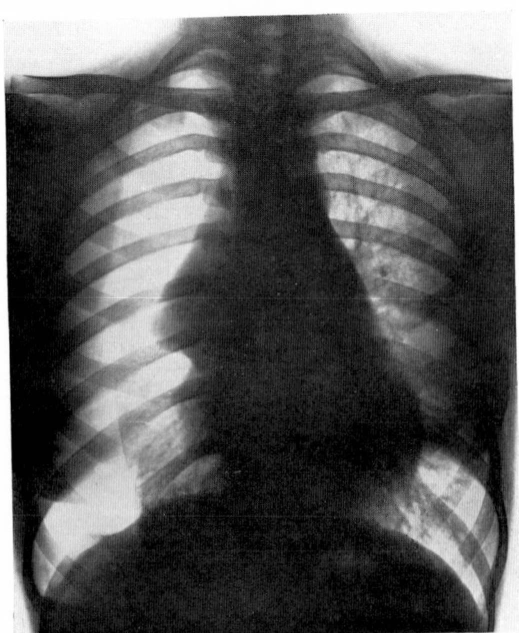

PLATE 2.—Same case Four Months after the Induction of Artificial Pneumothorax. Note the total collapse of the diseased lobe. There is slight displacement of the mediastinal structures with some resulting compaction of the lung tissue on the right side.

[*To face page* 123.

Intercurrent disease does not necessarily preclude treatment. For example, many patients who suffer from diabetes as well as tuberculosis derive benefit from collapse, and their insulin requirements may be notably reduced. Complications, however, such as tuberculous enteritis or tuberculosis of the kidney or the bones and joints are, with few exceptions, a contraindication to this mode of treatment. Ulceration of the larynx is an indication rather than a contraindication.

As there is still a significant mortality from extensive thoracoplasty, this major procedure must not be undertaken unless the patient's condition fully warrants its performance.

1. **Artificial pneumothorax** is the simplest means of producing lung collapse, and more complete collapse is attained by this than by any other method, provided adhesions between the visceral and parietal pleura are not present. In many cases it is only by trial that the efficacy of the method can be tested.

Artificial pneumothorax should be carried out in all but the very earliest cases of acute or subacute exudative tuberculosis of a unilateral nature, irrespective of whether there are gross physical signs or tubercle bacilli in the sputum. It should be used, too, in less acute cases in which activity persists in spite of rest in bed, or when the disease in the lung remains stationary, and especially if constitutional improvement is not satisfactory. Cavity formation is a common sequel of caseation and should be regarded as an indication for timely control by pneumothorax. There is less urgency in the more chronic and usually fibroid type of case, yet chronic invalidism need not be accepted as the inevitable culmination of the disease ; an attempt should be made to induce pneumothorax, though it may not always be possible nor completely effective ; not infrequently, if it is supplemented by other measures, such as division of adhesions, phrenicectomy or extrapleural pneumothorax, a successful issue may be attainable. With a successful pneumothorax the recovery of the patient may be accelerated and the risk of subsequent relapse diminished.

Enthusiasm for such treatment must be tempered with discretion because, on the one hand, there are certain early cases which may respond favourably to routine treatment and, on the other, fulminating types which are doomed from the outset. An experienced clinician will usually be able to anticipate the behaviour of any particular type of disease. A difficult problem arises when there is widespread acute disease in one lung and similar though less extensive disease in the other. The decision to induce pneumothorax on the worse side is based on the hope that reduction of toxæmia may bring about such improvement in the patient's general condition that the disease in the contralateral lung may improve. It is a reasonable gamble, but unfortunately the disease, especially if of the acute type, is often aggravated.

Bilateral Artificial Pneumothorax.—The decision to apply pneumothorax bilaterally may occasionally be justified if the pneumothorax on one side is already of a selective type with ample functioning lung remaining. The ideal is to secure a similar collapse on the opposite side. In acute cases with extensive disease induction of double pneumothorax often produces so much dyspnœa that it has to be abandoned. It may, however, succeed, and in selected cases is worth a cautious trial. There have been some striking successes.

The Induction and Management of Artificial Pneumothorax.—The simplest type of apparatus consists of two bottles, the one syphoning fluid into the other. Air is thereby displaced from the second bottle through a rubber tube and needle into the pleural cavity. The second bottle is graduated in hundreds of cubic centimetres, and the amount of air displaced can, therefore, be read off by the rise of the fluid level in the bottle. A water-manometer is always in connection with the apparatus so that the intrapleural pressure can be ascertained at any moment.

The technique of induction follows the lines of paracentesis in general and is carried out under local anæsthesia (2 per cent. novocaine), particular care being taken to infiltrate the sensitive pleura. The point of initial puncture is decided by the distribution of the disease as portrayed in the X-ray film. The fourth intercostal space in the mid-axillary line, or the sixth or seventh space in the scapular line, are favourite sites. A special pattern of needle is employed.

A successful entry into the pleural space is registered by the respiratory oscillations in the manometer, and in no circumstances should air be allowed to enter until an unequivocal oscillation is obtained. Continued failure to procure such oscillations is an indication to try elsewhere. When, from the manometer readings, it is certain that the needle is between the pleural layers, 50 to 100 c.c. of air are allowed to enter by aspiration ; confirmatory pressure readings are taken before a total of 300 c.c. are admitted. The intrapleural pressure should remain negative. A positive reading suggests adhesion of the lung and should be a signal for caution or for abandoning further attempts.

If induction has been successful and the X-ray appearances and pressure readings are satisfactory, a refill may be given the following day. Thereafter, refills are continued at short but gradually lengthening intervals. It is usually about a month before the optimum collapse is established. Then the interval between refillings varies with each patient according to the rate at which the air is absorbed. The X-ray appearances are the most reliable guide in arriving at a decision. In an average case refilling at ten or fourteen day intervals is necessary at first, but as the rate of absorption decreases the interval can often be extended to three weeks or a month.

Treatment should be continued, even in the most favourable cases, for at least two years, and for three or more when the disease has been extensive or cavities present. Sometimes termination of treatment is decided by the behaviour of the pneumothorax itself—either by its progressive shrinkage or its obliteration by adhesions.

When the lung is allowed to re-expand it is safer to let it be gradual by spacing the refills at longer intervals and by reducing the amount of air given. Six to twelve months are usually necessary to achieve full re-expansion, and the patient should be kept under careful clinical and radiological observation throughout.

Incidents during Treatment.—Pleural shock is a very rare but disturbing effect of puncture of the parietal pleura. The symptoms vary from faintness and pallor to profound collapse, with, in exceptional cases, sudden death. Its occurrence has been attributed to incomplete anæsthesia of the pleura, but proof of this is lacking. The phenomenon is seldom witnessed after the initial puncture of the pleura. Treatment is on the same lines as for shock.

Air (gas) embolism resembles pleural shock in its manifestations, but is quite different in origin. It results from the entry of air into the pulmonary veins and its passage as emboli to the coronary or the cerebral arteries. Death may be immediate, or there may be epileptiform fits, hemiplegia or profound unconsciousness. In rare cases it may be survived. Air embolism should be extremely exceptional if it is always ascertained that the pneumothorax needle is within the pleural cavity by the characteristic oscillations in the manometer.

Interstitial emphysema is due to escape of air into the subcutaneous tissues via the puncture in the pleura. It produces a characteristic " crackling " sensation to the examining hand ; but apart from the mild discomfort and annoyance it occasions, it calls for no concern. It is prevented if the induction of a positive pressure within the pleura is avoided, following upon a refill, and coughing discouraged.

Displacement of the mediastinum may occur when the

mediastinal septum is more yielding than is usually the case in chronic inflammatory diseases of the chest. It may develop even when a negative pressure is present in the pleural cavity. The common effects are dyspnœa, tachycardia and loss of weight. The condition seldom calls for interruption of treatment. It can usually be corrected by reducing the volume and shortening the interval between each refill.

Pleural effusion is the most frequent complication of artificial pneumothorax. It is the expression of a tuberculous pleurisy. It is more common when adhesions are present, and though it may appear at any stage of treatment it generally occurs in the early months. The onset of an effusion is indicated by malaise, pain and a sharp rise of temperature which may last for a few days or sometimes weeks. If the effusion is copious there may be dyspnœa. A pleural effusion is not necessarily an untoward occurrence, and in the majority of cases it disappears spontaneously. In consequence, expectant treatment is usually indicated. Aspiration of a pleural effusion is required in the following circumstances :—

1. When there is long-continued pyrexia.
2. When it is of such bulk that it produces pressure symptoms.
3. When its delayed absorption is likely to cause obliteration of the pneumothorax.

Following aspiration of a large pleural effusion, re-expansion of the lung should be prevented by replacing the fluid with air (see p. 138).

In a small proportion of cases an effusion becomes purulent —pyopneumothorax. This is a serious occurrence and is usually an indication to abandon the pneumothorax. Periodic aspiration of the fluid should be carried out and re-expansion of the lung encouraged. Expansion of the lung may be long delayed and may not occur completely. It may be necessary finally to obliterate the persisting cavity by thoracoplasty.

A graver situation arises when there is a superadded pyogenic infection of the pleura (infected pyopneumothorax). Toxæmia is severe and persistent and cannot be checked by repeated aspiration. It is necessary to carry out an air-tight drainage of the pleural cavity and to attempt its disinfection by irrigation. The outlook is generally (though by no means always) unfavourable. Prolonged drainage may bring about remarkable improvement in the general condition of the patient, so much so that a successful thoracoplasty may ultimately be undertaken.

2. **Intrapleural Division of Adhesions (Internal Pneumolysis).**

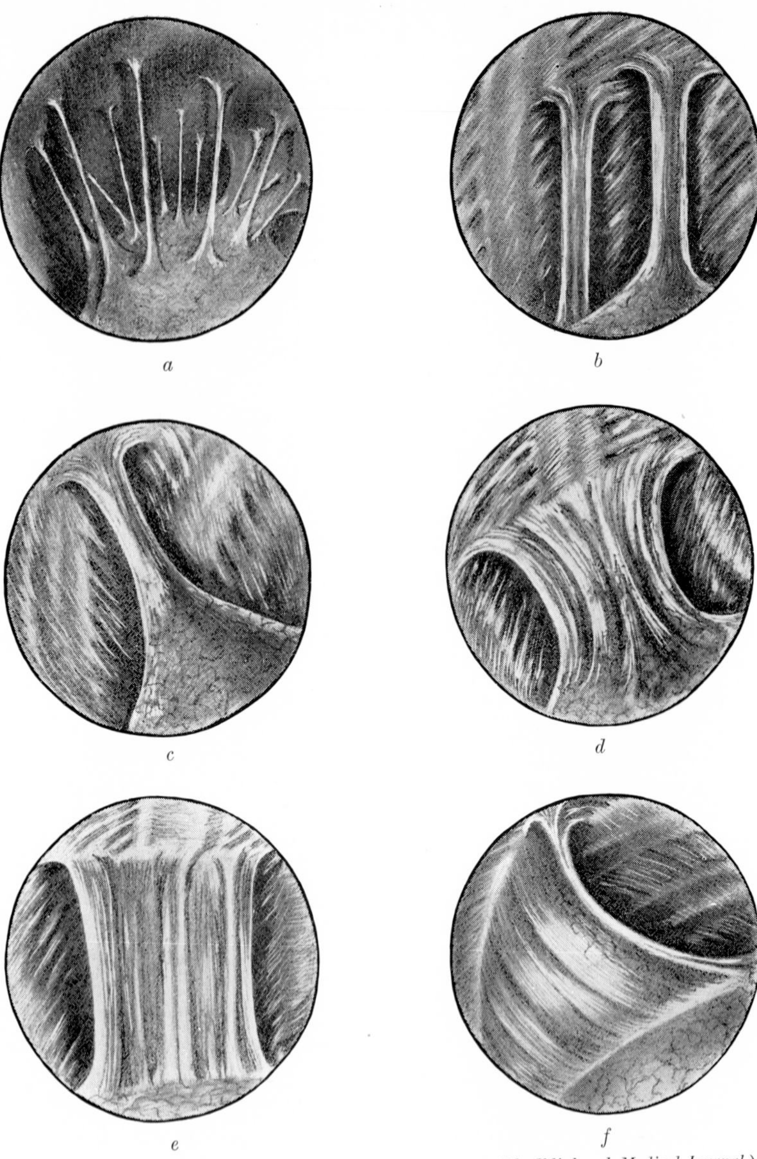

(*By courtesy of the Edinburgh Medical Journal.*)

PLATE 3.—Types of Pleural Adhesions.

a. Multiple string adhesions.
b. Cord adhesions.
c. Cone-shaped adhesions.
d. Spool or capstan adhesions.
e. Band adhesions.
f. Curtain adhesions.

[*To face page* 127.

—Adhesions may be unimportant, but often they prevent relaxation of the diseased parts of the lung or closure of cavities. In such cases artificial pneumothorax may have had promising effects in the early stages of treatment, but disappointment follows because continued activity of the disease is suggested by such symptoms as cough, expectoration, hæmoptysis or by persisting systemic disturbance.

If, after a reasonable time (say four to six months), it can be demonstrated that adhesions interfere with an otherwise satisfactory collapse, and especially if cavities persist or increase in size, the division of the adhesions should be considered. This is a most valuable supplementary method in pneumothorax work. Serial radiograms afford most help in recognizing the position and extent of adhesions. It should be kept in mind, however, that even gross adhesions may not be obvious radiographically, and even when portrayed, their number or complexity cannot be gauged with accuracy. Therefore the most exact method of deciding the possibility of operation is direct examination of the pneumothorax cavity by the thoracoscope, a procedure which should be painless and certainly without risk.

The common types of pleural adhesions are illustrated in Plate 3. To avoid accidents it is important that the operator should ascertain their vascularity and their relationship to the underlying lung as well as to important blood vessels.

Division of adhesions is carried out through an instrument like an operating cystoscope—the thoracoscope. The instrument is inserted through an intercostal space at a point which has been selected as most likely to give the best view of the adhesions, and one from which they will be more accessible for subsequent cutting. Division should be performed as close to the chest wall as possible. It is done with the electric cautery at a dull red glow. Cutting should be done slowly, avoiding blind or lavish sweeps. Bleeding, when it occurs, is almost always from the parietal stump; it is usually controlled promptly by light touches of the coagulating diathermy electrode.

It is surprising how little upset usually accompanies or follows operation. Some degree of pleural effusion is to be expected. It is usually slight and transient, but occasionally it persists, and in a few cases becomes purulent. The perfection of the technique has made hæmorrhage a rare occurrence.

3. **Phrenicectomy.**—Permanent paralysis of the diaphragm on one side can be produced by division at the root of the neck of its main and accessory nerve fibres, or evulsion of the entire nerve. Temporary paralysis, by crushing the nerve, lasts for

six or more months and may meet the requirements of a case, because if the desired effect (usually fibrosis or closure of cavities) is not forthcoming within that period it can scarcely be expected later. Operation is carried out under local anæsthesia without much discomfort and without untoward sequelæ. The result of phrenicectomy is elevation of the diaphragm with consequent reduction in lung volume, the combination of which favour healing throughout the lung, more especially those parts already undergoing fibrosis. The apical regions may derive benefit, but usually to a less extent than the middle and lower zones.

The indications for operation are numerous, but require exact specification if disappointing results are to be avoided. The prospect of success can be decided only by a studious consideration of the influences which delay resolution in the diseased parts of the lung. Haphazard operations are to be deprecated. It is for unsuccessful pneumothorax cases that the help of phrenicectomy is usually sought. In acute cases it is seldom of assistance unless multiple soft-walled cavities are present. In more fibroid types, especially if there are cavities in the central and lower parts of the lung, great benefit, and sometimes cure, may be anticipated. The results are usually very disappointing in those common cases of stiff-walled cavities in the apical zones of the lung, and alternative methods of collapse are preferable.

Phrenicectomy may be employed with value in combination with artificial pneumothorax, especially when diffuse adhesions are an obstacle to effective collapse, and also when additional collapse is required at the base of the lung. As a preliminary to complete thoracoplasty, it may be helpful (never—in the writer's experience—harmful) in that it may permit of a more circumscribed operation being effective.

Phrenicectomy is sometimes indicated at the completion of treatment by artificial pneumothorax, so that the healed lung may not be exposed to undue strain as it re-expands. Troublesome symptoms, in otherwise untreatable cases, may be relieved by phrenicectomy ; *e.g.*, dry, spasmodic cough due to irritation of the diaphragm from the pull of an adherent lung can be abolished, and also the pain and dragging along the attachment of the diaphragm when there is old-standing basal pleurisy.

4. **Thoracoplasty : Total and Subtotal (including Apicolysis).**—Thoracoplasty on the drastic lines once in vogue has given place to much more selective forms of rib resection and pneumolysis. Operation is usually considered only in chronic types of disease when less severe measures are impracticable on account of widespread pleural adhesions and the excessively indurated

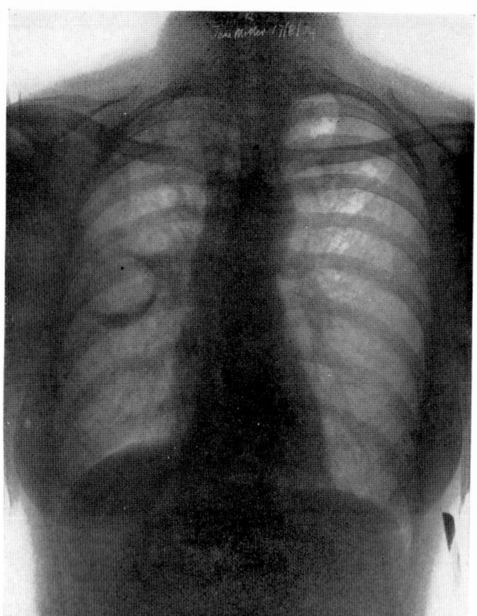

PLATE 4.—Single Large Cavity, involving Middle Zone of Right Lung.

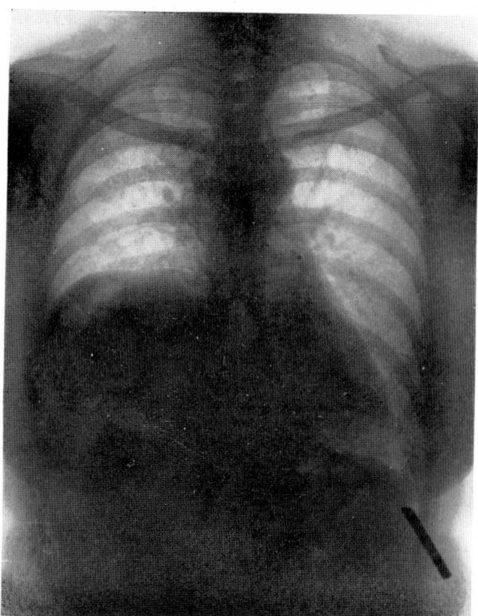

PLATE 5.—Same case a Year after Phrenicectomy. Note the elevation of the diaphragm and the disappearance of the cavity.

(*By courtesy of the Edinburgh Medical Journal.*)

[*To face page* 128.

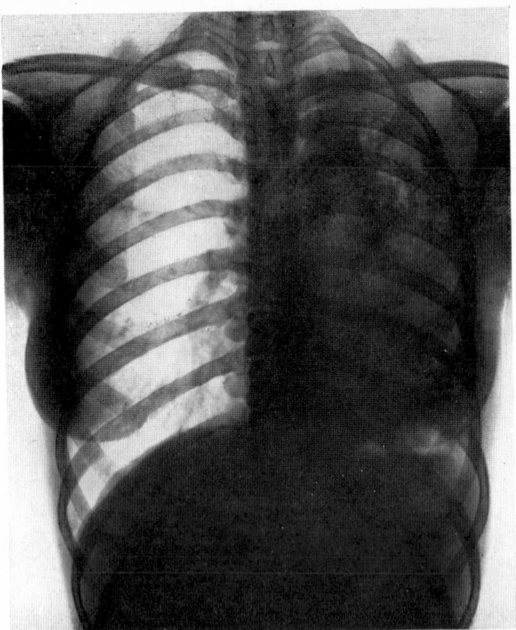

PLATE 6.—Extensive Old-standing Fibro-cavernous Disease confined to the Left Lung in a Female Patient aged Twenty-five. There is notable retraction of the mediastinal structures towards the diseased side.

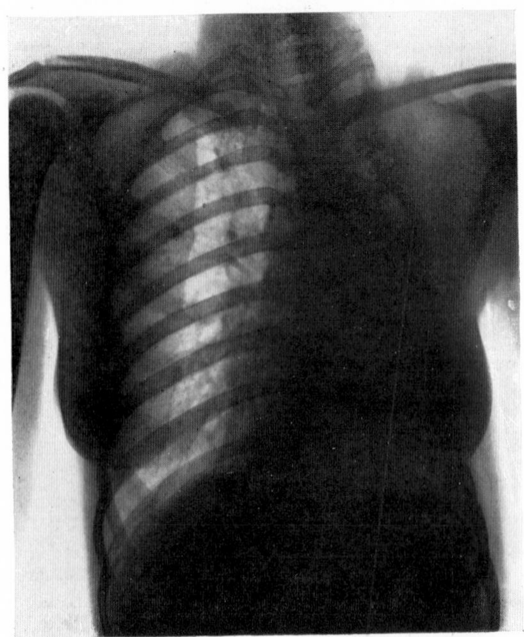

PLATE 7.—Same case Five Years after an Extensive Thoracoplasty. Patient is well and working.

[*To face page* 129.

condition of the lung. It is specially valuable when there are multiple rigid-walled cavities, provided there is no active or uncontrolled disease in the other lung, and provided the circulatory system is not seriously impaired. Plate 6 illustrates the type of case which is likely to benefit from operation.

Thoracoplasty entails excision of lengths of bone from the posterior parts of the ribs as far back as (and sometimes including) the transverse processes of the vertebræ. The number of ribs and the amount of each removed varies according to the extent and character of the disease : it varies from four to ten ribs and should always include a liberal portion of the first and second. A manœuvre now commonly combined with thoracoplasty, and especially for upper lobe cavities, is extra-fascial stripping of the lung (apicolysis of Semb). It affords a free relaxation of the diseased parts and is usually successful in bringing about closure of stiff-walled cavities ; indeed, extrapleural pneumothorax (to be described later) is simply an evolution of the same practice.

Considerable shock may follow thoracoplasty ; therefore it should be done in two or more stages. Cyclopropane, on account of its non-asphyxial properties, has proved the best anæsthetic, though chloroform is almost as good. Operation during the winter months in a general hospital may expose the patient to the risk of a superadded respiratory infection.

5. **Extrapleural Pneumothorax.**—This method promises to be of value in promoting retraction of diseased and excavated areas of lung when artificial pneumothorax fails and when the age or condition of the patient contraindicates thoracoplasty.

The operation consists in stripping the parietal pleura from the deep surface of the chest wall and mediastinum to allow collapse of the underlying lung. The result is to leave a large raw space into which air can be introduced under pressure to maintain collapse.

The most troublesome complications have been hæmorrhage, effusion and infection. Thoracoplasty may be required later to obliterate the cavity in the chest. A considerable time will have to elapse before the merits of this method can be assessed.

Summary.—Collapse therapy should not be regarded either as a short cut to cure in pulmonary tuberculosis or as a final and desperate resort when all other forms of treatment have failed. It should be emphasized strongly that it is not a substitute for the general methods of treatment. It is true that collapse therapy may bring about a spectacular improvement in an acute case and may remedy the otherwise permanent mechanical effects of chronic disease. Yet, the various methods of collapse are merely factors in a fight which is the ultimate concern of the natural resistance of the body, and general methods calculated to increase this natural resistance are just as important in patients receiving collapse treatment as in those being treated by conservative methods.

Artificial pneumothorax may shorten the duration of treatment by rest, and indeed this is one of the acknowledged advantages of the method. Too early a resumption of activity, however, can mar what might otherwise have been a permanent success, and it is much better to "hasten slowly" in this respect.

When the disease has reached the stage that a drastic operation, such as thoracoplasty, is recommended, success is unlikely unless the general treatment of the patient receives careful consideration at the same time. Operation should only be contemplated when the maximum beneficial effect has accrued from symptomatic treatment and an extended period of rest in a sanatorium environment is imperative after the operation. Surgical interference is, indeed, only an incident in the course of treatment. It is usually six to nine months before the patient appreciates its full benefit.

THE TREATMENT OF SYMPTOMS

Cough.—Cough is the most common symptom requiring treatment in pulmonary tuberculosis. A certain amount of coughing is often beneficial, especially in cases with pulmonary cavitation, in order to free the air passages from secretions which are frequently toxic. A dry unproductive cough, however, serves no purpose and may be a factor in preventing the lesion in the lung from healing. Even when the cough is productive, it should not be so frequent as to exhaust the patient; it should not be allowed to disturb sleep unduly, nor should it cause vomiting after meals. It is better for secretions to be allowed to accumulate for some time and to be coughed up at intervals rather than to be coughed up in small quantities very frequently throughout the twenty-four hours.

It is often unnecessary and undesirable in the treatment of pulmonary tuberculosis to administer drugs to stop the cough. Rest in fresh air which is free from dust is frequently all that is required to allay unnecessary coughing. Coughing is often a bad habit and patients can be trained to resist it. The cough may be very acute for a few days, but if it is voluntarily suppressed it tends to wear off rapidly; indeed, in a sanatorium for early cases one hears the visitors coughing a good deal more than the patients!

Patients who do not have numerous large cavities in their lungs full of secretion can usually get their air passages cleared of sputum after waking in the morning, and need have no more coughing throughout the twenty-four hours. A warm alkaline drink on waking assists the loosening of such secretions and makes coughing easier, *e.g.*:

℞			
℞	Sod. Bicarb.		gr. xv
	Sod. Chlorid.		gr. v
	Sp. Chlorof.		♏x
	Aq. Anisi dil.	ad	oz. ½

To be taken in a glass of hot water on waking.

Patients with pulmonary cavitation often find a certain position in bed in which the secretion from their cavities drains most easily into their bronchial tubes. They learn to get into this position at certain times during the day and to empty their cavities by coughing.

Where the above simple measures fail, and the cough is excessive and disturbs sleep unduly, or where the cough is unproductive and useless, a sedative should be prescribed. Codein is the drug of choice; it has a strongly depressant action on the cough centre and has few of the undesirable effects of the other alkaloids of opium. It may be given in tablet form in doses of ¼ to ½ gr., or as syrup codein phosphate in doses of 1 to 1½ teaspoonfuls. This dose may be given at night only, or three or four times in the twenty-four hours as required. In patients with large cavities and a severe cough which prevents sleep, a stronger sedative may be necessary. Mixtures containing morphine should, if possible, be avoided on account of their constipating effects and a linctus of heroin is preferable:

℞		
℞	Heroin. Hydrochlor.	gr. $\frac{1}{16}$
	Glycer.	♏x
	Syr. Pic. Liq.	ʒi

This should not be given sufficiently often to suppress the cough entirely during the night, as this will only result in increasing the toxæmia and will produce an undue amount of coughing the next day.

An "emetic" cough is a very troublesome complication which is often extremely resistant to treatment. When it is present, meals should be simple and frequent rather than few and large. The patient should keep very still for some time after eating and should not be allowed to talk. A codein pill or sedative linctus can be given before the meal. Severe cases, however, may continue to vomit all food taken in spite of these measures. Under such circumstances cocaine is the only drug likely to give relief: a 5 per cent. cocaine solution should be sprayed on the larynx before and after meals. Occasionally a pastille, such as is prescribed below, sucked immediately after a meal may be sufficient:

℞	Menthol	gr. $\frac{1}{4}$
	Cocain. Hydrochlor.	gr. $\frac{1}{20}$
	Glycogelat. B.P.C.	q.s.

Hæmoptysis.—Of all the complications of pulmonary tuberculosis, hæmoptysis is probably the one which is most dreaded by the patient. Actually it is not usually a serious complication. Death as the immediate result is uncommon, and in the majority of cases it is not followed by an extension of the disease. Patients, therefore, should be encouraged to believe that hæmoptysis is a trivial incident in tuberculosis, in spite of the fact that this is not invariably the case.

Slight streaking of the sputum with blood need not affect the general course of treatment in any way provided it is not accompanied by other signs of increased activity of the disease. There is no need to confine the patient to bed on this account alone.

Where the hæmoptysis is rather more severe, the patient should be kept resting quietly in bed and should be confidently told that the bleeding will stop spontaneously in the course of time and that there is no cause for undue alarm. With moderate bleeding this is all the treatment which is necessary.

Profuse hæmoptysis is an indication for complete rest and careful nursing. An injection of $\frac{1}{6}$ or $\frac{1}{4}$ gr. of morphia should be given to calm the patient's anxiety and restlessness, to render the breathing quiet and peaceful and to allay excessive cough. The physician has to steer a somewhat difficult course in respect of the subsequent administration of morphia. When given in large and frequent doses it will so inhibit the cough reflex that the blood may accumulate in the air passages and cause pulmonary atelectasis or aspiration pneumonia. Morphia should, therefore, be used to control undue cough, restlessness and apprehension, but not to the extent of rendering the patient semi-conscious with extremely shallow breathing and a completely suppressed cough reflex.

It is inadvisable to keep the patient flat in bed or to frighten him with the suggestion that the slightest movement will cause further bleeding. This will only increase the danger of atelectasis in the posterior parts of his lungs. He will be more comfortable moderately propped up in bed, and in this position it will be much easier for him to get rid of blood clots and sputum from his air passages.

No solid food should be given for twenty-four hours after a severe hæmoptysis, and thereafter feeding should be started cautiously. The patient may drink fluids as he wishes, but these should not be hot.

The indications for transfusion with blood or salines are the same as for severe hæmorrhage in any other part of the body (see p. 475). The blood of all patients with profuse hæmoptysis should be typed and a suitable donor procured and kept at hand.

Large numbers of drugs have been recommended from time to time for the treatment of tuberculous hæmoptysis. Emetin, pituitrin, congo-red, the nitrites, calcium, adrenalin, thromboplastin and many others have had their advocates. It would be irrational to suppose that any of them could influence a severe pulmonary hæmorrhage, and in our opinion they are quite worthless in practice. The only form of active treatment likely to be successful is collapse of the affected lung by artificial pneumothorax if it can be effected (see p. 123). It is not always possible to say from which lung the hæmorrhage is occurring, but when this is known and the case is sufficiently serious, the feasibility of securing a rapid collapse of the lung as an emergency measure should always be considered. When a satisfactory collapse can be induced the bleeding is often dramatically arrested.

The after-treatment of a patient who has been exsanguinated by pulmonary hæmorrhage is the same as for hæmorrhage in other parts of the body, and the anæmia should receive appropriate treatment with iron (see p. 471).

Gastro-intestinal Symptoms.—*A poor appetite and dyspeptic symptoms* are common in untreated cases of pulmonary tuberculosis. They are often due to the general toxæmia which is present, and disappear with rest and fresh air treatment, which are much more efficacious in this respect than bitter tonics and stomachics. Irritation due to swallowed sputum is sometimes responsible for gastritis and enteritis, and for the much greater danger of tuberculous ulceration of the bowel. The patient must be impressed with the importance of expectorating all the sputum coughed up. Overfeeding is another common cause of dyspeptic symptoms, which should always necessitate a review of the patient's diet (see p. 110), and when the symptoms are severe a day of virtual starvation may be beneficial.

Hypochlorhydria and achlorhydria are common in tuberculosis, as they are in all debilitating conditions. Where a flatulent dyspepsia persists in spite of attention to the points already mentioned, a fractional test meal should be performed and where achlorhydria is discovered suitable treatment should be instituted (see p. 541). Less commonly the characteristic symptoms of hyperchlorhydria are present and should receive appropriate treatment (see p. 542).

Constipation is common in tuberculosis, where an atonic state of the intestinal musculature may be present in association with the atony of the skeletal and cardiac muscles. Its treatment differs in no respect from constipation in general (see p. 573).

Diarrhœa may be due to toxæmia, to tuberculous ulceration of the intestine or, occasionally, in advanced cases of long duration, to amyloid disease. Where ulceration is present the benzidene test for occult blood is usually positive, and pus cells are present in the fæces. Because a patient is getting two or three loose stools a day it should not be concluded hastily that tuberculous ulceration of the intestines is present.

A dose of castor oil is the best treatment for simple diarrhœa, and the patient should be kept warm in bed. Where symptoms persist the diet must be suitably altered. A low residue high vitamin diet should be given similar to that described for chronic dysentery (see p. 27). Milk and excessive fats may have to be omitted where the stools show that these are not well digested.

Tuberculous enteritis is a very grave complication of pulmonary tuberculosis, and in our experience the results in treatment have been singularly unsatisfactory. Three therapeutic measures have been advocated recently, particularly of America, as specifics for the condition: (1) Exposure of the abdomen to ultra-violet radiation from the mercury vapour lamp; (2) the administration of massive doses of cod-liver oil and tomato juice; (3) the injection of oxygen into the peritoneal cavity. We have treated many patients by the two former methods without observing any beneficial results. We have had no experience of treatment by means of pneumoperitoneum, but the published results are not impressive.

It is common for patients with tuberculous enteritis to be treated with a diet of milk and soft carbohydrate foods. This is a great mistake and results in the stools becoming excessively loose and offensive. If a dry low residue high vitamin diet (see p. 27) is prescribed the stools cease to be offensive and the diarrhœa and intestinal flatulence is often considerably relieved. In advanced tuberculous enteritis associated with severe diarrhœa and abdominal pain, the patient should be fed at frequent intervals with small meals of steamed fish, custard, jellies, bread and butter, and similar light food, milk being avoided. For the pain, tinct. opii (♏x) should be given three times a day, the dosage being liberally increased as required as there is no point in withholding sedative treatment from these unfortunate people. Occasionally we have found the intravenous injection of calcium chloride useful as a palliative measure, the pain and diarrhœa being sometimes dramatically relieved for some days. Five cubic centimetres of a 5 per cent. solution are injected slowly two or three times a week.

Care must be taken to get all the solution into the vein, for calcium chloride produces painful necrosis of the skin and subcutaneous tissues. The treatment is worth a trial and can do no harm if the injection is given carefully.

Attempts at surgical resection of the ulcerated portion of bowel are almost invariably unsuccessful and frequently fatal.

Pain.—Severe pain in the chest in the course of pulmonary tuberculosis is usually due to pleurisy. In emaciated patients with advanced disease it may be caused by fracture of a rib during the act of coughing, a complication which is much more common than is supposed and frequently overlooked. Occasionally pain may be due to spontaneous pneumothorax (p. 810).

The treatment of pain from dry pleurisy or a fractured rib is the same. Broad strapping is applied over the affected side, each strip overlapping the other. The strips must extend 2 in. beyond the middle line both in front and behind, and should be firmly applied when the patient's chest is fully collapsed in expiration. If this is insufficient to relieve the pain entirely, pyramidon (gr. v-x) or veramon (gr. vi) may be given. It is rarely necessary to administer morphia if the strapping has been correctly applied.

Sweating.—Sweating during sleep is the symptom which yields most rapidly to fresh air treatment. Even seriously ill patients rarely suffer from it if they are living under proper sanatorium conditions. When it occurs, therefore, it is usually an expression of the bad management of the case in respect of inadequate fresh air and excessive bedclothes. Exceptionally, however, "sleep sweating" persists in severely toxic patients in spite of excellent physiological conditions. Such cases should be given a glass of milk and a biscuit immediately before going to sleep, and a similar feed may be left by their bedside to be taken should they wake during the night. The use of atropine or any other drug has been, in our experience, quite useless in the control of sweating.

Scrupulous cleanliness is essential for all tuberculous patients, especially fevered patients whose skin is too often covered with a sweat rash. This will be prevented if ambulant patients take frequent baths, which should not be too hot, and if they dry themselves vigorously afterwards with a rough towel. Patients who are confined to bed should be washed completely night and morning.

Fever.—Absolute rest in the fresh air is the best treatment for fever. It is easy to reduce a tuberculous temperature by means of antipyretic drugs, but this procedure usually serves no useful purpose. Indeed, a helpful index of the progress of the disease is obscured, the tendency to sweating is increased and the temperature goes up again as soon as the drug is discontinued. If the fever is high and the patient is very uncomfortable on account of it, he may be relieved considerably by tepid sponging in bed.

TUBERCULOUS PLEURISY WITH EFFUSION

When an effusion in the pleural cavity is suspected it is wise to make a diagnostic puncture to confirm its presence. Some 15 c.c. of fluid should be removed for cytological and bacteriological examination. A clear sterile fluid containing a predominance of lymphocytes is almost certainly tuberculous in character. Tubercle bacilli, however, can rarely be demonstrated in the effusion, and even its inoculation into a guinea-pig may give negative results. The fact that it is often impossible to prove the tuberculous nature of the effusion bacteriologically should not influence the diagnosis. The serious nature of so-called "idiopathic pleural effusions" is often insufficiently appreciated by the doctor, or its significance minimized owing to his dislike of revealing the underlying tuberculous nature of the condition. A large percentage of such cases develop obvious pulmonary tuberculosis subsequently, often due to the fact that they have received insufficient care during the stage of effusion. Cases of tuberculous pleurisy with effusion should therefore be treated in the same way as early cases of pulmonary tuberculosis, with rest, fresh air and good food, according to the criteria laid down on p. 100, and should not be allowed to pass out of medical care and supervision as soon as the effusion and immediate symptoms have subsided. The true nature of the condition should not be withheld from the patient or his relatives, and any illness or symptoms which may occur subsequently should be interpreted with due regard to the tuberculous history.

Aspiration.—In the majority of cases it is unnecessary and unwise to aspirate the effusion, apart from a few cubic centimetres for diagnostic purposes. If left alone the fluid will usually be reabsorbed spontaneously, and while it remains it probably serves a useful purpose by keeping the lung collapsed and at rest as in therapeutic pneumothorax. This rule of non-interference is frequently broken with disastrous results. Even in teaching hospitals it is all too common for enthusiastic house physicians to remove at one aspiration some 30 or 40 oz. of fluid from the pleural cavity. The lung is thereby forcibly re-expanded and any small subpleural focus of disease which it may contain is liable to be activated. Acute pulmonary tuberculosis is not an uncommon sequel to such massive aspirations.

There are, however, certain occasions when careful aspiration of the fluid should be carried out. Occasionally the effusion is so large that serious dyspnœa or cardiac embarrassment may occur. Such pressure symptoms can be relieved by the removal of 8 to 12 oz. of fluid. Thereafter a slow, spontaneous absorption of the rest of the fluid may occur since the greatly increased intrapleural pressure may itself have been sufficient to inhibit absorption by compression of the blood and lymph vessels. It is better to aspirate an effusion by a Potain's, Dieulafoy's or Burrell's aspirator, using a very moderate suction, than by a two-way syringe, since it is difficult to keep the needle of the syringe steady in the pleural cavity while the aspiration and ejection of the fluid is being undertaken. In consequence, traumatization of the pleura and underlying lung may occur. Further, aspiration of an effusion by a two-way syringe is much more laborious for the operator and may be more uncomfortable for the patient than when an aspirator is used. The unpopularity of Potain's aspirator is largely due to the fact that the instrument is usually supplied with a set of fearsome and old-fashioned trocars and cannulas, which need only be used when very thick pus is present. A serum "record" needle of moderate bore is all that is necessary for the removal of serous effusions or thin pus, and can be fitted to any aspirator by means of a small metal adaptor.

A second indication for the removal of an effusion is its persistence for an unusual length of time, especially if pyrexia continues. It is difficult to lay down hard-and-fast rules as to how long an effusion should be left before aspiration is undertaken, but if there are no signs of spontaneous reabsorption after five or six weeks, aspiration should be considered. No more than 15 oz. should be removed at a time, as it is most undesirable to produce a markedly negative intrapleural pressure. Such negative pressures may cause pain, distressing cough and œdema of the lung in addition to the risk of activating any tuberculous lesion within the lung.

Air Replacement.—Where active pulmonary tuberculosis in the underlying lung is suspected, or known to be present owing to the discovery of tubercle bacilli in the sputum, it is best to remove the pleural effusion and to replace it with air. To do this two needles are inserted into the pleural cavity, the one low down and connected with an aspirator, the other higher up in the axilla and connected with a pneumothorax apparatus. This arrangement allows the simultaneous withdrawal of fluid and introduction of air to take place, and by keeping the intrapleural pressure about zero, practically all the effusion can be withdrawn without the risk of causing coughing, pain or œdema of the lung. Further, the therapeutic collapse of the lung is maintained, and can be controlled at will. The amount of air required to replace the fluid is usually about half the volume of fluid withdrawn. The management of the patient after a successful air replacement is the same as for an ordinary case of artificial pneumothorax complicated by an effusion (see p. 126). Unfortunately effective collapse is frequently impossible owing to pleural adhesions.

TUBERCULOSIS OF THE LARYNX

Tuberculosis of the larynx is a common complication of pulmonary tuberculosis. It is always secondary to the pulmonary disease and, though it is usually associated with advanced pulmonary tuberculosis, it may occur in early and curable cases. Contrary to the usually accepted belief, early laryngeal tuberculosis is quite amenable to treatment—provided the underlying pulmonary condition is not too far advanced. Severe laryngeal ulceration on the other hand, and especially ulceration of the epiglottis, are exceedingly recalcitrant to treatment, and their presence greatly increases the gravity of the prognosis in any case.

Thus the examination of the larynx at regular intervals should never be omitted as a part of the routine management of all cases of pulmonary tuberculosis. Too often this examination is neglected unless symptoms of hoarseness or aphonia manifest themselves, by which time laryngeal ulceration may have occurred. Whenever possible the examination should be carried out by an expert, as early tuberculosis of the larynx is difficult to diagnose without considerable experience of the condition and of the use of the laryngoscopic mirror.

No treatment of laryngeal tuberculosis can ever hope to be successful unless the underlying pulmonary tuberculosis is concurrently treated. Since the laryngeal disease is caused by infected sputum coughed up from the lung, every effort should be made to diminish the quantity of sputum and the amount of cough. Wherever it is feasible, artificial pneumothorax is the most useful measure at our disposal for this purpose. Tuberculosis of the larynx is, however, a contra-indication to thoracoplasty. Where the case is unsuitable for artificial pneumothorax, or where after a trial a satisfactory collapse of the lung cannot be secured, treatment with gold may be given a trial, as there is some evidence that this treatment on occasion has a distinct effect in diminishing the quantity of sputum and the number of bacilli expectorated.

Silence.—Apart from attention to the underlying pulmonary condition, the sheet-anchor of treatment in tuberculosis of the larynx is to procure rest for the part, just as it is the primary consideration in the therapeutics of tuberculosis affecting any other organ in the body. The treatment of excessive cough by appropriate sedatives (see p. 130) is a factor of importance in this respect. Apart from this, rest for the larynx may be secured to a great extent by insisting that the patient should maintain complete silence. This Trappist rule may have to be continued for many months and demands considerable resolution on the part of the patient. It is important, therefore, to explain fully at the beginning of the treatment that silence is of paramount importance and that serious consequences may ensue if the rule is broken. The patient should be provided with a pad on which to write out all his requirements, and sometimes a notice with " Silence " written on it, put up over the bed, may be a useful reminder and may prevent thoughtless people from asking the patient questions which might elicit a spontaneous reply. Many authorities allow patients with tuberculosis of the larynx to whisper. When this is carefully done and the sounds are produced by the lips and mouth only, and spoken so that they do not carry for more than a few feet, it probably does not interfere to a significant extent with laryngeal rest. In our experience, however, patients who are allowed such latitude soon become careless about the manner of their whispering. The whisper becomes louder and louder until it ends as a stage whisper, which is more of a strain on the larynx than ordinary speaking. We believe, therefore, that in curable cases speech in any form should be prohibited until the condition has subsided. Careful whispering should then be permitted, and only if the condition of the larynx has continued satisfactorily for a month should ordinary speaking be allowed. When the patient is allowed to speak after a long period of silence, he is usually unable to produce more than a hoarse whisper, as the vocal cords will not approximate to one another. He should be told, however, that this is only temporary and that he will regain his voice in the course of time.

Cauterization.—Apart from silence, the only treatment likely to prove of curative value in laryngeal tuberculosis is the cautious use of the galvano-cautery. The procedure known as ignipuncture is used for reducing the œdema of the arytenoids when they become unduly swollen. The cautery point at white heat is plunged into the turgid tissues at one or two points, and this may help to reduce the bulk of the swelling. The procedure is usually carried out through the direct laryngoscope, but it is possible to do so with the aid of the laryngeal mirror alone.

The cautery may also be used to remove small granulations or nodules within the larynx itself or on the vocal cords, and may facilitate the healing of the local lesion. It is to be understood that such procedures should only be undertaken after expert advice has been procured, and should only be performed by those practised in the art of laryngoscopy. They are simply incidents in treatment and are not a substitute for the general treatment of the tuberculous condition, nor do they dispense with the necessity for silence on the part of the patient. Although by no means a formidable operation in the hands of experts (for it only involves a few minutes' treatment which should be painless) great damage can be done by injudicious and inexpert interference.

Palliative Treatment.—Advanced tuberculosis of the larynx is a hopeless condition and calls only for palliative treatment. With ulceration, particularly of the epiglottis (which is very rarely involved in early disease), nerve endings are exposed and cause intense pain—especially on swallowing. The plight of such patients is a very dreadful one, and every effort must be made to relieve their sufferings. A 5 per cent. cocaine spray in aqueous solution, used before meals, is one of the most valuable palliative measures, or a cocaine pastille may be sucked (see p. 132). Alternatively, the insufflation of Orthoform (Bayer), a cocaine powder, often gives great relief. A suitable apparatus for introducing this preparation is a Leduc's insufflator. The powder is put upon a saucer and the patient inhales it into his larynx through the Leduc's apparatus. In extreme cases other methods can be tried, such as the superficial coagulation of the exposed ulcerated areas by diathermy, or the injection of the superior laryngeal nerve by Boulay's technique. These are both specialized procedures and require the collaboration of an expert.

Many patients suffering from dysphagia due to tuberculous ulceration of the epiglottis find it easier to take their meals while lying on their faces from a tray on their pillow. By raising the jaw and stretching the neck this procedure tends to lift the epiglottis forward and so to facilitate the passage of food past the ulcerated area.

We believe that all other methods of active treatment, such as the direct application of ultra-violet light to the larynx and attempts at surgical interference on the diseased parts, are contraindicated.

TUBERCULOSIS OF THE URINARY TRACT

RENAL TUBERCULOSIS

The kidney is the first part of the urinary tract to be involved in tuberculosis. It is not a primary and independent disease, but rather a local manifestation in a tuberculous patient, and is the result of blood-borne infection. Evidence or a history of previous or co-existing tuberculous disease is available in over 80 per cent. of cases. The common sources of the infection are the lungs, lymph glands in the thorax or abdomen and the epididymis (see p. 143).

Routine and careful examination of the urine in subjects undergoing treatment for tuberculosis may reveal a tuberculous bacilluria. It is usually symptomless, though occasionally there is frequency of micturition. The presence of leucocytes and a few red blood corpusles in the urine is invariable, and their detection should, therefore, suggest a full bacteriological examination. It is probably unnecessary to examine the urine for tubercle bacilli unless leucocytes are present. The underlying cause is an overt focus of disease in the cortex of the kidney which cannot be demonstrated at this stage by radiological investigation. Healing usually occurs, but in a few instances active and progressive disease of the kidney is manifest at a later date and this possibility should be kept in view in the after-care of tuberculous subjects.

When renal tuberculosis is suspected, a very thorough examination should be carried out in order to confirm the diagnosis and to ascertain the extent of the disease. Intravenous pyelography with uroselectan is often of great value, but it cannot be relied on in every case because when the lesions are small the kidney may appear normal. Cystoscopy may be negative or may show a diminished bladder capacity, mild cystitis, miliary tubercles or ulceration. Finally, and especially when the diagnosis is in doubt, catheter pyelograms should be obtained; they give the clearest definition of structural changes in the kidney and ureter.

Early renal tuberculosis can be cured by general treatment alone, but this is only possible if the disease is in its initial stages, *i.e.*, when the lesion is so small that it cannot be detected by pyelography and is only demonstrable by a few leucocytes, red cells and tubercle bacilli in the urine.

Once the disease has progressed beyond the early stage, and can be demonstrated by retrograde pyelography, spontaneous cure is found from experience to be exceedingly rare, and the question of nephrectomy has to be considered. It should be emphasized, however, that surgery will not benefit the patient fully until he has developed his resistance to tuberculosis, and this is best promoted by a period of residence in a sanatorium. It is remarkable how under sanatorium treatment the general health is improved, symptoms relieved and ulceration of the bladder diminished. Following constitutional treatment operation is more easily borne, convalescence more rapid and the risks of complications, such as generalization of the disease or affection of the remaining kidney, reduced. An active lesion in the lungs is a definite contraindication to operation, for this focus will probably remain active and may be a source of infection to the remaining kidney. When severe disease affects both kidneys surgical interference is obviously contraindicated.

As in tuberculosis generally, the operative procedure is merely an incident in treatment. Many of the unsuccessful results of nephrectomy can be attributed to insufficient postoperative care. Responsibility does not end with the immediate recovery of the patient from the operation. A period of from three to six months' convalescence in a sanatorium, or under sanatorium conditions at home, should be enforced, no matter how well the patient may appear.

Following operation the bladder, if it has been affected, may recover with remarkable rapidity, but in many cases a considerable time (even years) may elapse before this takes place. Unfortunately, there are many cases in which ulceration of the bladder persists and leads to great contraction of its walls. In these cases pain and frequency of micturition may be very distressing. Little relief is secured by local treatment, and generally resort must be made to increasing doses of anodyne drugs. Occasionally transplantation of the ureter may be feasible.

A review of statistics suggests that nephrectomy for tuberculosis of the kidney results in cure in about 60 per cent. of cases. One of the chief objects of nephrectomy is to safeguard the bladder from extension of disease, and when it is affected to facilitate its healing.

TUBERCULOSIS OF THE EPIDIDYMIS

It is not appreciated sufficiently how readily the disease at this site yields to conservative treatment by rest and constitutional measures, provided there is not progressing tuberculosis elsewhere. A period of rest in bed—say eight weeks—and not necessarily in a sanatorium, usually results in a rapid subsidence of the testicular swelling and relief of symptoms such as aching and "dragging." In the majority of cases fibrosis or calcification occurs within the diseased area. A suspensory belt is a useful appliance to support the diseased testicle and to protect it from jolting movements.

In a number of instances a localized cold abscess develops. If rupture has not occurred spontaneously an incision should be made to evacuate it. A sinus may persist for many months but, except in a few cases, healing may be anticipated.

Radical surgical treatment, especially orchidectomy, should be avoided wherever possible, because it is a common experience that the remaining testicle may subsequently become the seat of disease. Frequently concomitant lesions elsewhere in the genito-urinary tract preclude radical measures. Surgery may, however, be advised in a few cases where the prospect of natural resolution is very remote, and to relieve the discomforts incumbent upon extensive suppuration and persistent sinus formation.

GLANDULAR TUBERCULOSIS

Any group of lymphatic glands may be the seat of tuberculous infection. The mucous surfaces of the pharynx, bronchi and the small intestine are the usual portals of entry. Accordingly, the cervical, tracheobronchial and mesenteric systems are most commonly involved. The general treatment is on the lines already outlined (see p. 100) and the strictness of the regimen imposed should be governed by the presence or absence of constitutional signs and symptoms.

TUBERCULOSIS OF THE CERVICAL GLANDS

Tuberculous enlargement of the cervical glands may be localized or diffuse, acute, chronic or recurring. These varying pathological features, together with the age of the patient, will govern to some extent the type of treatment adopted.

In childhood the disease often pursues an acute course, culminating in caseation or suppuration of one or several glands. In such cases a varying degree of constitutional upset is often present and requires appropriate general treatment according to the criteria laid down elsewhere (see p. 100). No local treatment is required except in the event of suppuration, when evacuation of the pus by a small incision should be undertaken. Early healing without sinus formation or secondary infection may be anticipated—provided the general measures of rest, fresh air and good feeding are continued during a sufficient period.

The ready accessibility of the glands of the neck has made them a tempting object for surgical attack. As a routine practice it is to be deplored. Surgery removes the obviously enlarged glands, but does nothing for the underlying tuberculous disease. The response to general methods of treatment is usually as gratifying in glands in the neck as it is in the treatment of those in the abdomen or thorax ; no surgeon would attempt to deal with glands in these latter situations. With few exceptions, surgery should be employed only for the evacuation of cold abscesses and in those rare cases in which the disease proves unusually indolent and an unsightly swelling or sinus persists in the neck.

Institutional treatment, or rest in bed, is impracticable and unnecessary for all cases, and is only imperative in the few who exhibit significant constitutional symptoms. The state of the child's general health will decide the advisability of keeping him away from school. The parents should be instructed as to the necessity of providing ample rest, fresh air and good food and the avoidance of over-fatigue in work and play. Town children will frequently benefit by a long holiday in the country, though this is unfortunately often impracticable.

Treatment by tuberculin (see p. 116) may augment the

child's resistance, and is worthy of trial. Its weekly administration by the doctor at least ensures constant medical supervision.

In older children, and in adults, the disease usually assumes a more chronic form, and may affect a single or several groups of glands. The risk of general infection is slight. The disease may remain stationary for a long time, or one or several glands may undergo caseation and suppuration and require surgical treatment. An indolent mass of glands should be removed, especially if it is responsible for a persistingly discharging sinus.

Heliotherapy.—In glandular tuberculosis, heliotherapy is a valuable means of improving the general resistance, and for this purpose the exposure of the whole body to the carbon-arc light is most suitable. It is also of great service in the local treatment of the glandular swellings, especially if there are ulcers and sinuses. The mercury-vapour lamp is preferable for local treatment.

The time of exposure to the carbon-arc lamp should be carefully regulated. In the first days of treatment seven to ten minutes is sufficient. As tolerance is acquired, the exposure is gradually increased to half an hour or more. Particular care should be taken not to increase the time of exposure too rapidly in blonde subjects, since such patients may blister very readily. It is very important that the patient's eyes be protected with dark glasses or an acute conjunctivitis may result.

In using the mercury-vapour lamp for local treatment the face, neck and chest are protected with linen, and only the part undergoing treatment is left exposed, and the exposure should, on the first occasion, be no longer than five minutes. Each exposure should produce a mild erythema of the skin. Treatment is repeated twice weekly and may extend over a period of from six to twelve months.

TUBERCULOSIS OF THE MEDIASTINAL GLANDS

The mere radiological demonstration of enlarged mediastinal glands is not necessarily an indication for active treatment of any kind. Indeed, the fact that tuberculous glands in this region are easily demonstrable radiologically is usually an index of their satisfactory healing by calcification. The diagnosis of active tuberculosis of the mediastinal glands is always a difficult one, and depends to a large extent on the constitutional symptoms presented by the patient. Treatment is limited to the general measures already described. In addition, a careful clinical and radiological search must be made for an associated pulmonary lesion which, when discovered, should receive appropriate treatment.

TUBERCULOSIS OF THE MESENTERIC LYMPH GLANDS

Enlargement and caseation of the mesenteric glands is a very common outcome of milk-borne infection in childhood. It may be, and commonly is, a primary source of infection in the body. The glands most commonly affected are those of the ileocæcal region. They may reach such bulk as to be readily palpable through the abdominal wall. Gradual healing is the rule and calcification the usual dénouement. In rare instances a gland may soften and rupture into the peritoneal cavity, giving rise to acute—though not necessarily fatal—peritonitis. Inflammatory adhesions quite frequently occur and are one of the common causes of acute intestinal obstruction in adults.

The effects of the disease may be so mild that it is not suspected, but in young children it may be responsible for chronic digestive upsets, malnutrition and frequent and obscure febrile attacks. Sometimes there are more acute attacks, like appendicitis, and, unless the glands are palpable, differentiation is practically impossible. In practice it is wiser to ignore the possibility of tuberculous glands being the source of acute pain in the lower abdomen lest an early opportunity be lost of removing a diseased appendix. The diagnosis of appendicitis will usually prove more acceptable to anxious parents than that of tuberculosis.

When the diagnosis of tuberculosis of the mesenteric glands can be established, treatment should be on general lines to increase resistance. In very young children the disease may be the source of a more generalized infection, and this possibility should be kept in view when any subsequent illness arises. However, in the majority of cases the infection remains localized, the glands become calcareous and no permanent ill-effect remains.

In the course of operations for appendicitis discovery of caseous mesenteric glands is very common. It is both unnecessary and unwise to interfere with them unless rupture seems imminent. It may be more prudent to withhold knowledge of the incidental discovery from nervous parents, as an uneventful recovery may be anticipated. When constitutional symptoms are present, however, general treatment must be instituted along the lines already mentioned, including a course of heliotherapy and tuberculin, provided the symptoms are not very acute.

PERITONEAL TUBERCULOSIS

The treatment of the other manifestations of abdominal tuberculosis such as tuberculous enteritis and tuberculosis of the mesenteric glands has been respectively discussed on pp. 133, 146; in addition, tuberculosis may involve the peritoneum; sometimes the various lesions are combined in different degrees. The disease is commonest in childhood, but not confined to that period.

In the peritoneum the disease may assume a miliary form—blood borne or from an active glandular or other lesion in the abdomen. In such cases the general illness may overshadow the abdominal features. It usually progresses to a fatal issue, but when the disease is confined to the abdomen it may be survived. More often the infection is of a chronic nature and is manifest pathologically by (1) multiple and diffuse subperitoneal infiltrations and a profuse serous effusion, or (2) by an accumulation of gelatinous or caseous exudate upon or between mesenteric and intestinal surfaces—which may become confluent in an inextricable mass. Both types may be associated with a severe and continued systemic disturbance. In the early years of life the outlook is grave, but in older children the prognosis is very favourable, especially in the ascitic type.

In all cases sanatorium treatment should be enforced. A very rapid and striking improvement is usually witnessed, as evidenced by a diminution of the systemic intoxication and of the abdominal swelling from absorption of the effusion, though disappearance of the masses within the peritoneum is more gradual. The sanatorium regimen may, with advantage, be supplemented by heliotherapy when the disease has reached a stage of comparative quiescence. The once common practice of evacuating the effusion by operation should be abandoned; it deals with a beneficent expression of the disease and does not influence the underlying and still active sources of toxæmia. Occasionally the ascites may reach such dimensions as to cause serious embarrassment, and relief by tapping may be required (see p. 1087).

The exudative form of infection follows a more protracted course. The prognosis is less favourable than in the ascitic form because cold abscesses may occur with eruption at the umbilicus, commonly causing a fæcal fistula. Further, when healing occurs the diffuse adhesion of bowel and mesenteries entails a continued menace of obstruction. It is remarkable, however, how seldom the obstruction reaches such a degree as to demand its relief by surgery. After reaching a certain degree the obstruction usually relieves itself spontaneously. Should operation become necessary, the universal adhesions may render the operative manœuvres more than usually difficult.

TUBERCULOSIS OF THE SKIN

Infection of the skin with *B. tuberculosis* causes a chronic inflammation, the clinical appearance of which varies according to the depth of the infection and the route by which it has gained access. Thus, lupus vulgaris results from a blood-stream infection or an extension from a diseased mucous membrane, scrofuloderma from underlying glandular tuberculosis, and tuberculosis verrucosa cutis from external infection through an injury. The treatment is essentially the same for all types of tuberculosis of the skin with minor differences to meet conditions in individual cases. The ideal treatment is a combination of local irradiation with the Finsen-Lomholt lamp, and general irradiation from the carbon arc. Unfortunately the Finsen-Lomholt apparatus is not generally available and other methods have also to be considered.

In the first instance the affected area must be put in the best possible condition to receive treatment, and this can easily be done by the practitioner in charge of the case. Secondary impetiginization must be dealt with (see Impetigo), ulceration as far as it is due to secondary infection must be reduced and the secondary warty development on the surface, which is seen from time to time, removed by the application of 10 per cent. solution of sodium hydroxide and subsequent scraping with a sharp spoon.

The Finsen-Lomholt lamp is devised to concentrate the ultra-violet portion of the spectrum while at the same time removing the infra-red rays. The concentrated beam of ultra-violet rays is applied direct to the diseased area which is irradiated systematically until it has been completely treated. Only a small area can be dealt with at a time. An inflammatory reaction is produced, and this is associated with disintegration of the tubercular foci and their replacement by fibrous tissue. The treatment is repeated until no sign of the disease remains. Irradiation of the entire body surface with light from a carbon-arc source can be used in conjunction with this treatment, and almost all cases benefit from carbon-arc irradiation alone. General irradiation is carried out daily over a period of months.

If irradiation is not available, resort must be made to caustic applications. Coagulation of the diseased area with diathermy is the most efficient method, because the destruction can be carried to any desired depth. A patch may be painted with trichloracetic acid, acid nitrate of mercury or pure carbolic acid once or twice weekly, the application being made to a small area at a time. These substances can also be introduced directly into isolated nodules by means of a dental burr.

Recently a number of cases have been successfully treated by infiltrating the diseased area with ethyl hydnocarpate. A small area is injected at each treatment, using from 1 to 2 c.c. of the solution. The injections may be performed once or twice weekly. The results of this treatment have so far been encouraging, and it has the advantage of being easily and cheaply carried out.

It should be deeply impressed on patients suffering from lupus, firstly that regular attendance for treatment is essential, and secondly that they must keep in touch with their doctor for two years after an apparent cure. Thereafter advice should be sought immediately there is any suspicion of recurrence.

D. M. Dunlop.
B. M. Dick.

COMMON DISEASES OF THE SKIN

INTRODUCTION

A LARGE proportion of the skin diseases which are met with in general practice lend themselves more readily to treatment than the common disorders of most other organs. Disease of the skin can be recognized as soon as it develops and remedies can be applied directly to the affected area. Response to treatment can be ascertained by direct observation. In spite of such ideal conditions the cure of skin diseases, and by that is meant the complete disappearance of an eruption but not freedom from recurrence, is in many instances exceedingly slow. The tendency for skin diseases to recur is notorious.

One feature of therapy in dermatology deserves emphasis, namely, that almost without exception it is possible to achieve by treatment the complete disappearance of an eruption, so that if recurrence does take place it is a true recurrence and not an exacerbation of an incompletely treated disease. The problem of recurrence as it affects skin disease is no different from that involved in diseases of other organs, and it resolves itself into speculations on biological peculiarities or idiosyncrasies, which are for the most part theoretical. From the biological standpoint it is probable that more concrete facts regarding the human aspects of idiosyncrasy have been gathered from the observation of skin diseases and their response to treatment than by any other method of study.

CAUSE OF DISEASE AND RESPONSE TO TREATMENT

Skin eruptions and alterations in cutaneous function and structure can be produced by the action of noxious substances which reach the skin either from the outside or from within via the blood stream. It is the possibility of this direct external contact with irritants and poisons which renders the skin vulnerable to types of injury which are unknown in other organs.

Since disease of the skin may be produced by internal causes, it may suffer in conjunction with disorders of the internal organs. In these circumstances the visceral disease usually gives rise to the more serious manifestations and the skin eruption is regarded as secondary. In addition to such eruptions there exist a number of skin diseases obviously due to some internal factor which appears to poison the skin alone. Here treatment is directed against the cause if this is known, or is governed by the principle of free elimination and the administration of some drug which experience has shown to be beneficial.

One important point must be noted in connection with skin disease, namely, that the interference with skin function which is bound to result from an extensive eruption does not necessarily produce any grave systemic symptoms or upset in general health such as accompanies the derangement of function associated with disease of other organs. Nevertheless extensive destruction of the skin surface may prove fatal. Modification of function plays a great part in the treatment of disease of certain organs other than the skin, but physiological variation in the skin can only be produced to a limited extent, and the employment of methods calculated to produce such changes is not rewarded with much success in the treatment of skin diseases.

From what has been said it may be gathered that the treatment of skin disease solely by internal methods, while often desirable on theoretical grounds, is not entirely satisfactory from the practical point of view. With the exception of syphilis and leishmaniasis there exists no specific internal cure for any skin disease. Nevertheless, internal measures are valuable aids in a number of conditions, but, unless combined with external methods of treatment, they are, generally speaking, insufficient. In some cases a combination of both external and internal treatment is essential.

Before discussing separately the treatment of the common skin diseases, it will be an advantage first of all to give a detailed description of the technique employed in the application of external remedies, for this is a subject of particular importance.

It may be said without fear of contradiction that but for external treatment few skin diseases would ever be cured. Yet criticism is still levelled against dermatologists by some internists because of this dependence on external remedies. This is hard to understand, for if the drug employed acts unchanged on the diseased organ, it would seem to matter little whether it reaches the organ via the blood stream or as a result of direct application. Moreover, direct application ensures that the drug reaches the cells of the organ to be treated more quickly, more certainly, and in a more controlled concentration than is possible by the blood-stream approach.

A large variety of chemical substances are applied externally in the treatment of skin diseases and each one of them may be observed to have an almost specific healing action in individual examples of each disease. Certain chemicals or groups of chemicals are indicated in the majority of cases in each disease group, but there is invariably a small number of patients in each group whose skins will not tolerate the applications which are generally employed. Again, different chemicals are suited to the different phases of the same disease. Two types of cutaneous intolerance to chemical applications may therefore be revealed in the treatment of any one skin disease ; firstly, a general cutaneous idiosyncrasy to the chemical applied, and secondly, a temporary intolerance dependent on the phase through which the disease is passing. Both types may depend to some extent on the concentration of the drug applied, and by reducing the concentration the intolerance may disappear. On the other hand, the idiosyncrasy may be towards the chemical irrespective of its concentration. Intolerance of the first type may be considered an example of individual variation, whereas in the second type it constitutes a true idiosyncrasy. No matter what may be the nature of the intolerance, it can act as a very great obstacle to treatment, for it may be exhibited to such universally employed substances as fats and mineral oils.

Only general statements can be made regarding the pharmacological actions of the numerous remedies applied externally in the treatment of skin diseases. Some are absorbent ; some, by evaporation, have a cooling and decongestive action ; alteration of the fluid balance of the epidermal cells may be produced by wet dressings ; osmotic effects, surface tension changes and alterations in electrical conditions at cell surfaces may be induced ; epidermal growth may be stimulated or inhibited. Such actions are bound to occur, but the effect of a given drug cannot definitely be ascribed to any one of them. All that can be said with certainty about the common chemical applications is that they have antiseptic properties, and in high concentrations act to a greater or less extent as irritants, and even cause the death of living cells. Their successful manipulation depends not on a knowledge of their pharmacological action but on a knowledge of skin disease in each and every one of its phases, an experience of the effect of a chemical substance on any one of these many phases, and an appreciation of cutaneous idiosyncrasy.

Since our accurate knowledge of the pharmacological action of the substances applied externally to the skin is so limited it will serve no purpose to tabulate them in a list which could not be arranged in any significant classification. Their consideration, both as to method and strength of application, will therefore be deferred to the discussion of the treatment of individual diseases. In the majority of cases, however, the chemical substance is applied to the skin diluted in a vehicle, and the type of vehicle may profoundly influence the result obtained. It will be advantageous to give at this point a detailed description of such vehicles and the technique of their application, in order to avoid subsequent repetition.

The response of any skin disease to a suitable form of treatment depends on the efficiency with which it is carried out, and on the facilities available for doing so. It is not infrequently noted that a treatment which is eminently successful in hospital has proved of little value when carried out by the patient in his home. Skin applications are unfortunately expensive, and as a result treatment is sometimes unsatisfactory and prolonged because of false economy.

LOCAL TREATMENT

Generally speaking, the use of soap and water is indicated in the treatment of all skin diseases for purposes of general cleanliness, and for assisting the removal of surface therapeutic applications and the products of the disease process, such as crusting and scaling. Washing may cause a temporary increase in the symptoms of itching and burning, but this can be ignored in the majority of cases as it is generally very transient. Occasionally, however, very sensitive inflamed skins will not tolerate the use of soap and water because the reaction which is produced does not subside rapidly, and the condition is aggravated. In such cases cleansing has to be carried out exclusively with olive oil, almond oil, or peach kernel oil. It may be necessary to use these oils prior to washing with soap and water in order to soften crusts and certain therapeutic agents which have been applied to the skin. Occasionally patients complain of a feeling of irritation and dryness after the application of olive oil, but this is rarely a serious drawback to its use.

Baths may be given in all skin diseases and may on occasion cause irritation in the same way as when soap and water is used for washing purposes. The bath should not be more than 100° F., and a patient may soak in it for fifteen to twenty minutes. A number of drugs may be added to the bath, but it is very doubtful if such medicated baths have any real value, although patients with an extensively inflamed skin may find a starch bath more comfortable than an ordinary one. The following are the common drugs which may be added to a bath of approximately 40 gals.

Starch bath : $\frac{1}{2}$ lb. of starch is first mixed with cold water in a basin to make a paste, and the bath is filled by allowing the hot water to run into the basin and overflow from it into the bath.

Potassium permanganate bath : Potassium permanganate crystals are added in sufficient quantity to make the water a bright pink colour, and the patient is immersed for ten minutes before soap is used.

Bran bath : 4 lb. of bran contained in a muslin bag are placed in the bath which is then filled by allowing the tap to run on to the bag.

Sulphur bath : 2 to 4 oz. of potassa sulphurata are put in the bath prior to filling.

The cleaning of the bath contaminated by medicaments added to the water, or by pastes or exudations from the patient's skin, is a matter of importance. Sulphur, potassium permanganate, tar, chrysarobin, silver nitrate and the aniline dyes will stain a bath if it is not cleaned immediately and thoroughly after use. For a greasy bath, vim, Brooke's soap or paraffin may be used ; for chrysarobin, a mixture of paraffin and bath-brick ; for the aniline dyes, turpentine or methylated spirit.

Powders.—For ordinary purposes starch, talc or kaolin, used either singly or mixed in equal parts, form suitable bland powders which can be dusted on as a protective and cooling application to an inflamed surface, *e.g.*, in erythemas, in dry scaly dermatitis and in herpes zoster. They are only useful when the eruption is of a dry nature, because if there is any discharge the powder cakes and acts as a mechanical irritant. Drugs such as boric acid, salicylic acid and iodoform may be added to these inert powders in a proportion of 1 to 2 per cent. They are dredged on the skin and form a clean preparation which is cooling and easy to remove. At certain stages in inflammatory skin diseases the best results may be obtained from the application of powders alone.

Watery Pastes.—Powders may be mixed with water to form a substance having the consistency of a paste, and these watery pastes are sometimes useful in acutely inflamed erythematous eruptions, particularly in acute sunburn.

Poultices.—The only poultice which is really efficacious and of outstanding value in the treatment of skin diseases is the starch poultice. It is made up in the following way, using either wheaten or maize starch:—

To make a starch poultice for the scalp, four tablespoonfuls of starch, one teaspoonful of boracic and one pint of water are required. Double this amount is needed for a poultice for the hand and arm. The starch is put into a basin and the boracic, after being crushed to a powder, is added to it. It is then mixed with cold water until it forms a thick cream. Boiling water is added until the diluted cream sets into a jelly. During this addition the mixture is stirred continuously with a wooden spoon. The jelly so obtained is then beaten with the spoon for a few minutes until the starch is smooth, and then it is left until quite cold.

The cold jelly is spread in a layer about $\frac{3}{4}$ in. thick on a piece of strong calico, leaving a margin all round. It is then covered with gauze and the margin folded in. The poultice should be of such a size that it extends 1 in. beyond the margin of the affected area. Where the use of a poultice spread in this way is not possible owing to anatomical difficulties such as are met with in a body fold, the starch jelly should be rolled in a single layer of gauze and this bandaged on. When a whole limb is being treated with starch poultices, two should be made and applied to the upper and under surface so as to overlap at the sides.

The ordinary washing starches do not produce such a good jelly as do the wheaten, maize, or even potato starches. If desired, the initial paste may be made with 2 per cent. aqueous solution of gentian-violet or 1 : 1,000 aqueous solution of acriflavine instead of ordinary water. A charcoal starch poultice may be obtained by adding 1 to 2 drachms of charcoal to the cold-water paste before the addition of boiling water.

The application of starch poultices is a universally safe treatment for all exudative forms of skin disease, and with ingenuity they can be applied and retained in position on any part of the body. Their disadvantage is their weight and sometimes the feeling of clamminess which they produce. When starch poultices are being used it may be necessary to keep the patient in bed in order to allow applications to be made and to be kept in position. It is particularly important to avoid a hard edge of linen or calico coming into contact with the eruption. The starch poultices should lift off easily and leave, practically speaking, no starch adherent to the skin surface. They absorb exudate into their substance and thus reduce the chance of the dressing causing a spread of infection by the retention of discharges in contact with the skin, or by their extension to adjacent areas as is liable to happen with ordinary occlusive wet dressings. Starch poultices are difficult to make, and if not made properly they may either be lumpy, too moist, or may dry to a cement-like consistency after an hour or two, and in consequence do considerable harm. They should be renewed every four or five hours, and as good poultices come cleanly off the skin, washing the part once daily is all that is required. In this way a minimum of interference with an inflamed surface is necessary.

Lotions.—Lotions may contain medicinal substances either in solution or in suspension. A lotion commonly employed is one containing glycerin and an inert powder in addition to the medicinal substances dissolved or in suspension in the fluid vehicle. Lotions are usually made up with water, but spirit may be added to the water, and some lotions are entirely spirituous. Lotions may be applied either by dabbing or painting them on the surface with a pledget of cotton wool or a brush, or by applying strips of calico or linen soaked with the lotion which are then covered with some occlusive material such as oiled silk or jaconet. If the surface to be treated is extensive, the lotion should be brought to blood heat before use. A powdery lotion when painted or applied to the surface has a cooling effect due to the evaporation of water, and after evaporation has taken place a thin layer of powder is left on the skin surface and this remains adherent on account of the glycerin contained in the lotion.

Lotions are useful because they are easy to apply, they are clean, and in virtue of their cooling effect they are efficient in allaying itch. They are used in inflammation of the skin in all its forms, and they may be applied, even as occlusive dressings, to large areas of the body surface. Lotions are removed by gentle washing with soap and water, if necessary after a preliminary softening with olive oil. Should some of the lotion become adherent to an irritable surface it should be allowed to remain, because vigorous rubbing will only further irritate and inflame the area.

Ointments and Pastes.—Ointment bases may be either

animal fats or mineral oils of suitable consistency. For practical purposes lard, hydrous wool fat and soft paraffin are all the bases which are required. The addition of wax, eucerine, spermaceti, stearines, etc., is quite unnecessary; these substances merely giving a smoother feel to the base. Ointments are used as a vehicle for the application of all types of chemicals to the skin. They may be rubbed in, or applied spread on strips of linen or calico which are then bandaged on to the part. When rubbing is carried out the palm of the hand should be used in preference to the finger tips, the inunction being performed with steady even pressure and in a unidirectional manner if the part is hairy.

An ointment may be stiffened by the addition of an inert powder such as zinc oxide or starch to give it the consistence of a paste. The same medicinal substances may be incorporated in pastes as in ointments. Pastes cannot easily be rubbed in unless they are very thin, that is to say, containing about 10 to 15 per cent. of powder, and if they are stiffer they must be applied spread on strips of calico or linen varying in width from ½ in. for the fingers to 3 in. for the limbs. If the trunk has to be dressed, material is shaped to fit, overlapping the shoulders and sides and cut to clear the axillæ. For the head and face a mask is used, and this should always cover the head, even when the face only is being treated. The material is pinned at the back and sides of the neck and kept in position with a bandage. A mask which only covers the face and is not carried over the head will invariably slip out of position and be uncomfortable. Pastes cannot conveniently be applied to surfaces covered with hair, and should their application be necessary to such areas the part must be shaved. Pastes are, generally speaking, more useful than ointments, although they are more difficult to apply. Being stiffer in consistence than ointments, they lend more support to the area to which they are applied, and a certain amount of exudate may penetrate into the interstices of the paste. Although it cannot be demonstrated that a paste is capable of absorbing water or serum, there is no doubt that pastes can be applied to exudative lesions with benefit, whereas ointments are unsuitable applications if there is much exudation from the skin.

Pastes should not be made too thick because of the difficulty in removing them. Before removal the part is saturated with olive oil; it is then wiped gently with dry cotton wool. If a great deal of rubbing is required to remove any application from a diseased skin surface, the irritation so produced may undo any good which has been brought about by the treatment.

In this country from 15 to 20 per cent. of inert powder added to an ointment base will give a paste which is easily applied and easily removed. In warmer climates it may be necessary to increase the amount of powder in pastes for general use, and in certain circumstances a larger amount of powder may be required even in colder climates.

The amount of ointment or paste required for a single dressing of different areas in an adult is approximately as follows when spreads are used: (1) face, head and neck; (2) hand, fingers and whole arm; (3) back or front of trunk; 2 oz. Complete dressing of the entire skin surface, 1 to $1\frac{1}{2}$ lb.

Paints.—Some antiseptics, and particularly the aniline dyes, are applied to the skin in the form of paints which dry on the surface. These drugs may be dissolved in water, in spirit, or applied undiluted. Paints in common use are: (1) the aniline dyes in watery or spirituous solution, (2) ichthyol and silver nitrate, either alone or combined, in watery solution, or (3) silver nitrate dissolved in spirits ether nitrosi. Crude gasworks tar in the form of a thin varnish is applied as a paint which, after five minutes, is powdered with talc or starch. This preparation dries in about fifteen to twenty minutes and is allowed to remain on the skin for from twenty-four to forty-eight hours. It may then be removed with olive oil. It is usually advisable to apply a paste for from twelve to twenty-four hours before repainting with the tar. Wherever possible paints should be applied in watery solution to avoid any irritant effect which might be produced by spirit.

Permanent fixed dressings are not of great value in dermatology except in artefact dermatitis and as a final dressing in varicose dermatitis. The preparation which is least likely to irritate an inflamed or recently inflamed skin is Unna's ichthyol zinc gelatin.

Choice of Treatment

The choice of drug and its strength depends entirely on the type and stage of the eruption which is under treatment. Generally speaking, substances such as ichthyol, ammoniated mercury, boric acid and tar may be used in concentrations of $\frac{1}{2}$ to 1 per cent. in the treatment of acutely inflamed conditions. If much scaling is present, drugs which have a solvent action on scales are indicated, and of these salicylic acid in a strength of 2 to 5 per cent. and tar in a strength of 3 to 5 per cent. are the most useful applications. Stronger applications for scaly and hyperkeratotic conditions are undiluted crude tar, 20 per cent. salicylic acid and 5 to 20 per cent. chrysarobin. If there is a great deal of thickening of the skin, painting with alkaline caustics may be necessary.

The use of X-rays and radium in the treatment of skin diseases requires special apparatus and special training, so that only the indications for advising such treatment need be given here. This applies also to the local treatment of lupus vulgaris with ultra-violet light.

Diathermy, carbon dioxide snow and various other destructive methods are commonly employed in dermatology, but they will not be discussed, as they play very little part in the treatment of those skin conditions to which the term medical may be applied.

Formulæ for Common Local Applications

Baths (see preceding text).

Lotions.

Calamine—

Acid. Boric.		5
Calamin.		15
Zinc. Oxid.		15
Glycer.		10
Aq.	ad	200

Sulpho-Calamine—

Sulphur. Præcip.		5
Zinc. Oxid.		10
Calamin.		10
Glycer.		5
Aq.	ad	200 or 210

Ichthammol Calamine Cream—

Ichtham.	1 part
Calamin.	1 ,,
Zinc. Oxid.	1 ,,
Ol. Oliv.	1 ,,
Liq. Calc. Hydrox.	1 ,,
Adip. Lan.	4 parts

Lead and Tar—

Liq. Pic. Carb.		10
Liq. Plumb. Subacet. Fort.		10
Zinc. Oxid.		20
Glycer.		20
Aq.	ad	200

Zinc Sulphate—

Zinc. Sulph.		7
Potass. Sulphur.		7
Aq.	ad	200

(Note on application of powdery lotions.—The bottle must be thoroughly shaken and a sufficient quantity of the lotion poured into a saucer. This is further stirred with cotton wool, and then painted on the part with the wool.)

Gentian violet—

Gentian violet		2
Aq.	ad	100

To be painted on.

Carbol Fuchsin—

Carbol fuchsin		2
Aq.	ad	100

To be painted on.

Pastes.

Base.	Zinc. Oxid.		15
	Vaselin.	ad	100
	or		
	Zinc. Oxid.		15
	Vaselin.		50
	Lanolini.	ad	100

Tar Applications.

Paste.	Pic. Carb. Præp.		1 to 10
	Zinc. Oxid.		15
	Vaselin.	ad	100
Paint.	Pic. Liq.		15
	Benzen.		30
	Aceton.	ad	100

To be painted on.

Paint. Crude gasworks tar.

To be painted on in a thin varnish and powdered.

Ol. Cadin.		10
Lanolin.		10
Vaselin.	ad	30

Apply to scalp.

Ichthyol and Silver Nitrate—

Argent. Nit.		10
Ichtham.		20
Aq.	ad	200

To be painted on.

Silver Nitrate—

(*a*) Aqueous.	Argent. Nit.		1
	Aq.	ad	200

To be applied as a wet dressing.

(*b*) Spirit.	Argent. Nit.		2 to 5
	Sp. Æther. Nitros.	ad	100

To be painted on.

Scalp Lotions—

(*a*) Resorcin.	Resorcin.		4
	Acid. Salicyl.		4
	Ol. Ricin.		3 to 4
	Sp. Meth. Indust.	ad	100
(*b*) Lactic.	Acid. Lact.		12
	Ol. Ricin.		6
	Sp. Meth. Indust.	ad	100

Scalp Ointment—

Acid. Salicyl.		0·5 to 1
Vaselin.	ad	30

Chrysarobin—

Ointment.	Chrysarob.		5 to 10
	Vaselin.	ad	100
Paste.	Chrysarob.		5 to 10
	Zinc. Oxid.		15
	Vaselin.	ad	100

Dreuw's Ointment—

Chrysarob.		20
Acid. Salicyl.		10
Ol. Rusc.		10
Sap. Moll.		30
Vaselin.	ad	100

To be rubbed in (never apply spread on calico).

Peeling Paste—

Betanaph.		2
Sulphur. Præcip.		4
Balsam. Peruv.		15
Vaselin.	ad	30

Zinc Ichthyol Jelly.—Place solid cubes of jelly in pan and heat till cubes liquefy. Allow to cool sufficiently and then paint on skin. Flick over lightly with cotton wool so that wool fibres adhere to painted surface. Apply a second coat of jelly and repeat flicking with wool. To remove, peel off.

BACTERIAL INFECTIONS

Impetigo Contagiosa.—This is a superficial inflammatory condition produced by infection with a streptococcus. It is one of the commonest skin diseases and as a rule its treatment presents no difficulty, but from time to time cases are encountered which run a prolonged course and require more than ordinary care. The lesion in impetigo is a bulla, the fluid content of which is capable of producing fresh lesions. Crusting due to the coagulation of the bulla fluid is a marked feature. The aim of treatment is therefore to kill off the infecting streptococcus without damaging the skin in the process, to absorb the exudate, thus minimizing the risk of the development of further lesions, and to render the skin in the neighbourhood of the disease as aseptic as possible.

Starch poultices should be applied at the commencement of treatment in every case which is at all extensive. The effect of the poultice is to soften the crusts and so permit of their easy removal; it also absorbs infectious exudate, thus lessening the possibility of the development of fresh lesions. The poultices should be renewed three times daily and should be continued until exudation has become much reduced or has ceased altogether. It is often an advantage to use a 2 per cent. aqueous solution of gentian violet in conjunction with the poultices. This solution is painted on once daily, the application being made both to the lesions and to the surrounding skin. The part should be washed at least once daily to remove any crusts and to prevent the accumulation of medicaments on the skin.

When the exudative phase has ceased a 1 per cent. ammoniated mercury paste should be used, and it is advisable to employ a fairly stiff paste, *i.e.*, containing at least 30 per cent. of powder in the greasy base.

The poultices will, of course, have to be bandaged in position, and in the case of the face, which is the region most commonly affected, a mask will be necessary. It is usually advisable to apply the ammoniated mercury paste spread on strips of calico or linen or as a mask. The main risk of spread in impetigo arises from scratching and from the contamination of the sheets and pillows with infected discharge. It is therefore of the utmost importance that the affected part should be covered at night even in cases in which it may not be convenient to have bandages applied during the day.

In young children impetiginous lesions situated on the upper lip and on the chin may be difficult to eradicate because of persistent nasal discharge, salivation and contamination with food. It is in these areas that elastoplast is useful. The part should first be painted with 2 per cent. gentian violet, the elastoplast being applied afterwards. The area may also be dabbed with a 10 per cent. solution of silver nitrate in water two or three times daily. Children suffering from impetigo also tend to infect the nail folds, and here occlusive wet dressings with 1 per cent. boric lotion are most suitable in the early stages, and an ammoniated mercury paste in the healing stages.

The treatment of impetigo of the scalp is similar to that on non-hairy areas, but it is essential to clip or shave the hair on and around the affected areas. In severe cases the entire scalp should be shaved, and in children this might almost be advised as a routine procedure in all but the most limited eruptions. It is not easy to apply starch poultices to the scalp unless a fairly large area of hair is clipped or shaved. In the occasional cases of impetigo affecting the adult scalp, this can sometimes be avoided by dabbing on frequently an antiseptic astringent of 5 per cent. silver nitrate and 10 per cent. ichthyol in water in the exudative stage, the hair being clipped only in the immediate vicinity of the lesions. A 1 or 2 per cent. ammoniated mercury vaseline can be used when the lesions have been dried by the lotion. In a certain number of cases of impetigo of the scalp there is also an infection with the pediculus capitis, and until the parasitic element is eradicated the impetigo will persist. The pediculosis must first be treated with paraffin soaks before commencing to deal with the impetigo. Severe cases of impetigo of the scalp, especially when associated with pediculosis, are sometimes complicated by adenitis of the cervical glands, but incision is seldom required and the glands usually subside under hot wet dressings of 10 per cent. ichthyol in water.

In the average case of impetigo no general treatment is required, and vaccines are never necessary. A proportion of children, however, tend to have frequent recurrences affecting the face, scalp, hands, knees and feet, and when this occurs the general condition of the child must be taken into consideration and measures adopted to improve the nutrition and general health. In the poorer classes one need not hesitate to hospitalize such children over a period of weeks. It should be remembered that the home surroundings may be the main factor in the causation of such recurrent cases, and the help of the Public Health Authorities may have to be sought to improve them. In such recurring cases an underlying scabies must not be overlooked.

Furunculosis.—By furunculosis is meant a recurring deep staphylococcal infection of the hair follicles and sebaceous glands. The inflammatory reaction produced by such infections may eventually extend to involve the whole of the true skin, and adjacent lesions may coalesce, resulting in a greater or less degree of tissue destruction. Scar formation is an invariable result.

This brief pathological summary has been given in order to define the condition from a similar, more superficial staphylococcal infection affecting the same areas, which is more appropriately termed folliculitis, and is dealt with under the heading " Sycosis."

The treatment of individual furuncles is a simple matter. The overlying skin can be painted with 2 per cent. aqueous solution of gentian violet once daily, and hot wet dressings of 10 per cent. ichthyol in water can be applied every two to three hours. This is continued until the furuncle bursts or has been opened surgically and the core of dead tissue has been extruded or removed and the discharge has subsided. In addition to this treatment, cupping of the lesions may be performed twice daily, and this procedure, although painful, very materially accelerates the course of the furuncle. Commencing furuncles are often successfully aborted by the application of elastoplast in the following way: A ring of the plaster is cut and fitted round the small swelling and then a circle of the plaster is applied to cover the entire surface. Such a dressing protects the lesion to a great extent from friction and pressure and affords it some support.

A full skin dose of X-rays is often successful in causing the rapid disappearance of a furuncle, and may be given with benefit any time up to the period when the lesion is obviously subsiding.

Difficulty arises when the lesions recur. If recurrence takes place more or less on the same part of the body, the treatment is easier than in cases where the lesions keep on appearing at widely separated sites. In the former case, keeping the infected area continuously painted with a mild antiseptic such as gentian violet will reduce surface contamination and lessen the risk of re-inoculation with organisms. Avoidance of friction to the area is most important. If the part is covered with hair, it should be kept shaved, and this applies to the scalp as well as to the covered areas. The commonest sites for recurring furuncles are the back of the neck, the forearms, the buttocks and the axillæ. In the axillæ the lesion is quite commonly situated in the sweat glands and not in the pilo-sebaceous system.

When the furuncles continue to appear irregularly on widely separated sites, local antiseptic prophylaxis is of less value than general measures calculated to increase the skin resistance to the organism. Vaccines are useful in a number of cases, and a mixed stock staphylococcal vaccine, containing a number of different strains, is usually as efficient as an autogenous or toxoid one. Injections of manganese are widely used, but their value is doubtful and the injections are painful. A liberal supply of vitamins must be included in the diet, and it is advisable for the patient to rest as much as possible. Daily, or twice daily, immersion in a potassium permanganate bath is useful, and avoidance of friction is most important.

In spite of these active and prophylactic measures, cases may drag on for a period of months, and if this occurs it is justifiable to give a period of complete rest in bed if the patient's circumstances allow him to do so.

In every case of furunculosis the patient should undergo a general medical examination to determine whether the furunculosis may not be dependent on some chronic constitutional disorder, particularly diabetes.

Sycosis.—Sycosis is a staphylococcal infection of the orifices of the hair follicles, and it occurs exclusively on areas where the hair is well developed, *i.e.*, the condition does not affect areas covered with lanugo hair. The characteristic feature of sycosis is the repetition of multiple superficial pustules on a localized area, and this is a constantly recurring phenomenon which persists for months and sometimes for years. As a result of the prolonged inflammation and contamination of the skin surface, an infective dermatitis becomes early associated with the pustular eruption, and in its fully developed state sycosis is a combination of infective dermatitis and folliculitis. The term sycosis is usually reserved for this type of eruption when it affects the beard region, but an exactly similar condition can affect the scalp, eyebrows and any other region covered with strong hair, and treatment is the same for all areas. The follicular lesions develop much less readily if the affected area is kept shaved, and they cease to develop if epilation of the area is performed. Unfortunately when the hair commences to regrow after epilation the infection may reassert itself and the follicular lesions recommence.

Treatment consists in keeping the area shaved or in producing complete temporary epilation and thereafter applying mild antiseptics. Unfortunately an area of skin affected with this type of eruption is often in a hypersensitive condition, so that it does not tolerate chemical applications in the same concentration as the normal skin, and in addition to this, grease is not the most suitable application because it tends to favour pustulation.

During the first few days of treatment the removal of hair may have to be limited to clipping, as it may not be possible to shave the acutely inflamed skin, but shaving should be performed at the earliest opportunity and the area should be kept shaved. As grease is not well tolerated by the majority of cases, the local treatment is limited to painting with one or other of the aniline dyes, and the application of starch poultices ; in fact, it is that already outlined for the early stages of impetigo (see p. 162). When the inflammation has begun to subside with treatment, and this may take weeks to achieve, crude gasworks tar is a very useful application. It is to be noted that tar frequently produces pustulation, and it might be thought that it would be definitely contraindicated in sycosis. Certainly if it is applied in the form of an ointment or paste, pustulation is almost always aggravated, but its application in the crude form as a paint is much less frequently attended by pustulation, and in most cases is beneficial. Probably the reason why the inflamed skin can tolerate crude tar is that the tendency to follicular infection has subsided and the actual lesion which benefits from the tar is the complicating dermatitis.

Although grease is as a rule an unsatisfactory application, there is one ointment which is found to be beneficial in early cases, and it is also useful in dealing with commencing recurrences. This is a proprietary preparation, Ung. Quinolor Co. (Squibb), containing chlorquinilin and benzoyl peroxide. It is probable that it is the quiniline which is effective, as ointments containing benzoyl peroxide alone are not efficient.

Epilation with X-rays is necessary in a large percentage of cases affecting the beard region, and a full epilating dose is given. There is often an increase in the severity of the symptoms during the first week after X-ray treatment, but by the third week, when epilation has commenced, there is a very marked diminution in the inflammation and usually a return of the skin surface to a slightly pink but otherwise normal appearance. It will remain in this condition for a few weeks, but when the hair commences to grow again a small area of pustulation may recur and spread to involve the whole of the area originally affected. Such small areas can be again X-rayed, care being taken to screen the surrounding skin up to the edge of the area of recurrence. If the area of sycosis is a very limited one, epilation may be carried out with forceps.

Vaccine therapy has not proved useful in this condition, probably owing to the fact that the lesions are superficially situated as compared with furunculosis. Staphylococcal anti-virus applications do not seem to have any specific effect on the disease, but in some cases they act as soothing dressings in the same way as starch poultices.

PARASITIC INFECTIONS

Ringworm.—Infection of the skin with the various types of ringworm fungus produces a number of eruptions which are more or less characteristic for the type of infecting fungus and for the site affected. The treatment of such conditions is simply directed towards the destruction of the parasite, and the difficulties encountered are due to its situation in the skin, its normal resistance to antiseptics and the susceptibility of the skin—and particularly the inflamed skin—to chemical irritation.

Ringworm of the Body.—When a fungus infects the non-hairy non-flexural surfaces its destruction is a fairly easy matter. With the exception of the palms and soles where the stratum corneum is thick, the fungus is situated on and very close to the surface, is easily accessible to antiseptics and the area can readily be cleansed. In tinea corporis, therefore, repeated painting at daily intervals or every second day with a $2\frac{1}{2}$ per cent. tincture of iodine is usually all that is required to eradicate the condition in from ten days to a fortnight. Ungentum iodidi rubbed in twice daily is equally efficient. In infections with virulent fungus derived from an animal source, it may be necessary to commence treatment with starch poultices and gentian violet to allay the acute and often purulent inflammation, and to use iodine in the later stages. As an alternative to the iodine treatment an ointment containing 6 per cent. benzoic acid and 3 per cent. salicylic acid may be prescribed, to be rubbed in twice daily.

Ringworm of the scalp presents a much more difficult problem because the fungus is present inside and surrounding the hair shaft in its intra-follicular portion, and in this situation it is exceedingly difficult for antiseptics to reach it. It is therefore necessary to epilate the scalp either by means of X-rays or thallium in order to get rid of the infected hairs, and so to permit the entrance of antiseptics into the follicles. The technique of X-ray treatment of the scalp is difficult, and as it requires considerable knowledge of superficial X-ray therapy it need not be dealt with here.

Epilation with thallium acetate is an easy procedure in children, but one which must be carried out with scrupulous attention to detail, because thallium is a dangerous drug producing severe constitutional symptoms and possibly death if wrongly used. Thallium has gained an unfortunate reputation in some parts of this country because of one dispensing error which had a fatal result. A similar error in the dispensing of arsenic or strychnine might have led to equally disastrous results without these drugs falling into disrepute, and the toxic properties of thallium need not, therefore, contraindicate its use. The criticisms which have been levelled against thallium are applicable to all poisonous substances employed in medicine.

The dose of thallium is calculated for each individual case, the child being given 8·5 mgm. of thallium acetate for each kilogram of naked body-weight. The calculated amount is given in a single dose and is not repeated. Following its administration a mild constitutional upset is noticed three or four days afterwards in about 30 per cent. of children. This takes the form of temporary lassitude associated with rheumatic pains in the legs. The symptoms last only for a few days. From seventeen to twenty-one days after the administration of the epilating dose the hair commences to loosen and can be plucked out painlessly all over the scalp; the eyebrows are not affected. Compared with X-ray epilation the fall of hair due to thallium occurs earlier and is less complete, and the regrowth of hair takes place more rapidly. With thallium it is therefore essential to supervise the epilation of the scalp to make certain that it is thorough, and to carry out antiseptic measures in a most careful and vigorous fashion. Thallium should not be administered to a child weighing over 30 kg. unless in very special circumstances, when a dose may be given to children weighing up to 36 kg. It is a drug which must never be given to adolescents or adults for purposes of epilation because of the severe toxic symptoms which result.

Following a dose of thallium, epilation will occur and regrowth of the hair to a length of about half an inch will take place during a period of approximately three months. In addition to epilating measures, antiseptic treatment has to be applied to the scalp twice daily and the scalp must be washed once daily during the entire period of depilation and regrowth.

The treatment of a case of ringworm of the scalp would therefore be as follows :—

After a diagnosis has been made, the hair is clipped short all over the scalp, and this may reveal the presence of hitherto unsuspected patches of disease. The scalp is then treated twice daily with a 10 per cent. sulphur ointment, and it is an advantage to paint on 2 to 5 per cent. tincture of iodine twice weekly in place of the ointment. Epilating measures are carried out as soon as possible. The antiseptic treatment is continued during the period of epilation and regrowth until the new hair has reached a length of about half an inch. Treatment and washing are then both stopped altogether for a period of three weeks, at the end of which time the scalp is examined. If any fungus has escaped destruction by the antiseptic the disease will become apparent during the three weeks in which treatment has been discontinued. During the entire course of treatment the child should wear a paper lining inside the cap, and this should be renewed daily, the old lining being burned. All contacts should be carefully examined for the presence of disease, and, of course, an infected child must not attend school.

The infiltrated lesions produced by infection with virulent fungi derived from animals do not require epilation because they cure themselves in from three to four months' time by the production of a natural immunity to the fungus. All that is necessary in treatment is the relief of pain by starch poultices or wet dressings in the early stages, and the limitation of secondary infection by means of a 1 per cent. ammoniated mercury paste when the phase of infiltration is subsiding. Similar measures are used for ringworm of the beard, a condition which has to be differentiated from sycosis, and one which, like kerion, runs a self-limiting course calling only for palliative treatment.

Ringworm of the Body Folds (Epidermophytosis).—Infection with the epidermophyton fungus occurs in the areas between the toes, in the groins and less frequently in other body folds. The infection may extend from the interdigital areas to involve the soles of the feet, and the palms of the hands may also become affected. A great variety of antiseptics have been used in the treatment of this particular type of fungus infection, but while many are efficient it cannot be said that any one of them is outstanding. Tincture of iodine in strengths from 0·5 to 5 per cent. may be used according to the tolerance of the individual skin, and swabbing the area with a 3 to 5 per cent. solution of silver nitrate in spirits ether nitrosi is a clean and useful method. If there is marked secondary infection with pyogenic organisms, a 2 per cent. solution of gentian violet may be used in the early stages. When the condition has reached a dry scaly stage, an ointment containing 6 per cent. benzoic acid and 3 per cent. salicylic acid should be used in preference to lotions. Should the fungus produce an intense inflammation of the skin, the more vigorous remedies may have to be withheld for the time being.

Soothing applications such as starch poultices or wet dressings of boric acid solution or a solution of 10 per cent. ichthyol in water should be used until the acute inflammation — which is often associated with secondary pyogenic infection—has subsided.

In the acute vesicular pompholyx-like eruptions which affect the soles, palms, and the sides of the fingers, wet dressings of ½ per cent. silver nitrate in water are most beneficial. They are applied twice daily for three or four days, and usually cause rapid desiccation of the vesicles and prevent the appearance of fresh ones. At the end of that time a 1 per cent. ichthyol paste is used and finally the benzoic and salicylic vaseline should be applied. Infections of the feet are extremely stubborn and resistant to treatment, and it is doubtful whether the infection can ever be completely eradicated from this area. When the condition seems to be in abeyance the individual should be advised to apply an antiseptic, such as tincture of iodine, periodically to the affected areas.

Ringworm of the groin is much more amenable to treatment than ringworm of the feet, and if thoroughly treated its disappearance can be assured. In all cases of epidermophyton infection, care must be taken to disinfect wearing apparel, and especially all the articles with which the infected person comes into contact in the bathroom, *i.e.*, bath mat, floor, etc. In a private house there is no need to anticipate a spread of the infection, provided reasonable precautions are taken. The disease is usually acquired from the floor of dressing rooms, swimming baths, Turkish baths, *plages* and, in the case of the groin, from lavatory seats. When an object or room has once become infected it is often a difficult matter to secure complete destruction of the parasite even by the use of strong disinfecting measures. The condition is so prevalent that no attempt at isolation of cases can be made as the number of very slight unrecognized cases far outweighs the number of cases which exhibit active signs of disease.

Ringworm of the Nails.—Infection of the toe nails and finger nails may occur as an isolated event, or the nails may become infected from already existing ringworm lesions on other parts of the body. The difficulties in treatment are comparable to those met with in ringworm of the scalp, and as in the case of the hair, removal of the nail is essential to rapid cure. Surgical removal is probably best, although it may be difficult in some cases on account of the friability of the nail plate. After surgical removal strong antiseptic paints, such as 5 per cent. tincture of iodine, are applied to the nail bed and nail fold as soon as possible, and are continued during the whole period of regrowth of the nail. The patient must be informed of the difficulty of destroying the fungus and of the risk of reinfection of the new nail plate. He should be advised to take this risk, however, because if the nail is not removed there is no chance of the disease being cured or disappearing spontaneously. Infection of other parts of the body from an infected nail, although a possibility, is uncommon, and experience shows that an individual suffering from ringworm of the nails need not be considered a grave source of danger to others.

Scabies.—Scabies is a disease which, if neglected, can produce considerable incapacity in large masses of people. The accompanying irritation alone is often a serious feature on account of loss of sleep and consequent loss of efficiency, and the impetigo and furunculosis which may complicate the disease can cause incapacity of a major type. The economic effect of this is self-evident, and under war conditions the consequences of the disease may be serious from a military point of view.

During an epidemic the requirements of treatment are speed, efficiency and cheapness, and treatment with sulphur ointment meets these better than any other method. There are a number of alternatives designed to shorten treatment which are admirable in individual cases but unsuitable for all, and the sulphur treatment alone will be described.

The full treatment is as follows: The patient steeps in a bath for twenty minutes, lathers all over with soft soap and scrubs the affected areas with a soft nail brush to open up as far as possible the burrows of the acarus. Thereafter a 5 per cent. sulphur ointment is rubbed in thoroughly all over the body with the exception of the head. The inunction is repeated at intervals of twelve hours, till six applications have been made. If convenient the ointment may be spread on strips of calico, which are then bandaged on to legs, feet, arms and hands, the lethal effect on the parasite being thus enhanced. Twelve hours after the last treatment a bath is given, clean underwear worn and the bedding disinfected. In mild cases four, or in urgent circumstances two, inunctions only may be given.

If there is a severe complicating impetigo it should be treated in the usual way for a few days before sulphur ointment treatment is begun.

The patient is usually free from itch after the first or second inunction, and he remains so unless the sulphur irritates his skin. A few patients develop a mild dermatitis after the six applications, but this yields readily to a calamine or lead and zinc lotion used for a few days after cessation of the sulphur treatment. Recurrence of the irritation in a week to ten days after treatment has been completed means a recurrence of the disease, either due to inefficient treatment or to reinfection.

It is important to examine and, if necessary, to treat all contacts and also to make sure that the infected bedding has been adequately disinfected.

Pediculosis.—*Pediculosis capitis* is much less common now than formerly. It is best treated with paraffin soaks. The forehead, ears and neck are first protected with zinc ointment, then, with no preliminary washing, the hair and scalp are soaked with paraffin. Strips of calico soaked in paraffin are applied to the scalp and covered over with an improvised cap of jaconet or with a rubber bathing cap. The soaks are repeated after twelve hours, and according to the result they may be reapplied at twelve-hourly intervals for a further twenty-four hours. After the last application has been removed the scalp is washed. The adult parasites are readily killed by this method, and the nits can later be removed by combing with a small tooth comb which has been dipped in weak acetic acid.

If the infection is severe, the nits numerous, and an extensive impetigo present, it may be necessary as a preliminary measure to cut, and subsequently shave, the scalp (see Impetigo). No matter how impetiginous the scalp may be or how severe the accompanying adenitis of the cervical glands, the pediculosis should be dealt with in the first instance. The associated impetigo and adenitis are treated in the ordinary way, but it is seldom necessary to incise the glands.

Pediculosis pubis is treated by one or two inunctions of unguentum hydrargyri, and it is advisable to shave the hair at the commencement of treatment. It should be remembered that the hair of the natal fold, trunk, axillæ and eyebrows and lids can be infected with this parasite.

Pediculosis corporis is treated in the same manner as scabies, and a bath followed by one or two inunctions of sulphur ointment, and disinfection of the underwear, is usually sufficient to eradicate the infection.

ACNE

While there is little doubt that the development of acne is ultimately dependent on the functions of the endocrine glands, the main treatment of the condition is essentially local. Overactivity of the sebaceous glands seems to be the important local predisposing factor in the development of the condition. It results in the formation of the comedones, fosters the growth of pyogenic organisms and so predisposes to pustule formation.

The local treatment of acne consists of (1) methods to keep the skin surface as free from oil as possible, (2) the external application of drugs which seem to have an inhibitory effect on oil formation, (3) the administration of X-rays to diminish the activity of the sebaceous glands, and (4) internal treatment for the reduction of the functional activity of the sebaceous glands. Frequent swabbing of the affected area with ether or surgical spirit may be advised to remove the surface grease. Once daily, preferably at night, the face is very thoroughly washed with hot water and sulphur soap and the lather massaged into the skin for a few minutes. The lather is then removed, the face dried gently, and thereafter the following lotion dabbed on :—

℞	Zinc. Sulph.		ʒi
	Potass. Sulphur.		ʒi
	Aq.	ad	℥iv

The lotion leaves a powder on the skin and this is allowed to remain on over night and is washed off in the morning. After a week or ten days of this treatment the following peeling paste may be used :—

℞	Betanaph.		2 gm.
	Sulph. Præcip.		4 ,,
	Balsam. Peruv.		15 ,,
	Vaselin.	ad	30 ,,

The paste is smeared on the affected areas at night and removed in the morning with olive oil. Immediately after its application it causes a good deal of nipping and burning, which lasts for about a quarter of an hour and then subsides. The effect of the paste is that of an antiseptic and counter-irritant, and it causes the skin to become slightly inflamed and subsequently to peel. This desquamating effect clears the mouths of the follicles, thus facilitating the removal of black-heads and dammed-up sebaceous material, and, in virtue of the antiseptic action of the paste, surface infection is reduced. It is not as a rule possible to apply the peeling paste for more than two consecutive nights because of the amount of inflammation it produces, and to allay this an ichthyol paste is used every third night. After about three weeks' preliminary treatment on these lines X-ray treatment may be commenced, and while this is being given it is better to stop all active local treatment and merely to use mild applications such as calamine lotion. It may be said that X-ray therapy is essential at some stage in the treatment of all but the mildest cases of acne. X-rays are best administered in fractional doses once weekly, and a course consists of four to six doses spread over a period of six weeks, the total amount of X-rays given during that period being not more than one and a half skin doses. The X-rays have an inhibitory action on the sebaceous glands, thus reducing the amount of oil secretion, a stimulating action on the epidermal cells and an antiseptic action on the whole of the exposed surface. This antiseptic action is, of course, only partial, but the inhibition of organismal growth must be beneficial and play some part in the effect produced.

Internal measures are limited to the administration of iron, the regulation of the digestion and the reduction of carbohydrate intake, especially the actual sugar content of the diet.

Vaccine therapy is only useful in cases in which deep-seated pustulation is a feature and is of no value when comedones, superficial pustules and seborrhœa are the main features.

Recently, extracts of anterior pituitary, notably Antuitrin S. (Parke Davis), have been used with some success, especially in those cases occurring in girls where there is a history of exacerbation of the eruption just before or during a period.

It is important to see cases of acne at frequent intervals whether or not X-ray treatment is being given, because, to achieve rapid improvement, all large blackheads should be removed from the affected area and pustules incised with a narrow-bladed knife.

It is also necessary to see that the scalp is washed regularly because it is invariably greasy, and often scaly. Organismal contamination in these circumstances is abundant, and the chance of pustulation due to infection from the scalp is increased.

ROSACEA

Rosacea is almost always associated with one or more of the following conditions: A certain amount of seborrhœa of the face; seborrhœa and pityriasis of the scalp; a mild degree of gastric indigestion; symptoms indicating slight ovarian dysfunction. The local predisposing factors are a marked tendency to capillary flushing, very open pores and an increased virulence in the organisms which normally contaminate the surface. Treatment may therefore have to be directed towards the correction of one or all of these contributing causes. A sulpho-calomin lotion is probably the best local application, and it may be helpful to alternate it day about with either a 1 per cent. sulphur paste or a 1 per cent. ichthyol paste. In addition to daily treatment, weekly fractional doses of X-rays given in the same way as for acne are almost essential for rapid cure. If possible the individual should avoid undue exposure to sunlight, heat and cold winds. The scalp must be kept clean by frequent washing, and, if necessary, the application of a 2 per cent. salicylic vaseline or a lotion containing 1 drachm each of salicylic acid, resorcin and castor oil in 6 oz. of spirit.

The diet should be plain, all spicy foods should be eliminated from it, and the patient should be instructed to allow all hot fluids to become cool before they are ingested. Some cases will be found to improve if alkali is given after their main meals, and in others the administration of dilute hydrochloric acid is helpful. Neither the eruption nor the history may give any indication as to which of these remedies will be efficacious, and it is hardly worth while to carry out a test meal to ascertain the exact state of the gastric secretion.

Vaccine therapy is of little value in rosacea even when pustulation is marked.

If rosacea is treated in its early stages the affected skin will return to normal and the vascular dilatation will subside. If, however, the eruption has been present for some time a permanent capillary dilatation is almost inevitable, and the only way to diminish the redness in such cases is to obliterate as many of the dilated vessels as possible by diathermy coagulation. The results of diathermy coagulation in suitable cases are often most satisfactory to the patient if the treatment is persevered with over a period of months.

DERMATITIS

Dermatitis is a specific type of skin reaction characterized by superficial inflammatory œdema of the epidermis associated with vesicle formation. After a longer or shorter time this reaction passes through a scaly phase towards healing. It is an exceedingly common type of eruption and one which requires the utmost care in its treatment. A skin which is affected by dermatitis is one which has shown an idiosyncrasy to some irritant. This being so, a further idiosyncrasy to one or more of the drugs which are commonly used in the treatment of the disease is encountered in a number of cases. The irritant factor which has caused the eruption may continue to act for a considerable time after treatment has been instituted, and for this reason the fact that treatment has been commenced does not ensure that the eruption will from that time forward proceed towards healing. Sometimes the patient carries out the treatment prescribed in a most inefficient way, or else he exposes the eruption to irritation with dust or liquids or mechanical trauma while treatment is being carried out, and these injuries, however slight, will counteract any beneficial effects which may have been obtained. There is no reason why a large proportion of cases should not be fairly easily and quickly cured if treatment is commenced soon after the appearance of the rash, and provided a correct diagnosis of the type of dermatitis has been made. Recrudescence and recurrence are common features of dermatitis. In a number of cases they might be avoided if an existing eruption were treated till complete cure was obtained, and if adequate precautions were taken to protect the area of skin which had recently been affected from obvious sources of irritation. It is only too common to observe a patient who applies treatment enthusiastically until the rash has almost disappeared, and then, satisfied with the partial result obtained, he discontinues treatment, neglects the care of his skin, and wonders why the eruption flares up again. It is important to ensure a period of rest and protection for an area of skin which has been the seat of dermatitis for some weeks or even months after it has been cured.

Dermatitis can be divided into two main groups, first, those cases in which an irritant affects an idiosyncratic skin from the outside, and secondly, cases in which the irritant reaches the idiosyncratic skin via the blood stream. Fortunately the external cases predominate numerically, for when the irritant is derived from within, treatment is much more difficult and the tendency to recurrence greater.

Dermatitis due to External Causes.—*Dermatitis due to Light.*—This is a most distressing condition, for obviously it is difficult for an individual to avoid entirely exposure to sunlight. The local treatment consists in the application of a 1 per cent. ichthyol paste at night as a healing measure, and during the day an ointment containing 1 to 2 per cent. quinine sulphate may be used as a protection against the sun's rays. Another application which sometimes affords protection in mild cases is a 2 or 3 per cent. solution of tannic acid in equal parts of spirit and water. Apart from treating the skin, all reasonable precautions must be taken to avoid direct exposure to sunlight.

Internal Treatment.—A proportion of mild cases are greatly relieved by a course of peptone injections in early or middle spring, a procedure which seems to increase the skin resistance to light irritation and one which should be tried in all cases. A 10 per cent. solution is used and the injection given twice weekly subcutaneously over a period of three weeks, the initial dose being 0·5 c.c., and this is gradually increased to 2 c.c. A small number of cases benefit if wheat is excluded from the diet, and in them it would appear that some chemical complex in the wheat sensitizes the epidermal cells to sunlight. Other dietary modifications do not seem to have any influence on the condition.

Dermatitis due to External Chemical Irritation.—If the external application of a chemical to the skin has produced dermatitis, the eruption, if left to itself, may take as long as two months to subside, provided all further contact with the irritant has ceased. Under treatment the rash should disappear in a much shorter period. If, however, it has been present for some considerable time prior to the commencement of treatment, the skin may have undergone anatomical and probably functional changes due to the prolonged inflammation, and these changes retard the healing process. The object of treatment is to provide a protective soothing covering to the affected area. If the eruption is in an acute vesicular exudative stage, starch poultices are indicated. Whenever the exudative phase has subsided the application of a 1 per cent. ichthyol paste spread on linen or calico is all that is required. If secondary infection is present the methods used in the treatment of infective dermatitis will have to be instituted (see below). If hypertrophy of the skin has taken place as a result of a long-continued inflammation, it will be necessary to use crude gasworks tar, and perhaps X-rays as well, to aid the dissipation of the chronic dermal infiltration.

Every effort should be made to determine accurately the chemical cause of the eruption, and for this purpose a careful history is necessary followed by patch tests with all the likely irritants suspected of being of ætiological importance. Specific desensitization to a discovered irritant, while it has been successfully carried out in isolated cases, is not as yet a procedure which is generally serviceable.

Infective Dermatitis.—As the cause of this condition is almost always a streptococcus, staphylococcus or yeast, the treatment is essentially antiseptic and is in many ways similar to that employed in impetigo and sycosis. The type of rash varies according to the situation of the dermatitis, but on any area it may present an exudative stage followed by a dry scaly stage. In the exudative phase gentian violet and starch poultices may be used, or wet dressings of ½ per cent. silver nitrate in water. Crude tar may be tried as soon as the exudative phase has subsided. An ichthyol paste can be used for a day or two between the discontinuation of the starch, gentian violet, or wet dressings, and the commencement of the crude tar. It is remarkable how an acutely inflamed but only slightly exudative patch of infective dermatitis will tolerate crude tar treatment and improve under it. It is important in infective dermatitis situated in the flexures to continue treatment until every vestige of inflammation in the deepest part of the fold has disappeared. X-ray treatment is useful for patches of infective dermatitis affecting the backs of the hands and the dorsum of the feet, but it is not very helpful in flexural infective dermatitis. It is to be noted that flexural fungus infections will stand much stronger concentrations of antiseptics than dermatitis of the flexures due to bacterial infection (see Ringworm). Infective dermatitis, like sycosis, may be intolerant to grease for considerable periods during the course of treatment.

Dermatitis due to Internal Causes.—It is extremely rare to discover the exact cause of a dermatitis which, from its distribution, course and history, is obviously of internal origin. Occasionally one single article of diet is found to be responsible, but usually no causal relationship can be established between the diet and the rash. The removal of areas of focal sepsis may be followed by the rapid disappearance of the rash, but this is noted only in isolated cases. While the diet should be investigated and attention paid to areas of focal sepsis in every case, active general treatment may resolve itself into carrying out procedures to ensure free elimination, *i.e.*, the administration of fluids in quantity, saline diuretics and colon lavage. Local treatment consists in the application of tar preparations in the form of lotions or pastes, and later as crude tar, and the avoidance of friction which tends to localize the eruption and possibly to precipitate fresh patches. Grease sensitivity is much less marked in dermatitis arising from internal causes. When it is noted in the more acute phases of the eruption which would otherwise be treated with pastes, the use of a lead and tar lotion or ½ per cent. silver nitrate soaks may be necessary until it is in a condition deemed suitable for crude tar. Localized patches of internal dermatitis sometimes respond in a most satisfactory way to X-ray therapy, and this is especially so in the chronic lichenified patches of dermatitis seen in elderly people usually situated on the nape of the neck, the sacral region, the thighs or the outer aspects of the forearms.

Infantile Dermatitis.—Although a great deal of work has been done to ascertain the role of diet in the production of this type of eruption, it is only in exceptional instances that a specific protein can be legitimately incriminated as the cause. Nevertheless the condition seems to be undoubtedly associated in some vague manner with the gastro-intestinal tract, and while gastro-intestinal symptoms are by no means a frequent accompaniment, alteration or modification of the diet seems to be necessary in many cases as an adjuvant to local treatment. In practice it is advisable to change the diet completely in every case, and to ensure that the feeds are given properly and at regular intervals. As a substitute for fresh milk a dried milk preparation, either human or bovine, is probably the best type to use. If goat's milk is available it should be tried, and increasing the fat content of cow's milk by adding 1 oz. of suet in a muslin bag to 1 pint of milk and boiling for twenty minutes makes a mixture which is often well tolerated. The addition of a little citrate of magnesia to the milk may also help. Orange juice aggravates the eruption in a number of cases, and it is perhaps wise to omit it from the diet and substitute grape fruit juice, tomato juice or spinach strainings. The daily supply of vitamins A and D should be ensured by suitable additions. Syrup of figs should be given twice weekly, and in older babies the bowel may be washed out.

The local treatment consists in the application of tar preparations, the protection of the affected skin with bandages and the immobilization of the arms and legs with splints. Such restraint is a most important feature because a scratch habit is almost always present in infantile dermatitis, and scratching with the hands and feet and rubbing on the bedding greatly aggravates the eruption. In the vesicular stage a lead and tar lotion should be used as a wet dressing, and when the eruption has dried the lotion may be replaced by a 1 per cent. tar paste. Crude tar may finally be used, and it may be applied to large areas of skin, for it is unusual to find infants suffering from infantile dermatitis intolerant to tar.

Besnier's Prurigo.—By this term is meant the chronic recurrent dermatitis which develops in childhood and adolescence often as a sequel to infantile dermatitis, and which affects the flexures of the knees and elbows, the forehead and the sides of the neck. In some cases it develops imperceptibly from an infantile dermatitis, and it is the type of skin eruption which is associated with asthma. Skin tests and elimination diets have proved most disappointing in the investigation of such cases. Occasionally the eruption has been shown to be due to contact substances such as hair, fur, flock or feathers, but in the majority of cases the cause remains as much a mystery as the cause of the asthma which so often accompanies the skin eruption or alternates with it. A definite and striking feature of the condition is the well-marked nervous irritability and suppressed anxiety which is exhibited by many of the cases. In addition to this nervous element, the skin has the capacity to develop dermatitis if it is scratched.

Local treatment resolves itself into the application of crude tar as soon as the state of the eruption will permit, and this must be continued for a number of weeks until the maximum thinning of the affected skin has been obtained. It is hardly ever possible to bring the skin completely back to a normal texture if the disease has been present for any length of time. X-ray treatment is almost always successful in reducing the irritation and scratching, and it may be used from time to time. It must not be forgotten, however, that these patients have recurrences over a period of years so that there is a limit to X-ray therapy on account of the cutaneous atrophy which would result if X-rays were depended on for the alleviation of every attack.

Non-specific desensitization methods may be tried in an attempt to prevent recurrence, but the results of this treatment are not encouraging.

An individual suffering from this type of skin eruption should lead as regular and quiet a life as possible, because overwork, worry, lack of sleep and dietary indiscretions predispose to recurrence (see Asthma, p. 826). Change of climate or a change of locality is in some cases followed by relief, and it is remarkable how rapidly an acute exacerbation will subside if the patient is hospitalized.

Dermatitis due to toxic states comparable to those found or envisaged in " rheumatism " is seen to occur with increasing frequency as age advances after middle life. The eruption may be widespread or localized, and is characterized by its extreme itchiness and tendency to exacerbations and remissions. The treatment is no different from that of Besnier's prurigo, but the response to it is much more satisfactory. Free elimination is particularly beneficial, and in cases where the eruption is chronic and localized X-rays are more useful than in any other form of dermatitis.

Varicose Dermatitis.—When varicosity of the cutaneous venules of the legs has become established, the affected area is particularly prone to develop either chemical or infective dermatitis. In such cases treatment is hampered by the inefficient circulation, and the usual methods of dealing with these types of eruption must be supplemented in the majority of cases by rest in the horizontal position. Complicating ulceration is treated by wet dressings applied to the actual ulcer, a 1 per cent. ichthyol paste being applied to the surrounding skin. Adhesive plaster dressings should not be used when dermatitis accompanies ulceration.

Varicose dermatitis, when it heals, leaves the skin stretched, glazed and pigmented, and the recurrence which tends to take place when the patient starts to walk about can sometimes be avoided by the use of Unna's zinc ichthyol gelatin.

Occupational Dermatitis.—Cases of dermatitis directly due to the individual's occupation are becoming increasingly common, and such cases often take a very long time to heal, even when the extent of the eruption is limited. They may be due to chemical irritation or they may be due to mechanical or caustic injury with dust or liquids, which allows infection to gain access to the deeper layers of the epidermis with the production of an infective dermatitis. In any case, whether due to external chemical irritation or bacterial infection, internal toxic factors may commence to play a part in the production of the rash, thus prolonging its course and increasing its resistance to treatment. All these factors must be taken into account when assessing a case and deciding the line of treatment to be adopted. When a case has been cured, the question of returning to work and the risk of recurrence must be considered. The individual should be warned to take every possible precaution to avoid prolonged contact with dust or liquids and to avoid all forms of minute injury to his skin. The skin should be kept as clean as possible, and emollients, such as cold cream, mixtures of lanolin and vaseline, or glycerin and water should be used regularly after washing. No strong soaps or grease solvents should be used for cleansing purposes.

After an attack of occupational dermatitis has subsided it is wise to keep the individual off work for a period of one to two months in order to allow the previously inflamed skin to return as far as possible to normal and to recover from the effects of previous long-continued inflammation. Recurrence is practically certain when the dermatitis has been caused by a chemical irritant acting on a skin which is highly sensitive to it, and in these circumstances return to the employment in which the dermatitis was acquired may be impossible.

PRURITUS

Pruritus is a sensation which is only experienced in the skin, and we are entirely ignorant of its cause. It may accompany a local pathological change which is in its essential structure similar in detail to a condition which is not associated with pruritus. Again it is not infrequently observed that the same disease may cause intense pruritus in one patient but not in another. Pruritus is rarely continuous, and as a rule it comes in spasms at intervals of one to many hours, often without any apparent precipitating cause. Like the skin diseases with which it is associated, it can be profoundly influenced by external applications so that its point of origin is presumably superficial.

Pruritus occurs most commonly in conjunction with visible pathological changes in the skin. It may, however, arise spontaneously in areas of skin having a normal appearance and texture, and it is then presumably due to the action of some internal irritant on the cutaneous nerve endings, to some irritant acting reflexly on these, or to central nervous causes.

Pruritus associated with obvious skin disease is most intense at the onset of the eruption, or just prior to an exacerbation. It is usually alleviated when the disease itself begins to subside, and the treatment of the disease is the treatment of the pruritus. Thus in parasitic, bacterial or fungus infections antiseptics are used, in inflammation due to chemical irritation protective and cooling measures usually suffice, and in conditions due to some internal poison the removal of its source combined with free elimination relieves the pruritus. It is sometimes necessary, however, in addition to such lines of treatment, to employ specific measures to relieve the pruritus, which, on account of the scratching it causes, may be a serious obstacle in the treatment of the condition responsible for it. The symptomatic treatment of pruritus is limited to the application of lotions or pastes containing tar, with or without the addition of 1 per cent. phenol or menthol. Such applications are made frequently, and whenever possible the parts should be guarded from friction and changes in temperature. Exposure to X-rays is sometimes helpful, and in severe cases there is no objection to the administration of sedatives of the basal hypnotic class. Morphine and its derivatives should be avoided because they have a tendency to aggravate an itch after affording initial relief. The mode of action of X-rays is often a mystery, but in some cases the effect is undoubtedly psychological. Apart from obvious disease of the skin, generalized pruritus is usually seen as an isolated symptom in elderly subjects due to some internal disorder or toxæmia. A careful examination is therefore necessary in every case to discover if possible any such factor, and its rectification is usually followed by disappearance of the pruritus.

The pruritus of the elderly is frequently associated with slight atrophy of the skin, and thorough lubrication with grease or creams, along with a liberal supply of vitamins and attention to elimination by kidneys and bowel, usually brings about a cure. Here, again, X-ray exposures may be given for troublesome areas, and sparking with a high-frequency current, using a flat glass electrode, may be helpful. It is important to avoid sudden changes of skin temperature, and all garments worn next the skin must be smooth in texture. The diet in these cases must be of an easily digestible type and all spices and condiments should be forbidden. Measures should be taken to rectify any digestive errors. Hot fluids should be allowed to cool before drinking, and it is preferable to forbid alcohol.

A few cases of pruritus are met with in hysterical young women and in both men and women under middle age, associated with some definite or incipient mental disorder, including that brought about by drug habit.

Pruritus without any accompanying skin change may occur on localized areas, and the sites most commonly affected are the peri-anal region, the scrotum and the vulva. In such cases it is important to exclude the presence of any systemic disorder, and also to examine the immediate surroundings of the affected areas for any abnormality which might, by causing reflex nervous impulses, produce a sensation of pruritus. Psychological factors should not be overlooked in cases which are resistant to treatment. Any local abnormality, such as piles or enlargement of the prostate, should be dealt with. In cases of pruritus ani the bowel should be washed out because overloading of the rectum or pelvic colon may, by causing slight peri-anal venous congestion, produce the symptom. The stools may have to be examined bacteriologically and chemically, and any suggested abnormality rectified by dietary measures or lavage. In cases of pruritus vulvæ the patient may have to undergo a thorough gynæcological as well as a general medical examination.

The prolonged scratching associated with localized pruritus eventually leads to hypertrophy of the skin of the affected area.

The local treatment of pruritus consists in the application of lead and tar, carbolic or menthol lotions, the use of crude gasworks tar and the administration of X-rays. It is wise to ensure that only the smoothest material comes into contact with the affected area, and it is often helpful to keep contiguous skin surfaces from rubbing together by interposing a non-irritant silk or linen material. If hair is shaved, the shaving must be repeated because the growing hairs themselves can cause severe irritation.

Pruritus, whether localized or generalized, presents a much greater therapeutic problem when it is an isolated symptom than when it accompanies some visible cutaneous manifestation.

URTICARIA

The majority of cases of urticaria are due to intolerance to some article of diet. The eruption occurs suddenly in an acute form, and the cause is usually indicated by the history. A drastic purge and a light diet are sufficient to clear the eruption in the course of a day or two, and recurrence does not as a rule take place. Local treatment is limited to the application of an antipruritic lead and tar lotion, and the existing eruption can almost always be made to disappear rapidly by the injection of from 0·5 to 1 c.c. liq. adrenalin hydrochlor. Cases of urticaria which have persisted for weeks or months are much more difficult to treat, and often the cause is never determined. In dealing with such cases a series of simple diets must be given to eliminate the possibility of food being the cause, and if necessary a period of starvation may be advised as an aid to dietary investigation. Areas of focal sepsis must be sought and dealt with if present. Free elimination must be encouraged by diuretics and an adequate supply of fluids, and colon lavage should be carried out thoroughly over a period of two to three weeks. If no cause is discovered, non-specific desensitization may be attempted, either by giving 5 to 10 gr. of peptone powder half an hour before each meal, by a course of peptone injections, or by autohemotherapy. Ephedrine is sometimes useful, and in a few cases calcium administered by mouth is of service. Mixtures which contain the intestinal ferments may be added to the diet and will occasionally give relief, but when we are driven back upon such measures therapy has assumed a " hit or miss " aspect. It must be remembered that a certain number of chronic urticarias are really cases of dermographism for which little can be done, although they occasionally respond to alterations in diet even although the skin eruption is not dependent on the ingestion of any particular food. Every now and then a case of urticaria is met with which seems to be due definitely to nervous influences, but this type, like that due to heat and cold, is extremely rare.

Cutaneous scratch tests with foreign proteins seldom provide any evidence which cannot be obtained by the more direct means of history taking, elimination diets, a complete physical examination and the results of therapy. The tests are tedious to carry out, often extremely difficult to interpret, and positive reactions may have no relation to the case. Occasionally they demonstrate rapidly the protein to which an intolerance has been developed, but whatever indication is given by the tests it must be verified by therapy, and frequently the results of therapy do not correspond to the results of the test.

Specific desensitization to a protein which is definitely the cause of the eruption is not worth while. It is highly improbable that specific desensitization can be achieved, although over a period of years desensitization may occur naturally and spontaneously.

DRUG ERUPTIONS

These, including enema rashes, are by no means uncommon. The majority of them do not itch, so that no treatment is required beyond the discontinuance of the causative drug. Morphine and its derivatives, however, can cause a very irritable type of erythematous and urticarial rash which may require the application of a lead and tar or a 1 per cent. carbolic lotion to allay the itching. The rashes due to the organic arsenical compounds or to gold run a very prolonged course, and their treatment is the symptomatic treatment of dermatitis.

BULLOUS ERUPTIONS

These include dermatitis herpetiformis, the pemphigoid eruptions, iodide eruptions and certain forms of insect bites. In all cases it is advisable to snip the roofs of the bullæ and to use starch poultices until the exudative phase of the lesion has subsided. Starch poultices have the advantage that they are easily applied, and no special cleansing procedures are necessary after their removal. In addition they absorb exudate better than any other type of application. Once exudation has subsided a 1 per cent. ichthyol or ammoniated mercury paste may be applied in the form of spreads.

HERPES SIMPLEX

At the commencement of an attack, dabbing the irritable tingling area of skin with 5 per cent. silver nitrate in spirits ether nitrosi is often sufficient to prevent the further development of the lesions. Unfortunately this treatment produces a black stain on the skin, and as the eruption almost always affects an exposed area it may not be feasible to carry it out in every case. After the eruption has developed a 1 per cent. ammoniated mercury paste is the most suitable application, and should be continued until the crusts have separated. Such treatment will undoubtedly shorten the course of the eruption. There is no method of preventing recurrences with certainty, but sparking the area of skin which is the usual site of the eruption with a high frequency current, using a flat glass electrode, may prevent further attacks. Vaccination with calf lymph as for smallpox, and also cutaneous vaccination with the fluid obtained from the early vesicles of herpes, seems to stop the recurrences in a proportion of cases.

HERPES ZOSTER

In the early stages of this condition the injection of pituitrin is extremely useful, both in allaying the pain and in shortening the duration of the eruption. Doses of $\frac{1}{2}$ to 1 c.c. can be given once or twice daily for the first two or three days. The affected skin should be powdered with talc and covered with a thick layer of cotton-wool. When crusting has occurred, a 1 per cent. ammoniated mercury paste can be substituted for the talc. In cases of zoster affecting the first division of the fifth nerve, great care must be taken of the eye. If lesions develop on the conjunctiva or lids, cold compresses should be used for a day or two and atropine instillations given daily. In ophthalmic zoster involvement of the conjunctiva may not occur until five or six days after the onset of the skin lesions. The after-pain of herpes zoster is treated with the usual methods suitable for neuritis.

ALOPECIA

The treatment of alopecia depends on the cause of the condition. That following febrile illnesses or traumatic shock requires no treatment, as the hair grows in normally in due course. Patches of alopecia due to scar formation from whatever cause are permanent and no treatment is of any avail. In alopecia seen in the early stages of syphilis the hair grows in naturally, but regrowth is accelerated by antisyphilitic treatment. The only forms of baldness which definitely benefit from treatment are alopecia areata and alopecia due to deficiency of thyroid secretion.

In alopecia areata counter-irritation either with chemical applications or with ultra-violet light definitely limits the disease and accelerates regrowth. The following lotion is widely used :—

℞		
	Acid. Lact.	ʒvi
	Ol. Ricin	ʒiii
	Sp. Meth. Indust. . . . . ad	℥vi

Painting the patches with tincture of iodine or liquid carbolic acid is always useful and may be carried out once weekly. Ultra-violet light may be tried, using a mercury vapour lamp. Short courses lasting over a period of from four to six weeks, giving an erythema dose twice weekly, are as efficient and less tedious to the patient than a prolonged continuous course lasting for several months. Such short courses can be given at intervals of two months. In addition to local treatment, small doses of thyroid and a liberal supply of all the vitamins may be given for their properties as general growth stimulants. Attention to the general health and removal of all septic foci should, of course, be considered in addition to the local measures.

PITYRIASIS ROSEA

This condition is self-limited, and if it does not cause any discomfort it may be left untreated and allowed to disappear spontaneously. There is no doubt, however, that a daily potassium permanganate bath followed by the application of a 2 per cent. sulphur and salicylic acid vaseline greatly accelerates the disappearance of the rash. If there is much irritation a 1 or 2 per cent. tar paste may be used in preference to the salicylic vaseline. Most cases will clear up quickly under the influence of one or two erythema doses of ultra-violet light, but as there is often a certain amount of irritation produced by this treatment, it is questionable if it serves any useful purpose. Pityriasis rosea seems to produce a lasting immunity and recurrences are practically unknown.

LICHEN PLANUS

Nothing is known regarding the ætiology of lichen planus, although it has all the characteristics of an eruption due to internal toxic causes, and in addition to this it seems to have some curious association with the nervous system. In treating a case, one has to combat the itch, which may be intense, with suitable anti-pruritic lotions, such as a lead and tar lotion, with or without the addition of 1 to 2 per cent. phenol, or the application of 1 to 5 per cent. tar paste. If the eruption is localized a full skin dose of X-rays will almost invariably relieve the itching and cause the rapid absorption of the lesions. X-rays are, of course, not practicable in extensive eruptions involving a large area of the skin surface, and their use in widespread cases has to be carefully judged. For some unknown reason, radiation of the spinal cord with X-rays relieves itching in a large proportion of cases and also causes the eruption to disappear with moderate rapidity. The area of the spine to be treated is that which gives rise to the nerves going to the area of skin affected with the rash.

Internal treatment consists in the administration of perchloride of mercury in doses of $\frac{1}{20}$ gr. three times daily. Arsenic is also useful, and intramuscular injections of enesol, a preparation containing mercury and salicylarsonate, have recently been found to give good results. In cases which are very resistant to treatment and in which the irritation is severe, lumbar puncture and the withdrawal of 10 to 20 c.c. cerebrospinal fluid may be followed by symptomatic relief.

PSORIASIS

Success in treatment in psoriasis depends to a large extent on how much time a patient is willing to devote to the cure of the disease, and how much inconvenience he is willing to undergo during the treatment. Any attack of psoriasis can be cured if a patient will give up his whole time to it, and but for the fact that almost every case recurs, it would be as satisfactory to treat as any other disease. In giving advice to a patient about the treatment of his psoriasis it is necessary to consider whether the amount of eruption present is sufficient to justify putting him to considerable inconvenience and expense, bearing in mind the certainty with which recurrence will almost always take place. This problem does not arise if a patient insists that he must be made spotless, nor when the eruption is so extensive as to cause a great deal of inconvenience from scaling, cracking and general discomfort. The treatment which will be described applies to any case of psoriasis no matter how scanty or how extensive the eruption, and in addition to this a modified ambulatory treatment will be outlined.

External Treatment.—The treatment should commence with twice daily applications of a 1 per cent. tar paste, and the strength of the tar should be increased at intervals of two days up to 5 per cent.; the increase might be graded 1, 3, 5 per cent. The tar pastes should be spread on calico. Thereafter a 5 per cent. chrysarobin paste should be applied twice daily, and it may also be spread on strips of calico or merely rubbed into the skin. When it is found that the skin will tolerate chrysarobin, and very few psoriatics seem to be intolerant to it, Dreuw's ointment can be used.

This should be rubbed in twice daily and should not be applied spread on strips unless to localized hypertrophic patches. If spread on strips and bandaged on, there is a very definite risk of blistering due to the high percentage of salicylic acid present in the preparation. Dreuw's ointment causes a blackish-brown discoloration of the skin, and it is superfluous to continue when a thick blackened surface layer has been formed. It is then an advantage to interrupt the treatment for two or three days and to use an ichthyol paste; first, to allow the removal of the black surface skin, and secondly, to give the patient relief from the heat and irritation which almost always accompanies the application of this preparation. The Dreuw's ointment, alternating with the ichthyol paste, is continued until the whole skin surface has become smooth and only staining marks the site of the psoriasis lesions. It is an advantage to give a week or ten days' treatment with crude gasworks tar after the Dreuw's ointment has been discontinued, because if this is done there is less chance of recurrence at an early date. Dreuw's ointment and 5 per cent. chrysarobin paste can be applied to the scalp provided it is kept shaved, and provided the chrysarobin applications are washed off at night and replaced with tar paste. There are two possible dangers associated with the application of chrysarobin, one being the production of conjunctivitis, the other, the occurrence of an erythematous and later a vesicular dermatitis. Provided the treatment is carefully supervised, the onset of either of these complications need not be considered a serious matter. The conjunctivitis can be treated with instillations of castor oil, and the dermatitis will settle very quickly after the chrysarobin is removed with olive oil, and a 1 per cent. ichthyol paste substituted. Another drawback to chrysarobin treatment of which the patient must be warned is staining of bedding, clothing and the bath. A bath need only be given every second or third day when chrysarobin is being used, and care must be taken to clean the bath immediately after use, particularly when the strong applications are being used.

If a case of psoriasis, or even a patch of psoriasis, is not treated in the fairly drastic manner outlined above, a longer period of treatment will be required. The same sequence of treatment can be employed in ambulatory cases, but in them it is only applied at night, a bath being taken in the morning, and no application made during the day.

Short of drastic treatment carried out at least once daily it seems barely worth while to advise less active methods, for they rarely meet with much success. Clothing is ruined, and the patient frequently becomes disheartened and stops all treatment. In view of this some patients suffering from a mild attack of psoriasis, which is not causing any inconvenience, may be advised merely to apply a tar paste, or even plain vaseline, one or two nights weekly, and to take a bath the following morning. This type of treatment need only be considered as a toilet procedure designed to keep the patches supple and in a state which is not troublesome. There is justification for the attitude that psoriasis is such a chronic skin affection that as little attention as possible need be paid to it unless it becomes so severe as to interfere with æsthetic feelings and personal comfort.

Recurrences take place in a most erratic way. Sometimes only a few weeks' freedom follows the complete cure of an attack, and sometimes the eruption does not recur for years.

In very generalized cases it may be necessary to begin treatment with plain vaseline or an ichthyol paste, and then work on to the tar pastes and finally to chrysarobin. In cases which show intolerance to tar or chrysarobin or to both, a 2 or 3 per cent. paste of oxidized pyrogalic acid, or a similar concentration of resorcin, or ammoniated mercury, may be used.

Chronic isolated patches which are resistant to local treatment, and also psoriasis affecting the nail folds, may be treated with X-rays, but, as in the case of Besnier's prurigo, the X-rays must never be repeated indiscriminately. Ultra-violet light sometimes helps a patient, sometimes spreads the eruption, and generally has no effect. Medicated baths have no advantages over ordinary baths.

Internal Treatment.—As in the case of external treatment a large number of drugs have been advocated from time to time in the internal treatment of psoriasis, but there are only three which are of proved value, namely, salicin and salicylates, arsenic, and thyroid.

Stated briefly, salicin and salicylates (both gr. x, t.i.d.) are given in a spreading case, arsenic (liq. arsenicalis, ♏iii to ♏v, t.i.d.) in a chronic stationary case and in cases which are responding to local treatment satisfactorily, and thyroid (gr. ½ to 1 daily) to psoriatics past middle age. Various forms of diet have been advocated from time to time, but there is no one diet which is of universal help in psoriasis, and diet need hardly be considered as an aid to treatment. There is no doubt that alcohol is contraindicated when psoriasis is spreading.

G. H. PERCIVAL.

VENEREAL DISEASES

Introduction

THE prevention of venereal infections is a social and public health problem of considerable magnitude, and progress will be made by better education, increased recreational facilities, improved housing conditions and reduction of unemployment.

Improved methods of treatment should result in a marked decrease in the percentage of patients who cease treatment before cure is achieved. The individual physician has a considerable public responsibility in securing the co-operation of the infected person until he is cured.

Individual Prophylaxis.—The measures advised must be carried out as soon as possible after coitus. Where possible the treatment should be carried out by a trained orderly or nurse, but it is within the powers of the average person. To be effective, prophylaxis must be undertaken within twenty-four hours.

Male.—The patient is instructed to wash thoroughly with soap and water the genitals, the lower abdomen and perineum. He then irrigates the urethra with one pint of potassium permanganate solution (1 : 10,000). As an alternative he may instil into the urethra with a syringe 10 c.c. of 5 per cent. argyrol or 5 per cent. neo-protosil. This solution should be retained in the urethra for three minutes by the pressure of his fingers on the glans penis. On releasing this pressure, the surplus lotion flows out, and the patient places a pad of wool or gauze over the penis to prevent staining his clothing. He is advised not to pass urine for several hours after this instillation. The final part of disinfection is the thorough application of a mercurial ointment to the pubes, penis and scrotum. An ointment of 10 per cent. hydrarg. ammoniat. or $33\frac{1}{3}$ per cent. calomel cream is reliable for this purpose.

Female.—It is more difficult for a female to carry out efficient self-disinfection after coitus, for she can rarely disinfect the urethra without the services of a nurse. She should wash the lower abdomen, vulva and perineum, then douche the vagina with 1 quart of 1 : 10,000 potassium permanganate or 1 : 500 dettol. She then inuncts the pubes, vulva and introitus vaginæ with mercurial ointment (10 per cent. hydrarg. ammon.). If treatment by a nurse or doctor is available, 10 per cent. neo-protosil is introduced into the cervical canal by a dressed probe, and 5 per cent. neo-protosil is instilled into the urethra by a syringe or dressed probe. Argyrol is equally effective but is liable to stain her clothing.

Where prophylactic treatment is carried out under medical supervision the patients should be urged to return for examination and bacteriological tests one week later, and again after three months. On the last visit the blood is tested by Wassermann and Kahn tests to exclude syphilis.

GONORRHŒA

General Measures.—The patient should be informed of the diagnosis and instructed regarding his mode of life. The contagious nature of the disease should be explained, and indulgence in sexual intercourse forbidden until he is proved to be cured. Strict instructions must be given that the discharges from the infected areas must not be allowed to come in contact with articles likely to be used by other people, such as towels and lavatories. Soiled dressings and sanitary pads must be burned at once. The patient must wash his hands after contact with the genitals or soiled dressings. Personal clothing should be soaked in 2 per cent. lysol or dettol, or boiled if the material permits this treatment. A male patient should wear a "Jock strap" or suspensory bandage, and surround the penis with gauze. A female should wear external sanitary pads as long as there is vaginal discharge. The use of the tampon type of sanitary pad (*e.g.*, tampax) is not advisable during gonorrhœa. The patient should be encouraged to take baths, but must disinfect the bath thoroughly after use. He should not frequent public baths or swimming pools.

The patient should rest as much as possible during the acute stage of the illness. Tennis, cycling, dancing, heavy manual labour and strenuous exercise are not advisable.

Diet.—Alcohol is forbidden, and all highly seasoned foods, curries, mustard and spices, should be avoided. Large quantities of water, tea, fruit drinks, etc., should be taken. It does not seem necessary to forbid meat. While under treatment with sulphanilamide compounds, all sulphates and foods containing much sulphur are avoided; these are eggs, onions, peas and beans. Sulphur and sulphates are mainly taken as constituents of aperients.

Protection of Contacts.—At the first interview inquiry should be made if other parties (*e.g.*, his wife) have been infected by direct or indirect contact. If the circumstances make this seem probable such individuals should be advised to be medically examined and have prophylactic treatment.

Nursing and Isolation.—The attendant should wear rubber gloves when carrying out treatment of a patient. All soiled dressings should be destroyed at once. Rubber gloves may be sterilized by heat, or soaked in antiseptic. Bedpans, catheters and douche nozzles should be sterilized after use by heat. Bed linen and personal clothing may be soaked for one hour in 2 per cent. lysol, rinsed, and then treated by the usual laundry methods.

It is unnecessary to sterilize cups, cutlery, etc., if the patient suffers from gonorrhœa. Towels must be kept strictly separate from those belonging to others. They must be changed frequently, and the patient should use a separate towel for the face, as there is a danger of carrying gonococcal pus to the eyes. In maternity hospitals patients with gonorrhœa should be treated and nursed apart from all other cases, and special care is required to prevent ophthalmia neonatorum (see p. 205).

In children's hospitals, schools, orphanages, etc., cases of gonococcal vulvovaginitis should be isolated from other female children.

The bath should be rinsed with lysol, sanitas or a similar antiseptic, immediately after the patient vacates it. The patient should sleep alone.

Relief of Symptoms.—The common symptoms of gonorrhœa are pain on micturition, with frequency and urgency of micturition, and occasionally painful erections.

Women very often have very slight symptoms, but may have dysmenorrhœa. The administration of an alkaline diuretic and sedative mixture usually relieves such symptoms rapidly. The following prescription may be given every four hours until the symptoms are relieved :—

Pot. Cit.	gr. xx
Sod. Bicarb.	gr. xx
Sod. Brom.	gr. x
Tinct. Bellad.	♏vii
Aq. . . . . ad	℥ss

Sandal-wood oil and similar preparations are useless.

The symptoms of gonorrhœa are also relieved by heat, and this shortens the course of the disease. Hot baths and the application of fomentations or hot-water bottles to the pubis and perineum relieve pain. Short-wave diathermy and general hyperpyrexia are very effective, but are required only on rare occasions for the most resistant cases. Diathermy may be applied by special electrodes to the cervix in females, to the prostate and scrotum in males, or to joints.

Specific Treatment.—*Sulphonamides.*—The advent of sulphonamide compounds has revolutionized the treatment of gonorrhœa. The published reports show that a rate of cure between 70 and 90 per cent. may be expected. A dramatic reduction in the incidence of the major complications and in the duration of disability due to the disease has been observed. Established complications of gonorrhœa recover more rapidly and usually more completely.

Sulphapyridine (M. & B. 693) has proved the most potent curative drug in gonorrhœa and the other members of this group, such as sulphanilamide, uleron and albucid are decidedly inferior and are seldom required. Accordingly, the use of sulphapyridine alone will be described in this section. The drug may be used in all types of cases at any stage of the infection. In early acute cases it acts with great rapidity; the purulent secretions diminish and the gonococci disappear in about three days. In chronic cases more prolonged treatment or repeated short courses of the drug are required and local antiseptic and instrumental treatment may be necessary to sterilize or evacuate foci of gonococcal infection.

Sulphapyridine is given in tablets of 0·5 gm., and an adult requires 3 gm. per diem continued for five days as a minimum course of treatment. An effective tissue concentration is reached rapidly, and a suitable scheme of dosage is one tablet at 8 A.M., 12 noon, 4 P.M., and 8 P.M., with a bed-time dose of two tablets. The tablets may be swallowed whole or crushed. The patient's usual fluid intake should be continued. Young children can take the drug powdered and mixed with milk or glucose solution.

In the treatment of gonorrhœa, the toxic effects of sulphapyridine are relatively infrequent and slight, though about 50 per cent. of patients suffer from slight nausea. This nausea can sometimes be relieved by taking small doses of alkali, *e.g.*, sodium bicarbonate, along with the tablet. A few individuals may suffer from severe nausea and vomiting, and in such cases injections of sodium sulphapyridine may be given intramuscularly. The patient should be advised to take only the exact dose prescribed. The administration should not continue for longer than ten consecutive days, and prescriptions should limit the amount of the drug to be supplied. If repeated courses are required, an interval of a week should separate them. Adequate doses should be administered from the outset. If sub-curative doses are given for some time the organism often becomes drug-resistant and maximum doses thereafter may prove ineffective.

Female patients tolerate the drug well, and treatment should be commenced as soon as the diagnosis has been established. It is an advantage to give an additional course of sulphapyridine during the first menstrual period after treatment has commenced.

A small percentage of patients fail to respond to sulphapyridine. In such cases it is futile to give larger doses or prolonged administration. A few patients (about 5 per cent.) relapse shortly after stopping sulphapyridine. Such cases may respond to a second or third course of the drug, but search must be made for a deep-seated or enclosed focus of infection, and prolonged observation is essential.

Vaccines.—Gonococcus vaccines are now seldom required. Their action is probably non-specific, and protein shock treatment may be equally effective. A stock vaccine of gonococcus combined with " secondary " organisms (staphylococci, *B. coli*, diphtheroids, etc.) is most likely to prove effective. Vaccines may be required in cases of chronic urethritis and prostatitis following neglected gonorrhœa, or in the interval between " courses " of sulphanilamide treatment. They should be used to supplement other forms of therapy and cannot alone be trusted to control or cure the infection.

Antiseptic Irrigations and Installations.—When the patient does not respond to sulphapyridine, or when discharge due to secondary organisms continues, irrigations may be required. Irrigation of the urethra with warm antiseptic lotions reduces the amount of discharge and accelerates recovery, but the treatment must be carried out with care, using the correct apparatus, with aseptic precautions.

Irrigation should not be attempted in the acute stage of gonorrhœa, but may be required if there is a purulent urethral discharge after ten days' treatment with sulphanilamide drugs.

If the urethral secretion then contains gonococci, or definite pus, the patient is taught to irrigate the urethra.

The apparatus required is a 1-quart douche container, rubber tubing with a spring clip, and a glass or metal urethral nozzle of the "Janet" type—*i.e.*, with a rounded blunt end. The nozzle is sterilized by boiling, or it is stored in a wide-mouthed bottle containing surgical spirit or 1 : 20 carbolic acid solution. The irrigation lotion should be used at a temperature of 115° F. The patient empties his bladder, cleans the meatus, and allows the lotion to flow into the urethra. When the urethra feels distended he stops the flow of lotion by pressure on the rubber tube, and on withdrawing the nozzle the lotion flows out from the urethral meatus. In this way the anterior urethra is irrigated gently about ten times. He then fills the urethra again and, keeping the nozzle firmly pressed against the meatus, he strains as if starting the act of micturition. This generally relaxes the urethral sphincters and the lotion flows through the urethra into the bladder. The patient meantime experiences the sensation of micturition, but in a few minutes he feels the urge to empty his bladder, so after he has allowed about 1 pint to flow in he withdraws the nozzle and voids the bladder contents. He repeats the process several times and bladder irrigation per urethra may be done thrice daily.

Failure to carry out posterior irrigation properly may be due to: (*a*) the use of cold lotions; (*b*) irritant antiseptic; (*c*) insufficient or excessive pressure of the fluid; (*d*) nervousness of the patient. If there is much discomfort or spasm of the sphincters, posterior irrigation is facilitated by instillation into the urethra by a syringe of 10 c.c. local anæsthetic which is retained in the urethra by pressure on the glans for two minutes. The anæsthetic recommended is 1 : 1,000 percaine or ½ per cent. cocaine.

Potassium permanganate (1 : 10,000) is the most suitable antiseptic for routine use in gonorrhœa. If a tablet (2 gr.) is dissolved in 1 quart of water it forms approximately the correct solution.

In cases with superadded infection with staphylococci, diphtheroids and *B. coli*, irrigation with chloramine T—1 : 5,000 is more effective, or silver compounds may be used (*e.g.*, albargin 1 : 6,000).

Silver nitrate (1 : 10,000) or zinc sulphanilate (1 : 2,000) may be used if there is a persistent mucoid urethral discharge without active infection.

Acriflavine and mercurochrome do not possess superior curative powers and they have the disadvantage of staining clothing and utensils.

Instillation of the Urethra.—This is a less efficient method of antiseptic treatment of the urethra. A syringe of 15 c.c.

capacity, with a blunt nozzle, is required. It is sterilized, filled with an antiseptic (*e.g.*, 5 per cent. argyrol) and this is gently pressed into the urethra. The antiseptic is retained in the urethra for five minutes by pressure on the glans. The surplus lotion is then allowed to escape, a pad of gauze is applied to the meatus and the patient is instructed not to micturate during the next two hours. Instillations may be repeated twice or thrice daily. The antiseptics most frequently employed for instillation are :—

Collosol argentum.
Argyrol, 5 up to 10 per cent.
1 per cent. picric acid in 50 per cent. glycerin.
Neo-protosil, 10 per cent.

Management of a Male Case of Gonorrhœa

The diagnosis is confirmed and the general mode of life, the diet and the necessary precautions regarding spread of the infection are explained to the patient (see p. 193).

Drugs of the sulphonamide series—preferably sulphapyridine—are prescribed, and the patient's progress is assessed by daily observation of the amount of discharge and of pus in the urine and bacteriological examination of the urethral secretion.

If gonococci are present after the first course of sulphapyridine an interval of one week is allowed in which the patient irrigates thrice daily with potassium permanganate. The course is then repeated. This mode of treatment is repeated until urethral and prostatic secretions have been normal for two weeks. Treatment is then stopped and tests of cure begun.

If there are no gonococci and few pus cells present the patient is kept under observation, and smears and cultures of urethral and prostatic secretion are examined every seven days for one month. The urethra is then examined by endoscopy, and if it is healthy the patient is allowed to resume his normal mode of life, except that sexual intercourse is forbidden. The examination of the urethral and prostatic secretion is repeated one month and two months later. Three months after the onset of the disease the blood should be examined by Wassermann test and gonococcus complement fixation test, and in addition to urethroscopy a large urethral sound should be passed. If no evidence of gonorrhœa is revealed by these tests the patient is cured.

Complications of Gonorrhœa in Male.—The local complications most frequently encountered are : Peri-urethral abscess, prostatitis and seminal vesiculitis and epididymitis. These complications have been greatly reduced in incidence as the result of sulphonamide therapy.

Local extensions of the disease are favoured by sexual excitement or coitus, strenuous exertion and faulty methods of urethral irrigation.

In all the local complications of gonorrhœa, drugs of the sulphonamide group (*e.g.*, sulphapyridine) have a very beneficial action and they should be administered in maximum doses, and repeated courses given if necessary.

Epididymitis.—This is usually unilateral. There is severe pain, and general constitutional upset, with increased severity of the urinary symptoms.

The patient should rest in bed for a few days. The scrotum should be supported by a "T bandage" or "Jock strap," and applications to the scrotum of hot antiphlogistine or 10 per cent. glycerin of ichthyol relieve the pain. In the subacute and chronic stages stimulating dressings such as ungt. hydrargyri co. may be applied. Irrigation of the urethra should be suspended during the acute stage.

The associated infection of the prostate and seminal vesicles requires treatment as detailed below.

Gonococcal epididymitis practically never suppurates and surgical operative treatment is unnecessary. Epididymitis due to staphylococcal infection or *B. coli* frequently suppurates and demands surgical drainage. Tuberculous epididymitis should be excluded in less acute cases as the treatment of this condition is principally the treatment for tuberculosis (*q.v.*).

Prostatitis and Seminal Vesiculitis.—Rest in bed and cessation of urethral irrigation are advised during the acute phase. If there is severe pain, great frequency of micturition or hæmaturia, relief will follow the use of a suppository containing :—

Morphine sulph.	$\frac{1}{4}$ gr.
Atropine sulph.	$\frac{1}{75}$ gr.

This may be inserted into the rectum three times a day. Frequent hot baths and hot fomentations applied to the perineum and suprapubic area soothe the pain.

If retention of urine occurs the urethra should be irrigated gently with antiseptic lotion (*e.g.*, 1 : 10,000 potass. permang.), anæsthetized by an instillation of 1 : 1,000 percaine and then a gum elastic catheter of the Coudé type passed. After the urine has been evacuated the bladder should be irrigated through the catheter with 1 : 10,000 potassium permanganate. A prostatic abscess usually points spontaneously into the urethra and then clears up rapidly. Surgical drainage is rarely required.

In the subacute and chronic phases of prostatitis and vesiculitis, the prostate and vesicles should be emptied by thorough but gentle massage per rectum. The urethra should be irrigated with a hot antiseptic lotion immediately after prostatic massage. This is required twice per week. Progress should be assessed by the size and consistence of the gland on rectal examination, and by examination of films and cultures of the fluid expressed, and of the urine voided immediately after the massage. These fluids should not contain pus or pathogenic organisms.

Where chronic infection persists in the prostate and seminal vesicles in spite of thorough treatment by massage, irrigations, etc., benefit may be obtained from dilatation of the urethra by passing large sounds, and from instillations into the posterior urethra.

If a seminal vesicle is chronically infected and is the source of metastatic complications such as arthritis, or if it causes recurrent epididymitis, then the operation of vasostomy may be required. The vas deferens is opened at the inguinal region, and 10 to 30 c.c. of an antiseptic solution such as 10 per cent. argyrol is instilled towards the vesicle.

Vaccine treatment may prove beneficial where there is a chronic resistant infection. The vaccine should contain a mixture of gonococci and the secondary organisms.

Peri-urethral Abscess.—The abscess should be aspirated on one or two occasions, and if it persists it should be drained by a small longitudinal incision and then packed. After the acute infection has subsided the urethra will require dilatation to prevent stricture formation in the abscess area.

Arthritis and Synovitis.—In acute arthritis the joint is treated as in rheumatic fever. The gonococcal infection is attacked vigorously by administration of sulphonamide compounds, and later by treatment of the focus of gonococcal infection—*e.g.*, in the prostate and seminal vesicles of a male, or the cervix and uterus of a female.

The main points of difference in treatment between gonococcal arthritis and acute infective arthritis due to other organisms are :—

1. Direct and vigorous attack on the organism is the main line of treatment.

2. Gonococcal arthritis very rarely suppurates. It is seldom necessary to aspirate or drain the joint.
3. It is generally wise to commence massage and passive and active movement of the joint at an early stage—as soon as the pain abates.
4. The condition is amenable to hyperpyrexia. A pyrexia of 106° F. for six to eight hours on four to six occasions is required.

The treatment of chronic arthritis and synovitis is essentially similar to that of rheumatoid arthritis (see p. 894), but more active massage, movements and exercises are possible from the beginning. An effort to detect and clear up the focus of infection should precede forcible manipulation of partially ankylosed joints. In the absence of bony ankylosis the prognosis is usually very good and complete recovery of joint function is possible.

Spurs on the plantar surface of the calcaneus disappear very slowly, but surgical removal is unwise.

Iritis.—Acute iritis and iridocyclitis may be unilateral or bilateral, and may recur on several occasions, and may accompany arthritis.

If the iridocyclitis is acute the patient should rest in a dim light or wear dark glasses and refrain from reading. The pupils are kept fully dilated by instillations night and morning into the affected eye of two drops of 1 per cent. atropine sulphate solution.

With vigorous treatment of the gonococcal infection iritis resolves rapidly and completely. Recurrences of iritis are frequent, so every effort should be made to secure complete cure of the focus of gonococcal infection. If the iris has formed adhesions and the pupil is fixed or occluded, iridectomy may be required.

Management of a Female Case of Gonorrhœa

General Measures.—The patient should follow the same general instructions given to male patients (p. 193), with the addition that she should rest and avoid sport and exercise during the menstrual period. All local treatment must be suspended during menstruation, but sulphonamide compounds should be taken throughout the period, as there is then an increased liability to complications. Rest in bed is rarely necessary, unless the patient has severe pain.

In the acute stages the patient should receive sulphapyridine compounds for ten days, but no local antiseptic treatment is attempted. She should wear a sanitary pad of the external type, and should wash the vulva or have a daily hot bath, but she must not douche the vagina.

After ten days the administration of sulphapyridine is suspended and the urethra and cervix uteri are treated with antiseptics. The patient is placed in a semi-lithotomy position, the vulva are cleansed with 1 : 1,000 dettol or 1 : 1,000 lysol, and a vaginal speculum is inserted. The bivalve type of speculum is likely to be the most convenient. Local antiseptic measures are only required if symptoms and signs persist or if smears still contain pus and organisms.

The vagina, the fornices and the vaginal portion of the cervix are swabbed clean with either dettol (1 : 1,000) or a warm solution of sodium bicarbonate (1 : 100), and with dry sterile gauze swabs. The endocervix may then be treated by inserting a dressed probe, previously dipped in antiseptic, into the cervical canal for a distance of 1 to 2 in. This must be done gently.

One per cent. solution of picric acid in glycerin, or 10 per cent. argyrol, may be used for application to the cervix.

As the speculum is withdrawn an astringent absorbent dusting powder should be applied to the vaginal walls and vulva. A suitable powder is :—

Zinc Oxid.	. . . . . .	ʒi
Bism. Subgall.	. . . . . .	ʒij
Mag. Carb. Lev.	. . . . . .	ʒij
Pulv. Amyli	. . . . . ad	℥i

At the same time the urethra may be treated by instillation, from an appropriate syringe, of 10 per cent. argyrol (or neo-protosil). Such local antiseptic treatment may be given daily at first, but in the subacute or chronic stages twice per week is sufficient.

When the menstrual period is expected, local treatment is stopped and sulphanilamide drugs are prescribed. Smears and cultures of the urethral and cervical secretions and the urine are examined twenty-four hours after the cessation of the period. If the patient is pregnant or after the menopause, progress is assessed by bacteriological examinations each week, and the sulphonamide drugs are given again only if the infection persists, or if there is much pus in the secretions.

Complications of Gonorrhœa in the Female.—*Cystitis.*—As the bladder is seldom infected, bladder lavage is seldom required. If cystitis is present the bladder should be irrigated daily with 1 : 10,000 pot. permang., followed by instillation of $\frac{1}{2}$ oz. argyrol solution in a strength of 1 per cent. gradually increased up to 10 per cent. as the severity of the symptoms abates.

Bartholinian Gland.—Infection of these glands occurs frequently and often proceeds to abscess formation. Repeated aspiration of the abscess, followed by instillation of either collosol argentum or 1 : 20 dilution of liquor iodi mitis (B.P.), may cure the abscess, but frequently incision is required. General anæsthesia is advantageous and the abscess should be incised freely—the cavity is disinfected with liquor iodi mitis and then packed with gauze. The packing is changed daily till healing is complete.

Salpingitis.—Acute salpingitis is the most serious complication of gonorrhœa in a female. There is usually a high temperature with great malaise, abdominal pain and vomiting. The patient is confined to bed, and she is nursed in the sitting position. All local antiseptic treatment or douching, etc., is suspended.

Sulphapyridine is given in full doses. Hot poultices (*e.g.*, antiphlogistine) applied over the lower abdomen give relief.

Morphine ($\frac{1}{4}$ gr.) and atropine ($\frac{1}{100}$ gr.) are often given by hypodermic injection to relieve severe colic or pain. The bowel should be emptied by enemata. If the right Fallopian tube is acutely infected, and particularly if there is pyosalpinx, the surgeon may be unable to exclude acute appendicitis, and an operation is advisable.

In the majority of cases of acute salpingitis all the symptoms subside rapidly, but if pyosalpinx does not resolve, an operation undertaken after ten days is easier and safer, for the pus in the tube is then sterile and there are fewer adhesions.

Chronic salpingitis is treated by the insertion each night of a vaginal tampon soaked in 20 per cent. glycerin of ichthyol or 20 per cent. magnesium sulphate in glycerin. This is withdrawn next morning and the patient is given a hot douche (115° F.) at low pressure.

The douche can must not be more than 2 ft. above the pelvis, and at least four pints of 1 : 10,000 pot. permang. are used.

Tests of Cure.—The treatment is continued until all symptoms and signs disappear, and until all bacteriological tests of urethral and cervical secretions are negative for one month. The tests are repeated after three successive menstrual periods, or on three occasions at intervals of four weeks. The blood should also give a negative Wassermann reaction and a negative gonococcus complement fixation test.

Trichomonas Vaginalis.—Every case of leucorrhœa must be investigated for the presence of tr. vaginalis. This parasite is found in about 50 per cent. of cases examined for gonorrhœa. A swab of vaginal secretion is collected, one film is covered by a cover-glass and is examined immediately by oblique illumination and the high-power $\frac{1}{6}$ in. lens, or by dark-ground illumination and $\frac{1}{12}$ in. lens. The parasite is easily seen with the $\frac{1}{6}$ in. lens, as a motile flagellate oval body. A second film is stained with Leishman's stain. Cultural methods are also available.

Trichomonas infection usually requires prolonged treatment. After a cleansing douche with sod. bicarb. (1 drachm in 1 pint of water) a vaginal tablet of stovarsol is inserted into the vaginal fornices. Devegan pessaries (Bayer) are very effective. The patient inserts one or two pessaries each night, and has a douche once per week. It is also beneficial to powder the vulva with dusting powder containing stovarsol.

Silver picrate is also curative and is conveniently used as picragol pessaries (Wyeth). Carbasone (Lilly) pessaries are also effective.

Treatment must be continued for a considerable time—usually more than three months—otherwise relapse may be expected.

Vulvovaginitis of Children

The vulva and vagina are readily infected by the gonococcus before puberty, and such infections prove very resistant to treatment.

In children the cervix uteri and Bartholinian glands usually escape infection, but the anal canal and rectum may be infected. The child should be isolated from other female children, as epidemics of vulvovaginitis occur readily in hospitals, crêches, orphanages, etc.

Sulphapyridine is given in doses appropriate to the weight of the child, and several short treatments at intervals of fourteen days seem to be advisable.

If there is tenderness of the vulva and pain on walking, the child should be confined to bed and she should be given frequent antiseptic hip baths, or the vulva may be irrigated with 1 : 10,000 pot. permanganate, and then dried and powdered with bismuth subgallate powder (see p. 202).

If the gonococci persist after sulphonamide treatment, local antiseptic treatment must be given in addition. The vulva and vagina are irrigated each day and then dried and powdered. Treatment must be continued till all bacteriological tests have been negative for gonococci for one month. The period of stay in hospital is greatly reduced, and cure is achieved in a much shorter time than previously. As a rule clinical recovery occurs within one month.

Observation, however, must be prolonged. Tests should be made each week for one month and then at intervals of one month until six months have elapsed. The infection is very liable to relapse after several months.

Ovarian extracts are not necessary—they usually produce a temporary cessation of the acute symptoms, but do not cure the gonococcal infection.

Gonococcal Infection of the Eye

Ophthalmia Neonatorum.—Any inflammation of the eye accompanied by a purulent discharge within twenty-one days of birth should be notified to the Medical Officer of Health. This discharge should be examined for gonococci and other organisms.

Ophthalmia neonatorum may be prevented by careful cleansing of the eyelids of the new-born child, followed by instillation of two drops of 1 per cent. silver nitrate solution into each eye. The silver nitrate solution is washed out after two minutes with warm saline. Instead of 1 per cent. silver nitrate solution, 10 per cent. argyrol may be used which should not be washed out afterwards. If ophthalmia has developed, sulphapyridine is given for five to ten days in doses of 0·05 gr. thrice daily. With this treatment recovery is rapid ; in over 95 per cent. of cases the swelling and redness subside within a week, and complications are very few.

If only one eye is infected with gonococci the child is turned on the affected side, and the hands are confined in a shawl so that they cannot be lifted to the face. Smears from the apparently healthy eye are taken and a prophylactic instillation of silver nitrate solution is given. The affected eye is bathed every hour with warm normal saline, irrigating the conjunctival sac gently but thoroughly. Then 10 per cent. argyrol is instilled into the eye thrice daily. The edges of the eyelids are smeared with sterile vaseline to prevent accumulation of pus inside the lids.

Corneal ulceration and perforation of the cornea with

consequent loss of vision are common in neglected cases. If this occurs the condition of the eye is hopeless.

Gonococcal conjunctivitis in adults is rare and it is treated in the same way.

SYPHILIS

Principles of Treatment

In early syphilis the treatment is designed first to secure very rapid healing of contagious surface lesions by intensive dosage at intervals of a few days, and later the eradication of *Spirochæta pallida* by prolonged administration of smaller doses of antisyphilitic drugs. In every case both arsenical drugs and bismuth or mercury are required. Prolonged observation after treatment is essential—a minimum period is two years.

Treatment can be conducted according to a schedule.

In late syphilis of several years' duration, the patient does not require and will not tolerate intensive antisyphilitic treatment. The gummatous lesions will heal rapidly and completely with moderate doses. There will be no risk of the therapeutic paradox where rapid improvement is followed by aggravation of the symptoms and signs due to contraction of fibrous tissue.

In late syphilis serological improvement is less important than clinical improvement. Prolonged treatment is inevitable and observation may be required throughout life. Every case is an individual problem—a schedule of treatment cannot be applied.

Drug Treatment

Drugs Used.—" 606 " *Arsphenamine.*—Stabilarsan (arsphenamine diglucoside) (Boots) is given in doses of 0·15 to 0·6 gm. by intravenous injection. It is sold in ampoules dissolved in 50 per cent. glucose. The solution should be diluted with 5 to 10 c.c. sterile distilled water, then injected immediately.

" 914 " *Neoarsphenamine.*—Neokharsivan (B., W. & Co.), novarsenobillon (M. & B.), neo-salvarsan (Bayer). The dose is 0·15 to 0·6 gm. The drug is dissolved in 10 c.c. cold sterile distilled water, and is injected intravenously. Injections are usually given every seven days until ten doses have been given, when an interval of four weeks is advised. The total dose in a course is 6 gm. for a male and 4·5 gm. for a female of average weight. This drug has to be used with great caution if there is hepatic disease, albuminuria or dermatitis, and in cases of syphilitic cardiac disease.

Sulpharsphenamine.—Sulphostab (Boots), kharsulphan (B., W. & Co.) sulpharsenol, etc. This has an identical action to neoarsphenamine, and equal curative power. It is given by intramuscular injection, dissolved in 3 c.c. of sterile distilled water. The dose is 0·15 to 0·6 gm.

Acetylarsan (diethylamine acetarsone) is sold in ampoules—3 c.c. each—equivalent to 0·15 gm. of arsenic for adults ; also 2 c.c. each, equivalent to 0·04 gm. arsenic for children. It is given by intramuscular or subcutaneous injection twice weekly. It is painless, of low toxicity and is suitable for the treatment of children or cases of late syphilis.

Tryparsamide (tryparsone) is specially suitable for syphilis of the nervous system. It is given intravenously, dissolved in 10 c.c. sterile distilled water. The dose is 1 to 3 gm. per week and 30 gm. may be given in a course.

The toxic effects are few, but special precautions are necessary to observe the action on the optic nerve. Occasionally toxic amblyopia or blindness follows its use and this is more likely in cases of primary syphilitic optic atrophy. The fields of vision should be recorded before giving tryparsamide and at intervals throughout treatment. Warning symptoms of a toxic action on the optic nerve are dimness of vision, coloured lights and flashes of light before the eyes.

The maximum benefit from tryparsamide is obtained after prolonged use, and bismuth or mercury should be given simultaneously.

Acetarsone (stovarsol, spirocid, orarsan) is supplied in tablets containing from 0·01 to 0·25 gm. It is given orally in doses of 0·06 gm. per diem, increased gradually up to 0·5 gm. per diem, giving about 14 gm. in seven weeks, followed by a six weeks' rest period. The above dosage is for a child aged three, but it is modified for age and weight.

Toxic Sequels to Arsenical Compounds.—The injection of drugs of the neoarsphenamine series may be followed by an immediate "anaphylactoid" or vasodilator effect.

The treatment consists of the stoppage of the injection, and the subcutaneous injection of 0·5 to 1 c.c. of a solution of 1 : 1,000 adrenalin. Before subsequent injections the patient should be given glucose by mouth, and a hypodermic injection of atropine sulph. ($\frac{1}{100}$ gr.) half an hour before the treatment reduces the risk of severe reactions. If the patient continues to have vasodilator reactions it is wise to give another drug, such as acetylarsan.

Jaundice.—Jaundice occurs quite frequently in the course of treatment with organic arsenical drugs, and alcoholism, constipation, cirrhosis or syphilis of the liver predispose to it. Pains in the joints and general malaise may precede the appearance of jaundice. Treatment consists in stopping all arsenical drugs, the prescription of a diet appropriate for jaundice, and the daily administration for one week of sodium thiosulphate by intravenous injection in doses of 1 gm. in 10 c.c. of sterile distilled water. Glucose should be taken freely. Vitamin C by mouth in doses of 1,000 units per diem accelerates recovery (see below). The patient should not receive arsenical treatment for six months. If there has been severe liver damage, arsphenamine should not be given again.

Dermatitis.—The eruption may appear rapidly and become an acute exfoliative dermatitis in a few days, or it may have a more chronic course. Patients with seborrhœic dermatitis or widespread psoriasis should be given arsenical drugs with caution.

The patient should be confined to bed in a warm but freely ventilated room. Every care must be taken to prevent chills, as there is considerable risk of pneumonia and bronchitis. Starch poultices may be required for impetiginous areas around the mouth, nose and ears.

The diet should be simple and a brisk saline purge should be given daily during the acute stage. Warm baths of potassium permanganate (1 : 20,000) are helpful if there is a tendency for the eruption to become moist.

Sodium thiosulphate may be given daily for one week by intravenous injection in doses of 1 gm. dissolved in 10 c.c. sterile water.

Ascorbic acid (vitamin C) has proved in our hands the most effective remedy for this type of dermatitis. For the first three days a subcutaneous injection of 4,000 units is given, then it is given by mouth. It is supplied in tablets each containing 5 mg.=500 units vitamin C. Two tablets are taken thrice daily for two weeks.

Patients who have had severe arsenical dermatitis should never be given arsphenamine again, and frequently they do not tolerate other arsenical drugs.

Purpura and Aplastic Anœmia occur rarely after prolonged antisyphilitic treatment. They are best treated by blood transfusions and large doses of vitamins.

Bismuth.—The action of bismuth is partly curative and also inhibitory to the development of *Sp. pallida*. The action of most bismuth preparations is slow and prolonged—their speed of action is determined by the solubility of the preparation and also by the vehicle in which it is suspended or dissolved.

Practically all cases of syphilis should be treated by a combination of arsenical drugs and bismuth. The two drugs may be given on the same day. Bismuth is always given by intramuscular injection.

Bismuth preparations in common use may be classified :—

(*a*) Suspensions of bismuth metal.
(*b*) Suspensions of bismuth salts.
(*c*) Oil-soluble bismuth.

Bismuth metal is most frequently given as injectio bismuthi (B.P.)—a suspension in isotonic glucose solution. One cubic centimetre equals 0·2 gm. bismuth and the average dose varies from 0·2 to 0·4 gm. per week.

Bismuth oxychloride and bismuth salicylate may be suspended in oil or in glucose solution. The suspensions in oil produce less pain on injection, but are more slowly absorbed.

The oil-soluble preparations of bismuth (dose, 1 to 3 c.c.) are represented by such preparations as neo-cardyl and stabismol. They are absorbed very rapidly but their action is of relatively short duration as excretion is also rapid. To produce an intensive bismuth effect, injections should be given twice weekly. Oil-soluble preparations are particularly valuable where it is essential to avoid a Herxheimer reaction, or where rapid action is desired, or where the excretory organs may be damaged, *e.g.*, in cardiac or renal cases.

While a patient is under treatment with bismuth it is essential to test the urine frequently for the presence of albumen, and the mouth requires very thorough care. A blue line forms rapidly around any septic teeth, and the gums become tender and spongy. In neglected cases a severe stomatitis may develop.

After prolonged bismuth treatment patients may become anæmic, with malaise and loss of weight. Gastro-intestinal disturbance, particularly diarrhœa, may occur.

Treatment of Toxic Effects.—The toxic effects following the use of bismuth disappear rapidly when the administration of the drugs is stopped. One gramme of sodium thiosulphate should be injected daily for five days, as it appears to have some beneficial effect in hastening recovery. Stomatitis and gingivitis should be treated by frequent mouth washes of hydrogen peroxide and by painting the gums with an astringent paint, *e.g.*, Mandl's paint. When the condition is subacute, dental attention will be required for the eradication of septic roots and carious teeth.

Mercury. — Bismuth has almost completely supplanted mercury in the parenteral treatment of syphilis. Mercury given by injection is more painful and more toxic than bismuth, and the inunction of mercury is dirty and absorption is uncertain.

Mercury is of value in cases of syphilis of long duration where the Wassermann reaction remains positive after prolonged treatment with neoarsphenamine and bismuth. Many such patients appear to benefit from the prolonged administration of small doses of mercury. This is generally prescribed as a pill, such as Hutchinson's pill (hydrarg. cum cret. : pulv. ipecæ co., āā 1 gr.). Another useful pill is hydrarg. perchlor., $\frac{1}{16}$ gr. ; pot. iodide, 5 gr. The patient is advised to take one of these pills three times a day for a period of three weeks in each month, and may continue to use the drug in this way for three months. The course may be repeated after an interval of a month or longer.

Iodides.—Iodides are used in late syphilis, particularly for gummata and for the cardiac and central nervous system manifestations of syphilis. Sodium iodide or potassium iodide are most frequently prescribed :—

Pot. Iod.		gr. x
Sod. Bicarb.		gr. v
Aq.	ad	℥ss

Few patients are intolerant of iodides, but large doses, up to 20 gr. three times a day, are frequently tolerated better than small doses, and the mixture should be taken in very dilute form. For patients who will not tolerate iodides, colloidal iodine or organic iodine preparations may be administered, but these are not so active therapeutically.

Liquor iodi mitis (B.P.) may be given thrice daily in doses of 5 to 20 minims mixed in 2 oz. of milk or water.

Management of a Case of Early Syphilis

Until the diagnosis is established no antiseptics should be applied to the primary ulcer. Saline dressings, changed frequently, are usually sufficient to control superadded pyogenic infection. Skin and mucous membrane lesions do not require special treatment.

The patient should observe some measure of isolation until all the surface lesions have healed—this usually occurs within fourteen days. If there is a primary ulcer on the genitals this should be covered with a gauze dressing and soiled dressings should be destroyed immediately. Application of eusol dressings expedites healing.

He should be warned of the danger of infecting others, either by direct contact or by the use of common utensils, cutlery, etc. After the patient has received two or three weeks' treatment and when all the skin and mucous membrane lesions have healed, this danger disappears.

If possible the source of the infection should be traced, and all others who may have been infected should be advised to undergo a medical examination.

In the case of a married person coitus is forbidden entirely at first, but after three months may be permitted if efficient contraceptive measures are adopted.

The diet need not be altered drastically, but it is advisable that the patient should avoid alcohol entirely and he should not allow himself to become constipated. The teeth and gums should receive treatment from a dentist, if this is required, and the patient is urged to brush the teeth regularly and thoroughly.

He is instructed not to take a heavy meal within two hours before or after an arsenical injection, but he may take glucose or eat boiled sweets.

Specific Treatment.—Our practice has been to adopt the interrupted method of giving " courses " of treatment in which the drugs are given once per week for ten successive weeks. Both neoarsphenamine (i.v.) and bismuth (i.m.) may be given on the same day.

SPECIMEN COURSE OF TREATMENT FOR ADULT PATIENT

Week.	Neoarsphenamine (i.v.).		Bismuth (i.m.).		Observations.
	Male.	Female.	Male.	Female.	
	Gm.	Gm.	Gm.	Gm.	
1	0·6	0·45	0·3	0·2	Right side.
2	0·6	0·45	0·3	0·2	Left side.
3	0·6	0·45	0·3	0·2	Right side.
4	0·6	0·45	0·3	0·2	Left side.
5	0·6	0·45	0·3	0·2	Right side.
6	0·6	0·45	0·3	0·2	Left side.
7	0·6	0·45	0·3	0·2	Right side.
8	0·6	0·45	0·3	0·2	Left side.
9	0·6	0·45	0·3	0·2	Right side.
10	0·6	0·45	0·3	0·2	Left side.
Total	6·0	4·5	3·0	2·0	

After this course of treatment there is an interval of four weeks, during which the patient does not receive injections, but he may with advantage take iodides and if he is anæmic iron is indicated (see p. 471).

A case of primary syphilis requires four such courses of injections. Where the blood has become Wassermann positive or where secondary manifestations have appeared, five such courses of treatment are considered necessary.

A Wassermann and Kahn test should be made before each course is commenced and these tests usually remain consistently negative after the completion of the first course.

After these courses have been administered the patient may be regarded as provisionally cured, but he must be kept under observation for a period of at least one year. During this period there should be a clinical examination and serological examination of his blood every three months.

Before the final course of treatment is administered, or at any convenient time after the first course of treatment, it is advisable to examine the cerebrospinal fluid. If the cerebrospinal fluid is normal, further lumbar punctures are not necessary.

It is frequently advantageous to substitute acetylarsan for neoarsphenamine in the fourth and fifth courses. This is particularly indicated if the intravenous injections are not well tolerated.

The prognosis in early syphilis is extremely satisfactory, and after the treatment outlined above the patient may be regarded as cured.

Further observations are not necessary, but certain individuals who are very apprehensive regarding relapse may be permitted to return for clinical and serological examination once a year, but more frequent examinations are likely to produce unnecessary anxiety.

Management of a Case of Late Syphilis

The treatment of late syphilis presents quite distinct problems from early syphilis, for each patient has a different pathological picture, and widely varying powers of spontaneous recovery and of tolerance to antisyphilitic drugs are observed.

In every case prolonged treatment is necessary. Very intensive treatment is less frequently required, but observation for several years after treatment is wise.

Gummatous ulcers are not very contagious and they heal

rapidly with dressings of eusol and later elastoplast, in conjunction with antisyphilitic treatment.

A patient with syphilis affecting the heart or nervous system may be considered non-contagious, and may be nursed without special precautions. Gummatous ulcers in the mouth benefit by frequent antiseptic mouth washes, such as glycerin of thymol or phenol sodique. Leucoplakia should be treated by soothing and non-irritant applications, such as glycerin boracis used as a paint. If the appearances of a patch of leucoplakia suggest the possibility of malignant change a biopsy should be performed.

Iodides are of great value in the treatment of late syphilis. They produce resolution of gummata very rapidly, and a mixture containing potassium iodide (10 gr.) may be given thrice daily for two weeks before injections are commenced, and its administration is continued for two months. Iodides should be given during the intervals between courses of injections.

Arsenical drugs—especially arsphenamine—are not well tolerated by patients who have impairment of their liver function, due either to the syphilitic infection or to alcoholism or other causes.

The kidney is damaged less frequently, but if there is albuminuria, hæmaturia or a failure of the power of renal concentration, mercury and bismuth must be given with caution. Alcoholic patients who have reduced hepatic efficiency are treated with iodides and bismuth for three months, then moderate doses, *e.g.*, 0·3 or 0·45 gm., of neoarsphenamine may be given each week for ten weeks. Two such courses of 4·5 gm. neoarsphenamine and 3 gm. bismuth may be given each year. Cases of renal disease are given iodides for several weeks, then small doses of an arsenical drug, *e.g.*, 3 c.c. acetylarsan or 0·3 gm. neoarsphenamine weekly for ten weeks. At the same time appropriate dietetic and other treatment is prescribed. As recovery occurs tolerance may be acquired to moderate doses of oil-soluble bismuth preparations, *e.g.*, 2 c.c. neo-cardyl or 2 c.c. stabismol per week.

If the excretory powers of the kidney and the liver functions are not impaired, the patient will tolerate a scheme of treatment in which he receives in three months 4·5 gm. neoarsphenamine and 2 gm. bismuth, and iodides.

Four such courses may be given each year and treatment will be required for two years. If the Wassermann reaction is then negative, small doses of mercury and iodides are given by mouth for three periods of two months each year, or the patient may receive two courses of 3 gm. bismuth each year. After four years the antisyphilitic treatment is stopped, but clinical and serological examinations are made twice each year for at least three years thereafter.

The general health is regarded as the principal guide to treatment, rather than the result of the Wassermann test. Elderly patients with a persistently positive Wassermann test should not be subjected to the risks of intensive or prolonged antisyphilitic treatment. They benefit greatly, however, by a course of treatment of moderate intensity, *e.g.*, 3 gm. neoarsphenamine and 2 gm. bismuth, twice a year, and in the intervals small doses of iodides should be prescribed.

If the heart or nervous system are affected by syphilis, then treatment is modified, and details will be found on pp. 654, 216.

Syphilitic disease of the liver benefits by prolonged administration of iodides. Small doses of bismuth are given at first, but the dose is soon increased and 2 or 3 gm. may be given in ten weeks, and four courses of 3 gm. bismuth may be given in the first year. If progress has been satisfactory and if there is no evidence of impaired liver function, 3 gm. neoarsphenamine may be given along with 3 gm. bismuth in each of four courses in the second year's treatment. Iodides are prescribed during the intervals between courses.

Syphilis during Pregnancy

Pregnancy modifies the course of syphilis favourably so that the clinical manifestations may be trivial or absent.

In early syphilis it is desirable to institute intensive treatment. During the last three months of gestation drugs must be given cautiously. The dose of neoarsphenamine and of bismuth must be limited to 0·3 and 0·15 gm. respectively at weekly intervals for a period of five or six weeks.

Syphilis of the Cardio-vascular System

The details of treatment are given on p. 654.

Antisyphilitic treatment must go hand in hand with cardiological treatment. The best results are obtained by a judicious combination of all available remedial measures.

The principles of treatment are :—

1. The cautious administration of iodides, and later, bismuth or mercury.

2. Arsphenamine should only be given in small doses if there has been cardiac failure, and then only after several months' treatment with bismuth and iodides.
3. Treatment and observation must be prolonged.
4. The patient must adjust his life to the capacity of a heart that is permanently damaged.

Congenital Syphilis

Congenital syphilitic infants may be treated from birth, even if marasmic.

In very small infants it is advantageous to give arsenic and bismuth in minute doses twice a week. Sulpharsphenamine is given by intramuscular injection, in doses of 0·01 gm. per kilogram of body-weight. Bismuth is given in doses of 0·005 gm. per kilogram of body-weight. This is conveniently measured by preparing a 1 : 10 dilution of the usual suspensions of bismuth employed for the treatment of adults.

Hydrarg. c. cret. by mouth and the inunction of mercurial ointments are not efficient methods of treatment for syphilitic infants.

Later in childhood the dosage is calculated according to the body-weight. As a rule children tolerate antisyphilitic treatment very well.

Very prolonged treatment is unnecessary in every case, but a minimum of two years is advised and an attempt should be made to secure complete eradication of the syphilitic lesions and a return of the Wassermann reaction to negative. The patient must be kept under observation for many years, as it is not uncommon for clinical or serological relapses to become apparent at puberty or during early adolescence.

In general the prognosis is extremely good in congenital syphilis, but certain lesions require individual treatment.

Interstitial keratitis should be treated by instillation of 1 per cent. atropine drops—night and morning—and both eyes should be shaded by wearing close-fitting dark glasses. Nerve deafness may occur suddenly. It is frequently complete and bilateral and does not respond to treatment. Such children should receive special education, lest they become deaf mutes.

Congenital syphilitic infants showing ulceration of the mouth or skin eruptions are very contagious and must be isolated. This is unnecessary with late manifestations.

Syphilis of the Central Nervous System

The treatment of syphilitic lesions of the nervous system varies to some extent according to the tissues mainly affected—and the lesions may be considered under the terms :—

1. Meningo-vascular syphilis.
2. Cerebral vascular syphilis.
3. Tabes dorsalis.
4. General paralysis of the insane.

Meningo-vascular Syphilis. — Meningo-vascular syphilis occurs relatively early in the course of syphilitic infection, and if treatment is instituted early the prognosis is good and complete recovery is usual.

After treatment for one month with iodides by mouth and injections of bismuth, tryparsamide should be administered in doses of 3 gm. per week along with bismuth until a course of 30 gm. tryparsamide and 3 gm. bismuth has been given.

After four weeks' interval this course of 30 gm. tryparsamide and 3 gm. bismuth is repeated, and four such courses may be given in a year. Progress is estimated by regular clinical examination and by examination of the cerebrospinal fluid before each course. After one year the cerebrospinal fluid may return to normal, in which case the patient is treated as for late syphilis.

Vascular Syphilis.—Vascular syphilis manifests itself mainly as cerebral thrombosis and hemiplegia or hemiparesis (see p. 995). The general treatment advocated for these conditions is applicable to syphilitic cases. It is important to avoid intensive treatment with antisyphilitic drugs early in such cases—a slight reaction in the diseased cerebral vessel may cause a great increase in the area of nervous tissue affected or may cause permanent destruction of nerve cells.

Iodides are prescribed and often mercury is administered as liq. hydrarg. perchlor. (15 to 30 minims three times a day). After two weeks bismuth is given in doses of 0·1 gm. per week, and iodides are taken continuously. After one month neoarsphenamine may be given in moderate doses, *e.g.*, 0·3 or 0·45 gm. per week for ten weeks. Thus a suitable scheme of treatment in the first three months is iodides by mouth, with bismuth (2 gm.) and neoarsphenamine (4 gm.).

The paralytic symptoms and signs usually disappear rapidly and completely, but prolonged treatment is advisable to safeguard against a recurrence. The treatment is essentially that of long-standing syphilis, but it must be continued until the cerebrospinal fluid returns to normal.

Gumma.—Cerebral gumma is a rare lesion, and it responds very rapidly to treatment with iodides, bismuth and tryparsamide. In a few instances surgical operation is required to remove meningeal adhesions or to relieve intracranial pressure.

Tabes Dorsalis.—The general mode of life of the patient should be reviewed and an effort should be made to reorganize his régime so that he does not have undue physical strain and fatigue. He may have to change his work on account of ataxia or visual failure. Before treatment is commenced the visual fields should be measured accurately. He should also be examined for foci of chronic infection as these frequently accentuate the symptoms.

Tabes dorsalis responds well to prolonged treatment with tryparsamide and bismuth—courses of treatment consisting of 30 gm. tryparsamide and 3 gm. bismuth are given four times a year. In the intervals iodides should be given, and occasionally iron should be prescribed.

The treatment of tabes dorsalis will inevitably extend over two or more years, but in the majority there is a great improvement in the symptoms—the pains are relieved, ataxia disappears, bladder control is restored and his general physical state improved.

Observation of the visual fields is necessary every three months when tryparsamide is being given. If the patient has pale optic discs or any restriction of the visual field at the onset, very frequent perimetric examinations are necessary—every two weeks at first and later on every three months. If rapid visual failure occurs after tryparsamide, the use of the drug is discontinued. Sodium thiosulphate is injected intravenously in doses of 1 gm. per diem for one week, and vitamin B_1 is given in doses of 2,000 units per diem for fourteen days. Tryparsamide should never be given again to patients who have shown definite toxic amblyopia following its use.

The progress of the patient is assessed by clinical examinations and by examination of the cerebrospinal fluid twice a year. Certain symptoms may also demand special treatment.

Ataxia.—The psychic factor in tabetic ataxia must be clearly recognized, and success in treatment will depend largely on the degree to which the patient's self-confidence can be restored. A tabetic should not be confined to bed unless this is absolutely necessary. If he is confined to bed an effort should be made to restore the tone of the muscles and to re-educate the sense of position and joint and muscle senses. Simple exercises carried out in bed are of value, and massage and passive movements will assist in restoring weak muscles.

As soon as possible he is encouraged to get up, to stand and to try to walk, being supported and given confidence by sympathetic helpers. He is urged not to watch his feet, but to step forward with confidence and look at some object straight in front.

At first re-education will progress more rapidly if he has a level, smooth, firm and non-slippery surface on which to practice, and he should not have to endure the gaze of critical spectators. When he has achieved some degree of proficiency he may be encouraged to display with pride his daily progress, and he may venture first in quiet streets and then in traffic.

If there is pronounced hypotonia the joints should not be exposed to hyperextension or undue trauma. It is usually unwise for an ataxic tabetic to drive a motor vehicle.

Complete recovery from ataxia is possible except in the most advanced cases.

Incontinence of Urine.—The patient is taught to attempt to empty the bladder at regular intervals, *e.g.*, every four hours. He should empty the bladder completely before retiring to bed at night and again in the morning on waking. If the bladder is overdistended and there is overflow-incontinence, the hypodermic injection of 1 c.c. doryl (Merck), a choline preparation, will produce evacuation in most cases. This may have to be repeated on several occasions.

If catheterization is required the bladder should be emptied completely and then irrigated with one quart of 1 : 10,000 silver nitrate solution at a temperature of 112° F. The urine is often loaded with pus and organisms and in such cases urinary antiseptics are advised, and bladder irrigation either through a catheter or by per urethral irrigation is carried out daily until the pyuria is relieved.

Lightning Pains and Crises.—These are among the most intractable symptoms, but a great measure of relief is usual after prolonged treatment with tryparsamide, bismuth and iodides.

The initial dose of bismuth or tryparsamide may provoke severe bouts of pains or crises, and in this event the patient should take iodides and mercury by mouth for at least one month and then the injections may be resumed. If the pains remain severe or crises frequent after prolonged antisyphilitic treatment, it is justifiable to advise fever therapy. During the course of fever therapy the patient usually suffers severely from pains, but he later gains a great measure of relief which may last for a considerable time.

For temporary relief of an attack of pain, any mild sedative drug may prove successful. A combination such as :—

Acid. Acetylsalicyl.	gr. v
Phenacet.	gr. v
Codein.	gr. $\frac{1}{2}$

In powder or tablet form.

This may be repeated every four hours. Some patients get relief from large doses of phenacetin, *e.g.*, 20 gr., repeated in two hours if necessary. Atropine frequently gives rapid relief in doses of $\frac{1}{100}$ gr. by hypodermic injection, or $\frac{1}{75}$ gr. by mouth or in a suppository. Ephedrine (1 gr.) by mouth may abort an attack. A very severe attack is often terminated by lumbar puncture and withdrawal of 30 to 40 c.c. of cerebrospinal fluid.

Attacks of pains are often associated with wet weather, so residence in a dry and sunny climate usually has a favourable influence on the course of the disease.

Optic Atrophy.—The prognosis in regard to vision in primary syphilitic optic atrophy is always grave. Treatment with mercury, neoarsphenamine, bismuth, fever and intraspinal injections of neoarsphenamine have all proved practically powerless to arrest the course of the atrophy. Treatment with iodides and bismuth and tryparsamide gives a moderate measure of success—in 30 per cent. there is no further loss of vision, in 20 per cent. the atrophy proceeds more slowly, and a useful standard of vision is retained for several years or permanently. The remaining 50 per cent. progress to blindness. Tryparsamide must be used cautiously and carefully when optic atrophy is present, or if the optic fundus is abnormal in any way. A detailed chart of the fields of vision is prepared and the visual acuity measured.

The specific treatment is commenced with iodides by mouth and 0·2 gm. bismuth per week for four weeks. The visual fields are then measured again. Tryparsamide is given in small doses at first, *e.g.*, 1 gm. per week for two weeks, then 2 gm. per week for two weeks. The visual fields are observed each week at this time. If there is a sudden or rapid progress of the atrophy, or if a central scotoma appears, tryparsamide treatment is stopped. If there is no rapid change in the fields, tryparsamide is continued in doses of 3 gm. per week till 30 gm. have been given. Bismuth (3 gm.) is given during the course. The visual fields are again observed, and during an interval of four weeks the patient takes iodides by mouth. The routine course of tryparsamide (30 gm.) and bismuth (3 gm.) is then given again. The visual fields are charted at the end of each course, and many courses are required—at least two years' treatment in every case.

The cerebrospinal fluid should be examined every six months and treatment should continue till the blood and cerebrospinal fluid give a negative Wassermann test ; or in the event of the tests remaining positive, treatment should be continued for two or three years.

The patient should be very moderate in his use of tobacco, and refractive errors should be corrected. The patient may have to change his occupation, *e.g.*, it is often unsafe for him to drive a motor vehicle or to work on a railway. Vitamin B_1 may be administered and a diet rich in this vitamin prescribed (see p. 406).

The patient should remain under observation after treatment stops—his fields of vision should be checked at least once a year.

If tryparsamide causes rapid shrinkage of the visual field the patient may have to depend on intensive treatment with neoarsphenamine, bismuth and iodides. This delays the failure of vision, but the prognosis is unfavourable.

Arthropathies.—The arthropathies of tabes dorsalis are Charcot's disease of the joints, pathological fractures and perforating ulcer of the foot.

Perforating ulcers of the foot respond to a combination of antisyphilitic treatment, and local measures such as surgical removal of the deep layers of thickened, soft, horny material and scraping of the sinus. Mild antiseptic dressings such as eusol or bismuth iodoform paste, and a pad applied to the foot to relieve pressure on the affected joint are required.

Pathological fractures in tabetics are treated according to the usual surgical methods, but much less traction is required on the fragments, as the muscles and ligaments of the limb are usually hypotonic. At the same time treatment with tryparsamide and bismuth is administered.

Charcot's disease of the larger joints responds well to antisyphilitic treatment and orthopædic measures if treated early. The joint should be manipulated into the best possible position, and then fixed so that it is subjected to the minimum of weight or trauma on the joint. A great measure of recovery is possible, and after three months the joint is re-examined clinically and radiologically. If there is less swelling and deformity and if there is improvement in function, the patient may be permitted to use the joint in moderation, but it should not be exposed to the strain of normal use for six months, even under the most favourable circumstances.

In designing orthopædic appliances for such patients it is important not to place additional strain on the other joints, otherwise they may develop similar arthropathies.

If great disorganization of the joint has occurred the best possible result may be firm ankylosis in a good position. This can be secured by surgical operation to remove extraneous masses of irregular bone and to fix the joint in a suitable position. The joint is fixed by plaster bandages for three to six months. Antisyphilitic treatment should precede and follow surgical measures in all cases.

General Paralysis of the Insane.—The treatment of general paralysis of the insane offers a considerable measure of hope provided treatment is started at an early stage in the disease. The shorter the duration of the disease the better the prognosis irrespective of the severity of the symptoms or the type of mental disorder. Manic and grandiose patients in general show more improvement than the depressed and demented type. The prognosis in juvenile general paralysis of the insane is much worse than in the adult type of disease, but considerable improvement is possible and further deterioration of intelligence can be prevented.

Specific Treatment.—Tryparsamide and bismuth administered in full doses and continued for long periods produce considerable improvement in many cases. The risk of optic atrophy is slight but is guarded against by preliminary examination of the fields of vision and by subsequent observation at intervals of two months.

If optic atrophy is present, treatment should be given as advised on p. 219 and then fever treatment instituted.

The great majority of cases require fever treatment to supplement the specific treatment, but one course of tryparsamide and bismuth is considered a useful preliminary to fever therapy.

Fever Therapy.—Two methods of fever therapy are available —malaria inoculation and physical methods.

The inoculation of malaria is most frequently employed in this country, but the induction of pyrexia by physical means is now gaining popularity as improved technique has increased the reliability and safety of this method.

Malaria Therapy.—Blood from patients with benign tertian or quartian malaria is used. The benign tertian type is more readily available.

A supply of malarial blood may be obtained on application to The Ministry of Health, Room 44, V., Whitehall, London. The blood may be defibrinated or citrated and is transmitted in a sterile tube placed in a thermos flask containing ice. Inoculation will be successful up to twenty-four hours after the specimen has been collected. Infection by infected mosquitoes is also practised, but this method is not in general use. Malarial blood may be inoculated either intravenously or subcutaneously: 2 to 5 c.c. are required. After intravenous inoculation the incubation period ranges from three to fifteen days. After subcutaneous injection the incubation period is ten to thirty days. Wide variations are occasionally experienced. The patient should be kept under close observation after inoculation, preferably in hospital, and after the first rise of temperature blood films are examined for the presence of malaria parasites. When malarial pyrexia commences the temperature should be recorded every half hour until the temperature has returned to normal. In many cases a daily rise of temperature is experienced. If this proves exhausting to the patient, 2 gr. of quinine may be administered by the mouth and this usually modifies the course of the fever and often allows it to resume a true tertian form, but sometimes it stops the malaria or reduces it to too low a level.

Extremely careful nursing is necessary during malaria therapy. If the skin temperature rises above 105° F. the patient should be sponged with tepid water until the temperature falls to 102° F. Abundant supplies of fluids and glucose should be given throughout the course of the fever and the blood pressure should be estimated daily. A rapidly falling blood pressure is a warning of impending cardiac collapse and the fever should be terminated by quinine therapy.

As a rule the patient is allowed to have eight to ten rises of temperature to 104° F. or over, before the malaria is cured by the administration of quinine. Artificially inoculated malaria is very easily cured and is not liable to relapse or become chronic. During the later part of the course the patient may require cardiac stimulants and it is advantageous to administer iron.

Contraindications to malaria therapy are :—

Serious cardio-vascular disease with failure of compensation.
Severe anæmia.
Active tuberculosis.
Severe diabetes.
Idiosyncrasy to quinine.

The indications for stopping the course of malaria are :—

Cardiac failure.
Low blood pressure (systolic, 80 mm. or less).
Hyperpyrexia (over 106·5° F.).
Broncho-pneumonia.

The mortality from the malaria therapy is about 10 per cent. if advanced cases are included. This can be reduced to about 4 per cent. if cases presenting severe cardio-vascular disease are excluded.

After cessation of malaria treatment the patient is allowed a period of one month for convalescence and then vigorous antisyphilitic treatment is resumed with tryparsamide and bismuth. It may be advantageous for the patient to spend several months of his convalescence in a mental home or quietly resting in the country away from the strain of ordinary life. The maximum improvement may not be observed until six months after the cessation of the malaria.

Physical Means of Pyrexial Treatment.—Physical methods of securing fever therapy demand very elaborate and costly apparatus and can only be undertaken in hospitals where suitable equipment and a specially trained staff are available.

At present two main methods are available :—

(*a*) The inductotherm, where elevation of the patient's temperature is produced by high frequency currents from a coil placed a short distance away from the patient's body. The patient has to be enclosed in a special cabinet in which the air is heated, humidified and circulated. The temperature can be raised to 105° F. in about two hours. The patient's temperature is recorded every thirty minutes and this is regulated by variations of the temperature inside the cabinet, which can be controlled by a thermostat. In this way the temperature can be maintained between 105° and 106·5° F. for six or eight hours.

The patient's temperature and pulse are measured every half hour, and he must be carefully supervised during this time. Very large amounts of water and salt are lost by the very profuse perspiration and this loss should be restored by the administration of normal saline, ice drinks and probably stimulants.

(*b*) In the Kettering hypertherm the patient's temperature is raised without the assistance of diathermy, but exclusively by the temperature and humidity of the air in the cabinet. The patient's temperature rises rapidly and the pyrexia induced is controlled by alterations in the temperature and humidity of the air inside the cabinet. Accurate and sensitive control of the patient's temperature is possible, especially if an electric recording thermometer is used to register rectal temperature. Of the various types of apparatus for inducing artificial pyrexia, the Kettering hypertherm is the one most commonly employed.

With any physical method of inducing pyrexia the treatment may be given on alternate days or at longer intervals if the patient appears unduly exhausted.

In general paralysis of the insane a temperature of 105·5° F. should be maintained for six to eight hours on ten occasions to obtain the maximum benefit. Further, fever therapy may be again given after an interval of at least six months.

The advantages claimed for physical fever therapy are :—

1. It is more readily available—the pyrexia can be produced on any day or hour.
2. It is suitable for non-syphilitic patients.
3. The exact degree of pyrexia and the duration of the fever are readily regulated.
4. In skilled hands the risk and mortality are negligible.
5. Better results are obtained.
6. It is suitable for patients who are immune to malarial inoculation.

After fever therapy the patient should have prolonged treatment with tryparsamide and bismuth. In this way the blood and cerebrospinal fluid frequently return to normal and coincident syphilitic lesions are healed. The patient should revisit the physician for observation once a year.

Chancroid (Soft Sore or Ulcus Molle)

The diagnosis should first be established by Reenstierna's test, in which 0·2 c.c. of dmelcos vaccine (90 million B. Ducrey) is injected intracutaneously in the forearm and a pronounced local reaction indicates chancroid infection. Syphilis should be excluded. Dressings of eusol should be applied to the ulcer every four hours. It is essential to secure free exposure of the ulcers and circumcision or dorsal slit may be necessary. Buboes should not be incised, but sometimes require aspiration.

Sulphanilamide has proved very effective in chancroid, and should be given in doses of 4 gm. per diem for seven days. If healing is not then complete, smaller doses of sulphanilamide, *e.g.*, 2 gm. per diem, should be continued for another five days. Sulphapyridine is equally effective in doses of 3 gm. per day continued for seven to ten days.

Treatment with dmelcos vaccine (1 c.c. equals 225 million *B. Ducrey*) by intravenous injection is also effective, but has been superseded by the success of sulphanilamide treatment.

Lympho-granuloma Inguinale (Climatic Bubo, Poro-adenitis, Esthiomene)

Lympho-granuloma inguinale is common in tropical and sub-tropical countries but rare in Britain, except in the larger seaports. The diagnosis is established by Frei's test, in which material derived from a bubo is injected intracutaneously and gives a positive skin reaction in cases of lympho-granuloma inguinale.

There is no specific treatment. The condition responds fairly well to non-specific protein shock, *e.g.*, to a series of injections of T.A.B. vaccine, or dmelcos vaccine. A fairly severe temperature and general reaction seems to be necessary to secure recovery.

Material derived from a bubo may be used in the same way for curative inoculations. Organic preparations of antimony, such as fouadin, are of some value in resistant cases.

Rectal stricture may occur many years later in women and this requires surgical relief.

Warts (Condylomata Acuminata, Venereal Warts)

Warts occur frequently in association with venereal infection and are due to a virus infection. They grow rapidly and spread quickly in moist and dirty areas, so that the patient should wash frequently, dry the part affected and apply dusting powder. A single wart may be ligated if it has a definite pedicle. Painting the warts with 20 per cent. salicylic acid in collodion may produce a cure.

In most cases the area should be anæsthetized by infiltration with 1 per cent. novocaine and the warts removed by electro-cautery or diathermy. The area is kept clean and dry and the patient is re-examined one month later, as small areas of warty growth may escape the first treatment. Very extensive warty growths may require X-ray treatment.

Herpes Genitalis

This is a source of annoyance to the patient. The vesicles on small ulcers heal rapidly if bathed every four hours with saline. Recurrence of the herpes is minimized by keeping the surface of the prepuce clean and dry and by occasional applications of surgical spirit.

Balanitis

Balanitis heals rapidly with frequent saline baths and dressings. Strict attention to cleanliness is required, and many patients will benefit from circumcision at a later date.

R. Lees.

COMMON TROPICAL DISEASES

INTRODUCTION

THE selection of the tropical diseases, the treatment of which is discussed in this section, was made to meet the requirements of students and practitioners in this country, for whom this book is primarily intended. In the course of their practice they may meet with examples of the diseases listed from time to time; further, as modern methods of communication with tropical countries increase in frequency and speed, they may expect in the near future to meet with such diseases more frequently than at present. The omission of other tropical diseases has been made not because they are unimportant but because they will not be met with at all in this country—or extremely rarely. For those who propose to devote themselves to a career in the tropics, a specialized training is essential. Some diseases that are usually included in textbooks of tropical diseases will be considered in other sections of this book, *e.g.*, deficiency diseases, beriberi, pellagra, scurvy, bacillary dysentery, certain parasitic skin diseases; climatic bubo, etc.

In all diseases an accurate diagnosis is an essential preliminary to treatment. In the case of tropical diseases it is specially important because a number of specific drugs are available, which, if administered early, give very striking therapeutic results.

The practitioner will be asked by patients, proposing to go to the tropics, what steps they should take to prevent infection. To help him to answer this question, a short account of personal prophylaxis is given under the diseases discussed. It will be noted that among other measures, some specific drugs employed in the treatment of the disease can also be used prophylactically to prevent attacks.

Perhaps it might appear that too many preparations of specific drugs have been mentioned, which might rather confuse the practitioner. However, it has been found that the same infection, *e.g.*, leishmaniasis, malaria, trypanosomiasis, etc., in different parts of the tropics respond differently to the same preparation. Consequently, it may be necessary for the practitioner to try other preparations. This is the reason for listing a number of drugs.

MALARIA

Specific Therapy.—*Drugs Employed.*—Quinine, an alkaloid derived from the bark of different species of cinchona. The constituents of cinchona bark are certain acids, tannin and cinchona red with the following alkaloids: cinchonine, cinchonidine, cuprein, cinchonamine, quinamine, quinine, quinidine, hydroquinine. A cheap and largely used preparation is cinchona febrifuge, which contains all the alkaloids in the bark. It has the disadvantage, however, that the alkaloid content is liable to vary in different samples. Accordingly, a standard preparation called totaquina has been produced containing 70 per cent. of crystalline alkaloids, of which not less than 15 per cent. must be quinine. Three recent synthetic Bayer preparations are also used—plasmoquine, atebrin and certuna.

Treatment of an Acute Primary Attack of Malaria.—It has been suggested that it might be advantageous, in order to allow of the development of immunity, to permit the patient to have several rigors before arresting the infection. This might be permissible and perhaps advisable in an infection with the benign forms, but it would be too dangerous in the severe malignant tertian malaria.

In an ordinary case without complications, a useful scheme of treatment for an adult is to give calomel (3 gr.) at night, followed by a saline purge (sod. sulph., ½ oz.) in the morning. Quinine is then given by the mouth, combined with an alkali in the following prescription :—

℞		
	Quinin. Sulph.	gr. x
	Pulv. Acid. Cit.	gr. xx
	Mag. Sulph.	gr. x
	Sp. Anis.	♏iii
	Syr.	dr. i
	Aq. . . . . . ad	oz. i

Sig.—One oz., t.i.d., two and a half hours after food for one week. Dose then reduced to ½ oz., b.i.d., for further two weeks. Totaquina, which contains all the alkaloids, may replace the quinine in the above prescription.

On the completion of the course of quinine, plasmoquine simplex (one tablet, containing 0·01 gm.) may be given twice daily after food for a week. Children require smaller doses than adults, and the taste has to be disguised. One-twentieth of the adult dose is given for each year up to fifteen years; above this the adult dose is given. A useful method of administration to children is to make an emulsion of quinine sulphate in olive oil, or liquid paraffin (32 gr. to the ounce). This should be well stirred and the required amount floated on a little cold, sweetened milk followed by a further drink of milk. Tablets of quinine made by good firms are satisfactory, but solutions are preferable.

In cases where administration of quinine by the mouth is contraindicated—*e.g.*, severe vomiting—the drug may be given intramuscularly. For this purpose the best salt is the quinine bihydrochloride (10 gr.) dissolved in sterile saline and put up in 2 c.c. ampoules ready for use. The best site for injection is the gluteus maximus muscle at a point on a line horizontal with the tip of the great trochanter. It is very important to avoid the neighbourhood of the large nerves, otherwise serious damage may be done. The injection may be repeated on three consecutive days. For children, proportionately smaller doses are given. After the injections the part should be carefully massaged to help the dispersion and so to prevent local necrosis of muscle. Atebrin musonat in a dose of 0·3 gm. can be given instead of quinine, and has been found very useful.

In severe cases of malignant tertian malaria, where a rapid and powerful action is required, quinine may be given intravenously. The salt employed is again the quinine bihydrochloride (10 gr. in 10 c.c. sterile aq. dest.). The injection is made into the median basilic vein at the front of the bend of the elbow. It should be made *very* slowly, at least five minutes being spent over the injection. If given too quickly, there may be a rapid and alarming drop in blood pressure. One dose is usually sufficient to control the symptoms and administration by mouth may follow. For children, the dose is again adjusted according to age.

In some cases there is an apparent failure of quinine to check the infection. This may be due to a wrong diagnosis or, on the other hand, the patient may not be taking the quinine prescribed. To settle the latter question, a convenient test is available. Quinine is excreted in the urine, and a reagent, Mayer-Tanret, can be used for its detection. The reagent is made up as follows :—

Hydrarg. perchlor. . . . . gr. 1·3
Aq. . . . . 75 c.c.
Mix with
Pot. iod. . . . . . gr. 5
Aq. . . . . 20 c.c.
in a 100-c.c. flask.

Add a few drops of this reagent to the urine, and if quinine is present a white deposit occurs. If albumin is present, heat and filter whilst warm, then apply test. It is important to make certain that the patient is taking no other alkaloid than quinine. If this is done, the test is very reliable and useful.

The introduction recently of atebrin, plasmoquine and certuna has improved the treatment of malaria considerably. Atebrin, like quinine, acts specially on the asexual stage of the malaria parasite ; it is this stage which causes the clinical symptoms. It has much less action on the sexual stage. Plasmoquine, on the other hand, acts on the sexual stage, especially that of the malignant tertian parasite. Hence, the ideal for the complete treatment of malaria is a combination of quinine, or atebrin and plasmoquine. Atebrin (Bayer) is dispensed in tablets of 0·1 gm. each. For treatment the adult patient is given one tablet thrice daily after food for five to seven days. This is followed by plasmoquine simplex (0·01 gm. in each tablet), one tablet twice daily after food for five to seven days. This course may be repeated. It is not advisable to give atebrin and plasmoquine simultaneously. Atebrin is well borne by children and by pregnant women. One tablet divided into two may be given to young children. One tablet daily of plasmoquine is the suitable dose for children.

Very recently (1938) an account of a new synthetic drug, certuna (Bayer), was published. It is a dialkylamino-oxychinolylaminobutan. The results recorded show that it is a potent gametocide and superior to plasmoquine. It can be given at the same time as atebrin. It is especially useful in malignant tertian infections. In severe cases, after an initial intramuscular injection of 0·3 gm. atebrin musonat, give tablets of atebrin (0·1 gm.) thrice daily, and at the same time tablets of certuna (0·01 gm.) thrice daily for three successive days. In persons of heavier weight and in all cases with numerous crescents in the blood, certuna may be given in doses of 0·02 gm. thrice daily. No toxic symptoms have been observed during its use.

Treatment of Relapses in Malaria.—Whatever course of treatment is adopted in the primary attack, a relapse will probably occur in a certain proportion of cases at a later date. As there is little danger to life from a relapse, the patient may be allowed to have several febrile paroxysms before treatment is started as this allows the natural process of immunity to develop without interference, and makes the subsequent treatment more effective and less prolonged. Quinine sulphate (6 gr., three times a day) in solution for a few days will be sufficient as a rule. It is essential, of course, to make certain that the patient is suffering from a relapse and not a primary attack.

Toxic Effects of the Specific Drugs.—Quinine as a rule only causes slight tinnitus, but in some persons with an idiosyncrasy to the drug other symptoms may develop. These are: urticaria, hæmorrhages, bradycardia, gastric disturbance and amblyopia (which has to be distinguished from malarial amblyopia). Even death from syncope may occur. Atebrin is comparatively free from toxic effects, but colicky pains may be complained of, and a yellow discoloration of the skin generally follows its administration; this is not due to jaundice but to a yellow pigment, and is harmless. Plasmoquine may give rise to cyanosis, which is seen at first especially in the lips. It is probably due to the conversion of hæmoglobin into methhæmoglobin. Sometimes pains in the abdomen are felt by the patient.

Malaria in Pregnancy.—Atebrin is well tolerated even in comparatively large doses by pregnant women, and is indicated when pregnancy is present in preference to quinine.

Non-specific Treatment.—In severe cases of cerebral malaria, after intravenous injection of quinine, lumbar puncture may be performed and 20 c.c. of cerebrospinal fluid withdrawn. This may greatly relieve the cerebral symptoms. If vomiting is persistent, 10 minims adrenalin, 1 : 1,000, may be given by the mouth in a little water. This has given good results in practice. For hyperpyrexia, cold packs or baths are essential if the temperature is over 106° F. The rectal temperature should be taken, and when it falls to 102° F. the patient should be removed from the cold pack, or bath, and warm blankets applied. In malarial cachexia with marked splenomegaly, counter-irritants (ung. hydrarg. biniodide) should be rubbed in over the splenic area. If anæmia is very severe (*i.e.*, below 30 per cent. Hb.) and the patient very collapsed, a blood transfusion should be given. In the majority of cases full doses of iron in the form of ferrous salts will rapidly restore the blood to normal. Helminthic infections are frequently present in malaria and should be treated on lines that will be discussed later under this heading. The disinfestation of the patient greatly assists the specific therapy (quinine and synthetic drugs).

General Management.—Every case of malaria with fever should be treated seriously and carefully nursed in bed, as severe symptoms may develop without warning in the malignant form. The patient should be given plenty of water and lemonade to drink, as he may be very dehydrated by the profuse sweating. The addition of glucose to the lemonade is useful, since in many cases of malaria a toxic hepatitis occurs. Food at first should be fluid and easily digested. In convalescence, if the appetite is good, a full diet may be given.

Blackwater Fever

This is a very serious and urgent complication of malaria, most frequently of the malignant tertian infection. The first essential in the treatment is to put the patient at once at complete rest, no matter how unsatisfactory his surroundings may be. Transportation is very badly tolerated. As there is a rapid destruction of blood with intense anæmia in severe cases, a transfusion of compatible blood should be given as early as possible. This may be followed by an intravenous injection of a pint of distilled water containing sod. bicarb. (150 gr.), to which glucose, in strength of 5 per cent., may be added. If the urine is made alkaline by massive doses of pot. cit. (60 gr.) every four hours, early suppression, which is frequent, may be prevented. In all cases—whether mild or severe—the patient should be urged to drink freely, irrespective of thirst. This is most important. When there is much vomiting, a Murphy's rectal drip with warm saline may be used. Morphia ($\frac{1}{4}$ gr.) should be given, especially if there is restlessness or vomiting. Good nursing is extremely important, but in certain cases this may not be available in the tropics. As a rule parasites are very scanty in the blood. If present, a course of atebrin as outlined above may be administered. Quinine itself should not be used.

Personal Prophylaxis of Malaria and Blackwater Fever

Chemoprophylaxis.—There is no such thing as a causal prophylaxis, because none of the drugs, quinine, atebrin or plasmoquine in medicinal doses can destroy sporozoits, which the mosquito injects into man, but all of them can prevent the development of clinical signs by acting on the schizont stage which develops from the sporozoits in the red cells of man. They are, therefore, called "clinical prophylactics" and are in this respect of very great value, since their regular administration enables persons to continue their work in malarial areas in which otherwise they would be incapacitated by fever. Whilst living in such an area, it is recommended that quinine (6 gr.) should be taken daily and for two or three months after leaving the district. It is best taken in tablets after the last meal in the evening. Atebrin, given in doses of 0·2 gm. (two tablets) on two successive days in each week has been found useful, particularly in persons with an idiosyncracy to quinine. Plasmoquine has also been found valuable because of its effects on the sexual phase of the parasite, and it has the further great advantage that it acts as a communal prophylactic by preventing the mosquitoes of the district from becoming infected. A dose of 0·02 gm. on two successive days of the week is recommended.

Protection against Bites of Mosquitoes.—The best personal prophylactic is a good mosquito curtain on the bed. It must be free from holes and in good condition. It should be well tucked under the mattress before sunset. It is advisable, as a precaution, when the person has got into the net to examine the interior carefully with an electric torch to see that there are no mosquitoes enclosed. Apart from the use of the net, repellents may be applied to the skin of the exposed parts. Of these an ointment recently introduced by Bayer, called mitalin, is useful. It should be rubbed freely on to the hands, ankles and face. Other measures are the removal, or oiling, of collections of water in which mosquito larvæ may breed. The dwelling-house should, if possible, have the doors and windows screened, and should not be built in the neighbourhood of native quarters. Persons who have had severe attacks of blackwater fever should, if circumstances permit, avoid returning to the tropics.

AFRICAN TRYPANOSOMIASIS

Specific Therapy. — *Drugs Employed.* — Bayer 205 (Germanin); French equivalent, Fourneau 309. Tryparsamide; French equivalent, Fourneau 270. Other drugs less frequently employed at present are atoxyl and preparations of antimony.

Treatment of an Early Acute Infection.—In the early stages treatment with Bayer 205 may be sufficient. It is given intravenously, 1 gm. being dissolved in 10 c.c. sterile distilled water and injected slowly into a vein at the bend of the elbow. This is repeated until a total of 5 gm. have been given. If this quantity is given within a week, a maximum effect is produced on the organisms. In some parts of the tropics a single dose of 1 gm. of 205 is administered and followed by a course of tryparsamide.

Treatment of Relapses.—If the case is seen in the later stages, especially when the cerebrospinal system is invaded by the trypanosome, then Bayer 205 is not alone sufficient, and a combined treatment with tryparsamide is indicated. A preliminary course of 5 gm. of 205 is given as above, and after an interval of a week or ten days, depending on the condition of the patient, tryparsamide injections are begun. The initial dose is 1 gm. in 10 c.c. of distilled water injected intravenously. The next dose is 2 gm., and the later doses may have to be increased to 3 gm.—depending on the stage of the disease. The injections may be given twice weekly till a total of 24 gm. have been administered. The dosage of tryparsamide for children is 0·07 gm. per kilogram of body-weight ; 0·055 gm. per kilogram for young adolescents ; and 0·045 gm. per kilogram for adults. For children, Bayer 205 may be given in doses of 0·4 to 0·6 gm. Children tolerate these drugs well.

Toxic Effects of Drugs.—At the end of the course of 5 gm. of Bayer's 205, some signs of irritation of the kidneys are often observed, as indicated by a temporary albuminuria with a few granular casts in the urine. This usually clears up quickly. A toxic dermatitis not infrequently appears, but this also disappears on cessation of the treatment. Tryparsamide may produce ocular symptoms in some patients, *e.g.*, photophobia, lachrymation, pain in the eyes and dimness of vision. Hence, in every case, before beginning treatment with tryparsamide, the eyes should be carefully examined, especially the fields of vision and the fundus oculi. In suspicious cases the drug should be stopped and an intravenous injection of ametox (May & Baker) given. It is put up in 5 c.c. ampoules containing 0·45 gm. of thiosulphate of soda, and should be repeated on alternate days till six injections have been given. Other toxic effects of tryparsamide, *e.g.*, the Herxheimer reaction and the nitritoid reaction, are rare in the treatment of trypanosomiasis.

Drug Resistance.—It has been shown that trypanosomes become readily drug-fast to the arsenicals. Moreover, these drug-fast strains retain this property even after passage through the tsetse fly. This opens up a question of great importance in connection with the prevention of the disease. Although the trypanosome can be rendered drug-fast to Bayer's 205, this, fortunately, occurs much less frequently than with arsenicals ; hence the value of the treatment with 205 described above.

General Management.—An important preliminary to specific therapy is the disinfestation of the patient of helminths, *e.g.*, ancylostomes, bilharzia, etc., as will be described later.

During the earlier stages of the treatment the patient may be kept in bed, but the later courses of tryparsamide may be given at the out-patient clinic. The diet should be as generous as possible, if the digestion is not impaired. In the later stages of untreated cases the patient will be completely bed-ridden and will have to be fed and nursed ; fortunately, this stage is not so frequently seen nowadays owing to the great advance in methods of treatment.

Personal Prophylaxis.—*Chemoprophylaxis.*—It has been found that a single intravenous dose of Bayer's 205 will give protection for 115 days. It is particularly applicable to infections with *T. rhodesiense.*

Avoidance of Flies.—Flies bite during the middle of the day ; thus, by avoiding the fly belts in the daytime, the individual can protect himself against infection. Tsetse flies, except *Glossina swynnertoni*, are not found in dwelling-houses as a rule. For protection against *G. swynnertoni* the same precautions in dwelling-houses should be instituted as for malaria.

LEISHMANIASIS

Kala-azar

Specific Treatment.—*Drugs Employed.*—Pentavalent compounds of antimony : stibosan, known formerly as von Heyden 471 (Bayer) ; neostibosan, known formerly as von Heyden 693, which contains 40 per cent. antimony and is comparatively non-toxic ; urea stibamine, introduced by Brahmachari of Calcutta ; Solustibosan 561 (Bayer) ; trivalent compounds of antimony, such as tartar emetic (sodium-antimony tartrate) ; Neo-antimosan or Fouadin.

Treatment of Acute Attack.—Neostibosan has proved a useful and efficient drug. It is given intravenously as are nearly all antimony preparations, owing to the intense irritation which they cause in the subcutaneous or muscular tissues. Neostibosan is made up in a 25 per cent. solution in sterile fresh distilled water. The initial dose for an adult is 0·1 gm., which is given slowly intravenously. It is very important to avoid any leakage into the surrounding subcutaneous tissue, as this will cause severe pain and inflammation. The second dose will be 0·2 gm. and the third

0·3 gm. The injections are given on alternate days until a total of 2·7 to 4 gm. have been given. Children stand antimony compounds well, but smaller doses are required. At three years the initial dose would be 0·025 gm. Intravenous injections are often difficult in children, but recent antimony preparations — fouadin, solustibosan or neoantimosan — can be given by intramuscular administration. They are manufactured by Bayer and are put up in ampoules ready for injection. For a course of fouadin there are ten ampoules, one containing 0·5 c.c., one containing 1·5 c.c. and eight containing 3·5 c.c. The injections are given every second day.

Solustibosan 561 (Bayer) has been recently introduced and is a pentavalent antimony hexonate. It is issued in ampoules and appears to be quite stable. The clinical trials suggest that the drug is in the same class as neostibosan, and the fact that it can be given intramuscularly without damage to the tissues constitutes a distinct advance in the treatment of kala-azar. Each cubic centimetre contains 20 mg. antimony (metal) as compared with 21 mg. in a 5 per cent. solution of neostibosan. The initial dose for an adult is 2 c.c., increased up to 6 c.c., which is administered on alternate days or daily till a total of 59 to 84·5 c.c. has been given. It is relatively non-toxic and it has succeeded in certain cases which had proved resistant to a full course of neostibosan.

Tartar emetic is still used, and it has the advantage of being cheaper than the other compounds. A sterile 2 per cent. solution in fresh distilled water is prepared. An initial dose for an adult is 2 c.c., and this is gradually increased to 5·8 c.c., which is the maximum individual dose for an adult. It is injected slowly intravenously. For young children, in whom intravenous medication is difficult, a dose of 12 mg. in 60 c.c. sterile saline may be given intraperitoneally in the middle line of the abdomen just below the umbilicus. The injections are given bi-weekly and the total dose for an adult is 30 gr. It is very important that the solutions should be made up daily as required, with fresh distilled water, as they are liable to undergo deterioration on standing.

Treatment of Relapse.—Some cases become resistant to the drug that is being used, in which case it is advisable to change to one of the other preparations of antimony mentioned. Where the relapse takes the form of a skin lesion, called dermal leishmanoid or post-kala-azar leishmaniasis, it will usually be found that the patients have suffered from kala-azar about a year previously and have been insufficiently treated with antimony. Biopsy of the skin shows the presence of the

Leishman-Donovan body. They respond well to a course of treatment as described above, using solustibosan, neostibosan or urea stibamine; for this reason it is very important to recognize the true nature of the skin lesion.

Toxic Effects of Drugs.—An early sign is coughing, and a feeling of constriction in the chest may occur immediately after, or even during, an injection. This is an indication for the reduction of the subsequent dose. In some cases vomiting and purging may develop during the course of treatment, the symptoms being not unlike those of cholera. Towards the end of the course cramps in the muscles of the leg may be felt, and occasionally arthritic pains are experienced. Jaundice may also be noted occasionally. If toxic symptoms arise, the drug should be temporarily discontinued. In some resistant cases it may be necessary to push the administration to the limit of tolerance, and these cases require careful watching. Occasionally the patient is unable to tolerate a sufficient quantity of the drug to ensure destruction of the parasite.

General Management.—The expulsion of helminths and the treatment of coincident infections, such as malaria, are very important. The anæmia should be treated with full doses of iron in the form of ferri et ammon. cit. or Blaud pills (see p. 471).

The appetite in cases of kala-azar is generally unimpaired and the digestion is good, so he should receive a nourishing, well-balanced diet with plenty of fluid in the form of glucose lemonade. He should be kept in bed and carefully nursed during the acute phase. Cancrum oris may be treated by bathing the ulcer with hot permanganate solution.

Personal Prophylaxis.—*Chemoprophylaxis.*—So far this has not been employed in kala-azar.

Other Methods of Protection from Infection.—Domestic and personal cleanliness is important. In some areas dogs are also infected, so any infected animals should be destroyed. Mosquito curtains of a fine mesh and repellents, as indicated in malaria, should be used to prevent the bites of sand-flies. It is an advantage to live in the upper storey of the dwelling, as sand-flies do not usually leave the lower parts of the house.

Oriental Sore

Specific Treatment.—*General.*—The antimony preparations already mentioned are used in the same way as for kala-azar.

Local.—Berberine sulphate, which is put up by May & Baker as a 2 per cent. solution in ampoules under the name of "orisol," is given in doses of 2 to 3 c.c., injected at points round the periphery of the sore. Two to three such injections at weekly intervals are usually sufficient to cure the sore. Emetine hydrochloride has also been used. Doses of 0·13 to 0·75 gr. in sterile distilled water have been injected round the edges of the sore. Treatment with X-rays, ionization and carbon dioxide snow have all been recommended, as has the scraping of the sore with a Volkmann spoon, followed by the application of pure carbolic, after which the sore is covered with elastoplast. Berberine sulphate is the most efficacious treatment in such a condition and may be tried initially, but if it is not successful the other alternatives may be employed.

Personal Prophylaxis.—As for kala-azar.

INFECTIOUS JAUNDICE (WEIL'S DISEASE)

Specific Treatment.—If the diagnosis is made within seven days of the onset, a polyvalent serum should be given as soon as possible. In advanced cases in which jaundice and uræmic symptoms have developed, it is of little value. The serum is given intravenously or intramuscularly. An efficient serum is prepared by Burroughs, Wellcome & Co. Twenty cubic centimetres should be given at six-hourly intervals for twenty-four hours, and then once daily until the temperature is normal.

General Management.—As the liver is generally severely attacked, glucose in orange or lemon juice should be given freely by the mouth.

The patient should be kept at rest and carefully nursed. A milk diet should be given in the early stages. If vomiting is marked, nutrient enemata may be required and 10 minims of 1 : 1,000 adrenalin in a little water may be given by the mouth.

Personal Prophylaxis.—All food should be carefully protected from contamination by rats, which are the carriers of the parasite. The urine and fæces of patients should be disinfected. Swimming, especially using the " crawl " stroke, in bathing pools, canals or rivers suspected of being the source of infection should be avoided.

Infectious jaundice may be regarded as a disease of certain industries. Sewer workers, miners, fish curers and workers in certain sugar-cane plantations are particularly liable to become infected and should be warned to take special precautions, *i.e.*, protect their food and drink from the excreta of rats and to protect themselves from abrasions.

The Japanese have used—with success—killed cultures of the *leptospira icterohæmorrhagiæ* as a prophylactic. This is probably unnecessary in this country.

RAT-BITE FEVER (SODOKU)

Specific Treatment.—*Drugs Employed.*—Salvarsan and its derivatives.

Treatment of Acute Attack.—Neoarsphenamine is given intravenously in doses of 0·4 to 0·6 gm. dissolved in 10 c.c. of sterile distilled water. One dose is sometimes sufficient to effect a cure, but as a rule it is necessary to repeat the injections on several occasions at short intervals.

Treatment of Relapses.—Some cases may relapse, but, fortunately, this is rare. A case seen by the author recently continued to have relapses over a long period, in spite of repeated courses of neoarsphenamine, and died from a complicating pneumonia. In this case the parasite had become drug-fast.

General Management.—A bite by a rat or cat should be cauterized by pure carbolic after the wounds have been freely opened up.

During the attack of fever the patient should be kept in bed on a light diet.

Personal Prophylaxis.—Protection against bites by rats and cats. As in plague, the most important protection against this disease is efficient rat destruction.

PLAGUE

Specific Therapy.—In plague, specific therapy plays a less prominent part in the treatment than in the other diseases discussed. There is no specific drug, the two specific agents employed being antisera and bacteriophage.

Recently a potent serum has been prepared in the Bombay laboratory, which has given promising results in some cases. Injections should be begun early in the disease and given intravenously in doses of 30 to 40 c.c., repeated as required.

Bacteriophage is injected into the bubo in doses of 2 to 3 c.c. on the first day and again on the second. In septicæmic cases 3 c.c. or more have been given intravenously. A preliminary injection of 5 to 10 c.c. of the patient's own blood (autohæmotherapy) is recommended.

Non-specific Therapy.—Mercurochrome, 220 soluble, as in other septicæmic conditions, has been tried with some success in plague. Twenty c.c. of a 1 per cent. solution are given intravenously, and this dose can be increased in subsequent injections. For pain and sleeplessness, the injection of $\frac{1}{4}$ gr. of morphia is indicated. It is important to accelerate the bursting of the bubos, for when this occurs the general symptoms improve and there is less risk of the blood becoming infected. Frequent poulticing is useful, and as soon as softening occurs the bubo should be incised and packed with iodoform gauze. Indolent bubonic swellings may be treated with liniment of iodine.

General Treatment.—This is a very important factor in the treatment of the various forms of plague, of which nursing forms a large part. In the earlier stages tepid sponging and the application of ice caps for the high fever and headache are indicated. Sponging the body every hour is a much safer method of lowering the temperature than the employment of antipyretic drugs. Vomiting may be controlled by sucking ice or by giving adrenalin (10 minims of a 1 : 1,000 solution in a little water by the mouth). For collapse, stimulants such as strong ammonia to the nostrils, or ether subcutaneously, are indicated.

Personal Prophylaxis.—The most important measure is prophylactic inoculation with Haffkine prophylactic vaccine. A dose of 4 c.c. is given to an adult. The dose is reduced for children. No unnecessary visits to a person suffering from plague should be made, and areas in which plague is occurring should be avoided. Nurses should be careful to cover any abrasions which they have on their skin, and those engaged in plague duty should wear boots and have their legs protected by puttees to prevent access of infected fleas. Attendants on cases of pneumonic plague should be inoculated with anti-plague vaccine. In addition, they should wear masks of absorbent cotton wool (16 cm. by 12 cm.) enclosed in muslin and retained by a many-tailed bandage, goggles and rubber gloves. All houses should be made rat-proof.

UNDULANT FEVER

Melitensis Type

Specific Therapy.—In this disease there are no specific drugs available. Autogenous vaccines have proved useful, and a serum is also marketed by Mulfords. Stock vaccines are less effective than the autogenous types. The serum may be given intravenously in doses of 50 to 100 c.c. in the early stage of the disease and may be repeated at twenty-four hour intervals. At a later stage the vaccine can be usefully employed. Starting with a dose of 10 to 15 million organisms it may be increased gradually till a dose of 200 million is reached.

Non-specific Therapy.—Recently the administration of sulphonamide-P (British Drug Houses) has been followed by satisfactory improvement. Two tablets of $7\frac{1}{2}$ gr. are given four-hourly till twelve tablets in all have been taken. Intravenous injection of mercurochrome 220, in doses of 20 c.c. of a 1 per cent. solution, has been followed by favourable results, but the reactions may be severe. Other dyes have also been employed—*e.g.*, 2 per cent. trypflavine (10 c.c.) intravenously at two-day intervals. In resistant cases protein shock therapy should be given a trial, using T.A.B. vaccine, starting with a dose of 5 to 10 million and working up to 100 million.

General Treatment.—This is very important. Careful nursing is essential in this usually long drawn-out illness. The nurse should be instructed to keep the temperature below 103° F. by sponging with tepid water and vinegar, which is more efficacious than the use of antipyretics. If hyperpyrexia threatens, the wet pack or cold bath should be used. For pain and sleeplessness, morphia ($\frac{1}{4}$ gr.) may be employed, but care must be taken that a habit is not formed by too continued use. Clothing should be frequently changed if there is much sweating. Diet should at first be composed of milk and then gradually increased. Care must be taken to avoid overfeeding. The patient should have plenty of fluid in the form of orange juice glucose, and marmite is a very useful addition to the diet. Rest in bed for at least three weeks after the temperature has become normal should prevent a relapse.

Personal Prophylaxis.—As the chief method of spread is by milk (goat's milk in the case of the militensis type, and cow's milk in the abortus type), all milk in endemic areas should be boiled before use. Unfermented cheese is also a frequent but unsuspected source of infection and should be avoided. Man is probably naturally more resistant to the abortus than the militensis type. Prophylactic injections of dead vaccines have been tried with encouraging results for both types.

Abortus Type

Treatment is on the same lines as for the melitensis type, but protein shock therapy has given particularly good results in cutting short the abortus infection.

CHOLERA

Specific Therapy.—There is no specific treatment for cholera, hence non-specific therapy has to be employed and has been developed on scientific lines.

Non-specific Therapy.—The very serious symptoms of cholera are mainly due to profound dehydration of the tissues. Consequently, it is most important to replace the fluid as rapidly as possible, or the case will end fatally in a very short time. The scheme of treatment in a moderately severe case is as follows: first the blood pressure and specific gravity of the blood is estimated. The latter is quite easily carried out. A series of small bottles can be purchased containing glycerin and water, the specific gravity of which increases by two degrees in each bottle from 1,048 to 1,070. The finger is pricked and the blood is sucked into a capillary pipette. A drop is added to each bottle, and the bottle in which the drop remains stationary in the middle of the fluid for a minute or two gives the specific gravity of the blood. The normal specific gravity of the blood of a European is 1,058 and that of an Eastern native is 1,056. A specific gravity of 1,063 in cholera indicates a fluid deficiency requiring an injection of 3 to 6 pints of fluid to restore it to normal. A systolic blood pressure below 70 mm. is a very serious sign. The fluid is best replaced by using a hypertonic saline solution containing the following: sodium chloride (120 gr.); potassium chloride (6 gr.); calcium chloride (6 gr.); sterilized water (1 pint). This is injected by the intravenous route; owing to the collapsed state of the veins it will be necessary to expose the vein and insert a canula. If the rectal temperature is below 99° F., the saline should be heated to 100° F. If it is above 100° F., the solution should be given at a temperature between 80° and 90° F., as there is a risk of hyperpyrexia. The fluid is run in at the rate of not more than 2 oz. per minute; if there is distress or headache, it should be slowed down to 1 oz. per minute. From 3 to 6 pints should be administered, the amount being controlled by the specific gravity of the patient's blood. If the specific gravity rises and the blood pressure falls, it will be necessary to repeat the transfusion. In severe cases several transfusions may be required. If there is a tendency to suppression of urine, a rectal injection of hyperalkaline solution should be given—sod. bicarb., 150 gr. to 1 pint of isotonic saline, to be given slowly every two to four hours in cases where collapse has been overcome but suppression persists. At the same time the patient should be encouraged to drink water freely, and calcium permanganate may be added to the water so that it is just slightly pink in colour. A suspension of 7 oz. of kaolin in 14 oz. of water may be given in 1-oz. doses at frequent intervals even if there is vomiting, as it helps to adsorb the toxin. Atropine ($\frac{1}{100}$ gr.) given morning and evening is useful. Morphia ($\frac{1}{4}$ gr.) may be required if the pain is associated with muscular cramps. For milder cases of cholera without collapse a mixture of essential oils has been used with success. The mixture is as follows :—

℞ Sp. Æther. . . . . . . ♏xxx
Ol. Anis. . . . . . . ♏v
Ol. Cajuput. . . . . . ♏v
Ol. Junip. . . . . . . ♏v
Acid. Sulph. Aromat. . . . ♏xv

Sig.—Half a drachm in $\frac{1}{2}$ oz. of water every fifteen minutes. Total dose in four to six hours should be 8 to 10 drachms. To be given immediately symptoms start.

Pregnancy is a serious complication of cholera, as the fœtus almost invariably dies of toxæmia. Lovell in the Philippines reduced the mortality rate by watching for evidence of death of the fœtus or commencement of abortion ; he then removed the fœtus without anæsthetic. Pneumonia is a further serious complication (see p. 782).

Bacteriophage has been employed in the treatment of cholera. In an acute case its action will not be sufficiently rapid, so that it cannot replace the use of hypertonic saline, but it may be a useful adjuvant. A polyvalent bacteriophage may be given in drachm doses by the mouth every thirty minutes till symptoms improve, or 5 c.c. may be given intravenously along with the hypertonic saline. This form of therapy in cholera, and other diseases, has aroused much interest and requires mention. It is at present on trial, and some time will elapse before a definite opinion can be expressed on its value.

General Management.—*During the Acute Phase.*—Nursing is very important during this stage. The patient should be kept strictly in the horizontal position in a warm bed and in a well-ventilated room. The surface heat should be maintained by hot-water bottles, or warmed bricks placed alongside the feet, legs and flanks. The patient must not be allowed up to pass his stools, but a warmed bed-pan should be available. The foot of the bed should be raised. All food should be withheld for some hours whilst the disease is active. Nurses must see that all discharges, soiled linen, etc., are disinfected with a $2\frac{1}{2}$ per cent. cresol solution.

During Convalescence.—Alcohol may be of benefit to those accustomed to it. Great care is necessary in beginning to give food for fear of producing a relapse. To begin with, farinaceous foods such as arrowroot, cornflour and milk whey should be given, and this diet should be continued until the kidneys act freely. The recumbent position should be enforced for about two weeks to avoid sudden cardiac failure. Convalescence, however, is usually surprisingly rapid.

Personal Prophylaxis.—Inoculation with a dead cholera vaccine has been widely employed with good results. The initial dose of ½ c.c., given subcutaneously, should contain 4,000 million cholera vibrios. The second dose of 1 c.c. should be given ten days later. Bacteriophage has also been recommended as a prophylactic, and if this is used, 30 c.c. of potent bacteriophage should be added to the well (see note above). During cholera epidemics great care should be taken to maintain the general health. All attacks of diarrhœa should be treated at once. Purgatives, especially salines, should be avoided. All drinking water and milk should be boiled. All food should be protected from flies, and uncooked vegetables, as well as raw and unripe fruit, should be avoided. Visits to cholera districts should if possible be postponed.

AMŒBIC DYSENTERY

Specific Therapy.—*Drugs Employed.*—Emetine and its various preparations (alkaloid of ipecacuanha), yatren (an iodine preparation of Bayer), quinoxyl (Burroughs, Wellcome & Co.), carbarsone (Lilly) and stovarsol.

Treatment of Acute Attack.—The best treatment is to begin at once subcutaneous injections of emetine hydrochloride (1 gr.) dissolved in 1 to 2 c.c. sterile distilled water. This dose is given daily for ten days, or it may be given in divided doses (½ gr.) morning and evening. Another useful method is to give emetine in the form of emetine bismuth iodide (which is made up in gelatine capsules) by the mouth, combined with irrigation of the bowel with yatren. At 8.30 A.M., after a cleansing enema of sodium bicarbonate, 8 oz. of a 2½ per cent. yatren solution is run into the bowel and the patient encouraged to retain it as long as possible. At 9.30 P.M. give a sedative, such as luminal (1 gr.). At 10 P.M. give emetine bismuth iodide (1 gr.); later this dose may be increased to 2 gr. It is not necessary to give more than a total of 19 gr. in about twenty-one days. The last food and drink should have been taken at 6 P.M. Some vomiting and diarrhœa may be expected and are not contraindications. Alcohol in any form should be prohibited. Such a combined course of treatment tends to prevent relapses.

Treatment of Relapses.—A course of yatren by the mouth and by enema may be tried. Three to four yatren pills (0·25 gr. in each) are given thrice daily after meals for ten days. After a cleansing enema of sod. bicarb., 8 oz. of $2\frac{1}{2}$ per cent. yatren are run into the bowel and the patient is asked to retain it as long as possible. The injections are continued each day for about ten days. Some diarrhœa and flatulent distension may be expected. Then two pills of yatren may be given after food daily for a period of three weeks, after which the patient should continue to take one pill daily after food for a further period of one month. Carbarsone (Lilly), an organic arsenic preparation, may be given in the same way as yatren ; it has the additional advantage of being non-toxic. The average daily adult dose is $7\frac{1}{2}$ gr., and this should be given for ten days.

Toxic Symptoms.—Emetine affects the heart and may cause fibrillation if given in excessive doses or for too long a time. Neuritis may be produced, and in some cases paralysis of the diaphragm and intercostal muscles may occur with serious respiratory embarrassment. The skin may show a fine brawny desquamation and the finger-nails an atrophic condition with marked increase in the size of the lunule. Emetine is particularly toxic in bacillary dysentery when it is administered in cases which have been wrongly diagnosed. This toxic action occurs easily in young children, and emetine should be administered to them with the greatest care.

Non-specific Therapy.—Bismuth subnitrate by the mouth in large doses has been found useful in combination with emetine. It is given in doses of 180 gr. suspended in aerated water, every three hours day and night for ten days. Kurchi bark and its derivatives have been used. Kurchi bismuthous iodide (Anabin) which contains the total alkaloids of the kurchi bark is given by the mouth in doses of 10 gr. twice daily for ten days. In some persistent cases it may be necessary to perform cæcostomy and irrigate the large bowel daily with $2\frac{1}{2}$ per cent. yatren solution. The wound is kept open till the lesions in the bowel are completely healed, as determined by sigmoidoscopic and X-ray examination. Ileostomy is perhaps better, as it puts the large bowel at complete rest. The risk of all surgical measures in this condition is, however, very considerable.

General Management.—*During the Acute Phase.*—Nursing is most important during the acute phase. As already noted, emetine is a toxic drug, and during its administration the patient should be kept in bed under supervision. The mouth should be carefully washed and any excess of saliva removed.

The patient should not be allowed to get out of bed to pass a stool, but a bedpan should be used. The diet should consist of easily digested food having a low residue—milk, orange-juice glucose, baked apples, tea and toast.

During Convalescence.—The patient may be allowed to get up to go to the bathroom. The diet may be gradually increased, but potatoes, carrots, etc., should be used sparingly. It is not necessary to starve the patient. The best guides are the appetite and tongue of the patient. Alcohol should be forbidden for a month or two after treatment is completed.

Personal Prophylaxis.—As the infection is acquired through food or drink contaminated by cysts of *Entamœba histolytica*, precautions must be taken to prevent this. In areas where the disease is endemic, food should be carefully protected from flies; all milk and water should be boiled before consumption. Uncooked vegetables should be avoided. One yatren tablet taken at night acts as a prophylactic and also as an aperient.

Complications of Amœbic Dysentery

Amœbic Hepatitis.—For this the best treatment is a course of injections of emetine hydrochloride for ten days as for amœbic dysentery. If the diagnosis is correct, the symptoms quickly clear up with this treatment, but if they do not, then at the end of this time the diagnosis must be revised. The course is frequently used in this condition as a "therapeutic diagnosis."

Amœbic Liver Abscess.—When symptoms suggest the presence of pus, it is necessary—in addition to the administration of emetine—to explore the liver, and, if pus is found, to evacuate it by aspiration. For this purpose, a full-sized aspiration needle is used, as the pus is thick. Local anæsthesia should be employed. In the absence of localizing signs, the best point to insert the needle is in the right anterior axillary line in the eighth or ninth interspace. The needle should be introduced inwards and slightly upwards for 3 to 3½ in. At least six explorations in different directions in the liver should be made before abandoning the attempt to find pus. If pus is found, the needle is connected up with a Potain's aspirator and the pus evacuated. A further ten-day course of injections with emetine is then given. The combination of aspiration and administration of emetine is by far the best method of dealing with a liver abscess, and the earlier these are carried out the better. In some cases it may be necessary to do an open operation, either by the transperitoneal or pleural route.

The drawback to this in the hot moist climate of some parts of the tropics is that there is a very great risk of the abscess becoming secondarily infected. When a liver abscess opens through the lungs, the pus may be completely evacuated by the patient coughing it up. In some cases the drainage may fail, and in these cases surgical measures are indicated.

Pulmonary Amœbiasis.—This condition is not secondary to liver abscess. The infection has been conveyed by the blood stream to the lungs from the primary lesion in the large intestine, causing broncho-pneumonia. These cases respond very rapidly to a course of emetine.

Patients who have suffered from any of the above complications should not, if possible, return to the tropics. Before giving permission to return, a careful examination of the stool should be made to determine if it is, or is not, free from amœbæ. In the latter case he should be treated with emetine bismuth iodide and yatren bowel washes as described above.

SPRUE

Specific Therapy.—In the case of sprue there is no specific drug or other therapy. Recent biochemical investigations, however, have placed the treatment of the disease on a much more scientific basis.

Non-specific Therapy.—The principles of treatment are :—

(*a*) Alimentary rest by suitable diet, viz., high protein, low fat and carbohydrate.

(*b*) Treatment of existing anæmia.

(*c*) Replacement of demonstrable deficiencies. If achlorhydria is present, full doses of hydrochloric acid should be given. The addition of bile salts is useful in facilitating the absorption of fats.

The following scheme is recommended for the management and treatment of a case of sprue :—

1. On admission, cases are kept on a milk dietary, or one similar to that which they have been having until preliminary investigations are completed.

2. The routine examinations before treatment are :—

(*a*) Estimation of serum calcium and phosphorus.

(*b*) Estimation of van den Bergh reaction.

(*c*) Analysis of fat in fæces.

(*d*) Fractional test meal and histamine response.

(*e*) Complete hæmatological examination. In severe cases gastric analysis may be postponed. The patient should be weighed regularly, as body-weight is an important factor in the control of treatment. Weighing of the stool is also of importance. A normal stool weighs from 6 to 8 oz., but in sprue this may be doubled or trebled.

3. Ol. ricini (2 drachms) is given as a routine and the patient is put on Diet I (*vide* below).

4. Acid. hydrochlor. dil. ($\frac{1}{2}$ to 1 drachm), with or immediately after the 8 A.M., noon and 6 P.M. feeds, where gastric analysis shows deficiency in hydrochloric acid. Tabloid fellis porcini purificati (B., W. & Co.) (4 gr.), four of which may be taken thrice daily after food to supply the deficiency of bile salts which is said to exist.

5. Where the blood examination shows deficiency of serum calcium, calcium lactate (20 to 30 gr.) should be given thrice daily. Vitamin D in the form of tabloid calciferolis (B., W. & Co.) may also be given daily, as well as ultraviolet radiation.

6. Water should be drunk freely between meals. No condiments or pepper may be added to food, but salt is allowed.

7. If constipation occurs, liquid paraffin should be given, but no other aperient. Excessive diarrhœa is checked by the special diet (*vide* later), but in severe cases tinct. opii (10 minims) twice or thrice daily, along with 15 gr. of pulv. bataviæ co. (a cuttle-fish bone powder combined with an iron compound) in wafer cachets, four times daily, will prove beneficial.

8. The patient must be kept warm in bed both during the day and night. Sprue cases are very susceptible to chills. Nursing is very important. The nurse should supervise the special diet and keep careful records of the body-weight, etc.

9. Where anæmia is present, liver extract must be given in full doses. Campolon (Bayer) (2 c.c.) should be given by intramuscular injections daily, or 10 c.c. weekly or fortnightly. Liver soup is also valuable, Liver Extract No. 343 (Lilly), one to three phials daily as soup. One phial equals $3\frac{1}{2}$ oz. liver.

In the construction of the diets, sprulac will be found to be valuable and simple. It is a dried high protein milk product prepared by Cow & Gate. Milk has always been recognized as very valuable in the treatment of sprue as its fat is easily assimilable. Sprulac is an advance on ordinary milk, especially on that supplied in the tropics. It is pure and free from bacteria, the vitamins have not been destroyed and its composition has been adjusted to the requirements of a sprue case, the fat and carbohydrate content being low. The ratio is protein : fat : carbohydrate=1·0 : 0·3 : 1·0. The calorific value of 1 oz. is 125. Buffalo milk, which is commonly used in some parts of the tropics, should be avoided owing to its high fat content.

The following diets are recommended :—

Diet I (Calorific value=697. P. : F. : C.=1·0 : 0·3 : 1·3).—One and a half ounces sprulac made up to 8 to 12 oz. with water every two and a half hours, for six feeds.

Diet II (Calorific value=1,117. P. : F. : C.=1·0 : 0·3 : 1·4).—One and a half ounces sprulac made up to 8 to 12 oz. with water every two and a half hours. Juice of orange. Calf's foot jelly, 1 oz.

Diet III (Calorific value=1,536. P. : F. : C.=1·0 : 0·3 : 1·5).—Two ounces sprulac made up with 12 to 16 oz. water every two and a half hours, for six feeds. Juice of two oranges. Calf's foot jelly, 2 oz.

Diet IV (Calorific value=2,001. P. : F. : C.=1·0 : 0·3 : 1·5).—Sprulac as in Diet III. Juice of two oranges. Calf's foot jelly, 3 oz. Two baked apples. Baked custard, 2 oz. Underdone lean beef of good quality, 4 oz. Half a rusk.

Diet V (Calorific value=2,516. P. : F. : C.=1·0 : 0·3 : 1·4).—Sprulac as in Diet III. Juice of two oranges. Calf's foot jelly, 3 oz. Two baked apples. Baked custard, 2 oz. Two rusks. Underdone lean meat, 10 oz.

Weight will be lost on Diets I and II, but Diet III meets basal requirements, and a gain of weight may be expected on Diets IV and V. The changes from the lower to the higher diets will be guided by the improvement in symptoms. As far as possible the feeds should be given six times a day, but latitude to suit individual requirements may be allowed. If the progress is satisfactory, there will be a diminution of diarrhœa, intestinal flatulence and distension, and the character of the stools will also improve. During convalescence a more liberal diet may be allowed, including fresh fruit and well-cooked vegetables (passed through a fine sieve), such as celery, marrow and cauliflower. Lean steak, chicken, fish and eggs may also be allowed. Carbohydrates such as potatoes and milk puddings are gradually added. Articles to be avoided are overdone and twice-cooked meat ; foods cooked or fried in fat ; condiments such as pepper, mustard, chillies, sauces, chutneys, curries and spiced foods ; duck, salmon, trout, mackerel and herring ; new bread ; salad dressings and sauces of all kinds ;

suet puddings ; cakes with icing ; raisins and pastry ; sweets and chocolate ; alcoholic drinks and aerated water. Smoking in moderation is allowed when convalescence has commenced.

For painful tongue and mouth, boroglycerine is useful, or, if severe, the small ulcers may be painted with cocaine solution (2 gr. to the ounce). For abdominal distension, charkaolin (one to two heaped teapoonsfuls in water, t.i.d.) is useful. If the weight does not increase, glucose (2 oz.) and insulin injections (10 units twice daily) will help. If the patient becomes very anæmic one or more blood transfusions may be required, 300 to 400 c.c. being given intravenously on each occasion, but with modern liver extracts this is less frequently required. Iron may also be necessary. Dermatitis, which is frequently observed in elderly persons, may be treated at first with calamine lotion, followed by the application of a pigment containing ½ to 2 per cent. cignolin (Bayer, a chrysarobin preparation). The teeth should be thoroughly examined and pyorrhœa treated, but wholesale extraction should be avoided. Any complicating diseases, *e.g.*, malaria, syphilis, active amœbic dysentery, helminthic infestations, appendicitis, etc., should be treated on the usual lines. The latter is not uncommon and the sprue patient stands appendicectomy well. Patients who have had sprue should, if possible, not return to the tropics, but if they have to do so, they should be told to resume the strict diet should there be any recurrence of symptoms and remain on such a diet until the symptoms have disappeared. Should they fail to respond to treatment they should leave the tropics permanently.

LEPROSY

Specific Therapy.—In recent years it was thought that in chaulmoogra oil and its derivatives we had a specific remedy for leprosy, but further experience has not confirmed this view. The position of the treatment of leprosy is very similar to that of tuberculosis. No one measure is sufficient, but a general building up of the patient's resistance by diet, improved personal hygiene, etc., is of the greatest value. Chaulmoogra oil has a place in this treatment. It is a very old remedy for leprosy in India, the best oil being obtained from the seeds of the *Hydnocarpus wightiana*. The oil itself is used and has the advantage of being both cheap and effective. The proprietary preparations, which are more expensive, are the ethyl esters. Originally Bayer produced one called antileprol ; others prepared by Burroughs, Wellcome & Co. are moogrol and alepol. The latter contains the less irritating, lower melting-point fatty acids of hydnocarpus oil. It is much cheaper than the ethyl esters. A good method of administration is to inject the oil itself intradermally into the skin lesions. Muir recommends 0·5 c.c. as the initial dose of the oil and thereafter it is increased by 1 c.c. until 5 to 10 c.c. are injected at one time. When the latter large dose is given, it should be divided over a number of lesions of the skin. The injection is given once a week. A reaction may occur with a rise of temperature, swelling and redness of skin nodules and thickening of nerves. When this occurs, treatment should be suspended until the reaction has subsided, and the next dose should be reduced by 0·5 c.c.; thereafter the dosage should be increased as before and usually no further reaction will occur. Four per cent. creosote is added to the oil to preserve it.

Moogrol is given in doses of 1 c.c. intramuscularly and this is increased up to 5 to 6 c.c. At the same time iodicin (B., W. & Co.) tabloids are given. The dose is 0·25 gm. per 100 lbs. of body-weight and this is increased every two weeks up to 1 gm. per 100 lbs. Alepol is given intravenously. If an equal quantity of blood is mixed with it in the syringe before injection, thrombosis of the vein is prevented. As severe reactions may in some cases follow intravenous injections, it is well to commence with intramuscular and subcutaneous doses of 1 c.c. of a 3 per cent. solution (increased by 0·5 to 5 c.c. or more) twice weekly. The intravenous injections of 1 c.c. of a 1 per cent. solution may be given alternately with the intramuscular injections.

It is advisable to control the injection of chaulmoogra oil and its derivatives by observations on the blood sedimentation rate. A high reading indicates an active lesion and caution should be adopted in administering the oil. Other drugs are used for the treatment. Potassium iodide is recommended in large doses twice weekly; the initial dose of 10 gr. may even be increased up to 120 gr. This is used as an adjunct to the chaulmoogra-oil treatment, but great care must be exercised and the patient must be very carefully watched, as a severe reaction may occur. Ephedrine (2 gr.) in hard gelatine capsules relieves the severe nerve pain in leprosy. Various dyes have been used recently, *e.g.*, trypan blue is given intravenously in 25 c.c. doses of a 4 per cent. solution.

Protein shock therapy has been tried and found useful. T.A.B. vaccine is given intravenously, commencing with a dose of 5 to 10 million, repeating it twice weekly with increasing doses until a 100-million dose is reached—or more if reactions are insufficient. In the neuritic form of the disease it has been suggested that there is a vitamin B_1 deficiency and injections of this are recommended, such as betaxan (Bayer). Surgical measures of various kinds may be required, *e.g.*, eye operations, tracheotomy, removal of dead bone, amputations, etc. It is very important to locate and remove foci of septic infection. Massage and electrical treatment for muscular wasting are useful. It is essential to recognize and treat complicating infections, *e.g.*, particularly syphilis (*vide* p. 206). Intestinal parasites should be dealt with; malaria, kala-azar and any other infection must be treated.

General Management.—Scrupulous and systematic attention must be paid to personal and domestic hygiene and cleanliness; frequent bathing and free use of soap; changes of underclothing; good food; fresh air; light work; avoidance of fatigue—all these points should be insisted upon. Europeans who have contracted leprosy invariably show improvement on return to a more bracing climate from the tropics. It should be noted that improvement frequently occurs without the administration of any drug when the patient is placed under favourable conditions, hence great care is necessary in assessing the value of a drug in the treatment of leprosy.

Personal Prophylaxis.—As children are much more susceptible to infection than adults, they should always be removed from leprous parents and from all contact with lepers. Leper colonies with facilities for modern treatment, and run on humanitarian lines, are very important for the prophylaxis of leprosy. Particular care should be taken to disinfect the nasal discharge of lepers and also their eating and drinking utensils. Contact with discharging lesions of the skin should be avoided as these often contain very large numbers of bacilli. Native washermen, cooks and other servants should be carefully inspected for any signs of leprosy, and if found to be infected, should be suspended from their work and put under treatment.

YAWS

Specific Therapy.—*Drugs Employed.*—Salvarsan, neosalvarsan (neoarsphenamine); stovarsol; halarsol (May & Baker); carbarsone (Lilly); sodium and potassium tartrate; sodium-bismuth tartrate (Sobita); bismostab (Boots); casbis (Bayer); bismuth arsanilate (Martindale); bismuth arsphenamine sulphonate.

Treatment of Early Stage.—The best treatment is a combination of arsenic and bismuth. In the tropics the natives improve so rapidly with the first few doses of the arsenicals that they often do not return for completion of the course, and only appear when a relapse sets in. Neosalvarsan is given intravenously to adults, but may be given to children intramuscularly suspended in oil if the intravenous route is not possible. The initial dose for adults is 0·6 to 0·9 gm. in 10 c.c. sterile distilled water. For children under two years the dose should be 0·1 gm., and for those up to ten years old it should be 0·3 gm. It may be given intramuscularly, alternating with bismuth in weekly injections. In this way severe reactions are avoided. The dose of sodium-bismuth tartrate for an adult is 3 gr. dissolved in 3 c.c. sterile distilled water or in oil; for children up to two years, ½ to 1 gr.; from two to eighteen years, 1 to 2 gr. A course of about twelve weekly injections, alternating neosalvarsan and bismuth, may be considered suitable for the treatment of a case of yaws. Stomatitis may be avoided if the bismuth is injected into the deep subcutaneous rather than the muscular tissue. The other bismuth preparation, viz., bismostab (Boots), which is metallic bismuth suspended in glucose solution, is given weekly into the deep subcutaneous tissue in doses of 3 gr., with a total of 60 gr. in refractory cases, casbis (Bayer), which is a sterile oily suspension of bismuth hydrate in very fine dispersion, is given to adults in 0·5 to 1 c.c. doses with a total of 12 to 15 c.c. The following are given orally: stovarsol (May & Baker), starting with a dose of two 4-gr. tablets for an adult, and increasing to three on the second and four on the third day; miss a day and repeat in reverse order. The dose for children is ½ to 1 gr. It is said to cause slight diarrhœa, but it is a convenient method for mass-treatment. Carbarsone (Lilly) is another drug given by mouth in gelatine capsules (pulvules). The average dose for an adult is 7½ gr., which may be given daily for ten days. The course may be repeated after a short interval.

Treatment of Relapse.—In cases which relapse, a second course of the combined treatment will be required.

General Management.—For the painful "crab" yaws of the feet a local application of a 2 per cent. tartar emetic ointment in vaseline is very useful. The name is given because the patient walks like a crab on account of the lesion in the feet. Perchloride of mercury solution (1 : 1,000) may be used to cleanse the sores.

The general health should be improved by good food, tonics and occasional aperients. Daily bathing and stimulation of the skin by abundance of demulcent drinks are also helpful and in the colder season warm clothing is indicated.

Helminthic and other complicating infections should be dealt with.

Personal Prophylaxis.—The protection of wounds and abrasions from infection by contact, or by flies, is the most effective measure. Public bathing places liable to pollution by discharges should be avoided.

RABIES

Cases of rabies present themselves for treatment when the symptoms of the disease are already manifest, or because they have been recently exposed to infection by the bite of a rabid animal. In the former, a fatal termination invariably occurs and treatment is only palliative.

Palliative Treatment of the Developed Case.—The violent and painful spasms may be best controlled by inhalations of chloroform. Subcutaneous injection of curare may be tried, using tabloid hyp. curarinæ chloride (B., W. & Co.), $\frac{1}{120}$ gr. up to a maximum of $\frac{1}{2}$ gr. When swallowing becomes impossible, rectal alimentation is required. Nurses should do all they can to reassure the patient and allay fear and excitement.

Treatment of those who have been Exposed to Infection.—Local treatment is most important and the sooner it is undertaken the better is the outlook for the patient. The wounds should be opened up freely, if necessary, so that access may be gained to every part. Then apply pure carbolic acid to every part systematically. Carbolic acid is better than nitric acid as it is not so painful and it destroys the virus. If this treatment is carried out within an hour of the exposure, the risk of contracting rabies is slight. The most serious bites are those on the face. An animal which has bitten a person and is suspected to be rabid should not be killed, but kept securely under observation. If it is alive and well ten days later, it is very unlikely to have been suffering from rabies at the time it bit the person, and the latter is therefore not at risk. Persons who have been licked on the unbroken skin or on abrasions which are not recent are not in danger.

After the local treatment has been applied, and if the person is definitely at risk, he should undergo a course of anti-rabic inoculations. The nature of the vaccine may be briefly indicated here. First, a fixed virus is prepared ; this is done by injecting an emulsion of the brain of a rabid dog intracerebrally into a rabbit. When the rabbit dies, some of its brain is injected intracerebrally into a second rabbit, and so on through a succession of rabbits until the virus becomes exalted and kills the rabbit in exactly ten days ; the virus is now known as the " fixed virus " and is used for the preparation of the vaccine. Some strains of the virus have better antigenic properties than others ; for example, it was found that a fixed virus obtained from Paris was a better antigen than one that had been in use in India for some time. There have been various methods of preparing the vaccine with the fixed virus, and the technique has gradually evolved. At present a dead carbolized virus is commonly employed. This is made by emulsifying the brain of an infected rabbit, or sheep, in 1 per cent. carbolic saline. This is allowed to stand in the incubator for twenty-four hours at 37° C. to kill the virus. The strength of the brain emulsion may be from 1 to 5 per cent. The former being used in the less severe cases and the latter for severe bites about the face and head, which require intensive treatment. The course usually lasts fourteen days, daily injections of 4 c.c. of the vaccine being given subcutaneously on each side of the abdomen. During the course the patient is instructed to abstain from all alcohol and vigorous exercise. These precautions are very important, and if not taken the treatment may prove ineffective and the patient die of rabies. In a small percentage of cases certain " accidents," as they are called, may occur during the treatment, *e.g.*, paraplegia, a condition like Landry's paralysis, etc. They are rare and the mode of production is not clear. The carbolized vaccine has reduced the frequency of these unfortunate occurrences.

Personal Prophylaxis.—All animals suspected of rabies should be avoided. Dogs showing signs of choking should be handled with great care as this is often the first sign of rabies, and fingers should never be put into the mouth of the dog. Muzzling is important, especially if cases of rabies in dogs are occurring.

TROPICAL NEURASTHENIA

Far too often the medical man does not know what neurasthenia is and tells the patient there is nothing the matter with him and that all that is required is for him to " pull himself together." Such advice is usually ill-advised. The patient feels ill and his doctor cannot find out what is the matter with him, and so he thinks he must have a very obscure malady which is incurable. If an infection, *e.g.*, malaria, dysentery, etc., is detected, the patient should be assured that with suitable treatment he will improve quickly. This will allay his anxiety. If, after dealing with exciting and predisposing causes, there is no definite improvement, then long leave to a good climate must be prescribed. Alcohol probably plays a more important part than climate in causing neurosis in the tropics and therefore it should be forbidden. Smoking, if carried to excess, should be reduced or prohibited. If insomnia is marked it should be treated by such measures as a hot bath and a cup of hot milk at bedtime, or, if necessary, mild hypnotics such as soneryl (May & Baker), two tablets of 1½ gr. half an hour before retiring. Hobbies should be encouraged, such as golf, fishing, etc., which will take the patient's attention away from himself and take him into pleasant surroundings in the fresh air.

It is very important to seek carefully for any underlying infection and if found treat it thoroughly.

Prophylaxis.—Certain types of individuals never adjust themselves to tropical conditions and are very liable to develop this form of anxiety neurosis. In examination of recruits for work in the tropics it is necessary for the medical examiner to have had considerable tropical experience and to have paid particular attention to the reaction of individuals to tropical environment. It is not easy to lay down definite rules, but particular attention should be paid to the family and personal history; independent reports on the character and conduct of the applicant may also be helpful.

HELMINTHIC INFECTIONS

(*a*) SCHISTOSOMIASIS

1. **Specific Therapy.**—(i) *Drugs Employed.*—Tartar emetic (sodium antimonyl tartrate); fouadin (neoantimosan) (Bayer); emetine.

(ii) *Treatment of an Acute Attack.*—*Tartar emetic* is given intravenously. For convenience it may be put up in a sterilized vaccine bottle with a rubber cap in a strength of ½ gr. to 1 c.c. of distilled water. For use, dilute each cubic centimetre with 5 c.c. sterile distilled water. The technique is the same as that described in the treatment of kala-azar (see p. 235). The injections are given on alternate days and the dose gradually increased till 2 to 2½ gr. are given at one injection. The total amount of tartar emetic required for a course is 25 to 30 gr. For children, 10 gr. is sufficient for a total course with a maximum of 1 gr. for a single dose. The course should occupy four to six weeks. *Fouadin* is given intramuscularly and therefore is convenient for administration to children. It is put up in a 7 per cent. solution in ampoules and the dosage recommended for an adult is: first day, 1·5 c.c.; second, 3·5 c.c.; third, 5 c.c.; fifth, 5 c.c.; seventh, 5 c.c.; ninth, 5 c.c.; eleventh, 5 c.c.; thirteenth, 5 c.c.; fifteenth, 5 c.c. For children the initial dose should be 0·5 c.c. rising to 2 to 3 c.c. according to age. *Emetine* can be given to children who are intolerant to antimony, or whose veins are too small for intravenous therapy. It is given intramuscularly and the initial dose should not exceed ½ gr., and a maximum dose for a child is 1 gr. and the total for a course is 15 to 20 gr. The heart must be carefully watched during treatment with emetine.

(iii) *Treatment of Relapses.*—Relapses generally occur if the full course of treatment has not been completed. When they do occur, the treatment outlined above must be repeated.

(iv) *Toxic Symptoms.*—The toxic symptoms of the antimony preparations and emetine have already been described in connection with leishmaniasis and amœbic dysentery (see pp. 235, 245). The specific therapy is applicable to all three forms of schistosomiasis, viz., *schistosoma hæmatobium* (urinary form), *schistosoma mansoni* (intestinal form) and *schistosoma japonica* (Far Eastern schistosomiasis).

2. **Non-specific Therapy.**—In the urinary form, stone and papillomata of the bladder require to be removed by operation. Hyperplasia of the vagina and cervix is best treated by scraping. In the intestinal form with extensive papillomata of the rectum, removal of the whole tube of mucous membrane is recommended—as much as 12 to 15 in. have been successfully removed. There is little tendency to contraction of the rectum, and control of the anal sphincter is regained. When splenomegaly is a marked feature, as is frequently the case, splenectomy for so-called Egyptian splenomegaly is recommended. In the late stage of the Far Eastern variety, hepatic cirrhosis becomes a marked feature and little can be done when this stage is reached (see Cirrhosis, p. 610).

3. **Personal Prophylaxis.**—In endemic areas, drinking from or bathing in rivers, ponds and canals should be avoided. Children should be carefully and repeatedly warned about this. Sportsmen should be carefully warned also against wading, especially when snipe shooting in infected localities; even fishing in canals in Egypt is not free from risk. All drinking water should be boiled. The reason for these precautions is to avoid infection from snails harbouring the parasite. The schistosome undergoes part of its life cycle in certain species

of fresh water snails from which the parasite emerges in the form of actively swimming cercariæ, and when they meet the human host they infect him by penetrating through his skin or mucous membrane.

(*b*) CESTODIASIS

A. Tænia Saginata

Specific Therapy.—(i) *Drugs Employed.*—Filix mas, which is the rhizome of the male fern; carbon tetrachloride and oleum chenopodium.

(ii) *Treatment of Intestinal Form.*—The adult worms are present in the intestine and the following scheme of treatment is recommended. Preliminary starvation is necessary for two days. Food should be restricted to weak tea, toast and a lightly boiled egg; for clearing out mucus from the bowel, sodium bicarbonate (20 gr.) should be given thrice daily. In the morning sodium sulphate (½ oz.) is given. Extractum filicis liquidum is put up in gelatine capsules containing 15 minims in each. On the day of treatment at 8 A.M. give two capsules of 15 minims, repeat at 8.30 A.M. and 9 A.M. The dose for an adult male is 1½ drachms; for a female, 1 drachm. The patient must then lie perfectly quiet in bed sipping water. At 10.30 A.M. give sodium sulphate (½ oz.). When the bowels move freely, segments of the worm begin to appear. They must all be carefully preserved and a search made for the head. In cases where the filix mas has failed to eradicate completely the worm, a useful anthelminthic is a combination of carbon tetrachloride and oil of chenopodium in the following mixture:—

℞		
	Carbon Tetrachlor. . . .	3·5 c.c. (ʒi)
	Ol. Chenopod.	1 c.c. (♏xv)
	Paraff. Liq.	28 c.c. (℥i)

Adults should receive a full dose; children under six, 2 drachms; up to eight years the dose should be 3 drachms; and up to fourteen, 4 drachms. The mixture should be made up fresh. After half an hour the patient is given sodium sulphate (½ oz.).

If the head has not been recovered, efforts should be made to prevent the further growth of the helminth, and for this purpose betanaphthol (15 gr.) in 5-gr. tablets should be taken first thing in the morning on an empty stomach for ten days.

B. Tænia Solium (Cysticercosis)

Normally the cysticercus stage of *Tænia solium* takes place in the pig, but sometimes the development occurs in man with very serious results, as it selects for its location the muscles and the central nervous system in particular, causing epilepsy and other manifestations varying with the location of the parasite. The cysticerci, when they become dead and calcified, can be demonstrated in the tissues by X-ray examination; before calcification, cysts under the skin may be felt on palpation, excised and submitted for examination. Unfortunately the treatment of this condition is very unsatisfactory and is purely symptomatic. For the epilepsy, luminal and bromides may be given as in the case of idiopathic epilepsy. Unless there are very definitely localizing signs, surgery is not indicated.

Personal Prophylaxis.—This is very important. A patient with intestinal tapeworms should be treated thoroughly and at once, since he may acquire the visceral form of cysticerosis if he harbours *T. solium* in his intestine. As the pig is normally the intermediate host of *T. solium*, the flesh—particularly in the East—(where the disease is very common amongst them)—should not be eaten unless it has been obtained from a well-supervised slaughter house and has been thoroughly cooked. Raw vegetables should be avoided as in the tropics they are frequently contaminated with the eggs and ripe segments of tapeworms. Nurses and attendants should handle with great care the ripe segments of *T. solium* and take every precaution to avoid infection of their hands and food.

C. Tænia Echinococcus Granulosus (Hydatid)

The sexually mature worm occurs in the dog as the definite host and is a small tapeworm. Man is its intermediate host and in him it may form large cysts in various organs, particularly in the liver and lungs. Aspiration should not be attempted either for diagnosis or treatment, as the fluid is often under great pressure and is toxic; further, it contains scolices which, if they escape, may disseminate the disease widely in the tissues. Drug therapy is valueless and surgical treatment by open operation is the only method indicated. In the case of the liver, the incised cyst may be stitched to the abdominal wall and allowed to fill up by granulating (marsupialization). Aspiration of cysts is dangerous because fluid may escape suddenly from a pulmonary cyst into the lungs, or into the peritoneal cavity from a cyst in the liver, and in the former case death from suffocation may result. The fluid which escapes into the tissues is toxic and symptoms of collapse, or even death, may result. An open operation with adequate drainage is therefore required.

Personal Prophylaxis.—Close association with the sheep-dog, the host of the adult worm, must be avoided.

FILARIASIS

Specific Treatment.—There is no drug known to destroy filaria in the tissues ; consequently the disease manifestations are treated on non-specific lines. The principal types of filarial infections are *Filaria bancrofti*, *Filaria Malayi* and *Filaria loa* (Loa Loa).

The bancroftian and *Malayan infestations* may produce a series of clinical manifestations which require treatment. The principal of these are :—

(*a*) *Filarial lymphadenitis*, *lymphangitis*, *orchitis* and *funiculitis*. In the acute stage the treatment is rest in bed with elevation of the parts. Calamine lotion should be applied and in cases of fever hydrotherapy is useful. A careful search should be made for bacterial septic foci. Autogenous vaccines made from the vesicles in the skin have been found useful in combating the secondary bacterial infection.

(*b*) *Filarial Abscess.* Pus should be evacuated and hot boracic fomentations applied. Autogenous vaccines containing staphylococci and streptococci may be used.

(*c*) *Lymph scrotum*, *hydrocele* and *varix*. Surgical measures are required in these cases. Suspensory and pressure bandages are useful.

(*d*) *Elephantiasis.* Again a careful search should be made for focal infections. Non-specific shock therapy is of value in these cases and T.A.B. vaccine should be given intravenously, commencing with doses of 5,000,000 to 10,000,000, increasing gradually up to 100,000,000. The limb should be carefully guarded against injuries and elastoplast bandages may be found helpful. The limb should be massaged and kept elevated. Various operative procedures have been proposed, but none are entirely satisfactory. Kondoleon's operation consists of free incision of the fascia lata of the leg and removal of a large section of aponeurosis ; this assists the anastomosis of lymph channels and veins.

(*e*) *Synovitis.* This is not an uncommon complication of filariasis, and as there may be no very evident trauma to account for it, the condition may be rather puzzling, especially if it occurs in this country. The treatment is on the usual lines for synovitis.

(*f*) *Chyluria.* This is not an unusual complication and the treatment should consist of rest in bed with the foot of the bed elevated. Restriction of fats and fluids in the diet, gentle purgation and the washing out of the bladder with warm boracic lotion should all be carried out. If blood is present the following mixture may be used for irrigation :—

℞	Liq. Adrenal. Hydrochlor. (B.P.)	.	ʒi
	Zinc Sulph.	.	gr. v
	Lot. Acid. Boric (B.P.C.) . .	ad	℥i$\frac{1}{4}$

To be used with equal quantities of warm water.

Personal Prophylaxis.—In practice this amounts to anti-mosquito measures and protection from mosquito bite—as have been detailed under malaria (see p. 233).

Filaria Loa (Loa Loa)

The condition known as Calabar swellings is caused by this worm. There is no specific treatment. Should the adult worm appear under the conjunctiva or under the skin, it may be removed. There are generally a number of worms. For the relief of the swelling an injection of 1 c.c. of adrenalin (1 : 1,000) is sometimes useful. An abscess may be produced by a dead worm. The pus should then be evacuated and hot boracic dressing applied. Occasionally the worm moves in the subcutaneous tissue to near the larynx and may give rise to the serious complication of œdema glottidis, in which case a tracheotomy will be required at once.

Personal Prophylaxis.—Protection is required against the bites of the vector, a horse-fly (*Chrysops dimidiata*), which comes into houses and bites during the daytime. Therefore the dwelling houses in endemic areas should be protected with wire gauze.

Other Forms of Filariasis

Dracunculus Medinensis or Guinea Worm.—The adult female worm is found in the subcutaneous tissue, generally of the leg. In the early stages the patient may suffer from urticaria, vomiting and purging due to toxins produced by the worm. There is a marked eosinophilia. These symptoms are frequently very puzzling, as the existence of the worm may not be obvious. Administration of 1 c.c. of adrenalin (1 : 1,000) frequently gives relief. Later the worm penetrates the skin and the diagnosis is then clear. A simple form of treatment is to tie a small piece of silk thread to the worm as it protrudes from the opening of the skin. The thread is attached to a piece of stick. The worm is then wound round the stick daily with very gentle traction; if too much force is applied, it may rupture the worm and a disastrous cellulitis may result. Recently Fairley has devised an operation for removal of the worm *en masse* at once. If cellulitis and other septic complications have occurred, then these should be dealt with on ordinary surgical lines.

As infection is conveyed by drinking water from wells containing infected cyclops (water flea) which is the intermediate host of the worm, all water for drinking purposes should be strained through clean calico, such as villagers use for clothing. This removes the cyclops and is the simplest and most practical method of avoiding infection. No one should drink water from wells which are approached by steps, as this kind of well is the greatest source of infection. Wells should be closed and the water pumped from them.

Onchocerca Volvulus.—These worms cause small subcutaneous tumours in various parts of the body. Those about the head are often associated with ocular symptoms which may be very severe, leading finally to complete blindness. Consequently, in South America this worm has been known as the "Blinding Worm." Brumpt considers that the eye lesions may be due to a distinct species, *O. cæcutiens*. The tumours may be removed under local anæsthesia, and removal of those on the head are said to be followed by improvement in the ocular lesions.

Personal Prophylaxis.—As the sand-fly is probably the vector of the infection, anti-sand-fly measures, as described under Leishmaniasis, should be instituted.

ANCYLOSTOMIASIS (HOOKWORM)

1. **Specific Therapy.**—(*a*) *Drugs Employed.*—Thymol, carbon tetrachloride, oil of chenopodium, tetrachlorethylene.

(*b*) *Schemes of Treatment.*—Thymol was introduced by Bozzolo in 1880. It is a phenol derived from the oils of *thymus vulgaris*. It is only slightly soluble in water, but freely soluble in fats, oil and alcohol. Before administration the patient is put on a light diet containing no fats, oils or alcohol for a day or two, and given sod. bicarbonate (20 gr.) thrice daily. The bowels are well cleared out with sodium sulphate ($\frac{1}{2}$ oz.) in the morning. The thymol should be given on an empty stomach. The total dose for an adult man is 60 gr.; adult woman, 45 gr.; in pregnancy, 30 gr.; children under five, 5 gr.; ages 5 to 10, 15 gr.; ages 10 to 15, 30 gr.; ages 15 to 20, 34 gr. It is best given in rice-paper cachets in three doses of 20 gr. at hourly intervals. The thymol should be well ground and mixed with an equal quantity of sod. bicarb. The patient should be kept in bed during the administration and not allowed up till the bowels have moved freely. If necessary, a saline aperient is given two hours after the last dose of thymol. Alcohol and all solvents of thymol must be avoided during treatment. It is regarded as the safest and most effective of the anthelminthics by those who have had a very large experience of the treatment of ancylostomiasis (Clayton Lane). If ova are found in the stools after an interval of ten days the treatment may be repeated.

The combined treatment of *carbon tetrachloride and oil of chenopodium* gives better results than using the two drugs separately. After the preliminary treatment, as described above, the following mixture is given in the morning, either in one or divided doses.

℞		
	Carbon Tetrachlor	3·5 c.c. (ʒi)
	Ol. Chenopod.	1 c.c. (♏xv)
	Paraff. Liq.	28 c.c. (℥i)

Glucose and carbohydrates should be included in the diet and calcium lactate (20 gr.) given thrice daily for a few days previous to the administration of the mixture, as carbon tetrachloride has a specially toxic action on the liver. A saline aperient should follow the mixture if there has been no movement of the bowels. The dose of carbon tetrachloride for children is 3 minims for each year of life. Chenopodium should not be repeated for at least a week.

(*c*) *Toxic Signs.*—Thymol may cause vertigo and considerable excitement, and the urine becomes dark as in carbolic acid poisoning. Carbon tetrachloride causes damage to the liver and jaundice may occur. Chenopodium may cause depression of the respiratory centre.

2. **Non-specific Therapy and Management.**—During convalescence from a heavy infection with ancylostomes the patient should be carefully supervised. A full dietary should be avoided as it is liable to cause enteritis. For anæmia iron should be given as in secondary anæmia (see p. 471).

3. **Personal Prophylaxis.**—To prevent the larvæ from getting access to the skin, the universal use of boots in infected areas should be advised. All latrines should be kept in good

condition. Salt spread over the soil in sufficient quantities to form brine will prevent the development of larvæ and the washing of latrines with a 30 per cent. salt solution is also a valuable prophylactic measure.

ENTEROBIASIS (THREADWORM)

1. **Specific Therapy.**—This infection, especially in adults, is often very difficult to treat. Butolan (Bayer)—carbamic acid ester of p. oxydiphenyl methan—is given in doses of one to three tablets (0·5 gm.) daily for adults ; for children over ten years the dose is the same and for younger children the dosage is proportionately smaller. The treatment should continue till twenty tablets have been taken. Enemata of quassia are used to expel the worms per rectum ; the bowel is first washed out with a salt and water enema (one tablespoonful of salt to half a pint). Then 6 oz. of 1 : 100 solution of quassia are run slowly into the rectum and the foot of the bed raised. Along with the quassia injections, carbon tetrachloride combined with oil of chenopodium may be given by the mouth instead of butolan, in the same way as described under ancylostomiasis (see p. 263).

2. **General Management and Personal Prophylaxis.**—It is very important to prevent reinfection with ova ; nails should be kept short and the hands washed constantly. Sleeping drawers and gloves of cotton should be worn at night. For pruritis ani the anus should be smeared at night-time with ung. hydrarg. ammon. (B.P.). By adopting these precautions reinfection with the ova will be prevented, as the ova are conveyed by contaminated hands and clothing.

ASCARIASIS (ROUNDWORM)

1. **Specific Therapy.**—Santonin is very commonly employed in the treatment of this infection in doses of 3 to 5 gr. for an adult and ½ to 1 gr. for a child. It may be given combined with calomel (1 to 3 gr.) for three successive nights, followed by a saline purge, sod. sulph. (½ oz.), six hours later. Santonin may cause visual troubles and makes the urine yellow. The combination of carbon tetrachloride and oil of chenopodium in liquid paraffin, as described above, is very useful as an anthelminthic in this condition also.

2. **Personal Prophylaxis.**—In areas where this infection is common, uncooked vegetables and other raw food material should be avoided.

TRICHURIS TRICHIURA (WHIPWORM)

Fortunately this worm does not give rise to serious pathological lesions, as it is very difficult to dislodge by any known anthelminthic treatment. Thymol and a combination of carbon tetrachloride and oil of chenopodium may be administered as described under ancylostomiasis (see p. 263). Recently cases have been freed from ova within ten days by administration of ferri et ammon. cit., 4 to 5 gm. daily, but subsequent tests have failed to confirm this result.

Personal prophylaxis is the same as in ascariasis (see p. 264).

E. D. W. Greig.

SOME COMMON DISORDERS IN INFANCY AND EARLY CHILDHOOD

INTRODUCTION

N*URSING.*—The majority of diseases met with in infancy and early childhood are acute. Infections are more common and fraught with more serious consequences than in adults. Except where specific remedies are known, treatment is necessarily restricted to measures which help to tide the patient over the acute period. The recuperative powers of children, however, are great, and once an acute infection is overcome, convalescence is as a rule rapid. The most important therapeutic measures are nursing, the administration of a suitable diet and the giving of a plentiful supply of fluid. Drug treatment plays a minor part, though stimulants and sedatives may be of the greatest value on occasions.

The sick infant should, where possible, have a room to himself and on no account should a bed or cot be shared. The temperature of the room is best kept between 60° and 65° F. The child's clothing should be loose and comfortable. Harsh woollens next the skin are often irritating. After the umbilical stump is healed a binder is no longer required ; it impedes respiratory movement and is also a source of skin irritation. Great care should be taken to prevent skin infection ; a sweat rash which would not be more than a source of irritation in the adult may lead to widespread and serious skin infection in the infant. Frequently it is difficult to prevent a child from scratching or picking at an infected area on the skin. To prevent this the arms should be splinted so that the elbows cannot be flexed. The best method of doing this is to bandage strips of cardboard to the arms, extending from the axilla to the hand. The infant should be bathed in the morning and sponged at night. The buttocks require special attention and should be carefully sponged each time the napkins are changed. If there are any signs of irritation a bland ointment such as unguentum zinci et olei ricini may be applied freely. Tepid sponging for skin temperatures above 102·5° F. is valuable and often promotes sleep in addition to reducing the fever. The sick infant should not be allowed to lie in one position for too long, and in acute respiratory disease he should be propped up with pillows.

Diet.—A discussion on infant feeding is outwith the scope of this work but, generally speaking, in febrile conditions the food intake should be diminished as regards fat and protein, but an adequate supply of carbohydrate in the form of simple sugar (or glucose) is to be recommended. These principles can be put into practice by diluting the milk to half strength and adding sugar, while maintaining or even increasing the total fluid intake. Beef-tea, soup and cereals do more harm than good in acute illness. The first two have very little food value and limit the amount of fluid that can be taken as milk, while cereals are apt to upset digestion.

It is of the utmost importance to ensure that the ill infant receives an ample supply of fluid. Unlike the adult he cannot ask for a drink, so water must be offered at frequent intervals. There is no condition, except perhaps gastric or bowel perforation, in which unlimited fluid should not be given. It is not uncommon for a well-nourished infant weighing, say, 12 lbs. to lose 8 oz. (*i.e.*, one-twenty-fourth of his weight) in the first twenty-four hours of an acute diarrhœal disease. This loss of weight is almost entirely accounted for by loss of fluid from the blood and tissues. So prone is the young child to become dehydrated and so evil are the consequences that it is frequently necessary to give fluid by routes other than by the mouth. It is best given in the form of normal saline solution with or without the addition of glucose in a concentration of 10 per cent.

Drugs.—The administration of drugs is often difficult. It is better to give them in solution rather than as powders. It is impossible to give pills unless they are ground into powder and mixed with water. The infant's sense of taste is not well developed, and he will readily take medicine highly unpalatable to the adult. The dosage must be modified according to age, the usual formula being, adult dose $\times \frac{\text{age}}{\text{age}+12}$. Using such a formula there is little if any likelihood of overdosage and there are many drugs which may be given in much larger doses than the use of the formula would suggest—*e.g.*, chloral hydrate, belladonna and its active principle, atropine, and calcium or ammonium chloride. Preparations containing strychnine as well as opium and its derivative, morphine, must be given with caution. The most useful sedative for young children is chloral hydrate. It is particularly safe and has no cumulative effects. Aspirin and the bromides will also be found efficacious. The use of strong cathartics is seldom if ever necessary. Drastic purgatives are dangerous on account of the serious loss of fluid entailed. The brisk purge commonly given to an adult at the onset of an acute infection is neither necessary nor advisable in the infant. The most useful laxatives are fluid magnesia, syrup of figs and paraffin preparations ; frequent and long-continued use of mercurials such as hydrarg. cum cret. cannot be recommended.

A suitable method of giving medicine to an infant is to place the child in the semi-erect position with the arms enclosed in a blanket or shawl wrapped round the body. The mouth can be opened by gentle pressure on the cheeks with the thumb and forefinger of the left hand and the medicine poured from a teaspoon held in the right hand well into the back of the mouth. In order to get him to swallow, it is sometimes necessary to compress the nostrils for a few seconds.

Special Methods of Feeding

Sometimes on account of grave debility or deformity of the lips and mouth (hare-lip and cleft palate), the infant is unable to suck either the breast or the bottle. In those circumstances special methods must be employed. The commonest of these is spoon-feeding. This is often invaluable although time-consuming. Another method is to give the food by a pipette to which a small piece of rubber tubing has been attached. The food can be introduced drop by drop into the back of the throat. For the child too weak to swallow or for one whose swallowing reflex is in abeyance, resort must be had to feeding by stomach tube. This is known as gavage, and can only be adopted when skilled nursing is available. The child must be wrapped in a blanket enclosing his arms and laid on his side across the nurse's knees. The apparatus required consists in a glass funnel connected by rubber tubing and a short connecting piece to a small stomach tube (No. 8 to 10, English). The tube is lubricated with glycerin and inserted through the mouth into the stomach. A rough estimate of the length of tube to be passed in order to reach the stomach may be obtained by measuring the distance from the mouth to the xiphisternum. The tube may be marked by a thread tied round it at the appropriate distance from its point. After the tube has been inserted any residue of food lying in the stomach is withdrawn by siphonage and the food is then run into the stomach. When the tube is withdrawn it should be compressed between the finger and thumb to prevent reflux into the pharynx.

A similar apparatus may be employed for gastric lavage. The fluids commonly used for this are normal saline solution or a solution of bicarbonate of soda, a teaspoonful to the pint of water.

Special Methods of Giving Fluid

Fluid may be given to infants by the rectum or parenterally, *i.e.*, by routes other than the alimentary tract, such as into the subcutaneous tissues, the peritoneal cavity or by injection into a vein.

Rectal Administration.—A rubber rectal tube (size No. 10) to which a funnel is attached is, after lubrication, gently inserted into the rectum to a distance of 2 to 4 in. and the bowel washed out ; after the rectum has been emptied, 2 to 4 oz. of warm normal saline and 5 or 10 per cent. glucose solution are run in slowly and the tube withdrawn. The buttocks should be held together for a few minutes after withdrawal of the tube. This procedure may be repeated after an interval of four hours. Young infants cannot as a rule retain more than 2 oz. at a time. When there is diarrhœa or rectal irritation this method of giving fluid is impracticable.

Subcutaneous Route.—This is the simplest of the three methods of giving fluid parenterally, but it is painful, requires a considerable degree of exposure of the infant and the risk of infection is greater. Two needles connected by a glass Y-piece with a rubber tube leading from a funnel may be used. They are inserted into the subcutaneous tissue below the breasts or in the axillæ. The fluid is run in by gravity, and 100 to 150 c.c. of glucose in saline or normal saline can readily be given in this way in fifteen to thirty minutes.

Intraperitoneal Route.—This method has gained considerable popularity in recent years, and properly carried out is devoid of danger. It is more rapid in accomplishment than the subcutaneous method and the benefit is equally great. Any suspicion of acute abdominal disease of a surgical nature or tuberculous peritonitis must obviously be regarded as a contra-indication. Having made sure that the bladder is empty, a needle having a short bevel with a bore of 1·2 mm. and a length of 30 mm. is inserted into the peritoneal cavity at a point $\frac{1}{4}$ in. below and to one side of the umbilicus. Strict aseptic precautions must be observed. Normal saline at a temperature of 103° F. in the reservoir is run in by gravity and 100 to 200 c.c. can be given, depending on the age of the patient and the degree of dehydration. It is recommended that glucose solution be not used because of the increased risk of infection.

Intravenous Route.—This is the most direct, rapid and effective method of giving fluid. The principles involved are similar to those obtaining in the adult. Veins are much smaller, however, and it is frequently necessary to cut down and expose a vein under local anæsthesia. For this the internal saphenous vein, as it crosses the internal malleolous, will be found suitable. Employing very fine needles (0·8 mm. bore) scalp veins can often be utilized. In infants in whom the anterior fontanelle is still patent, fluid may be administered through the superior longitudinal sinus. The method is as follows: the child should have his arms pinioned by being firmly wrapped in a blanket or shawl. He should be placed with his head resting on a hard pillow at the end of the table. His head should be firmly held with a hand on each side of the face. The operator should be seated at the end of the table. The hair is shaved from the region of the fontanelle and the skin sterilized. A 2 c.c. saline infusion syringe is fitted with a hypodermic needle of 0·8 mm. bore. To the lateral opening a length of rubber tubing (about 8 in.) is fitted and this in its turn is connected by a 2½-in. piece of glass tubing with a second length of rubber tubing about 12 in. long. A funnel of a capacity of about 1 to 2 oz. is connected to this section of rubber tubing. The whole apparatus is sterilized by boiling. When all preparations have been made the funnel is filled with saline, or saline and 5 or 10 per cent. glucose, at a temperature of at least 106° F. and allowed to flow down the tubing to the syringe which has the piston fully withdrawn. The piston is then pushed home, care being taken to expel all air from the tubing and syringe. The needle with the syringe and tubing attached is then inserted through the scalp at a point immediately anterior to the posterior angle of the fontanelle in a downward and backward direction, the needle pointing towards the occipital protuberance. The sinus is reached at a depth of about 0·5 cm. As the needle is being inserted the piston of the syringe should from time to time be slightly withdrawn. When the sinus is entered a jet of blood will be drawn into the syringe. The piston is then withdrawn beyond the lateral opening and, with the operator holding the needle in position, the fluid from the funnel is allowed to run into the sinus by gravity. The funnel should not be held at a level of more than 12 in. above the child's head. Fluid should not be introduced at a rate greater than 10 to 15 c.c. per minute, and care should be taken that its temperature in the reservoir is not less than 106° F. Not more than 30 c.c. per kg. of body-weight should be given. Similar apparatus may be used in giving fluid by the other veins mentioned, but as a rule the reservoir has to be held at a rather higher level in order to get the fluid to flow at a reasonably rapid rate.

Fluid given by " continuous drip " has been found to be of considerable value in cases of severe dehydration. In infants it is necessary in employing this method to cut down on a superficial vein and to tie in a small cannula. It can be given roughly at the rate of 120 c.c. per kg. per day, that is 5 c.c. per kg. per hour.

NEO-NATAL CONDITIONS

Prematurity.—Any infant whose birth-weight is less than 2·5 kg. (5·5 lbs.) may be regarded as premature. The chances of survival in any given case depend on the weight of the infant and on whether disease or injury is present, *e.g.*, cerebral birth trauma. With experienced help and attention to detail much can be done even for very small and weakly babies. The first essential is to prevent heat loss. A severe chilling, which is most likely to occur in the first few hours after birth, may alone be responsible for the infant's death. In all cases in which it is suspected that the infant will be small, special preparation should be made for his reception. A bassinet with the necessary blankets and hot-water bottles must be in readiness, and someone must be detailed to care for the infant as soon as he is born. If there is cyanosis, artificial respiration should not be attempted, but one must make sure that the air passages are not obstructed. They may be cleared by a mucus extractor—a small bottle with a two-way stopper fitted with two soft rubber tubes, one of which is inserted into the throat, the other is used to create negative pressure, either with the mouth or a rubber bulb ; attempts to remove mucus by the finger wrapped in gauze are ineffective and dangerous. The infant should not be bathed ; it is sufficient to cleanse the body rapidly with olive oil. Indeed, all bathing should be avoided until his temperature becomes stabilized and he is thriving. All tight clothing is contraindicated. He should not be " dressed " but wrapped in a jacket made of gamgee with a hood to cover the head and fastened with tapes down the front. Instead of a napkin a square of gamgee placed under the buttocks should be used ; it can be discarded when soiled and is less irritating to the skin than the napkin. Even the binder should be loosely applied lest it interfere with respiration. The blanket over him should be as light as is consistent with sufficient warmth and an extra blanket can be placed over the bassinet as further protection. He can be carried about in this way without loss of heat or undue disturbance. Hot-water bottles to supply the necessary warmth are usually necessary, but the greatest care must be taken to prevent burns. The electric blanket may also be recommended and is of special value in institutions. He should have a room to himself, with ample fresh warm air. The room should be kept at a temperature of 70° F. Elaborate or complicated incubators are only practicable in institutions and cannot be recommended for general use.

Every possible care should be taken to prevent infection. Skin abrasions if present should be treated twice daily with a 1 per cent. aqueous solution of gentian violet and left, preferably without dressings, exposed to air as much as is practicable. The point should be stressed that any person who is even suspected of having a cold should have for the time being no access to the infant. All utensils, bottles and teats used for feeding must be cleaned and boiled with meticulous care each time they are used.

The feeding of the infant is greatly simplified if breast milk is available, and every attempt must be made to procure this, if not from the mother from a foster-mother. If it is not available, one of the half-cream dried milks or boiled and diluted cow's milk with added sugar may be used. One to two ounces of half-milk to which has been added ½ teaspoonful of cane sugar or dextro-maltose is a suitable feed to begin with.

If the infant is strong and breast-milk is available, he should be put to the breast in the ordinary way ; if he is too weak to suck, the milk must be exhausted and fed to him either by spoon or pipette. A valuable method is gavage. It has the great advantage of diminishing the time taken in feeding, thus allowing him more time to sleep. If he is fed by gavage a four-hourly interval will probably suffice ; if by any other method, in the early stages at any rate, it is better to feed him three-hourly. Only in exceptional circumstances is it advisable to feed a premature infant more often.

Premature infants are prone to develop rickets and nutritional anæmia. It is important that steps be taken to prevent this. About the end of the first month cod-liver oil, in doses of ½ teaspoonful night and morning, may be given and the amount must be increased, as he becomes accustomed to it, to 1 teaspoonful three times a day. Any of the numerous proprietary preparations in suitable doses (adexolin, ostelin, radiostol, etc.) is probably equally satisfactory. Iron may be given later, beginning about the tenth or twelfth week. A suitable formula is :

℞		
	Ferr. Sulph.	gr. i
	Cupr. Sulph.	gr. $\frac{1}{100}$
	Acid. Hypophosph. Dil. . . .	♏ ½
	Dextros.	gr. xv
	Aq. . . . . . . ad	℥i

Sig., ℥i, t.d.s.

It is important that ferrous sulphate be prescribed in this way to prevent oxidation. Ferri et ammonium citratis gr. x may be given in place of ferrous sulphate. There is good evidence to show that the hæmoglobin level will rise higher with the addition of copper than with iron alone. Iron need not be given continuously, but cod-liver oil and orange juice should be given throughout the first year.

Inanition Fever.—This condition is recognized by a sudden rise in temperature in an infant during the first week of life without there being any evidence of infection or cerebral trauma. It occurs at the period when the mother's milk is probably inadequate ; hence the name. Actually the *causa causans* is lack of fluid, *i.e.*, dehydration. The child should be given 4 to 8 oz. of water or normal saline during the course of a few hours. This will cause an immediate return of the temperature to normal : if it does not, the diagnosis should be reconsidered.

Sepsis Neonatorum.—This condition has greatly diminished in frequency. The infection usually gains entrance either through a skin abrasion or by the umbilical cord. Prevention consists in guarding all abrasions of the skin from infection by suitable antiseptic measures and by the use of sterile dressings for the umbilical stump. The best antiseptics are a 1 per cent. aqueous solution of gentian violet, acriflavine (1 : 1,000) or surgical spirit. Iodine is unsuitable. If the infection becomes generalized, *i.e.*, septicæmic, the outlook is grave and no form of treatment is likely to be of any avail. If pemphigus appears the dead skin must be carefully cut away and the raw area treated with antiseptics. Such patients must be isolated from other infants as this type of neonatal sepsis is extremely contagious.

Hæmorrhagic Disease of the Newborn (Melæna Neonatorum).—The diagnosis of this condition rests on the recognition of the occurrence of bleeding in an infant in the first twelve days of life. Bleeding may be from the bowel (melæna), from the umbilical stump, into the skin or into any of the viscera or body cavities, such as the meninges or the pericardial sac. If life is to be saved it is essential that the condition be recognized early. Ten to twenty cubic centimetres of whole blood should be withdrawn from a healthy donor and immediately injected into the loose subcutaneous tissue between the scapulæ, or it may be given intramuscularly. The procedure is repeated in four hours. This is sufficient in the majority of cases to control the bleeding. Blood-stained motions may continue to be passed and some difficulty may be experienced in deciding whether or not the bleeding has stopped; when in doubt a further blood injection should be given. A hæmoglobin estimation is useful in estimating the gravity of the condition. In cases where the loss of blood has been great, blood transfusion should be resorted to and can be relied upon to control the bleeding. Infants who have appeared moribund have recovered after transfusion. If given into a vein the blood must be carefully matched, and as this is a time-consuming process it is well to have available at hospital a universal donor for such cases and so avoid delay. When giving blood subcutaneously or intramuscularly it is of course unnecessary to group the blood. If there is extensive hæmorrhage into a vital organ, no form of treatment is likely to be of any avail.

Hæmolytic Anæmia and Jaundice.—Jaundice in the newborn is most frequently physiological. It is due to the destruction of erythrocytes in the first few days of life, during which the hæmoglobin content of 140 per cent. at birth falls rapidly below 100 per cent. It is probably correct to say that 30 to 60 per cent. of all newborn infants are to some extent jaundiced. The general health is unaffected and there are no signs of biliary obstruction. No treatment of the condition is required.

Under certain pathological conditions, the ætiology of which is at present unknown, this breaking down of red cells becomes excessive and gives rise to *congenital hæmolytic anæmia*. The rapidity of onset and development of such a condition is often alarming, and as soon as the diagnosis is made, resort should be had to transfusion, which may have to be repeated on successive days or every other day until the hæmolytic process is checked. Cessation of hæmolysis is marked by the return of the reticulocyte count to normal. Whole blood given subcutaneously or intramuscularly in the same way and in the same dosage as is given for hæmorrhagic disease of the newborn is of value, and if facilities for transfusion are not available this should be tried.

This pathological process of hæmolysis may in some cases be so acute that the bile ducts are unable to deal with the excess bile pigments excreted by the liver and become blocked. A true obstructive jaundice is then superadded (*icterus gravis*). The condition is recognized by bile pigment in the urine and the presence of severe anæmia with, as a rule, reticulocytosis. The hæmoglobin may fall as low as 20 per cent. and in such instances the prognosis is grave. The treatment is the same as for congenital hæmolytic anæmia, namely, repeated transfusion until hæmolysis is arrested.

Occasionally the condition develops during intra-uterine life (*hydrops fœtalis*). In such cases the infant is stillborn.

True obstructive jaundice also may arise from congenital atresia of the bile ducts. It is differentiated from icterus gravis by the absence of anæmia and of reticulocytosis. In the majority of cases the outlook is hopeless, although death may be delayed for several months or even years. If the presence of a gall-bladder can be demonstrated, operation may be considered. There are several successful results reported in the literature.

Sepsis, where the infection is generalized, may produce jaundice from hepatic involvement or from hæmolysis. The outlook, of course, is grave, and the usual measures for dealing with septicæmia should be adopted. Congenital syphilis is often mentioned as a cause of jaundice, but its incidence is probably casual and not as great as formerly believed. The treatment is that of congenital syphilis.

Birth Injuries.—Birth injuries are extremely common and, when involving nervous tissue, often serious. Their early recognition is most important if the best results from treatment are to be obtained.

A cephalhæmatoma which consists of an effusion of blood beneath the periosteum of one of the flat bones of the skull is often a cause of considerable apprehension to the mother. Any attempt to remove the blood clot by aspiration or by incision is to be condemned. The risk of infection is too great. If left untreated such swellings disappear in two or three months and leave no traces. The possibility of a cephalhæmatoma becoming infected even although not interfered with does, however, exist, and in such circumstances it should be dealt with surgically.

The commonest sites of *fracture* in the newborn are clavicle, femur and humerus. They are not, curiously enough, of the "green-stick" variety but complete. Displacement may be great, but in otherwise healthy infants healing readily occurs without deformity. Fractures of the clavicle require no special treatment; indeed probably only a small percentage of them are recognized. For the fractured femur a band of adhesive tape, $3\frac{1}{2}$ in. wide, is bound around the site of the fracture and the infant suspended by the legs from a light bar placed across the upper rail of the cot so that the buttocks are just free of the mattress. The weight of the child is sufficient to overcome any slight muscle spasm and produce satisfactory alignment. Another method is to flex the thigh on the abdomen and fix it there with adhesive plaster. The advantage of this method is that the child can be removed from the cot in order to be breast-fed or cleansed. The limb should be kept fixed by one or other of these methods for a fortnight or three weeks, following which free movement can be permitted. The fractured humerus should also be bound up with a band of adhesive tape and the arm bandaged across the chest for a fortnight. It has been claimed that without any immobilization such fractures heal well and that good alignment is obtained. Before fixing fractures of long bones the skin should be bathed with spirit and thoroughly powdered, special attention being paid to axilla, anticubital area and the groin.

Fractures of the skull are not common, but what is seen not infrequently is a gutter or funnel-shaped depression of the skull with no actual fracture, usually situated on the lateral aspect of the skull well forward. There have been many suggestions for dealing with such conditions surgically, but in the absence of signs of cerebral irritation they are much better left alone. The deformity, unless it is very severe, will disappear during the first year and the normal contour of the skull be restored.

Cerebral birth trauma is extremely common and often the diagnosis is not apparent. It occurs most frequently in premature infants. The trauma may result in cerebral hæmorrhage, œdema of cerebral tissues or rupture of the meninges with hæmorrhage. Among the manifestations of the condition may be mentioned convulsions, attacks of cyanosis, tense or bulging anterior fontanelle and inability to suck, shrill piercing cry and fever. Subtentorial lesions are more likely to result in death than those above the tentorium. The patients often present the picture of asphyxia pallida (shock). Rest and warmth in a quiet darkened room with a minimum of disturbance constitute an important part of the treatment. If there are signs of increased intracranial pressure, such as fullness of the anterior fontanelle or undue drowsiness, lumbar puncture should be performed to relieve the pressure and should be repeated if necessary. The injection of 1 to 2 oz. of 10 per cent. saline solution into the rectum has been advocated as a means of lowering intracranial pressure. The procedure may be repeated at four-hourly intervals. Chloral hydrate should be used freely if the infant is twitching or if he is restless. One or two grains three or four-hourly will be required; the dose must be increased until rest is obtained. If the signs and symptoms point to hæmorrhage over the vertex, surgical intervention may be considered. This is an extreme procedure, however, and the greatest difficulty is experienced in deciding on the case which offers a reasonable chance of success, especially as the lesions are so often multiple.

Certain authorities hold that cerebral hæmorrhage is often a result not of trauma but of hæmorrhagic disease of the newborn, and recommend that cerebral hæmorrhage in the absence of a history of birth injury, and coming on several days after birth, should be treated by subcutaneous injections of whole blood as in hæmorrhagic disease.

The seventh cranial nerve is often injured in newborn infants. This appears to be the result of pressure at the stylomastoid foramen; no treatment is required and certainly not electrical stimulation.

Brachial paralysis (Erb-Duchenne) resulting from injury to the brachial plexus and producing a flaccid paralysis of one or other arm should be treated as soon as it is recognized. The arm should at once be raised above the level of the shoulder with the forearm flexed at the elbow to a right angle and held there by pinning the sleeve to the pillow. In many mild cases that is all that is required, and after a fortnight or three weeks of such treatment full power may have been restored to the arm. Care must be taken during this time that the nerve trunks and affected muscles are not allowed to become stretched. During the bath, for instance, the affected arm must be carefully supported. In more severe cases some form of splint holding the limb in a position of abduction and external rotation at the shoulder and flexion and supination at the elbow will be required. The best material for a splint of this nature is vulcanized fibre. It should be remembered that at this age growth is very rapid, and too elaborate a splint is not advisable, as the baby will soon outgrow it. The further treatment of this condition belongs to the field of orthopædic surgery.

DISEASES OF THE DIGESTIVE SYSTEM

Disease of the digestive system is probably the commonest cause of illness in infancy and early childhood. In some of the acute conditions treatment must be carried out with promptitude if life is to be saved, while in certain of the more chronic disturbances a systematized plan of treatment which may have to be continued for a prolonged period has to be instituted. Hard and fast rules cannot be laid down for the treatment of individual cases, but there are certain general principles which should be borne in mind.

1. Breast feeding must be regarded as infinitely superior to artificial feeding. It may be taken for granted that a mother's milk is the most suitable food for the infant, and the practice of taking babies off the breast because of "upsets" is to be deprecated.

2. It is in the summer and autumn months that gastro-intestinal disturbance is most likely to occur. For this reason a correct system of feeding hygiene should be most carefully observed during this period.

3. Parenteral infection is a common cause of gastro-intestinal upset. In all cases of gastro-intestinal disturbance such extra-alimentary foci of infection should be sought for and dealt with.

4. In the chronic affections careful investigation of the previous feeding history and thorough physical examination are of great importance in affording a guide to treatment. In many cases cure may be effected merely by correcting errors in the diet, while in others careful examination may reveal unsuspected deformities or foci of infection which are the cause of the gastro-intestinal disturbance.

Stomatitis

Injury to the mucous membrane is commonly the cause of inflammatory conditions of the mouth and pharynx. The mouth of the infant requires no cleaning and attempts to do so may, by injury to the mucous membrane, give rise to stomatitis. Other causes are unclean rubber teats and comforters. In order to avoid mouth infection a mother should be warned against making any attempt to clean her baby's mouth after feeding, and in the case of the artificially fed infant the importance of sterilizing everything coming into contact with the mouth should be emphasized.

Parasitic Stomatitis (Thrush).—The condition is speedily remedied by painting the affected areas with 1 per cent. gentian violet in aqueous solution twice daily for a period of three to four days. Such preparations as glycerin and borax are more or less ineffectual. The condition is most frequently seen in marantic infants, and in addition to local treatment every effort should be made to improve the general condition.

Aphthous Stomatitis.—The child should be given potassium chlorate by the mouth at four-hourly intervals in doses of 2 to 7½ gr. according to the age, and the ulcers should be touched with a 1 per cent. solution of silver nitrate. *Ulcerative stomatitis* requires more energetic treatment on similar lines. In addition, the gums and buccal mucous membrane should be painted with a solution containing equal parts of liquor arsenicalis and tincture of ipecacuanha.

Bednar's Ulcers.—Sometimes ulceration of the pillars of the fauces and soft palate occurs in young infants. These ulcers are usually caused by misguided efforts to clear secretion from the mouth and pharynx of the newborn infant. They should be painted with a 1 per cent. solution of silver nitrate.

Vomiting

The treatment of vomiting depends on its cause. Mothers frequently seek advice because the baby brings up mouthfuls of milk after each feeding. In many cases this is not of serious significance, and if weight is being gained satisfactorily it may be disregarded. Sometimes, however, there is considerable loss of food and the infant does not thrive. In these cases there is probably some error in feeding technique. It may be that the child is placed flat on his back immediately after taking his feed, and in his endeavours to eructate ingested air brings up mouthfuls of food. To prevent this he should be held in the semi-erect position for some minutes after he has finished his feed. In other cases irregular feeding and unsuitable food are responsible for vomiting. In this the treatment consists in correcting the defects in the feeding regimen and the diet.

Rumination.— Some infants acquire the habit of purposefully regurgitating ingested foods. When this habit has become well established it is difficult to correct and may lead to severe inanition. Various mechanical devices, such as plugging the nostrils or gags which prevent the mouth from being opened, have been advocated, but they rarely meet with success. Probably the best results are obtained by getting the mother or nurse to occupy the child's attention after each feeding till he falls asleep. Thickened feeds, being more difficult to regurgitate, are also helpful. Any of the farinaceous foods, such as oat flour or Sister Laura's Food, may be used for this purpose.

Œsophageal Atresia and Cardiospasm.—The symptoms of atresia and cardiospasm which usually manifest themselves when the child commences to take solid food, may be treated by dilatation with gum elastic œsophageal bougies. Dilatation may have to be carried out daily at first and then, if improvement occurs, at gradually increasing intervals.

Mechanical Obstruction at the Pylorus.—This is a common cause of intractable vomiting in young infants. The obstruction may be due to spasm of the pyloric sphincter or to spasm combined with hypertrophy of the muscle (hypertrophic pyloric stenosis).

In *pylorospasm* treatment should be carried out on purely medical lines. Gastric lavage with normal saline solution should be used daily till the vomiting becomes less frequent. Whenever possible breast feeding should be employed. Failing this, cow's milk diluted with equal parts of water, to which is added half a drachm of sugar for each 3 oz. of the feed, should be given at three-hourly intervals, one feed during the night being omitted. Certain anti-spasmodic drugs have been used with success. Eumydrin (atropine methyl nitrate) given in doses of 2·5 to 5 c.c. of a 1 : 10,000 solution half an hour before each feed is probably the best. It is almost as efficacious as atropine sulphate and is fifty times less poisonous. The skin frequently becomes dry and there may be some rise in temperature. If these symptoms become unduly pronounced, the drug should be omitted before one or two feeds.

Hypertrophic Pyloric Stenosis.—The treatment of hypertrophic pyloric stenosis is, in our opinion, in the great majority of cases, surgical. Probably the best results are obtained when the physician is responsible for both the pre-operative and post-operative treatment. It is generally recognized that the greater the degree of emaciation and dehydration the less the chance of recovery. It is therefore of the utmost importance that the diagnosis should be made as soon as possible after the onset of symptoms and before emaciation has become severe.

The pre-operative treatment consists in measures aimed at restoring water and chloride to the infant's depleted tissues and in combating the condition of alkalosis which is always present. One hundred cubic centimetres of a solution of normal saline and 10 per cent. glucose should be given by a vein or the longitudinal sinus and 60 c.c. by the rectum, the latter at four-hourly intervals ; alternatively, saline without glucose may be given subcutaneously. Any septic focus should be attended to, and special care should be taken to ensure that the umbilicus is soundly healed. Both before and after operation the child should be guarded in every possible way from respiratory infection. He should be isolated from other children, and no one with any respiratory infection such as coryza or pharyngitis should be permitted to come near him. The stomach should be washed out daily with normal saline solution. Lavage with sodium bicarbonate solution is contraindicated. In the great majority of cases the operation should be performed as soon as possible, though when there is severe dehydration it may be delayed for forty-eight hours or longer while the tissue fluids are being restored. The Rammstedt operation is the operation of choice. Two hours after operation the child should be given saline solution or water by the mouth, followed two hours later by 4 drachms of milk acidified with lactic acid (see p. 287) and diluted to half strength with water ; alternatively, the same quantity of half cream dried milk, 1 part of the dried milk to 10 of water, may be given. During the next twelve hours water or saline alternating with the milk feeds in the above quantities should be given at two-hourly intervals. For the twelve hours thereafter double the quantity of saline and milk should be given at the same intervals. Twenty-four hours after the operation the child should be given 2 oz. of the feed seven times a day at three-hourly intervals, missing one feed during the night. The quantity of the feeds should then be gradually increased and about ten days after the operation their number should be reduced to five in the twenty-four hours. Sugar should be added with caution. For two or three days after operation, saline by the rectum at four-hourly intervals is extremely valuable but may not always be retained ; if there are signs of dehydration, fluid should be given parenterally. In very feeble infants blood transfusion may be of benefit. The danger of wound infection is very great in these infants and this should be most carefully guarded against.

Some children are only brought for advice when they are eight or nine weeks old ; as the disease as a rule cures itself by the age of three or four months, it may be advisable in these cases to endeavour to tide the patient over the intervening period by dietetic measures until spontaneous cure occurs.

Although we are in favour of operative treatment in the great majority of cases, non-operative treatment appears to have met with success in certain quarters. The chief objection to this is that it has to be continued for many weeks, during which time the enfeebled and emaciated patient may succumb to some intercurrent disease. This danger is specially to be feared in hospital practice where isolation cannot as a rule be carried out as efficiently as in the private home. Medical treatment consists of the administration of a suitable diet (diluted milk, acidified milk or dried-milk preparations with added sugar), gastric lavage once or twice daily with normal saline and the use of some antispasmodic drug. Eumydrin is probably the best of these and should be given in doses of 2·5 to 5 c.c. of a 1 : 10,000 solution half an hour before each feed. The correction of the dehydration and chloride loss is of primary importance. Saline should be given freely by the mouth and, if necessary, parenterally.

Vomiting in General Disease.—In children, vomiting very commonly occurs in general disease in which the stomach is not primarily at fault ; thus in pneumonia and pyogenic infection of the urinary tract it is often a prominent symptom. In these circumstances the treatment is that of the causative disease, but in infants care must be taken not to give too large feeds of milk, and it is usually wise to reduce its fat content by one of the recognized methods (see p. 286). Vomiting in conjunction with obstinate constipation should always raise the suspicion either of intestinal obstruction, *e.g.*, intussusception, or of increased intracranial pressure, *e.g.*, meningitis ; here, also, the treatment is that of the primary cause. Conversely, cyclic vomiting (see p. 297) may also give rise to symptoms suggestive of acute abdominal or cerebral disease.

Constipation

In infants and young children the most usual cause of constipation is insufficient food. The treatment consists in adjusting the diet. It is also commonly seen in cases of pyloric stenosis and meningitis in which the associated vomiting causes reduction in the amount of food entering the intestines. It rapidly passes off if the causative disease can be remedied. In this connection it should be mentioned that when there is great reduction in the amount of food entering the intestine, small, dark, rather loose slimy stools may be passed (starvation stools) and the mother may state that the child is suffering from diarrhœa. The stools consist largely of desquamated bowel epithelium and bile pigments and salts. Spasm of the anal sphincter, usually due to anal fissure, is sometimes a cause of constipation. The treatment consists in keeping the motions soft by suitable laxatives, *e.g.*, petrolagar, and, in the case of fissure, applying an ointment of ichthyol and tannic acid, in the proportion of 1 drachm of each to 1 oz. of vaseline, to the part on a pledget of cotton wool inserted into the anus. In many cases of anal spasm relief may be obtained by stretching the sphincter.

Gastro-enteritis

In its severe forms treatment must be prompt and energetic if life is to be saved. The main objects are to combat the toxæmia and to relieve dehydration and acidosis. Collapse may be severe, and in this case fluid must be given without delay by either the subcutaneous, intravenous or peritoneal routes. The child should be placed in a warmed cot, and if the temperature is subnormal heat should be applied by carefully guarded hot bottles or an electrically heated cage or blanket. As soon as the child's condition permits, the stomach should be washed out with a solution of bicarbonate of soda (ʒi to 1 pint) and the rectum with normal saline solution. Nothing but water should be given by the mouth for twelve to twenty-four hours and the child should be encouraged to drink as much as possible. As regards the all-important question of diet a bewildering variety of milk mixtures and other foods has been advocated, such as protein milk, curd mixture, lactic acid milk, peptonized milk, glucose, albumin water, apple puree and sweetened tea. Description of the method of preparation of some of these is given on p. 286. After trying many of these preparations we have come to the conclusion that a diet of diluted milk is as effective as any of the more complicated formulæ and has the advantage of being simple to prepare. After the preliminary period of starvation, small feeds of unsweetened milk diluted with an equal amount of water should be given at four-hourly intervals. Commencing with ½ oz. of milk and ½ oz. of water, the amount of the feed should be gradually increased until the child is receiving a quantity suitable for his age. The proportion of milk to water may then gradually be increased and, lastly, sugar added. During the first few days it may be necessary to give parenteral fluid repeatedly by one of the methods described previously. After the acute symptoms have passed off the greatest care with feeding must be observed, as relapse is very liable to occur if any liberties with the diet are taken.

Medicinal treatment is of little value. If the child comes under observation soon after the commencement of the illness, 1 drachm of castor oil may be given. In collapse, brandy is sometimes of benefit, while if there is great restlessness or if convulsions occur, chloral hydrate in doses of 2 to 3 gr. promotes sleep and depresses nervous irritability. Grey powder, the popular panacea for all infantile ailments, is of no value and may indeed be harmful.

In the less acute forms where gastro-intestinal disturbance may have been present for some days or weeks it is not advisable to subject the child to too rigorous starvation, and after attempting to replenish the depleted tissues with fluid by one of the recognized methods, small feeds of diluted milk may be started immediately. In these subacute cases relapse is particularly likely to occur. The gastro-intestinal tract seems only to be able to digest very small amounts of the simplest food, and whenever the diet is raised in quantity to a level sufficient to allow of a gain in weight, diarrhœa and vomiting recur. It is in intractable cases of this sort that we see the typical picture of marasmus or atrophy. Here we have to guard against enteral infection by a most careful feeding regimen and against parenteral infection by scrupulous attention to nursing hygiene. When gastro-intestinal disturbance has been of long-standing, iron deficiency anæmia is almost inevitable. This should be treated with appropriate doses of iron and copper or by blood transfusion.

Acute Ileocolitis (Dysentery)

Though the dehydration is not as severe as in acute gastroenteritis, toxæmia is as a rule very pronounced in ileocolitis. For this reason it may be necessary to administer fluid by one of the recognized routes. As vomiting does not usually occur, gastric lavage is seldom necessary. With a view to freeing the large bowel of muco-pus, magnesium sulphate in repeated doses should be given by the mouth. In a child of six months 15 gr. at hourly intervals for three or four consecutive hours will as a rule produce watery motions. This may be repeated daily for three or four days, by which time passage of blood, mucus and pus in the stools will probably have ceased. Tenesmus and colic are greatly relieved by this treatment. As the Flexner or Sonne organisms are commonly the causative agents, treatment with the appropriate serum has been advocated. The serum is injected intramuscularly in doses of 10 to 20 c.c. daily for several days. In our experience we have not found this form of treatment of any great value. The diet should at first consist of diluted milk. Commencing with 1 oz. at four-hourly intervals, the feeds may be gradually increased in quantity and strength as improvement in the condition of the stools occurs. As much water as the child will take should be given in the intervals between the feeds.

In the home strict precautions should be taken to avoid infection of other members of the family, and in institutions such precautions are doubly important.

Cœliac Disease

Of all the chronic diseases of childhood cœliac disease is probably the most difficult to treat successfully. Its essential chronicity, the tendency to relapse and the peevish and neurotic state of the patient impose an unenviable ordeal on the parents and medical attendant. As soon as the diagnosis is established, the nature of the disease should be explained to the parents, and it should be made clear to them that treatment will have to be continued for years before complete cure can be expected. The treatment is largely dietetic. As failure to absorb fat is the essential feature, and as the presence of this unabsorbed and decomposing fat in the bowel leads to general upset of the digestion, the first essential is to diminish the fat content of the food to a minimum. In the early stages carbohydrate must also be reduced. Associated with the general intestinal upset there is defective absorption of important vitamins and minerals, and this feature of the disease must not be overlooked.

To commence with, the diet should be restricted to skimmed milk, and if there is diarrhœa, it may be given in the form of curd mixture (see p. 286). As the stools improve, over-ripe pounded banana may be added to the diet, then calf's foot jelly sweetened with saccharin. After a variable period of two to three months, sieved fat-free meat may be allowed, then dextrinized or malted foods, such as corn flakes, Horlicks, Mellin's Food, may be added gradually. Only when convalescence appears to be fairly well established should the fat be increased, and that with the greatest caution. Throughout the whole course of treatment a teaspoonful of orange juice should be given daily as well as some non-oily form of vitamin D, such as ostelin or radiostol pellets in doses per day equivalent to 3 drachms of cod-liver oil, or, as a substitute, irradiation with ultra-violet light may be used to supply the necessary vitamin D. Anæmia is an almost constant finding, usually of the hypochromic variety; for this 1 to 3 gr. of ferrous sulphate thrice daily should be given. In the event of the anæmia being hyperchromic, campolon or one of the other liver extracts which can be given by injection should be used. Marmite, a teaspoonful twice a day, may also be of help. The child should be confined to bed until convalescence is well established, and the greatest care should be taken to guard him from intercurrent infection. In severe cases it may be necessary to give blood transfusions or saline and glucose by one of the recognized routes. If tetany should develop, 5 c.c. of calcium gluconate (sandoz) should be injected intramuscularly or into a vein and vitamin D pushed.

Should relapse occur a return must be made to the original diet and the whole process of gradually building it up must be gone through once more. The success of the treatment depends largely on the intelligent co-operation of the parents.

Milk Modifications

Protein Milk (Eiweissmilch).—Inoculate 1 pint of separated milk with lactic acid bacilli and incubate for eight hours. Curdle a second pint of milk with rennet and strain the whey from the curd through fine muslin for twenty minutes. Rub the curd through a fine sieve with the sour separated milk, and make up the whole to 2 pints with water. The preparation contains approximately 3 per cent. protein, 2 per cent. fat and 1·5 per cent. sugar and has a caloric value of 10 calories per oz.

Sweet Curd Mixture.—The curd is prepared in the same way as for protein milk and is then rubbed through a fine sieve with one-third of the whey, and the whole made up to 1 pint with water. It contains about 3 per cent. protein, 2·5 per cent. fat and 2 per cent. sugar.

Neither protein milk nor sweet curd mixture should be heated. The curd tends to settle on standing, and the preparation must be thoroughly mixed before measuring out the requisite feed.

Milk Containing a Low Percentage of Fat.—Milk separated by centrifugalization contains about 0·5 per cent. fat. The percentage of fat may be increased by adding to it a proportion of the separated cream.

Reduction of the fat may also be obtained by allowing milk to stand for four hours and skimming off the " top milk." If the top 12 oz. are removed the residue contains about 1 per cent. fat ; if the top 8 oz. are removed it contains about 2 per cent. fat. Dried-milk preparations containing a low percentage of fat can be purchased.

Peptonized Milk.—Dissolve one peptonizing powder (Fairchild) in 5 oz. of water. Add this to 1 pint of milk, warm gently to body temperature and allow to digest for twenty minutes ; then bring to the boil and allow to cool rapidly.

Lactic Acid Milk.—Stir into 1 pint of milk 45 minims of lactic acid (B.P.). The acid should be added drop by drop whilst the milk is being vigorously stirred. An egg whisk is useful for this purpose.

DISEASES OF THE RESPIRATORY SYSTEM

Infections

Disease of the respiratory system is caused mainly by " droplet " infection and is one of the major causes of death in young children especially in early infancy. Too much stress, therefore, cannot be laid on the prevention of infections of this nature. For example, any person with a head cold should, whenever possible, refrain from looking after an infant ; this may, of course, not be practicable in the case of a nursing mother, but she should be instructed to wear a mask of gauze or preferably a mask with one layer of cellophane or blotting paper between layers of gauze when nursing or caring for her infant.

" Colds."—The commonest respiratory infection is a " cold," and this may manifest itself in various ways : a nasal discharge, redness of the pharynx, tonsillitis, otitis media or cough. In all young infants, and especially during the neonatal period, upper respiratory infections should not be treated lightly. The patient should be confined to his cot in a cool room at a temperature between 60° and 65° F., and abundant fluid supplied. If fever be present the diet should be fluid, and in infants it is best to dilute the milk as their tolerance to food is usually diminished. If diarrhœa and vomiting are prominent features, treatment as for gastro-enteritis may be adopted, though the diet need not be so drastically restricted as in true gastro-enteritis. Local treatment for the throat is probably not advisable ; if the nasal passages are obstructed a few drops of liquid paraffin containing menthol and camphor (2 gr. of each to the ounce) may be instilled into each nostril ten minutes before feeding time. The head should be held slightly back to allow the liquid paraffin to run into the naso-pharynx. This clears the nasal passages, thus enabling the infant to breathe through the nose whilst sucking. If the cervical glands become involved it is advisable to protect them with a collar of gamgee.

Otitis Media.—The danger of spread of the throat infection to the middle ear must always be borne in mind. It is possible that this danger may in some degree be lessened if care is taken to have the infant nursed in the semi-erect position. This is particularly necessary whilst he is taking his feeds, for during the act of swallowing the pharyngeal orifice of the Eustachian tube gapes and may permit the entrance of infected material. In the event of infection occurring, a few drops of glycerin of carbolic (half strength of the B.P. formula) should be instilled into the auditory canal. This is useful in relieving pain. The tympanic membrane should be examined frequently and, if found to be bulging, incised. The introduction of the electric auriscope has greatly simplified this procedure.

Bronchitis and Pneumonia.—Upper respiratory infection may also spread to the lower respiratory passages, giving rise to bronchitis and broncho-pneumonia and adding to the gravity of the situation. It is often difficult to differentiate severe bronchitis from broncho-pneumonia, and in any case the treatment of both conditions is on similar lines.

Nursing.—Skilled nursing is the first requisite. The child should be nursed in a well-ventilated room, kept at a temperature of about 60° F. Nursing out of doors on a balcony or with the cot placed beside a widely open window regardless of climatic conditions has yielded good results. The clothing must be loose, especially round the neck. Tepid sponging, when the skin temperature exceeds 102·5° F., tends to the general comfort of the child and promotes sleep. Drinks of water or diluted fruit juice should be offered frequently in addition to the regular feeds. The child should be allowed to lie in the position in which he seems most comfortable, but it must be remembered that young children should not be permitted to remain in one position for too long a time. The diet should consist of diluted milk sweetened with sugar, which should be given at three-hourly intervals. In the presence of gastro-intestinal disturbance the amount of sugar in the feeds should be restricted.

Cough.—Cough can be a troublesome symptom and in very young infants it is probably unwise as well as useless to prescribe expectorant mixtures. A sedative, however, is often advisable. Fifteen to thirty minims of syrup of codeine to an infant of six months, and repeated if necessary, is helpful, or chloral hydrate will often produce a cessation of a troublesome cough and induce sleep. When secretion is abundant and the finer bronchi and bronchioles become obstructed, atropine in doses of $\frac{1}{150}$ to $\frac{1}{200}$ gr. should be given hypodermically at four-hourly intervals, or tincture of belladonna by the mouth in doses of 2 to 5 minims. Stimulants may be required; brandy four-hourly is valuable, and camphor in oil in doses of 10 to 15 minims has been recommended, though in our experience it has not proved of much avail. Elixir of ephedrine in doses of $\frac{1}{2}$ drachm at four-hourly intervals helps to dilate the finer bronchi and acts as a vasomotor stimulant. Strychnine and digitalis are better avoided.

Steam as an inhalant is sometimes of use when there is respiratory distress with a dry cough, severe stridor and difficulty in getting rid of bronchial secretion. In some cases its effect is dramatic in alleviating cough and inducing rest, in others it has the opposite effect, and in these circumstances should not be continued. A satisfactory tent can be devised by placing a screen round the head of the cot and covering this with a sheet with the side facing the foot of the cot open. Steam generated in a special kettle fitted with a funnel measuring $2\frac{1}{2}$ ft. in length is allowed to flow gently into the tent. It may be medicated by adding 1 or 2 teaspoonfuls of tincture of benzoin co. to the water in the kettle. The funnel should be adjusted so that there is no possibility of the steam impinging directly on the patient. The greatest precautions against fire must be taken. The funnel must be long enough to permit the kettle with its spirit lamp to be placed well away from the cot. Steam should not be used continuously, but only for a half or one hour every two hours. Occasionally it excites the patient or he fails to get any relief, and in such circumstances should be discontinued. Some authorities regard its value as doubtful; it is the antithesis of fresh-air treatment, and its use carries a risk of fire or burning which would not otherwise exist.

If there is reason to suspect pain on coughing, a poultice may be applied over the affected part of the lung. It is always well to warn the mother against the danger of burning the skin. If mustard is used, a concentration of 1 to 6 parts of linseed meal for infants and 1 to 4 for older children is suitable. After anointing the skin with olive oil, the poultice may be allowed to remain on the chest for twenty minutes to half an hour with safety.

Cyanosis.—If cyanosis is present, oxygen is indicated; nowadays this can be given readily by means of a small oxygen tent. Several types are available and can be purchased from the commercial houses. A simple tent is manufactured by The Condensed Gas Company, Manchester. The oxygen, which should in its passage from the cylinder be passed through a Wolff's bottle containing warm water, is allowed to run into the tent at the rate of 8 litres per minute. To estimate this the use of a flow meter is advisable. A rough method of ensuring a sufficient flow is to adjust the regulator on the cylinder so that the oxygen passes through the water in the Wolff's bottle in a steady stream. It has been calculated that bubbles passing through a glass tube of 1 cm. bore at the rate of two a second represent a flow of less than $\frac{1}{10}$ litre per minute—an amount that is quite ineffective. Failing an oxygen tent, the use of a small rubber catheter inserted to a distance of 1 to 2 in. into the nostril is recommended. It can be retained in position by fixing it with a small strip of adhesive plaster to the cheek. The rate of flow should be 3 to 4 litres per minute and the oxygen should be passed through a Wolff's bottle containing warmed water. The custom of giving oxygen by holding a funnel in front of the patient's nose and mouth is useless.

Specific Treatment.—As only 4 or 5 per cent. of young children with pneumonia are infected with Types I or II pneumococcus, and as the sera at present available are only effective against these two types, the indiscriminate use of serum cannot be recommended. Lederle Laboratories are now, however, producing immune sera for infection by other types. Should these come into general use specific serum therapy for pneumonia in infants may have a practical application. It may soon be possible to use polyvalent sera with the prospect of success.

The value of the sulphanilamide group of drugs in pneumonia in infancy and childhood is now proved. There have been many favourable reports of treatment with sulphapyridine (M. & B. 693), and our own experience is likewise satisfactory. For dosage see p. 808.

Empyema.—In the event of empyema developing, it is best in the first instance to persist with paracentesis at intervals as indicated by the physical signs and the temperature. Empyema is never a surgical emergency requiring immediate radical treatment. In infants under one year, conservative treatment by aspiration is likely to yield much better results than the more drastic procedures. In older children, however, when aspiration of the pus proves ineffective, the condition should be dealt with surgically. It is important to pay attention to the general health of small infants with empyema. Many of them develop severe anæmia and, as iron preparations administered by mouth in the presence of such an infection are seldom effective, blood transfusion may be required.

Pulmonary Fibrosis and Bronchiectasis.—Most frequently

this is the sequel to a pneumonia which has failed to resolve or of pulmonary collapse. Much can be done for such patients but improvement is slow, and in well-marked examples of the disease it must be recognized that cure in the sense of the lung returning to normal is impossible.

General hygienic measures are important, and abundant fresh air and a country life are of advantage, especially prolonged residence in a dry climate. The greatest care should be taken to prevent respiratory infections. Foci of sepsis in the sinuses or the tonsils should be dealt with. The antra are particularly liable to be affected and special attention should be paid to the examination of this part of the respiratory tract.

Two valuable methods of treatment are postural drainage and deep-breathing exercises. Every morning on rising, the patient should be placed over the side of a bed or a chair with the head hanging down and be made to cough up as much sputum as possible. If much is obtained, this procedure should be carried out twice or even three times daily. It is important that the bronchi should be emptied as thoroughly as possible. Following this, the patient should be instructed to breathe slowly and as deeply as he is able for a period of five minutes. If it can be arranged, it is best to have an adult do this exercise with the child. With patience even very young children can be taught these exercises satisfactorily.

Creosote, given by the mouth, inhalation of this or iodoform and eucalyptus from a mask and autogenous vaccines have been advocated, but their benefit is doubtful.

In certain cases in which less drastic measures have failed to bring about amelioration, resort should be had to surgery. Recent advances in the technique of thoracic surgery have made it possible to remove a part or the whole of a lung with good prospect of success. The extent of the disease must first be clearly defined by means of X-ray examination following lipiodol injection to outline the bronchial tree. After a period of medical treatment, and when the general condition of the patient warrants it, the affected lung or part of lung is removed. The operation still carries considerable risk in small children and the cases should be carefully chosen. Phrenic avulsion in certain cases in which lobectomy is impracticable may be considered. Artificial pneumothorax has been advocated, but in many instances, owing to pleural adhesions or because of the firm fibrotic nature of the lesion, it is not attended by any great degree of success.

Atelectasis

Failure of the lung to expand (atelectasis) is seen in very young children. Inhalations of oxygen with 10 per cent. carbon dioxide by means of a nasal catheter or a small tent are of great value. Quietness, rest and, if necessary, stimulants such as brandy or lobelin, in doses of $\frac{1}{6}$ gr., are indicated. In many instances the atelectatic lung becomes infected and as far as treatment is concerned the lesion becomes virtually broncho-pneumonia.

Thymic Enlargement

The subject of thymic enlargement and status thymico-lymphaticus is a most debatable one. Stridor, syncope and dyspnœa, cyanotic attacks or fits may be manifestations of the condition, and direct evidence of thymic enlargement may be obtained by the detection of dullness at the upper end of the sternum or by X-ray examination. If the existence of an enlarged thymus is established it is advisable to submit the patient to treatment by means of X-ray or radium in the hands of experts.

DISEASES OF THE NERVOUS SYSTEM

Convulsions

A convulsion is probably the commonest medical emergency in childhood. In the first instance efforts should be directed towards controlling the attack. There is general agreement that the hot bath or mustard bath (temperature 105° F.) is worth while if only to keep the mother or nursemaid occupied. If an anæsthetic such as chloroform or ether is readily available, its administration is the surest way of controlling the spasm. Chloral hydrate is satisfactory although it takes some time to produce its effect. If the child can swallow, a dose of 3 to 5 gr. to a child of one to two years should suffice ; subsequently smaller doses may be repeated four-hourly. If he cannot swallow, double the above dose may be given by the rectum. Some prefer to combine this with bromide, but there would not appear to be any particular advantage in doing so. If the fit has continued for some time and there is fear of a condition such as status epilepticus, morphine ($\frac{1}{24}$ gr. for a child of two years) given by hypodermic injection, or paraldehyde in doses of 1 drachm of paraldehyde in olive oil per stone of body-weight by the rectum is effective. It is frequently wise to perform a lumbar puncture and, if there are signs of meningitis, it is essential for diagnosis and subsequent treatment, although its value in controlling the convulsions may not always be apparent.

It is important to remember that having controlled the convulsions in the first instance it will be necessary to guard against their recurrence during the next few days. For this chloral hydrate is the most useful drug as it is rapidly eliminated and non-cumulative in its action. The dose and frequency should gradually be diminished during the succeeding three or four days.

To treat any case of convulsions intelligently one must ascertain the cause. The idea that sources of peripheral irritation such as teething, worms, constipation (or diarrhœa), adherent foreskin, enlarged tonsils and so forth are commonly the cause of fits is untenable. Such a suggestion may be comforting both to the physician and the parent in so far that one need never be at a loss to discover some source of peripheral irritation, but actual proof of their association as cause and effect is lacking. Actually convulsions in children may be classified under three main headings, those due to hypocalcæmia, those due to intracranial injury or disease and a group of unknown ætiology (idiopathic convulsions). Of these the convulsions due to hypocalcæmia are undoubtedly the most common. Other clinical signs of hypocalcæmia, such as tetany, may or may not be present, but not infrequently the only manifestation will be the convulsion. This is the case in many instances where the convulsion ushers in an acute infection and more likely is this to be so in the late winter and spring months when the incidence of tetany is at its maximum. Hypocalcæmic fits are readily controlled by chloral hydrate. For a child of one year an initial dose of 2 gr. should be given, followed by 1 gr. every two hours until he is thoroughly under the influence of the drug. Five cubic centimetres of calcium gluconate (sandoz) given intravenously or intramuscularly, by raising the blood calcium rapidly, will accomplish the same object; thereafter by the administration of a suitable vitamin D preparation, such as cod-liver oil, adexolin or ostelin, the retention of calcium can be restored to normal and maintained at this level. The sedative or the calcium gluconate should be continued for three days, by which time retention of calcium will be adequate. The antirachitic treatment must be continued for several months to prevent relapse. The blood calcium can also be quickly restored to normal and so prevent the possible recurrence of the fits by the administration of an acid-producing salt such as calcium chloride or ammonium chloride. These salts may be given to infants in doses of 15 to 30 gr. four-hourly, and by producing a compensated acidosis cause an increased amount of calcium to remain in solution in the blood stream. Here, too, acid treatment is only required for three to four days, but the antirachitic therapy which should be given along with it must be continued, as previously mentioned.

The group of convulsions frequently referred to as idiopathic, occurring later than the age of the cerebral birth trauma and earlier than that of frank tetany—*i.e.*, from second to fourth month—are also mainly hypocalcæmic in origin and may be treated successfully with chloral hydrate and vitamin D, as described above. One would emphasize the importance of diminishing the dose of chloral slowly once the condition has been brought under control.

Convulsions in the newborn, whether the result of cerebral birth trauma or not, should be treated with chloral hydrate four-hourly in doses sufficient to control them. A bulging anterior fontanelle points to the necessity of relieving the intracranial pressure by lumbar or ventricular puncture, procedures which may have to be repeated.

Convulsions which have been recurring over a period of weeks or months, such as those seen in mentally defective children and potential epileptics, are best treated with some sedative which can be continued over a long period. For this luminal or prominal will be found suitable. A child of two or three years can safely be given ½ gr. of luminal twice daily or twice this amount of prominal.

Finally, in all cases attention must be paid to the presence of other disease. Constipation should be treated, for while it may not be an ætiological factor, it tends to aggravate the condition.

Breath-holding attacks should never be treated lightly as seizures of this nature may end in true convulsions associated with loss of consciousness. The condition is said most commonly to be seen in spoilt only children ; this may be so, but it does not minimize the seriousness of the attack. With firm treatment, avoidance of " scenes " and the judicious use of a sedative, such as luminal, a satisfactory outcome can be expected.

Mental Deficiency

In the treatment of mental deficiency a proper understanding of the ætiology is important. Approximately half the cases may be included under the heading simple amentia, one-quarter are Mongolian imbeciles, and of the remainder such conditions as cretinism, amaurotic family idiocy, birth trauma, meningitis, encephalitis, etc., are responsible for the defect. The treatment of all save the cretins can only be palliative. As a general rule it is not advisable bluntly to tell the mother that her child is mentally defective. The phrase should be avoided in discussing the problem with her. It must be explained that the child is backward and will be difficult to bring up, but that the progress depends to a great extent on her efforts to educate him. With patience and unflagging care on the part of the mother many of the less afflicted children may be taught to feed and clothe themselves, to be cleanly in their habits and probably to perform simple household duties. As the child grows older it may be possible to send him to a special school where association with other children helps to stimulate his mental faculties. He should not be sent to school with normal children, for he is apt to be bullied and his sense of inferiority is increased. The child must be guarded from injury, convulsions may be controlled by sedatives, and where home conditions do not permit of proper care institutional treatment is advisable. In certain cases of cerebral diplegia, orthopædic measures which succeed in enabling the child to walk may lead to improvement in the mental condition.

Cretinism is the only form of mental deficiency where treatment holds out the hope of definite cure. The cretin does not as a rule show definite signs of the defect till he is about six months old, but the earlier treatment is commenced the greater the prospect of complete cure.

Thyroid extract (B.P.) should be given in small doses at first, commencing with $\frac{1}{4}$ gr. twice a day; the quantity should be increased fairly rapidly till the maximum therapeutic effect is obtained. It may be necessary to give a child of a year old as much as 5 gr. in the day. Signs of overdosage are nervousness, irritability, increased pulse rate and occasionally diarrhœa. The treatment should be continued throughout life and from time to time the dose increased and the effect noted. Improvement on the augmented dose suggests that it should be continued. Cretinism and Mongolian idiocy must be clearly differentiated. Thyroid has been recommended for the latter, but in our experience it is valueless.

Enuresis

Before commencing the treatment of this troublesome complaint it is essential that the presence of organic disease be excluded. The urine should be carefully examined for albumen, pus and sugar. Renal dwarfs, for example, often come under observation because of nocturnal incontinence, and if there is any dwarfing or sign suggestive of impaired renal function, the blood urea should be estimated. True enuresis is essentially a functional disease.

Many forms of treatment have been recommended, and it may be said at once that no one method is likely to succeed in more than a small percentage of cases. The principle of obtaining "dry nights" over a prolonged period of time by the simple expedient of getting the patient up to pass urine as frequently as is necessary is often effective. The child should be made to empty his bladder just before going to bed, an hour or two later and once between then and waking in the morning. After a month or two of "dry nights," the wakening in the early hours of the morning should be omitted. Relapses may occur and accidents will happen from time to time which may lead to abandonment of the treatment, but the parents should be encouraged to persevere, as their wholehearted co-operation is an important part of the treatment. Apart from the inconvenience entailed, which is not often an objection, the greatest drawback is the sleep lost by the child. Attempts should be made to restore his confidence by encouragement. Too often his anxiety not to wet the bed is his undoing. A calendar may be kept and a red star put on for each dry night. The habit should not be dwelt on too much, except to give encouragement, and the parents should never discuss his shortcoming in the presence of the patient nor show undue concern. An atmosphere of optimism is best. Scolding or punishment is to be deprecated. Such children are often unduly sensitive and punishment may be a prominent factor in keeping up the condition.

Whatever other treatment is adopted it is important that no fluid nor food should be given within two hours of bedtime. The general health must be seen to. Enlarged tonsils and adenoids may require removal. Rest must be adequate and, if possible, a rest in the middle of the day obtained. All undue fatigue and emotional disturbance are best avoided. The bedclothes should not be too heavy, and it may be of value to provide some device, such as a towel tied around the waist with the knot in the back, to prevent the child from lying on his back. Drug therapy is not of much value. Small doses of thyroid extract have been used by some. Others claim success with eserine. Belladonna, however, has the widest reputation, and its use with other methods can be recommended. Commencing with 5 to 10 minims of the tincture thrice daily, the dose should be increased until moderate dilatation of the pupils and dryness of the mouth indicate that the child is fully under the influence of the drug.

In intractable cases, and in mentally deficient children in whom it is impossible to obtain co-operation, the use of sphagnum moss is of value in making the nursing and care of these children less arduous. It can be placed under the child and between the thighs against the genitals at night. The urine is absorbed by the moss and the sheets are kept dry. The urinous odour which is so objectionable is also to a great extent dispelled.

Cyclical Vomiting

The ætiology of this condition is somewhat obscure and its diagnosis often open to criticism. There are varying shades of opinion as to what constitutes the clinical picture. Infection, often trivial, and emotional upset are regarded as the two most common predisposing causes. The outstanding clinical feature is the occurrence of more or less periodic attacks of intractable vomiting during which there is a marked ketosis and in most instances an acidosis. The age incidence is roughly from the second to the seventh year. The subjects of the disorder are often highly strung children. There may be a history of infantile eczema, and later asthmatic attacks or migraine are not uncommon.

The attack begins fairly abruptly after a few hours of lassitude. Dark rings appear under the eyes and vomiting sets in, even water being returned. The administration of water or saline with glucose and alkali are indicated. This can be accomplished readily by giving glucose in water or saline flavoured with orange or lemon juice by mouth. Big drinks are likely to be returned, and only sips from a spoon at frequent intervals should be given. It may be necessary to detail some person to be constantly in attendance for this purpose. Although much of the fluid may appear to be vomited, if the method is persisted with, a considerable amount will remain in the stomach and eventually be absorbed. The water and salt combat the dehydration and the glucose aids in the complete combustion of fat, thus controlling the production of ketone bodies. The best alkali to give is sodium bicarbonate. It should be dissolved in water and given separately in sips at the rate of 15 to 30 gr. four-hourly. It aids in the excretion of ketone bodies, provides alkali and acts as a stimulant to the secretion of gastric juices.

In all but the most severe cases administration of fluid by mouth will suffice. But when the vomiting is intractable and the dehydration and ketosis persist, 10 per cent. glucose in saline given by rectum is of the greatest benefit. The bowel should first be washed out and then 2 to 4 oz. of the glucose and saline solution run in four-hourly. If the patient is markedly dehydrated and presents alarming signs of acidosis such as air-hunger and a low CO_2-combining power, it is advisable to give the 10 per cent. glucose in saline intravenously. Care should be taken regarding amounts and rate of flow. It is probably unwise to exceed 30 c.c. per kg. of body-weight. If given by gravity, the funnel holding the fluid should not be more than 12 in. above the level of the vein ; if given by syringe, twenty to thirty minutes should be taken to give 200 to 300 c.c.

During the period of active vomiting all food save glucose should be withheld. Four to six hours after the vomiting has ceased diluted milk or weak sweetened tea or oat-flour porridge may be given. Recovery as a rule is rapid and the diet can be quickly increased.

Between attacks, a high carbohydrate intake is recommended, and the amount of fat in the diet should be reduced. Rich foods such as pastry and suet puddings should be avoided. All fruit and vegetables, because of their alkaline ash, are permitted. Sugar, as cane-sugar, barley-sugar or "boiled sweets," can be allowed. It is well to point out to the mother that chocolate and toffee contain a good deal of fat. Glucose or glucose D, a tablespoonful after each meal, has been recommended. It is doubtful if it is wise to use it thus as a medicine. The children often object to it and it is a constant reminder of their affliction. Cream, cod-liver oil tonics and fried foods are often given in large quantities to such children in an attempt to fatten them. This is a mistake. Such substances are better avoided. Butter should be allowed in reasonable quantities and milk in the usual quantities.

In addition to this dietary régime, a small ½ teaspoonful of baking-soda (sodium bicarbonate) in water each morning before breakfast should be given as a stimulant to the digestive juices.

PINK DISEASE (*Erythrœdema Polyneuritis*)

As the ætiology of pink disease is unknown the treatment is necessarily symptomatic. The first essential is to guard the child as far as possible from intercurrent infection. He should, whenever possible, live in good surroundings in the country. Institutional treatment is definitely contraindicated. Relief from many of the distressing symptoms of the disease can to some extent be obtained by careful nursing. Thus the intensely irritating sudaminous rash may be alleviated or prevented by ensuring that no flannel or woollen garments are placed next to the skin. The skin should be most carefully dried and powdered after bathing, and in some cases a soothing lotion such as

℞	Calamin.	ʒii
	Zinc. Oxid.	ʒii
	Phenol.	gr. x
	Glycer.	ʒii
	Liq. Calc. Hydrox. . . . . ad	℥iv

is useful in relieving irritation. The arms may have to be splinted to prevent scratching. When there is great irritation of the hands and feet, relief may sometimes be obtained by allowing the child from time to time to hold them in cold water. When photophobia is a prominent symptom it may be necessary to nurse the child in a darkened room or to provide an eye-shade. For sleeplessness sedatives are necessary, such as sodium bromide or chloral hydrate. The diet should be light and nourishing, and as anorexia is so commonly present the child must be coaxed to take his food and in some cases it may be necessary to feed by gavage. The child should be kept in bed at first, but as improvement takes place he may be taken out-of-doors in a perambulator. On the supposition that the disease is due to vitamin deficiency it may be advisable to give cod-liver oil or one of its derivatives, also orange juice and marmite or bemax. Though there is no proof that these accessary foods have any direct effect on the course of the disease, they may be of help in improving the general condition of the child. The parents should be warned that the disease usually runs a course of three to six months and that during this time incessant care and vigilance will have to be exercised. Complications such as otitis media, pyuria, respiratory and intestinal infections must be watched for and treated as they arise.

G. B. FLEMING.
S. G. GRAHAM.

INDUSTRIAL DISEASES

Introduction

" When a Handicrafts-man is taken ill, he must be cur'd by Vomiting, or Purging, or Searing, or Incision ; for if a Physician tells him of a long Diet, and Bolstering up his Head, and the like, he presently replies, That he has not leisure to lie by it, and that it will be of no use to him to lead an idle crazy Life, and neglect his Business. Upon this he takes leave of the Physician, and returns to his usual way of living."—Plato, quoted by Ramazzini (1705).

THE difficulties that beset the physician of Plato's Republic in the treatment of the diseases of tradesmen have persisted through the ages. Industrial disease is usually well established before advice is sought, and often, as in silicosis, progressive in nature ; the patient's financial resources are small and his family anxieties correspondingly great, while he is faced with eventual return to work that has been responsible for, or has contributed to, his illness. All these factors operate against the prospect of cure : as Ramazzini himself wrote of the diseases of potters :—

" . . . 'tis a hard matter to light upon such Remedies as will restore them to perfect Health. : For they seldom have recourse to the Physicians, till the use of their Limbs is taken from 'em, and their *Viscera* grown hard ; besides, they are commonly pinch'd with another Evil, viz., Extream Poverty."

In relation to industrial disease, prevention and treatment must essentially go hand in hand and it may be helpful to summarize the broad aims of prevention in this field.

1. The provision of properly adapted buildings, with facilities for keeping the workshops clean, and for effective ventilation.
2. Apparatus designed for its special purpose.

3. Appliances for the arrest of dust and gases at their place of origin and for their adequate removal and disposal.
4. So far as possible, avoidance of direct contact with poisonous materials: utmost possible reduction in hours of labour in dangerous employments.
5. Displacement of particularly dangerous methods and materials and the substitution of less dangerous materials.
6. Instruction of new workmen in the risks inherent in their work.
7. Constant supervision of all dangerous employments by expert and responsible persons.
8. Employment of appropriate means for personal protection—suitable work clothes, caps, goggles, etc.
9. Practice of personal cleanliness by workers concerned, and their utilization of facilities provided.
10. Immediate report of symptoms of illness and early attention to all wounds, however slight.
11. Employment of healthy working personnel, periodic medical examinations where necessary, and alternation of employment.

Some of these postulates, like measures for dust control, are essentially mechanical; some involve substitution of toxic agents by others less harmful, as in the classical replacement of yellow phosphorus in the manufacture of matches; while others involve close and continuing medical supervision in such matters as selection of personnel for particular work, alternation of employment, and painstaking search for the beginnings of disease. A great deal has been accomplished in Britain since the beginning of the present century towards the improvement of working conditions, mainly through the efforts of the Home Office, and the Factories Act (1937) should make possible yet further advances, notably perhaps by making more effective the medical supervision of young persons entering industry.

But, while industrial disease may conform to the clinical picture of a classical trade intoxication, certain classes of workmen suffer rather from an excessive incidence of incapacitating sickness of a type not peculiar to a specific occupation. The excess sickness falls chiefly into certain groups (injuries, rheumatic conditions, gastritis and dermatitis, for instance, in the case of coal-miners) and its association with employment, though real enough, is not always appreciated. Even unemployment, with its curious sequence of psychological changes, clearly influences health; while re-employment has problems of its own, such as increased liability to injury to the back and sepsis of the hands during the period of hardening.

Many factors quite outside the scope of factory control may influence the susceptibility of workers to industrial disease, and there is need for increasingly close co-operation between general practitioners and their professional colleagues charged with the more technical supervision of health conditions inside the factory. In this connection it is worthy of note that increasing numbers of industrial concerns are setting up within their factories efficient health organizations under the charge of a medical officer who is anxious to co-operate with outside practitioners in safeguarding the health of workers.

Another way in which the practitioner can further the prevention of industrial disease is by immediate compliance with his statutory duty to notify to the Chief Inspector of Factories, Home Office, London, all patients whom he believes to be suffering from the prescribed diseases (anthrax, toxic jaundice, compressed air sickness, epitheliomatous and chrome ulceration ; and poisoning by lead, arsenic, phosphorus, mercury, carbon bisulphide, aniline and benzol) contracted in the course of employment.

Apart altogether from exposure to toxic substances some occupations demand from the operatives unusually severe physiological response. Some, like iron moulding and certain kinds of labouring, must always call for heavy muscular effort, while it has been found necessary to control by law the weights that may be lifted by women and children.

EFFECTS OF HIGH TEMPERATURES

Other kinds of work expose operatives to the effects of high temperatures. Over a hundred years ago Thackrah recommended "for such as work at high temperatures" (1) diminution of muscular labour performed in hot rooms ; (2) the drinking of lemonade, or other diluent during the time of labour, rather than the noxious compound called ale ; (3) the use of stimulants with the food after labour ; (4) the reduction of the period of labour.

Heat disease may be classified into three clinical types : (1) Heat cramps ; (2) heat exhaustion ; and (3) heat retention.

Heat Cramps.—For the prevention of heat cramps saline waters (0·10 to 0·20 per cent.) chilled to a temperature of 45° to 50° F. should be made available to the workers : 5 gm. of salt added to a gallon of water is adequate to prevent heat cramps and is not unpleasant to drink. In the treatment of severe heat cramp intravenous injection of saline solution is invaluable.

Heat Exhaustion.—For prevention of heat exhaustion "jelly drops" containing approximately equal parts of glucose and granulated sugar are commonly used in America, while in this country many workers carry to work sweetened lemonade, which is useful both for maintaining blood-sugar level and for preventing acidosis. In the treatment of heat exhaustion the administration of glucose should be combined with sodium bicarbonate.

Heat Retention.—For the treatment of heat retention the essentials are (1) immediate reduction of the fever; (2) rest in the recumbent posture and (3) administration of fluids. The patient should be removed to cool surroundings, his head elevated, cool water sprayed over the body with, if possible, fans placed to evaporate the water, and cutaneous circulation maintained by gentle friction. Fluids should be given in abundance, orally, intravenously or subcutaneously. Artificial respiration may be necessary where there is respiratory failure. Adrenalin may be required to counter cardiac insufficiency, though it should be used only if strictly necessary because of its tendency to produce petechial hæmorrhage in these cases. Rest in bed should be prolonged, and the patient's subsequent work carefully supervised: convalescence is often slow.

I am indebted to Dr Bridge, H.M. Senior Medical Inspector of Factories, for the following note on a drink found useful in this country during hot weather by workers exposed to high temperatures:—

Sodium chloride	6 oz.
Potassium chloride . . .	4 oz.
Water	1¾ pints.

Seventeen fluid ounces of this concentrated solution to be added to 3 gals. of water for drinking: a flavouring agent may be added if required.

The drink can be made more palatable by modification as under:—

Table salt	1 lb.
Potassium chloride . .	10½ oz.
Citric acid	5½ oz.
Saccharin	3 gm.
Oil of lemon	22 c.c.
"Lemon squash" colouring .	A small quantity.
Water . . . . . to	3 litres.

Add 1 part of this concentrated solution to 30 parts of water.

WORK IN COMPRESSED AIR

Another type of strain on physiological adaptation is that involved by work in compressed air. Among the precautions taken to prevent compressed air illness are (1) medical supervision by physicians with experience of work entailing the use of compressed air; (2) preliminary medical examination of personnel; (3) limitation of hours of work in compressed air; (4) slow decompression, with rigid adherence to a prescribed technique; and (5) provision of a hospital lock for dealing with cases of caisson sickness. In selecting workmen the essentials are normal lungs, normal kidneys and a good heart; blood pressure should not be above normal. According to Singstad many American States have codes of regulations which require supervision by a qualified physician experienced in work with compressed air to secure (*a*) examination of each new worker; (*b*) test of each new man under actual working conditions; (*c*) re-examination of any worker absent from work for ten days or more; (*d*) periodic re-examination of all workers; (*e*) prohibition of employment of alcoholics; (*f*) complete record of all examinations and illnesses; (*g*) a medical lock 5 to 6 ft. in diameter, with a physician in constant attendance when pressures exceed 17 lbs. per sq. in. Adequate dressing-room facilities should be provided and hot coffee should be served to workers on their return from the air chamber.

In Britain the Committee on Regulations for Work carried out in Compressed Air recommended in 1936 that after 25 to 40 lbs. pressure men should be kept for forty minutes after decompression before leaving the works, and that with 40 to 50 lbs. pressure they should be kept for one hour.

Recompression and slow decompression is the recognized treatment of compressed air illness. It should be used as soon as possible after the onset of the illness. Some authorities advocate a return to maximum pressure, some to one-half the maximum absolute pressure, and others to two-thirds the maximum gauge pressure at which the patient worked. Shaw recommends first recompression to a pressure of 30 lbs. for two or three hours, then reduction of the air pressure to 20 lbs. for one and a half hours, during which time pure oxygen is breathed instead of air.

WORK WITH PNEUMATIC DRILLS

Though there is no effective method of preventing the functional nervous disturbance so frequently associated with the use of pneumatic drills, recent work suggests that something can be done for another trying disability of these workers—that associated with changes in the bones and joints and a pronounced vaso-constrictive effect leading to attacks of blanching and numbness in the fingers, with loss of power. Attempts have been made to prevent this condition by wearing protective resilient pads, though with indifferent success; but recently M'Laren[1] has described (with technical instructions for carrying out the treatment) a method of treating the spasmodic vaso-constriction by histamine ionization to the affected hands.

MINERS' NYSTAGMUS

Though there has been in the past a good deal of difference of opinion about the relative importance of faulty illumination and psychological disturbance in the production of miners' nystagmus, there is now fairly general agreement with the observations on prevention and treatment in the Reports of the Miners' Nystagmus Committee of the Medical Research Council published in 1922 and 1932. The Reports insist on the importance of adequate treatment.

> "Although it is of fundamental importance that every effort should be made to improve the lighting of mines . . . yet it is also of the utmost importance that the psychological aspects, not only of this disability but of similar conditions in other occupations, should be fully recognized.
>
> "*The Committee are strongly of opinion that the practical treatment of the disease from an administrative point of view should consist in the elimination of a hopeless dependence on compensation by the provision of opportunities for work of some kind, the end in view being complete restoration to full work underground, under conditions of proper illumination, even if this has to be preceded by a period of work in daylight.*"

More recently a Departmental Committee has reported along similar lines. It recommends that to improve lighting in mines the electric cap lamp should be given wider use; cases of nystagmus should not be certified unless oscillations have been present for a definite period, and Medical Boards should be set up in the coal districts to advise on all phases of the subject. As work plays a very important part in recovery and in preventing psycho-neurosis, each sufferer must be given a job and employers should co-operate in finding such work.

In their evidence to this Committee the British Medical

[1] M'Laren, J. W., *Lancet* (1937), **2**, 1296.

Association classified wholly incapacitated cases into (*a*) those likely eventually to resume their previous work (generally they should not be idle more than six months), and (*b*) those unsuited for the industry, though many are fit for training in vocational centres, especially if they have developed nystagmus within five years after becoming miners.

> "In the early stages change of work to other parts of the pit will often put off a threatened attack. If the symptoms continue the man should be put to work on the surface. Rest from underground work and surface employment are the only specifics for nystagmus, and medical treatment except that directed to the general health of the patient is of little avail."

Various alcohols and sedatives have been given with transient success, and recently the use of calcium salts has been advocated. Any refractive error should be corrected.

POISONING BY METALS

Lead.—The number of reported cases of lead poisoning has fallen enormously during the present century. Numerous preventive measures have contributed to this reduction. Innocuous materials have been substituted for those containing lead (as in paints and low solubility glazes). Steps have been taken for the control of lead-laden dust, the precise measures varying with the individual requirements of the industries concerned. The employment of women and young persons in certain processes involving the use of lead has been prohibited, and general hygienic measures have been introduced to minimize the risk of poisoning—prohibition of taking meals in workrooms for instance, and the introduction of adequate washing and dining facilities, together with strict insistence on the importance of personal hygiene.

Periodic medical examination by the Examining Surgeon (or other medical man appointed by the Chief Inspector of Factories) is required at intervals ranging from weekly (in the manufacture of compounds of lead) to quarterly (as in vitreous enamelling), the frequency varying with the risk involved. In carrying out these periodic medical examinations special attention should be given to a survey of the general health and to a search for early evidence of extensor paralysis. Lane has demonstrated the value of systematic blood examinations in the control of lead poisoning in industry; he believes that in general an increase in the degree of punctation of the red blood cells among workers exposed to lead indicates an increased risk.

Of recent years a number of cases of lead poisoning have resulted from the inhalation of lead vapour in the course of ship-breaking by the use of oxyacetylene. In this occupation preventive measures are difficult to apply and the clinical picture is more acute than that usually experienced in other forms of industrial lead poisoning. Periodic clinical examination has proved to be of little value in anticipating collapse in these cases, but it has been demonstrated that systematic examination of blood films in conjunction with clinical examination can be of real assistance. The ratio of large to small lymphoid cells has been found here to be a better guide to preventive action than the height of the punctate count ; very soon after starting this work there is an increase in the proportion of large lymphoid cells, the ratio of large to small commonly reaching 3 or 4 to 1 after two or three weeks, and a fall below 1·5 to 1 is to be regarded as a danger signal calling for a reduction in exposure to lead. A high degree of punctation may be found in these cases following a transfer to a minor risk, while punctate basophilia may be minimal in the presence of severe toxic symptoms.

It has long been the custom to encourage workers in lead industries to take drinks believed to be of service in the prevention of lead poisoning. Sulphuric acid orangeade is regarded as one of the best :—

Dilute sulphuric acid . .	12 parts.
Concentrated infusion of orange .	12 parts.
Syrup of orange . . .	40 parts.
Water	16 parts.

One part to be added to 32 parts of water. Daily dose, 3 oz.

The treatment of lead poisoning falls into two stages, first immobilization of the circulating lead, and later its elimination. It is believed that there is a close relationship between calcium metabolism and the behaviour of lead in the body. Lead can be immobilized in the bones by the administration of calcium given in large doses, either as lactate by the mouth (gr. xxx, t.i.d.) or as gluconate (10 c.c. daily of a 10 per cent. solution intramuscularly), supplemented by a diet rich in calcium (milk) ; and this immobilization relieves acute symptoms dramatically.

Deleading of the patient should be undertaken only after the acute symptoms have subsided and under the most careful clinical observation, with repeated blood examinations. To promote excretion of lead a low calcium diet (reduced intake of milk, cheese, egg yolk and green vegetables) is combined with the administration of dilute acid or ammonium chloride (gr. xx, t.i.d.). The effect of these can often be enhanced by the administration of parathormone (50 units daily), but it must be used with care, as acute lead poisoning has been produced by undue haste in deleading.

Sodium bicarbonate and potassium iodide have been used to mobilize stored lead, but both are liable to provoke symptoms of lead intoxication, particularly sodium bicarbonate.

Symptoms may call for palliative treatment, colic for an enema, hot application to the abdomen or even morphine. Goadby recommended for colic the administration of sodium nitrite (gr. i) or liquor trinitrini (♏ii) as in addition to the spasm of the intestine there is considerable vaso-constriction of all the vessels in the mesenteric area. Magnesium sulphate is useful in the treatment of constipation in these cases.

Splinting, massage and electricity, notably galvanism, have been found to be serviceable in the treatment of lead paralysis.

For the treatment of anæmia see p. 471.

Mercury.—Mercury poisoning has long had a direct interest for the medical profession. As long ago as 1705 Ramazzini wrote :—

> " Now a-Days, those who rub the Mercurial Ointments on Pocky Persons, are the meaner sort of Surgeons who undertake that Office to make a Penny by it ; for the better sort of Surgeons decline such a sordid Piece of Service, which is likewise accompany'd with Danger."

By that time even the meaner sort of surgeons had learned to let their patients do their own rubbing :—

> " But if such Surgeons have contracted any Harm by the Inunction, such as the Shaking of the Hands, a Giddyness in the Head, and Gripings of the Guts ; in this Case, as I said before, the Decoction of *Guaiacum* is the Remedy."

The preventive measures applicable to mercurialism in Ramazzini's time included the consumption of fat broth and generous wine : by the time of Thackrah (1833) they were more prosaic—personal cleanliness, change of dress and attention to ventilation, measures which are still commonly used.

It is important to secure limitation of the area of mercury exposed to the air and as low a temperature in the workroom as possible, since volatilization increases rapidly with temperature. Floors and work benches should be smooth and impervious and should drain to a collecting trough. All vessels containing mercury should be kept covered.

Frequent attention to the teeth is desirable: they should be examined regularly and necessary dental treatment undertaken. Regular brushing is important, and the use of a mouth wash, *e.g.*, hydrogen peroxide, or that recommended by Legge:—

Alum. . . . . . . gr. v
Pot. Chloras. . . . . . gr. v
Glycer. . . . . . . ʒss
Aq. . . . . . . to ℥i

For the prevention of ulcers from exposure to fulminate of mercury the use of a 10 per cent. solution of sodium hyposulphite has been recommended as a local application.

In the selection of workers there should be excluded those suffering from tuberculosis and nephritis, and those of inferior physique, as well as women and young persons.

The actual treatment of mercurial poisoning consists largely in removing the patient from exposure to mercury and in attention to his general health. Many medicines have been tried. Thackrah reported a hundred years ago that he found opium the most efficient remedy for the salivation from which most patients suffer; for the tremors he recommended rest, fresh air and aperients, treatment not yet improved upon. Potassium iodide has been used and baths designed to promote elimination of the mercury, but they are of little use.

In the treatment of conjunctivitis caused by fulminate of mercury Legge recommends the use of a 2 per cent. solution of sodium hyposulphite as an eyewash.

Arsenic.—Cases of poisoning by arsenical salts are nowadays rarely seen in industry. The general preventive measures that have been found most useful are substantially the same as those for the prevention of lead poisoning. The treatment of chronic arsenical poisoning consists in removal from exposure and improvement of the general health. There is no specific medicinal therapy.

The prevention of poisoning by arseniuretted hydrogen implies a knowledge of the extent of arsenical contamination of materials used in industry and recognition of the danger of this poisoning. Operations liable to produce arseniuretted hydrogen should be carried out only in closed apparatus or under good artificial exhaust ventilation. Strips of mercury bromide paper, which show by a yellow colour small traces of arseniuretted hydrogen, should be hung in the workrooms. In the face of a known risk of poisoning by arseniuretted hydrogen, it is a good plan to secure regular daily examination of the urine for the presence of blood.

In the treatment of acute poisoning by arseniuretted hydrogen the first essential is the administration of oxygen. Blood transfusion may be necessary. Convalescence is always slow and calls for prolonged care of the general health.

POISONOUS GASES

Henderson and Haggard illustrate the general type of precaution needed to prevent atmospheric contamination by noxious fumes and gases from industrial processes by reference to the rules applicable to an ammonia refrigerating plant.

1. The refrigerating equipment including valves and piping should be inspected at frequent and regular intervals, and suitable repairs made immediately when needed.
2. Every employee should be instructed regarding the dangers from ammonia and trained to avoid them.
3. No one should be allowed to sleep in rooms adjoining a refrigerating plant.
4. The rooms in which machinery is installed should have doors opening directly to the outside air. The position of these rooms should be such that escaping fumes cannot invade other parts of the factory or cut off the escape of persons in them. Regulations should be strictly enforced requiring that exits shall never be obstructed by temporary scaffolding or other impediments to escape.
5. Gas masks with canisters affording protection against ammonia should be provided. They should be stored in some locality readily accessible to, but outside the rooms in which there is a possibility of the escape of ammonia.
6. Every workman engaged in repair work on refrigerating apparatus should be required to carry a gas mask strapped to his body or hung round his neck in anticipation of the possible escape of ammonia.
7. A valve arranged to shut off the ammonia at the storage cylinders should be placed where it can be manipulated from the outside of the building.

Noxious gases encountered in industry may be classified according to their physiological action :—

(1) Asphyxiants : *e.g.*, carbon monoxide and cyanogen compounds ;

(2) Irritants : *e.g.*, sulphur dioxide, chlorine, sulphuretted hydrogen, nitrous fumes ;

(3) Volatile drugs and drug-like substances: anæsthetics, *e.g.*, tetrachlorethane, benzene, carbon bisulphide, nitrobenzene, carbon tetrachloride, trinitrotoluene.

Carbon Monoxide.—In the treatment of carbon monoxide poisoning the sheet anchor is the inhalation of oxygen containing 7 per cent. of carbon dioxide. The inhalation treatment by O_2 and CO_2 was introduced about 1921: originally the mixture recommended contained only 5 per cent. CO_2, but about 1929 the proportion was raised to 7 per cent. with excellent results.

The mixture of carbon dioxide and oxygen is available in cylinders of the compressed gases. It should be administered with a specially designed inhalator, the apparatus consisting of a cylinder of the mixed gas opening into a reducing valve from which the gas is passed under low pressure through a calibrated needle valve, and then into a collapsible reservoir bag. From this bag the gas is led by rubber tubing to a mask held lightly over the patient's face.

Artificial respiration may be necessary. If so, the oxygen-carbon dioxide mixture should be administered while it is being carried out. The inhalation of oxygen and CO_2 should be continued for at least twenty minutes after spontaneous respiration commences. It is important that the patient be kept warm by the use of blankets and hot-water bottles while inhalation treatment is being carried out.

Blood transfusion has been recommended, but it is useless unless performed within an hour of removal from the gas, which is seldom practicable under industrial conditions. Later the elimination of carbon monoxide renders transfusion unnecessary: the patient is by that time suffering from the late effects of asphyxia, which are not relieved by transfusion. German observers report that profuse bleeding is often of value in these cases.

Drugs are of little value in the treatment of asphyxia, though from time to time various respiratory stimulants have been advocated in this connection: in 1924 the German Imperial Health Office reported favourably on Lobelin Ingelheim as a respiratory stimulant (3 to 10 mg. intramuscularly). For some years the injection of methylene blue had a vogue, but it has now been discredited in the treatment of carbon monoxide poisoning.

Headache is apt to be persistent. It is due to increased intracranial pressure and is best treated by the intravenous administration of hypertonic saline (70 to 100 c.c. of a 15 per cent. solution). Phenacetin, aspirin, etc., should not be given to relieve headache, as severe attacks of heart failure have followed the giving of these in gas poisoning.

It is essential that persons who have been gassed should have prolonged rest. The patient should not be allowed to walk home from work after recovery. After-treatment consists of general measures designed to prevent the development of pneumonia.

Cyanogen Compounds.—Hydrocyanic acid should be used with the utmost precaution. Of recent years it has had an extensive vogue in the disinfestation of ships and premises, and accidents have occurred from failure to adhere to the necessary rigid instructions governing effective clearing of the atmosphere before re-entry.

Treatment of hydrocyanic acid poisoning is along lines similar to those described for carbon monoxide poisoning and consists essentially of artificial respiration and the inhalation of the oxygen-carbon dioxide mixture described above. Lobelin (0·01 gm. intravenously) has been found to be of service, and the consensus of opinion appears to be that methylene blue is of some value in the treatment of poisoning by hydrocyanic acid: the recommended dose is 50 c.c. of a 1 per cent. solution in physiological saline given intravenously.

After-care is the same as for carbon monoxide poisoning.

Nitrous Fumes.—When symptoms of poisoning from nitrous fumes occur while the patient is still at work, the appropriate first aid treatment is to make him lie down, keep him warm and, in the presence of cyanosis, to administer oxygen. Much of the danger of these nitrous gases lies in the fact that there is often a lag of several hours between exposure to them and the appearance of acute symptoms, which often rapidly assume the alarming clinical picture of pulmonary œdema. Medicinal measures contribute little to the relief of this condition, though sometimes it is improved by the intravenous administration of saline solution, combined with venesection where cyanosis is marked. Inhalation of oxygen, preferably through a suitable inhalator, as described above, is often of great value: a comparatively low concentration of oxygen in the inspired air may suffice to relieve the cyanosis. Bleeding, followed by the intravenous injection of glucose, is recommended by Professor Zangger. It is important to secure absolute quiet and rest; otherwise cardiac failure is liable to supervene.

Chlorine.—Chlorine is a typical irritant gas and its inhalation is apt to produce generalized inflammation throughout the respiratory tract. There is a tradition that the inhalation of low concentrations of chlorine are of value in the prevention of diseases of the respiratory tract, and over a hundred years ago Thackrah actually treated the bronchitis of flax-workers by the inhalation of chlorine, placing his patients for this purpose in a room artificially impregnated with the gas.

In first-aid treatment of chlorine poisoning it is important to keep the patient at rest, as exertion causes him to breathe more rapidly and deeply and thus inhale more of the irritant gas. The patient should be wrapped up warmly. Black coffee is a useful stimulant. Administration of oxygen is often soothing to the patient, but the main essential is to combat pulmonary œdema and this can probably best be done by profuse blood letting (up to 1,200 c.c.). Blood transfusions are of little use. The administration of strophanthin is desirable for a few days following exposure to the gas.

There has been considerable controversy as to the desirability of giving morphine for the relief of cough following the inhalation of chlorine; most authorities are agreed that it should not be used. Steam inhalations have been found serviceable in this connection.

Sulphuretted Hydrogen.—In the first-aid treatment of poisoning by this gas it is important to secure immediate removal of soiled clothes.

The treatment of acute poisoning by sulphuretted hydrogen consists in artificial respiration combined, where necessary, with the inhalation of oxygen containing 7 per cent. carbon dioxide. General symptomatic treatment and after-care are as for other poisonous gases.

For the irritation of mucous membranes which the gas is apt to produce when present in comparatively low dilutions, bland symptomatic treatment is all that is necessary. These local irritating effects tend to occur in epidemics which are best cut short by attention to workroom ventilation.

Benzene.—The absorption of even small amounts of benzene causes an increased proportion of the total sulphates of the urine to appear as organic salts. Experience has shown that the periodic determination of the inorganic fraction is a useful general measure in the supervision of the health of workers exposed to benzene. A progressive fall below the normal 80 per cent. points to the need for thorough clinical and hæmatological overhaul of all workers.

The treatment of acute benzene poisoning is similar to that described above for carbon monoxide.

The treatment of chronic benzene poisoning is unsatisfactory. It consists largely in removing the patient from exposure and in measures directed to improvement of the general health, and to safeguarding the patient from intercurrent infection which he is ill-equipped to meet. Repeated blood transfusions are of value ; they, and saline injections, are often necessary to tide the patient over periods of emergency.

Recently, liver therapy and a vitamin-rich diet (especially in vitamin C) has been recommended to combat the severe anæmia ; in this country liver treatment has proved disappointing.

Carbon Tetrachloride.—Carbon tetrachloride is widely used as a non-inflammable solvent for extracting grease (rapid cleaning processes) and as a fire-extinguishing fluid. Immediate mortality due to the acute narcotic effect of the fumes is of comparatively rare occurrence, but many cases have been recorded where death has followed at an interval of three to twelve days after severe exposure.

The treatment of acute poisoning by carbon tetrachloride is as described for carbon monoxide.

The treatment of subacute and chronic cases consists in removal from the causal work, plenty of fresh air and alkalization—with sodium carbonate, calcium carbonate or intravenous calcium gluconate ; calcium therapy may well be combined with the administration of dextrose or glucose drinks. Graham has recently described a case of poisoning by carbon tetrachloride in which acute abdominal symptoms predominated and in which he obtained striking improvement from the intravenous injection of 10 c.c. of a 10 per cent. solution of calcium chloride.

In the majority of cases the symptoms of renal injury overshadow those of damage to the liver. In these cases the early signs and symptoms—nausea, vomiting, jaundiced scleræ and tenderness of the liver region—are followed by the development of symptoms of uræmia, for the treatment of which see p. 862.

Tetrachlorethane.—Poisoning by tetrachlorethane was a major problem during the war (1914-18), and a drastic code of preventive measures was adopted to deal with it. These measures included effective local ventilation by exhaust fans placed at floor level, and also involved fortnightly medical examination of the workers. Willcox recommended in mild cases rest, a light diet rich in carbohydrates, but poor in fat and protein ; in cases with marked jaundice the administration of alkalis (sodium citrate and sodium carbonate, ʒss of each in solution four times a day), with in extreme cases venous, subcutaneous or rectal infusions of normal saline containing ʒii of sodium bicarbonate to the pint. Suppression of urine may call for hot-air baths.

Recently, Desoilles and Mélissinos have recommended injections of liver extract in daily doses corresponding to 60 gm. or more of fresh liver.

Nitro Derivatives of Benzene (Dinitrobenzol, trinitrotoluol, etc.).—The prevention of poisoning by these involves limitation of exposure to the toxic agent, as by mechanical ventilation, protective clothing and alternation of employment.

First-aid treatment consists in rest, removal of working clothes, cleansing of the skin, oxygen inhalation and, if necessary, artificial respiration. Hot black coffee is of value in the treatment of the headache and drowsiness that are common early symptoms.

For mild cases treatment consists in removal from work, correction of constipation (cascara sagrada), and a suitable diet (milk, milk puddings, fruit and vegetables). Patients with jaundice should be confined to bed, and to a rigorous milk diet, cautiously increased as above ; the tendency to acidosis should be counteracted by administration of alkalis (sodium citrate and sodium carbonate, ʒss of each in solution four times a day). Severe cases may require saline injections (rectally and intravenously) : in these cases blood transfusion is valuable.

INDUSTRIAL DUST DISEASES

The prevention of industrial dust diseases lies primarily in measures for efficient dust control. There are several ways in which this can be secured, and the choice of the method to be used must depend on such considerations as the nature of the dust in question, whether the process lends itself to enclosure or to wet working and so on : many industries of high dust exposure have adopted systems of artificial exhaust ventilation, and such systems are in some industries required by law. It occasionally happens that workmen are necessarily exposed to dust in processes that do not lend themselves to any of these measures of control ; then reliance must be placed on the use of respirators. Until recently it has been difficult to secure a respirator for industrial use that was at once efficient and comfortable, but after long tests it is hoped to make one available at an early date.

Since the war an interesting medical step has been taken in Britain towards the prevention of silicosis and asbestosis. In an effort to combat these diseases Medical Boards have been set up at different points in areas where these diseases are particularly prevalent: the headquarters of the Chief Medical Officer of the Board are at 37 Exchange Street, Sheffield. The examinations carried out by these special Boards fall into three groups, (1) Initial, (2) Periodic, and (3) Compensatory. All entrants to the scheduled industries must be examined within one month of commencing work and are prohibited from entering the industry if their physique falls short on the score of abnormality of the nose or throat, existing heart or lung disease or general under-development.

The periodic examinations cover workers employed in the specified industries (refractories, sandstone, pottery, asbestos), and their frequency varies with the risk of the several processes, examinations being carried out annually where the risk is greatest. The Board have power to exclude from the industries workers found to be suffering from tuberculosis, and power to recommend for compensation workers suffering from silicosis or asbestosis. In the case of younger men suffering from simple silicosis there is power to order them to leave the industry with the award of a small amount of compensation designed to tide over any financial loss involved in their change of occupation, the idea being that these men should seek more suitable work while yet their health is reasonably good. Older workmen found to be suffering from silicosis are advised to leave the industry and are offered compensation to enable them to do so.

It is open to any workman in the industries concerned to apply for medical examination by the Board with a view to obtaining compensation for silicosis, and it is open to the dependants of any deceased workman to make a similar claim, but this latter may involve post-mortem examination, and where such claims are contemplated it is advisable to communicate with the Chief Medical Officer of the Board before burial.

Silicosis and asbestosis tend to be progressive diseases, but their downhill course is accentuated by continued exposure to the causal dusts and by superadded infection. It follows that the aim should be to secure the withdrawal of affected workmen from exposure as early in the disease as possible. They should, so far as practicable, be protected from the rigours of strenuous work in unfavourable weather conditions. Many elderly stone-workers have found it serviceable to wear a layer of gamgee tissue on the chest. Otherwise the treatment is entirely symptomatic, though it is an extraordinary feature of silicosis that symptoms are often inconspicuous or absent even in the presence of advanced disease.

In general, exposure to dusts of organic origin produce more subjective disturbance of the type commonly associated with emphysema and bronchial asthma. In these cases symptomatic treatment for the relief of cough and dyspnœa is often necessary (see p. 794).

INDUSTRIAL DERMATITIS

The potential causes of dermatitis encountered in industry are legion. Among the chief are alkalis, oil, friction and heat, chemicals, degreasing agents and sugar, and the workers most affected are engineers, chemical workers, dyers and calico printers, painters and paint manufacturers, metal workers, metal platers and polishers and textile workers. But the number of occupations at risk and the risks involved are so many that only the most careful clinical examination, together with a consideration of individual and occupational history, can serve to decide whether there is an occupational element; and the clinical examination should be supplemented by such investigations as patch tests, wherever these are available.

In the prevention of industrial dermatitis certain general procedures are helpful.

In the examination of new workers it should be borne in mind that some are more susceptible to dermatitis than others and that one attack often predisposes to another. Experience has shown that workers with a good healthy skin, preferably not too dry, are least likely to develop dermatitis.

Systematic and frequent inspection of the hands and arms of workers, if carried out by a responsible person, can be of value in detecting early signs of dermatitis—redness, cracks, blisters, etc. Early treatment should be obtained for any commencing irritation, and if the condition does not immediately respond the causal work should be stopped or changed until the skin condition clears up. Care and cleanliness on the part of the worker can do much to prevent dermatitis and should be encouraged by the provision of adequate washing facilities. If alkalis or other similar agents are used to remove stains from the hands, they should be used as sparingly as possible—$\frac{1}{2}$ lb. of bicarbonate of soda to 2 gals. of water makes a suitable alkaline solution: for this purpose a weak solution of sodium hyposulphite is also useful. Where chloride of lime is used for the removal of dyes from the skin of the hands it frequently causes irritation; this may be avoided by dipping the hands in a 10 per cent. solution of bisulphite of soda after using the chloride, then rinsing them in water. Such substances as methylated spirits and turpentine, which are sometimes used to remove stains, are themselves liable to produce dermatitis if used too frequently and allowed to remain on the skin too long. Vegetable oils should be substituted for these wherever possible. After the use of any cleansing agent it should be the invariable practice to wash with soap and water, then to rinse the hands and arms thoroughly in running water. The application of cold cream to the skin after washing is of value in preventing irritation.

Gloves worn for the prevention of dermatitis should be used with care. It is important that they should be free from holes and sufficiently tight fitting at the wrist to prevent irritants from getting into them. Prosser White points out that the use of waterproof gloves encourages heavy sweating, especially when working in hot liquids; perspiration soddens and removes the horny layer and this renders the skin tender, thin and vulnerable to any active chemical. Before gloves are used they should be scrupulously dry and clean inside and the hands should be dusted with talc or other suitable dusting powder.

Early and careful treatment of all injuries, however trivial, is of importance, as dermatitis frequently originates round an untreated sore.

Experimental work continues to be done under the auspices of the Home Office towards the production of a satisfactory barrier substance that will be of value in the prevention of dermatitis. Lanolin has been found to be of service as a protective against mineral oil or tar dermatitis, and Henry has found pure liquid paraffin to be useful in the prevention of celery itch, a dermatitis occurring in the canning of celery.

The skin of men exposed to the dust of lime after it has been burned becomes dry and may fissure, with the formation of painful ulcers. Protection against these sores has been obtained from talc powder shaken over the skin from a pepper pot. It lessens sweating and forms a protective film on the skin: strips of lint worn under the collar save the skin of the neck from being abraded.

In the prevention of dermatitis from machine lubricants, it has been found of service to protect the oil from dust, to strain it free from extraneous material and to renew when it becomes contaminated; Bridge advises filtering and heating to a temperature of 300° F.

In the recognition of skin sensitiveness to trade irritants, *e.g.*, nickel, tests may be applied by patch or drop methods. In the case of nickel, for instance, 8, 4 and 1 per cent. alcoholic solutions of chemically pure nickel chloride are used, a drop of each being placed on the skin, usually that of the abdomen; the alcohol quickly evaporates and in sensitive cases a local reaction occurs in from six to eight hours.

For treatment of established cases the steps to be taken are: (*a*) removal from contact with the offending irritant; (*b*) attention to the general health (which is important); and (*c*) local treatment, the removal of crusts by the application of a boracic starch poultice and the application of an ointment containing 5 gr. to the ounce of ammoniated mercury in zinc paste. Where large areas are affected boro-calomine lotion may be used with advantage. In old-standing chronic cases the application of crude gas tar is worthy of trial.

Special agents have been found to be of service in dealing with dermatitis from particular sources. Thus Prosser White favours the treatment of all dermatoses caused by plants by the immediate application of watery solutions of alkalis. In the treatment of "tulip fingers" the use of biniodide spirit, along with the wearing of gloves, has been found to be effectual, while in the treatment of "grain itch" (due to pediculoides ventricosus) mere application of soap and water is sufficient treatment.

The prevention of chrome ulceration and dermatitis is facilitated by the care of cuts and abrasions and the protection of the hands with a suitable ointment (lanolin). Dressings should be protected from water by impermeable coverings. Skin ulcers can be treated by the application of boracic fomentations and the subsequent use of an ointment containing ichthyol gr. v to the ounce. Exposure to ultra-violet light has proved useful. For chrome ulceration of the nasal mucous membrane it is generally sufficient to apply a little liquid paraffin on plugs of cotton wool.

INDUSTRIAL CANCER

The measures for the prevention of industrial cancer may be regarded as falling into two broad groups: (*a*) those aiming at limitation of contact with carcinogenic substances; and (*b*) those involving medical supervision of the health of the worker. The first group includes such procedures as the substitution for carcinogenic oils of others not possessing those properties, and it has been demonstrated that there is considerable scope for substitution of this kind; alternation of employment; the provision of baths and of suitable changing facilities at the works; and the protection of the skin by suitable local application. Where the irritant is dusty, it has been found serviceable to dust exposed parts with zinc oxide and starch before commencing work. Where it is oily, as in work with paraffin, Scott has recommended smearing of the skin with either commercial castor oil or an ointment containing equal parts of olive oil and lanolin. A large jar of the protective substance is kept available or supplies issued to the men at weekly intervals, and they are encouraged to use it freely, *e.g.*, whenever they dry their arms after washing.

Thorough medical inspection of the skin of workers should be carried out at regular intervals (monthly to quarterly, depending on risk involved). It is important that accurate records should be kept of conditions found at each examination, so that deterioration can be promptly detected. New workers should be carefully observed, and those found to be particularly susceptible to papular dermatitis shortly after commencing work should be discouraged from continuing in the industry.

Successful treatment aims at the anticipation of malignant degeneration. Removal of warts by carbon dioxide snow and free excision, or other appropriate treatment (radium) of suspicious or malignant ulcers is indicated ; the results, if treatment is undertaken sufficiently early, are good. It has long been observed that the application of radium has a highly beneficial effect on warty conditions due to exposure to X-rays.

Brodie has reported good results from the electro coagulation of ulcers undergoing malignant degeneration.

To safeguard the health of workers exposed to the risk of bladder tumours (from contact with aniline and allied dyestuffs), clinical supervision of the workmen, reinforced by routine microscopic examinations of urine, are of value. If red blood cells are found in the urine, the worker should be examined cystoscopically. The further treatment is essentially surgical and should be instituted as early as possible.

INJURY FROM RADIO-ACTIVE SUBSTANCES

Of recent years much thought has been given to the protection of workers exposed to radio-active substances. The British X-ray and Radium Protection Committee (Sir Humphry Rolleston, Chairman) first issued recommendations on the subject in 1921, and issued its fifth revised report in 1938. The dangers of over-exposure to X-rays and radium can be avoided by the provision of adequate protection and suitable working conditions. Such protection is necessary to guard against injuries to the superficial tissues, changes in the blood and damage to other internal tissues, particularly the generative organs. It is recommended that for whole-time radium and X-ray workers hours of work should not exceed seven per day and five days per week, the off-days to be spent as much as possible out of doors; that there should be not less than four weeks holiday per year, preferably consecutively; that no person should be employed on this work whose blood condition (on complete investigation) or general health is unsatisfactory; and that the amount of X or γ radiation received by operators should be systematically checked to ensure that the tolerance dose is not exceeded, photographic films or small capacity condensers being carried on the person for that purpose.

Before the commencement of exposure to radio-active substances, the normal leucocyte level should be determined by making three total and differential blood counts in the afternoon. If none of the total counts reach 6,000 per c.mm. and none of the lymphocyte counts reach 1,200 per c.mm., the applicant should not be accepted for service. Periodical total and differential blood counts of the worker should be made during the afternoon once every six months in the case of X-ray workers and once every three months in the case of radium workers. If at any time there is found to be a decided and sustained drop in either the total leucocyte or the total lymphocyte count the worker should cease work and be placed under treatment for an adequate period. On resumption of work the health should be carefully supervised and working conditions thoroughly scrutinized to prevent a recurrence.

The British Report cited above contains precise directions on such matters as construction of workrooms, working temperatures, etc., and technical information about the nature of adequate protection from the action of radio-active substances.

Though these recommendations are framed primarily to safeguard the health of scientific workers, they apply with equal force to the industrial use of radio-active substances, *e.g.*, people working with luminous paints. Indeed, where X-ray screening is carried out continuously over long periods the protection afforded requires to be even greater than that specified for hospital practice. In any case the protective arrangements and working hours should be such that the radiation received by the operator does not exceed $0{\cdot}2\,\gamma$ per day.

It is well known that open and closed arcs yielding ultra-violet radiation are dangerous to the naked eye. During their use goggles of proved opacity to ultra-violet rays should be worn by patients and by operators. Their opacity can only be proved satisfactorily by a spectroscopic test, and goggles which transmit radiation shorter than 3,800 A.V. should not be used. Prolonged exposure to ultra-violet radiation produces pigmentation of the skin which may be prevented by wearing thin muslin over the face.

The ventilation of rooms used for ultra-violet therapy is of importance, since all arcs produce deleterious gases and open arcs also consume oxygen. It is generally necessary to secure artificial ventilation by exhaust fans.

The only effective treatment for the systemic disturbance of workers suffering from over-exposure to radio-active substances, lies in immediate removal from the working environment, attention to the general health under good open-air conditions and a prolonged holiday before return to work, with the subsequent preventive care noted above.

The treatment of injury to the superficial tissues depends on the nature and severity of the lesion. It should never be regarded lightly and may well call for consultation between dermatologist, radiotherapist, physician and surgeon.

T. FERGUSON.

METABOLIC DISEASES

DIABETES MELLITUS

DIETETIC TREATMENT

THERE are, perhaps, few diseases which the average doctor feels himself less qualified to treat than diabetes mellitus. Yet the wise management of a previously untreated case can almost be guaranteed to give the patient dramatic relief from his symptoms, and to produce a striking improvement in his general health, a therapeutic claim which can, unfortunately, be made with confidence in only a few other medical conditions. The reason for this disinclination to treat diabetes probably lies in the common belief that in order to do so efficiently a profound knowledge of dietetics is necessary, with an ability to calculate diets in terms of their total calories, their glucose : fatty acid ratio, and their fat, protein and carbohydrate content. Most doctors know perfectly well that even if they could, with the aid of a table of food values, calculate diets in this way, it would take them a considerable part of their working day to do one such diet accurately. In consequence, some resign themselves to the belief that the treatment of diabetes is the province of specialists or content themselves by advising their patients in a general way to cut down their intake of sugars and starchy foods, and where this is insufficient to abolish their glycosuria, insulin is prescribed in varying quantities.

Apart from the exceptional case, and apart from diabetes in children, this exaggerated belief in the difficulty of treating the condition is unfounded. Successful treatment demands, however, the possession of a good dietetic system with a knowledge of how to use it and how to adapt it to the requirements of the patient. The use of rigid standard diet sheets is to be deprecated, just as rule-of-thumb treatment is to be avoided in all therapeutics. This does not mean, however, that the doctor need work out the actual details of the diet himself. He does not, after all, gather his own herbs and prepare from them his own medicines. Rather he prescribes doses of certain drugs and his prescription is made up into the medicine by a pharmaceutical chemist. Similarly, he should be able to prescribe the dose of calories and carbohydrate suitable for his diabetic patient, and his prescription can be worked out for him by a dietitian.

A dietitian, however, is not always available, and in the following pages an attempt has been made to work out a simple dietetic system for the treatment of the average diabetic, which in all but exceptional cases should make the introduction of the dietitian or specialist superfluous. The system is capable of so many permutations and combinations that a considerable variety of diets can be prescribed from it. Further, by the use of exchange lists a great number of foodstuffs can be utilized, provided they are used in their proper proportions, so that there is no need to limit the diabetic to a dull and monotonous menu, and no need for him to use patent diabetic foods, which are often expensive and usually unappetizing.

The Calorific Value of the Diet.—The vast majority of people in this country eat more food than is necessary for them to maintain their weight and to give them energy for their various activities. This does not mean that many people are not undernourished; but they are undernourished from eating diets deficient in certain foods, rather than from eating too little food as a whole. Most of us, then, eat more calories than we actually require. In a few unfortunate individuals these excess calories are promptly stored in the form of fat, but in the great majority they are successfully burnt up and dissipated in the form of heat.

The diabetic individual has difficulty to a greater or less extent in metabolizing food, especially carbohydrate food. The first principle, therefore, of diabetic dieting consists in cutting out the luxus food consumption in which most of us indulge. In other words, we should only give the diabetic sufficient calories, and no more, to give him energy for his particular activities and to maintain him at his ideal weight or slightly below it. No diabetic should be allowed to be much overweight. In the case of grossly obese diabetics a reduction to within 10 per cent. of their standard weight is quite sufficient, but even this may be too drastic in certain individuals. Once the diabetic has become habituated to his diet he appears to be satisfied by fewer calories than normal people, probably because the quality of his diet in regard to protein, minerals and vitamins is so good, and possibly because the actual metabolic rate tends to fall when calories are reduced.

It is apparent that the number of calories required will vary considerably according to the age, sex, weight, height and particular activities of the diabetic concerned. For example, an elderly, small, fat diabetic female of sedentary habit will require considerably fewer calories than a young, tall, underweight, hardworking diabetic male. The first will probably benefit by being given a 1,000 or 1,200 calorie diet to bring her down to near her ideal weight, and will thereafter require not more than about 1,600 or 1,700 calories to maintain her at that weight and to satisfy her moderate energy requirements. The second, on the other hand, may need as much as 2,800 or even 3,000 calories to bring him up to near his ideal weight (though such high diets should only be given in exceptional circumstances), and he may thereafter require some 2,500 calories to maintain him at that new level and to give him energy for his strenuous life. In between these two extremes lie the majority of diabetics who will require diets varying in caloric value between 1,700 and 2,500, according to the particular circumstances of the case.

The Carbohydrate Content of the Diet.—Since carbohydrate is the food which diabetics have most difficulty in metabolizing, it would at first hand appear reasonable to reduce the carbohydrate content of the diet to the lowest possible limits, and this was indeed the aim of diabetic dietetics in the pre-insulin days and for a good many years after its discovery. A limit to carbohydrate reduction was set by the danger of inducing ketosis. If the carbohydrate content of a diet is reduced below a certain minimum, or if the proportion of available glucose to fatty acid in the diet is reduced below the ratio of 1 to 1·5, it is well known that the fats are inadequately burnt up and ketones make their appearance in the circulation with possibly disastrous consequences. The ratio between available glucose in the diet and its fatty acid content—the G : FA ratio—thus became a matter of importance, and up till a few years ago the aim of treatment in diabetes was to give a diet in which there was only just sufficient available glucose to ensure proper combustion of the fats and hence to prevent ketosis. We were then rather like yachtsmen attempting to sail just as close as possible to the wind without losing it altogether. Diets calculated in this way very rarely contained more than 100 gm. of carbohydrate, and seldom as much, and their high proportion of fat to carbohydrate made them unappetizing and somewhat nauseating. Thus the spectacle of the unfortunate diabetic balancing enormous quantities of butter on a small square of oatcake was well known.

Nowadays we realize that our diabetic patients do better if the carbohydrate in their diets is not quite so rigorously restricted. The patients feel better on a slightly more liberal allowance and the diets so constructed are much pleasanter to take. Further, modern research has shown that, for a variety of reasons which need not be discussed here, diabetics on a very low carbohydrate intake are less sensitive to insulin than they are when a more adequate allowance is made. Thus, if a diabetic is taking insulin the dosage is not necessarily higher on a carbohydrate intake of slightly over 100 gm. than it is on one of under 100 gm. This also applies to endogenous insulin secretion. In the healthy subject, for example, it is well known that the form and duration of the blood-sugar curve is conditioned by the constitution of the diet which the individual has been taking previously ; after a period on a low carbohydrate diet, ingestion of glucose leads to a much higher and more prolonged rise in the blood sugar than is the case when the subject has been taking a high carbohydrate diet. This suggests that carbohydrate is a stimulus to insulin formation, and if it is too rigorously controlled in the diabetic a further inhibition of an already poor supply may occur. The rationale of the high carbohydrate diet is based on this phenomenon, the advantages and disadvantages of which will be discussed later.

We believe that the average diabetic in this country requires for maintenance 115 to 145 gm. of carbohydrate a day, depending on his calorie requirements, though there are undoubtedly milder cases which can be controlled satisfactorily on a considerably higher allowance. Where the caloric requirement is low, 115 to 130 gm. of carbohydrate is usually sufficient ; where relatively higher calories, and therefore more fat is needed, 130 to 145 gm. of carbohydrate should be given to make the diet more palatable. With these more liberal carbohydrate allowances it is unnecessary to worry about the G : FA ratio of the diet, since it would be extremely difficult to eat sufficient fat to produce ketosis, provided these quantities of carbohydrate were properly metabolized.

When a patient, who is not very ill and who is not suffering from ketosis, first comes for treatment it is usually wise to attempt to get him " sugar-free " by dietetic means alone. With this object in view we usually prescribe a temporary low diet with a carbohydrate intake of 85 gm. and a caloric value of about 1,500, which approximates to the basal caloric requirements of the average individual (see Diet Sheet I). Should he become " sugar-free " on this diet his calories and carbohydrates are gradually built up to his required level, and insulin is only administered should he stick half-way up the dietetic ladder. If, after a fortnight on the initial low diet he still has glycosuria, no further attempt is made to get him "sugar-free" by further dietetic restriction, since if he is unable to tolerate such a diet he will invariably require insulin either temporarily or permanently. He is, therefore, given without more ado the calories and carbohydrate which it is thought he will need to maintain his weight and to give him sufficient energy to satisfy his requirements, and insulin is started in gradually increasing doses till he is "sugar-free." It is then often found that the patient has reacquired a good deal of his sugar tolerance, and the dose can sometimes be reduced and occasionally dispensed with altogether. It is a common fallacy to suppose that insulin once started will invariably be required permanently.

When the diabetic, on his first visit, is found to be emaciated and to have definite acetone as well as sugar in the urine, no attempt should be made to get him "sugar-free" without insulin on the drastically reduced calorie and carbohydrate intake mentioned above. The danger of producing an increased ketosis, and possibly coma, by such measures is a very real one, and insulin should be started at once with a diet containing 115 gm. of carbohydrate and a moderate fat content of 100 to 120 gm. When the sugar and acetone in the urine are controlled, the diet will be increased to meet the individual requirements.

Diet Sheet I

Test Diet

Unsuitable for prolonged use

Carb., 85. Prot., 69. Fat, 93. Cals., 1,451.

(If an extra ounce of meat is added :

Carb., 85. Prot., 77. Fat, 98. Cals., 1,530.)

Breakfast—

Bacon—45 gm. ($1\frac{1}{2}$ oz.).
Egg—1.
Tomato—100 gm. ($3\frac{1}{2}$ oz.).
Brown bread—30 gm. (1 oz.).
Tea or coffee.
Butter and milk from ration.

Dinner—

Clear soup, bovril or marmite if desired.
Cooked lean meat—60 gm. (2 oz.).
Vegetable from Group I—200 gm. (7 oz.), *or* vegetable from Group II—100 gm. ($3\frac{1}{2}$ oz.) (see p. 333).
Add butter from ration.

(*contd. overleaf*)

Orange—100 gm. ($3\frac{1}{2}$ oz.) or exchange (see p. 333).
Milk—120 c.c. (4 oz.) from ration } Custard.
$\frac{1}{2}$ egg.

Tea—

Cheese—22 gm. ($\frac{3}{4}$ oz.) or 1 egg.
Salad of vegetables from Group I—100 gm. ($3\frac{1}{2}$ oz.) (see p. 333).
Brown bread—30 gm. (1 oz.).
Butter and milk from ration.
Tea.

Supper—

1 egg or exchange (see p. 334).
Vegetable from Group I—100 gm. ($3\frac{1}{2}$ oz.) (see p. 333).
Brown bread—30 gm. (1 oz.).
Butter and milk from ration.
Tea or coffee if desired.

Daily Rations

Butter—30 gm. (1 oz.).
Milk—300 c.c. ($\frac{1}{2}$ pint).
Water—At least 4 glasses daily.

100 gm. ($3\frac{1}{2}$ oz.) of vegetable can be exchanged for 30 gm. (1 oz.) of orange or 60 c.c. of milk.

All food must be accurately weighed after cooking, except bacon, which is weighed before cooking—all the fat from it should be eaten.

The Fat and Protein Content of the Diet.—Of late years there has been a tendency in many schools to break away from the extremely meticulous dietetic directions of the past as regards protein and fat and to adopt a *laisser faire* attitude in regard to these constituents of the diabetic's diet. The rule of several dietetic systems has been "take care of the carbohydrate and the protein and fat will take care of themselves." We believe this attitude to be a wrong one, and that in order to get the best results at the beginning of treatment, the protein and certainly the fat in the diet should be as accurately calculated by the doctor as the carbohydrate.

It has already been shown that provided a really adequate amount of carbohydrate is taken in the diet and properly metabolized there is no great need to worry about the fat from the point of view of the G : FA ratio and the danger of ketosis, but the total calories of the diet are of great importance, and of the three foodstuffs, fat has the highest calorific value. Hence, if fat is eaten to excess, the calories will be increased over and above the patient's requirements and accordingly his endogenous and exogenous insulin needs will be increased, even although his carbohydrate intake is kept constant; for modern experience has suggested that the insulin requirements of a patient are by no means dependent only on his carbohydrate intake, but on his total calories as well. In addition, with an excessive fat intake the patient may go up in weight unduly, and we have seen that excessive weight is to be deprecated in the diabetic even more than in the normal individual. If, on the other hand, the fat in the diet is too low, the total calories are likely to be deficient, and the patient may lose weight unduly.

The same arguments apply to the protein content of the diet, but to a much less extent since protein is not such an important source of calories as fat. On the other hand, some of the protein of the diet can be converted into glucose; it would, therefore, seem inconsistent to make strict rules about the carbohydrate content of the diet unless some control is to be kept over the protein as well. A moderate variation in protein intake above or below the prescribed amount is unimportant. The greedy patient may, however, upset the balance of his diet by an excessive protein intake, while it is only too common for the impecunious patient to take insufficient of this more expensive foodstuff unless the amount which he has to take is definitely prescribed. The majority of diabetics require protein in amounts varying from 70 to 100 gm. a day. With low calorie diets, 70 gm. of protein will be sufficient to keep the patient in nitrogenous equilibrium and to give him a moderate meat allowance. With higher calorie diets, and especially where the patient is a male, a more generous meat ration should be given.

The Calculation and Prescription of the Diet.—From what has been said it will be apparent that if it is decided that a patient requires a diet of between 2,000 and 2,100 calories containing 130 gm. of carbohydrate, and a protein ration of, say, 80 gm., the remaining calories will be obtained at the expense of fat, and this quantity can easily be calculated. For clinical purposes the calories obtained from carbohydrate and protein can be calculated by multiplying the number of grams of each in the diet by four. In the example given this will equal 840 calories. On subtracting this figure from the total calories (*i.e.*, 2,055), 1,215 calories are left to be supplied by fat. Since each gram of fat gives on combustion 9 calories, the number of grams of fat required will be $\frac{1215}{9} = 135$. Thus the diet will be prescribed as 130 gm. of carbohydrate, 80 gm. of protein, 135 gm. of fat and total calories 2,055.

Table I

	Carb.	3 Per Cent. Vegetable.		10 Per Cent. Fruit.		Milk.		Brown Bread.		Cooked Meat.		Raw Bacon.		Cheese.		No. of Eggs.	Butter.		C.	P.	F.	Cals.	If 30 gm. Meat Added.
		Gm.	Oz.	Gm.	Oz.	C.c.	Oz.	Gm.	Oz.	Gm.	Oz.	Gm.	Oz.	Gm.	Oz.		Gm.	Oz.					Cals.
Ladder Diets	85	*500	17	100	3½	300	10	90	3	60	2	45	1½	22	¾	2½	30	1	85	69	93	1451	1530
	85	500	17	100	3½	300	10	90	3	60	2	45	1½	22	¾	2½	53	1¾	85	69	112	1624	1701
	100	500	17	100	3½	300	10	120	4	60	2	45	1½	22	¾	2½	30	1	100	71	93	1521	1598
	100	500	17	100	3½	300	10	120	4	60	2	45	1½	22	¾	2½	53	1¾	100	71	112	1692	1769
	100	500	17	100	3½	300	10	120	4	60	2	45	1½	22	¾	2½	75	2½	100	71	131	1863	1940
Maintenance Diets	115	500	17	100	3½	300	10	150	5	60	2	45	1½	22	¾	3	30	1	115	77	97	1641	1717
	115	500	17	100	3½	300	10	150	5	60	2	45	1½	22	¾	3	53	1¾	115	77	116	1812	1888
	115	500	17	100	3½	300	10	150	5	60	2	45	1½	22	¾	3	75	2½	115	77	135	1983	2060
	115	500	17	100	3½	300	10	150	5	60	2	45	1½	22	¾	3	97	‡3¼	115	77	154	2154	2231
	130	500	17	100	3½	300	10	†180	6	60	2	45	1½	22	¾	3	30	1	130	80	97	1713	1790
	130	500	17	100	3½	300	10	180	6	60	2	45	1½	22	¾	3	53	1¾	130	80	116	1884	1961
	130	500	17	100	3½	300	10	180	6	60	2	45	1½	22	¾	3	75	2½	130	80	135	2055	2132
	130	500	17	100	3½	300	10	180	6	60	2	45	1½	22	¾	3	97	‡3¼	130	80	154	2226	2303
	130	500	17	100	3½	300	10	180	6	60	2	60	2	22	¾	3	112	‡3¾	130	82	173	2405	2482
	145	500	17	100	3½	300	10	†210	7	60	2	45	1½	22	¾	3	30	1	145	83	97	1785	1862
	145	500	17	100	3½	300	10	210	7	60	2	45	1½	22	¾	3	53	1¾	145	83	116	1956	2033
	145	500	17	100	3½	300	10	210	7	60	2	45	1½	22	¾	3	75	2½	145	83	135	2127	2204
	145	500	17	100	3½	300	10	210	7	60	2	45	1½	22	¾	3	97	‡3¼	145	83	154	2298	2375
	145	500	17	100	3½	300	10	210	7	60	2	60	2	22	¾	3	112	‡3¾	145	85	173	2477	§2554
If required, *add extra meat*, 30 gm. (1 oz.), to any of these diets =																				8	5	77	...

* 100 gm. of vegetable can be exchanged for 30 gm (1 oz.) of orange or 60 c.c. (2 oz.) of milk.

† 1 oz. bread can be changed for 2½ oz. potato.

‡ 1 oz. butter can be changed for 2 oz. double cream.

§ Where higher calories are required, add thick cream; 1 oz. = 112 calories.

Diet Sheet II

Breakfast—

Bacon—........ oz. ; 1 egg or exchange (see p. 334).
Tomato—3½ oz.
Brown bread—........ oz.
Butter and milk from ration.
Tea or coffee.

Dinner—

Marmite, bovril or oxo, if desired.
Vegetable from Group I—7 oz. ; *or* vegetable from Group II—3½ oz. Add butter from ration (see p. 333).
Cooked lean meat—........ oz., or exchange (see p. 335).
Orange—3½ oz., or exchanges (see p. 333).
Milk from ration for curds, or as custard, using half or whole egg.

Tea—

Cheese—¾ oz.
Salad from Group I—3 oz. (see p. 333).
Brown bread—........ oz.
Butter and milk from ration.
Tea.

Supper—

Eggs—........, or exchanges (see p. 334).
Vegetable from Group I—3½ oz. (see p. 333).
Brown bread—........ oz.
Butter and milk from ration.
Tea or coffee.

Rations for Day

Milk—½ pint.
Bread—........ oz.
Butter—........ oz.
Thick cream—........ tablespoonfuls.
Water—at least 4 glasses.

All food must be accurately weighed after cooking, except bacon, which is weighed before cooking, and all the fat from it must be used.

In Table I a number of diets are worked out in terms of their carbohydrate, protein and fat and total calorie values. It will be seen that most of the foodstuffs are kept at a constant value in all the diets. Thus the quantity of vegetable, fruit, milk, meat, cheese and eggs (with only one small variation) are the same whether a diet of 1,451 calories or one of 2,554 calories are prescribed. The variations in carbohydrate and total calories are obtained simply by additions in bread, bacon and butter. It will be seen that there are only five variations in respect of carbohydrate, and these are made by adding 30 gm. (1 oz.) of bread, thereby increasing the carbohydrate from 85 to 145 gm. by increments of 15 gm. Once the quantity of carbohydrate and the total calories have been determined, all that is necessary is to look up the table and transpose the appropriate column on to the appended Diet Sheet II by filling up the blank spaces which have been left upon it.

The amount of bread allowed can be distributed among the various meals according to the circumstances of the case. If the patient is taking soluble insulin night and morning, most of the bread should be given at breakfast and supper. If he does not require insulin, or if zinc protamine insulin is being given, the bread can be distributed more evenly throughout the day. (Exchanges for bread will be found on p. 340.)

A diet consisting only of vegetables, fruit, milk, brown bread, beef or mutton, bacon, cheese and eggs, though adequate, would become extremely monotonous. The foodstuffs on the diet sheet, however, are only symbols for a large number of other foods of equal, or approximately equal, food value, both as regards their actual constituents and their total calories. Tables of exchanges for these symbols are therefore given, and by the intelligent use of these exchanges an extremely varied diet can be taken by the patient each day. In our experience patients very quickly learn how to make use of these exchanges, and indeed often make quite a hobby of working out their daily menu. This applies even to ill-educated people, but a certain amount of time must be spent in painstaking explanation and all instructions should be written out. In diabetes time and trouble spent initially in educating the patient in regard to the main facts of his disease are well worth while. Sometimes doctors are apt to think their patients more stupid than they really are.

Vegetables

(When fresh vegetables are unobtainable tinned ones may be substituted)

Group I—

1 *to* 3 *per cent. Vegetable* (*take the full quantity on Diet List*) :

Mushrooms (no food value).
Mustard and cress.
Watercress.
Lettuce.
Curly greens.
Celery.
Spinach.
Cabbage.

Cauliflower.
Artichokes.
Seakale.
French beans.
Eggplant.
Salsify.
Asparagus.
Radishes.

Cucumber.
Vegetable marrow.
Tomatoes.
Brussels sprouts.
Endive.
Leeks.
Rhubarb cooked with a pinch of baking soda.

Group II—

3 *to* 6 *per cent. Vegetable* (*take half the quantity on Diet List*) :

Turnips. Onions. Carrots.

Group III—

10 *per cent. Vegetable* (*take one-third of the quantity on Diet List*) :

Beetroot. Horseradish. Parsnip.

15 *per cent. Vegetable* (*take one-fifth of the quantity on the Diet List*) :

Peas, fresh or tinned.

20 *per cent. Vegetable* (*do not take without permission*) :

Potato. Cooked dried peas, beans, lentils.

Fruits

(No tinned fruits)

$4\frac{1}{2}$ *Oz.* =	$3\frac{1}{2}$ *Oz.* =	$2\frac{1}{4}$ *Oz.* =	$1\frac{3}{4}$ *Oz.*
$7\frac{1}{2}$ *Per Cent. Fruit.*	10 *Per Cent. Fruit.*	15 *Per Cent. Fruit.*	20 *Per Cent. Fruit.*
Grapefruit.	Gooseberries.	Apple.	*Not to be taken without permission :*
Strawberries.	Orange.	Pear.	Dried figs.
Blackberries.	Peach.	Apricots, dried (stewed).	Dried prunes (stewed).
Red currants.	Pineapple.	Plums, Victoria + stone.	Bananas.
Black currants.	Greengage + stone.	Grapes.	
White currants.	Cherries + stone.	Nectarine + stone.	
Cranberries.	Damson + stone.		
Raspberries.	Tangerines.		
Loganberries.	Apricots (fresh).		

Exchanges for Bacon and Egg

	Exchange for 1½ Oz. Bacon and One Egg.					Exchange for 2 Oz. Bacon and One Egg.				
	Gm.	Oz.		* Butter.		Gm.	Oz.		* Butter.	
				Gm.	Oz.				Gm.	Oz.
Herring . .	61	2	Add	22	Good ¾	75	2½	Add	28	1
Kipper	75	2½	Add	23	Good ¾	88	3	Add	29	1
Mackerel . .	68	2¼	Add	23	¾	80	2¾	Add	30	1
Cod roe . .	61	2	Add	26	1	73	2½	Add	32	1
Cold lean ham	68	2¼	Add	17	Good ½	80	2¾	Add	22	Good ¾
Kidney . .	68	2¼	Add	24	Good ¾	80	2¾	Add	30	1
Sardines . .	56	1¾	Add	17	Good ½	67	2¼	Add	22	¾
Finnan haddock .	50	Scant 1¾	Add	28	1	64	Scant 2¼	Add	35	1¼
White fish . .	65	2¼	Add	28	1	80	2¾	Add	35	1¼

Exchanges for One and Two Eggs

	Exchange for One Egg.					Exchange for Two Eggs.				
	Gm.	Oz.		* Butter.		Gm.	Oz.		* Butter.	
				Gm.	Oz.				Gm.	Oz.
Bacon	38	1¼	Omit	8	¼	76	2½	Omit	16	½
Bacon and one egg	...	...	...	...	...	38	1¼	Omit	8	¼
Tongue, tinned .	30	1	...	...	...	60	2	...	...	...
Cold lean ham .	30	1	...	...	...	60	2	...	...	...
Sardines . .	25	¾	...	...	...	50	1¾	...	...	...
Average cheese .	23	¾	...	...	...	46	1½	...	...	...
Salmon, tinned .	26	1	...	...	...	52	1¾	Add	6	¼
Salmon, fresh .	30	1	...	...	...	60	2	Add	8	¼
White fish . .	30	1	Add	7	¼	60	2	Add	14	½
Meat, average roast . .	24	¾	...	...	...	48	1½	...	...	...
Corned beef	...	...	...	...	...	48	1½	...	...	...
Chicken or rabbit	...	...	...	...	...	48	1½	Add	8	¼
Liver . .	...	...	...	...	...	60	2	Add	10	⅓
Kidney . .	...	...	...	...	...	60	2	Add	10	⅓
Herring, edible portion . .	...	...	...	...	...	55	1¾	Add	8	¼
Cod roe, steamed .	...	...	...	...	...	55	1¾	Add	12	½
Finnan haddock .	...	...	...	...	...	48	1½	Add	14	½
Kipper . .	...	...	...	...	...	67	2¼	Add	8	¼
Cutlet, grilled edible portion .	...	...	...	...	...	71	2¼	Omit	12	½

* The additions or omissions refer to the daily butter ration.

Exchanges for Two and Three Ounces Meat

	Exchange for 2 Oz. Lean Meat.					Exchange for 3 Oz. Lean Meat.				
	Gm.	Oz.	* Butter.			Gm.	Oz.	* Butter.		
				Gm.	Oz.				Gm.	Oz.
Grilled chop, edible portion	94	3	Omit	19	¾	141	4¾	Omit	29	1
Roast pork, very little fat	80	2½	Omit	10	⅓	120	4	Omit	15	½
Veal	64	2	Add	4	¼	96	3¼	Add	5	¼
Poultry	64	2	Add	4	¼	96	3¼	Add	5	¼
Liver	80	2½	Add	5	¼	120	4	Add	7	¼
Tripe	100	3½	...	...	...	150	5	...	...	...
Sweetbreads	80	2½	Add	8	¼	120	4	Add	13	½
Tongue, tinned	80	2½	Add	8	¼	120	4	Omit	13	½
White fish	80	2½	Add	10	⅓	120	4	Add	15	½
Salmon, tinned	70	2¼	...	...	...	105	3½	...	...	...
Salmon, fresh	80	2½	...	...	...	120	4	...	...	...
Cod roe	73	2½	Add	7	¼	107	3½	Add	11	½
Herring, edible portion	73	2½	...	...	...	107	3½	...	...	...
Corned beef	64	2	Omit	3	...	96	3¼	Omit	4	¼

* The additions or omissions refer to the daily butter ration.

Note.—It is unnecessary in all cases to make these meticulous omissions or additions of butter.

We believe it to be important that patients should buy scales and should get into the habit of weighing accurately the prescribed amounts of the different foodstuffs, and particularly the stated amount of bread and butter. If they are allowed to guess at the quantities to be used—taking 1 oz. of bread, for example, to be one thin slice—inaccuracies are bound to creep in, and these may become serious. Once a diabetic has been well trained in the hard school of food weighing, he may be able to relax somewhat, since by this time he will have got a very much more accurate idea of what 1 or 2 oz. of the various foodstuffs look like than if he had simply guessed from the first. Indeed, originally well-trained diabetics learn to guess food quantities with remarkable accuracy, and once they have achieved this facility they should be encouraged to go out to meals in their friends' houses and in restaurants like ordinary people, and on no account to regard themselves as invalids.

It is, of course, of the utmost importance to study the character of the patient concerned. There are many who require to be warned continually of the necessity of dietetic care, and may indeed occasionally have to be frightened into being more accurate by a lecture on the considerable risk which they run by non-observance of the rules. Such treatment in other patients would turn them into neurasthenic hypochondriacs. Some over-anxious diabetics require the disease and its dangers to be minimized rather than stressed. Such patients should be encouraged to regard diabetes as an inconvenient idiosyncrasy rather than as a dreadful and ever-present menace, and that the occasional occurrence of a positive reaction in their Fehling test must not be regarded as a disaster of the first magnitude.

The Treatment of the Obese Diabetic.—The mildly obese diabetic can be treated by the use of diets prescribed from Table I, with the caloric intake appropriately reduced. This can be done very simply by stopping the breakfast bacon. In this way a reduction of approximately 220 calories can be made, and the 1,641 calorie diet containing 115 gm. of carbohydrate can be reduced to approximately 1,400 calories, which is often sufficient to bring a moderately obese diabetic to more normal proportions. Where gross obesity exists, and in those cases which prove recalcitrant to the above milder method of treatment, it is advisable to keep the carbohydrate down to 100 gm. and to restrict the calories to 1,000 or 1,200. Examples of such diets are given on pp. 391-395.

Method of Adjusting the Diabetic Diets in Table I.—The chief disadvantages of standard diets are that the kinds or amounts of the various foods prescribed may not be acceptable to the individual patient, or that the arrangement of meals may not fit in with his hours of work. It may be necessary, for example, to plan a carried lunch and to arrange for dinner at 5 P.M. Many patients like a "high" tea and a light supper while others prefer to dine in the evening. Provided that the carbohydrate is distributed in accordance with the insulin dosage, the protein foods can be divided between the meals to suit the patient's convenience. The diet and the possible variations should be carefully explained and likes and dislikes must be considered. We have seen patients without teeth struggling with oatcake and lettuce, and a woman with cholecystitis faced with the problem of eating three eggs daily! By using the exchanges for two or more eggs at supper, fish, etc., can be given. On the lower diets the half-egg is meant to be used at dinner with one-third of a glass of the milk ration as a custard. Alternatively, it can be exchanged for a small teaspoonful of gelatine to make an orange jelly, or $\frac{1}{3}$ oz. of extra cheese or meat can be taken instead. The slight differences in fat involved by these changes are unimportant. Jewish patients do not eat bacon and some people cannot digest cheese, but a judicious use of the "exchange" lists will soon solve these difficulties.

Since on the standard diets the increases in carbohydrate are made by adding bread, the diet containing 145 gm. of carbohydrate involves the eating of 210 gm. (*i.e.*, 7 oz.) of bread daily. This is more bread than some people wish to eat, and 1 oz. of bread can be exchanged for 2½ oz. of potato. Similarly, where large quantities of butter are indicated in the high calorie diets, 1 oz. of it can be exchanged for 2 oz. of double cream. For economy, margarine can be substituted for part of the butter and can be used along with vegetables, or for scrambling eggs or cooking fish. Olive oil can be used with vinegar, or a home-made mayonnaise can be utilized. A scant tablespoonful of oil is equal to ½ oz. of butter.

The amount of vegetable may be too bulky for an elderly diabetic and a smaller quantity of the more concentrated kinds can be substituted ; if necessary they can be passed through a sieve. Tomato juice is a most useful substitute for vegetable, while an extra ounce of orange or 2 oz. of milk can replace a good 3½ oz. of 3 per cent. vegetable without materially upsetting the value of the diet.

In Scotland patients sometimes prefer oatcake to bread, and in pre-insulin days there is no doubt that many diabetics could be kept free of sugar with oatcake more easily than with bread. Oatcake and brown bread can be exchanged in equal quantities, though actually the fat in oatcake is so high that for every 2 oz. of oatcake eaten ¼ oz. of butter should be subtracted from the daily ration. If porridge is desired, 1 oz. of dry oatmeal will make 4 tablespoonfuls of thick porridge, and this can be taken in place of 40 gm. (1¼ oz.) of brown bread. Unless a light concentrated diet is required, we prefer brown bread to white, for, besides being a superior food, it is more satisfying. Malted and fancy brown breads should not be used. Clear meat soups, bovril, oxo, marmite, tea and coffee, which have no calorific value, can be taken as desired, and, if hungry, extra lettuce or other leafy vegetable can be taken, for they will add little carbohydrate to the diet.

Since the caloric value of the diets in Table I does not rise above 2,554, additions may have to be made to meet the nutritional requirements of certain patients. We have already mentioned that high calorie diets are undesirable from the diabetic point of view, but an unusually tall or emaciated patient, or one who has to undertake really hard manual work, may have to take a diet containing fully 3,000 calories. Merely to add fat is to make the diet unpalatable. An extra ½ pint of milk will probably give the best results, especially in the case of young people. This will increase the diet by approximately 200 calories, yielding carbohydrate, 15 gm.; protein, 10 gm.; fat, 12 gm. By substituting 6 oz. of oatcake for an equal quantity of bread, another 159 calories are added. For those who have to take carried meals, bread and cheese are useful. One ounce of bread gives carbohydrate 15 gm., protein 3 gm., fat 0·5 gm.; and 1 oz. of cheese gives protein 8 gm. and fat 9 gm. This combination would add 190 calories. Potato is satisfying—100 gm. (3½ oz.) give carbohydrate 20 gm. and protein 2 gm., calories 88. An extra 30 gm. (1 oz.) of cooked meat gives protein 8 gm. and fat 5 gm., calories 77.

With these higher calorie diets we find it is usually inadvisable to allow the carbohydrate to exceed 150 gm., and this amount is only prescribed when the lower diets have proved insufficient.

The Higher Carbohydrate, Low Fat Diet.—The diets shown in Table I represent the type of diabetic diet which we find most satisfactory in routine treatment, but a very different kind of diet is extensively used by some authorities and we have found it beneficial in selected cases.

Some years ago it was found that if the fat in the diet was reduced to a very low level (approximately 50 gm.) the diabetic could sometimes tolerate double his previous carbohydrate ration without increasing the insulin dosage, and, in some cases, even less insulin was required. The physiological processes involved are too complicated to be discussed here, but certain practical considerations must be taken into account in describing this modern development in diabetic dieting.

A big drop in fat naturally entails a reduction in calories, and this alone reduces insulin requirement. Moreover, the possible stimulus to the production of endogenous insulin by an increase in carbohydrate has already been referred to. How far fat in itself makes a demand upon the endogenous and exogenous insulin supply appears to vary in different individuals since, in our experience, the lowering of the fat does not always result in an increased tolerance for carbohydrate. Some authorities who favour the low fat diet in the treatment of diabetes do not do so merely because of its influence on the insulin requirement, but because they believe that a high fat intake is one of the factors in the production or aggravation of the arteriosclerosis so common in diabetes. Although this latter supposition is only a theory and by no means proved, many workers—especially in America—have,

TABLE II

Carb.	3 Per Cent. Veg.		10 Per Cent. Fruit.		20 Per Cent. Fruit.		Potato.		Bread.		Cooked Lean Meat (Fat Removed).		Cooked White Fish.		No. of Eggs.	Cheese.		Milk.		Butter.		C.	P.	F.	Cals.
	Gm.	Oz.	Gm.	Oz.	Gm.	Oz.	Gm.	Oz.	Gm.	Oz.	Gm.	Oz.	Gm.	Oz.		Gm.	Oz.	Gm.	Oz.	Gm.	Oz.				
150	330	11	100	3½	100	3½	100	3½	150	5	90	3	100	3½	1	22	¾	300	10	35	1¼	150	85	62	1498
150	330	11	100	3½	100	3½	100	3½	150	5	90	3	100	3½	1	22	¾	300	10	65	2¼	150	85	87	1723
175	330	11	100	3½	100	3½	150	5	180	6	90	3	100	3½	1	22	¾	300	10	35	1¼	175	88	62	1610
175	330	11	100	3½	100	3½	150	5	180	6	90	3	100	3½	1	22	¾	300	10	65	2¼	175	88	88	1844
200	330	11	200	7	100	3½	150	5	210	7	90	3	100	3½	1	22	¾	300	10	35	1¼	200	91	63	1731
200	330	11	200	7	100	3½	150	5	210	7	90	3	100	3½	1	22	¾	300	10	65	2¼	200	91	89	1965
225	330	11	200	7	100	3½	200	7	240	8	90	3	100	3½	1	22	¾	300	10	35	1¼	225	94	63	1843
225	330	11	200	7	100	3½	200	7	240	8	90	3	100	3½	1	22	¾	300	10	65	2¼	225	94	89	2077
250	330	11	200	7	100	3½	250	8½	270	9	90	3	100	3½	1	22	¾	300	10	35	1¼	250	98	63	1959
250	330	11	200	7	100	3½	250	8½	270	9	90	3	100	3½	1	22	¾	300	10	65	2¼	250	98	89	2193

for this and various other reasons, adopted for use in their routine treatment a carbohydrate intake approximating to that taken by a normal individual and a very low fat ration.

A normal diet usually contains from 200 to 500 gm. of carbohydrate (approximately 50 per cent. of the total calories); its protein varies from 60 to 120 gm. (from 10 to 15 per cent. of the total calories), while the fat averages about 100 gm., though more fat is usually eaten by the well-to-do. In the high carbohydrate, low fat diabetic diet, the carbohydrate content is usually from 200 to 250 gm. (or even more), the protein is about 90 gm. and the fat is fixed at the low figure of 50 gm. Such a diet has a caloric value of between 1,600 to 1,800 calories, which is insufficient for more active people, though as we have seen, it may meet the requirement of small persons engaged in sedentary occupations. If the carbohydrate is still further increased in order to raise the calories, the diet is not a "normal diet" as is sometimes claimed, but it is a badly balanced diet of the high carbohydrate, low fat type so often a factor in the production of infections. In our northern climate a fat intake of only 50 gm. has definite disadvantages. Sufficient whole milk cannot be given and the butter allowance has to be cut to $\frac{3}{4}$ oz. This is unpalatable and entails a shortage of fat-soluble vitamins which increases the risk of tuberculous and other infections, to which the diabetic is particularly prone. However desirable this very restricted fat may be from the diabetic point of view, the general opinion in this country is that it is wiser to prescribe a slightly higher fat—say, 60 to 80 gm.—even if this necessitates larger doses of insulin.

Exchanges for Bread

Three water biscuits *Or* 2 Rich Tea biscuits ,, 2 pieces ryvita ,, cooked potato—75 gm. = $2\frac{1}{2}$ oz. ,, rice, etc., dry weight—20 gm. = $\frac{3}{4}$ oz. ,, Benger's Food, dry weight—20 gm. = $\frac{3}{4}$ oz. ,, macaroni (boiled)—100 gm. = $3\frac{1}{2}$ oz. ,, orange or other 10 per cent. fruit—150 gm. = 5 oz. ,, apple or other 15 per cent. fruit—100 gm. = $3\frac{1}{2}$ oz.	= 30 gm. or 1 oz. bread.
Cooked potato—100 gm. = $3\frac{1}{2}$ oz. *Or* Kellogg's All-Bran — 2 heaped tablespoonfuls = 30 gm. ,, cornflakes—1 teacupful = 25 gm. ,, bananas, or other 20 per cent. fruit—100 gm. = $3\frac{1}{2}$ oz.	= 40 gm. or $1\frac{1}{3}$ oz. bread.
One shredded wheat biscuit *Or* boiled rice—100 gm. = $3\frac{1}{2}$ oz.	= 45 gm. or $1\frac{1}{2}$ oz. bread.

NATIONAL HEALTH SERVICE
SUPPLEMENTARY OPHTHALMIC SERVICES
MEDICAL RECOMMENDATION

To..

I certify that I have examined you and that, in my opinion, you require to have your sight tested.

Signature of doctor..

Date..

Please see overleaf

INFORMATION FOR THE APPLICANT

You may take this medical recommendation to any ophthalmic medical practitioner or to any ophthalmic optician who has undertaken to provide supplementary ophthalmic services under the National Health Service, and he will test your sight. If, after examination, he considers it necessary, he will give a prescription which will be forwarded to you later. You may then take the prescription to any ophthalmic optician or dispensing optician who has undertaken to supply glasses under the National Health Service. Lists of those who have undertaken to provide these services may be seen in doctors' surgeries, at opticians' premises, at Post Offices, or at the offices of Executive Councils set up under the National Health Service Act.

For office reasons, you will be asked to state your National Registration Identity Number when you visit the ophthalmic medical practitioner or optician.

We use these high carbohydrate, low fat diets chiefly for patients who cannot digest fat, or who dislike it, for those who will only adhere to a diet if it contains large amounts of bread, or for those few patients who may not respond well to treatment on the higher fat diets. It is obvious that these diets are unsuitable when generous calories are required, for in such cases patients do not maintain their weight and they miss the satiety value of the fat.

A word of warning is required regarding the use of high carbohydrate diets with unrestricted fat, especially where such foods as jam and sugar are allowed. Patients treated on these lines are seldom kept free from glycosuria and they often take unnecessarily large doses of insulin. We purposely omit jam and sugar from our diabetic diets, for patients agree that once they have forgotten the taste of sugar, they lose all craving for forbidden sweets. There are undoubtedly some patients who cannot remain consistently "sugar-free" throughout the twenty-four hours without showing symptoms of hypoglycæmia, and it is better that these patients should pass a little sugar. These are usually diabetics who have a low renal threshold for sugar, rather than a high threshold which is much more common in diabetes. Apart from these exceptional cases the majority of diabetics should aim at keeping their urine completely "sugar-free."

INSULIN TREATMENT

We have seen that insulin is required for those diabetics who, after a suitable trial on the test 1,500 calorie diet, continue to have a considerable glycosuria, and that insulin treatment should be instituted at once for those who, when first seen, are found to be much underweight and to have significant quantities of acetone as well as sugar in the urine. Those cases, also, who cannot climb to a sufficiently high rung on the dietetic ladder may require insulin to enable them to tolerate the calories and carbohydrate necessary to maintain their weight and to sustain their activities. In addition, we will see that all cases of diabetic coma or pre-coma require insulin in large doses; that diabetic children almost invariably need it, as do all cases of diabetes before and after surgical operations, and most cases complicated by infections or gangrene.

A large number of mild diabetic patients, however, particularly the obese and the elderly, are able to do without insulin altogether and to keep "sugar-free" by attention to diet alone. The expense of insulin to the individual or the state, the inconvenience of its hypodermic administration, and the fact that its use is not entirely free from danger, makes it desirable to do without it whenever possible. The attempt to dispense with insulin, however, should never be pushed to the extent of depriving the individual of carbohydrate or calories sufficient to make his diet palatable, to keep him free from ketosis or to maintain him in a good state of nutrition.

Many patients are averse to start insulin and doctors hesitate to prescribe it in the belief that once started it will have to be continued for life. In a large percentage of cases this permanent administration is, of course, necessary. Where this is so, however, delay in starting insulin is merely a matter of putting off the evil day, and in the meantime the patient will probably lose in condition, and his sugar tolerance will become progressively more and more impaired. Such a patient may, indeed, require eventually much larger doses than he would have done had insulin been given earlier. It is a fallacy to suppose, however, that insulin once started need in every case be permanently administered. After an initially severe hyperglycæmia has been well controlled by the use of insulin, the patient is often able to reduce the dose and even to do without it altogether. This phenomenon can be attributed to the effect of resting the damaged pancreas which may in consequence reacquire much of its lost function. The same principle seems to be involved in the gradual increase in tolerance for carbohydrate which follows a period of low feeding. The administration of insulin will, however, obviate unnecessary starvation with its ever-present risk of ketosis. Again, insulin may be required as a temporary measure because of some superadded infection, but when this subsides the sugar tolerance may once more improve so that the patient may be able to tolerate an adequate diet without the help of insulin.

Technique of Injection.—Soluble insulin is put on the market in single, double and quadruple strength preparations, containing 20, 40 and 80 units to the cubic centimetre respectively. Double-strength insulin should be used where more than 14 units have to be given in the dose, and quadruple strength should be prescribed where big doses of over 30 units are being employed, so as to avoid the necessity of giving uncomfortably large subcutaneous injections.

It is very desirable that an insulin syringe graduated in units (20 divisions per cubic centimetre), rather than an ordinary 1 c.c. or minim syringe, should be used, especially when the patient is going to administer the drug himself. It is a more accurate method and saves mistakes in calculation.

Most insulin syringes are graduated for single-strength insulin. This should be made perfectly clear to a patient who is being given the double-strength preparations. Thus, if 16 units of double-strength insulin are prescribed, he should only take 8 according to the graduations on his syringe.

Practically all patients can and should be taught to administer insulin to themselves. This is of the utmost importance, as it makes the patient much more independent and saves an infinity of bother. A great deal of encouragement, a little mild bullying and most patient explanations are sometimes necessary to begin with. If this initial trouble is taken, however, it is only very little children, the senile, the blind and the half-witted who cannot be taught to administer the drug to themselves accurately and efficiently. Most patients, in the course of time, come to regard their daily injection, or injections, with no more seriousness than they do other routine duties such as washing their teeth.

Cases of sepsis as the result of insulin injections are extremely rare. The patient should be taught to keep the needles in surgical spirit and to draw the syringe through with the spirit before use. Care should be taken to get rid of all the spirit from the needle and syringe before drawing in the insulin, as traces of surgical spirit in the injection will cause it to sting unpleasantly. Methylated spirit is often used instead of surgical spirit, the only drawback to the former being that needles left in it for a long time tend to become rusty. Many patients keep their syringe with needle attached all ready for use in a portable metal case with a screw top containing surgical spirit. This is an excellent plan, and the initial expense is not great, being only about 12s. 6d. We usually recommend our patients to boil their syringe once a week to ensure cleanliness.

When patients complain unduly of the pain of insulin injections, it is usually due to the fact that they are making the injections either too superficially just under the skin or too deeply into the muscles. We have sometimes seen patients who had caused multiple necrotic areas in the skin as the result of making what were practically intradermal injections. The injection should be made quickly and resolutely with a sharp fine needle (No. 17 to 20) into the loose fatty subcutaneous tissues. The best places for self-injection are the outer surfaces of the thighs and the loose tissues of the abdomen (see p. 1085). The site of the injection should be continually varied. Occasionally patients keep injecting themselves in practically the same spot for weeks on end, causing thickening of the skin in that site with painful nodules in the underlying tissues and even, on occasion, large areas of fat atrophy. These latter are probably due to the simple mechanical effect of repeated injections in the same place rather than to any specific effect of the insulin itself. Occasionally red, tender urticarial wheals make their appearance at the site of the injection. Such reactions are now uncommon, as they were due to sensitization to the protein fraction which insulin used to contain, but from which it is now almost entirely free owing to modern methods of purification in its preparation. When such local reactions do occur, they are usually only troublesome for a few days and tend to get less marked and to disappear entirely in the course of a week or a fortnight. When they persist, a different brand of insulin should be tried.

Soluble insulin should usually be injected half an hour before meals. This gives sufficient time for the insulin to begin to have its effect on the blood sugar in preparation for the meal, but not long enough to cause hypoglycæmic symptoms to develop before the meal is taken. In severe diabetics, with a high fasting blood sugar, the early morning injection, unless this is very inconvenient, is best given an hour before breakfast, the subsequent injection, or injections, being taken half an hour before meals.

Hypoglycæmia.—An overdose of insulin results in an undue lowering of the blood sugar causing the symptoms of hypoglycæmia to manifest themselves. The degree to which the blood sugar must fall to produce hypoglycæmic symptoms varies considerably. In a normal healthy individual a blood-sugar concentration of as low as 60 to 70 mg. per cent. is usually necessary to produce symptoms. In the diabetic, however, who has become accustomed to a high blood sugar, hypoglycæmic symptoms may occur at considerably higher concentrations. The level at which it occurs seems, indeed, to depend roughly on the average height of the blood-sugar previously. Thus, when a severe diabetic, who has had a high blood sugar continuously for some weeks, first comes under treatment and has his hyperglycæmia rapidly controlled, hypoglycæmic symptoms may occur when his blood-sugar concentration is still as high as 120 mg. or even 130 mg. per cent. Later on, however, after his tissues have become accustomed to a more normal blood sugar, hypoglycæmic symptoms may not occur unless the blood-sugar concentration falls to 70 or 80 mg. per cent.

Hypoglycæmia due to soluble insulin usually begins with a feeling of weakness and emptiness about the pit of the stomach. Tremor and tachycardia are common and diplopia occasionally occurs. The individual feels faint and dizzy and often experiences a strong desire for food. Clammy sweating is almost invariable, and, as the condition becomes more pronounced, mental symptoms are common, the patient sometimes becoming very hysterical—laughing, crying, shouting and struggling. Some most respectable diabetics, while hypoglycæmic, have run amuck in the streets and have been apprehended by the police as drunk and disorderly. At other times lassitude and somnolence are more marked features, especially in the case of children. The advanced stages of hypoglycæmia are characterized by muscular twitchings, deepening coma and eventually convulsions.

When soluble insulin has been used, the more severe hypoglycæmic symptoms seldom manifest themselves for at least a quarter of an hour after the initial sensations have been experienced. Thus, the patient has usually plenty of time to rectify matters. The treatment consists, of course, in raising the blood sugar by the administration of carbohydrate. This can be done most conveniently and simply by expediting the next meal, for in this way there is no upset of the patient's carbohydrate and calorie intake for the day. Hypoglycæmia does not, however, invariably occur under circumstances where a meal can be taken. All patients, therefore, who are taking insulin should invariably carry about with them some lumps of sugar. The patient should remain as quiet as possible till the symptoms have disappeared as exercise tends to exacerbate the tendency to hypoglycæmia. If the symptoms do not quickly disappear, or should they become worse, another two lumps of sugar can be taken, or preferably, 10 gm. of glucose. The object should be, however, to banish the symptoms with the smallest effective quantity of sugar, in order not to upset unduly the sugar intake for the day and to cause hyperglycæmia and glycosuria. When sugar is not at hand, as it always should be, any other carbohydrate food—such as orange juice or bread—can be taken. The latter, however, being more slowly absorbed, is less effective in dealing with the emergency of hypoglycæmia than sugar or orange juice. A drink of water should always be taken with the sugar in order to facilitate its rapid absorption.

In the great majority of cases these measures are rapidly effective. Occasionally, however, a case of severe hypoglycæmia is encountered who is in deep coma and unable to swallow. In such circumstances a subcutaneous injection of $\frac{1}{2}$ to 1 c.c. of adrenalin (solution 1 : 1000) should be given. This converts any available glycogen into glucose, thereby raising the blood sugar. This procedure is usually effective in rousing the patient from his coma sufficiently to permit him to swallow carbohydrate food, which should be given, if possible, in the form of glucose or sugar in orange juice. An intravenous injection of 400 c.c. of 10 per cent. glucose saline, or the giving of 2 oz. of glucose in 10 oz. of water by stomach tube, are measures which are seldom necessary, but may very occasionally have to be resorted to in exceptionally severe cases. The giving of rectal glucose salines, which is sometimes advocated, is a very slow and uncertain method of raising the blood sugar and is not to be recommended in such emergencies.

All patients taking insulin should have the symptoms of hypoglycæmia carefully explained to them, and should be thoroughly conversant with the methods of dealing with it. Some careless patients who do not take their disease sufficiently seriously may have to have the dangers of hypoglycæmia stressed to them. We believe, however, that many doctors overstress the dangers of hypoglycæmia, causing their patients to become unduly alarmed about it. This exaggerated terror of hypoglycæmia is responsible for much insufficient dosage, or even for insulin administration being withheld or stopped, with disastrous consequences. Thus the slightest, and often imaginary, feelings of discomfort are sometimes made the excuse by the patient for a debauch on sugar ; or again, if some gastric upset renders a patient temporarily unfit for his ordinary diet, insulin is often discontinued altogether from fear of hypoglycæmia. This is one of the most fruitful causes of diabetic coma. When a patient becomes unfit for his ordinary diet a light fluid diet should be substituted (see p. 386), and if necessary the ordinary dose of insulin may be appropriately reduced, but should never be discontinued as long as sugar is present in the urine. Where the digestion is upset as the result of an infection, the insulin requirements should be increased rather than diminished. It should always be remembered that while the number of deaths from diabetic coma are legion, those from hypoglycæmia are so rare as to be clinical curiosities.

Diabetics taking insulin are often recommended to suspend a card round their necks giving information as to their diabetic condition, along with their name, address and the name of their doctor or the clinic which they are attending, attached. This is a good plan in case they should be found unconscious by strangers, but before recommending it the temperament of the patient must be taken into consideration. The wearing of such a card will act as a psychological trauma to certain patients, continually reminding them that they are not as other men are and exaggerating in their minds the dangers which they run. For patients who are likely to look upon such a card as though it was the mark of the beast, it is much better to run the very slight risk of dispensing with it, than the more real risk of converting them into hypochondriacal neurotics.

Hypoglycæmia may be due to a natural improvement in sugar tolerance, to unaccustomed physical activity on the part of the patient, or to the fact that he has missed or been too late in taking his meal or that he has taken too little of it. When it is simply due to the dose of insulin being excessive, this should be reduced on the succeeding day by 2 or 4 units, depending on the severity of the symptoms, or alternatively the carbohydrate in the diet may be appropriately increased where this is desirable.

Insulin Dosage.—It is quite impossible to lay down rigid rules as regards the dose of insulin. Probably the majority of cases who require insulin take from 15 to 50 units a day, but the dosage depends on the severity of each individual's disease and his dietetic requirements. When less than 8 units are required, the adult diabetic can usually be controlled by making some slight modification in his diet without having recourse to insulin. When diets are properly controlled, it is exceptional for a diabetic to need more than 90 units a day, though occasionally refractory cases will be encountered who are extremely resistant to insulin and who may require, for a time at least, enormous doses.

Sometimes a single injection of from 10 to 15 units of soluble insulin a day, given before the principal carbohydrate-containing meal, is all that is required to keep the urine "sugar-free" throughout the twenty-four hours. The majority of diabetics, however, who require insulin need two injections a day—provided they are taking the soluble variety of insulin—one before breakfast and another before their evening meal, while severe cases will require insulin before breakfast, dinner and supper. It is no doubt true that where a very large total dose is required in the twenty-four hours, this can often be considerably reduced and the hyperglycæmia more efficiently controlled by giving the insulin four instead of three times a day. While this may be feasible in hospital, it is so extremely inconvenient to a patient attempting to live an ordinary life outside an institution, that any slight advantage to be gained by giving insulin so frequently is more than offset by its practical disadvantages. With the advent of zinc protamine insulin, the giving of frequent doses of soluble insulin should never be contemplated, except in emergencies such as severe diabetic ketosis.

When it has been determined that a patient requires insulin, and soluble insulin is to be used, it is well to start in the average case with 10 units before breakfast and 6 or 8 units at supper time—the greater part of the carbohydrate for the day being given at these two meals. For the next three days a mixed twenty-four hour specimen of urine is tested, and if this does not show a significant reduction in the glycosuria, the dose is gradually increased by 2 units at a time. In severe cases, of course, a larger initial dose and larger increases will be necessary. The breakfast insulin should be increased more freely than the evening dose, since it has to control the blood sugar throughout the day when meals are being taken. When the twenty-four hour specimen still contains some sugar, but in an obviously reduced amount, more frequent urine tests can be made to determine at what time or times in the twenty-four hours the leak of sugar is occurring. Once the time at which the glycosuria is appearing has been discovered, an increase in the preceding dose of insulin can be made, or the carbohydrate in the diet can be restricted or appropriately redistributed. In severe cases it may be found that the morning insulin does not control the hyperglycæmia in the afternoon and that the dose cannot be further increased owing to the occurrence of hypoglycæmic symptoms before the midday meal. In such a condition, the morning insulin should be somewhat reduced so as to abolish the midday hypoglycæmia, and a small dose of insulin can be given before the midday meal to abolish the glycosuria of the afternoon. As we shall see, however, the use of zinc protamine insulin should usually make the necessity of giving three doses of soluble insulin quite superfluous. Once the glycosuria is abolished, it is often possible in the succeeding weeks gradually to reduce the dose which was originally required to render the patient "sugar-free." In the absence of hypoglycæmia this reduction should, however, be done very gradually or hyperglycæmia will recur.

Just as the dose of insulin required by different patients varies very widely, so, to a slightly less extent, may the individual patient's insulin requirements vary from time to time. It is true that once certain cases have been stabilized on diet and insulin, they may go on satisfactorily year after year on the same diet and the same dose of insulin without requiring any modification of either. Such patients are usually middle-aged or elderly, for the sugar tolerance of younger diabetics is usually much less stable. We have already seen that improvement in sugar tolerance, and therefore in insulin dosage, may often take place during the first few months of treatment after an initial hyperglycæmia has been satisfactorily controlled. In some cases, however, whether as the result of inefficient control, intercurrent infections or, for no apparent reason, the sugar tolerance may deteriorate rather than improve, and the patient may require progressively larger and larger doses. In other cases the sugar tolerance fluctuates depending on the general state of the patient's health, mental stresses and strains, and physical activity, all of which may demand alterations in insulin dosage from time to time. It is a common experience, for example, for a diabetic business man who may take little exercise during the week to require rather less insulin during the week-ends when he may take very much more exercise than usual.

The Use of Blood-sugar Tests in Treatment

It is commonly believed that diabetes mellitus cannot be treated satisfactorily without the use of blood-sugar examinations. We believe, contrary to many authorities, that practically all the information required for treating the average case efficiently may be obtained by frequent urine examinations, without undertaking examinations of the blood, which are distasteful to the patient, frequently impracticable outside an institution or large centre, and which, in our opinion, need only be resorted to in certain exceptional circumstances. The method of examining twenty-four hour specimens, and, where necessary, each specimen of urine passed, until the suitable diet—and possibly the suitable dose of insulin—for the patient has been established, has a wide application, since any reasonably intelligent patient, after he has been taught to test his urine by Benedict's or Fehling's method, can make the necessary observations for himself. Nor do we think it necessary to estimate the amount of sugar passed in the urine by quantitative methods. It is held by some that in this way the amount of insulin required can be accurately calculated on the principle that 1 unit of insulin looks after 2 gm. of glucose. In practice, however, this is such a very approximate statement that with experience the dose of insulin can be gauged just as accurately by the appearance of the patient and the result of the Fehling test—whether brown, yellow or green. Once the diet and the insulin dosage suitable for the patient have been established by the method of frequent urine sampling, the testing of a urine specimen night and morning, with an occasional qualitative analysis of a twenty-four hour specimen, is sufficient for practical purposes.

The objection to the method of controlling dietetic and insulin therapy by analysis of the urine alone lies in the fact that it yields information only that the blood sugar is below or above the renal threshold of the patient. In diabetics this threshold may be raised very considerably, so that a significant hyperglycæmia may exist without any sugar being present in the urine. We have repeatedly observed, for example, in old-standing diabetics, fasting blood-sugar values of between 200 and 300 mg. per 100 c.c. without glycosuria being present. It has not yet been definitely established whether hyperglycæmia, moderate enough to show no glycosuria, should be treated as a matter of great significance. The majority of workers believe that it should be, holding that any degree of hyperglycæmia may cause further retrogression of sugar tolerance, and that it may be a factor in producing the arterial degenerations so common in the senile type of diabetic. On the other hand, it is possible that in diabetes of long standing the organs and tissues have become acclimatized to working at their optimal efficiency with a slightly higher blood-sugar level than normal, and that this hyperglycæmia may not, therefore, be entirely harmful. Certainly in many cases an attempt to keep the blood sugar of an old-standing diabetic within strictly normal limits causes, as we have seen, hypoglycæmic symptoms to occur, and the patient feels less well than when a moderate hyperglycæmia, though without glycosuria, is allowed to persist. Though occasional blood-sugar examinations may be ideal, we believe that for all practical purposes the diet and insulin should be so regulated that sugar does not appear in the urine, and that the treatment of the average case can be carried out perfectly satisfactorily by examination of the urine alone.

One of the exceptions to this rule is to be found in the case of a true diabetic with a low renal threshold for sugar. A high threshold for sugar is much more common in diabetics than a low threshold, but the latter is occasionally found and such cases are most difficult to treat, since any attempt to keep the urine entirely free from sugar is usually followed by hypoglycæmic symptoms. In such cases, therefore, glycosuria may occur even when the blood sugar is perfectly normal, and efficient treatment cannot be conducted by urine analysis alone, but demands blood-sugar estimations as well. These estimations should be carried out on the early morning fasting blood, which gives an indication as to the adequacy of the evening dose of insulin, and on a specimen of blood taken four hours after the morning dose, at which time the effect of the morning insulin should be maximal. The tests should be done once every two months, or more often while the case is being stabilized. A fasting blood sugar under 160 mg. per cent. should be looked upon as satisfactory, as should a midday specimen of under 130 mg. per cent. Higher figures suggest that the preceding doses of insulin can be increased. No attempt should be made to reduce the early morning blood sugar below 130 mg. per cent. or the midday specimen below 110 mg. per cent.

The Treatment of Diabetic Coma

Diabetic coma is practically always preventable, and should never occur where an intelligent patient is under efficient treatment. Occasionally it may occur in an undiagnosed untreated case; sometimes it is due to simple disregard of treatment by the patient or to grossly ineffective treatment on the part of the doctor; more often it is the result of gastro-intestinal upsets, infections or surgical operations in diabetics who are being adequately treated for all ordinary occasions, but whose treatment is not sufficiently elastic to cope with such emergencies.

Diabetic coma is a medical emergency whose treatment demands the constant attendance and care of the physician. In severe cases it requires skilled nursing and technical assistance, which are not easily procured outside a hospital or nursing home. It is a condition where expert treatment may make all the difference between the life and death of the patient. In the majority of severe cases, therefore, where skilled institutional treatment can be procured, it is well to transfer the patient to hospital after first-aid treatment in the form of an adequate injection of insulin has been given by the practitioner.

The sheet anchors of treatment in diabetic coma are to eradicate the ketosis by giving insulin and glucose, and to combat the invariable dehydration and circulatory collapse by giving fluids. In addition, it is often wise to wash out the stomach where vomiting is occurring; to clear the bowel where constipation is present, which is usually the case; and to search for and—when present—to evacuate pus, or to treat any associated infection which may have been the original cause of the coma.

Where the patient is still able to swallow and to retain fluids given by the mouth, the treatment of early diabetic coma is comparatively simple. Fifty units of soluble insulin should be given subcutaneously at once. Too often quite insufficient doses of insulin are administered in this emergency from fear of inducing hypoglycæmia. There is little danger of this in the early stages of treatment. If the means are not immediately at hand, it is not even absolutely essential to give glucose along with this original dose, though it is wise to do so. It is true that the blood sugar is high in diabetic coma, yet the body as a whole is depleted of sugar, and, theoretically, comparatively small doses of insulin ought to be sufficient to lower the blood sugar to hypoglycæmic levels unless adequate covering doses of glucose are given at once. In practice, however, a patient in diabetic coma is extremely tolerant to insulin, and in the early stages of treatment large doses can be given freely without any danger of the patient slipping imperceptibly from the coma of ketosis to that of hypoglycæmia, provided the urine is tested prior to each injection and sugar is always found to be present. After the initial large dose of insulin, at least 20 units should be given two-hourly as long as severe ketosis is present. These subsequent doses should be covered in each case by the oral administration of 20 gm. of glucose in solution or its equivalent. The use of zinc protamine insulin as an adjuvant to soluble insulin in the treatment of diabetic coma is referred to on p. 362. Feeds of common carbohydrate foodstuffs approximately equal to 25 gm. of glucose are given on p. 380. It should be remembered in selecting the appropriate food that strong sugar solutions are apt to cause vomiting, and, where this is a feature of the case, it is better to give—instead of glucose or ordinary sugar—feeds of Benger's Food. If possible, specimens of urine should be procured and tested prior to each injection of insulin, the dose being increased or decreased according to the reaction of the urine. The object to be aimed at is a rapid diminution of the ketonuria with a slow decrease of the glycosuria. It is, of course, ideal to have in addition frequent estimations of the blood sugar. Where this is possible, the suitable dose of insulin can be gauged with great accuracy.

When the patient comes out of coma, a light diet containing not less than 120 gm. of carbohydrate with a low fat content can be given for a day or two with appropriate doses of insulin three or four times a day. An example of such a diet is given on p. 381, and the same diet will be found suitable for severe cases of diabetic ketosis who are in danger of coma and for diabetics who may be temporarily unfit to take their ordinary diet owing to gastro-intestinal upsets or intercurrent infections. As long as the ketonuria is controlled, no serious attempt need be made at this stage to get the patient "sugar-free" till he is again fit to take his normal diet.

All patients in diabetic coma are profoundly dehydrated owing to the polyuria which has always preceded the condition, and to the vomiting with which it is so often associated. Evidence of this dehydration is to be found in the dry skin, leathery tongue, high blood urea and collapsed veins of the patient, and in the profound fall in blood pressure and intra-ocular pressure which also occur. The treatment of this dehydration and its associated circulatory collapse is almost as important as the treatment of the ketosis itself, but is often forgotten or treated inadequately. Not infrequently patients recover from their ketosis as the result of sufficient insulin and glucose treatment, but die from circulatory failure—the result of insufficient attention to their dehydrated state. Where the patient can swallow and retain fluid, very large quantities of water should be given by the mouth, with frequent drinks of hot tea or coffee. The retention of such fluids is frequently made possible by an initial gastric lavage, preferably with a weak solution of bicarbonate of soda. Where circulatory collapse is severe and the pulse is very feeble, the injection of 1 c.c. of coramine or 7 minims of adrenalin (solution 1 : 1,000) is often useful. In addition, salines should be given rectally or subcutaneously where it is not possible to give them intravenously, which is infinitely preferable.

Where the patient is in deep coma and unable to swallow, at least 80 units of insulin should be given as an initial dose, 20 to 50 of which can be given intravenously. In such cases, and in cases where intractable vomiting is present, it is ideal to give glucose and fluids intravenously. Two pints of 5 per cent. glucose saline solution (1 drachm of salt and 2 oz. of glucose in 1 pint of clean water, boil; cool to 108° F.) are run in slowly, using the technique described on p. 1075. In such cases circulatory collapse is usually a marked feature, and it is beneficial to add 3 minims of adrenalin (solution 1 : 1,000) to the transfusion. The veins of patients in deep diabetic coma are unfortunately so collapsed that it is generally impossible to administer the transfusion without cutting down upon one of them and inserting a cannula.

This procedure may have to be repeated in three hours if

the patient has not come out of coma sufficiently to permit of him being fed by the mouth, by the method described above.

The administration of subcutaneous glucose salines (for technique see p. 1070) is a poor substitute for intravenous therapy in such an emergency, but may have to be resorted to where, for one reason or another, intravenous treatment is impossible. It is, however, an additional method of introducing fluid and glucose, and may make a second intravenous transfusion unnecessary.

It is often recommended that as an alternative method glucose salines can be given per rectum, either in quantities of 8 oz. every few hours or by a Murphy drip. Except as another method of supplying fluid, we believe that this is of no service, and that the blood sugar is not affected to any significant extent by glucose given in this way.

Zinc Protamine Insulin

We have seen that the transient, if powerful, action of soluble insulin makes it necessary to give frequent injections to a severe case of diabetes in order to maintain the blood sugar at a relatively constant level throughout the twenty-four hours. As it is impracticable to give as a routine measure more than three injections in the day, patients with severe diabetes tend to oscillate between hyperglycæmia on the one hand and hypoglycæmia on the other. Some degree of hyperglycæmia is indeed almost unavoidable during the night, when such cases convert their endogenous protein into carbohydrate, thereby raising their fasting blood sugars.

Numerous efforts have therefore been made to prolong the action of insulin. These were all more or less unsuccessful till Hagedorn discovered that protamine prepared from the sperm of trout would combine with insulin to form protamine insulinate. When properly buffered this was found to be sparingly soluble in tissue fluids and, when given hypodermically, broke down slowly, gradually releasing insulin, which thus exerted an effect on the blood sugar for twelve to fifteen hours after its injection, in comparison to soluble insulin whose effect is not apparent for much more than six hours. Subsequently it was discovered by Scott that the addition to the insulin protamine mixture of minute traces of zinc, which is an essential constituent of the insulin crystal, still further prolongs the effect of protamine insulin. Thus a dose of zinc protamine insulin has a significant action for at least twenty-six hours after its injection. It is therefore still mildly effective at breakfast-time on the day subsequent to that of the injection, and the hyperglycæmia which tends to occur in severe cases during the night is more adequately controlled by its use.

At present Z.P. insulin is the only insulin besides soluble insulin generally used in this country, the use of Hagedorn's original protamine insulin having been largely discontinued. Z.P. insulin is dispensed in two strengths: the one most commonly used contains 40 units to the cubic centimetre, but where large doses have to be taken an 80-unit strength can be obtained. These two strengths are sometimes unfortunately referred to as "single" and "double" strength, but in comparison to soluble insulin, which is dispensed in 20, 40 and 80 unit strengths, it is apparent that they are really double and quadruple strength respectively. A confusion of terms is thus arising which is unfortunate and dangerous.

The varying actions of soluble and Z.P. insulin are best illustrated by their effects on the twenty-four hour blood-sugar curves of patients during the transition period from soluble to Z.P. insulin.

The first set of curves were taken from a relatively mild case of diabetes with sufficient endogenous insulin to regulate the fasting metabolism, but insufficient to deal with the added load of carbohydrate derived from meals. Such patients did comparatively well in the old days on Allen's starvation diets, as their blood sugars tend to fall during fasting. The second set of curves were procured from a severe case of diabetes with insufficient endogenous insulin to deal either with the fasting metabolism or with the added carbohydrate of meals. Such cases are intolerant of starvation and proved rapidly fatal in pre-insulin days as their blood sugars rise during fasting.

It will be seen from Chart I that the mild case, with a relatively low fasting blood sugar, was quite effectively controlled during the twenty-four hours by two injections of 10 units of soluble insulin given before the chief carbohydrate-containing meals of the day. The only disadvantage to soluble insulin in such cases lies in the inconvenience of the two injections, and perhaps in the fact that only very small amounts of carbohydrate can be allowed at the midday meal and at tea-time. When the two 10-unit doses of insulin are combined in a single dose of 20 units of Z.P. insulin, and the total carbohydrate allowance for the day is spread out uniformly throughout the various meals, the blood sugar is perhaps rather more evenly controlled, but the main advantage lies in the convenience of the single injection and possibly in the more natural distribution of the carbohydrate.

It will be seen from Chart II that for the first day or so after the transference to Z.P. insulin a transient glycosuria occurred after breakfast, owing to the fact that the action of Z.P. insulin is slow, and, to begin with, is insufficient to cope

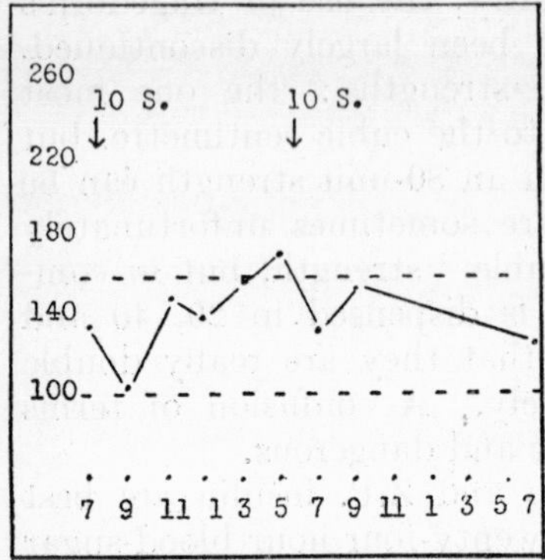

CHART I.—Twenty-four hour blood-sugar estimations on moderate case of diabetes adequately controlled by 10 units of soluble insulin given night and morning.

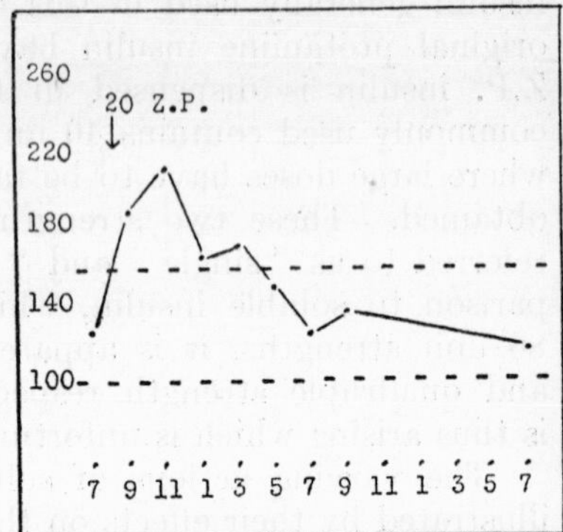

CHART II.—Same case on day of conversion to 20 units of Z.P. insulin. Note breakfast hyperglycæmia.

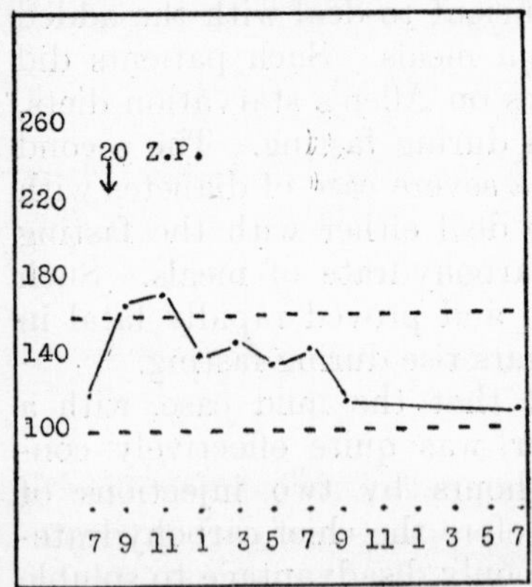

CHART III.—Same case a day later.

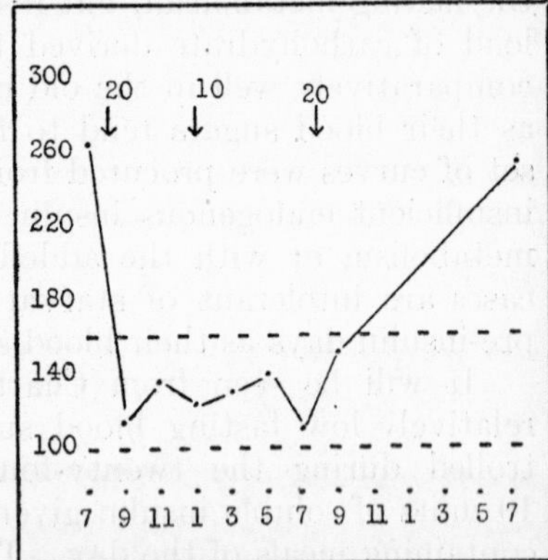

CHART IV.—Twenty-four hour blood-sugar estimations on a severe case of diabetes receiving three doses of soluble insulin. Note inadequate control during the night, resulting in a high-fasting blood sugar.

with the breakfast carbohydrate. On the third day, however, as is shown in Chart III, this hyperglycæmia was practically controlled, and after a few more days the dose of Z.P. insulin could be reduced so that the patient was eventually stabilized on a single dose of 16 units.

Chart IV represents the twenty-four hour blood-sugar curve of a relatively severe case of diabetes. The blood sugar was well controlled during the day by three injections of soluble insulin, but after the effect of the last dose had worn off hyperglycæmia occurred during the night. It is true that

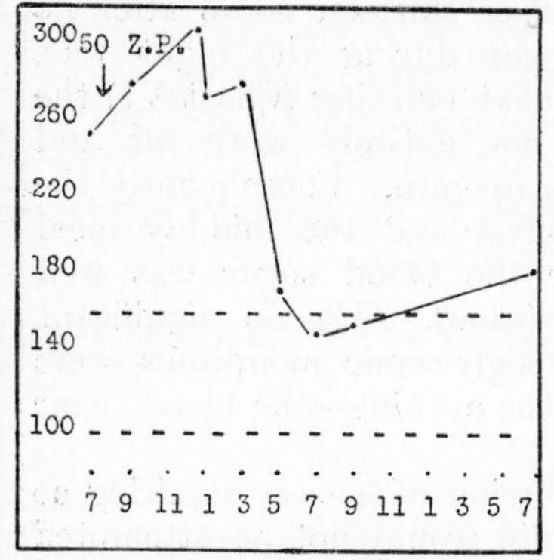

CHART V.—Same case on day of conversion to Z.P. insulin. Note severe morning hyperglycæmia.

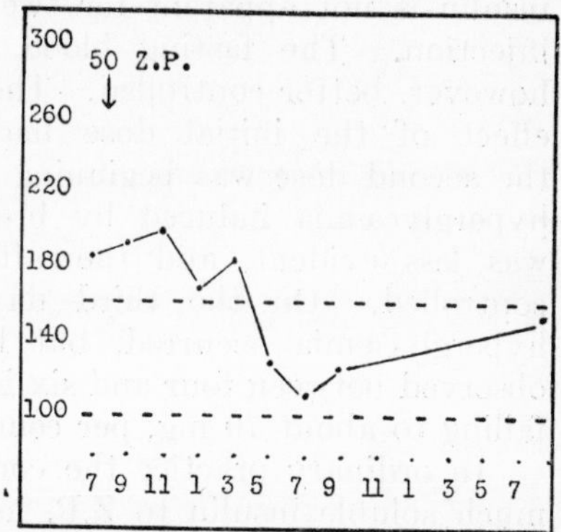

CHART VI.—Same case a day later.

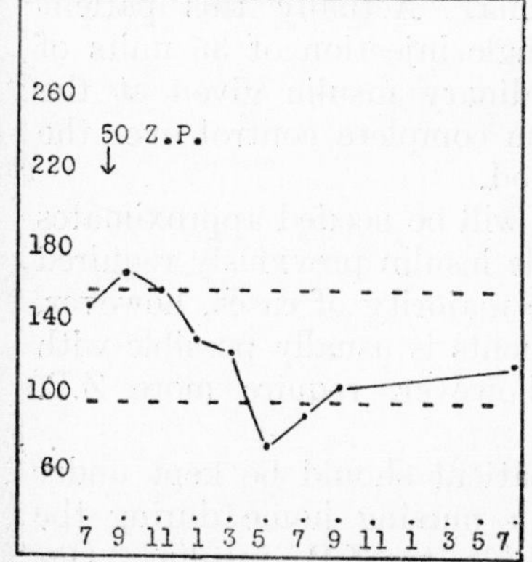

CHART VII.—Same case two days later. Note evening hypoglycæmia.

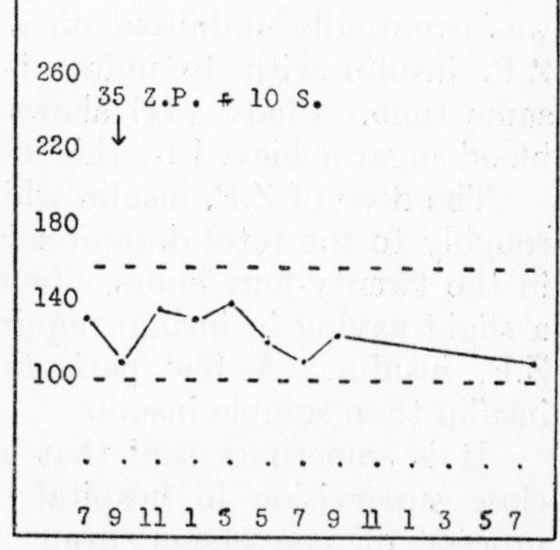

CHART VIII.—Same case eventually stabilized on 35 units of Z.P. insulin plus 10 units of soluble insulin.

a fourth dose of insulin given late at night would have solved the problem. Three injections a day, however, are bad enough, but four are apt to produce a hypochondriacal invalid, and the treatment is often worse than the disease. In such cases the use of Z.P. insulin is a blessing not only because of convenience, but because a superior control of the blood sugar can often be obtained throughout the twenty-four hours.

Chart V shows the blood-sugar curve of the same case on the day of conversion to a single dose of 50 units of Z.P. insulin, in place of three doses totalling 50 units of soluble insulin. It will be seen that a marked hyperglycæmia occurred during the first part of the day, as the maximum effect of the Z.P. insulin is not apparent for twelve or thirteen hours after its injection. The fasting blood sugar during the night was, however, better controlled. The next morning (Chart VI) the effect of the initial dose had not entirely worn off and the second dose was beginning to operate. Consequently the hyperglycæmia induced by breakfast and the midday meal was less evident, and thereafter the blood sugar was well controlled. On the third day (Chart VII) no significant hyperglycæmia occurred, but hypoglycæmic symptoms were observed between four and six in the evening—the blood sugar falling to about 70 mg. per cent.

In ordinary practice the conversion of a case requiring so much soluble insulin to Z.P. insulin would not be attempted in this way. Three-quarters of the total dose of soluble insulin would be given as Z.P. insulin and the other quarter would be given as soluble insulin, thereby diminishing to a large extent the morning hyperglycæmia. Actually this patient was eventually stabilized on a single injection of 35 units of Z.P. insulin with 10 units of ordinary insulin given at the same time. Chart VIII shows the complete control over the blood sugar achieved by this method.

The dose of Z.P. insulin which will be needed approximates roughly to the total dose of soluble insulin previously required in the twenty-four hours. In the majority of cases, however, a slight saving in insulin requirements is usually possible with Z.P. insulin. A few patients, however, require more Z.P. insulin than soluble insulin.

It is sometimes said that a patient should be kept under close supervision in hospital or a nursing home during the process of conversion from soluble to Z.P. insulin. Our experience does not suggest that this is necessary except in difficult cases who previously required very large doses of soluble insulin. Indeed, patients who have been stabilized on insulin in hospital frequently have to be stabilized afresh when they become out-patients, since the amount of insulin necessary to control them while leading a sedentary institutional existence is often considerably in excess of that required when they again take up active life.

It is necessary, however, to see out-patients at frequent intervals while the conversion from soluble to Z.P. insulin is being carried out. In individual cases the previous total dose of soluble insulin gives only a rough estimate of the amount of Z.P. insulin which will eventually be required; most patients, as has been said, require less, while a few require more. Where the total dose of soluble insulin was small—25 units or less—the patient can be started on the same dose of Z.P. insulin, to be altered as required later. Where a larger total dose of soluble insulin was needed, it is wiser, in order to avoid a morning and midday hyperglycæmia during the process of conversion, to start with three-quarters of the dose in the form of Z.P. insulin, the other quarter being given as soluble insulin. This latter can often be abandoned in a few days, the dose of Z.P. insulin being perhaps increased as the other is withdrawn. In severe cases, however, it is often impossible to give a dose of Z.P. insulin big enough to ensure absence of hyperglycæmia throughout the day without inducing hypoglycæmia at some time in the twenty-four hours. An example of this was shown in Chart VII. In such cases, therefore, a small dose of soluble insulin has to be continued to deal with the hyperglycæmia induced by the breakfast carbohydrate, the dose of Z.P. insulin being appropriately reduced to avoid hypoglycæmic symptoms in the evening or at night. As might be expected, the patients who require soluble insulin in addition to their Z.P. insulin are to be found mostly in the younger age groups.

Z.P. insulin should be given as early as is convenient before breakfast. Where soluble insulin has to be given in addition to Z.P. insulin it is injected first. The syringe is then disconnected from the needle, which is left sticking in the thigh, a new needle is fitted to the syringe and the dose of Z.P. insulin is sucked in. The syringe is then once more connected to the original needle and the Z.P. insulin is injected. Thus the two forms of insulin are not mixed in the syringe, but the patient only gives himself one prick with the needle. This technique has been adopted as experience has shown that it is difficult to measure accurately a dose taken from two rubber-capped vials into the same syringe.

A new case of diabetes when first seen can be started straight away on Z.P. insulin alone, provided the case is a moderate one and in no immediate danger of ketosis. Ten or twelve units can be given to begin with and the dose may be appropriately increased by 4 units at a time. Additions to the dose, however, should be made much more gradually than in the case of soluble insulin on account of the "hang-over" action of the Z.P. insulin.

It is probably wise to allow four days to elapse between each increase in dosage.

If the new case, however, is a severe one with a significant quantity of acetone in the urine, it is necessary to get the blood sugar under control more rapidly than is possible by the use of Z.P. insulin alone. This can be done by using soluble insulin entirely to begin with and then, when the patient is stabilized, conversion to Z.P. insulin, or to Z.P. insulin plus soluble insulin, can be carried out. An example of such a case is shown in the accompanying table.

Date	Sugar	Acetone	Insulin
19.5	+ +	+	20.10.15 = 45
20.5	+	tr.	18. 6.14 = 38
21.5	tr.	-	18. 8.14 = 40
22.5	-	-	20. 6.12 = 38
23.5	tr.	-	26 Z.P. + 10
24.5	-	-	24 Z.P. + 10
25.5	-	-	24 Z.P. + 6
26.5	-	-	20 Z.P.
27.5	-	-	20 Z.P.
28.5	-	-	18 Z.P.
29.5	-	-	18 Z.P.
30.5	-	-	16 Z.P.

To show method of controlling an acute case of diabetes by the use first of soluble insulin and then of Z.P. insulin.

The majority of patients express themselves as feeling better and more energetic on Z.P. insulin, and the beneficial psychological effect of having only one injection instead of two or three in the day is often very marked. No doubt much of the sense of well-being which severe diabetics experience on conversion to Z.P. insulin is due to the fact that soluble insulin tends in such cases to leave the night hours unprovided with the essentials for the complete combustion of food. Much of the available carbohydrate has already been burned, and the effect of the last injection of insulin has worn off. Thus an undue preponderance of protein and fat are burnt up at this time, and even these are often inefficiently metabolized. In consequence, excessive protein breakdown and mild ketosis occur, and the patient frequently feels weak and ill in the morning. Z.P. insulin in effective doses counteracts this tendency and the patients in consequence may feel considerably better.

Slight modifications have to be made in the diet on conversion of a patient from soluble to Z.P. insulin. If, for instance, a patient on soluble insulin night and morning is receiving 5 oz. of bread in the day, 2 oz. would be given at breakfast, 2 oz. at supper and 1 oz. at tea-time. When the same patient is given Z.P. insulin, the carbohydrate should be apportioned equally to the various meals.

The continuous gentle action of zinc protamine insulin is ill-suited to cope with the sudden strain of a high carbohydrate meal. Thus when large quantities of carbohydrate are being prescribed, it must be spread out in small feeds throughout the day—a little being given on waking, at breakfast, at 11 A.M., at the midday meal, at tea-time, at supper and on going to bed at night. Such frequent feeding is inconvenient to most patients, and it is probable that very high carbohydrate diets are less suitable for use with Z.P. insulin than those containing from 115 to 150 gm.

It is sometimes said that Z.P. insulin is ideal for the elderly diabetic, but is less effective in the young case with an unstable blood-sugar tolerance. It is, of course, true that elderly diabetics are more easy to control with Z.P. insulin than younger ones, but exactly the same can be said of soluble insulin. It is probable that there is no contraindication to Z.P. insulin as far as age is concerned. Children, indeed, respond well to it, and the great psychological advantage of giving only one injection a day to a child makes Z.P. insulin peculiarly suitable for such cases.

It is probably unwise to convert to Z.P. insulin elderly unintelligent diabetics who, year after year, have kept themselves sugar-free on two doses of soluble insulin a day. Such diabetics are frequently very conservative by nature, and object to an alteration in their routine which may have a temporary effect in upsetting their sugar tolerance. A few patients also, such as shepherds and gamekeepers who have extremely irregular meal times, are better with soluble insulin, since they do not take this until they are at home and ready for a meal. Z.P. insulin given to such patients in the morning may produce hypoglycæmic symptoms if they are unable to get home for their supper at the usual hour. Occasionally a case may be found who is definitely refractory to Z.P. insulin, due probably to some abnormality in absorption. Such cases are, however, extremely rare.

Hypoglycæmic reactions are rather less numerous with Z.P. insulin than with soluble insulin. The same patients who show a tendency to reactions with soluble insulin are most liable to reactions with Z.P. insulin and vice versa. When marked reactions *do* occur with Z.P. insulin they are, however, more severe than with soluble insulin and more difficult to treat, the patients tending to slip back again into coma after they have been brought out of it, unless large amounts of glucose are given.

The reactions produced by Z.P. insulin are very different symptomatically to those due to soluble insulin, and may be, to begin with, puzzling to patients accustomed to the ordinary insulin reactions. Failure to recognize the new symptoms as being due to hypoglycæmia may prevent the patient from taking appropriate measures and a severe coma may ensue. Many of the symptoms of soluble insulin hypoglycæmia are due to endogenous adrenalin which is secreted in an attempt to raise the blood sugar. In consequence sweating, palpitation and tremors are the characteristic features of such reactions. Hypoglycæmia produced by Z.P. insulin, on the other hand, comes on so slowly that this outpouring of endogenous adrenalin does not occur to the same extent, and general malaise, nausea, vomiting and, particularly, headache are the symptoms most commonly experienced—sweating, palpitation and tremor being much less usual. Patients should be suitably warned of these novel features of hypoglycæmia before being given Z.P. insulin. Reactions with Z.P. insulin may occur at any time during the twenty-four hours, but are more frequent in the evening and at night than during the morning.

As we have seen, exercise enables a diabetic to do with less insulin than when he is leading a sedentary existence, and unusual physical exertion is a common cause of hypoglycæmia. When soluble insulin is being taken, the dose immediately prior to strenuous exercise should be slightly reduced, but with Z.P. insulin it is wiser to eat a little more carbohydrate prior to such exercise rather than to reduce the morning dose.

It is apparent that Z.P. insulin alone, owing to its slow action, is unsuitable to cope with the emergency of diabetic coma. It is, however, a valuable aid to soluble insulin in dealing with such cases. An injection of about 40 units of Z.P. insulin given at the beginning of treatment along with 40 or 50 units of soluble insulin will cause a smoother fall in the blood sugar and a more rapid disappearance of the ketosis than when soluble insulin alone is given. The case is otherwise treated exactly as described on p. 351, though it may be found possible to give rather smaller quantities of soluble insulin. Charts IX and X show the blood-sugar concentrations of two very comparable cases of coma taken over two days, the one treated with soluble insulin alone, the other with soluble insulin combined on occasion with Z.P. insulin. It is apparent that the blood sugar is much more uniformly reduced in the latter case.

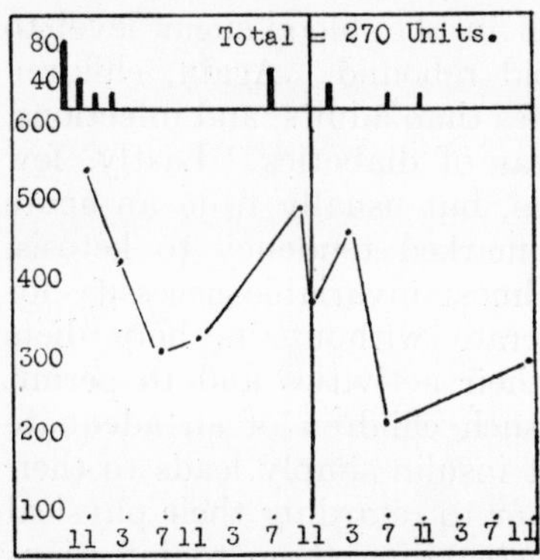

Chart IX.—Forty-eight hour blood-sugar estimations on a case of diabetic coma controlled by soluble insulin alone.

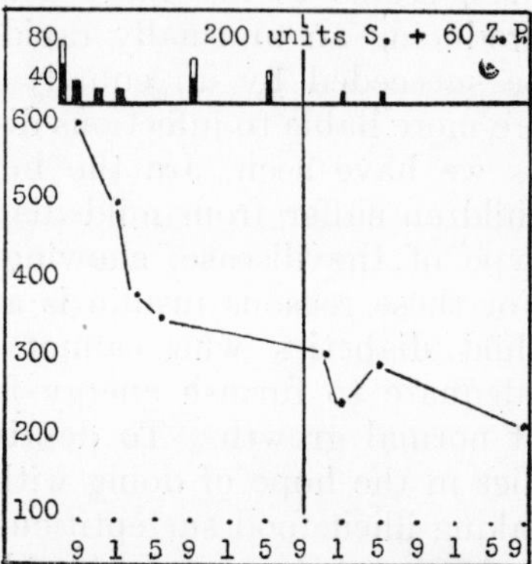

Chart X. — Forty-eight hour blood-sugar estimations on a case of diabetic coma, comparable to that shown in Chart IX., controlled by Z.P. insulin in addition to soluble insulin. Note more even reduction of the hyperglycæmia.

DIABETES IN CHILDREN

Diabetes may occur at any age, but it is relatively uncommon in children, especially in young children. This is fortunate, for the treatment of the diabetic child is much more difficult than that of the adult for a variety of reasons. It is impossible, for example, to stabilize a child for a long time on a standard diet and a fixed dose of insulin, as it is often possible to do in the case of an adult, for his nutritional needs are continually altering according to his changing development.

To provide for his growth and energy requirements, a child needs relatively much higher diets than an adult in respect of protein, carbohydrate and total calories, and a generous supply of milk must be given. A high fat intake, however, especially in young children, is often poorly tolerated, producing ketosis and fatty stools, and large quantities of green vegetables are often insufficiently digested. Further, just as a child's temperature is notoriously unstable, so his sugar tolerance is much more variable from day to day than that of an adult. This may be accounted for to some extent by the uncontrolled temper of children and by the great variation in their physical activity from one moment to another. Thus the passionate tears, the transports of joy, the wild excitements and intense activities, which characterize the life of children from time to time, have profound effects on their sugar tolerance. Insulin itself seems to act more acutely in children than in adults, producing an unusually rapid fall in the blood-sugar level to be succeeded by an equally rapid rebound. Again, children are more liable to infectious diseases than adults, and infections, as we have seen, are the bugbear of diabetics. Lastly, few children suffer from mild diabetes, but usually from an acute type of the disease, showing a marked tendency to ketosis. For these reasons insulin is an almost invariable necessity for child diabetics who cannot tolerate without its help diets adequate to furnish energy for their activities and to permit of normal growth. To deprive such children of an adequate diet in the hope of doing without insulin simply leads to their taking illicit food surreptitiously, or to retarding their physical and mental development and predisposing them to infections such as tuberculosis.

The difficulties in treating diabetes in children are, however, by no means insurmountable, and with the help of insulin and wise dietetics there is no reason why they should not live a normal life and grow into strong and healthy adults. It is very important to take the child himself into the doctor's and parent's councils, to treat him as an intelligent person and to give him a sense of responsibility in regard to his own health. Children respond well to such treatment and frequently become the best diabetic patients. Parents, indeed, may be to some extent comforted by the assurance that the self-control and discipline inculcated by their child's training in good diabetic habits will stand him in good stead in the future.

Calories.—In prescribing the calories for the diabetic child there are various aspects which must be kept constantly in mind. An excessive caloric intake is always harmful from the diabetic standpoint, since overeating will make an unnecessary demand upon the pancreas no matter whether the calories are derived from carbohydrate, protein or fat. On the other hand, the child must have sufficient food to satisfy his appetite, to meet his requirements for energy and to allow for growth. The diet must be regularly adjusted to meet these needs, since a normal rate of growth and increase in weight should be aimed at. Unfortunately, stunted growth in a diabetic

TABLE III (*a*)

Boys—

Age.	3 ft. 3	3 ft. 4	3 ft. 5	3 ft. 6	3 ft. 7	3 ft. 8	3 ft. 9	3 ft. 10	3 ft. 11	4 ft.	4 ft. 1	4 ft. 2	4 ft. 3	4 ft. 4	4 ft. 5	4 ft. 6	4 ft. 7	4 ft. 8	4 ft. 9	4 ft. 10	4 ft. 11	5 ft.	5 ft. 1	5 ft. 2	5 ft. 3	5 ft. 4
5	2 st. 7 *15·88*	2 st. 10 *17·24*	2 st. 11 *17·69*	2 st. 13 *18·6*	3 st. *19·05*	3 st. 4 *20·87*	*kilos.*																			
6		2 st. 8 *16·33*	2 st. 11 *17·69*	2 st. 13 *18·6*	3 st. *19·05*	3 st. 2 *19·96*	3 st. 4 *20·87*	3 st. 6 *21·77*	*kilos.*																	
7					3 st. *19·05*	3 st. 1 *19·51*	3 st. 4 *20·87*	3 st. 6 *21·77*	3 st. 7 *22·23*	3 st. 12 *24·49*	*kilos.*															
8							3 st. 3 *20·41*	3 st. 6 *21·77*	3 st. 8 *22·68*	3 st. 11 *24·04*	3 st. 12 *24·49*	4 st. 1 *25·86*	4 st. 3 *26·76*	*kilos.*												
9									3 st. 8 *22·68*	3 st. 11 *24·04*	3 st. 13 *24·95*	4 st. 2 *26·31*	4 st. 4 *27·22*	4 st. 6 *28·12*	4 st. 6 *28·12*	4 st. 9 *29·48*	*kilos.*									
10										3 st. 11 *24·04*	3 st. 13 *24·95*	4 st. 2 *26·31*	4 st. 4 *27·22*	4 st. 6 *28·12*	4 st. 9 *29·48*	4 st. 12 *30·85*	4 st. 13 *31·30*	5 st. 1 *32·21*	*kilos.*							
11													4 st. 5 *27·67*	4 st. 5 *27·67*	4 st. 9 *29·48*	4 st. 12 *30·85*	5 st. 1 *32·21*	5 st. 7 *34·93*	5 st. 7 *34·93*	5 st. 8 *35·38*	*kilos.*					
12														4 st. 7 *28·58*	4 st. 11 *30·39*	5 st. *31·75*	5 st. 5 *34·02*	5 st. 6 *34·47*	5 st. 9 *35·83*	6 st. *38·1*	6 st. *38·1*	6 st. 1 *38·56*	*kilos.*			
13															4 st. 11 *30·39*	5 st. 1 *32·21*	5 st. 5 *34·02*	5 st. 8 *35·38*	5 st. 10 *36·29*	6 st. 1 *38·56*	6 st. 2 *39·01*	6 st. 7 *41·28*	7 st. *44·45*	7 st. 1 *44·91*	7 st. 2 *45·36*	*kilos.*
14															4 st. 11 *30·39*	5 st. 1 *32·21*	5 st. 6 *34·47*	5 st. 9 *35·83*	5 st. 12 *37·2*	6 st. 2 *39·01*	6 st. 6 *40·82*	6 st. 10 *42·64*	6 st. 13 44	7 st. 5 *46·72*	7 st. 9 *48·54*	8 st. 2 *51·71*

Note.—Remove shoes and outdoor clothes before weighing.

TABLE III (*b*)

Girls—

Age.	3 ft. 3	3 ft. 4	3 ft. 5	3 ft. 6	3 ft. 7	3 ft. 8	3 ft. 9	3 ft. 10	3 ft. 11	4 ft.	4 ft. 1	4 ft. 2	4 ft. 3	4 ft. 4	4 ft. 5	4 ft. 6	4 ft. 7	4 ft. 8	4 ft. 9	4 ft. 10	4 ft. 11	5 ft.	5 ft. 1	5 ft. 2	5 ft. 3	5 ft. 4
5	2 st. 6 *15·42*	2 st. 9 *16·78*	2 st. 10 *17·24*	2 st. 13 *18·6*	2 st. 13 *18·6*	3 st. 3 *20·41*	*kilos.*																			
6		2 st. 7 *15·88*	2 st. 9 *16·78*	2 st. 11 *17·69*	2 st. 13 *18·6*	3 st. 1 *19·51*	3 st. 3 *20·41*	3 st. 6 *21·77*	*kilos.*																	
7				2 st. 11 *17·69*	3 st. *19·05*	3 st. 2 *19·96*	3 st. 3 *20·41*	3 st. 5 *21·32*	3 st. 8 *22·68*	*kilos.*																
8						3 st. *19·05*	3 st. 3 *20·41*	3 st. 5 *21·32*	3 st. 7 *22·23*	3 st. 9 *23·13*	3 st. 11 *24·04*	4 st. *25·4*	*kilos.*													
9									3 st. 7 *22·23*	3 st. 9 *23·13*	3 st. 11 *24·04*	4 st. *25·4*	4 st. 3 *26·76*	4 st. 7 *28·58*	*kilos.*											
10											3 st. 12 *24·49*	4 st. 1 *25·86*	4 st. 2 *26·31*	4 st. 6 *28·12*	4 st. 8 *29·03*	4 st. 13 *31·3*	*kilos.*									
11													4 st. 4 *27·22*	4 st. 6 *28·12*	4 st. 7 *28·58*	4 st. 12 *30·85*	5 st. *31·75*	5 st. 5 *34·02*	*kilos.*							
12														4 st. 7 *28·58*	4 st. 10 *29·94*	4 st. 13 *31·30*	5 st. 1 *32·21*	5 st. 5 *34·02*	5 st. 8 *35·38*	5 st. 13 *37·65*	6 st. 4 *39·92*	6 st. 10 *42·64*	*kilos.*			
13															4 st. 9 *29·48*	4 st. 12 *30·85*	5 st. 3 *33·11*	5 st. 6 *34·47*	5 st. 10 *36·29*	6 st. 2 *39·01*	6 st. 5 *40·37*	6 st. 10 *42·64*	7 st. 1 *44·91*	7 st. 6 *47·17*	*kilos.*	
14																		5 st. 8 *35·38*	5 st. 13 *37·64*	6 st. 4 *39·92*	6 st. 9 *42·19*	6 st. 12 *43·55*	7 st. 2 *45·36*	7 st. 6 *47·17*	7 st. 9 *48·54*	8 st. *50·8*

Note.—Remove shoes and outdoor clothes before weighing.

To face page 365.]

[*To face page* 364.

child cannot always be remedied by additions to the diet, for it is often glandular in origin. Some diabetic children, on the other hand, are abnormally tall for their age and this point must be taken into account when considering their caloric requirements. Other diabetic children tend to become unnaturally fat, especially if they are taking large doses of insulin, and overfeeding has to be carefully guarded against in these cases. It will be seen that age is not the only criterion as to the child's caloric requirements, but it is a useful guide.

By consulting Table III (*a*) and (*b*) it can be ascertained if a child is approximately the average weight for his height and age, and, unless he is very abnormal, he may safely be placed upon one of the standard diets given below. In constructing these diets we have chosen the lower rather than the highest caloric standards (except in the case of the younger children), for many children will be of smaller build than the standard we have taken, and, moreover, the urine can be cleared of sugar at this lower level and if really necessary the diet can then be increased. The diabetic child usually thrives on a number of calories rather below the usual intake of a healthy child. Children of the same age vary considerably in their capacity for food and it is impossible to gauge the appetite exactly. When fixing the child's theoretical requirements it is safest to base the calculation according to the *standard* weight rather than the actual weight for height and age. This will avoid overfeeding the short, fat child and underfeeding the tall lean one.

Protein.—It is obvious that adequate protein is extremely important for children of all ages and any attempt to keep the diabetic child on a minimum allowance is to be deprecated. An unnecessarily high protein intake is also undesirable since it will lessen the tolerance for carbohydrate, and, in children especially, large quantities of meat increase the tendency to acidosis.

Table IV (p. 366) shows the amount of protein believed to be advisable for the normal child. Slight deviations from this standard are immaterial.

Carbohydrate.—The benefit derived from a reduction in carbohydrate in the diabetic diet has already been discussed, and the undesirability of too low an intake has been emphasized. The same principles apply to the treatment of the child diabetic, but a comparatively higher carbohydrate allowance is here desirable. This is required to allow for the necessary pint of milk (which is responsible for 30 gm. of carbohydrate), and, moreover, high fat and low carbohydrate diets are unsuitable for young children.

Under modern treatment the diabetic child receives an adequate amount of fruit, bread and potato, though in our opinion it is advisable to avoid actual sugar and jam, for once a child has forgotten the taste of sugar he is less likely to indulge in sweets. The omission of sugar may be one of the factors responsible for the unusually sound teeth possessed by many young diabetics.

Many diabetic children are now given about 150 gm. of carbohydrate daily. The quantity prescribed in our standard diabetic diets is rather less than this, but has been found to satisfy the majority of diabetic children under our care. Others may require the higher figure and extra bread can then be given. The hungry child might be allowed extra vegetable, but care must be taken not to cause overdistension or gastro-intestinal irritation.

Fat.—Excessive amounts of fat are undesirable from a digestive point of view and also because of the tendency to acidosis which is common in children. On the other hand, the really low fat and high carbohydrate diets sometimes used in the treatment of adult diabetics are quite unsuited to children. Such diets are badly balanced for children and predispose to infections. The quantity of fat given in the standard diets for the younger children is very similar to that eaten by the normal child, while the allowance for the older children is somewhat higher.

TABLE IV

Age (Years).	Calories per Kilogram Body-weight.*	Grammes of Protein per Kilogram Body-weight.†
1, 2	90 to 100	3·5
3, 4, 5	80 to 90	3·0
6, 7, 8, 9	70 to 80	2·5
10, 11, 12, 13	Girls, 60 to 70 Boys, 65 to 75	
14, 15, 16	Girls, 40 to 60 Boys, 50 to 65	2·0
17, 18		1·5

* From Rose's "Laboratory Handbook for Dietetics."

† From the Report on the Physiological Basis of Nutrition drawn up by the Technical Commission of the Health Committee of the League of Nations.

Diets for Diabetic Children

Table showing the Three Main Diets

	Age.	3 Per Cent. Veg.	10 Per Cent. Fruit.	Potato.	Bread.	Milk.	Bacon.	No. of Eggs.	Meat.	Cheese.	Butter.	C.	P.	F.	Cals.
		Gm.	Gm.	Gm.	Gm.	C.c.	Gm.		Gm.	Gm.	Gm.				
Diet I . .	Three or four years.	150	180	75	105	600	30	1	30	...	22	120	52	70	1318
Diet II . .	Seven or eight years.	150	180	90	120	600	45	1	45	22	45	130	65	105	1729
Diet III . .	Eleven or twelve years.	300	120	100	135	600	45	2	75	22	75*	140	81	142	2162

* Some of this should be given as thick cream. Two tablespoonfuls of thick cream = ½ oz. butter.

For intermediate ages, see Notes for suitable additions.

Minerals and Vitamins.—It is very important that the diabetic child should have a generous supply of minerals and vitamins to provide for growth and to build up his resistance to infection. The calcium, phosphorus and iron content of the standard diets are all adequate, but children should be encouraged to eat extra cheese in place of eggs or bacon occasionally in order to improve the calcium intake. A helping of fish twice a week in place of meat or eggs ensures an adequate intake of iodine. The allowance of vegetable, fresh fruit, milk, eggs and whole grains in the standard diet provides all the necessary vitamins, except that during the spring and winter months cod-liver oil or some concentrated preparations of vitamin D (or A and D) is advisable.

The child should be encouraged to drink water freely ; this will help to prevent constipation and it is especially necessary if there is a tendency to acidosis.

The carbohydrate in the sample diets given is more or less evenly distributed over the four meals. This is suitable when zinc protamine insulin is being used, but if soluble insulin is given twice daily the carbohydrate should be redistributed.

Diet I

Type of Diabetic Diet for Child aged Two to Five Years

Child of Three or Four Years.—Carbohydrate, 120. Protein, 52. Fat, 70. Calories, 1,318.

Breakfast—

Bacon, 30 gm.—1 oz.
Brown bread, 45 gm.—$1\frac{1}{2}$ oz.
Butter, 7 gm.—$\frac{1}{4}$ oz.
Milk, 150 c.c.—5 oz.

Dinner—

Clear soup or marmite if desired.
3 per cent. vegetable (see Group I), 100 gm.—$3\frac{1}{2}$ oz.
Potato, 75 gm.—$2\frac{1}{2}$ oz.
Cooked lean meat, 30 gm.—1 oz.
* Milk, 150 c.c.—5 oz.
10 per cent. fruit, 90 gm.—3 oz.

* The milk may be used for curds or a custard can be made using 100 c.c. of milk and half an egg from tea. The other half egg can be exchanged for $\frac{1}{2}$ oz. of grated cheese. Milk jelly can be made with a small teaspoonful of gelatin and flavoured with saccharine and coffee, vanilla, etc. Bacon can be exchanged for an egg + 10 gm.—$\frac{1}{3}$ oz. butter.

Tea—

Tomato, 50 gm.—1¾ oz.
Lettuce, as desired.
Brown bread, 30 gm.—1 oz.
1 egg.
Butter, 7 gm.—¼ oz.
Milk, 150 c.c.—5 oz.

Supper—

Brown bread, 30 gm.—1 oz.
Butter, 8 gm.—¼ oz.
10 per cent. fruit, 90 gm.—3 oz. (or exchanges).
Milk, 150 c.c.—5 oz.

To increase this diet for *child of five years* :—

	Carb.	Prot.	Fat.	Cals.
Add Bread, 15 gm.—½ oz. .	7·5	1·5	0·25	38
Butter, 7 gm.—¼ oz. .	....	....	6	54
	7·5	1·5	6·25	92

Total : Carbohydrate, 128. Protein, 54. Fat, 76. Calories, 1,412.

Diet II

Type of Diet for Child of Six to Ten Years

Child of Seven or Eight Years.—Carbohydrate, 130. Protein, 65. Fat, 105. Calories, 1,729.

Breakfast—

Bacon, 45 gm.—1½ oz.
Brown bread, 45 gm.—1½ oz.
Milk, 150 c.c.—5 oz.
Butter, 10 gm.—⅓ oz.

Dinner—

Clear soup or marmite if desired.
3 per cent. vegetable (see Group I), 100 gm.—3½ oz.
Potato, 90 gm.—3 oz.
Cooked lean meat, 45 gm.—1½ oz.
Butter, 10 gm.—⅓ oz.
Milk, 150 c.c.—5 oz., for curds or custard, using an egg from another meal.
10 per cent. fruit, 90 gm.—3 oz.

Tea—

Tomato, 50 gm.—1¾ oz.
Lettuce, as desired.
Brown bread, 45 gm.—1½ oz.
Butter, 15 gm.—½ oz.
1 egg, Cheese, 22 gm. } or exchanges for 2 eggs (see p. 334).
Egg may be transferred to another meal.
Milk, 150 c.c.—5 oz.

Supper—

10 per cent. fruit, 90 gm.—3 oz.
Brown bread, 30 gm.—1 oz.
Milk, 150 c.c.—5 oz.
Butter, 10 gm.—⅓ oz.
Milk may be omitted at dinner and extra given at supper.

To reduce this diet for *child of six years* :—

	Carb.	Prot.	Fat.	Cals.
Omit Butter, 10 gm. . .	....	....	8·5	76
Cheese, 22 gm., or sometimes 1 egg . .	....	6	6	78
	0	6	14·5	154

Total : Carbohydrate, 130. Protein, 59. Fat, 91. Calories, 1,575.

To increase diet for *child of ten years* :—

	Carb.	Prot.	Fat.	Cals.
Add Meat, 15 gm. . .	0	4	2·5	39
Bread, 15 gm. . .	7·5	1·5	0·25	38
Butter, 15 gm., or thick cream, 30 c.c. . .	....	....	12·5	112
	7·5	5·5	15·25	189

Total : Carbohydrate, 138. Protein, 71. Fat, 120. Calories, 1916.

If hungry a little extra vegetable can be given.

Diet III

Type of Diet for Child of Eleven to Twelve Years

* *Child of Eleven or Twelve Years.*—Carbohydrate, 140. Protein, 81. Fat, 142. Calories, 2,162.

Breakfast—

Bacon, 45 gm.—1½ oz., and 1 egg (or exchange).
Butter from ration (use some for frying).
Brown bread, 45 gm.—1½ oz.
Milk, 100 c.c.—3½ oz. Weak tea.

Dinner—

Clear soup or marmite if desired.
3 per cent vegetable, 150 gm.—5 oz. (see Group I).
Potato, 100 gm.—3½ oz.
Butter from ration.
Cooked lean meat, 75 gm.—2½ oz.
10 per cent. fruit, 120 gm. (or exchanges).
Milk, 150 c.c.—5 oz. for curds or custard using egg from another meal.

Tea—

Tomato, 50 gm. Lettuce as desired.
Brown bread, 45 gm.—1½ oz.
Cheese, 22 gm.
Butter from ration.
Weak tea, with milk, 100 c.c.

Supper—

3 per cent. vegetable, 100 gm.—3½ oz.
1 egg (or exchanges).
Brown bread, 45 gm.—1½ oz.
(If preferred, replace 20 gm. of bread by 100 gm. of 10 per cent. fruit.)
Butter from ration.
Milk, 250 c.c.—one glass.

Daily butter ration, 75 gm.

If afforded, replace 15 gm. of butter by 30 c.c. of thick cream—2 tablespoonfuls.

* This diet will satisfy many diabetic children of twelve years, but the calories are below theoretical requirement and may have to be increased to satisfy the appetite or to maintain satisfactory weight. Unnecessarily high diets should be avoided.

Any of the following additions could be made according to the patient's appetite and the calories required.

	Carb.	Prot.	Fat.	Cals.
Meat, 15 gm.	...	4	2·5	39
Bread, 20 gm.	10	2	...	48
Bacon, 15 gm.	...	2·5	7	73
Cheese, 15 gm.	...	4	5	61
Milk, 300 c.c.	15	10	12	208

For children of fourteen years some or all of the above additions may be made to Diet III. If preferred, the diets for adults—Table I (p. 330)—may be used. Those with 115 or 130 gm. of carbohydrate should be selected and an additional ½ pint of milk must be included, giving calories suitable to the individual child.

DIABETES AND PREGNANCY

Diabetes may develop during pregnancy in women who have not previously suffered from the disease, but glycosuria at this time is not always associated with true diabetes. A blood-sugar curve is always advisable, and if it is a case where there is merely a lowering of the renal threshold for sugar, no special diet is indicated. Such patients should, however, be watched carefully as occasionally—though the blood-sugar level is normal—so much sugar is passed in the urine that ketosis may develop. In this case an intake of from 175 to 200 gm. of carbohydrate should be given with small doses of insulin, no attempt being made to keep the urine completely free of sugar, since hypoglycæmia might result.

The presence of lactose in the urine will give a positive reaction for sugar, and should be differentiated from glucose. Lactose may appear during the later months of pregnancy and during lactation, and its presence is of no importance.

A few cases of true diabetes of pregnancy clear up completely after delivery, when the blood-sugar curve should be repeated. It is possible that such cases are potential diabetics and they should be watched carefully, especially during subsequent pregnancies. They are probably of pituitary origin, but almost invariably require insulin at some time during pregnancy in order that an adequate diet may be given.

Pregnancy is always a serious complication in the true diabetic, for the diabetes becomes temporarily and often permanently more severe. During pregnancy the carbohydrate tolerance will fluctuate and the insulin must be regulated accordingly. The insulin requirement is usually considerably increased from the fourth or fifth month onwards, and it may fall considerably after delivery. In some cases there is an improvement in carbohydrate tolerance during the last month, so that hypoglycæmia must be watched for at this stage.

Hypoglycæmia must be avoided throughout pregnancy, and occasional glycosuria is preferable to insulin reactions. The urine should be carefully examined for sugar, acetone and albumin. A sudden increase in weight should be viewed with suspicion for œdema may occur even in the absence of albuminuria. Excess of salt should be avoided during pregnancy and in the presence of œdema it must definitely be omitted from the diet. Constipation should be guarded against and the diet should be regulated to ensure this. Bran will be found useful in these cases.

The babies of diabetics are often large and there is frequently hydramnios. Joslin and his associates, and also R. D. Lawrence, recommend a Cæsarean section for a first pregnancy in these cases.

The *dietary* requirements during pregnancy are rather similar to those of the growing child. Protein, minerals and vitamins being of the utmost importance. Little or no increase in calories is required during the first four months of pregnancy, though the diet should be modified to include a pint of milk.

After four months an increase of 10 to 20 per cent. in calories may be needed, but the diabetic, being used to a low caloric intake, seldom requires as many calories as the normal pregnant woman. Over-feeding is most undesirable, but patients who usually take 1,800 calories may need 2,200 during pregnancy, or those previously on 2,000 calories may require from 2,300 to 2,400.

The protein requirement during pregnancy is said to be about 1·5 gm. per kg. of body-weight. About 90 gm. is usually included in the diet, but this does not entail eating large quantities of meat since the necessary milk will provide the extra protein. Not less than 1 pint—preferably 1½ pints—of milk should be included and cheese should also be taken to ensure an adequate calcium intake.

The carbohydrate should not be less than 150 gm. ; it may

Diets for Pregnancy

Diet.	3 Per Cent. Veg.	10 Per Cent. Fruit.	Potato.	Bread.	Milk.	Bacon.	No. of Eggs.	Meat.	Cheese.	Butter.	Thick Cream.	C.	P.	F.	Cals.
	Gm.	Gm.	Gm.	Gm.	Gm.	Gm.		Gm.	Gm.	Gm.	Gm.				
I	300	210	75	120	900	30	2	60	22	45	...	150	85	119	2011
II	300	210	75	120	900	45	2	60	22	60	...	150	88	139	2203
III	300	210	75	120	900	60	2	60	22	76	...	150	90	160	2400
IV	300	210	75	120	900	60	2	75	22	76	60	150	94	186	2650

When diets III or IV are necessary to give adequate calories, nausea may occasionally be experienced, or acetone may be present in the urine. In these cases, extra bread and fruit can be added to diets I or II, increasing their carbohydrate to approximately 175 or 200 gm.

well be increased later in pregnancy, since the fœtus may demand some 50 gm. of carbohydrate during the last two months of pregnancy. Fat will make up the remaining calories, but some women tolerate fat poorly during pregnancy, especially during the early months, and it may often be necessary to increase the carbohydrate and to lower the fat.

The diet should be a well-balanced one with a generous supply of "protective foods." Iron may be required in medicinal form (see p. 471), and a preparation containing vitamins A and D is desirable, especially during the spring and winter months (see p. 414).

The standard diets given below should be modified to suit the individual patient, but they will serve as a useful guide. The lower fat, and therefore the lower caloric diets, are intended for the patient with a tendency to overweight or an intolerance for much fat. Insulin is required in all but the mildest cases and this may conveniently be given in the form of zinc protamine insulin, or a combination of zinc protamine and soluble insulin, before breakfast (see p. 359). If soluble insulin is used the carbohydrate should be rearranged in accordance with the times of injection.

Sample Diet for Pregnancy

(See Table on p. 374)

Carbohydrate, 150. Protein, 90. Fat, 100. Calories, 2,400.

Breakfast—

Bacon, 60 gm.—2 oz. (raw weight) } or exchange.
1 egg—cook with butter from ration }
Brown bread, 45 gm.—$1\frac{1}{2}$ oz.
Tea or coffee with milk from ration.

11 *a.m.*—

Milk from ration.

Dinner—

Vegetable from Group I, 150 gm.—5 oz.; *or* vegetable from Group II, 75 gm.—$2\frac{1}{2}$ oz.
Potato, 75 gm.—$2\frac{1}{2}$ oz.+butter from ration.
Lean meat, 60 gm.—2 oz. (or exchange).
10 per cent. fruit, 100 gm.—$3\frac{1}{2}$ oz. (or exchange).
Milk from ration for curds; *or* custard, using egg from another meal.

Tea—

Brown bread, 45 gm.—1½ oz.
Cheese, 22 gm.—¾ oz. (or see note at Supper).
Tomato, 50 gm.—1¾ oz. Lettuce, as desired.
Tea, milk from ration.

Supper—

1 egg (or exchange). (If cheese omitted at tea, take exchanges for two eggs now, *e.g.*, fish, etc.)
Vegetable from Group I, 100 gm.—3½ oz.
Brown bread, 30 gm.—1 oz.
10 per cent. fruit, 100 gm.—3½ oz. (or exchange).
Milk from ration to drink.

Daily—

Butter, 76 gm. = 2½ oz. (or 1 oz. of butter can be exchanged for 4 tablespoonfuls of thick cream).
Milk, 900 c.c.—1½ pints.

COMPLICATIONS OF DIABETES

Tuberculosis and Diabetes.—The liability of severe diabetic cases to develop tuberculosis should constantly be kept in mind. The possibility of this complication having occurred should always be suspected and excluded when, for no obvious reason, a previously controlled diabetic patient begins to require larger doses of insulin, to lose weight and to fail in general health. The danger is particularly present in patients who have suffered from diabetic coma and in diabetic children. Such cases should be examined at intervals for the specific purpose of excluding tuberculosis ; young diabetic patients particularly should be excluded from association with open cases of tuberculosis.

With early diagnosis of the tuberculosis and efficient treatment of the diabetes, our experience does not suggest that the prognosis is unduly gloomy or that the diabetes has a particularly adverse effect on the tuberculous process. A considerably higher calorie diet, however, should be given to such cases than to the average diabetic, and the high carbohydrate, low fat régime is manifestly unsuitable for them.

Gangrene.—A large number of cases of diabetic gangrene can be prevented by cleanliness, proper care of the feet and immediate treatment of the slightest abrasion of the feet which may occur. Diabetic gangrene is exceedingly rare under the age of forty. Its frequency advances as age increases, just as it does in non-diabetic gangrene. Hitherto, diabetics have grown older more rapidly than other people, but it is likely that with more efficient treatment diabetic gangrene will be less common in the future.

The first maxim in the prevention of gangrene is cleanliness. Joslin has said that if diabetics kept their feet as clean as their faces gangrene would be practically unknown. Elderly diabetics should therefore be encouraged to wash their feet night and morning with soap and water, to dry them thoroughly and to powder them afterwards. Warm socks, or stockings, should be worn and easy-fitting soft leather shoes. New shoes should only be worn for a few hours a day until they are broken in. Bed socks should be used instead of hot-water bottles. All corns and callosities should be treated with the greatest care, if possible by a competent chiropodist who should be warned that the patient has diabetes. Abrasions of the skin should not be dressed with strong antiseptics such as iodine, but with a simple spirit solution. The toe nails should be carefully cut in a good light, and any overlapping toes should be kept separate by inserting cotton wool between them.

The treatment of fully developed diabetic gangrene is discussed on pp. 735-740.

Neuritis, Retinitis, Cataract, Pruritus.—The adequate control of the underlying diabetic condition itself is the best treatment for the neuritis, retinitis and pruritus with which diabetes is so commonly associated. These complications frequently improve as soon as the glycosuria is controlled. When neuritis persists, however, large doses of vitamin B given parenterally seem to be of some service (see p. 979).

Failure of vision, the result of diabetic retinitis, is not greatly relieved by the prescription of glasses. Some patients suffering from diabetes waste a great deal of money in having their spectacles frequently changed, since what suits them on one day is often found to be unsuitable a few days later. The acuity of vision often tends to vary from day to day depending on the adequacy of the diabetic control. The onset of cataract demands a consultation with an ophthalmologist as to the feasibility of operative treatment and as to the correct time for its performance.

Pruritus usually clears up very rapidly with the disappearance of glycosuria. Its treatment when it persists is discussed on p. 182.

The Adjustment of the Diet in Complications.—The average diabetic diet is unsuitable in cases of gastro-intestinal disturbances or in acute disease, since it is usually bulky and high in residue and may contain considerable amounts of fat and fried foods. The newer type of diabetic diet which is low in fat and high in carbohydrate is no more suitable in these conditions, since large helpings of bread and potato are equally inadvisable.

It is impossible to give detailed diabetic diets suitable for every disease, but with the help of a table of food values and the fluid feeds and the light diets given on pp. 380, 381, 386 the standard diabetic diets already described can be adapted to suit various conditions. No attempt must be made to force unsuitable standard diets upon a patient unable to digest or to enjoy them.

Peptic Ulcer.—A diabetic may develop a peptic ulcer and there is no reason why the two conditions should not be treated satisfactorily at the same time. An ulcer régime can be given containing a definite amount of carbohydrate and calories. In such cases about 150 gm. of carbohydrate are necessary to allow for milk to be given between meals and to include fine cereals and orange juice. Protein should be higher than usual (probably about 100 to 120 gm.) to permit of sufficient eggs, fish, finely divided meat and milk being taken. The amount of fat will depend upon the calories required, but unless the patient is overweight, cream and butter are desirable from the ulcer standpoint. Sugar should be omitted, fruit and vegetables must be sieved, while white bread, and later fine brown bread, should take the place of coarse cereals. Bacon and other fried foods, highly seasoned foods, meat soups and strong tea and coffee should be omitted.

In cases of hyperacidity or in chronic gastritis any of the above adjustments can be made according to the severity of the symptoms.

Cardiac Disease.—In cardiac cases, or for any patients with flatulence, bulky vegetable should be omitted or given in the form of a purée, fluids should be given between meals only, and white toast should replace bread. Only a light supper is indicated. Diabetic patients showing signs of œdema should curtail their salt intake.

Cholecystitis.—Disease of the gall-bladder is not uncommon in diabetics, and here the higher carbohydrate and low fat diet is suitable. Eggs should be omitted and also flatulent-forming vegetables, while hot water should be taken between meals.

Diarrhœa.—Diarrhœa is sometimes troublesome, especially in elderly diabetics, and drastic purges should never be given to those patients. When an attack of diarrhœa occurs the fat in the diet should be reduced and the fruit and vegetables and the coarse cereals should be omitted temporarily. The carbohydrate should be increased by the addition of boiled milk, fine cereals and white toast. Symptoms of hypoglycæmia must be watched for in these cases. Should the diarrhœa become chronic, care must be taken to give adequate vitamins, and a colitis diet may be necessary (*e.g.*, low residue, low fat, moderate carbohydrate and high protein).

Fevers.—In cases of acute illness such as influenza, pneumonia or any septic condition, the patient may develop ketosis rapidly and pass into diabetic coma if prompt treatment is not given. In such cases the treatment already described for impending diabetic coma may be necessary, but if the doctor is summoned in time less drastic doses of insulin may suffice. In the event of a severe cold, fever, sickness, abdominal pain or any infection, the diabetic should be warned to stay in bed and to call in the doctor. If present, constipation must be treated.

Patients who are taking insulin must on no account omit it even if they cannot take their usual food. They are advised to divide the usual dose or doses into three or four smaller doses. It has already been mentioned that soluble insulin is more suitable than zinc protamine insulin in emergency work, though a small dose of zinc protamine insulin can be given in addition before breakfast. In acute diseases three or four doses of soluble insulin will be required daily and the increase in total insulin requirement may be considerable. If severe vomiting is present, hospital treatment is essential since intravenous glucose will be needed. In the case of patients who live far from a doctor it is advisable to give them a note of suitable feeds to be taken in times of emergency.

In all cases of fever and acute illness the diet should be mainly fluid and the feeds on pp. 380, 386 should be given with due regard to the patient's preferences. About 120 gm. of carbohydrate should be included daily ; this will be given in four feeds, preceded by soluble insulin. Diluted milk, unsweetened orange juice, weak tea, chicken tea and bovril can be given between meals (reckoning the carbohydrate of the milk and orange juice). Water should be taken freely. When the acute stage is over, the light diet on p. 381 should be given and the usual diet gradually resumed.

When a temporary fluid or light diet is ordered for a diabetic it is a common error to prescribe too many calories and this may entail a nauseating amount of cream, which is most unsuitable when acetone is present or threatening. If, on the other hand, the fat is kept low, concentrated glucose and orange drinks or sweetened milk are often included to give the number of calories ordered, which may readily cause sickness. Provided a reasonable amount of carbohydrate and plenty of fluid are given *the question of calories are of no consideration in acute diseases of short duration* and overfeeding is definitely harmful.

Fluid Feeds

(Each feed contains approximately 25 gm. carbohydrate.)

	Carb.	Prot.	Fat.
Benger's Food, dry weight, ½ oz.—15 gm.	12	1·5	0
Milk, 6 oz.—180 c.c.	9	6	7
Sugar, 1 teaspoonful—5 gm.	5	0	0
	26	7·5	7
Orange juice, 3½ oz.—100 c.c.	10	0	0
Glucose, ½ oz.—15 gm.	15	0	0
Squeeze of lemon juice	...	...	...
	25	0	0
Strained porridge, 3 tablespoonfuls = ¾ oz. or 22 gm. dry meal	15	3·75	1·5
Hot milk, 3½ oz.—100 c.c.	5	3·3	4
Orange juice, 2 oz.—60 c.c.	6	0	0
	26	7	5·5
Bread, ¾ oz.—22 gm.	12	2	0
Milk, 6 oz.—180 c.c.	9	6	7
Sugar, 1 teaspoonful—5 gm.	5	0	0
	26	8	7
Ovaltine, ⅓ oz.—10 gm.	7	1·5	1
Milk, 8 oz.—240 c.c.	12	8	9·5
Sugar, 1 teaspoonful—5 gm.	5	0	0
	24	9·5	10·5

Light Diabetic Diet (see also p. 386)

(Carbohydrates, 120. Protein, 57. Fat, 98. Calories, 1,590.)

	Carb.	Prot.	Fat.
Breakfast—			
Tea, with thin cream, 2 tablespoonfuls—30 c.c. .	1·2	0·7	6
White bread, 1 oz.—30 gm. (toast after weighing)	16	3	0·5
Butter, ⅓ oz.—10 gm.	0	0	8·5
Lightly boiled egg	0	6	6
Pulp of orange or juice, 3 oz.—90 gm. . .	9	0	0
10.30 *a.m.*—			
Milk, 5 oz.—150 c.c.	7·5	5	6
Bovril or marmite can be added or the egg from breakfast can be switched.			
Dinner—			
Steamed white fish, 3 oz.—90 gm.	0	18	0
Butter, ½ oz.—15 gm. (use some with vegetable)	0	0	12·7
Flower of cauliflower or French beans, or sieved spinach, or other suitable vegetable, 3 oz.—90 gm.	2·7	1·5	0
Floury potato, 2½ oz.—75 gm. ; *or* bread, 1 oz.—30 gm.	15	1·5	0
Milk, 5 oz.—150 c.c. (as curds, or make custard, using egg from breakfast)	7·5	5	6
Apple purée (cooked without sugar), 3 oz.—90 gm.	9	0	0
Serve with thin cream, 2 oz.—60 c.c. . .	2·4	1·5	12
Tea—			
Tea, with thin cream, 1 oz.—30 gm. . . .	1·2	0·7	6
Thin white bread, 1 oz.—30 gm.	16	3	0·5
Butter, ⅓ oz.—10 gm.	0	0	8·5
One Tea biscuit ; *or* extra bread, ½ oz. . .	7	0·6	1
Supper—			
Milk Soup :			
Milk, 5 oz.—150 c.c.	7·5	5	6
Tomato or spinach purée, 3 oz.—90 gm. .	2·7	1·5	0
Stock, if desired.			
Cornflour, ¼ oz.—7 gm.	5	0	0
Thin cream, 1 oz.—30 c.c.	1·2	0·7	6
Or, in place of Soup :			
Serve the milk and cream to drink with one Tea biscuit.			
Orange Jelly :			
Orange juice, 3 oz.—90 c.c.	9	0	0
Water, 2 oz.—60 c.c.			
Gelatin, 1 teaspoonful	0	3	0
Serve with 2 tablespoonfuls of thick cream, whipped	0·6	0·4	12
Total . . .	120	57	98

Total Calories, 1,590.

Variations for the Light Diet

Breakfast.—When disinclined for other foods many patients will take porridge, this can be sieved if necessary. The ounce of bread can be exchanged for 3 tablespoonfuls of thick porridge ($\frac{3}{4}$ oz.—20 gm. dry oatmeal), or the bread and fruit can be exchanged for 5 tablespoonfuls of porridge ($1\frac{1}{4}$ oz.—37 gm. dry oatmeal). Serve with milk from dinner.

Dinner.—The fish should be varied with tripe, chicken, rabbit, sweetbread or, in some cases, minced beef can be given. The slight change in food value is not very important but the protein may fall, since in cases of illness not more than $1\frac{1}{2}$ to 2 oz. of chicken or meat can usually be taken—an egg could therefore be added to the milk to make a custard.

Supper.—Patients soon tire of milk soup, and the alternative feed of milk and biscuit can be used.

The orange jelly can be changed for other suitable fruit.

As the appetite improves, an egg or a little fish or chicken can be served at this meal or at tea-time to improve the protein value of the diet.

As the patient's appetite and general condition improve, the diet can be increased gradually—since the food value of each serving of food is given above this is a simple matter.

If the bread is increased this allows more butter to be given, and each ounce of butter gives 225 extra calories.

An extra $\frac{1}{2}$ pint of milk is a useful addition and gives carbohydrate 15 gm., protein 10 gm., fat 12 gm., calories 208.

Care should be taken not to serve exactly the same foods each day, and the patient's preferences should be considered.

THE CARE OF THE SURGICAL DIABETIC

The discovery of insulin and the introduction of various anæsthetics as substitutes for chloroform and ether have greatly lessened the dangers of surgery in diabetes. Nevertheless, the risk of an operation is still considerable if the patient falls into inexperienced hands. Successful treatment depends upon close co-operation between the surgeon and the physician, and, if possible, a nurse who is experienced in the care of diabetic patients should be employed.

The chief danger in diabetic surgery is ketosis, which may be caused by giving an unsuitable anæsthetic, by prolonged starvation, by sickness or by failure to control the glycosuria and blood sugar with sufficient insulin either before or after the operation. The routine measure of testing every patient's urine before operation is an obvious necessity, since it may be too late to give adequate treatment if the diabetes is only discovered after the operation. A general anæsthetic, especially chloroform or ether, is well known to be toxic to the liver and has a tendency to cause some degree of ketosis even in the normal individual. This danger is greatly increased in diabetics owing to the poor store of glycogen in the liver, hence the necessity for giving glucose covered by an adequate dose of insulin *prior* to giving an anæsthetic.

Chloroform should never be given to a known diabetic, and ether should also be avoided if possible. Gas and oxygen, avertin or a spinal or local anæsthetic are suitable from the point of view of the diabetes. Even with a well-chosen anæsthetic sickness may occur after operation and if this is prolonged dehydration will follow, thus increasing the dangers of ketosis and collapse from shock.

When the patient is taking fluids by the mouth, sickness is sometimes caused by giving too strong a solution of glucose or by giving orange juice to patients who cannot tolerate it. In cases of severe vomiting a definite amount of glucose is administered by the intravenous route and a suitable insulin dosage must be given. Extra fluid can also be administered as saline per rectum. The old idea of giving glucose by the rectum in such cases is to be deprecated as the absorption of the glucose cannot be relied upon. In addition, in female patients the urine may become contaminated with glucose, and this will lead to confusion.

Apart from the hyperglycæmia which occurs after a general anæsthetic, the nervous shock which is inevitable in any operation tends to raise the blood sugar and to cause a return of glycosuria. In the presence of sepsis the carbohydrate tolerance is still further diminished and the insulin requirement is considerably increased until the infection subsides. As the patient recovers the decrease in insulin requirement is often marked, and care should be taken to ensure that hypoglycæmia does not occur at this stage.

In surgical cases it is too often assumed that the diabetes is the cause of all unusual signs and symptoms, and that drowsiness is necessarily due to ketosis, or that symptoms of collapse are always caused by an overdose of insulin. In a well-managed case these emergencies seldom occur. It should be remembered that the toxæmia caused by a large carbuncle or a severe gangrene is very great and may in itself result in drowsiness, while the senile diabetic with marked arterial degeneration may readily collapse from cardiac failure or go into coma as the result of a cerebral hæmorrhage.

It is neither desirable nor possible to outline a routine to be followed in all cases of diabetic surgery. Experience is the only sure guide to treatment. The method of preparing the patient will vary according to whether the operation is undertaken as an emergency measure or if there is time to prepare for some days beforehand, and the treatment must be modified to suit the surgical condition. The severity of the diabetes, the presence or absence of ketonuria and the choice of an anæsthetic are decisive factors governing insulin dosage. The advisability of operation cannot be discussed here, but all severe infections should be dealt with as soon as possible without waiting to clear up the glycosuria.

In cases which are not surgical emergencies the patient is stabilized for several days on a satisfactory diet, insulin being given if necessary. The carbohydrate of the daily diet should not be less than 115 gm. and preferably more should be given. The urine should be free from acetone and no appreciable amount of glycosuria should be present.

On the day of operation 30 gm. of carbohydrate should be given in the form of glucose in lemon, orange or grapefruit juice three hours before operation ; sickness at the time of operation may occur if this is given one and a half to two hours before operation as is sometimes advocated. The dose of insulin will depend upon the patient's usual insulin requirement. In a mild case not previously on insulin, 10 units of soluble insulin may be enough ; 15 units is a fairly common dose, but in more severe diabetics accustomed to larger doses of insulin, 20 to 30 units may be required, and in such cases 40 gm. of carbohydrate may be necessary. Those patients who are accustomed to zinc protamine insulin can have a reduced dose of this before the operation, but any subsequent glycosuria should be controlled with soluble insulin. In all cases of sepsis and unless the patient has been under observation for a considerable time, it is simpler to use soluble rather than zinc protamine insulin, as the latter cannot be adjusted so easily from day to day.

If the operation takes place in the morning the patient may feel inclined for a cup of tea with a lump of sugar (5 gm.) in the late afternoon, depending upon what anæsthetic he has had. In the evening a fluid feed of 30 gm. of carbohydrate (see p. 380) can usually be taken (unless this is contraindicated by the nature of the operation). Patients are often tired of glucose and orange juice and they prefer Benger's Food. Unless zinc protamine insulin has been given before the operation, this feed is preceded by insulin as before, but rather a smaller dose should be given, especially if a specimen of urine can be obtained and is found to be "sugar-free." If sickness occurs, it may be necessary to administer the glucose intravenously. If the nature of the operation makes feeding by the mouth impossible or inadvisable, a measured quantity of glucose is usually given by the continuous drip method and small doses of insulin will be required at regular and stated intervals.

Where there is no ketosis and the patient has been well stabilized before operation there is no necessity to give more glucose and insulin during the subsequent night, but in the case of an emergency operation on a diabetic with acetonuria more intensive treatment is required, as in impending coma. In such cases there may be no time to give glucose by the mouth before operation, and insulin and intravenous glucose should be given in the theatre and repeated later by the continuous intravenous method or at four-hourly intervals until the acetonuria is controlled.

When only a local anæsthetic is given, as in diabetic cataract or for minor operations, the patient is allowed a light breakfast prior to operation, *e.g.*, tea, toast and butter and grapefruit or orange juice. If he has not previously been taking insulin, it is unnecessary to administer it unless glycosuria is present. If the usual diet can be taken after operation a patient on insulin will have his customary dose.

Whenever the usual number of calories are not given, insulin must be reduced even though the usual carbohydrate allowance is prescribed. The diet for a case of cataract must be served in such a form that no mastication is necessary until the patient is discharged from hospital. It is very important that the urine should be kept free from sugar, but any risk of insulin reaction must be avoided or the eye may be damaged during a hypoglycæmic fit.

Post-operative treatment will depend upon the individual case, but after an amputation of a leg, for example, the following would be suitable for the day after operation, the subsequent diet being built up on the lines of the light diet given at the end of the chapter, until the patient is taking his usual diabetic diet.

Fluid Diet for Day following Operation

e.g., Amputation

(Also suitable for patient recovering from Diabetic Coma)

	Carb.	Prot.	Fat.
Early Morning—			
Cup of tea ; milk, 2 tablespoonfuls—30 c.c. .	1·5	1	1
Soluble Insulin, 7.30 *a.m.*			
Breakfast, 8 *a.m.*—			
Strained porridge, 4 tablespoonfuls = dry meal, 1 oz.—30 gm.	20	5	2
Hot milk, 5 oz.—150 c.c.	7·5	5	6
10.30 *a.m.*—			
Milk, hot or cold, 5 oz.—150 c.c.	7·5	5	6
Soluble Insulin, 12.30 *p.m.*			
Dinner, 1 *p.m.*—			
Milk Soup :			
Milk, 4 oz.—120 c.c.	6	4	5
Sieved carrot, 1½ oz.—45 gm.	2·7	0·6	0
Or Tomato juice, 3 oz.—90 c.c.			
Stock or bovril, as required.			
Milk Pudding :			
Dry cereal, ⅓ oz.—10 gm.	8	1	0
Milk, 6 oz.—180 c.c.	9	6	7
Milk to serve, 2 oz.—60 c.c.	3	2	2·4
Tea, 4 *p.m.*—			
Tea, with milk, 1 oz.—30 c.c.	1·5	1	1
One Tea biscuit ; or ½ oz. thin bread with butter to cover	7	0·6	1
Soluble Insulin, 6.30 *p.m.*			
Supper, 7 *p.m.*—			
Benger's Food, ½ oz.—15 gm.	12	1·5	0
Milk, 6½ oz.—200 c.c.	10	6·6	8
Sugar, 1 teaspoonful—5 gm.	5	0	0
9 *p.m.*—			
Orange juice, 3 oz.—90 c.c.	9	0	0
Sugar, 1 teaspoonful—5 gm.	5	0	0
Total . . .	115	39	39

Total Calories, 967.

OBESITY

Introduction

Perhaps it is nothing less frivolous than fashion which has of late years focused medical interest on the subject of obesity, and has directed particular attention to the more serious aspects of excessive corpulence. Quite apart from æsthetic considerations, however, long-continued obesity has as its almost invariable concomitants more or less grave disturbances of most of the systems of the body. Thus, the statistics of Life Assurance Companies all go to show that mortality rates rise steadily in proportion to the extent to which people are overweight. Flat foot, varicose veins, osteo-arthritis of the knees and hips, postural backache, ventral herniæ, cholecystitis and gall-stones, diabetes, degenerative changes in and overstrain of the myocardium, angina pectoris, hypertension and bronchitis are all evils to which the corpulent are heirs more often than the lean. It is far too often forgotten that the more specific treatment of these ailments is likely to be unsuccessful if the associated obesity is allowed to continue. Indeed, reduction in weight is sometimes the only treatment required to banish the symptoms arising from the milder forms of such conditions.

Just as the maintenance of a constant body temperature and a constant blood pH, under widely varying exogenous and endogenous conditions, form striking facts of human physiology, so the maintenance by the healthy adult of an almost constant body-weight over long periods of time is a remarkable phenomenon, when it is remembered that this constancy may be maintained in spite of great variations in physical activity and food intake. The glutton does not necessarily become overweight, nor is the ascetic necessarily emaciated. It is certain that most of us eat in excess of our calorific requirements, but this excess, in the normal person, may not be absorbed or is easily burnt up and dissipated in the form of heat. Did this capacity not exist obesity would be almost universal, for a daily intake of 200 calories in excess of actual requirements, such as would be represented by an extra glass of milk or two slices of bread, would have the result of increasing the weight by some 24 lbs. a year; and this is actually what may occur to some extent in certain unfortunate individuals, in whom the mechanism for regulating body-weight is less flexible than in the normal person. On the other hand, some individuals become obese simply because they put their regulating mechanism to a strain which no ordinary mechanism is capable of withstanding.

Two types of obesity have, therefore, been distinguished: an exogenous type involving some dietetic error or some environmental factor, such as lack of exercise; and an endogenous type involving an abnormality of the weight-regulating mechanism, which is usually taken as synonymous with some endocrine disturbance. In practice, however, it is impossible to make such an arbitrary and clear-cut distinction in the majority of cases. The two extremes are obvious enough: on the one hand, there are the few cases showing the typical stigmata of deficient pituitary, thyroid or ovarian function with an increased sugar tolerance, a lowered metabolic rate or absent menses; on the other hand, there is the individual who has habitually sacrificed his figure to his appetite and his indolence. In between these two extremes, however, lie the great majority of cases which are hardly susceptible of classification into one or other type. It is probable that in these latter no single factor is responsible, but rather a mixture of mild exogenous factors combined with some small degree of endocrine upset, as yet unrecognizable by the means at our disposal.

As far as the treatment of obesity is concerned it is unnecessary to distinguish between endogenous and exogenous obesity, since both types respond to the same therapeutic methods. In each case income exceeds expenditure and rational therapy must consist in correcting the balance. Further storage may be prevented by cutting down the intake of food, or by causing the body to metabolize more rapidly, so that the stores of fat may be depleted. Dieting has long been recognized as a successful method of treatment, and many régimes have been recommended. An increased combustion of foodstuffs can be encouraged in two ways: by raising the general level of metabolism; or by increasing physical effort. In popular imagination lack of exercise bulks large as a cause of obesity, and hard exercise is looked upon as a specific weight reducer. Severe and sustained muscular work is, however, necessary if any significant increase in the expenditure of calories is to be attained. This will be appreciated when it is recalled that a man of average size only consumes about 60 extra calories while walking a mile on the level, and very often increases his appetite thereby to the extent of adding several hundred calories to his subsequent meal. Further, owing to the disabling effects of his obesity it is rarely possible for a fat person to take really hard physical exercise. The alternative to exercise is to employ hormone or drug therapy to influence the activity of tissue metabolism. Drastic purgation by hypertonic salt solutions and the encouragement of profuse sweating by Turkish baths have had, and still have, their vogue as treatments of obesity. Quite apart from the fact that long-continued use of these methods, especially the former, may be exceedingly deleterious to the general health, their effects—though considerable at the time—are transient and short lived, being almost entirely due to a temporary loss of water from the body. The two most practical procedures are, therefore, the use of rationally constructed subcaloric diets and occasionally the administration of a metabolic stimulant.

DIETETICS

Calories.—In constructing a diet for obesity, certain physiological principles must be taken into account. The most important consideration is the total calorific value of the diet. In really obese people the total calories should not exceed 25 calories per kilogram of the standard body-weight, which represents the requirement of the healthy individual under basal conditions. In practical therapeutics, however, it is quite superfluous to enter into such elaborately meticulous dietetic refinements. None the less some consideration should be paid to the height, age and nutrition of the patient concerned. For ordinary purposes the prescription of a diet of 1,000 or 1,200 calories is all that is necessary. Occasionally, a hard-working man may require one of 1,500 calories, but it must be remembered that unless the patients are under close supervision in hospital, it is safe to estimate that they will tend to be liberal in interpreting their diets and, therefore, that diets of 1,500 calories or over are usually singularly unsuccessful in reducing the weight of an out-patient, though they may well do so in hospital. On the other hand, diets with a value of less than 1,000 calories are unsuitable for patients who are not confined to bed. They are seldom adhered to and if they are observed in the letter they cause weakness, faintness and an unduly rapid loss in weight.

Fat.—Consideration is not only to be given to the total number of calories provided, but also to the proportion of the basic foodstuffs (carbohydrate, protein and fat). In deciding the quantity of fat to be allowed it is assumed that, as the body will call upon its own stores, this substance can be reduced to a minimum in the diet. Some régimes allow no added fats, the patients merely getting the fat which is inseparable from other foods (such as meat) and, in consequence, the daily intake of fat may be as low as 20 gm. To compensate for the absence of fat, soluble vitamins in specially concentrated preparations have to be added. This extreme reduction of fat makes the diet difficult and unpalatable and is, moreover, unnatural, since the content of fat in a diet does not seem to affect weight reduction to the same extent as its content of carbohydrate, provided the total calories are kept unchanged.

Carbohydrate.—Since excess carbohydrate eating is the most important single ætiological factor in obesity, the carbohydrate should be restricted as far as possible in obesity diets. Sufficient carbohydrate must, however, be given to avoid the feeling of weakness and faintness which severe curtailment of carbohydrate intake so frequently occasions, and to avoid the occurrence of ketosis with its concomitant headaches. In addition, carbohydrates are the most powerful sparers of protein and their too severe restriction leads to excessive loss of body nitrogen. These effects can be avoided by giving not less than 100 or more than 130 gm. of carbohydrate a day. The greater part of the carbohydrate should consist of fruit and green vegetables. These give bulk to the diet and a considerable quantity of such foods can be taken without causing much addition to the patient's calorific intake. This has the double effect of causing a feeling of satiety and at the same time of providing the roughage to combat constipation, which subcaloric diets always tend to produce.

Protein.—Because of its stimulating action on metabolism, protein is often given in large quantities in reducing diets (*e.g.*, Banting and Salisbury diets), but as this means a higher calorific intake its advantage is somewhat doubtful, and such diets are ill-balanced and unnatural. If, on the other hand, the protein of the diet is too low, a negative nitrogen balance will result from excessive destruction of tissue protein. The optimum intake of protein for a subcaloric diet should vary from 60 to 80 gm. per day.

Salt.—Apart from alcohol and sweetened drinks, no attempt need be made to restrict fluids, but the intake of sodium chloride should be curtailed. Salty foods should be avoided and as little table salt as possible should be taken.

Obesity Diets

Notes.—The following notes apply to all the sample obesity diets given :—

The helpings of food are expressed in ounces instead of in grammes, since a reducing diet is most often used in the patient's home. If weighing on gramme scales, 1 oz. may be reckoned as 30 gm.

Bread and butter should be weighed and milk must be measured. It is convenient to measure the butter and milk in the morning and use them as desired throughout the day.

No foods are " slimming " foods.

Toast is no less fattening than bread.

Salt is to be taken in moderation.

Foods to be Avoided.

Sugar, sweets, jam, etc.
Scones, cakes, pastry, cereals.
Thick soups and sauces made with flour or butter.
Fried foods, cream and salad dressings.
Pork, duck, goose, fat meat and bacon.
Sweet wines, beer, stout, spirits or sweet aerated waters.
Nuts.

Fruits—

Dried, canned in syrup, bananas.
Grapes and plums allowed in moderation only.

Vegetables—

Potato, dried or fresh peas, dried beans, parsnips.
Beetroot allowed in small quantities only.

Foods with no appreciable Caloric Value.

Oxo, bovril, marmite, clear soups. (Avoid excess of meat extracts because of their salt content.)

A dessertspoonful of sugarless marmalade or jam (as sold for diabetics).

Gelatin, egg-white, green vegetables, vinegar, tea, coffee, unsweetened pickles.

Mineral oil, *i.e.*, liquid paraffin, can be used in place of fat for frying or instead of olive oil to make mayonnaise dressing.

No. 1. Inexpensive Obesity Diet. Calories, 1,000.

Carbohydrate, 100 gm.
Protein, 60 gm. (approximate daily average).
Fat, 40 gm. (approximate daily average).

Breakfast—

Orange or ½ a grapefruit without sugar.
Wholemeal bread, 1 oz. (1 thin slice); *or* 2 pieces of ryvita or vitaweat.
Butter from ration.
1 egg, *or* 1 oz. *lean* cold boiled ham or tongue.
Tea or coffee with milk from ration.

Dinner—

Clear soup, or marmite, or oxo, or bovril, if desired.
A medium helping (2 to 3 oz.) of cooked *lean* meat, chicken, rabbit, tripe or white fish. (If fish is taken, ¼ oz. butter may be used for cooking).
A large helping of vegetables, preferably from Group I (see p. 333). (See list of those to be avoided.)
1 apple, or pear, or other fruit (except those forbidden).

Tea—

(Now or at supper)—1 egg, *or* ¾ oz. cheese, *or* medium helping of white fish, lean meat, chicken, *or* 1 oz. cooked lean ham or tongue.
Fresh salad or tomato.
Wholemeal bread, 1 oz.
Butter from ration.
Tea or coffee with milk from ration.

Supper—

Wholemeal bread, 1 oz.; *or* 2 pieces of ryvita or vitaweat, *or* 3 water biscuits.
Butter from ration.
Skim milk from ration; coffee, if desired.
1 medium-sized orange, or choice from the list.

Rations for Day—

Butter, ¾ oz.
Skim milk, ½ pint.
No sugar. Saccharine or saxin can be used.
Water, 4 glasses, preferably not with meals.

To increase this diet to 1,100 calories give whole milk in place of skim milk.

To increase further to 1,200 calories add ½ oz. butter.

No. 2. Obesity Diet

Carbohydrate, 116 gm.
Protein, 70 gm. (approximate daily average).
Fat, 52 gm. (approximate daily average).
Calories, 1,200.

Breakfast—

1 orange or ½ grapefruit—saccharine may be used, but no sugar.
Tea or coffee with milk from ration.
1 egg, *or* 1 oz. cold lean ham or tongue.
1 oz. brown bread (1 thin slice).
1 small pat of butter, ¼ oz.

Dinner—

Clear soup, if desired.
An average helping of lean meat, poultry or game (2 to 3 oz.), *or* white fish.
No goose, pork or duck.
A large helping of any vegetable, except potato, dried peas, beans or lentils.
Fresh salad when possible (no oil or cream in dressing).
¾ oz. cheese.
½ oz. (½ thin slice) brown bread, *or* 2 plain biscuits—no butter.
Fresh fruit, except bananas, grapes or plums.
Coffee with milk from ration.
No sweet wine, beer, stout, spirits or sweet aerated waters.

Tea—

Tea with milk from ration—saccharine instead of sugar, if wanted.
Brown bread, 1½ oz. (1½ thin slices).
Tomato, lettuce or cress for a sandwich.
Small pat of butter, ¼ oz.

Supper—

Clear soup, if wanted.
Fish, 3 oz. (cooked weight), *or* 1 egg, *or* 1 oz. boiled lean ham or tongue.
Vegetable or salad as at dinner.
Fruit as at dinner.
Milk from ration for curds, *or* with coffee, *or* make a custard, using the egg from breakfast.
Bread, ½ oz.; *or* 1 piece of ryvita.

Rations for Day—
Butter, $\frac{3}{4}$ oz.
Milk, $\frac{1}{2}$ pint.
Water, 4 glasses, preferably not with food.
No sugar.

If preferred tea and supper can be interchanged.

To increase this diet to 1,500 calories :

	Cals. Approx.
Add Butter, $\frac{3}{4}$ oz.	171
Cheese, $\frac{3}{4}$ oz., *or* 1 egg . . .	78
Bread, $\frac{3}{4}$ oz.	56
Total extra cals.	305

In the case of women or young people extra milk is often preferred.

	Cals. Approx.
Milk, $\frac{1}{2}$ pint	200
Butter, $\frac{1}{2}$ oz.	112
Total extra cals.	312

No. 3. Expensive Obesity Diet

This diet allows for greater variety than Diets 1 and 2. It includes more expensive foods and has a higher protein content.

Carbohydrate, 100 gm.
Protein, 84 gm. (approximate daily average).
Fat, 52 gm. (approximate daily average).
Calories, 1,204.

Breakfast—
Tea or coffee, with milk from ration.
Ryvita or vitaweat, 2 pieces ; *or* bread (preferably brown), 1 oz. (1 thin slice).
Butter, 2 small balls ($\frac{1}{3}$ oz.) from ration.
Fresh peach, slice of melon, $\frac{1}{2}$ grapefruit or orange.
1 egg ; *or* 1 oz. cold lean ham or tongue. (If preferred, use this for custard or serve as a savoury at dinner.)

Lunch—
Tomato juice cocktail, if desired.
Meat : Medium-sized helping of cooked *lean* meat (2 to 3 oz.), or chicken, or game, or white fish—a good-sized fillet, grilled or baked with $\frac{1}{4}$ oz. extra butter.

Or 2 eggs as omelette, with butter from ration. Mushroom or kidney can be added, also herbs and seasoning.

Or Aspic jelly with cold shell-fish, chicken, game, or egg.

Vegetable: Salad of lettuce, cucumber, tomato, radishes, asparagus tips, etc. Vegetable, as desired, except those forbidden (see List).

Fruit, *e.g.*, apple or pear, etc. (see List to be avoided).

Cheese, one section, $\frac{3}{4}$ oz.

Ryvita or vitaweat, 2 pieces; *or* 3 water biscuits.

Coffee, if desired, with milk from ration.

4 *p.m.*—

Tea, if desired, with milk from ration.

Dinner—

Clear soup, if desired.

* Fish: Fillet of sole (approximately $2\frac{1}{2}$ oz.) grilled with butter from ration.

Or lobster or crayfish (mineral oil mayonnaise). Salad as desired.

Or 1 doz. oysters—lemon juice.

* Meat: Noisettes of mutton (centre of 2 grilled cutlets = 2 oz. meat).

Or chicken, game or braised sweetbread.

Vegetable, except those forbidden.

Fresh fruit as before.

Ryvita, 1 piece; *or* $\frac{1}{2}$ slice thin toast.

Milk from ration can be used for curds, milk jelly custard (using egg from breakfast, or omitting fish); or sauce can be made with butter from allowance and 1 teaspoonful of flour (omitting ryvita, 1 piece). Flavour with vinegar, lemon juice, tomato purée, anchovy essence, parsley, mushroom or a few oysters.

Rations for Day—

Milk, $\frac{1}{2}$ pint.

Butter, $\frac{3}{4}$ oz.

No sugar. Saxin or saccharine, if desired.

To increase this diet, add extra butter which will greatly add to the palatability. Each $\frac{1}{2}$ oz. butter = 112 calories.

* If both fish and meat are not desired, a large helping of either could be taken, *e.g.*, 2 fillets of fish or $\frac{1}{4}$ lb. grilled fillet steak.

If fish only is taken, $\frac{1}{4}$ oz. extra butter may be allowed for cooking.

Diet in Complications.—Obesity is often associated with complications, and some modification of the above diets may be necessary.

Constipation.—If constipation is present larger helpings of green vegetables should be taken. Two tablespoonfuls of Kellogg's All-Bran can be given at breakfast (calories, approximately, 100).

Shredded agar-agar is useful, a dessertspoonful taken with meals as required.

Buttermilk is helpful, and the ration of sweet milk can be reduced. One pint of buttermilk gives 200 calories.

Cholecystitis.—If the obesity is complicated by cholecystitis or gall-stones, egg yolks should be omitted and extra fish or chicken substituted. The more gas-forming vegetables should be omitted, *e.g.*, cabbage, brussel sprouts, peas, turnip, onions. If necessary, other vegetables may be served in purée form. Hot water should be given before breakfast, at bed-time and between meals.

Cardiac Diseases.—Bulky diets are unsuitable in cardiac cases. Very little fluid should be given with meals. The vegetables should be sieved and only served with the mid-day meal, and supper should be light and taken early in the evening. If œdema is present salt should be restricted.

Hypertension.—Low protein diets are sometimes prescribed for obesity with hypertension, but there is little evidence that restriction of protein reduces the blood pressure. There is no doubt, however, that a reduction in the patient's weight helps to accomplish this. If the hypertension is associated with renal insufficiency of the azotæmic type the cooked protein may be omitted from the evening meal, especially in the higher protein diets. Unlimited amounts of tea, coffee and highly salted meat extracts are undesirable in these cases.

THYROID

The well-known stimulating effects of thyroid on the metabolism have been utilized in the treatment of obesity since the end of the nineteenth century. Its popularity has waxed and waned. Formerly large doses were given, but as its limits and dangers have become recognized, more conservative tendencies have prevailed. Many modern writers warn against its promiscuous use in obesity and some consider it irrational and dangerous, since it may cause a degree of hyperthyroidism resulting in an overstrained myocardium.

This latter extreme view is far too narrow. The mere fact that a drug is dangerous when improperly used is not an argument for its banishment from the pharmacopœia. It is true that most obese patients can be treated quite satisfactorily by careful dieting, and for them thyroid is as unnecessary as insulin for the mild diabetic. It is also true that many obese persons with overstrained hearts are intolerant to thyroid, even in minute doses, and rapidly develop tachycardia and palpitation when it is given to them. For them, also, the use of thyroid is contraindicated. In any case, the patient should never be given a prescription for thyroid and be allowed to continue to take the drug indefinitely without medical supervision. Serious permanent damage, especially to the myocardium and nervous system, may result from such methods. Patients taking thyroid should be seen once a fortnight at least and any evidence of tachycardia, such as a resting pulse-rate of over 90, should be an indication for reducing the dose or for withdrawing the drug altogether. Sometimes its use seems to cause tremor, nervousness and, occasionally, diarrhœa, symptoms which again indicate an intolerance to the drug. While thyroid should, therefore, only be prescribed with caution, it is undoubtedly of service when definite subthyroidism is present, or when the weight lost with a subcaloric diet alone is unsatisfactory. It is a useful drug if properly handled and, when definitely indicated, is invaluable.

If it were possible to be certain which endocrine gland was mostly at fault in certain cases of obesity, more specific hormones than thyroid might be used. Endocrine preparations other than thyroid, however, have either no effect, or very inconsistent effects, on the obesity itself—whatever other beneficial results may accrue from their use. Further, it is doubtful to what extent other endocrine preparations, apart from thyroid, are active when given by the mouth, and it is impracticable—or at least inconvenient—to treat obesity by daily injections. Lastly, all other potent and properly standardized endocrine preparations are exceedingly expensive.

Unfortunately, thyroid is procurable in a large number of different forms, giving rise to an inconvenient and possibly dangerous confusion as regards dosage. It is, therefore, much better to confine oneself to the prescription of the standardized pharmacopœial preparation (thyroideum (B.P.)). Unstandardized thyroid preparations, whether of fresh gland or dried extract, may vary more than sixfold in their content of active material. The average dose of thyroideum (B.P.) is 1 gr.

twice a day, which can be increased or decreased as found necessary, the pulse-rate being the chief guide to the size of the dose. As it takes at least a week for a daily dose of thyroid to produce its full effect, some time should be allowed to elapse between each increase in dosage.

Synthetic preparations of thyroxine are expensive and have no particular advantages over the pharmacopœial preparation. Other metabolic stimulants such as dinitrophenol, which had a transient and disastrous popularity, should never be used. Dinitrophenol has powerful toxic effects, especially on the liver, and is no substitute for thyroid in myxœdematous states.

THE CONTROL OF TREATMENT

Patients undergoing reduction in weight should be seen frequently by the doctor, even if they are not taking thyroid. Their dietetic enthusiasm tends to wane unless they receive constant encouragement, and occasionally mild bullying. It is important to warn them against taking sweets and chocolates and sweet drinks between meals. Unless they are so warned, many patients take these oddments quite innocently, thinking that there is little or no food value in such things. Again, many patients become careless about their diet when they go on holiday, or may be unable to procure it accurately in hotels or lodgings. The labour of months may be undone in this way in a few weeks. We have known, for example, one patient who regained 7 lbs. during the course of a week's holiday, and this is not an exceptional example.

Patients should be weighed weekly, and an average loss of between 2 and 3 lbs. a week should be aimed at. If the weight loss is constantly more rapid than this the diet should be slightly increased. When the loss on the other hand does not average 2 lbs. a week, the patient should be carefully questioned as regards her strict observance of the diet, as slackness in this respect is far the most common cause of failure to lose weight satisfactorily. Occasionally, however, it may be necessary in such cases to modify the diet still further from perhaps 1,200 to 1,000 calories, or to give thyroid.

The rate of weight loss from day to day varies considerably. Such fluctuations are of little importance, though they occasionally make it difficult to ascertain the real rate of loss over short periods, and make it unnecessary to weigh the patient more than once a week. Some of these fluctuations may depend on whether or not urine or fæces have been evacuated before weighing, but changes in water balance probably account for most of them. In addition to these daily variations a disturbance in weight loss often accompanies menstruation. For two or three days before the period weight loss usually ceases, and a slight gain may occur, to be followed about the middle of the period by an increased rate of weight loss.

The influence of a subcaloric diet usually falls into three stages. During an initial period of a few days there is a rapid fall in weight, which is probably largely due to fluid loss. Then follows a steady but diminishing loss, and lastly there may occur a phase in which the weight falls very slowly or is even maintained at a new level. Several explanations may be offered for this decreasing rate of weight loss. In part it may depend on the altering relationship of food intake to the body needs, for as the weight falls the total caloric requirements also diminish, and the discrepancy or deficit between these and the food supplied constantly becomes less. To some extent the phenomenon is due to a reduction in the metabolic rate, which invariably occurs on low caloric diets, and which is shown in its greatest degree in the completely fasting individual. This slowing of metabolism is an unavoidable disadvantage when attempting to effect weight reduction by means of a subcaloric diet alone, and justifies the use of small doses of thyroid to counteract its effects. Except in obviously subthyroid patients, it is wise to withhold thyroid till this flattening of the curve of weight reduction becomes obvious. The patients should be warned that the drug is not to be looked upon in any way as a substitute for dietetic treatment, but simply as a subsidiary measure.

No attempt should be made to reduce a very fat woman to her " ideal " weight for her height and age, nor should girls in search of a fashionable figure be allowed to reduce themselves to unduly exiguous proportions. The practitioner must use his common sense in these respects.

It may be said that with practically no exceptions all patients who keep to the régime outlined above lose weight satisfactorily, though they vary considerably in the rate at which this is done. Thus, those who are initially grossly overweight lose on the average more rapidly than those in whom the initial excess weight is only moderate. It might be expected that those cases who show an obvious disturbance of endocrine function would not respond satisfactorily to simple dietetic treatment. This, however, is not the case, since the vast majority of cases of endogenous obesity seem to lose weight satisfactorily with dietetic treatment alone, though endocrine treatment may be advisable for other reasons. Again, the response to treatment is very comparable in those who have been a long time fat, and in those who have only been fat for a few years. Long-standing obesity is, therefore, no drawback to successful treatment.

Unfortunately, once the weight has been satisfactorily reduced, there is usually a tendency for corpulence to return when treatment is entirely discontinued, though the gain in weight is not nearly so rapid as the loss under treatment. Usually a slightly modified normal diet is sufficient to counteract this tendency. The patients have learned dietetic discretion and are usually able to maintain their weight at the new low level by the exercise of a little care, and very strict dieting is no longer necessary. In a few unfortunate people, however, the slightest relaxation in dietetic care is followed by a rapid gain in weight. This tendency is most marked among patients with some definite endocrine disturbance. It is also frequently evident in those who were originally grossly obese and who have lost weight rapidly under treatment. Indeed, the greater the original obesity and the greater the response to treatment, the greater must be the care in relaxing treatment.

In conclusion, it may be said that there are few therapeutic measures in medicine so certain to produce results as the prescription of a subcaloric diet to an obese patient, provided the prescribed diet is strictly observed. In addition, there are few purely medical measures so likely to restore health or to prevent disability as the controlled weight reduction of excessively obese persons. Like so many other forms of therapy, however, much harm can be done by excessive enthusiasm; by an attempt to produce in a few weeks a result which should only be attained in many months, or by attempting to slim people of already normal proportions. It must also be remembered that there is no royal road, nor even a short cut, along which an obese person may travel safely to an ideal weight; but only along the thorny path of dietetic restriction, assisted, perhaps, in the steepest places by the stimulating influences of a little thyroid.

D. M. Dunlop.
R. Pybus.

DEFICIENCY DISEASES

Introduction

Deficiency disease may be defined as a morbid condition caused by the lack of a sufficiency of one or more factors present in a good mixed diet. Prophylaxis, therefore, consists in making certain that the food contains all the proximate principles, minerals and vitamins in sufficient amounts ; here we are concerned specially with the vitamins. Naturally, the requirements will vary with age, rate of growth and special conditions, such as pregnancy. As a general rule, it may be stated that anything which raises the metabolism will also increase the demand for the vitamins, and in this connection infection, toxæmia and pregnancy must be specially noted. Accordingly, when any extra strain is put on the organism, care must be taken that the supply of vitamins is sufficient.

Much has been written about the prevalence of what has been called subclinical hypovitaminosis. There is no doubt that milder degrees of vitamin deficiency may and do pass unrecognized because of cursory clinical examination and lack of appreciation of their early manifestations. This is specially liable to occur in infancy and childhood, during periods of active growth and also in the female during pregnancy and lactation. It is possible that mild degrees of hypovitaminosis may frequently be found when special technical measures are used for their recognition. It is doubtful, however, whether the results of many of these can be taken as evidence of vitamin deficiency. Nevertheless, most authorities are agreed that the incidence of hypovitaminosis, which cannot be recognized by a careful and competent clinical observer, has been much overrated. Furthermore, when a deficiency state exists it can easily be eliminated in the majority of cases by the provision of an adequate mixed diet without having resort to special vitamin preparations. Although a platitude, it seems necessary to keep on reiterating that proximate principles and calories are as essential as vitamins. With good food everything essential is supplied, whereas with attention devoted exclusively to vitamins there is more than a risk that energy-yielding and body-building materials may be insufficient.

For the prophylactic treatment of hypovitaminosis little need be done for the individual with a healthy digestive system except to provide a good mixed diet. Care, however, must be taken when for any reason there is some interference with the processes of digestion or absorption. Thus the problem of hypovitaminosis C (see p. 410) may easily arise in patients with gastric ulcer, or hypovitaminosis B (see p. 404) in subjects suffering from chronic alcoholism. In these and similar cases special measures are required in order to ensure an adequate provision of the various vitamins.

The therapeutics of any deficiency disease is based on a knowledge of three things: (*a*) the clinical picture of the disease in question; (*b*) the diet required to make good the deficiency; (*c*) the highly concentrated preparations which are available for the supply of large amounts of the missing factor.

Generally, the administration of the vitamin required is a matter of little difficulty since oral administration suffices to replenish the supplies of the missing factor. It may be stated that in most cases the treatment of the less severe degrees of deficiency disease requires only natural food products, including cod-liver oil, and that expensive concentrates and proprietary articles achieve no additional purpose. With the severer forms of deficiency disease, highly concentrated products do offer a more rapid and at times a much more effective line of therapy. Occasionally, indeed, it may be necessary because of a very severe deficiency to supply the factor at a rate which cannot be accomplished by the oral route. Parenteral administration may also be required when intestinal absorption is defective, as may occur in cœliac disease (p. 285) or in alcoholic neuritis (p. 978).

It is important to remember that in deficiency diseases the deficiency is frequently multiple. Accordingly, in addition to supplying the vitamin, the lack of which is apparent, it is necessary to provide food containing an abundance of all essential factors.

The table on p. 403 indicates some foodstuffs which contain relatively large amounts of various vitamins.

VITAMIN A DEFICIENCY

The most important function of vitamin A is to promote the nutrition of epithelial surfaces, and the regeneration of visual purple in the retina, and possibly also to maintain the healthy function of the nerve cells. In its absence the epithelial cells tend to atrophy, become keratinized and desquamate. As a result, epithelial ducts become choked with the fragments of dead and dying cells which afford a nidus for the growth of micro-organisms, which cause a low-grade inflammatory reaction in the devitalized epithelial layer. All epithelial surfaces are liable to be involved, but one may mention particularly the cornea, skin and urinary tract. Recent work has shown that one of the first manifestations of hypovitaminosis A is defective vision in dim light (nyctalopia), which apparently is more widespread than is commonly realized. In the less severe types of deficiency the administration of vitamin A in adequate amounts rapidly leads to revitalization of the affected tissues, usually within two or three weeks.

Vitamin A (or its precursor).	Vitamin B.	Vitamin C.	Vitamin D.
Liver.	Liver. Kidney. Lean meat.		
Herring, eel and sardine. Herring roe. Fish liver oils. Egg-yolk.			Herring. Fish liver oils. Egg-yolk.
	Whole-meal bread. Oatmeal. Nuts. Peas and beans. Rice bran. Yeast. Marmite.		
Tomatoes. Spinach. Carrots.		Tomatoes. Oranges. Lemons. Grapefruit. Watercress. Asparagus tips. Parsley. Black currants.	

The ingestion of an adequate diet is without doubt quite sufficient to prevent any deficiency of vitamin A. Consideration of special measures for supplying this factor only arises when the diet is deficient as a result of poverty or idiosyncrasy, or when requirements are increased as is likely in the presence of infection, etc. It should be noted, however, that it is not yet certain whether a curative effect on infection is exerted by a greatly increased supply. Ordinarily, a healthy adult requires about 3,000 international units of vitamin A daily. This is contained in rather more than a teaspoonful of cod-liver oil. A child needs about double the adult requirement, because of the demands resulting from active growth. In pregnant and lactating women the demand for vitamin A is also increased; for them a daily intake of 5,000 international units (contained in 2 teaspoonfuls of cod-liver oil) has been recommended. A good general diet, however, containing some of the following —egg, liver, carrot, spinach and tomato—is all that is generally necessary to meet these requirements. If for financial or other reasons an adequate diet cannot be obtained it is advisable to give cod-liver oil. When the patient is unable or unwilling to take cod-liver oil, a vitamin A concentrate must be prescribed, such as avoleum (B.D.H.) or prepalin (Glaxo).

The actual dose varies with the intensity of the deficiency. When the manifestations of hypovitaminosis are severe, as much as 600,000 international units should be given daily. For milder degrees of deficiency 1 capsule of one of the above preparations three times daily generally suffices. Usually, however, there is an associated hypovitaminosis D, in which case capsules of adexolin (Glaxo), radiostoleum (B.D.H.) or halibut-liver oil (Crookes) are to be preferred. Each of these preparations contains both vitamins A and D ; in mild degrees of deficiency they should be given in doses of 3 capsules daily, one with each meal.

In addition to the administration of the necessary vitamin, appropriate local treatment, for the lesions in the eyes, skin and mucous membranes, must be given. Drops of cod-liver oil can be instilled into the conjunctiva every morning and evening, and $\frac{1}{4}$ per cent. atropine ointment every night. For the skin a simple preparation such as zinc ointment suffices, while for mucous membranes a non-irritant antiseptic lotion such as hydrogen peroxide or euflavine 1 : 1,000 may be used.

BERI-BERI

Beri-beri is prevalent in those countries where the common dietary habits result in a marked deficiency in the intake of vitamin B1. In its frank form, characterized by severe multiple neuritis or signs of cardiac failure, it is very rare in this country. Within the past few years, however, clinical studies have shown that minor degrees of hypovitaminosis B1 are not infrequent, even in regions where the diet of the population had previously been considered satisfactory. Especially is this the case when for any reason absorption in the alimentary tract is defective. Thus, in chronic alcoholism there appears to be no doubt that vitamin B1 deficiency plays a very important part in the causation of polyneuritis. In some of the other forms of polyneuritis also, it is possible that an insufficiency of B1 has at least an aggravating influence. The growing popularity of special diets renders it likely that minor degrees of B1 deficiency will tend to increase and in this connection the dietary régimes so commonly advocated for gastric or duodenal ulcer, obesity and diabetes, have specially to be remembered.

Vitamin B1 can now be obtained in a chemically pure state from natural sources, such as yeast, and can also be prepared synthetically. In this country it is sometimes called aneurin, in the United States, thiamin.

The daily requirement in the healthy adult is said to be amply met by 500 international units (contained in about 2 oz. of marmite or 1 tablet of betaxan (Bayer) or benerva (Roche)). Infants and children require relatively more, as much as 250 units being considered necessary.

It is important, however, to remember that vitamin B1 requirements in man are dependent on body-weight, carbohydrate content of the diet and general metabolism. A high intake of carbohydrate necessitates an extra supply of the vitamin. In addition, the demand for vitamin B may be increased up to fivefold during pregnancy and lactation. Indeed, anything which increases the metabolism, *e.g.*, infection or hyperthyroidism, by raising the need for B1, may precipitate an attack of acute B1 deficiency. Accordingly, in areas where beri-beri is rife, the onset of pregnancy or the presence of infection, as well as the appearance of early symptoms, is a signal for increasing the administration of vitamin B1.

The onset of hypovitaminosis B1 is insidious. Its manifestations are varied and include general muscular weakness, loss of appetite, vague abdominal pain with constipation, neuralgic pains and odd sensations of tingling in the limbs. Later, there is frank peripheral neuritis with circulatory disturbance indicated by dyspnœa, hypotension and œdema. It is obvious that many of these symptoms may be found in association with conditions other than defective B1 intake or utilization. They should not therefore be attributed to hypovitaminosis without a complete investigation of the patient's history and condition.

In this country, at any rate, there is little need to worry about the intake of vitamin B1, unless the dietetic history suggests that the patient has been living on a diet consisting largely of highly refined foodstuffs. It should be remembered, however, that vitamin B1 is rapidly destroyed in an alkaline medium. Accordingly, it seems probable that in conditions where the gastric secretion of hydrochloric acid is defective (primary or secondary hypochlorhydria and achlorhydria) the administration of B1 must be carefully supervised, and on the first indication of hypovitaminosis parenteral therapy adopted. This is specially necessary when there is any history of alcoholism. Alcohol renders B1 very susceptible to destruction in an alkaline medium and in addition lessens and even completely prevents its absorption by the intestinal mucosa. Furthermore, disease of the liver (cirrhosis) or other organ may prevent the utilization of B1 after its absorption.

The vitamin is found in relatively high amounts in yeast, wheat germ, bran, peas and beans, liver and kidney. It is destroyed by prolonged heating, but enough is left in these foods after the ordinary cooking processes to supply the needs of the body. In rice-eating countries much has been done by changing the diet from one of highly polished rice to one in which the rice is boiled and dried prior to the removal of the pericarp. Another method which has been used with some success in India is the daily administration of a freshly prepared infusion of rice bran or of a commercial extract of rice, ryzamin B, (B., W. & Co.) in doses of 20 gr. thrice daily; in addition, attempts are made to insist on the use of unhulled rice with as much vegetables and fruit as can be afforded. The adoption of this procedure suffices not only to prevent the onset of beri-beri but even to effect a cure in the milder cases.

Special diets used for the treatment of gastric or duodenal ulcer, cœliac disease, sprue, or obesity may produce a mild degree of hypovitaminosis. It is of great importance to make certain that the diet contains a sufficiency of B1, or, if this is impracticable for financial or medical reasons, to provide a concentrate of the vitamin. For this purpose 1 oz. of bemax, a stable preparation of wheat germ, or 1 teaspoonful of marmite can be given daily; yeast tablets (Phillips) may also be used, 2 being given three times daily before meals. When there is reason to suspect defective intestinal absorption, betaxan, benerva or other similar preparations can be injected intramuscularly: 1 ampoule containing 2 mg. of synthetic vitamin B1, equivalent to 1,000 international units, is the usual daily dose, but more may be given if it is thought necessary.

When obvious clinical manifestations of vitamin B1 deficiency are already present no time should be lost in commencing treatment, since there is always the danger of circulatory failure. Rest in bed is essential, care being taken, if neuritis is present, that the weight of the bedclothes is removed from the patient's limbs by a cage. While too much work should not be imposed on the digestive tract, it is important so to arrange the diet that a large amount of vitamin B1 is ingested with a minimum quantity of carbohydrate. The feeds, therefore, should be small and frequent, consisting largely of the foodstuffs rich in the vitamin (see Table). Yeast tablets, 2 to 4 three times a day before food, or marmite, 1 to 2 teaspoonfuls three times a day, is a suitable method of giving large doses of B1 when there is no evidence of defective absorption. These substances have the advantage that they contain all the factors present in the vitamin B complex. A more certain method of ensuring an adequate supply of the vitamin is the intramuscular or intravenous injection of " crystalline B1." This overcomes the possibility of defective absorption which is apparently not infrequent in cases of B1 deficiency. Numerous preparations are available. Two to five milligrams (1,000 to 2,500 international units) of a crystalline preparation should be given daily for a fortnight by one of the parenteral routes. Betaxan (Bayer) and benerva (Roche) are preparations of vitamin B1 supplied in ampoules each of which contains 2 mg. of the crystalline substance. Thereafter, treatment can be continued by the oral administration of vitamin B1 preparations in the quantities already mentioned (2 to 5 tablets). When large amounts of vitamin B1 are to be given parenterally it is wise to use special strong solutions available in the form of betaxan or benerva forte, each ampoule (1 c.c.) of which contains 10 mg. In very severe cases 50 or even 100 mg. intravenously may be required, followed by daily intramuscular injections of 20 mg. for two weeks. After a period of intensive therapy the oral route can be adopted, the same amounts of B1 being used until the patient is free of symptoms.

Great improvement and even complete recovery may take place within a few weeks of the commencement of B1 therapy, provided the polyneuritis is not severe.

If paralysis is present, wrist and foot drop must be treated with appropriate splinting to maintain the extremities in the correct positions. Massage should be withheld until pain or tenderness have already disappeared, when it can be gently commenced along with galvanism. As improvement progresses, active as well as passive movements must be undertaken. All forms of muscular exercise must be very carefully graduated, and, in view of the risk of cardiac failure, should be carried out by the patient in bed until a considerable degree of recovery is manifest. Improvement is slow, at times very slow. With the severer cases months are required before appreciable restoration of function is noted. Regeneration of the axone is said to take place at the rate of about 1 mm. per day: accordingly, it is necessary to persevere with treatment and not be disheartened if the degree of recovery is slow.

Circulatory failure is an urgent feature in some cases. If cardiac decompensation is present it should be dealt with (p. 665). Generally the response of patients with circulatory failure to B1 therapy is fairly rapid. Within a few days the pulse-rate falls, the strength of the heart-beat is increased and a large output of urine occurs, so that within two weeks the patient may lose the bulk of his œdema.

It may take two months or longer before all the signs and symptoms of cardiac failure disappear. The longer the previous duration of the disease the more prolonged will be the convalescence, since the myocardium may be seriously weakened in long-standing cases. Of the other manifestations of vitamin B1 deficiency constipation is frequently troublesome, but will usually respond to the specific treatment, assisted when necessary by one or other of the saline purgatives.

During convalescence attention must continually be paid to the diet which should be rich in vitamin B1 and poor in carbohydrate, and should contain a sufficiency of other essential factors.

PELLAGRA

Pellagra is a disease associated with some dietary defect resulting from poverty, disorder of the gastro-intestinal tract or refusal to take certain articles of food. The diets of pellagrins are poor in the foodstuffs which are relatively rich in B complex; another characteristic is a deficiency of protein of high biological value. In this country pellagra occurs chiefly among insane persons but is also found among alcoholics, individuals with cirrhosis of the liver and gastritis, and patients who have had short-circuiting operations on the alimentary tract. Mild degrees are probably not infrequent and may be recognized by pigmentation, dryness and scaliness of the skin.

Prophylaxis consists in the supply of foods rich in pellagra-preventing vitamin, *i.e.*, milk, lean beef, liver, chicken, rabbit, salmon, green peas, spinach, tomatoes, turnip greens and yeast. In areas of the U.S.A. where pellagra is endemic, home gardening and the distribution of powdered yeast have yielded good results.

When the pellagrous symptoms are already manifest the diet should immediately be changed to one rich in protein and poor in carbohydrate and fat. Restriction of the latter is advisable in order to avoid the production or aggravation of the digestive disorder which is so frequently associated with pellagra. The caloric intake should be high, amounting to at least 3,000 calories. Furthermore, the diet must be presented in a form which is easily digested by the alimentary tract. Lastly, it is most important to make certain that the prescribed foodstuffs are taken, and for this purpose individual nursing is very often necessary. Broths made from liver, lean meat and beef juice, and fresh vegetable soups have all yielded good results. If milk is to be the chief source of the antipellagra factor it is best given in the form of buttermilk in amounts of not less than 2 pints per day.

Dried powdered yeast in amounts of 1 to 7 oz. per day has been found valuable. Liver extracts in large doses parenterally have also been used with success, especially when there is any disturbance of intestinal absorption. Achlorhydria is very frequently present and hydrochloric acid should be given in doses of 1 drachm of the dilute acid (B.P.) three times a day.

One of the features of the disease is dermatitis which is chiefly confined to regions of the body exposed to light. Patients should therefore be protected from direct sunlight, and, where necessary, a soothing ointment, such as unguentum zinci oxidi (B.P.), can be applied to the skin. For stomatitis, which is frequently present, a bland antiseptic paint such as glycerinum acidi borici (B.P.) can be used.

Reports are now available of the successful use of nicotinic acid in the treatment of pellagra. This substance, which is a constituent of the vitamin B complex and has been isolated from yeast and liver, can be produced synthetically. It may be given in a solution of normal saline in daily amounts of 60 mg. by the intravenous or intramuscular route or in the form of tablets in larger doses of 500 to 1,500 mg. per os. In all the cases so far reported rapid improvement was observed. Within twenty-four hours the desire for food returned, while in two days there was a distinct betterment of the mental condition. Shortly afterwards the dermatitis and inflammatory lesions of the tongue and buccal mucosa disappeared and the excess porphyrinuria characteristic of pellagra subsided. Within a fortnight the lost peripheral reflexes were again elicited. Spies, who is responsible for much of the clinical investigation, recommends nicotinic acid in doses of 100 mg. five times daily, and states that it is rarely necessary to give the drug by a parenteral route. If the latter is necessary it is to be noted that, in every case, injection of more than 50 mg. has caused some slight discomfort, such as sensations of heat and tingling with peripheral vasodilatation and a slight fall of blood pressure.

Spies further stresses the fact that nicotinic acid is only one of the essential substances and urges that this drug should only be used as a supplement to a well-balanced diet in the treatment of pellagra.

SCURVY

Frank scurvy, which is due to an inadequate supply of vitamin C or ascorbic acid, is in this country a comparatively rare condition. It is occasionally met with in infants and young children, especially those fed on some of the dried milks without supplements of some vitamin-C-containing food. It is also to be found among subjects with chronic alcoholism and old people living in lodging houses, whose diet has been extremely poor. It is possible that mild degrees of hypovitaminosis C are more frequent than has hitherto been supposed but it is unlikely that such conditions are as widespread as some authors have stated.

Prophylaxis and treatment consists in ensuring an ample supply of ascorbic acid. Among the common articles of diet containing large amounts of vitamin C are oranges, lemons, grapefruit and tomatoes. Carrots, potato-juice (uncooked) and sprouted vegetables are also fairly rich in ascorbic acid, a moderate amount of which is present in fresh beef and liver broth. Cooking leads to a destruction of ascorbic acid, and even storage of food is associated with a gradual diminution in this substance. Tinned fruits, however, retain their vitamin C potency. Pasteurization may, and often does, lead to a destruction of the ascorbic acid of milk. The vitamin C content, however, even of fresh milk is insufficient by itself to meet the requirements of infants or children, so that its destruction is of little import, since under all circumstances more has to be provided.

The best preventive measure is undoubtedly the provision of a good mixed diet, taking special care that there is a plentiful supply of fruit and vegetables. There is no necessity for the wholesale distribution of tablets of ascorbic acid. An orange contains about 25 mg. of ascorbic acid—the daily amount required both by adult and child. Relatively higher amounts are required during periods of rapid growth or when infections are present. In pregnancy and during lactation vitamin C requirements are also increased, as is the case when much muscular exercise is being undertaken. There is no doubt that during febrile states there is a greater utilization or destruction of vitamin C. Accordingly, a larger intake is required, especially if the fever is continued for more than a few days. This has long been, and can still be, quite efficiently accomplished by the administration of large amounts of fresh fruit juices (orange and lemon drinks). During the course of a prolonged illness, especially when associated with some infective process, great care must be taken to provide a sufficiency of vitamin C in the food. This is also necessary when for any reason a patient is on a restricted diet, such as occurs in the treatment of gastric ulcer and various forms of dyspepsia. In these cases it may be necessary to give vitamin C in the form of ascorbic acid itself, which is available as tablets, *e.g.*, redoxon (Roche), each containing 50 mg. ascorbic acid: 2 tablets per day usually suffice. The infant's requirements of vitamin C are also high and it is necessary to provide this factor for the breast-fed as well as the artificially-fed baby. Orange juice, or some similar vitamin-C-containing fluid, should, therefore, always be included in the infant's dietary. The *minimal* daily amounts recommended are 1 teaspoonful of sweetened orange juice in the first month of life, gradually increased to 4 teaspoonfuls by the end of the third month. Tomato juice in double these amounts is equally efficacious.

When the symptoms and signs of scurvy have already appeared it is essential to give large doses of vitamin C. Here special standardized preparations of ascorbic acid are preferable to fruits whose content of vitamin C is variable. Occasionally, the writer has encountered cases where the scorbutic condition has proved refractory to treatment, possibly as a result of the poor quality of the oranges supplied. Furthermore, the use of a concentrated preparation of ascorbic acid enables much larger doses to be administered than could conveniently be done with fruit juice.

One hundred and fifty to two hundred and fifty milligrams of ascorbic acid (3 to 5 redoxon tablets) should be given daily. When the condition is very severe, or when there is any reason to suspect imperfect intestinal absorption, a parenteral route of administration may be chosen. Generally, an intramuscular injection is given, but if the patient is very ill, the intravenous route should be used. For parenteral injection a 2 c.c. ampoule of redoxon, containing 100 mg., may be given once or twice daily. The special *forte* preparation containing 500 mg. in 1 ampoule may be necessary when there is an urgent demand for vitamin C in large amount.

In addition to the administration of vitamin C general hygienic measures are required. Careful nursing in the acute stage is of very great importance, special care being taken to handle the patient as little as possible. Indeed, owing to the possibility of myocardial weakness, movement in bed should be reduced to a minimum. Clothing should be so arranged that it can easily be removed and changed. The limbs, which are painful as a result of subperiosteal hæmorrhages, should be lightly wrapped in cotton and the weight of the bedclothes avoided by a cage. If the arms are tender they may be bandaged to the chest. For the lower limbs light splinting may be used. Frequently, there is diarrhœa, but this has not to be taken as a contraindication to the administration of either ascorbic acid or orange juice, which indeed usually cures an apparently severe gastro-enteritis. If necessary, a sedative antidiarrhœal mixture (chalk-mixture or bismuth with or without opium) can be given. For the bleeding from the mouth, bowel or urinary tract no special treatment is required, since it rapidly ceases with the administration of vitamin C. If there is marked anæmia, a blood-transfusion may be necessary (see p. 478). Frequently the gums and mouth are fœtid with patches of ulceration : a simple antiseptic mouth wash such as hydrogen peroxide should be used. If the ulceration is severe the affected parts may be painted with 1 per cent. gentian violet.

Within twenty-four hours of the administration of vitamin C the pains diminish greatly, movement becomes easier and the patient brighter. Bleeding from the mouth and bowel rapidly stops, as does the hæmaturia, the cessation of which is accompanied by an increased output of urine. Subperiosteal hæmorrhages generally persist for a considerable time. Shortly after the initiation of vitamin C therapy, the X-ray reveals a rapid deposition of calcium in the hæmatoma. Repeated skiagrams, however, show that it may take months before conditions in and around the bone return to normal. Indeed, a permanent arthritis may result.

Once the stage of convalescence has been reached, the diet should be increased, steps being taken to make certain that it contains ample vitamin C. At the same time attention has to be given to the necessity for dealing with other deficiency conditions, among which anæmia may specially be mentioned. The anæmia of scurvy responds to vitamin C alone, but as iron stores may also be depleted it is wiser to give iron as well. In this connection it is worth remembering that in certain cases of microcytic anæmia, when the hæmoglobin ceases to rise with iron therapy, the use of vitamin C has resulted in a steady improvement as judged both by clinical and hæmatological standards.

As in the case of most other new drugs, ascorbic acid has

been recommended as a panacea for many widely different diseases. Apart from scurvy and the anæmia which accompanies it, the administration of ascorbic acid has led to insignificant results. Accordingly the indiscriminate use of proprietary preparations of ascorbic acid is to be deprecated.

RICKETS

It is important for everyone responsible for the care of infants and young children to remember that while florid rickets may have all but disappeared, mild degrees of the rachitic process are still frequently found in the first two years of life by careful clinical, radiological and biochemical examination. A recent investigation, in which the writer took part, revealed the fact that about 50 per cent. of the infants admitted to the wards of a large municipal hospital showed definite signs of rickets, although only 3 per cent. were diagnosed as such on admission. The significance of mild degrees of rickets in relation to the future health of the child is not clear, but it seems reasonable to avoid any possible effects by ensuring an adequate retention of lime, especially during periods when growth of bone is very active.

The most important factors in the ætiology of rickets are lack of sufficient exposure to sunshine and a diet defective in vitamin D. Although breast-milk is undoubtedly the best type of infant food, it does not necessarily contain enough vitamin D to prevent rickets. The action of vitamin D is to promote the retention of calcium and phosphorus, and this is particularly important if the supply of these minerals is defective. In infancy milk is the staple food, so that an inadequate intake of lime must rarely be a factor in the production of rickets, unless human milk of a poor quality or a very dilute cow's milk mixture is supplied. During childhood, however, there appears to be no doubt that a dietary deficiency in calcium may be quite marked.

It is obvious that the prophylaxis and treatment of rickets resolves itself into ensuring an ample supply of calcium and vitamin D. Phosphorus may be left to look after itself, since it is hard to conceive of any human diet likely to be deficient in this element if a diet adequate in calcium is being taken. Milk, cheese and other milk products are the only satisfactory sources of lime, but it must be remembered that, quite apart from its bone-forming substances, milk contains elements of high biological value, capable of stimulating growth. With the promotion of growth produced by a good milk intake, the development of rickets may actually be favoured, unless vitamin D is given in sufficient amount.

Before discussing the measures to be adopted in the prevention and treatment of rickets, it is necessary to consider the various forms in which vitamin D may be supplied, viz., cod-liver oil and other fish-liver oils, concentrated preparations of vitamin D, irradiated milk and other irradiated foodstuffs, and the irradiation of the skin of the patient.

Cod-liver Oil.—This is probably the easiest and certainly the cheapest method of administering vitamin D. It has the additional advantages of containing vitamin A, and is itself of high caloric value. The infant is well able to assimilate cod-liver oil without digestive disturbance unless there is an idiosyncrasy to fat such as occurs in fat dyspepsia and cœliac disease. In some districts there is a tradition that cod-liver oil is harmful during warm weather, but there is no evidence to substantiate this view. Up till the past few years a valid objection to the use of cod-liver oil might have been that its content of vitamin D was not guaranteed. Nowadays, however, the British Pharmacopœia insists on a minimum content of 85 international units per ml. of the oil. Good brands of oil usually contain 100 units per ml. Another objection frequently raised was the rancid odour and the fishy taste of the oil. The rancid odour is no longer present in modern preparations. The objection to the taste is not instinctive but acquired, usually as a result of the parents' or nurse's stupidity. It need hardly be said that even if the mother or nurse has a profound abhorrence of the taste and smell this should not be revealed to the child. It is neither necessary nor advisable to add orange juice or any flavouring agent to the oil, since with continuous administration infants and young children rapidly begin to like the taste and look forward to the oil. Care must be taken that the oil is entirely swallowed. With the child this is not difficult, but during the administration of the oil to an infant the baby's mouth should be kept open by pressing the cheeks inwards with the thumb and forefinger of the left hand, while the oil is slowly poured into the mouth from a spoon held in the right hand. The mouth must be kept open until the oil has been swallowed : otherwise some may be expelled. There are possibly a few young children with an idiosyncrasy to cod-liver oil, but the one real contraindication to its use is the presence of fat intolerance, especially cœliac disease.

For prophylactic purposes, then, cod-liver oil is quite adequate. It should be given in doses of 10 minims daily at two weeks, 30 minims at four weeks, 60 minims at six weeks, gradually increasing to 2 drachms at three months and 3 drachms at four months. Although many rachitic infants have been completely cured by the use of cod-liver oil alone it is probably wise in the treatment of active rickets to fortify the oil by the addition of some vitamin D concentrate.

There is no advantage in preferring a cod-liver-oil emulsion or a cod-liver oil and malt mixture. If sanely handled, the young child does not require to have the taste disguised, and the use of these preparations simply makes it necessary for the patient to swallow larger amounts of medicine. Cod-liver oil emulsion may contain only 25 per cent. of oil and cod-liver oil and malt only 10 per cent.

Halibut-liver Oil has yielded excellent results in the prophylaxis and treatment of rickets. It is available in the form of Crookes collosol brand halibut-liver oil, haliverol (Parke, Davis) and other preparations. Other fish-liver oils have also been used successfully in the treatment of rickets, and some form the basis of vitamin D concentrates, but none have achieved the popularity of cod-liver oil.

Vitamin D Concentrate.—Numerous brands are available, all being prepared from calciferol (crystalline vitamin D). The chief advantage obtained from the use of one of these concentrates is the ability to administer large doses of vitamin D in relatively small bulk. This is highly desirable in the treatment of a patient with active rickets and in the prophylactic treatment of those children with fat dyspepsia or an idiosyncrasy to cod-liver oil. At one time it was said that the vitamin D contained in a natural product such as cod-liver oil was more potent than calciferol in the treatment of rickets in the human subject. More recent work has shown that this is not the case, and carefully conducted clinical studies indicate that calciferol and cod-liver oil are equipotent, unit for unit, both prophylactically and therapeutically. An objection that has been put forward to the use of vitamin D concentrates is the danger of hypervitaminosis D. This will be discussed later : here it need only be said that if the administration is kept within the recommended dosage there is certainly no more risk of poisoning than with any other drug in the pharmacopœia.

For prophylactic purposes a daily intake of 5 to 10 minims of liquor calciferolis, equivalent to 1,000 to 2,000 international units, is to be recommended for the infant, and 2,000 units for the child. The therapeutic dose should not be less than 10 minims of the liquor (2,000 units). The wide variations in these amounts are due to the differences in the diets of the individual patients.

Various other preparations of vitamin D concentrate are available, such as radiostol or ostelin. For prophylaxis in infants 6 to 15 drops daily should be given, and for active treatment 15 to 20 drops, which may be added to the milk. For older children radiostol pellets or ostelin tablets, two or three daily, can be used. In some cases the concentrate is made up with calcium, but these preparations do not present any advantage as the amount of lime given is relatively insignificant. If there is any reason to suspect a vitamin A deficiency in the diet it is advisable to choose a preparation containing this factor. For this purpose adexolin (10 drops) or radiostoleum (30 drops) daily can be given to infants with manifest signs of rickets. Capsules or pellets can be used for older children.

Irradiated Milk.—An increase in the antirachitic activity of milk may be obtained either by adding a vitamin D concentrate to the milk, feeding the cows on irradiated yeast or irradiating the milk. The last variety has been used successfully both in the prevention and cure of rickets. It has the advantage of supplying other factors of prime importance. Its disadvantages are the inconstancy of the vitamin D content which varies with the efficiency of the irradiating plant and the care with which the irradiation is done. It is only adapted for cities where pasteurization and irradiation can be combined and carefully supervized. There is a risk of inefficient therapy since the antirachitic potency of the milk cannot be determined prior to its use, whereas cod-liver oil and vitamin D concentrates can be and are standardized before they are marketed.

Heliotherapy.—Since the work of Huldschinsky the efficiency of direct irradiation of the skin with ultra-violet rays has been recognized. These rays lead to the formation of vitamin D in the skin.

Only radiations with wave-lengths of less than 310 Angström units have any antirachitic potency. Quite apart from the pall of smoke which overhangs industrial areas, the atmosphere itself absorbs a large proportion of these short-wave radiations. Accordingly the greater the thickness of the atmosphere through which the sun's rays have to pass, the fewer the ultra-violet radiations that reach the earth's surface. It has been shown that the angle of inclination of the sun must be greater than 35 degrees before any ultra-violet rays get through. Thus direct sunlight in the winter months has little or no antirachitic potency in northern countries. Fortunately skyshine, which is composed of the sun's radiations that have been reflected and scattered, has considerable antirachitic power. In the winter months the ultra-violet radiations of skyshine may far exceed those of direct sunshine. It should be emphasized, however, that in order to obtain the full value of skyshine nothing must intervene between the skin of the patient and any portion of the sky. Thus an infant at an open window facing open country will at best receive but half of the available ultra-violet irradiations. In a city street only a small fraction of rays of skyshine will fall even on those out of doors. Hence to get full value of either direct sunshine or skyshine it is necessary to take the child to an open space such as a park.

Since ordinary window-glass absorbs ultra-violet rays and renders them ineffective, the use of special glass with the property of being permeable to these rays has been strongly recommended. The generalized use of this form of window, however, would entail very considerable expense without corresponding advantage, since the amount of ultra-violet irradiation even through an open window diminishes rapidly as one moves inwards. This special glass may be of use in large institutions where it is impossible to take the infants out every day, but is certainly not worth while where they can be exposed daily to sun or skyshine, because on the days when weather conditions prevent children being taken out, very little ultra-violet light can get through the atmosphere.

The formation of vitamin D in the skin as a result of ultra-violet irradiation takes place only in the exposed areas. Fortunately the exposure of a comparatively small area can, if sufficiently prolonged, have a marked antirachitic action. The smaller the area and the less intense the irradiation the longer must be the duration of the exposure. If heliotherapy is to play a significant part in the supply of vitamin D the young subject must be taken into the open air, preferably in a field or park, for as long as possible and in all weathers except fog, storm or heavy rain. The presence of snow on the ground increases by reflection the intensity of the ultra-violet irradiation. The antirachitic potency of sunshine cannot be measured by the intensity of "sun-burn." This fact is worth stressing in view of the tendency noticeable in recent years to a return to sun-bathing. Indeed, prolonged exposure to the sun's rays, unless carefully regulated, may be followed by exhaustion, quite apart from the destruction of the skin by burning.

In conclusion, it may be said that exposure to sunshine or skyshine is a valuable adjunct in the prophylaxis of rickets, but in this country other measures in addition are generally necessary.

Artificial Ultra-violet Irradiation can be obtained from a mercury-vapour lamp. This is an expensive apparatus requiring the services of a trained operator, luxuries far beyond the means of most parents. In order to bring the benefits into almost every home, ultra-violet clinics have been established where efficient treatment is given. These clinics suffer from the disadvantage that they form admirable means for the dissemination of infection, thereby counter-balancing the good results of ultra-violet therapy which can be obtained more cheaply by the wise use of cod-liver oil. It must be admitted, however, that when there is some form of fat intolerance, such as cœliac disease, artificial ultra-violet therapy is invaluable.

For prophylactic purposes irradiation should be given for five minutes on alternate days. When active rickets is already present, daily irradiation should be given at first for thirty seconds, the time being increased by one minute at each session until the treatment lasts ten minutes. The distance of the lamp may be cautiously diminished. Some form of dark glass must be used to protect the eyes.

Prophylaxis.—This consists in the supply of vitamin D by one of the above-mentioned methods together with the provision of a suitable diet containing an abundance of lime, and the institution of a satisfactory general hygiene. Open air provides a stimulus to the general metabolism, so that the child should be taken out every day unless weather conditions render this unwise. The diet will vary with the age of the individual, but as soon as possible it should contain eggs, dairy foods, vegetables and fruits, and for older children the supply of milk should not be stinted, being kept at a level of 2 pints per day or even higher. It may be mentioned that neither pasteurization nor boiling of milk has any deleterious effect on the vitamin D content. Carbohydrates should not be given in excess. The fact that cereals have a rachitogenic effect which can be abolished by irradiation has led to the advocacy of irradiated cereals. The use of these expensive foods is quite unnecessary, nor is it necessary to stop the consumption of untreated cereals, since any rachitogenic effect that they possess can be effectively overcome by the provision of adequate vitamin D. The actual amounts of vitamin D which should be specially supplied depends on the diet, the daily exposure of the infant to skyshine or sunshine, and, most important of all, the rate of growth. The more rapid the increase in weight the more ample must be the supply of vitamin D.

Maternal Treatment.—It seems undoubted that the supply of milk and vitamin D to the expectant and nursing mother increases the calcium content of the newborn infant and raises the quality of the breast milk both as regards its concentration of lime and its antirachitic potency. During pregnancy and lactation care should therefore be taken of the mother's diet and hygiene, because in this way the susceptibility of the infant to rickets may be considerably reduced. It is wise, for this reason and also because of the demands made on the expectant and nursing mother for the supply of lime, to give her a diet containing abundant milk and a generous amount of vitamin D. This will prevent osteoporosis and osteomalacia, minor degrees of which are probably much more frequent than is suspected, and is particularly evident in some forms of dental hypoplasia and caries.

Since there is definite evidence that the rachitic process may commence in the first month of life, prophylactic treatment should be commenced within two weeks of the infant's birth and ought to be continued for at least the first three years of life and preferably till much later. It must be carried on throughout all the seasons. Although the maximum incidence of rickets is in late winter and spring, it may occur at any time when growth is taking place and when the child is not supplied with a sufficiency of vitamin D.

Treatment of Patient with Active Rickets.—The essence of the therapeutic attack on rickets is the provision of an ample supply of lime and vitamin D. This can be achieved by a diet rich in milk and milk-products, and the administration of one or other of the preparations with a high content of vitamin D. Elementary phosphorus, whether as phosphorated oil or in other form, is of no value, since it has no effect on the rate of healing of the rachitic process : it may induce deposition of lime in the juxta-epiphyseal region of the bone, but it does not promote the calcification of proliferating cartilage. Nor is there any need for other drugs. It must be remembered, however, that the rachitic infant frequently suffers from other defects besides that of vitamin D, so that it may be necessary to supply iron to cure an attendant anæmia or vitamin C for associated scurvy.

It should be emphasized that while dietetic measures may prevent rickets it is certainly not sufficient to cure this disorder. Overfeeding should be avoided. In the first place the infant with rickets is liable to be affected by alimentary disorders, and, secondly, a high caloric diet may act as a stimulus to the growth process with the result that more lime is required and the rickets becomes more acute. Consequently, during the active phase of rickets, the diet, while rich in minerals, should contain a limited amount of carbohydrates and cereals.

The bones, owing to their low content of lime, tend to be easily deformed. Accordingly as little strain as possible should be put on the skeletal system. The infant should be kept in bed and handled as little as possible, but he should not be allowed to lie for too long in one position in case curvature of the spine or other deformity should result. The older child should be kept off his feet and discouraged to use his upper limbs until the acute stage is passed. Once treatment has been initiated gentle massage and passive movements may be started, but it is generally found that as the rachitic process is cured the natural activity of the child increases, and voluntary movements soon restore the natural tone to the muscles. Special medicated baths are quite unnecessary, although the stimulus of the ordinary bath is as valuable for the rachitic as for the healthy infant. Commencing deformities are often reduced by exercises specially adapted for each case. Particular care has to be taken, especially in the case of infants with deformities of the thorax, to prevent upper respiratory infections, which are liable to progress to a severe bronchopneumonia (see p. 287).

One of the commonest accompaniments of rickets is tetany, which is specially liable to occur in the very early stages of healing, particularly if inadequate doses of vitamin D are being given. The treatment of this condition is dealt with elsewhere, but here it is worth stating that if there is any reason to suspect a tendency to spasmophilia, extra calcium should be given in the form of gluconate or other easily assimilable salt (see p. 425).

Results of Treatment.—The rachitic patient begins to react to vitamin D administration within one week. By that time an increased retention of calcium and phosphorus can be demonstrated. Signs of healing cannot, however, be seen on the X-ray picture for two to three weeks, and about the same time is required before any alteration in blood chemistry (increase of serum inorganic phosphate and reduction of plasma phosphatase) is noted. Clinical improvement is rapid—the child becomes less irritable and fractious, ceases to perspire so profusely and is handled more easily. Soon an improvement in muscle tone is observed and the patient becomes more active. Cranio-tabes disappears quickly, but many of the bony deformities may be permanent. For some of the latter, such as contracted pelvis, nothing can be done, but considerable improvement of the less severe of the limb deformities may be obtained by a combined process of softening of the bones and suitable splinting. The bones are softened by means of ammonium chloride, given by mouth in large doses (15 to 30 gr. five times daily). The compensated acidosis thus produced leads to a greatly increased excretion of lime and consequent decalcification of bones which become more capable of being moulded. The rachitic state itself must be completely healed before this form of treatment is commenced.

Hypervitaminosis D.—Ever since it has been shown that massive doses of irradiated ergosterol could produce toxic symptoms and pathological changes in animals, reports have appeared of symptoms of overdosage in the human subject. There seems to be no doubt that some infants and children show an idiosyncrasy to vitamin D preparations—in one case even a single drop of a concentrate was sufficient to produce a violent attack of vomiting. In such patients recovery from these symptoms is rapid after the administration of the vitamin is stopped. More serious is the statement that administration of vitamin D in high doses produces calcinosis affecting specially the kidneys. The case reports demonstrating this are not convincing, while records are available showing that even colossal doses of vitamin D continued for months have not caused any untoward symptoms. It is necessary to emphasize this fact, since a few odd case-records may tend to limit quite unjustifiably the use of one of our most valuable remedies. Renal calcinosis was described by pathologists long before vitamin D was discovered, and will continue to occur for reasons quite unconnected with this vitamin. It may therefore be confidently asserted that vitamin D, in amounts considerably exceeding the usual therapeutic dosage, is not fraught with any ill-effect apart from the digestive disturbances that may occur in individuals with an idiosyncrasy.

Refractoriness to Treatment.—The presence of infection prevents the usual reaction to antirachitic therapy. Frequently recurring mild infections have a greater inhibitory effect than single acute attacks. Catarrh of the upper respiratory passages is particularly prone to favour the development of rickets and prevent its cure, possibly because the young patients are so frequently confined indoors. Every effort, therefore, should be made to keep these patients in the open air as much as possible, a procedure which will be of benefit in the management of the respiratory infection as well as for the prevention and treatment of rickets. Occasionally, even in the absence of infection, the rachitic state does not yield to treatment with the usual amounts of vitamin D. Increase in the dosage will generally overcome this refractory state unless there is some underlying constitutional abnormality.

Cœliac Rickets.—Essentially there is no difference between cœliac and ordinary infantile rickets. The important point to remember is that rickets is specially prone to occur when the growth impulse becomes active during a period of remission of the cœliac disease. Care must be taken in treatment that calcium and vitamin D are supplied in forms that are likely to be utilized. For calcium, useful forms of administration are skimmed milk or dried milk with a low percentage of fat: these are available in the form of Cow & Gate separated milk food (white label), prolac or buttermilk powder (G.L.). Vitamin D should be given with a minimum amount of oily substance. For this purpose concentrates in the form of tablets are particularly suitable, but it is here that ultra-violet irradiation finds one of its most beneficial applications.

Renal Rickets.—The pathogenesis of this condition has not been elucidated, but the rickets is merely a secondary feature of some profound underlying disturbance. Treatment, which at best can be merely palliative, is rendered extremely difficult by the fact that the mechanism regulating acid-base equilibrium is greatly impaired. Where renal inefficiency is marked the metabolism rapidly swings from acidosis, with its attendant uræmia, to alkalosis and tetany and vice versa. Although the administration of large amounts of vitamin D leads to an increase in the retention of lime it appears to do little to alter the course of the disease. Recently it has been shown that the use of an alkaline diet supplemented by alkalis and the addition of lime salts, such as calcium gluconate, may improve the renal condition. It may therefore be of advantage to give vitamin D with the object of increasing the retention of lime. The outlook in these cases is so gloomy that such a form of therapy is well worth trying, although it has been pointed out that the administration of vitamin D with a diet rich in calcium may lead to metastatic calcification.

Osteomalacia.—This disease may be defined as rickets occurring after osseous growth has been completed. It is therefore the result of vitamin D and calcium deficiency. The belief is still widespread that the ovarian secretions play a mysterious but important part in its pathogenesis. This is probably due to the fact that exacerbations are caused by pregnancy and lactation. This is not surprising when one remembers that the fœtus makes a great demand on the calcium stores of the mother in the later months of intra-uterine life. It is necessary to emphasize these points in order to stress the fact that therapy is identical with that advised for ordinary infantile rickets. The diet must be ample and care must specially be taken to ensure an adequate supply of lime, in other words, milk, cheese and other milk-products. Vitamin D must be supplied either as cod-liver oil or calciferol or by means of ultra-violet irradiation.

At least 4 pints of milk or its equivalent must be present in the daily diet. Should there be a scarcity of milk foods calcium can be given in the form of *lactate* or *gluconate* (2 drachms or more thrice daily). Cod-liver oil, in amounts of 2 oz. per day, generally relieves the pains of the osteomalacic patient, but it is preferable to fortify the calcifying action of the oil by the addition of calciferol. Thus ostelin or radiostol can be given in doses of 30 drops daily. As in rickets, phosphorated oil has no value. Steps should also be taken to make good other deficiencies in the diet.

If labour has to be conducted in an osteomalacic patient, it is probably best to advise Cæsarean section. A repetition of pregnancy is very inadvisable until the osteomalacic condition is cured. Oophorectomy, although still holding a place of honour in many textbooks, is no longer necessary; it probably received its place in the treatment of osteomalacia merely because of its action in preventing pregnancy. If calcium metabolism is restored to normal by an adequate dietary and vitamin D there is no reason why the patient should lose the benefit of the ovarian secretions.

TETANY

Introduction

An appreciation of the pathogenesis of tetany is of great advantage when one is faced with the choice of suitable therapeutic measures. Clinical varieties of tetany are conveniently divided into two groups according as the serum calcium is or is not reduced. In the first, or hypocalcæmic group, are included cases associated with rickets, cœliac disease, hypoparathyroidism and renal dysfunction; in the latter, or eucalcæmic group, are tetanies due to gastric disorder, bicarbonate administration and hyperventilation. While it is not conclusively proved, it is helpful from the therapeutic point of view to accept the hypothesis that the cause of the increased neuromuscular excitability is a reduction in the amount of ionized calcium. In hypocalcæmic tetany this fraction is diminished because of the fall in total calcium, while in the eucalcæmic group the ionized calcium is below normal limits as a result of an increase in the alkaline reaction of the blood.

The level of serum calcium can be raised in one of four ways : (1) by the parenteral administration of calcium ; (2) by the administration of vitamin D together with a diet rich in lime ; (3) by the injection of parathyroid extract ; (4) by the administration of an acid-producing salt. Parenteral administration of calcium, especially if accomplished by the intravenous route, provides the most rapid method of raising the serum calcium level. It has, however, but a transient effect and is therefore suited only for tiding over an emergency such as a prolonged convulsion. Furthermore, if the tetany is of the eucalcæmic variety the beneficial effect of the increase in serum calcium may be almost immediately rendered null by the fact that little addition is made to the ionized fraction.

The second method, that of supplying vitamin D, is undoubtedly most satisfactory in all types where hypocalcæmia is the result of defective retention of lime. It takes some days, however, before the increased retention produced by vitamin D makes itself effective in raising the serum calcium. Accordingly, if there are active manifestations of tetany such as laryngismus or carpo-pedal spasm, some method must be adopted to tide over this latent period.

The supply of parathyroid extract would appear to be the ideal method of treatment where there is defective secretion of the parathyroid hormone, such as occurs after parathyroidectomy or in idiopathic hypoparathyroidism. Even in this type of case there are disadvantages. The preparation is expensive and, in addition, prolonged use of the extract leads to a gradual weakening of its effect so that larger doses have to be employed with diminishing effect. In infantile tetany due to vitamin D deficiency the use of this expensive preparation is neither necessary nor desirable. Its prolonged use, indeed, is contraindicated, since it produces its effect on the serum calcium by decalcifying osseous tissue.

The fourth method of raising the serum calcium by the use of acid-producing substances is also dependent on an increased flow of calcium from the bones, and therefore should not be used for more than a few days when there is osteoporosis, unless steps are taken to make good the lime deficiency. This method has, however, one great advantage : not only does it lead to a rise in total calcium, but it also produces an increase in the ionized fraction so that it can be used in tetany of the eucalcæmic variety. Acid-producing substances can be given in therapeutic doses without risk to healthy children and to most infants and children with rickets. It has to be remembered that some children, particularly of the latter group, suffer from intestinal and other disorders that render them easily liable to disturbances of acid-base equilibrium so that a severe acidosis may be, and occasionally is, produced. This liability to acidosis is even more marked in the patient whose tetany is due to chronic interstitial nephritis. In this latter condition a small addition of acid may suffice to precipitate a very severe attack of uræmia.

These, then, are the methods in common use for raising the level of serum calcium and for the prevention and cure of the tetany syndrome. It will now be convenient to consider the treatment of each type of tetany in more detail.

TETANY ASSOCIATED WITH DEFICIENCY OF VITAMIN D

Rachitic Tetany.—Efficient prevention and treatment of rickets is undoubtedly the best prophylactic. In this connection the biphasic effect of vitamin D on the retention of lime should be kept in mind. It has been shown by the writer and others that shortly after beginning the administration of vitamin D there may occur a rapid fall in the retention of calcium which may precipitate an attack of tetany. It is therefore advisable to make certain that ample calcium is available by giving large doses of an easily assimilable calcium salt (gluconate or lævulinate).

Once the signs of tetany are detected, active treatment should be initiated as soon as possible. Calcium gluconate (10 c.c. of a 20 per cent. solution) may be given intravenously where the symptoms are urgent, *e.g.*, convulsive seizures or painful carpopedal spasm. If this degree of urgency is not required, the gluconate may be given intramuscularly. It is doubtful whether even large doses of gluconate or lævulinate are efficacious when given by the mouth. If it is desired to avoid parenteral administration, calcium or ammonium chloride (10 to 20 gr. every four hours) should be given. For tetany of the newborn a dose of 7½ gr. suffices. This treatment depends for its effect on the fact that there is a net increase in acid ion in the body fluids. The calcium of the calcium chloride is retained in large part in the gut, while the ammonium ion is rapidly converted into the neutral urea, in both instances leaving an excess of uncompensated chloride ion to enter the tissue fluids. As has already been mentioned, the risk here is the production of a dangerous degree of acidosis and great care should be taken to stop the drug before this develops. Thus vomiting, diarrhœa and increased depth or rate of breathing are indications for the prompt cessation of the drug. Even when these signs do not appear, the administration of calcium or ammonium chloride should not be continued for more than three days, from the very commencement of which vitamin D should be given in full therapeutic doses.

When convulsions occur in rapid succession, and it is not feasible to administer calcium intravenously, it may be necessary to give a sedative. For this purpose chloral hydrate is generally satisfactory, although in very severe convulsive states chloroform inhalation may be required, but it must be emphasized that the use of these sedatives is a very temporary measure designed to act on the nervous system until the serum calcium is raised.

Tetany Associated with Cœliac Disease.—Essentially this demands the same treatment as that outlined for the tetany of rickets. It is advisable, however, in view of the tendency to the passage of large bulky fluid motions to refrain from the use of acid-producing salts. The administration of calcium gluconate intravenously, intramuscularly or orally, depending on the urgency of the symptoms, and the institution of a fat-free diet with an adequate supply of vitamin D rapidly leads to a disappearance of the manifestations of tetany.

PARATHYROID TETANY

(Considered in the section dealing with Parathyroid Disorders.)

THE TETANY OF CHRONIC RENAL DISEASE

In this condition, which is due to the hypocalcæmia engendered in chronic renal disease, the difficulty of treatment lies in the very unstable acid-base equilibrium. The metabolism sways between the Scylla of alkalotic tetany and the Charybdis of acidotic uræmia. The administration of large amounts of alkali, while facilitating the urinary excretion of acid substances, reduces the ionized fraction of calcium. Nevertheless, renal function is in some cases so impaired that without the addition of alkali there is too great a call on the calcium stores of the body with resultant fall in the level of total serum calcium. On the whole, it is much better to make certain of a sufficient intake of alkali since it is comparatively easy to deal with symptoms of tetany should they arise, whereas the acidotic state of uræmia is much more serious and likely to prove fatal. The best method of dealing with the tetany of chronic renal disease is the parenteral administration of calcium gluconate. Even after the symptoms have disappeared, it is wise to continue the oral administration of this substance.

ALKALOTIC TETANY

Tetany due to Vomiting.—This condition is the result of an alkalosis produced by the excessive loss of chloride in the vomitus. It is best dealt with by the injection of large amounts of sodium chloride as normal saline intravenously, subcutaneously or rectally depending on the severity of the vomiting. Rarely is it necessary to give any other medication, although calcium gluconate or ammonium chloride may be used. If the underlying cause is high intestinal obstruction, laparotomy may be necessary.

Tetany due to Alkalis.—In the alkaline treatment of pyuria and gastric ulcer, tetany occasionally supervenes. In these cases cessation of the alkaline medication usually suffices to remove the manifestations of spasmophilia. Only occasionally will it be necessary to give acid-producing substances such as ammonium chloride.

Hyperventilation Tetany.—This type is the result of alkalosis caused by overbreathing. The attack itself is rapidly alleviated by the inhalation of a gaseous mixture containing 5 per cent. CO_2, 21 per cent. O_2 and nitrogen. This, however, is only a temporary remedy: the underlying causes of the hyperventilation should be removed if at all possible. In some, if not all instances, there is a very large neurotic element. Some form of psychotherapy is often helpful: the patient, who is usually high-strung, should be told how the attacks are produced and encouraged to control the impulse to overbreathe. The use of mild sedatives such as bromide, chloral or luminal is often of considerable value.

N. Morris.

DISEASES OF THE DUCTLESS GLANDS

THE THYROID GLAND

Simple Goitre

Prophylaxis.—In areas where goitre is endemic, prophylactic administration of iodine is carried out on a nation-wide scale. This is practised extensively in Switzerland, around the Great Lakes in the United States, and in other goitrous regions of the world. The results of such prophylaxis are excellent, and endemic goitre now ranks as one of the few diseases which medical science has mastered. Though such prophylaxis does not require to be practised in this country, some details of the iodine dosage necessary may be of interest, in view of the light shed on iodine requirements in general and in relation to the doses of iodine used in the treatment of thyrotoxicosis.

Two methods of iodine administration are practised: (*a*) The admixture of a small percentage of iodine with table salt, the exact proportion being fixed by law, to ensure that all members of the community ingest a sufficiency of the element; and (*b*) the administration of iodine to school-children for a week or two in each year, and similar iodine therapy for women during pregnancy.

The amount of iodine added to salt is based on a knowledge of the quantity required per day by a human being. Estimates of this vary, but all agree that the amount is extremely low, somewhat less than 100 gamma per day (1 gamma=0·001 mg.). Assuming an average daily salt intake of 10 gm., the addition of 1 part of iodine in 100,000 of salt will yield a daily intake of 100 gamma, which is ample for health. In actual practice the concentration of iodine added varies from 1 : 5,000 to 1 : 250,000 in different countries. It is probable that the higher concentrations are wasteful, and in excess of requirements.

Where iodine is given only over a short period in the year,

the dosage is usually in the region of 0·2 gm. (3 gr.) of potassium iodide daily for ten days in autumn and spring. This represents a total yearly intake of 4 gm. potassium iodide, equivalent to about 3 gm. of iodine element, or an iodine intake of about 8 mg., or 8,000 gamma, per day, which is very much in excess of the amount given in iodized salt. Probably a good deal of the excess is lost by rapid excretion at the time of administration. The question arises as to whether excessive doses of iodine have any untoward effects. This will be discussed below (see next paragraph).

Curative.—The treatment of established simple goitre is less satisfactory than the results of prophylaxis. Prevention is once again better than cure. Administration of iodine is worthy of trial, and may prove successful, but diminution in the size of the gland is by no means the rule. Continental and some American writers are insistent on the danger of provoking hyperthyroid symptoms by the ingestion of excessive quantities of iodine (Iodine-Basedow). In Vienna the fear of this complication is so great that it is not usual to prescribe potassium iodide for arteriosclerosis or in cough mixtures, and our reckless administration of potassium iodide to such cases in 15-gr. doses provokes consternation. Physicians in this country, who see relatively few cases of simple goitre, can hardly judge whether this is a common complication, but general opinion here is against its frequency. The existence of Iodine-Basedow is, however, denied by some American observers who work in areas of high goitre endemicity, where iodine is given freely. Means quotes an impressive array of syphilitic cases in such an area, all presumably receiving massive doses of iodide, without a case of hyperthyroidism occurring amongst them. Though the case for the occurrence of hyperthyroidism after iodine is " not proven," it is well to proceed with caution in our treatment of simple goitre, particularly in cases with nodular glands.

The dosage of iodine given in cases of simple goitre is governed then by our beliefs regarding the reality of Iodine-Basedow. In Switzerland, where such belief is strong, an additional ration of 10 mg. iodine per day is given to established cases of simple goitre. In Britain, where the menace is regarded lightly, the usual dose is of the order of 0·1 to 0·2 gm. (usually in the form of Lugol's solution, ♏xv to ♏xxx per day).

When iodine fails to effect improvement, as it so often does, thyroid extract is sometimes tried. It is difficult to understand the rationale of its administration unless symptoms of subthyroidism are present. The results of thyroid treatment on the size of the gland are disappointing.

The majority of simple goitres yield only to surgical treatment. This is not indicated in the average mild case in a young subject, but should be considered if pressure symptoms arise, if the swelling is disfiguring, if the gland becomes nodular, if hyperthyroid symptoms develop, or if any suspicion of malignant change arises.

Cretinism

Cretinism in this country, being sporadic and relatively rare, is more liable to escape detection in the first few months or years of life than in areas where it is endemic and common. This is unfortunate, since the results of treatment are most satisfactory when substitution therapy is started at a very early age. The prospects of complete relief of symptoms diminish steadily with increase in the age at which treatment is started. Marked improvement, however, may be looked for if treatment is begun at any time during early childhood, though treatment initiated in the teens or after twenty confers little benefit. Authorities with wide experience have noted in fact that treatment started in older children may rouse the placid cretin to a state of peevish irritability, and that thyrotoxic symptoms are readily induced. On the other hand, treatment instituted in the first few months of life, and maintained steadily, will promote normal physical and mental development in children devoid of functioning thyroid tissue.

The quantity of thyroid required is usually gauged by the response of the patient. The correct dose is that which will allow of normal growth and development without producing signs of hyperthyroidism. The amount required varies with the age and weight of the child from about $\frac{1}{10}$ gr. in early infancy to doses of 1 to 3 gr. in late childhood. (All references are to the B.P. preparation, thyroideum. This is a dried extract, standardized to contain 0·1 per cent. of iodine in combination as thyroxine. Non-official preparations vary considerably in potency, and unless this is stated by the manufacturers in terms of the B.P. standard, such preparations should not be used.)

It is most important that thyroid administration should be continuous. A break of months or years will inevitably impair the final state of development attained. This point should be impressed on the parents, in whom ignorance or prejudice may undo a great deal of the good which has resulted from previous careful treatment.

Myxœdema

There are few conditions in which the response to treatment is so gratifying as in hypothyroidism in the adult. Judicious treatment will not only restore the myxœdematous patient to normal health, but will maintain him in that state throughout a long life. Reports have recently been published of some of the earliest cases treated by thyroid. Two of these at least lived to advanced ages, ninety-five in Murray's case, eighty-four in Burgess's case. They prove that intolerance or refractoriness to thyroid do not occur even after thirty or forty years' treatment, and that under proper treatment life is not shortened.

In treating cases of myxœdema it is advisable to use a thyroid preparation of known potency, such as the official B.P. thyroideum. If other (proprietary) preparations are used, their potency in terms of the B.P. standard should be known. Great confusion and some accidents have resulted in the past from substitution of one preparation for another, for differences of six-fold in strength exist between brands of thyroid extract marketed by different firms. In this article all doses are in terms of the B.P. extract, standardized to contain 0·1 per cent. of iodine combined as thyroxine.

Since oral administration of thyroid extract is effective and in every way satisfactory, there is no justification for its administration by other routes. Thyroxin is of great theoretical interest, and its use in research is justified, but its value in practice is negligible. Its cost and its great potency, as well as the necessity for intravenous injection, render it a needlessly complicated way of attaining a simple end.

The dosage of thyroid extract required varies somewhat from case to case, depending on a number of factors, among them the initial level of the B.M.R. before treatment. The final selection of a maintenance dose is governed by the reaction of the patient. In general from 1 to 3 gr. of extract will be required per day. It is wise in any case to start with small doses, and to work up gradually till a satisfactory response is obtained. By this method there is less risk of producing cardiac symptoms (*e.g.*, angina) in susceptible cases. It is customary to give the main dose of thyroid in the evening, so that the patient is in bed at the time when palpitation and weakness are apt to occur. This rule is not absolute, for some patients prefer to take the main dose in the morning, since they suffer from sleeplessness after a large dose taken before retiring.

When symptoms have been relieved, the maintenance dose which will keep the patient in normal health must be found. This is not infrequently less than the amount required to relieve symptoms, and can only be assessed by the patient's continued freedom from symptoms and signs of myxœdema. The patient must be instructed to take the extract daily without intermission, and on no account to alter the dose without medical advice. Many patients cease to take the drug when they feel that their health is restored, under the impression that they no longer need assistance. Others may increase the dose to dangerous levels in an attempt to reduce weight, or to secure added vigour. All patients taking thyroid extract should be seen by a doctor at regular intervals, and the adequacy of dosage assessed. A careful watch should be kept for signs of over and under dosage. The occurrence of tachycardia, palpitation, loss of weight, nervousness or sweating indicates that dosage is too high ; and conversely increase in weight, lethargy, sensitivity to cold, or changes in skin, hair or voice demand increase in the daily dose.

In cases where anæmia is marked it may be necessary to give iron as well as thyroid in order to restore the blood to normal. Ferrous iron, as ferrous sulphate (9 to 12 gr. daily), or ferri et ammon. citras. (90 gr. daily) are usual preparations. Rarely myxœdema is associated with a macrocytic hyperchromic anæmia, for which appropriate treatment is required (see p. 482).

The cardiac symptoms of myxœdema yield as a rule to the specific hormone therapy, and do not require treatment by digitalis or diuretics. Persistence of œdema, etc., after the B.M.R. has returned to normal, indicates cardiac decompensation of other ætiology, for which appropriate treatment should be instituted. In some cases the restoration of metabolism to normal levels is accompanied by the development of anginal pain. Slight reduction in the dose of thyroid may abolish the symptom, but when pain is obstinate and easily provoked it may be necessary to keep the patient continually in a state of moderate hypothyroidism. Considerable judgment is necessary in selecting a dose of thyroid sufficient to relieve the worst features of myxœdema without producing anginal symptoms.

Hyperthyroidism

General Management.—The management of cases of thyrotoxicosis may on occasion be simple, but in general involves a nicety of judgment and a degree of experience which render it as difficult a field as any in therapeutics. Simple cases are those where either mild symptoms of Graves' disease in a young girl disappear readily on solution of some family or emotional problem, or where moderate hyperthyroidism with a nodular gland in a woman of forty-five is referred at once for operation. But the majority of cases require full study and careful assessment before the line of treatment can be decided upon. The question of therapy is probably best solved when surgeon and physician see the case together at the outset, discuss the pros and cons, and decide on a line of treatment planned to suit the individual needs of the case. In many cases the considerations involved in deciding for or against operation are complicated, and demand a wide experience of similar cases. The general practitioner with an experience of necessity more limited than that of the specialist, should therefore seldom be required to decide the matter for himself. His duty lies in the early diagnosis of the case (itself often no easy matter), the determination of the exciting factor and its elimination where feasible, and the careful observation of the case under simple treatment till he can reach a decision whether response is satisfactory or whether hospital treatment and specialist advice are necessary.

The treatment of a case of moderately severe Graves' disease in a young adult should therefore include an initial period of treatment at home by the family doctor. During this period, which should last at least a month but which should not exceed three months, the patient should be off work and on a régime of rest, with sedatives and probably iodine, and with a carefully regulated diet. In the mildest cases it is probably sufficient to arrange that the patient does not rise till after breakfast, has two hours rest in bed or on a couch after lunch, and retires to bed in the early evening between 7 and 8 P.M. In more severe cases complete rest in bed is essential, especially for a week or two at the outset.

During this period of conservative treatment every effort should be made to find the cause for the development of hyperthyroid symptoms. Unhappiness at work or in the home, an unhappy love affair, the fear of an undesired pregnancy in a young woman, or some similar psychological disturbance may be discovered in the course of investigation, and may be dealt with. In many cases the doctor cannot interfere in respect of such a matter even if it be unearthed; but in others a doctor's advice may smooth things out. In the elucidation of the cause of the disorder, and in exercising his tact and judgment in its elimination, the family doctor can render a service beyond the scope of the hospital specialist. The general practitioner who enjoys the trust of his patient is more likely to meet with success than the stranger who attends the patient in hospital or sees her for a few minutes in consultation. A complete change of environment is often helpful. A holiday with relatives may suffice, if their society is congenial, but may aggravate the trouble if home difficulties are the subject of " improving " discourses by pharasaical busybodies. When the environment is obviously at fault it is often wiser to advise hospital treatment at the outset, and it may be necessary to prohibit visitors and letters.

Sedatives.—The attainment of mental rest is facilitated by the use of sedatives, of which one of the most effective and probably the most convenient is phenobarbitone. In doses of ½ to 1 gr. twice or thrice daily this drug is valuable in the restless anxiety of hyperthyroidism, and may be given safely for long periods. Potassium bromide (in 10-gr. doses) is as efficacious, but less convenient and certainly more unpleasant to take.

Diet.—During this period the diet should be generous, and in most cases unrestricted in variety. The increased metabolism of the body demands a fuel intake in excess of that usual for people of the same age and sex and build. A total calorie intake of 2,500 to 3,000 is desirable, a high intake for a woman, especially if she be at rest in bed. Carbohydrate and fat are allowed *ad libitum*, but protein should not exceed 100 gm. per day. Protein in fair quantity is required to make good the tissue waste inevitable with high metabolism, but excessive protein intake is undesirable, since its specific dynamic action tends to raise still further the already excessive metabolic activity. The patient should be encouraged to partake freely of the milk-egg-cream type of diet which is widely recognized by lay people as " fattening," and a diet on the lines of that below meets the requirements.

High Calorie Diet for Thyrotoxicosis

Calories, 3,000. Carbohydrate, 330 gm. Protein, 80 gm. Fat, 150 gm. (All values approximate.)

Early Morning—

Juice of 1 orange and ½ lemon, with 2 tablespoonfuls glucose. Water if desired.

Breakfast—

1 teacup of freshly made tea or coffee with cream and sugar.
Porridge or other cereal, with cream.
Wholemeal bread (not new) ; ryvita or vitaweat.
Butter plentifully. Marmalade or honey or jelly.
Cooked egg or bacon.

Forenoon—

Malted milk, or ovaltine, or switched egg and milk, or fruit drink as before.

Dinner—

Milk soup, adding cream.
An average helping of any kind of meat or poultry, but no twice-cooked meat.
A good helping of vegetable, adding butter or white sauce.
Fresh lettuce and tomato salad in season, with dressing made with cream, yolk of egg, lemon juice, etc. Oil dressing good if it can be taken.
Any simple pudding desired.
Always fresh or stewed fruit with cream.

Tea—

1 cup freshly made tea, with cream and sugar.
Brown bread sandwiches, with egg, banana, date, lettuce
Butter in plenty. Honey, jelly, marmalade.
Any simple cake.

Supper—

Glass of milk with cream.
Lightly cooked egg ; or fish, or other light supper dish.
Brown bread and butter.
Stewed fruit with cream and sugar.

Bedtime—

Ovaltine or malted milk, or fruit juice and glucose.

NOTE.—Calorie values approximate, since quantities are not specified.

Increase in weight is always a reassuring and satisfactory sign. It is a sound plan in all cases of thyrotoxicosis, even those in whom symptoms have apparently subsided and where the disease is regarded as " cured," to make the patient keep an accurate weekly record of body-weight. In active cases an increasing weight is a valuable sign of improvement; in quiescent cases, a stationary weight is equally reassuring. In all cases, a fall in weight of even a few pounds, especially if steadily maintained week by week for a month or so, is disquieting, and is the signal for a review of the whole treatment of the case.

Iodine.—Though many milder cases may improve strikingly on rest, diet and sedatives alone, it is usual to find that improvement is hastened by administration of iodine in small doses. The mode of action of iodine is entirely obscure, and the details of its effects are still in dispute, but there is no doubt that it does cause remission of symptoms. So firmly established is this belief in the minds of some doctors that the writer once came across a young woman who had taken Lugol's solution daily for ten years under her doctor's orders, and without other treatment for her thyrotoxicosis! At the end of that time she was still mildly toxic, and considerable cardiac damage had resulted.

Iodine continues to be widely prescribed in the familiar Lugol's solution. This contains a mixture of iodine (5 per cent.) and potassium iodide (7½ per cent.) in water. The iodine content of potassium iodide is approximately 75 per cent., so that the total iodine content of Lugol's solution works out at approximately 10 per cent. On this basis 10 minims of the solution contain the equivalent of 1 gr. of iodine. There seems no valid reason for prescribing iodine in this cumbersome form, exactly similar results being obtained by giving potassium iodide in appropriate doses: in fact, the substitution of potassium iodide for Lugol's solution in practice is long overdue. The dosage of potassium iodide required in cases of hyperthyroidism is small by ordinary expectorant or antiluetic standards, and the substitution of 10 or 15 gr. doses for an equal number of minims of Lugol's solution is liable to give rise to unpleasant symptoms, and is not without danger. A usual dose of potassium iodide in cases of thyrotoxicosis is ½ gr. twice daily. In some cases this may be increased to as much as 2 or 4 gr. twice daily, but such large doses are rarely called for. The drug may conveniently be prescribed in a solution containing 4 gr. to the fluid ounce (*i.e.*, ½ gr. per fluid drachm) flavoured as desired.

The iodine content of even the smallest of these doses (1 gr. per day) has been shown to be considerably in excess of the quantity required for full iodine effect. It appears from the careful work of Means, Lerman and others that 6 mg. of iodine daily produces the maximum effect on pulse-rate,

B.M.R., and symptoms. This quantity of iodine is contained in about 1 minim of Lugol's solution per day. The larger doses commonly employed do no harm, provided their use does not lead the physician into the fallacy of believing that 90 minims per day will produce a more dramatic effect than 5 or 15 minims a day.

The trial of di-iodotyrosine and allied compounds in substitution for inorganic iodine has not shown them to possess any activity in excess of what might be anticipated from their iodine content. Their administration is therefore wasteful in view of the complicated synthesis necessary in their preparation.

Whatever be the mechanism of iodine action, it appears to run a definite time-course. The action is at its height in from ten to fourteen days, the B.M.R. showing an initial sharp fall which diminishes in its steepness as the low (iodine) B.M.R. level is approached. The dose of iodine, provided it is over 6 mg. per day, appears to exert no influence either on the steepness or the depth of the fall. During this period of falling B.M.R. there is a marked decrease in the intensity of all symptoms, with a gain in weight, and a slowing of the pulse-rate. The latter naturally is not to be expected in cases with auricular fibrillation. This iodine response occurs in the great majority of cases, though now and then a patient fails to respond in the classical manner.

Opinions differ as to the course of the disease when iodine administration is prolonged beyond the ten to fourteen day period. In general, the opinion of physicians and surgeons is that the pulse and B.M.R. start to rise again, the symptoms become aggravated, and a general deterioration in the patient's health occurs. Such a patient is considered to have escaped from iodine control, and to be refractory to further dosage. There is no doubt that such deterioration under iodine frequently occurs in cases allowed to go on taking the drug after the first ten to fourteen days. Means and Lerman, however, consider that such cases are not really iodine-resistant, but are still under the control of iodine though their state grows worse. The disease is known to pursue a cyclic course, and it is claimed that such cases may be on the up-grade of a cycle of activity during the period of observation. If iodine be stopped when such a case is growing steadily worse there is a sharp acceleration of the deterioration, which is claimed to represent the escape from iodine control consequent on the cessation of the administration of the drug. Iodine is considered to hold the symptoms and B.M.R. in check at a level somewhat below that which they would attain in the uniodized case.

The question of iodine resistance is of considerable practical importance, since pre-operative preparation with iodine is so important. There is no doubt that when operation is contemplated the first abrupt fall in the B.M.R., etc., should be the signal for carrying out the operation. The difficulty arises in the pre-operative management of cases who have been treated medically with iodine for prolonged periods. If iodine resistance is considered to be real and not imaginary, then the patient should be sent away *without* iodine for a period of two to three months before operation. At the end of this period iodine refractoriness will have disappeared, and the drug may be restarted and operation carried out as in the freshly iodized case. On the other hand, if it is believed that the climbing B.M.R., etc., under iodine does not denote iodine escape but a natural cycle of activity, then the giving of the drug should be continued, secure in the knowledge that the peak of the crisis will be lessened by its control. Operation may then be carried out when the crisis of the cycle has passed and the metabolic rate is once more upon the down-grade. Evidence at the moment is not conclusive, but it is safe to say that, in general, surgeons prefer freshly iodized cases, and will not operate on patients who have taken iodine for prolonged periods unless an iodine-free period of six to eight weeks has elapsed immediately before the pre-operative iodine preparation.

Management of Mild Cases.—A mild case of recent onset treated with rest, sedatives, diet and probably iodine, may respond well, and after some four to eight weeks may be allowed more liberty. If after three months of careful medical treatment a patient with thyrotoxicosis is unfit for return to a normal routine, then operation should be seriously considered. If the patient's economic circumstances permit, a further three months' trial of the strict régime may be made, but in the average wage-earner no such luxury is permissible. In no case should month be allowed to succeed month without a decision being reached. One has seen too many cases come to the surgeon eventually, often in poor condition, where so-called medical treatment had been indulged in over periods of three, or even of ten years. True, some patients will refuse operation, especially if it be suggested to them at a time when symptoms are acute, but the wise doctor will usually carry his point if he explains the prospects clearly when a remission renders the patient more reasonable. Frequently the fear of operation has been sown by a warning from a doctor whose acquaintance with thyroid surgery dated from the days of nearly 100 per cent. mortality. One patient was warned by an old family physician that some young doctor would one day advise operation to which she must on no account submit. She nursed her goitre for many years, in constant ill-health, till she was eventually restored to health by a belated but successful operation.

It is essential in the management of any mild case that the response of the patient to normal environment and to the strain of normal occupation be tested. Cases which respond to a régime of rest but relapse on return to normal employment should be referred for specialist advice, and probably for operative treatment. An early decision that the patient is unable to stand the stress and strain of everyday life and that surgical treatment should be instituted means a great saving of time and hardship for the patient. It may be permissible to allow a young lady of leisure to fritter away a couple of years in semi-invalidism if thereby an operation can be averted. But such a course is not good practice when the patient is the usual twentieth-century working girl, often supporting herself, and even shouldering the responsibilities of her family, on a typist's slender income. This economic factor is equally important when the patient is a young mother, or a man whose family are dependent on his earnings. It is ethically unsound to deny such patients the undoubted benefits of operation on the ground that spontaneous recovery in two or three years may occur.

Radiation.—Radiation by X-rays or radium has been used for many years in the treatment of hyperthyroidism. There is much controversy as to its usefulness. In America such radiation treatment is held to be of little value, and is seldom employed ; operation is the method of choice in treating all but the mildest cases. In some continental countries a very high percentage of successful results with radiation is claimed, and the method is widely used. In this country there is no doubt that radiation is not now nearly so popular as it was ten or fifteen years ago, and general dissatisfaction with the results has led to the earlier and more general employment of surgery. Radium treatment has now been largely abandoned in many centres, though X-radiation is still employed. It appears that some 60 per cent. of cases of Graves' disease improve on radiation, about the same proportion as recover under a general medical régime without its aid. The treatment as formerly practised, by weekly exposures to small doses of 500 *r* units, necessitated long hospitalization for all cases living outside a short radius of the hospital where treatment was given, and even now, with intense radiation over a short period (2,000 *r* in ten days), X-ray treatment demands close observation of the patient over many months and prolonged disability. The results of radiation cannot be accurately assessed for some three months after exposure, and it is obvious that repetition of the course on three or four occasions, as is frequently necessary, may drag out the duration of disability over a number of years. In cases which do well, the period off work varies from six months to two years : in those which do not respond satisfactorily, it is not uncommon for operation to be performed finally after three or four years, or more, of chronic invalidism. In general it may be said that the results of radiation treatment are not very satisfactory, and a great deal of avoidable economic hardship is caused by the prolonged nature of the treatment. X-rays have been found useful in cases with recurrence of mild symptoms after operation, but with good surgery such cases are not very common. X-rays have no place in the treatment of nodular goitres in the middle-aged.

Septic Foci.—Many cases of thyrotoxicosis are noted to follow acute infections, and this observation has led to debate as to the possible rôle of sepsis in aggravating the symptoms of the disease. In many cases obvious septic foci are present, particularly in the upper respiratory tract (accessory sinuses, tonsils) or in the teeth (pyorrhœa, apical abscesses). Removal of such foci is frequently advocated as a preliminary to a course of medical treatment, and is even demanded by some surgeons before they will undertake operation on cases of hyperthyroidism. However desirable it may be to get rid of such foci, there is no doubt that their removal is fraught with danger in any but mild cases. It is not sufficiently appreciated that tonsillectomy and similar operations carry nearly the same risk of post-operative hyperthyroid crisis and death as the major operation on the thyroid gland itself. Pre-operative preparation with sedatives and iodine, etc., must be as thorough and careful as when partial thyroidectomy is contemplated, and the choice and manner of administration of the basal narcotic and anæsthetic are just as vital as in the radical operation. Neglect of such preparation, or even an ill-timed operation on a patient otherwise well prepared, have led in our experience to fatal results. As the risks of operative interference, therefore, are the same as in thyroidectomy, and may be even greater if adequate pre-operative care is omitted, it seems unwise to subject a patient with any significant degree of thyrotoxicosis to the surgical removal of minor foci of sepsis. If the patient is in such a state that minor operations can be carried out safely, then the time is also safe for partial thyroidectomy, which should be the operation of choice. If partial thyroidectomy is judged to be dangerous, then *ipso facto* small operations on tonsils, etc., are likewise dangerous, and no surgical treatment whatever should be attempted till a favourable moment arrives. When such a propitious time does come, the operation of choice should again be thyroidectomy, a safe opportunity for which may not arise again. The dangers of operative interference of whatever kind in cases of thyrotoxicosis is illustrated by the extremely high mortality which follows acute abdominal operations in these patients.

Thyroidectomy.—Some twenty years ago the mortality from operation in cases of toxic goitre was appalling: few cases were operated on, but nearly all died. This was changed completely when the pre-operative use of iodine was introduced by Plummer, and with improved operative and anæsthetic technique and skilled pre-operative care the mortality is now very low. In this country the mortality figures vary from 2 to 5 per cent. in the hands of good surgeons. High mortality figures (12 per cent. or so) may occur where late or neglected cases are referred for operation. In addition, the mortality is high where goitre surgery is performed by those unfamiliar with its special dangers, and where medical co-operation is inadequate.

In general, the results of operation are excellent. As already stated, the mortality in good hands is low, certainly under 5 per cent.; recurrences after operation are probably not over 5 per cent., and the remaining 90 per cent. are rid once and for all of their disorder. Improvement is dramatic within a few days of operation, and the total period of disability from the pre-operative period till the patient is fit to return to work is about three or four months. The patients after operation are frequently fit for strenuous work, and one's personal experience includes instances of men returning to arduous or exacting duties—farm labourers, drivers of heavy road-transport vehicles, night express service men, fishermen, etc. The short period of disability, the very high prospect of economic rehabilitation and the rarity of recurrence, render surgery by far the most advisable treatment for all but the mildest cases.

All cases of toxic nodular goitre in people of forty or over should be submitted to surgical treatment as soon as pre-operative medication has been carried out, because of the known danger of subsequent cardiac failure in such cases.

The presence of congestive failure and/or auricular fibrillation merely renders operation the more imperative. In these cases, however, the pre-operative treatment must include adequate attention to the cardiac disability.

It does not always follow that the decision to resort to surgery is to be followed by operation within a few weeks. Many patients are in no state for immediate operation, as, for example, cases who are gravely ill, where in spite of iodine the B.M.R. and pulse-rate rise or remain fixed at a high level, and where the weight continues to fall despite treatment. In such cases any operative interference, even simple ligation of a superior thyroid artery under local anæsthesia, is likely to be fatal. These cases must be treated medically till a natural remission of the disease brings about some improvement, and a favourable moment for operation is seized when it arises. It is a grave mistake to force the hand of the surgeon into operation against his better judgment, on the grounds that "something must be done." The risk to life is much less when conservative measures are pursued than if operation is rashly undertaken on a patient who fails to respond to medical measures.

Pre-operative Treatment.—Careful medical preparation over a period of two to three weeks is an essential preliminary to operation. During this time the patient should preferably be in the hospital or nursing-home in which the operation is to be performed, though not necessarily in the surgical ward. The date of the proposed operation should be left indefinite to the patient. Complete rest in bed should be maintained and phenobarbitone ($\frac{1}{2}$ to 2 gr. b.i.d.) or other sedative should be administered. Visitors should be few, and every measure taken to ensure that the patient is mentally at ease. A generous diet of the type already described (p. 434) should be allowed, with the addition in the few days before operation of glucose and orange juice (4 oz. of orange juice with $\frac{1}{2}$ oz. of added glucose) once or twice daily. In cases who are emaciated and fail to gain weight, the administration of insulin (5 to 15 units hypodermically twice daily) is often worthy of trial, while the glucose in the diet may be increased. Not uncommonly diabetes occurs along with thyrotoxicosis and in cases with glycosuria, therefore, blood-sugar analyses should be carried out. These will decide whether the condition is simply due to the hyperthyroidism or whether a true diabetes mellitus is present. In the latter event treatment should be modified accordingly (see p. 323).

Digitalis is of no value in cases with simple tachycardia

without failure and should not be given. Its use in cases with fibrillation is discussed below. If the patient on admission has had no iodine for two or three months, a fall in pulse-rate and B.M.R. may be expected after a week as a result of rest in the new surroundings and careful nursing. Iodine should then be given, preferably as potassium iodide in doses of $\frac{1}{2}$ gr. b.i.d., though usually Lugol's solution continues to be employed (15 to 30 minims per day). After ten to fourteen days of iodine treatment, the pulse and B.M.R. will have fallen to a new low level, and the most favourable moment for operation has arrived. The general state of the patient leaves no doubt as to the improvement, of which the low pulse-rate and B.M.R. are merely reflections. The body-weight frequently falls slightly during the first week after admission, but should have risen appreciably before operation is due. Daily estimations of the B.M.R. are a luxury, and need not be carried out if careful attention is paid to the bedside signs of pulse, weight and general well-being. Explanation to the patient that the improvement which she feels indicates that operation is now safe will allay the apprehension with which many regard the ordeal.

Pre-operative Treatment with Cardiac Failure and Auricular Fibrillation.—The pre-operative treatment of a case with congestive failure and auricular fibrillation does not differ, so far as the thyrotoxicosis is concerned, from that of an uncomplicated case. The congestive failure should, however, be treated along the usual lines with digitalis and diuretics, salt and fluid restriction, etc. It will often be found that relatively larger doses of digitalis are required to control the ventricular rate in cases of fibrillation with hyperthyroidism than in those of other ætiology, probably on account of the increased rate of destruction of the drug. Operation should be undertaken only after adequate control of the failure, at a precise time dictated by the hyperthyroid condition. Digitalis should be maintained right up to the day of operation, and should be continued in the post-operative period. It is not good practice to attempt to restore normal rhythm by means of quinidine before operation, for even if this be successful, the resumption of normal rhythm deprives digitalis of its chief action in controlling the ventricular rate, and robs the physician of his main weapon against excessive tachycardia. In any case, patients so restored to normal rhythm often relapse into fibrillation at operation or during the post-operative phase.

Immediate Pre-operative Treatment.—The patient should be under the influence of a basal narcotic from the early morning of the day of operation. Paraldehyde, given *per rectum*, in a dose of 1 fluid drachm per stone of body-weight, with a maximum of 8 to 10 drachms, is generally effective and can be given without disturbance to the patient. Nembutal ($1\frac{1}{2}$ gr.) by the mouth the night before and again on the morning of operation may be substituted. Scopolamine-morphine " twilight-sleep " is equally effective, $\frac{1}{4}$ gr. morphine and $\frac{1}{100}$ gr. hyoscine hydrobromide being given subcutaneously two hours before operation, and half quantities of each repeated one hour before going to the theatre. Avertin per rectum, in half the anæsthetic dose, is also a useful drug. Each surgical service has its preference, and whichever method is adopted it is wise to master it thoroughly and to use it exclusively. Whatever the drug employed, the patient should be thoroughly drowsy on leaving the ward, and in well-managed cases may fall asleep before the anæsthetic is started. In no case should operation be attempted if the patient is acutely conscious and distressed, or where the pulse-rate on the table rises to 130 or more. It is wiser to postpone the operation for a day or two than to risk a post-operative thyrotoxic crisis. For anæsthesia, nitrous oxide and oxygen is generally used, and is most satisfactory in skilled hands.

Post-operative Treatment.—The critical stormy period after thyroidectomy occurs in the first forty-eight hours after the operation. During this period the patient should be nursed in absolute quiet and seclusion, either in a room by herself, or screened off in a corner of a general ward. Visitors and letters should be forbidden and medical examinations reduced to an absolute minimum. It is desirable that one day and one night nurse, specially trained or experienced in this work, should have charge of the patient. Their duties will include keeping an hourly record of pulse and temperature for the first twenty-four to thirty-six hours.

Owing to the high metabolism after the operation the temperature rises in most cases, and few bed-clothes are necessary or desirable. Heat loss is facilitated by cool air and light coverings, and chills are very rare. Quiet is assured by hypodermic administration of morphia ($\frac{1}{4}$ gr.) or omnopon ($\frac{1}{3}$ gr.) which is repeated as required. Heroin ($\frac{1}{6}$ gr.) is frequently used for this purpose, but in our experience has occasionally led to a rather disquieting depression of respiration.

The administration of adequate amounts of fluids is most important, and rectal glucose-salines (6 per cent. glucose in saline, 4 to 6 oz.) should be started at once and continued four-hourly till the patient is able to swallow. Glucose and orange drinks by mouth may then be substituted or used as adjuvants. In severely toxic cases subcutaneous salines may be given with advantage, or an intravenous drip saline injected.

Iodine is frequently given post-operatively, up to a fluid drachm of Lugol's solution being added to the first glucose saline per rectum or potassium iodide being added (5 to 10 gr.) to one of the intravenous infusions. If the patient has been thoroughly iodized before operation this is less necessary, but it is usual to continue iodine in the same dosage as in the pre-operative period for a week or two.

In many cases soreness of the throat is a troublesome post-operative feature. This is best controlled by steam inhalations, rest to the voice and sedatives. A watch must be kept for the occurrence of post-operative complications—crisis, tetany or hæmorrhage. These demand special treatment, to be considered below.

In an uncomplicated case such measures are sufficient to carry the patient over to the third or fourth day, when rapid improvement has as a rule been established. Further progress is uneventful, and slowing of the pulse, fall in temperature, subsidence of excitement and general well-being indicate that strict measures of isolation and sedative therapy can safely be relaxed. Transference to a medical ward may be allowed when the clips or stitches are removed on the fourth or fifth day, and in many cases the patient is fit to get up for a short period some seven days after operation. Severe reaction, or the presence of cardiac failure, may delay progress considerably. Convalescence should be gradual and a holiday of one to two months enforced after discharge from hospital before a return to work is sanctioned.

Hyperthyroid Crisis.—This may occur post-operatively, or may supervene at any time in severe cases under medical treatment. A common precipitating factor is a pulmonary infection (*e.g.*, broncho-pneumonia). In all cases its recognition is only too easy—the high fever, extreme tachycardia, and great restlessness of the patient composing an unforgettable clinical picture. The condition, once it has developed, is very intractable, and is attended by a very high death rate. The essence of its treatment is in its *prevention.* It should very rarely occur after operation in cases properly treated pre-operatively and in which the time of operation has been well selected. Nor should it occur in well-supervised medical cases, for it is seldom that a case of moderate severity suddenly goes into crisis. It arises usually in cases which have been deteriorating for some time, or which have run a severe course for months or years, and which therefore have not had timeous and efficient treatment. It frequently occurs in cases of moderate or severe toxicity who have drifted out of medical supervision, and in our experience has been more common in such "medical" cases than after thyroidectomy. It may also occur, with fatal results, after ill-timed operations for focal sepsis (tonsillectomy, etc.) in moderately toxic patients.

Established cases of hyperthyroid crisis should be treated on the lines detailed for the management of cases after thyroidectomy. Quiet and seclusion with adequate sedatives (morphia, etc.) are essentials. The promotion of heat-loss and avoidance of hyperpyrexia can be aided by hydrotherapy. Tepid sponging may suffice or in more desperate cases cold packs and applications of ice-bags to the head and precordium may be required. Fluids must be administered per rectum and intravenously, a saline intravenous drip (2 to 4 pints) being probably the most efficient method. There is a danger of waterlogging and pulmonary œdema if large quantities of fluid are given *quickly* intravenously, and this is obviated by the use of the drip method, whereby the administration of a pint of fluid takes about sixty minutes. Iodine can be given, as 5 to 10 gr. of potassium iodide in the intravenous saline, or as a fluid drachm of Lugol's solution per rectum in 4 oz. of saline.

The efficient administration of oxygen (by tent if available, or by intranasal catheter) is an important part of the treatment, and should be instituted early. Too often oxygen is administered only when the patient is already moribund. Digitalis does not control the tachycardia, and is useless unless auricular fibrillation is present. Even then the drug appears less efficacious than in auricular fibrillation of other ætiology.

Tetany.—The treatment of this complication is dealt with on p. 447 *et seq.*

Hæmorrhage. — While the treatment of post-operative hæmorrhage must remain a surgical problem, it is necessary for the physician who may be looking after a patient to recognize the indications for calling surgical aid. It is seldom that massive hæmorrhage occurs, with the symptoms of collapse, etc., due to blood loss. Much more commonly hæmorrhage into the wound causes local tension and may bring about symptoms from pressure on the trachea, etc. It should be remembered that oozing of serous fluid frequently occurs, and may cause swelling in the region of the wound. In all cases of doubt as to the nature of such a swelling the opinion of the surgeon should be sought.

Myxœdema.—Cases of myxœdema arising after thyroidectomy must be treated with thyroid extract. The treatment does not differ from that in cases of myxœdema of other ætiology, and should be along the lines suggested on pp. 431-432.

I. G. W. Hill.

THE PARATHYROID GLANDS

Tetania Parathyropriva

Clinically this condition may result from a parathyroidectomy undertaken for generalized fibrocystic osteitis or from a total or subtotal thyroidectomy. The symptoms, which may become manifest as early as twenty-four hours after the operation or may be delayed in their onset for a week, rapidly become serious and demand urgent treatment. If carpo-pedal spasm or laryngismus is already apparent when the patient is seen, an intravenous injection of calcium gluconate or lævulinate should immediately be given. Ten to twenty cubic centimetres of a 20 per cent. solution should be injected slowly into one of the veins, five to eight minutes being allowed for the injection. Shortly afterwards a similar amount should be administered intramuscularly. The intravenous injection causes an almost immediate disappearance of the symptoms of tetany while the intramuscular administration helps to prolong the effect. The whole procedure may be repeated if the symptoms reappear. It is wise, however, to begin parathyroid medication as soon as possible.

In mild cases the intramuscular injection of 20 units of parathyroid hormone (para-thor-mone (Lilly), euparatone (Allen & Hanbury) or paroidin (Parke, Davis)) will produce a rise in serum calcium which begins within six hours of the injection and is maintained for about eighteen hours : the dose should be repeated every eight hours for the first day, after which 30 units daily will usually suffice. For the more severe type, when the serum calcium has fallen below 5 mg. per cent., 60 units may be given intravenously, followed in six hours by an intramuscular injection of 30 units : thereafter, the daily dose should be reduced to 30 units unless the acute symptoms have not disappeared. It is wise in all cases, where parathyroid hormone is used, to obtain serial estimations of the serum calcium as a protection against overdosage. The earliest indication of this is hypercalcæmia (serum calcium higher than 13 mg. per cent.) Some time later the patient begins to show signs of listlessness which gradually deepens into coma. In such a case the parathormone injections must be stopped, venesection performed and an intravenous injection of 1 litre of normal saline given. These last two measures reduce the high viscosity of the blood produced by the hypercalcæmia and accelerate the blood flow.

Once the maintenance dose of parathyroid has been determined it is advisable to give calcium (2 drachms of calcium gluconate daily, together with a diet rich in milk and milk products) by the mouth in order to counteract the decalcification of the bones produced by parathormone.

Tetany following removal of a parathyroid tumour does not generally last longer than two or three days, after which time the remaining parathyroid glands are usually capable of producing a sufficiency of hormone. When, however, the condition has resulted from thyroidectomy there may be little or no parathyroid tissue left in the body and treatment with parathyroid hormone may have to be continued for some months or even years.

Parathyroid hormone accompanied by an adequate intake of lime can maintain the serum calcium at a sufficiently high level to prevent the symptoms of tetany for many weeks. The routine use of an efficient extract is expensive and, in addition, there is a tendency for its effect to be diminished by long continued use in any one patient. It is therefore important that steps should be taken to maintain the level of the blood calcium without relying indefinitely on injections of parathyroid extract. Successful results are often obtained by the use of ammonium chloride or hydrochloric acid. The former can be given in 30-gr. doses every four hours: its taste, which is very disagreeable, can be disguised fairly efficiently by the addition of liquid extract of liquorice to the mixture.

℞	Ammon. Chlorid.	gr. xxx
	Ext. Glycyrrh. Liq.	ʒi
	Aq. . . . . . . ad	℥fs

Hydrochloric acid is probably best given incorporated in milk—300 c.c. of N/10 HCl to 2 litres of milk. Another method that has been successfully tried is the administration of vitamin D in massive doses. In one instance daily doses of 650,000 units were given for fifty days, resulting in an increase of serum calcium and the disappearance of symptoms, the patient remaining well for at least three months without further treatment.

The calcium content of the diet should be high. In addition to milk, lime can be given as calcium gluconate or lactate, the sedative effect of which is said to be potentiated by the addition of lactose: two teaspoonfuls of lactose with 1 drachm of calcium lactate may be given before each meal and at bed-time.

Idiopathic Hypoparathyroidism.—This rare condition is treated on the same lines as those outlined for post-operative tetany.

Hyperparathyroidism

The clinical picture designated as generalized fibro-cystic osteitis is the result of overaction of the parathyroid glands. It is characterized by pains in the limbs and fractures; occasionally attention is drawn to the condition by renal colic produced by the formation of calculi in the urinary tract. X-ray examination reveals the presence of multiple cystic tumours of the bones, especially the long bones. Biochemical examination of the blood is of considerable importance in differentiating this disease from other pathological conditions of the bones such as focal osteitis fibrosa. In the generalized form the serum calcium is high, the serum phosphorus is low and the plasma phosphatase is greatly increased. These findings are important as indications of hypersecretion of the parathyroid hormone. They should immediately lead to an examination of the thyroid region of the neck for the presence of a tumour of the parathyroid. Frequently, however, even a most careful examination of the neck fails to reveal the presence of any tumour. In such a case, the finding of a high serum calcium and increased plasma phosphatase renders it necessary to perform an exploratory operation: although prolonged search is often required this is generally successful in detecting an adenoma of parathyroid tissue which should, of course, be removed. The biochemical findings are important because if they are within normal limits it is useless to undertake any surgical interference—local osteitis fibrosa has apparently no connection with the parathyroid secretion even when the cystic tumours of the bones are multiple.

Prior to operation, the patient's calcium stores should be replenished by the administration of a diet rich in milk and the giving of calcium salts (gluconate).

The post-operative treatment is carried out on general lines, but one must be on the lookout for prodromal symptoms of tetany. In any case abundant calcium should be given both in the diet (milk) and as calcium gluconate or other salt. If tetany makes its appearance it is necessary to begin the intensive therapy noted under post-operative tetany.

The results of surgical treatment of generalized osteitis fibro-cystica are good. Very soon the pains in the limbs disappear, and there is a great improvement in health with disappearance of digestive and urinary symptoms. Naturally it takes very much longer for the bones to recover their normal texture and months may elapse before there is much reduction of the plasma phosphatase. This emphasizes the necessity for continuing a high calcium diet with abundance of vitamin D.

THE SUPRARENAL GLANDS

Addison's Disease

The syndrome of Addison's disease is largely, if not entirely, the result of deficiency of the hormone produced by the adrenal cortex. The functions of this internal secretion are still a matter of dispute but it would appear that, as a result of removal or destruction of the adrenal cortex, sodium and water are lost in excess from the blood while potassium is retained. In association with these changes in blood chemistry a significant reduction in blood volume takes place together with a diminishing rate of blood flow, an increasing muscular weakness and possibly some fundamental disturbance of carbohydrate metabolism. The therapeutic technique at present generally adopted is based on these findings. The loss of sodium is made good by the administration of an abundance of sodium chloride ; restriction of potassium intake is also advocated since it is believed that decrease in the sodium-potassium ratio is of importance in producing the manifestations of cortical insufficiency. A plentiful supply of carbohydrate is important if for nothing else than to act as an easily utilized source of energy for the weakened myocardium.

Since the preparation of an active extract of adrenal cortex, the employment of cortical hormone has taken an important place in the treatment of Addison's disease, although its success has not perhaps been as great as was originally anticipated. The reports in the literature are conflicting and the cost of its regular use is still high, so that it is necessary to make as much use as possible of all other methods of treatment. At present the mainstay of treatment in Addison's disease is undoubtedly sodium chloride, the chief use of cortical extract being to tide over the crises.

Treatment in Crises.—During the crises that occur in the course of the disease the patient should be put to bed, kept warm with an electric blanket or hot-water bottles and prevented from moving more than is absolutely necessary. As has already been mentioned, the use of cortical hormone preparations such as eschatin (Parke, Davis), eucortone (Allen & Hanbury) or cortin (Organon) is specially to be recommended. An initial dose of 30 c.c. of extract should be given intravenously together with 500 c.c. of 10 per cent. glucose and normal saline: this should be followed by intramuscular injections of 20 c.c. of the extract at six-hourly intervals until a remission is induced, which generally becomes apparent within three days. As the crisis passes the need for the hormone gradually becomes less so that the amount of extract should be slowly reduced and, if it is to be continued, the maintenance dose determined for the particular patient. During crises patients appear very commonly to react severely to any parenteral injection, especially by the intravenous route, so that a sharp febrile attack with a rigor may follow the administration of extract. In spite of the severest reactions it is necessary to persevere with this line of treatment, after which rapid clinical improvement frequently occurs. The intensity of the reactions usually diminishes *pari passu* with the disappearance of the acute symptoms. Adrenalin may also be given, but at best it has only a very transitory effect.

Maintenance Treatment.—The basis of maintenance treatment is the administration of sodium salts. Some physicians, indeed, assert that, in the absence of a crisis, the injection of cortical extract does not yield any better results than sodium medication. Whether or not this is the case, it is certainly true that an ample supply of this element is essential and that it lessens the requirement of cortical hormone when this is used. The emetic action of large amounts of salt when given by the mouth constitutes a difficulty. Fortunately, however, patients with Addison's disease tolerate sodium chloride much better than most healthy subjects. In order to prevent the local irritant effect on the gastric mucosa, salt may be given in 1 gm. capsules and may of course be added to the general diet. Fifteen grams of sodium chloride daily are recommended. Although there is a diminution in blood chloride as well as blood sodium the deficiency of the latter is by far the more important, since with return of the sodium content to normal level the chloride content almost automatically increases. Accordingly the sodium can be supplied with some other acid radicle, such as phosphate, citrate or bicarbonate.

The prevention of an excessively high concentration of

potassium in the blood is also of importance. Because of this a diet containing minimal amounts of potassium is of great advantage. Abrahams and Widdowson ("Modern Dietary Treatment," 1937) give the recipe for such a diet, which contains eggs, white bread, rice, macaroni, butter, cheese, honey, marmalade, stewed beef without gravy and vegetables. They point out, however, that vegetables lose their potassium when cut into small pieces and boiled in a large volume of water. Generally, low potassium diets contain too little protein so that extra protein should be supplied in the form of a low mineral casein bread to which sodium chloride has been added. Directions for preparing this bread are contained in Abrahams and Widdowson's book mentioned above. Furthermore, the diet should be of high caloric value and should contain an abundant supply of carbohydrate, since there is a tendency to hypoglycæmia in Addison's disease.

In some patients the continued administration of cortical extract may be found to be advantageous or even necessary. The level of dosage, which may vary from 1 to 20 c.c. per day naturally depends on the severity of the condition. Generally the intramuscular route is chosen, since this is easier than the intravenous and less likely to produce a severe reaction. With small amounts subcutaneous injection may be employed, but oral administration for the present is ineffective.

In 1937 an essential principle of the adrenal cortex was isolated. This was named corticosterone, and it has since been found possible to synthesize a closely allied compound, desoxycorticosterone-acetate (D.O.C.A.) (Organon & Ciba), which also possesses the essential biological properties of corticosterone. D.O.C.A. is available in an oily solution for injection and also as tablets for implantation. As far as can be determined, 5 mg. of D.O.C.A. is approximately equivalent to 10 c.c. of cortical extract (Cortin-Organon). Preliminary observations have demonstrated the value of D.O.C.A., but it is probable that it is not the only constituent of the active cortical extract.

The general treatment of the patient should be conducted on the usual lines, but special note must be taken of the heightened sensitivity to cold. During a crisis and whenever asthenia is marked, confinement to bed should be insisted on and care must be taken that the patient is kept warm. In view of the fact that the underlying cause of the destruction of the adrenal cortex is usually tuberculosis, fresh air, rest and a good diet are necessary. A careful search should be made for other tuberculous foci, especially in the lungs and kidneys.

Digestive symptoms are occasionally troublesome and should be dealt with as they arise. A bitter acid mixture is sometimes of value as a stomachic in promoting appetite. If vomiting supervenes, food should be withheld and glucose and saline given per rectum or parenterally. The rest given to the stomach, together with the replenishment of the water and sodium stores of the body, usually suffices to allay the vomiting. For constipation, which sometimes is present, only liquid paraffin or the mildest purgatives (senna, rhubarb) should be used since the stronger remedies may lead to violent and intractable diarrhœa.

It should be the aim of treatment to maintain the blood sodium at a normal level, to prevent a rise of blood potassium and urea and to keep the fasting blood sugar above 60 mg. per cent. The estimation of the weight of the patient would seem to be the best and simplest index of the efficacy of treatment. When this shows a tendency to fall, the administration of cortical extract may be started or increased and steps may be taken to insure that the sodium intake is sufficient and the potassium intake minimal. In cases successfully treated the patient exhibits a normal appetite, an improvement in the general physical condition and almost a state of euphoria in contrast to the previous depression and listlessness. The presence of digestive symptoms, persistent loss of weight, and muscular weakness suggest that treatment is inadequate. It is unnecessary, however, to begin the administration or to increase the dose of cortical extract merely because the blood pressure is low if health is otherwise satisfactory.

Tumours of the Adrenals

Tumours of the Adrenal Cortex.—These may give rise to changes in the sexual organs and the secondary sexual characteristics. Surgical removal of the neoplasm should, if possible, be attempted. If there is any indication of malignancy on histological examination deep X-ray treatment should be given. In view of the fact that the removal of one adrenal gland may give rise to symptoms of adrenal insufficiency because of hypoplasia of the remaining gland it is wise to anticipate this event by the administration of large amounts of salt and glucose and, if available, adrenal-cortical hormone.

Hyperplasia of the Adrenal Cortex.—According to Broster and Gardiner-Hill benefit may result from removal of one adrenal gland.

Tumours of the Adrenal Medulla.—If a diagnosis is made

sufficiently early, surgical removal of the neoplasm offers some chance of success. In the case of neuroblastomata treatment does not seem to be of any avail.

THE GONADS

In spite of the vast output of work relating to internal secretions arising from and affecting the gonads, very little can be stated with even a moderate degree of certainty about the appropriate therapeutic measures required for the numerous clinical conditions of gonadal dysfunction.

Hyperfunction of the gonads when due to tumours of the sex or other glands may be dealt with by removal of the neoplasm. The success of the treatment generally depends upon the extent to which the new growth can be extirpated.

Gonadal hypofunction has been the subject of a large number of quite unwarranted statements with reference to therapeutic procedures, especially as regards the use of the sex hormones. Although much of the experimental work on the sex glands appears to be satisfactory there are not enough records of controlled therapeutic trials to permit of accurate statements being made as to the use of these preparations. All that can usefully be done at present is to consider briefly the main classes of preparations which are available, and to state those clinical conditions for the treatment of which there seems some *prima facie* evidence. First, however, one must utter a word of caution as to the use of any preparation that has not been standardized and issued by a commercial firm of repute.

Gonadal hormones are at present divided into four groups :—

1. Gonadotropic Hormones. Prolan A : Prolan B.
2. Œstrogenic Hormone. Œstrin.
3. Corpus Luteum Hormone. Progesterone.
4. Male Hormone. Androsterone.

Gonadotropic Hormones.—These are of two types, one originally named prolan A, able to stimulate the growth of graafian follicles in the ovaries, and the other, prolan B, capable of producing luteinization of mature follicles. The follicle-stimulating hormone has a stimulant effect on both male and female germ cells, whereas the luteinizing factor acts chiefly on the theca cells of the ovary and the interstitial cells of the testis. Originally detected in the anterior lobe of the pituitary, they are also present in the urine of women during pregnancy and after the menopause. The substance derived from pregnancy urine is chiefly luteinizing in effect although it has a slight follicle-stimulating action. Menopausal urine, on the other hand, yields a substance which is entirely follicle-stimulating in effect.

Most of the preparations available for clinical use are derived from the urine of pregnant women and therefore contain both follicle-stimulating and luteinizing fractions although the latter predominates. Among such preparations may be mentioned gonan (British Drug Houses), antuitrin S. (Parke, Davis), prolan (Bayer) and pregnyl (Organon, London). Standardization is in terms of rat units, a common concentration being 100 units per ampoule of 1 c.c. They have been used in the treatment of amenorrhœa, dysmenorrhœa, menorrhagia, sterility and habitual abortion. In the male they are said to be of advantage in the treatment of undescended testes. In this latter case it should be remembered, however, that with the onset of puberty the testes frequently descend into the scrotum without the aid of hormonal injections or surgeon's traction. One hundred units of antuitrin S. or other preparation are recommended to be given three times weekly.

Preloban, a Bayer preparation biologically standardized, contains the follicle-stimulating factor (Prolan A). It is recommended in doses of 1 ampoule injected three times weekly for sterility in the male due to defective spermatogenesis.

As regards the method of administration, there is no evidence that even large doses of the gonadotropic hormones possess any activity when given orally. Accordingly they should only be administered subcutaneously or intramuscularly, the latter route being preferable owing to the frequency of local reaction such as redness, swelling and tenderness. These reactions tend to diminish in intensity with repeated injection.

Œstrogenic Hormone (œstrin).—This is present in the growing ovarian follicle but is also found in the placenta, the amniotic liquor and urine of pregnant women. Its function would appear to be to stimulate the development of both primary and sexual sex organs and after puberty to produce the periodic increase in vascularity of the lining membrane of the uterus. Accordingly it has been used for the treatment of ovarian hypofunction, uterine infantilism, functional amenorrhœa and sterility both in the male and female. It is to be noted that its administration is contraindicated whenever there is hyperplasia of the endometrium.

Preparations are available both for oral and parenteral administration. For the former, tablets of œstroform (British Drug Houses), capsules of theelol (Parke, Davis) or dragées of progynon (Schering), among others, are available, but the dosage required is about five times the amount required for parenteral use. For injection aqueous or oily solutions contained in ampoules are used.

There would appear to be some advantage in using an oily rather than a watery preparation because absorption is more continuous and prolonged and, owing to the very poor solubility of the hormone in water, large amounts can be given in much smaller bulk. Thus with oil as much as 50,000 units can be dissolved in 1 c.c. (progynon-B oleosum forte (Schering); œstroform B. (British Drug Houses)). Oily preparations are generally given intramuscularly with very little resulting irritation. Administration of œstrogenic hormone by means of vaginal suppository and nasal spray has also been recommended, but these methods are much too uncertain.

Corpus Luteum Hormone (progesterone).—This is said to bring about the endometrial changes occurring prior to the commencement of the menstrual flow and in the early days of pregnancy. The clinical indications for the employment of preparations containing this hormone are still ill-defined, but in general it may be said that its use is indicated whenever there is uterine hæmorrhage resulting from ovarian dysfunction. It has been strongly recommended in some quarters for the treatment of threatened or habitual abortion. Of the preparations available proluton (Schering) and progestin (B.D.H.) may be mentioned.

Male Hormone (Androsterone).—This has been obtained from the testes of large mammals and from human urine. It has also been prepared synthetically. Its function would appear to be the control of the secondary sex characters and the stimulation of spermatogenesis. At present there are no well-defined indications for its clinical use, although it has been recommended for the treatment of retarded puberty, premature senility and hypertrophy of the prostate. Perandren (Ciba) and testoviron (Schering) are among the preparations available.

THE PITUITARY

Diabetes Insipidus

Diabetes insipidus, characterized by marked polyuria and thirst, is generally attributed to a lesion in the floor of the third ventricle anterior to the tuber cinereum. The nature of the lesion varies in different patients, often being the result of syphilis; neoplasm, trauma and post-encephalitic changes have also been reported as causal factors, while there is a group of patients in whom there appears to be a hereditary or familial tendency.

If there is evidence of syphilis, vigorous anti-luetic treatment should be instituted. A neoplasm causing this lesion is at present almost always inaccessible to surgical treatment, although deep X-ray therapy has been said to yield promising results. In most cases treatment should be directed to the relief of the thirst and polyuria. For this purpose intramuscular injections of posterior pituitary extract (extractum pituitari liquidum, B.P.) or, preferably, a solution of the pressor fraction of the extract (pitressin, Parke, Davis & Co.) are often of value. The usual dose of either is 1 c.c. twice daily, but this may have to be increased or reduced as found necessary in different individuals. Occasionally patients become very pale and rather nauseated after an injection of posterior pituitary extract, but this is only a transient phenomenon: prolonged use does not appear to be attended by any untoward effects. It must be remembered that the antidiuretic action of the drug is transient, lasting usually about four hours, but sometimes considerably longer. It is thus advisable to give an injection late in the evening so as to permit as long a period as possible of undisturbed sleep. Posterior pituitary extract is absorbed when applied to the nasal mucosa and successful results have been reported from the use of an intranasal spray, or from the insertion of a pledget of cotton wool soaked in the extract. This method is, however, less efficacious than the intramuscular injection and requires more pitressin to produce a significant effect. Insufflation of a dry powder consisting of 1 gr. of dried posterior lobe extract (pituitarium posterium, U.S.P.) in lactose three times daily has also proved beneficial in mild cases.

The posterior pituitary hormone probably increases tubular reabsorption in the kidney. This leads to an increase in the specific gravity of the urine and marked diminution in urinary volume with consequent retention of water in the tissues and alleviation of thirst.

Reduction in the intake of sodium chloride may produce some amelioration of the symptoms, but it is almost impossible to restrict the ingestion of fluid to any significant extent until polyuria is diminished owing to the intense thirst.

Adenomata of the Pituitary

Adenomata of the pituitary body are restricted to the anterior lobe and may be classified as (*a*) chromophobe or agranulocytic, (*b*) eosinophil and (*c*) basophil according to the staining reactions of the cells composing the tumour. The symptoms and signs produced depend upon the pressure exerted on the remaining tissue of the anterior lobe and the surrounding structures, upon the extent of actual destruction and the nature of the secretion produced by the tumour cells.

The Chromophobe Adenomata.—A tumour of the chromophobe cells, to which no secretory function has yet been attributed, manifests itself by the effects of pressure on and destruction of pituitary tissue and such structures as the optic chiasma and hypothalamus. The only treatment which holds out any hope is surgical removal, since the chromophobe cells do not appear to be sensitive to X-rays. Increasing loss of eyesight is an important indication for surgical interference which should be attempted as soon as possible before the destruction of tissue is advanced. If there is evidence of deficient secretion of pituitary hormones replacement therapy should be instituted.

The Acidophil or Eosinophil Adenoma.—This gives rise to the clinical conditions of gigantism or acromegaly according to the age of the patient. In addition, signs of pressure on the optic paths are generally present. Deep X-ray therapy is frequently successful in arresting the growth of this type of tumour and should always be tried before resorting to the rather desperate expedient of attempting to remove the adenoma surgically.

The Basophil Adenoma.—This produces the clinical manifestations generally known by the term " Cushings's syndrome." Deep X-ray therapy has been found beneficial in some cases. In those cases where such treatment has failed it is possible that the syndrome was caused not by a basophil adenoma but by an adenoma or hyperplasia of the adrenal cortex, which may produce an almost identical syndrome.

Pituitary Infantilism

Pituitary infantilism, which generally becomes manifest before the tenth year of life, is associated with defective production of the growth hormones and is frequently associated with a failure of the gonadotropic secretions. The clinical picture is one of dwarfism with defective development of the primary and secondary sex characters. The mental processes, although sometimes unaffected, generally remain childish. Successful results are reported following the use of the pituitary growth hormone. Antuitrin G. (Parke, Davis & Co.) may be used in doses of 1 to 3 c.c. subcutaneously two or three times weekly. It is advisable at first not to use an extract prepared from the entire anterior lobe of the pituitary, since the gonadotropic hormones which such extracts contain may lead to closure of the epiphyses before a sufficient degree of growth has been obtained. Later, when the growth hormone has achieved the desired result or its maximum effect, a preparation containing gonadotropic secretions may be given in an attempt to promote the development of the sex organs. Improvement has also been claimed from the use of stimulant doses of X-rays. The treatment of infantilism is still, however, in the experimental stage.

Simmond's Disease

Simmond's disease, characterized by marked wasting, premature senility and sexual dystrophy, results from gradual destruction of the anterior lobe of the pituitary body with consequent deficiency of its hormones. The causal factor may be syphilis, tuberculosis, cystic degeneration, thrombosis or embolism. The latter has been observed following the termination of pregnancy. Treatment depends to some extent on the nature of the lesion. If the Wassermann reaction is positive, antisyphilitic measures should be instituted. The administration of anterior pituitary extract has been tried, but it is doubtful whether much benefit accrues. Attempts have also been made to stimulate the anterior pituitary cells to increased activity by means of X-ray radiations. For combating the progressive emaciation large quantities of glucose should be administered.

N. Morris.

DISEASES OF THE BLOOD

INTRODUCTION

IT is universally agreed that in all diseases, treatment, to be successful, must be preceded by accurate diagnosis. This is particularly the case in diseases of the blood. In the diagnosis of the anæmias it is not sufficient to rely solely on the symptoms complained of or on the appearance of the patient. The symptoms of all types of anæmia are dependent mainly on the anoxæmia present, and their magnitude varies according to the degree of anoxæmia and the rapidity with which it is produced. Similarly, no sign by itself can be held to be diagnostic, and it is unwise to rely solely on the appearance of the skin, especially of exposed surfaces, for diagnosis of the type or degree of the anæmia present. Hence no short cut to correct diagnosis exists, and a careful blood examination should always be performed when anæmia is suspected. If the general practitioner is unable or unwilling to do this, he should send a blood smear and a sample of oxalated blood to a laboratory. This should be done prior to the institution of treatment, otherwise essential diagnostic features in the blood picture may be altered to such a degree that the pathologist may have great difficulty in reaching a correct diagnosis. This is particularly likely to occur if the practitioner uses a shot-gun prescription of both iron and liver extract, in which case the unfortunate patient will have to carry on both forms of treatment indefinitely when only one or neither is required.

That general practitioners still rely largely on a physical examination for the diagnosis of the type of blood disease present, and not on a blood examination, is fully recognized by medical men with special experience in hæmatology. Not infrequently patients report at our blood clinic who have been treated for months or years, at great expense, with liver extract, and who could have been cured with iron in a few weeks at the cost of a few shillings. On the other hand, the majority of cases of pernicious anæmia entering hospital have been diagnosed as hypochromic anæmia and have been treated with iron for months.

Lastly, we wish to stress the need for a thorough investigation into the underlying causal factors. The value of making such investigations is twofold: first, if the causal condition is not removed, treatment of the anæmia may fail even if the appropriate hæmatinic is given; second, pathological conditions causing the anæmia may advance to an incurable stage if symptomatic treatment for the anæmia alone is prescribed. This is particularly true of malignant disease of the gastro-intestinal tract, where a considerable temporary improvement in the blood picture may result from the administration of iron, despite the progress of the cancer.

So far we have made a plea for full blood examination in every case in which the doctor suspects the presence of anæmia from the symptoms and physical signs, but certain clinical features in the absence of anæmia call equally for blood investigations. In chronic leukæmias, hæmolytic anæmias, the hæmorrhagic diatheses and agranulocytic angina, anæmia may be absent or mild in degree at certain periods. Accordingly, the presence of enlargement of the spleen, liver or lymph nodes, and unexplained hæmorrhage, sepsis or icterus, indicate the need for a blood examination which should include, in every case, a red and white cell-count, hæmoglobin estimation and examination of a stained blood film, and in some cases a differential white cell-count, thrombocyte count, reticulocyte count and other special investigations.

CLASSIFICATION

Treatment can be placed on a more rational basis if the practitioner has some simple but clear conception of the classification of diseases of the blood. The classification submitted below places the various blood disorders into two main groups: (A) the anæmias, and (B) a miscellaneous group of diseases, some of which are not necessarily accompanied by anæmia, but which are generally dealt with in textbooks of hæmatology.

Group A is divided into three subdivisions. The obvious advantage of this classification is that cases in Group A (I) are treated by appropriate substitution therapy, namely, iron, liver extract and vitamin C; cases in Group A (II) by removal of the hæmolytic agent, where possible, or by splenectomy; and cases in Group A (III) by removal of the causal agent, where possible, and by blood transfusion. In Group B the treatment varies in each individual disease.

A. THE ANÆMIAS

I. Anæmias due to Deficiency of Factors essential for Normal Blood Formation

(*a*) Iron.

1. Chronic nutritional hypochromic anæmia, including the Plummer-Vinson syndrome, chlorosis, and the hypochromic anæmia of pregnancy.
2. Nutritional hypochromic anæmia of infancy and childhood.
3. Post-hæmorrhagic anæmia, acute and chronic.

(*b*) The antipernicious anæmia factor.

1. Addisonian pernicious anæmia.
2. Pernicious anæmia of pregnancy.
3. Macrocytic anæmia complicating pathological conditions of the gastro-intestinal tract, *e.g.*, intestinal anastomoses, sprue, idiopathic steatorrhœa, etc.
4. Tropical macrocytic anæmia.
5. Macrocytic anæmia of liver disease.

(*c*) Vitamin C.

Scurvy (dealt with in the section devoted to Deficiency Diseases).

(*d*) Thyroxin.

The anæmia of myxœdema (dealt with in the section devoted to the Endocrine Glands).

II. Anæmias due to Excessive Blood Destruction

(*a*) Primary hæmolytic anæmia.
Familial and acquired acholuric jaundice.
(*b*) Secondary hæmolytic anæmia.
(*c*) Paroxysmal hæmoglobinuria.
(*d*) The acute hæmolytic anæmia of Lederer.
(*e*) Sickle-cell anæmia.
(*f*) Hæmolytic anæmias of infancy (dealt with under "Diseases of Infancy").

III. Anæmias due to Aplasia or Hypoplasia of the Bone-marrow

Aplastic and hypoplastic anæmia.

1. Idiopathic.
2. Secondary.

B. MISCELLANEOUS DISEASES OF THE BLOOD

I. Splenic Anæmia (Banti's disease).

II. Polycythæmia.

- (*a*) Polycythæmia vera.
- (*b*) Enterogenous cyanosis.

III. Hæmorrhagic Diseases.

- (*a*) The purpuras.
  1. Primary.
  2. Secondary.
- (*b*) Hæmophilia.

IV. The Leukæmias.

V. Diseases of the Lymphatic System.

- (*a*) Hodgkin's disease.
- (*b*) Lymphosarcoma.

VI. Agranulocytic Angina.

VII. Infectious Mononucleosis (dealt with in the section of Infectious Diseases).

VIII. Diseases of the Reticulo-endothelial System.

- (*a*) Reticulo-endotheliosis.
- (*b*) Gaucher's disease.
- (*c*) Niemann-Pick's disease.
- (*d*) Hand-Schüller-Christian's disease.

There are certain forms of treatment of particular value for, and commonly employed in, widely differing types of anæmia. In order to save needless repetition regarding technique and dosage, we have dealt with such procedures in great detail in certain sections, and merely refer the reader to the appropriate pages, where they are advised in other forms of anæmia. A full description of iron therapy and the general measures required for the care of a case of anæmia will be found in the section on Chronic Nutritional Hypochromic Anæmia; the indications for, and dangers of, blood transfusion in the section on Acute Post-hæmorrhagic Anæmia; while liver and liver extract therapy is described under the heading "Pernicious Anæmia and other Macrocytic Anæmias."

THE ANÆMIAS DUE TO IRON DEFICIENCY

I. Chronic Nutritional Hypochromic Anæmia.

Chronic nutritional hypochromic anæmia is the name given by us to the iron-deficiency anæmia occurring chiefly among women of the child-bearing age belonging to the poorest classes of the community. The fundamental factor in its causation is the ingestion of a diet, the iron content of which is insufficient to meet the demands of menstruation and pregnancy. (This form of anæmia has been given many names, of which "idiopathic hypochromic anæmia," "chronic microcytic anæmia," "simple achlorhydric anæmia" and "chloranæmia" are the most frequently used.) Our investigations in Aberdeen indicate that anæmia is present in some degree in 50 per cent. of working-class women, 15 per cent. of whom are severely anæmic. The same factors operating in adolescent girls produce an identical anæmia to which the name "chlorosis" is given. In pre-war days chlorosis occurred with great frequency and severity, but to-day, owing to improved working conditions, it is relatively infrequent and mild in degree. When a woman becomes pregnant, anæmia may develop or become accentuated because of the reduced intake and assimilation of iron from alteration of appetite and diminished gastric secretion of hydrochloric acid, and also because of the fœtal demands for iron. Since exactly the same measures for the prevention and treatment of these three forms of hypochromic anæmia are indicated, it is unnecessary to deal with them individually.

Prophylaxis.—The first step is improvement of the diets of women of the poorest classes. While in theory this is easy, it is in practice often extremely difficult, since the principal cause of dietary deficiency lies in the economic field. Hence the family doctor should know the relative values of the different foodstuffs in regard to their iron content and its availability and their cost. Table I gives a list of some of the commoner foods rich in iron and indicates which are the cheapest sources of this mineral. As will be indicated in the section devoted to dietetics, it is far more economic and more efficient to buy medicinal iron from the chemist than to buy food iron from the butcher and the greengrocer. From the point of view of prophylaxis, however, this is not to be recommended, since our dietary surveys have clearly shown that iron is only one of many deficiencies in the diet of the poorest classes. When the iron intake is improved by a selection of foods rich in iron, *e.g.*, liver, meat, fruits and green vegetables, the deficiency of animal protein, calcium, phosphorous, and vitamins is simultaneously corrected. It is only when such a diet is found to be unable to maintain a normal blood level that the administration of medicinal iron is indicated. In women past the menopause we have found that a normal blood level and iron balance can be maintained on an intake as low as 4 mg. of iron daily. Approximately 10 mg. will supply the needs of the majority of women whose menstrual periods are moderate to scanty, or in whom child-bearing is infrequent and not attended by excessive post-partum hæmorrhage. In women with more profuse periods and more frequent pregnancies a dietary intake of 10 mg. daily, or even considerably more, may not maintain a normal blood level. In such cases the administration of medicinal iron for one week in each month is a cheaper and more efficient method of achieving this result than increasing the iron intake further by dietary means.

The second factor requiring consideration is pregnancy. Since approximately 50 per cent. of women of the poorest classes suffer, during pregnancy and the early puerperium, from some degree of anæmia conditioned by the fœtal demands for iron, and post-partum hæmorrhage, it is obvious that the family doctor should be continuously on the outlook for the occurrence of anæmia by examining the conjunctival mucous membrane and by inquiring into such symptoms of anæmia as weakness, dyspnœa and palpitation. Our experience of hæmoglobin estimations at the ante-natal clinic at Aberdeen strongly suggests the desirability of making this procedure part of the routine examination at all such clinics. In all cases of anæmia, no matter how mild, a month's treatment should be instituted with curative doses of iron, as indicated below, and this should be followed by a maintenance dose (one-third of the curative dose) for the duration of pregnancy and one month afterwards. By such means it should be possible to prevent labour occurring under the dangerous conditions not infrequently seen, where the hæmoglobin level may be 30 per cent. or less. Moreover, should a severe post-partum hæmorrhage occur, the patient might be able to withstand it without being precipitated into a dangerous state of shock.

The third factor to be considered in relation to prophylaxis is menstruation. In women whose diet has been corrected as far as possible in keeping with their economic circumstances, and in whom anæmia develops without any obvious cause, such as pregnancy, post-partum hæmorrhage, abortion or infection, the most likely cause of the anæmia is menstrual blood loss. In some persons a clear history of menorrhagia is obtained, whereas in others the periods are stated to be normal. Little reliance, however, can be placed on a woman's assessment of her menstrual loss. If it is believed that excessive menstrual blood loss is occurring, it is essential to exclude organic disease of the uterus or adnexæ, and to consider the question of endocrine dysfunction in addition to prescribing prophylactic doses of iron. Before advising curettage for menorrhagia in women already anæmic, a course of iron therapy should be instituted, since correction of the anæmia not infrequently leads to more normal periods. In other cases menstrual loss of blood may not be reduced or may even become more profuse. In such cases either curettage or endocrine treatment may be indicated. If the woman is approaching the menopause, the hastening of this process by radium treatment may be advisable.

Curative Treatment.—Treatment may be considered under the following heads :—

(*a*) General measures.
(*b*) Symptomatic treatment.
(*c*) Dieto-therapy.
(*d*) Iron treatment.

(*a*) *General measures* include the provision of physical and mental rest, good nursing, fresh air and sunshine if possible, the avoidance of chills and a satisfactory diet. If the hæmoglobin level is 40 per cent. or less, the patient should be confined to bed. Since the blood level falls very slowly and the blood volume is maintained in chronic nutritional hypochromic anæmia, the patients become to a considerable extent acclimatized to a low level of hæmoglobin. (This is in contrast to the state of shock which occurs in patients with a sudden external loss of blood, even though the hæmoglobin has fallen only to 50 or 60 per cent.) Hence it is unnecessary for the patient to be at complete rest in bed ; she may assume the position she finds most comfortable and sit up in bed for her meals. Usually such patients defæcate more regularly if they are allowed to go to the lavatory, and this may be permitted if it is in close proximity to the bedroom and on the same floor. Alternatively a bedside commode may be used. When the hæmoglobin has reached 50 per cent., the time allowed out of bed should be increased and graduated exercise should be ordered, particular care being taken to avoid undue fatigue or chilling owing to the liability of anæmic individuals to develop infections. Until iron treatment has corrected the anæmia, rest in bed is the best form of treatment for alleviating the symptoms of anoxæmia, circulatory instability, and myocardial weakness, namely, dyspnœa, palpitation, giddiness, etc.

(*b*) *Symptomatic Treatment: Gastro-intestinal System.*—Gastro-intestinal disturbances are frequently present. Anorexia, often of many years' duration, occurs in many patients. A feeling of weight and discomfort in the epigastrium after meals, nausea, vomiting, flatulence, constipation and periodic attacks of diarrhœa are other symptoms. A rapid improvement in all such symptoms may be expected within a week or two of the start of iron therapy, especially if the patient is confined to bed on a light diet. Nevertheless it is often desirable to give symptomatic treatment while awaiting the effects of iron therapy. In some patients with dyspepsia and flatulence associated with achlorhydria and chronic gastritis, beneficial results occur from the administration of an alkaline powder (sod. bicarb., bismuth. carb., mag. carb. pond., āā oz. ii; sig. drachm i ex aq. t.i.d. p.c.). In other cases a teaspoonful of the powder in a tumblerful of warm water should be taken on awakening in the morning and before going to sleep at night, with the object of loosening the excess of mucus in the stomach, and dilute hydrochloric acid and pepsin should be taken with meals in the following proportions:—

Acid. Hydrochlor. Dil. . . .	1 part
Glycer. Pepsin B.P.C. . . .	2 parts

One teaspoonful in a tumblerful of water flavoured with orange juice should be sipped during meals three times daily, and the dose should be increased to two or three teaspoonfuls three times a day, particularly if the type of diarrhœa sometimes associated with achlorhydria is present. The majority of patients, however, are constipated owing to the poor tone of the musculature of the alimentary tract and lack of vitamin B and roughage in the diet. When the patient is very anæmic and is suffering from anorexia, it is not advisable to treat the constipation by adding large amounts of fruits and vegetables to the diet, because this may cause dyspepsia; nor is it advisable to give purgatives, because they increase small-intestinal hurry and so reduce the absorption of iron. Mineral oils with the addition of agar, with or without a small amount of cascara sagrada or senna (lixen), should be prescribed. Proprietary preparations such as Agarol and Petrolagar are suitable for this purpose. Occasionally it may be necessary for the first few days to wash out the colon with saline in the morning, a few ounces of olive oil having been introduced into the rectum the night before. For the atonic constipation so frequently present in these anæmic women we have found yeast to be of considerable value. Vitamin B not only helps constipation by improving the tone of the bowel, but promotes appetite and improves absorption. Two or three yeast tablets three times a day before meals are in our experience an excellent tonic. Many doctors think that iron has a constipating effect, and this may be the case with the small doses of iron formerly used. In the dosage used to-day iron usually has a laxative effect and may even cause pain and diarrhœa if maximal doses are taken from the start.

The Tongue.—In the majority of cases the lingual changes are those of an atrophic glossitis with little or no pain. For this condition no symptomatic treatment is required and regeneration of the epithelium may be expected to occur as a result of iron treatment. In some cases, however, painful fissures or ulcers of the tongue and fissuring at the corners of the mouth are present. These also will disappear during treatment with iron, but while awaiting this effect painting the lesions of the tongue with 2½ per cent. (10 gr. to the ounce) solution of chromic acid in water is recommended, and application of carbolised resin (B.P.C.) to the corners of the mouth twice daily will relieve the painful fissures. In some cases the tongue is red, inflamed, and painful, a condition of generalized glossitis being present. Under such conditions the diet should be bland and fluid, and the use of a glass tube to enable the patient to take the food directly to the back of the pharynx may be helpful. Painting with chromic acid may be tried, but is not very successful. Fortunately the condition usually settles down rapidly when the blood begins to improve.

Dysphagia.—A mild degree of dysphagia frequently occurs. This requires no special treatment as it improves *pari passu* with the hæmoglobin level. Should the dysphagia be more severe and persistent, the passage of a mercury bougie may be necessary. In a small proportion of cases difficulty in swallowing is due to a mechanical cause, namely, a web occluding the inlet to the œsophagus. In at least half a dozen of our patients an œsophagoscope had to be passed and the membrane ruptured or cut.

Nervous System.—Numbness and tingling in the extremities are common complaints. In the majority of cases no special treatment is required, since the condition disappears as a result of iron therapy. In more severe cases the parenteral and oral administration of vitamin B preparations is of value.

Suitable preparations of vitamin B for oral and parenteral use can be obtained from any first-class chemist. For oral treatment yeast in tablet form, marmite or bemax are satisfactory preparations, and for parenteral treatment 1 c.c. subcutaneously of a vitamin B concentrate daily for one or two weeks is usually sufficient.

In view of the anoxæmia of the central nervous system and the anxiety state resulting from the struggle for existence to which many women of the poorest classes are submitted, it is not surprising that many patients are nervous, worried, easily upset, suffer from headaches and sleep badly. Small doses of bromide and chloral (pot. brom. and chloral hydrate āā gr. xv m. *et* n.) or phenobarbitone (gr. $\frac{1}{2}$ to i m. *et* n.) are of great value in obtaining the mental and physical relaxation which is so desirable.

(*c*) *Dieto-therapy.* — In severely anæmic patients with anorexia, nausea and possibly vomiting, no attempt should be made at this stage to give a diet rich in iron or roughage. A bland, easily digested diet is recommended, divided into small meals at two to two-and-a-half hourly intervals. The basis of the diet should be milk and milky foods, jellies and custards, lightly boiled or scrambled eggs, pounded fish, purées of fruit and vegetables and small amounts of thin bread and butter. Patients in the severely anæmic stage with marked gastric disturbances require hospitalization for nursing and dietetic reasons. With the rise of the hæmoglobin level appetite and digestion improve, and the diet should be cautiously increased by the addition of chicken and meat, vegetables and raw fruit. Our aim is to reach a diet containing at least 10 mg. of iron a day. The optimal intake of iron is stated to be 15 mg. daily, but the economic circumstances of the poor classes will not in general permit the purchase of such a diet. Should it be found that the normal requirements for iron conditioned by pregnancy or menstruation cannot be satisfied by a maintenance diet containing approximately 10 mg. of iron a day, the administration of medicinal iron for one week in each month must be advised after the normal hæmoglobin level has been restored.

No attempt should be made to bring the hæmoglobin level to normal by dietetic measures alone, since we have shown that this is both uneconomic and unsatisfactory. This does not mean that we should be content with low iron diets (5 to 8 mg. daily), since a figure of at least 10 mg. daily can be attained cheaply and easily by a proper selection of foods. In addition, an improvement in the protein, mineral and vitamin content will result. Accordingly Table I is submitted in order to indicate the articles of diet most suitable for this purpose, and Table II is a diet sheet which will serve as a guide. A study of Table I shows that the flesh foods, eggs, oatmeal, lentils and split peas are articles of food particularly rich in iron. It does not follow, however, that the efficacy of any foodstuff in promoting hæmoglobin regeneration depends solely on its iron content. The availability of the contained iron which in turn depends on the ease with which ionizable iron is liberated by the processes of digestion is a factor of great importance. Fortunately it has been found that in general the foods richest in iron have also the highest content of available iron, and accordingly all that the family doctor need know is the list of the foods of a high total iron content included in Table I.

Table I

Iron Content of the Cheaper Foodstuffs

	Total Iron (mg. per 100 gm.).	Ionizable Iron (mg. per 100 gm.).	Cost per lb.	Mg. of Iron for 1d.
(1) *Flesh Foods*—				
Liver (ox: raw) . .	6·70	5·96	1s. to 1s. 2d.	2·7
Sausage (beef: fried) .	4·18	3·01	4d. to 8d.	3·7
Beef or mutton (raw) .	3·54	0·35	6d. to 10d.	2·0
Corned beef (tinned) .	3·34	1·17	7d. to 10d.	2·3
Rabbit meat (stewed) .	1·89	0·79	2½d. to 5d.	2·0
Herring (fried) . .	1·02	0·75	1d. each	1·0
Haddock (stewed) .	0·75	0·75	8d. to 10d.	0·38
Skate (raw) . .	0·33	0·33	4d. to 6d.	0·28
Eggs . . .	2·50	2·50	1d. to 1¼d. each	1·7
Cheese . . .	1·50	...	6d. to 8d.	1·25
(2) *Cereals, etc.*—				
Oatmeal . . .	4·15	3·98	1½d. to 2d.	8·3
White bread . .	1·07	0·94	2½d.	2·14
Rice	0·45	0·38	2d. to 3d.	0·8
Golden syrup . .	1·68	1·60	3d. to 4d.	2·1
(3) *Vegetable Foods*—				
Lentils (raw) . .	7·63	5·04	2d. to 2½d.	15·3
Split peas (raw) .	5·41	4·38	2½d. to 3½d.	8·8
Cabbage . . .	0·98	0·71	1d. to 1½d.	4·0
Leeks . . .	0·77	0·70	1½d. to 2d.	2·5
Potato . . .	0·60	0·59	½d. to ¾d.	4·0
Carrot . . .	0·50	0·50	2d. to 3d.	1·0
Onion . . .	0·40	0·40	2d.	1·0
Turnip . . .	0·33	0·22	¼d. to ½d.	4·0
Apple . . .	0·23	0·23	1d. each	0·23
Orange juice . .	0·20	0·17	1d. each	0·12

TABLE II

	Iron Content (mg.).	Cost in Pence.
Breakfast—		
Porridge (1½ oz. oatmeal)	1·87	0·16
2 oz. white bread	0·64	0·31
Dinner—		
2 oz. meat	2·12	1·0
3 oz. potato	0·40	0·10
3 oz. cabbage	0·88	0·25
Milk pudding (½ oz. rice)	0·07	0·10
2 oz. white bread	0·64	0·31
Tea—		
1 oz. oatcakes	1·25	0·11
Supper—		
Fish : 1 herring (fried in oatmeal : 3 oz. flesh)	0·92	1·0
1 oz. white bread	0·32	0·15
1 oz. oatcakes	1·25	0·11
Rations per Day—		
10 oz. milk	0·72	1·50
2 oz. margarine	...	0·90
1 oz. syrup	0·40	0·22
1 oz. sugar	...	0·16
½ apple	0·12	0·50
Total	11·60	6·88
Alternatives to Meat or Fish Dishes—	Iron.	Cost.
(1) Lentil soup (2 oz. lentils per person)	4·56	0·50
(2) Sausage (3 oz.)	4·18	1·13
(3) Cheese (2 oz.)	0·90	0·50
(4) 1 egg	1·88	1·0

Specimen Diet—Total calories, 2,200. Protein, 80 gm. Iron, 10 to 14 mg. Cost : approximately 7d.

As the economic factor is of such importance we have shown in column 4, Table I, the amount of iron in milligrams which can be purchased for one penny, and we draw particular attention to the cheapness of "food iron" in oatmeal, lentils and split peas. The costs of the different foods, on which the figures in column 3 are based, were obtained directly from the shops used by the poorest classes in Aberdeen.

(*d*) *Iron Treatment.*—It is now generally agreed (*a*) that iron is absorbed in the ferrous state, mainly from the duodenum and upper jejunum ; (*b*) that the ferrous salts are more efficacious than the ferric salts ; (*c*) that organic preparations of iron (*e.g.*, hæmoglobin and bone-marrow, etc.) are valueless; (*d*) that much larger doses are required to obtain optimal results than was formerly believed; and (*e*) that parenteral iron therapy is attended by considerable danger and discomfort, and at present should seldom, if ever, be advised. While many preparations of iron are now known to be satisfactory, a comparison of their efficacy, their dosage and cost, is a matter of great interest and importance.

Provided that inhibitory factors such as sepsis, toxæmia or hæmorrhage are absent, a rise of at least 1 per cent. per day in the hæmoglobin level should result from efficient iron therapy. Our investigations have definitely shown that the following preparations in the dosage mentioned may all be considered satisfactory, since a rise in hæmoglobin value of more than 1 per cent. daily resulted from their administration. Of the preparations we have tried, the following are very satisfactory :—

1. Ferri et ammon. citrat., gr. xxx t.i.d.
2. Tab. ferrous sulphate (fersolate: Glaxo Co. Ltd.), 1 t.i.d.
3. Ferrous carbonate (bipalatinoids No. 501A: Oppenheimer Son & Co. Ltd.), 1 t.i.d.
4. Ferrous sulphate and yeast (plastules plain: John Wyeth & Brother Ltd.), 1 b.i.d.
5. Tab. ferrous chloride (ferronyl: H. R. Napp Ltd.), ii, t.i.d.
6. Colliron (Evans Sons Lescher & Webb), drachm i t.i.d.

Since all the above preparations are of equal potency in the doses mentioned, it would seem not unreasonable to base one's selection on their convenience, palatability and cost. With regard to convenience, all the tablet or capsule preparations are equal and are superior to the fluid preparations, because they are more portable and do not blacken the teeth and tongue. In addition, a small bottle containing 100 ferrous sulphate tablets will last a month, whereas equivalent treatment with iron and ammonium citrate in the form of a mixture would require renewal of the prescription several times, resulting in inconvenience and repeated payment of the dispensing fee. From the point of view of palatability all are satisfactory, and the choice depends on individual preference. If dysphagia is present, fluid mixtures are obviously preferable. Although cure of the anæmia may be achieved with any of these products at a cost of a few shillings, preparations 1, 2 and 3 appear to be the most economical at present market costs.

When the preparation of iron to be administered has been selected, it is inadvisable to start treatment with the full curative dose, since in some individuals this may result in dyspepsia, vomiting or diarrhœa. Accordingly a test dose of one-third of the curative dose should be given for a day or two, and if no gastric symptoms result this should be increased to the full dosage. If some dyspepsia occurs the final dose should be reached by gradual increases over a few days. If dyspepsia persists and is considered not to be functional in origin, it may be necessary to try another preparation of iron. In this connection it is important to realize that the dyspepsia may be a symptom of the anæmia itself, in which case persistence of iron medication is the correct way of accomplishing its relief.

Lastly, iron should always be prescribed to be taken after meals and followed by a drink of water, as by this means the irritating effects of the mineral on the gastric mucosa are reduced to a minimum.

Duration of Iron Therapy.—The period which will elapse before a normal blood count is attained will vary from one to three months in individual cases, depending on the initial blood level. Treatment should be continued in full therapeutic doses for one month thereafter, in order to provide adequate stores of iron. In women past the menopause maintenance treatment is in general not required, because of their decreased demands for iron. In individuals still menstruating a tendency to relapse is frequently present. If the periods are profuse or pregnancy occurs, iron treatment on the lines laid down in the section devoted to prophylaxis should be instituted. In those with normal or scanty periods it is unnecessary to continue iron treatment, provided that re-examination for the appearance of anæmia is undertaken at six-monthly intervals. By these means the administration of iron with its attendant cost and trouble to many women who would not relapse is avoided. The recommendations regarding diet, and the factors causing anæmia outlined in the section on Prophylaxis, are equally applicable to the prevention of relapse.

II. Nutritional Hypochromic Anæmia of Infancy and Childhood.

Since an adequate store of iron in the fœtal liver is of some importance in maintaining a satisfactory blood level in infancy, careful attention should be directed to the provision of a well-balanced diet for the pregnant mother, and the administration of iron should be undertaken if anæmia is present during pregnancy. Such measures are desirable not only from the point of view of prevention of anæmia in the infant but probably also as a means of improving its general nutrition.

A rapid fall in the hæmoglobin level occurs during the first two months of extra-uterine life. No method of treatment can prevent this fall, which appears to be physiological. Recovery normally occurs during the next eighteen months, but there are two factors of particular importance which may prevent or retard this improvement. The first of these is low birth weight occurring as a consequence of prematurity or otherwise. All children of low birth weight should receive iron therapy from the second month. The second indication for prophylactic iron therapy in infancy is the presence of infections. Even mild infections may cause anæmia and retard blood regeneration—hence the administration of iron for some weeks following infection is a sound general rule. Since mild degrees of anæmia have been shown to be frequent in infants of the poorer classes between six and eighteen months, even in the absence of low birth weight and obvious infections, it is probable that at this age-period nutritional factors are also of importance, namely, undue delay in the change from a milk to a mixed diet and the poor quality of the mixed diet which is given. Accordingly the practitioner would be well advised to institute iron therapy in all cases where the infant appears to be pale, easily fatigued and not thriving.

Iron.—A palatable, efficient and non-irritating preparation of iron in liquid form which can be added to the infant's feeds is the ideal. For a child of three to six months, $1\frac{1}{2}$ gr. of iron and ammonium citrate in water sweetened with glycerin, three times a day, is a satisfactory preparation for prophylactic use. The dose should be 3 gr. three times a day if anæmia has already developed. For children of six to eighteen months the prophylactic dose is 3 gr., while the curative dose varies from 5 to 10 gr. thrice daily. The ferrous salts of iron have been shown to have a higher percentage utilization than the scale preparations, and in our opinion are preferable, since they are equally efficacious in smaller doses. It must be remembered that their efficiency is rapidly reduced if oxidation to the ferric state occurs. Accordingly they must not be prescribed in simple watery solutions but should be mixed with 50 per cent. glucose, which retards oxidation. According to Helen Mackay, the addition of a trace of hypophosphorus acid enhances this effect. She has found the following prescription to be both palatable and efficient :—

℞ Ferrous sulphate . . . . $1\frac{1}{2}$ gr.
Dilute hypophosphorus acid . . $\frac{1}{4}$ m.
Dextrose . . . . . . 15 gr.
Chloroform water . . . to ℥i

Sig., ℥i three times daily.

Whatever preparation of iron is used, treatment should be started by giving doses of one-third to one-half of what is ultimately desired, and the material should be mixed with the feed or given at the end of a feed.

Copper, manganese and some other minerals are believed by certain workers, on the basis of laboratory research in animals, to be necessary for normal hæmopoiesis. Of these minerals the claims of copper alone may be said to have received complete acceptance. It promotes the full utilization of iron in the formation of hæmoglobin by a catalytic action. Because only traces are required it is extremely doubtful if there is any need for its addition to preparations of iron, since our investigations have shown that even in the diets of the poorest classes adequate quantities are present for this purpose. There is some evidence, however, that certain cases of nutritional anæmia in infancy respond better to iron and copper than to iron alone, though this is not the experience of Helen Mackay or ourselves. Should the practitioner desire to give copper as well as iron, certain proprietary preparations are available, such as the ferrous sulphate tablets marketed under the name of fersolate by Glaxo Laboratories, which contain traces of copper and manganese. The difficulty of giving iron in tablet form to infants may be overcome by crushing the tablet immediately before use and mixing it with a feed.

III. Post-hæmorrhagic Anæmia.

Extra-vascular blood loss may be acute or chronic. It is necessary to describe the treatment of these two conditions separately, because the mechanism of their symptomatology and treatment is entirely different.

Acute post-hæmorrhagic anæmia is due to the sudden loss of a large amount of blood or to repeated smaller hæmorrhages occurring in rapid succession.

Treatment.—This will be described under the following headings: (*a*) Arrest of Hæmorrhage and (*b*) Treatment of Shock.

Arrest of Hæmorrhage.—In some cases hæmostasis may be secured by ligature of or pressure on the bleeding point—for example, a severed artery, extra-uterine gestation or the bursting of a superficial varicose vein. In other cases, such as in hæmorrhage from a peptic ulcer, it may be possible to ligature the ruptured vessel, but usually this procedure is not indicated. Lastly, the hæmorrhage may be part of a general blood disease such as thrombocytopenic purpura, hæmophilia or acute leukæmia, where mechanical arrest of the hæmorrhage may be impossible. In summary, it may be stated that where the bleeding point can be secured, this should be undertaken at once.

Treatment of Shock.—The degree of shock which follows a sudden loss of blood depends on several factors. The principal ones are : the amount and rate of blood loss, the age and previous health of the patient and, in accidents and major operations, the concomitant effects of tissue trauma and previous exposure to cold. Since the decision to give intravenous fluids depends on a proper appreciation of these factors, it is desirable that they should be elaborated.

The sudden loss of 500 c.c. of blood will not produce symptoms of shock in a healthy adult, as is clearly indicated from everyday experience with blood donors. When symptoms arise they are usually psychological in origin rather than the result of lowered blood volume. Definite symptoms of shock appear when 1,000 c.c. of blood is lost rapidly, and a fatal result may occur if the figure approaches 2,000 c.c. If the loss is spread over twenty-four hours the symptoms are less severe and the prognosis correspondingly better. Infants and old people stand acute hæmorrhage relatively badly, and this is particularly true if there is a history of previous debility or ill-health.

A patient suffering from acute post-hæmorrhagic anæmia and shock should immediately be placed in bed between blankets. A suitable dose of morphia should be injected subcutaneously and repeated in two hours if necessary. The amount required is the minimal quantity necessary to allay apprehension and restlessness, and to control pain if present. Excessive doses of morphia are harmful because of its depressant effect on the respiratory centre. A quarter of a grain for an adult and $\frac{1}{6}$ to $\frac{1}{12}$ gr. for a child is sufficient for the initial dose. The foot of the bed should be raised on blocks, the patient being kept flat on his back except for a low pillow under his head. In severely exsanguinated patients awaiting blood transfusion, the limbs should be bandaged from below upwards. The body heat should be restored by placing hot bottles along both sides of the body, due care being taken not to burn the patient, whose threshold for pain may be lowered owing to collapse, by ensuring that the bottles are well covered by flannel and are not too hot. When available, a radiant heat cradle should be used, as a more even warming of the body can be obtained without the danger of burning the patient. The temperature should be controlled so as to avoid excessive sweating, which would increase the fluid loss and thus further deplete the blood volume. Cardio-respiratory stimulants are frequently ordered in cases with severe collapse while awaiting the assembly of the apparatus necessary for intravenous transfusion. Pituitrin 1 c.c. subcutaneously, strychnine $\frac{1}{30}$ to $\frac{1}{60}$ gr. subcutaneously and coramine 2 c.c. intramuscularly are used for this purpose, and the dose may be repeated in two to four hours. These preparations may also be used alternately. Consideration of the mechanics of the circulation in post-hæmorrhagic shock suggests that these drugs are unlikely to be of value and may actually be harmful. As a compensation for blood loss, generalized vasoconstriction occurs in an attempt to maintain the blood pressure at a level which will ensure adequate blood supply to the vital centres. Accordingly there appears to be little object in giving the vasoconstrictor drugs adrenalin and pituitrin. Likewise, the stimulants coramine and strychnine are unlikely to be efficacious since the heart and vital centres of the brain are already doing their utmost to maintain a satisfactory circulation and respiratory exchange.

Since the essential cause of shock in acute hæmorrhage is the resulting low blood volume, the restoration of the blood volume is undoubtedly the most important therapeutic procedure required. When shock is only mild in degree, all that may be necessary is adequate amounts of water by mouth. One pint of fluid in an hour, for three or four hours, may make good the deficiency. If the degree of shock is more severe, fluid must be given intravenously (*vide* Technique). For this purpose saline, glucose saline, gum saline and blood are available. Of the fluids mentioned, blood must take first preference, since it is of the correct viscosity and osmotic pressure and the contained corpuscles effectively increase the oxygen-carrying capacity. Second in order of merit is gum saline (6 per cent. gum acacia in normal saline), because the gum holds the fluid within the vessels for a considerable time. On the other hand, saline and glucose saline pass into the tissue spaces within a few minutes of their injection and hence cannot be recommended for the restoration of blood volume, although they are of the greatest value in correcting the dehydration with loss of chlorides, which occurs in excessive vomiting and diarrhœa. A pint of blood will raise the hæmoglobin level and blood volume by approximately 10 per cent. with a concomitant rise of blood pressure. One, two, or more pints of blood should be introduced, the amount depending on the severity of the shock and the degree of anæmia present. Similar quantities of gum saline are indicated if blood is not available.

Blood transfusion should preferably be given by the continuous drip method, as by this means 1,000 to 2,000 c.c. of blood can be introduced over twenty-four hours with complete restoration of the blood volume and with the lowest possible risk of producing acute heart failure and pulmonary œdema, or causing aggravation or recurrence of the hæmorrhage due to a sudden increase in the blood pressure. If only a tube and funnel are available, it is advisable to limit the amount of blood to 1 pint, to introduce the fluid very slowly (forty-five minutes) and to repeat the operation if necessary in from four to six hours.

When the bleeding point has been effectively secured and the state of shock adequately treated, recovery will occur without further intravenous therapy. On the other hand, when the bleeding point cannot be secured it is usually desirable to make immediate arrangements for finding a suitable donor even if the initial degree of shock is not marked, since recurrence or increase in the severity of the hæmorrhage may suddenly precipitate the patient into a dangerous state of collapse.

It is now necessary to discuss the indications for blood transfusion. First, it is unwise to rely solely or mainly on a blood count, since for some hours after acute hæmorrhage the hæmoglobin and red cells per c.mm. of blood may be little altered. Accordingly an estimation of the degree of shock with its concomitant fall in blood volume should be based on the following clinical signs : sighing respiration, coldness and clamminess of the skin, pallor, general weakness, impairment of mental faculties, rapidity and reduced volume of the pulse and fall in the blood pressure. When the pulse-rate is over 100 and the systolic blood pressure below 90 mm. Hg., a considerable degree of shock is present. It has been calculated that the blood volume is less than 60 per cent. of normal when the systolic blood pressure falls below 80 mm. Hg., and the prognosis is very grave unless immediate blood transfusion is given.

It should be remembered that the great strain on the

cardio-vascular system, which occurs in severe post-hæmorrhagic anæmia, necessitates the continuation of complete rest in the recumbent position, warmth and good nursing for at least a week after restoration of the blood volume. Thereafter treatment comprises removal of the causal condition where possible and the application of the measures already given in detail in the section devoted to chronic nutritional hypochromic anæmia under the headings General Measures, Dieto-therapy, and Iron.

Chronic Post-hæmorrhagic Anæmia

Treatment.—The treatment of chronic blood loss is considered under two headings: (*a*) Removal of the Causal Condition, and (*b*) Treatment of the Anæmia.

Removal of the Causal Condition.—The most frequent cause of this form of anæmia, especially in males, and the one most likely to be missed, is occult bleeding from the gastro-intestinal tract. We have not infrequently seen patients with hæmoglobin levels below 30 per cent. who were unaware that they were losing blood by this route. The occult bleeding may come from varicose veins in the œsophagus and stomach, peptic ulcers of stomach or duodenum, malignant tumours or polypi of the gastro-intestinal tract, hæmorrhoids or infestation with animal parasites, particularly ankylostomata. Attention is drawn to the great value of the benzidine reaction for the recognition of occult blood in the stools. More obvious causes of chronic blood loss are repeated nose-bleedings, excessive hæmorrhage from the uterus resulting from the presence of tumours, polypi or endocrine dysfunction, and chronic blood diseases such as purpura, hæmophilia and scurvy. In the great majority of cases of obscure hypochromic anæmia the gastro-intestinal and urogenital tracts should first be investigated as possible sources of hæmorrhage. When the cause of the hæmorrhage has been discovered, treatment directed to its removal must be instituted. It should be noted that the diet frequently prescribed for diseases of the gastro-intestinal tract is often low in iron and may accentuate the anæmia if not adequately reinforced with medicinal iron.

Treatment of the Anæmia.—This consists of the administration of full doses of iron together with the general measures outlined under chronic nutritional hypochromic anæmia (see pp. 466-473). If the source of bleeding has been removed, the chances of relapse after the blood count has been brought to normal are insignificant and therefore, in general, maintenance treatment with iron is not required.

PERNICIOUS ANÆMIA AND OTHER MACROCYTIC ANÆMIAS

It is necessary to emphasize that there are many types of macrocytic anæmia which differ widely one from another in their ætiology, response to treatment and blood picture, excluding the common factor of increased diameter of the erythrocyte. For convenience, however, it is possible to divide all macrocytic anæmias into two groups.

Group I contains the macrocytic anæmias which develop from a megaloblastic bone-marrow consequent on a deficiency of the factor necessary for normal blood formation. This factor, often described as the "specific anti-anæmic factor," is produced in the stomach as the result of the action of a gastric enzyme on food and is absorbed from the intestine, stored in the liver and supplied as required to the bone-marrow. Anæmias developing consequent on a deficiency of the specific anti-anæmic factor belong to the category of megalocytic anæmias.

Group II consists of those anæmias in which the macrocytosis results from causes other than a deficiency of the specific anti-anæmic factor; it is a more ill-defined and heterogeneous group of relatively rare macrocytic anæmias resulting from widely differing causes. The macrocytosis is secondary, in the majority of cases, to prolonged stimulation or irritation of the bone-marrow. Blood formation proceeds on a normoblastic basis, but owing to its excessive activity the parent cells in the bone-marrow are primitive normoblasts and as a result many of their offspring entering the peripheral circulation are larger and more immature than normal erythrocytes. Macrocytic anæmias belonging to Group II are present in (*a*) some cases of hæmolytic anæmia—for example, acholuric jaundice, sometimes of the congenital but more usually of the so-called "acquired" type; (*b*) occasionally in malignant malaria and lead poisoning; (*c*) not infrequently in acute leukæmia and in the terminal stages of chronic leukæmia; and (*d*) in cases of Hodgkin's disease and malignant disease, in which the bone-marrow is irritated by metastatic deposits. These macrocytic anæmias are differentiated from the true megalocytic anæmias on three main grounds: (*a*) the finding of the ætiological factor; (*b*) by full examination of the blood picture, which differs in important details in regard to red cells, white cells and platelets; and (*c*) by their failure to respond to the ingestion or injection of the specific anti-anæmic factor and by their response to appropriate treatment (splenectomy, X-rays, etc.).

It is hoped that the preceding remarks make it clear that all megalocytic anæmias are macrocytic, but that all macrocytic anæmias are not megalocytic. The following discussion will be restricted to the treatment of pernicious anæmia and other megalocytic anæmias.

CLASSIFICATION OF THE MEGALOCYTIC ANÆMIAS

It is obvious that a deficiency of the specific anti-anæmic factor may arise in one of three ways : (A) by a failure in its manufacture in the stomach ; (B) by defective absorption ; and (C) by ineffective storage, mobilization, or utilization. On this basis a simple classification of the megalocytic anæmias can be produced.

Under (A) are included : (1) Addisonian pernicious anæmia and the pernicious anæmia of pregnancy. In the former the loss of the specific gastric enzyme is permanent, while in the latter it is temporary. (2) The megalocytic anæmias which result occasionally from extensive resection of the stomach or its widespread destruction by cancer. (3) The tropical macrocytic anæmias of Indian women (Wills), which arise from nutritional deficiency and not from a failure of gastric secretion.

Under (B) is included the megalocytic anæmia which occurs in many cases of tropical and non-tropical sprue, and in some cases of pellagra. In certain instances, dietary deficiency and impairment of gastric secretion are factors to be considered in addition to a failure in absorption. Occasionally absorption is so seriously affected in individuals suffering from intestinal stenosis, from multiple anastomoses and from prolonged diarrhœa, as to result in a megalocytic anæmia.

Under (C) are included cases of severe liver diseases, particularly cirrhosis, in a proportion of which, estimated by various authors at from 5 to 25 per cent., a megalocytic anæmia occurs. In some of these cases, cell-volume measurements show that this is really a false macrocytosis, due to a flattening of the cells produced mechanically during the spreading of the blood film. It is suggested that the physical state of the plasma in cirrhosis conduces to this effect. In other cases, however, cell-volume measurements are in agreement with cell-diameter measurements, and it is presumed that the damage to the liver prevents it from functioning efficiently as a storage organ for the specific anti-anæmic factor, thus allowing a megalocytic blood picture to occur. In such cases, the administration of the specific anti-anæmic factor, by mouth or by injection, may cure or improve the anæmia, but will not alter the underlying disease of the liver. Lastly, it has been suggested that a failure in the mobilization or utilization of the specific anti-anæmic factor arises occasionally, since in certain cases of megalocytic anæmia production and storage of the active principle have been shown to be satisfactory and yet the bone-marrow fails to respond to the naturally produced factor or to its parenteral administration. Before this group of megalocytic anæmias, called by Wilkinson the " achrestic " anæmias, can be fully accepted and its clear demarcation from partial aplasia of the bone-marrow be fully distinguished, further studies of the bone-marrow are required.

The value of such a classification lies in the fact that all cases of megalocytic anæmia falling under (A) and (B), and some under (C), are examples of anæmias due to a specific deficiency and as such can confidently be expected to be relieved by supplying the missing factor. Since Addisonian pernicious anæmia is the most common and the most important of the megalocytic anæmias, it will be used as the example on which treatment of all the megalocytic anæmias can be modelled, with minor modifications.

Treatment.—The aim of treatment is (1) to restore the blood picture, qualitatively and quantitatively to normal as quickly as possible ; (2) to maintain a normal blood level ; and (3) to replenish and stock adequately the depots of the body with the factors necessary for blood formation. Minot has rightly pointed out that the individual who receives only just enough of a nutritional factor, such as a vitamin or a mineral, to maintain health, may be precipitated into the zone of partial deficiency with the advent of infection : hence the importance of adequate reserves.

It would appear advisable to consider the treatment of pernicious anæmia according to the stage of the disease present when the patient is first seen.

The Severe Relapse Stage.—The patient is critically ill and in a collapsed state, with a blood count of approximately 1 million red cells and a hæmoglobin content of 20 to 30 per cent. Before 1926, patients were frequently seen in this terminal stage, but to-day there can be no possible excuse for allowing such a state to develop. The question of blood transfusion immediately arises, and the clinical condition of the patient, as judged by the degree of circulatory failure rather than by the blood level, must be the deciding factor (see p. 478). If it is concluded that the delay of four or five days which must elapse before improvement can occur as a result of treatment entails a risk to life which should not be taken, a blood transfusion should be given at once.

One pint of blood from a suitable donor should be run into the recipient's vein, very slowly in order to avoid a reaction which the weakened system may be unable to tolerate (see p. 478). Five cubic centimetres of a liver extract specially prepared for intravenous injection (*e.g.*, Hepatex P.A.F.) should be added to the blood and an extract suitable for intramuscular injection should be injected into the gluteal region (*e.g.*, 4 c.c. campolon, or 2 c.c. anahæmin, hepastab, neo-hepatex, or Lederle's Liver Extract). In less urgent cases, in which some doubts exist regarding the need for immediate transfusion, a suitable donor should be procured and arrangements made to have him available immediately an emergency arises. The intramuscular injection of liver extract in the doses mentioned above should be continued daily for three or four days, by which time the reticulocyte increase and a marked subjective improvement will be noted. Within ten days the blood count should have risen by nearly 1 million red cells and the patient should be out of all danger.

Iron.—A preparation of iron (see p. 472) should be given twice a day after meals and continued for two months, in all cases receiving treatment by the parenteral route, since an iron shortage is apt to arise owing to the exceedingly rapid production of erythrocytes.

Hydrochloric Acid.—Hydrochloric acid, combined with glycerin of pepsin (see p. 467) is of value if dyspepsia or diarrhœa is present.

It should be pointed out that the most efficacious treatment for all the symptoms of pernicious anæmia and for the prevention of such serious complications as spinal cord degeneration and disease of the gall-bladder is the administration of adequate amounts of the anti-anæmic factor. Dyspepsia, diarrhœa, sore tongue and general weakness all disappear in the majority of cases without any symptomatic treatment.

General Measures.—Diet, rest, nursing, etc.—see pp. 466-469 for full details.

Stage of Moderate Relapse.—The patient complains of weakness, palpitation, exhaustion, dyspepsia and dyspnœa on effort, but there is no danger to life. The blood count may be from $1\frac{1}{2}$ to $2\frac{1}{2}$ million red cells and the hæmoglobin 40 to 60 per cent. In such a case a choice must be made between parenteral and oral treatment.

Parenteral Treatment.—An intramuscular injection of liver extract in the doses already mentioned should be given on three or four consecutive days, deeply into the gluteal region, alternating daily from side to side. Following the injection, firm massage should be applied to the site for a few minutes (for a full description of the technique of intramuscular injections, see p. 1086). By this means subsequent pain and stiffness are greatly reduced. Thereafter, a weekly injection must be given until the blood count is normal. It not infrequently happens that the blood level tends to become stationary around 3½ to 4 million red cells and 80 to 85 per cent. hæmoglobin, and the patient looks and feels perfectly well. This is sometimes due to the presence of factors inhibiting blood regeneration such as arteriosclerosis, or chronic sepsis and hæmorrhage. It is essential to restore the blood level completely to normal (5 million red cells and 100 per cent. hæmoglobin), as this is important in preventing degenerative changes in the spinal cord. It may be necessary to double or treble the number of weekly injections before normality is attained.

No special diet is required. The patient should take a plentiful, well-balanced, mixed dietary, containing red meat, liver or kidney and green vegetables in at least one meal a day.

Drugs.—Iron and hydrochloric acid as already indicated.

Oral Treatment.—Liver extract by mouth was the treatment of choice until about three years ago. The extract from 500 gm. of liver daily is generally needed to obtain maximal regeneration of the blood. As the cost of treatment works out at from 20s. to 30s. weekly, compared with 2s. to 3s. when parenteral treatment is given, liver extract by mouth can no longer be recommended, for economic reasons. In addition, in resistant cases and in those in whom absorption is poor, oral treatment does not compare with parenteral, on the grounds of efficiency. Half a pound daily of lightly cooked liver is the average dose required, if liver is taken in the crude state. Since the specific anti-anæmic factor is moderately heat stable, there is no point in prescribing raw liver. There are several reasons why the ingestion of liver cannot be recommended as the treatment of choice : first, there is an ever-increasing difficulty in obtaining regular and adequate supplies ; secondly, the cost of liver has risen very greatly ; and thirdly, many persons fail to continue to take the amount required to attain and maintain a normal blood level, owing to the nausea and disgust engendered by the constant sight, taste and smell of the article.

Hog's Stomach Preparations.—These preparations are insoluble and contain the gastric enzyme, which is thermolabile; hence they must not be heated. Excellent results can be obtained from the use of such preparations as ventriculin, pepsac, ektomak, etc., in doses of a tablespoonful three times a day, in water, milk, orange juice, etc. English preparations such as pepsac are cheap (8s. 6d. a pound), but they have an unpleasant taste and smell, which can be improved, however, by exposing the next day's ration to the air for twelve hours, in a saucer covered with muslin.

Pre-operative Measures.—Should an emergency arise during the relapse stage of pernicious anæmia, requiring an operation which cannot be delayed, intensive parenteral treatment should be undertaken immediately (10 c.c. of liver extract intramuscularly, repeated in six hours), and a suitable donor should be procured in order that a blood transfusion can be immediately given if required. Patients in the remission stage of pernicious anæmia, particularly if they show signs of neurological disease, should receive double or treble the usual quantity of liver extract for a few days before undergoing any major operation, since the blood level tends to fall and neurological degeneration to progress after serious surgical procedures.

Chronic focal sepsis (in tonsils, teeth, or accessory sinuses) should not be treated radically until there has been an adequate response to specific anti-anæmic therapy. On the other hand, localized and easily accessible collections of pus should be evacuated, since they tend to inhibit or retard the therapeutic response.

Maintenance Treatment.—Since liver treatment does not produce a cure, but is a form of substitution therapy, maintenance treatment must be continued for life.

The amount of material required to maintain a normal blood level varies greatly in different individuals, often for no apparent reason. Only by trial, checked by blood counts, can the problem of dosage be satisfactorily settled, and this applies equally to the stages of remission and relapse. For maintenance treatment the necessary number of intramuscular injections of liver extract varies in different individuals from one a week to one every six weeks. In our experience an average dose is 5 c.c. of campolon given every three or four weeks or 4 c.c. of anahæmin or the other more concentrated extracts already mentioned at intervals of four to six weeks. Iron is not required if it has already been prescribed during the first two months of treatment. Hydrochloric acid and pepsin are necessary only for the purposes already mentioned.

An ordinary mixed diet is all that is required. The maintenance dose of liver and hog's stomach preparations is also extremely variable in different individuals; on the average it may be said to be 2 lbs. of liver or 4 oz. of dried hog's stomach preparation weekly.

The depot storage method of treatment, whereby 5 to 10 c.c. of a liver extract is injected intramuscularly on two consecutive days, is of value to patients proceeding on holiday or on business to places where facilities for treatment are not available. By this method a satisfactory blood level may be maintained over periods up to three months.

In our experience, parenteral treatment is the method of choice at all stages of the disease, on the grounds both of efficiency and of economy. Should the patient object to injections, however, cooked liver and hog's stomach preparations may be taken on alternate days, in the doses mentioned above, as by this means the distaste engendered by both articles, if taken continuously over long periods, is reduced.

Subacute Combined Degeneration of the Spinal Cord

Prophylaxis.—Lesions of the cord rarely if ever develop in pernicious anæmia if the blood level is maintained within normal limits. It must be emphasized, however, that the symptoms of a patient having maintenance treatment for pernicious anæmia cannot be relied upon as an indication of the blood level. Many patients receiving inadequate maintenance therapy complain of no symptoms although the blood count may be definitely subnormal, *e.g.*, Hb. 80 per cent., R.B.C. 3·5 to 4 millions. It is in such cases that the incidence of subacute combined degeneration of the cord is highest. It is of great importance, therefore, that blood counts should be done at regular intervals (preferably every three months) during maintenance treatment, unless the expensive policy of giving excessive amounts of liver extract is followed. If the red cell count falls below 4·5 millions in the case of women or 5 millions in men, or, if examination of a blood film shows the presence of macrocytes although the blood count is above these levels, maintenance treatment is inadequate and should, therefore, be increased. Our experience has convinced us that the danger of degeneration of the spinal cord is obviated by observance of these precautions.

The treatment of established subacute combined degeneration is discussed in the section devoted to diseases of the nervous system (see p. 986). All that need be said here is that cases of pernicious anæmia with signs of neurological involvement should receive from two to three times as much of the anti-anæmic factor as cases with a comparable blood picture but without neurological changes. In addition, it is wise to supplement parenteral treatment with whole liver, hog's stomach preparations and vitamin B (yeast, marmite, etc.). This intensive treatment should be continued for at least six to twelve months after the blood count has reached normal and should be combined with remedial exercises. By these means many cases which are bedridden may be able to lead a useful life, while patients with less severe involvement of the spinal cord may return to full employment.

Megalocytic Anæmias other than Addisonian Anæmia

The scheme of treatment outlined above is satisfactory for the treatment of the anæmia present in the other conditions mentioned, with the following modifications.

Pernicious Anæmia of Pregnancy

In the majority of cases treatment can be discontinued after parturition.

Tropical and Non-tropical Sprue and Pellagra

In these conditions multiple deficiencies are present which must be corrected. In addition to supplying the anti-anæmic factor, the deficiency of vitamins and minerals must be repaired by the administration of marmite (one teaspoonful in water or in a bread and butter sandwich thrice daily); radiostoleum or adexolin (5 minims thrice daily); calcium (calcium lactate, 30 gr. thrice daily) and iron (as above). For the control of the fatty diarrhœa restriction of fatty foods, especially cream, butter, milk, bacon and fatty meat, must be made. A high intake of Grade A protein—for example, liver and butcher's meat—is recommended, while starchy food should be taken in small quantities only. For details, the reader is referred to the sections devoted to the dietary problems in the above deficiency diseases. When the condition has been cured by diet and anti-anæmic treatment, the maintainance dose of the specific anti-anæmic factor may be steadily reduced, many cases being able thereafter to maintain a normal blood level by diet alone.

Diseases of the Liver and Achrestic Anæmia

With regard to the megalocytic anæmias occurring in cases of severe liver disease, the results of anti-anæmic treatment are less satisfactory, since prognosis depends on the degree and progress of liver damage. Lastly, in the so-called " achrestic " and semiplastic anæmias with a megalocytic blood picture, the response of the formative tissues to the treatment outlined above is absent or very poor. Repeated blood transfusions can, however, maintain the patient alive, but in a poor state of health, for long periods.

HÆMOLYTIC ANÆMIAS

The hæmolytic anæmias include a group of anæmias of widely differing causation, the essential diagnostic feature of which is the presence of excessive blood destruction as demonstrated by the finding of bilirubinæmia, urobilinuria and an excess of immature circulating erythrocytes (reticulocytes), in the presence of a stationary or falling blood count. This term should not be applied to the mild hæmolytic phenomena which occur in the severe relapse stage of the megalocytic anæmias, such as pernicious anæmia, sprue, etc. In such diseases the anæmia is not mainly due to hæmolysis, but to disturbed erythropoiesis, whereas in the true hæmolytic anæmias hæmolysis is the essential factor in the production of the anæmia.

True hæmolytic anæmias can be divided into two groups :—

Primary.—Where the fault lies in the formation of defective erythrocytes which are peculiarly susceptible to destruction by the cells of the reticulo-endothelial system, especially in the spleen.

Secondary.—Where the hæmolysis results from direct injury to normal cells by extraneous toxic or infective factors, and where it occurs, often from unknown causes, as an accompaniment of certain diseases such as carcinomatosis.

The need for this subdivision is apparent if intelligent treatment is to be prescribed, because in the first group the abnormal erythropoiesis cannot be altered by any known method, and treatment consists essentially of reducing blood destruction by splenectomy ; while in the second group the aim is the removal or neutralisation of the toxic or infective factors, together with symptomatic treatment of the anæmia.

Primary Hæmolytic Anæmias

Under this heading are included the familial and acquired forms of acholuric jaundice (hæmolytic icterus, congenital hæmolytic anæmia, acholuric family jaundice). In no other blood disease is there a greater need for accurate diagnosis than in the primary hæmolytic anæmias, since the course is not influenced materially by drug or dietetic treatment, but only by splenectomy. The reader is referred to textbooks of hæmatology for details of the blood investigations necessary to establish the diagnosis. The problem of treatment resolves itself into a simple one, namely, whether splenectomy should be undertaken and if so, when. Considerable divergence of opinion exists in this matter, particularly in mild forms of the disease, where the patient is "more jaundiced than ill." Many authorities believe that splenectomy should be advised in every case when the diagnosis is made, because of the occurrence of serious complications in a high percentage of cases, at some later period in the disease. The principal complications which may endanger life and greatly enhance the risk of operation are cholelithiasis and cholecystitis, severe hæmolytic crises and a terminal exhaustion of the bone-marrow. On the other hand, since the familial form of the disease has been recorded in successive generations in individuals who were able to carry on their occupations with little or no ill-health, other authorities do not consider that splenectomy is indicated in the milder cases of this group. Our own feeling is that, since it is impossible to foretell with certainty the future of even the mildest case of acholuric jaundice, it is wiser to advise operation while the patient is in good health than to risk the serious complications already mentioned. We have no hesitation in offering this advice if the anæmia is in any way affecting the patient's physical and mental health, and causing a loss of efficiency. Additional reasons for advocating splenectomy are a past history of hæmolytic crises or a history of the disease occurring in a severe form in relatives, since it has been shown that the course of the disease runs fairly true to type in different members of the same family. When the hæmolytic anæmia commences in infancy and early childhood, the dangers of biliary complications are remote for many years to come, and provided health is not impaired by anæmia, splenectomy may be safely postponed until the child is ten or twelve years of age, when the procedure is attended by less risk.

Should acute inflammation of the gall-bladder, necessitating laparotomy, occur in a patient with acholuric jaundice, it is generally advisable to limit the operative procedure to the gall-bladder, and to undertake splenectomy at a subsequent suitable date. The interval between the operations should not, however, exceed a few months, since the excessive hæmolysis will continue until splenectomy is performed and, therefore, formation of calculi in the bile ducts may occur. On the other hand, if a chronically diseased gall-bladder with or without stones is found during an operation for splenectomy, the opportunity should then be taken to correct the biliary disease.

The so-called acquired form of acholuric jaundice in which the familial taint cannot be discovered occurs mainly in adult life and usually in a severer form. We have had two patients in whom a fall in the red cell count from approximately 5 to approximately 1 million occurred within twenty-four hours, and was accompanied by severe gastric pain, vomiting, collapse, and a temperature of 105° F. In cases of such severity, blood transfusion must immediately be given, for by this means one does not merely improve the oxygen-carrying capacity of the blood, but may, for reasons at present unknown, break the hæmolytic cycle. Blood transfusion during hæmolytic crises is fraught with great danger and should be advised only when the risks are considered to be less than the dangers of a fatal termination from anæmia. Particular care should be given to the selection of a suitable donor (see p. 1079) and the blood must be introduced extremely slowly. The use of the drip transfusion method, by means of which several hours can be taken to introduce 1 or 2 pints of blood, marks a real advance in the reduction of the dangers of transfusion in the hæmolytic anæmias. Before, and for twenty-four hours after transfusion, 1 drachm of bicarbonate of soda should be given every two hours, as by this means, should hæmolysis of the transfused cells occur, precipitation of hæmoglobin in the tubules of the kidneys, with the production of anuria, is prevented or is materially reduced.

In the majority of cases the results of blood transfusion are satisfactory as judged by improvement in the clinical condition of the patient, rise in the blood level and a reduction in the evidences of hæmolysis. A second or a third transfusion at intervals of a few days may be required to bring the patient to a suitable condition for the safe removal of the spleen. Unfortunately, blood transfusion is ineffective in a small proportion of cases, the gain in the blood level from the transfused corpuscles being more than counterbalanced by the excessive destruction of the patient's own cells. Should this be the case, emergency splenectomy followed by another transfusion, despite its obvious dangers, offers the only chance of saving life. A quarter of an hour before the splenic artery is tied, 0·5 c.c. of 1 : 1,000 solution of adrenalin should be injected subcutaneously, and after the artery has been tied an interval of three minutes should elapse before tying the splenic vein. As a result of these procedures we have found, from making blood counts at the operation, that a gain of half a million red blood cells per cubic millimetre may result from the passage of erythrocytes from the congested spleen into the general circulation. When splenectomy has been satisfactorily accomplished in hæmolytic anæmias the principal source of blood destruction has been removed, although the fundamental defect in erythropoiesis remains unchanged. Since the bone-marrow is extremely hyperplastic, a rapid rise in the blood level occurs after splenectomy, and a gain of $\frac{1}{2}$ to 1 million cells per week may be confidently expected. The rapid rate of regeneration begins to slow down as the count approaches 3·5 to 4 millions, and at this stage iron and whole liver are of value as hæmatinics. The general measures regarding rest, nursing, diet, etc., in a case of hæmolytic anæmia, are identical with those required in any case of anæmia of similar severity and will be found on pp. 466-469.

Secondary Hæmolytic Anæmias

The treatment of this group differs widely from that of primary hæmolytic anæmia and consists, not of splenectomy but of removing the causal condition together with attempts to relieve the anæmia by blood transfusions and hæmatinics. Accordingly, a suitable classification of the conditions producing a secondary hæmolytic anæmia facilitates an understanding of the problem.

Classification

Infections and Intoxications.—Sepsis, streptococcal and staphylococcal septicæmia, gas gangrene (clostridium welchii infection), malaria, oroya fever.

In sepsis and in streptococcal and staphylococcal septicæmia, it is now recognised that when severe anæmia develops it is, in most cases, due mainly to toxic inhibition of the bone-marrow, and that a direct hæmolytic action, resulting from the bacterial infection, plays only a minor rôle in the production of the anæmia. In gas gangrene, however, a severe anæmia may occur which is definitely due to increased hæmolysis.

Drugs and Industrial Hazards: *e.g.*, lead, phenylhydrazine, potassium chlorate, the arsenicals, arseniuretted hydrogen (particularly in submarine crews), dinitrobenzene (used in the manufacture of explosives), methyl chloride (used in domestic refrigerators), certain snake venoms. In view of the present wide use of sulphanilamide preparations it is important to note that several cases of acute hæmolytic anæmia due to this drug have been reported. This complication is so rare, however, that it should not be considered a contraindication to the employment of the drug in suitable cases.

Occasionally in Other Diseases: *e.g.*, Hodgkin's disease, syphilis, tuberculosis, reticulum-celled sarcoma, carcinomatosis, etc.

Treatment of Secondary Hæmolytic Anæmias.—Treatment is considered under three headings :—

Removal of the Cause.—In infections this may mean the evacuation of local collections of pus, the administration of antibacterial or antitoxic sera, or the use of special drugs such as prontosil, quinine, or atebrin. When the hæmolytic process is due to drugs, cessation of administration must be immediately ordered and, where possible, measures to increase elimination should be advised. If the poisoning is part of an industrial hazard, removal of the individual from the occupation is essential and the Inspector of Factories must be notified so that the hazard may be modified or eliminated by measures specially adopted to meet the circumstances. For details of the specific treatment of individual infections and poisoning with drugs and chemical substances, the reader is referred to the appropriate sections.

Blood Transfusion.—If the hæmolytic anæmia is chronic and mild to moderate in degree, blood transfusion is generally found to be unnecessary. On the other hand, if the infection is severe, the exposure to the poisonous substance is heavy, or idiosyncrasy is present to a marked degree, a rapid and severe hæmolysis may occur, which will precipitate the patient into a state dangerous to life. In such cases, blood transfusion should be immediately given, and repeated if necessary. At the same time, large doses of alkalis should be given orally, as described on p. 490, because of the danger of hæmoglobinuria and anuria.

Hæmatinics.—In all forms of Secondary Hæmolytic Anæmia, iron, whole liver, yeast and dieto-therapy as already described, should be ordered.

Paroxysmal Hæmoglobinuria

The several varieties of paroxysmal hæmoglobinuria are best considered separately.

Cold Hæmoglobinuria.—In this type, rapid hæmolysis leading to hæmoglobinæmia and hæmoglobinuria occurs when the patient enters a warm atmosphere after having been exposed to cold. In such cases there is an abnormal lysin in the patient's serum. Preliminary cooling is essential for the union of lysin and red cells and the action of complement occurs when the body is subsequently warmed. Syphilis is the principal ætiological factor.

Treatment.—Prophylaxis, which should include avoidance of all forms of chilling, *e.g.*, washing the hands in cold water or drinking cold fluids, is an important part of the treatment.

Thorough and prolonged antisyphilitic treatment should be instituted and it is claimed by some authorities that this is usually successful and may cause disappearance of the autohæmolysin from the blood.

During an attack the body should be kept warm, and alkalis (see p. 490) and plenty of fluids should be given by mouth. If anæmia results, iron therapy (see p. 472) should be instituted. These measures are equally applicable to all types of hæmoglobinuria.

Hæmoglobinuria on Exertion.—This type occurs in young males and is probably analogous to postural albuminuria.

Treatment.—Usually no treatment is necessary since it is a mild disease which disappears when adult life is reached.

Nocturnal Hæmoglobinuria (Marchiafava-Micheli syndrome). —Ætiology is obscure although recent work suggests that it may be due to an autohæmolysin, which acts when slight lowering of the hydrogen-ion concentration of the blood occurs consequent on reduced pulmonary ventilation during sleep.

Treatment.—There is a divergence of opinion regarding the value of splenectomy, and some authors believe that blood transfusions are contraindicated because they tend to aggravate the hæmolysis. Probably treatment should be symptomatic as outlined above. If, however, severe anæmia results, one may have to employ blood transfusions in an effort to tide the patient over a crisis.

The Acute Hæmolytic Anæmia of Lederer

Since the ætiology is obscure, this form of anæmia is considered separately. The presence of leucocytosis, high fever and anæmia, has led many authorities to suggest that the hæmolytic process is due to an unknown infective agent, a view with which we are unable to agree since identical manifestations are found in any severe hæmolytic anæmia.

Treatment.—The treatment to be adopted is blood transfusion, which should be repeated if recovery does not rapidly occur. Beneficial effects may result from blood transfusion in any type of hæmolytic anæmia, but the rapid and lasting improvement which occurs in Lederer's anæmia, appears to be much more marked than in other hæmolytic anæmias. Indeed, it is mainly this characteristic which has been responsible for the description of Lederer's anæmia as a separate entity.

The general measures described regarding nursing, diet, and hæmatinics on pp. 466-472, are equally necessary in this condition.

Sickle-cell Anæmia

Sickle-cell anæmia, which occurs in negroes, is a very rare disease in this country.

Treatment.—Treatment is purely symptomatic.

APLASTIC AND HYPOPLASTIC ANÆMIA

Aplastic and hypoplastic anæmias result from a loss, complete or partial, of the erythroblastic, leukoblastic, and thromboblastic cells in the bone-marrow.

In certain cases, especially when the disease occurs in an acute form in young persons, the cause is unknown and the name " idiopathic or primary aplastic anæmia " is used, while in others—the disease may occur at any age—it is usually more chronic and is frequently secondary to some recognizable infective or toxic element.

Accordingly, it is desirable to have a clear conception of the causes known to produce an aplastic or hypoplastic state of the bone-marrow.

Causes of Secondary Aplastic or Hypoplastic Anæmia

Drugs and Physical Agents.

(*a*) The heavy metals. Gold, mercury, silver, bismuth, arsenic, lead.

(*b*) The benzol compounds. Benzol, trinitrotoluol, dinitrophenol, etc.

(c) Poisonous gases. Carbon monoxide, methane, mustard gas.
(d) Radio-active materials and X-rays. Radium, radon gas, thorium.

Hazardous Occupations.
(a) Benzol. In the following occupations benzol is used for its solvent properties : rubber workers, dry cleaners, tanners, varnish and paint workers, gilders, feather workers, milliners, printers and tinners.
(b) Lead. Painters, plumbers, etc.
(c) Munition workers. Trinitrotoluol.
(d) Gases. Soldiers, sewer workers, mine workers.
(e) Radio-active substances. Luminous-paint workers, workers with X-rays and radium.

Infections and Intoxications.—While aplasia is rare, hypoplasia of the bone-marrow not infrequently results from infections and intoxications. Occasionally, particularly in children, inhibition of the bone-marrow may rapidly result if the infective process is extremely severe, as may occur in typhoid fever, diphtheria, miliary tuberculosis, malignant endocarditis, influenza and pneumonia. More usually, a hypoplasia occurs insidiously and as the result of long-continued chronic infections, such as chronic pulmonary tuberculosis, osteomyelitis, rheumatic fever, malaria and other chronic tropical diseases. The relationship of hypoplasia of the bone-marrow to focal sepsis (in teeth, tonsils, appendix and gall-bladder) is far from clear. In some cases, no improvement of the blood picture occurs until the focus of infection has been removed, while in others, this procedure effects no beneficial change, thus suggesting that the focus of infection was the result rather than the cause of the anæmia. Accordingly, wide experience and sound judgment are required in making a decision as to when and whether foci of infection should be removed, in view of the particular dangers associated with this procedure in the presence of aplasia and hypoplasia of the bone-marrow.

Terminal States of Certain Diseases.—The bone-marrow becomes progressively exhausted towards the termination of many diseases of long standing. This is particularly true of the blood diseases, such as pernicious anæmia, pellagra, leukæmia, erythræmia, myelophthisic anæmia and rarely in chronic post-hæmorrhagic anæmia, but it also may occur in diseases of the endocrine glands such as myxœdema or as the result of severe and long-continued deficiency of nutritional factors, both vitamin and mineral, essential to health.

Lastly, bone-marrow inhibition may be very severe in the terminal stages of hepatic and renal failure, especially in chronic kidney disease with nitrogen retention, in which a progressive anæmia develops which is little influenced by liver or iron.

A study of the list submitted above of factors which can cause aplasia or hypoplasia of the bone-marrow might lead one to suppose that severe types of anæmia from these causes are of frequent occurrence. In actual practice, however, aplastic anæmia, whether primary or secondary, is extremely rare, although mild degrees of bone-marrow inhibition are not uncommon. Since only a small minority of individuals exposed to risk actually suffer from aplastic anæmia, an unexplained idiosyncrasy of that individual's bone-marrow to toxic and infective processes is probably the most important factor in its production, as is also evidenced by the fact that the severity of the anæmia may bear no relationship to the dosage of the toxic agent. Since, however, excessive exposure of the bone-marrow to influences known to be toxic increases the liability to inhibition, it is a sound rule to remember which drugs have this peculiar selective action on the formative tissues and to be on the outlook for such changes by recognition of the early clinical symptoms (purpura, sepsis and exhaustion), and changes in the blood (anæmia, leucopœnia and thrombocytopenia).

Treatment. — In all cases of aplastic and hypoplastic anæmia, the patient should be confined to bed and the general measures suitable for the degree of anæmia, as outlined on p. 466, instituted.

Where the blood level is so low as to endanger life (see p. 478), blood transfusion should be undertaken at once and repeated at intervals as required in order to keep the blood at a level at which the patient is free from risk to life. At the same time iron, yeast and whole liver by mouth and liver extract by injection should be given. By these means symptomatic relief is given and time is secured to enable the physician to search for and if possible remove the causal factor.

A consideration of our classification of the ætiological factors as outlined above will indicate the investigations and treatment required in individual cases.

Where no obvious cause can be found other than the presence of focal sepsis in the teeth, tonsils, sinuses, etc., it is wise to try the effects of rest, diet, hæmatinics and blood transfusions before resorting to the removal of the focus in the hope that improvement in the local condition may occur concomitantly with the raising of the patient's resistance and the improvement in the anæmia resulting from the general measures described.

Should the patient continue to go downhill, however, it may be necessary to eradicate such foci despite the recognized danger of resultant sepsis, necrosis and hæmorrhage at the site of the operation. This danger is obviously connected with the failure in production of leucocytes and thrombocytes, whose function is to control infection and bleeding.

The minimal amount of operative interference should be undertaken at one time and should generally be preceded and followed by a blood transfusion and the administration of prontosil (1 to 2 tablets three times a day).

If a diagnosis of idiopathic aplastic anæmia is made because at the end of some weeks the patient's condition and the blood picture continue to deteriorate and the fullest investigation fails to produce any evidence of any causal condition, or if a cause is discovered which is found to be irremediable, blood transfusions should be discontinued and the patient allowed to die under the influence of morphia.

In cases of hypoplasia of the bone-marrow for which no cause can be found and in cases of aplasia or hypoplasia where a cause is discovered which can be removed, the patient should be kept alive with blood transfusions and the other remedies mentioned should be continued, if necessary for months or even years, in the hope that bone-marrow regeneration will occur in the interval. The method of drip transfusion is particularly valuable, because by this means a massive transfusion of 3,000 to 4,000 c.c. of blood may be given over forty-eight hours and may maintain a satisfactory blood level for several months thereafter.

SPLENIC ANÆMIA

Splenic anæmia is more a syndrome than a disease and in its commonest form may be described as a chronic condition characterized by splenomegaly and hypochromic anæmia, with leucopenia, no enlargement of lymphatic glands, a tendency to gastro-intestinal hæmorrhages, and, in the late stages, a liability to cirrhosis of the liver.

Before the diagnosis of splenic anæmia (Banti's disease) is

accepted the following conditions, in which anæmia and splenomegaly occur, must be eliminated :—

1. Acute and chronic infectious diseases with splenomegaly, *e.g.*, infective endocarditis, malaria, schistosomiasis and syphilis.
2. Pernicious anæmia and the leukæmias (see pp. 480, 524).
3. The hæmolytic anæmias (see pp. 488-493).
4. Idiopathic thrombocytopenic purpura (see p. 508).
5. Chronic nutritional hypochromic anæmia (see p. 464).

When this is done a residue of cases is left, in some of which the splenomegaly has obviously occurred secondary to cirrhosis of the liver, whereas, in others, enlargement develops concomitantly or apparently prior to the disease of the liver. The name " Splenic Anæmia " should be confined to this latter group, which forms the subject of this section.

Treatment.—Treatment will be considered under two headings :—

Splenectomy—indications for and against.
Symptomatic treatment.
(*a*) Diet and iron.
(*b*) Blood transfusion.

Splenectomy.—Splenectomy is definitely contraindicated when the splenomegaly is secondary to cirrhosis of the liver and the treatment of this group is considered in its appropriate section (see p. 610).

Since the rationale of splenectomy as a form of specific treatment in splenic anæmia depends mainly on the assumption that the spleen is the primary locus of the causal factor, it is necessary to consider this hypothesis further.

The principal evidence advanced by supporters of this hypothesis is the occurrence of splenomegaly for a considerable time before the development of cirrhosis of the liver, as judged by the presence of the accepted clinical manifestations of this condition, or even macroscopic signs at operation.

The reasons for not accepting this hypothesis may be summarized as follows :—

1. The histological picture of the spleen is that of long-standing passive congestion and is identical with the pathological features found in the spleen in cases of primary cirrhosis of the liver, and hence is in keeping with the hypothesis that the splenic changes are secondary to portal obstruction.

2. When histological examination of the liver has been undertaken in cases of splenic anæmia, evidence of some degree of cirrhosis has almost invariably been found.
3. Even when the macroscopic appearance of the liver at operation appears to be normal, gross dilatation of the splenic veins is nearly always present. This is strong presumptive evidence of portal obstruction.
4. Cirrhosis of the liver may progress and hæmorrhages from the stomach and œsophagus recur, or even start for the first time subsequent to removal of the spleen.

Accordingly, we are unable to agree that there is substantial evidence in favour of the disease starting primarily in the spleen.

There is no evidence that the anæmia in splenic anæmia is due to blood destruction or that the spleen has some toxic or inhibiting effect on blood formation. Hence the beneficial effects claimed for splenectomy must rest only on anatomical and mechanical foundations. Splenectomy or ligature of the splenic artery may be of value in reducing portal congestion, thus lessening the chance of hæmorrhage from the dilated œsophageal veins. Unfortunately, statistics show that at least 50 per cent. of patients who had hæmorrhages before operation continue to have them subsequently, and cirrhosis of the liver may progress.

The principal reason generally advanced for advising splenectomy is the claim that improvement in the blood condition and prolongation of life result from the operation.

Before this claim can be substantiated it would be necessary to compare a series of cases subjected to operation with a series adequately treated by medical measures including efficient iron therapy, and then followed up for many years. Unfortunately, such information is not available. The fact that individual cases have survived operation for periods of five, ten or twenty years may be of little significance, since splenic anæmia is recognized to be a very slowly progressing disease and many physicians have had patients under their charge who have survived for ten years or longer without any surgical treatment.

Lastly, because reduction of portal congestion and ascites sometimes occurs after splenectomy, it does not necessarily follow that this is due to removal of the spleen, since it may result from formation of a collateral circulation in the post-operative adhesions which we can testify from personal experience may become widely developed. If this is the object desired it is more simply and more safely achieved by a Talma-Morrison operation than by splenectomy.

Since the beneficial effects of splenectomy are, to say the least, questionable, and since the operative mortality rate is high, varying from 5 to 10 per cent. in the early to 30 per cent. in the late stages of the disease, our own feeling is that splenectomy should never be advised in splenic anæmia except in the very rare case when the patient is suffering serious inconvenience because of the splenic tumour, or has repeated attacks of severe pain from infarction or perisplenitis. While we must admit that medical opinion is sharply divided on the question of splenectomy, we are satisfied, from personal experience and a study of the literature, that the operation is certainly of little value once definite signs of liver cirrhosis have appeared and particularly if hæmatemesis has occurred and œsophageal varices can be demonstrated by X-rays. However, if our views are not accepted and a decision to perform splenectomy is made, it is essential that prior to operation the patient's blood should be brought to a safe level (hæmoglobin, 70 to 80 per cent.) by iron and repeated blood transfusions if necessary, and a suitable donor held in readiness to combat the severe hæmorrhages which are so liable to occur during the operation.

Where technical difficulties discovered during the operation make splenectomy a highly dangerous procedure, ligation of the splenic artery has been recommended. We have no experience of this method, but we understand that those who believe in the beneficial effects of splenectomy consider that ligation of the splenic artery is not an entirely satisfactory substitute. Although the operative risk is less, very severe reactions may result.

Another operative procedure, which we have tried in two advanced cases with repeated hæmatemeses, is ligation of the coronary vein of the stomach, but in neither case was a permanent beneficial effect produced.

In the few cases reported in the literature in which splenectomy was performed in individuals with thrombosis of the splenic vein the results appear to have been satisfactory. Unfortunately, we know no means by which the splenomegaly associated with thrombosis of the splenic vein can be differentiated from that of classical Banti's disease. Even hæmatemesis, a symptom so characteristic of portal obstruction, has been reported to occur in cases of thrombosis of the splenic vein.

Irradiation of the spleen is of little value in splenic anæmia.

Symptomatic Treatment.—The general treatment of the anæmia in splenic anæmia is on the lines indicated on pp. 466-467. When a large hæmatemesis occurs, the patient is suffering from acute post-hæmorrhagic anæmia, for the treatment of which see pp. 476-479. In other cases a chronic hypochromic anæmia results from continuous occult bleeding from the gastric and œsophageal varices, and the measures outlined on pp. 469-473 will be found to be suitable.

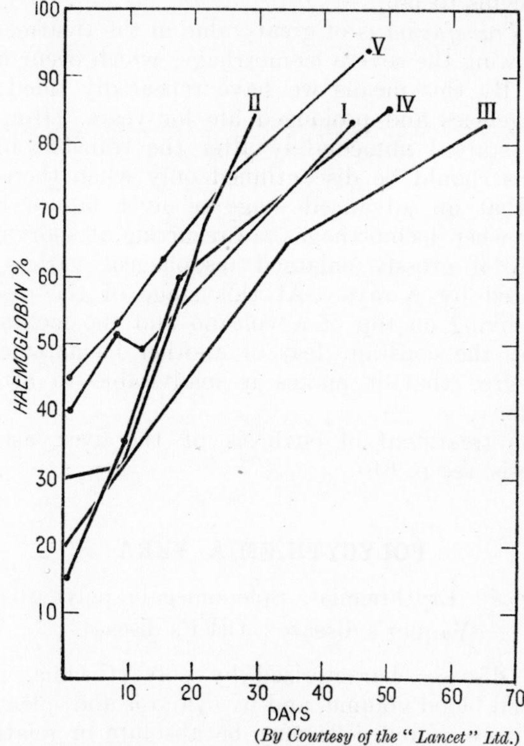

(*By Courtesy of the "Lancet" Ltd.*)

Graph illustrating the hæmoglobin percentage increase in five cases of splenic anæmia treated with iron.

A diet should be prescribed rich in the food factors valuable for blood formation, in particular, liver, kidney and butcher meat. Indigestible articles of food which are liable to injure mechanically the gastric and œsophageal varices should be excluded from the diet or their irritating components removed. The following articles should be excluded—highly seasoned and indigestible foods, condiments and pickles, the skins and pips of fruits, nuts, etc., and coarse vegetables and fruits should be passed through a sieve and served as purees or fools.

Iron.—A study of the best-known textbooks of medicine suggests that iron is of little or no value in the treatment of splenic anæmia. Our experience of the excellent results which may frequently be obtained leads us to protest against this view. The Graph on p. 501 illustrates the rapid rise in the blood level which may be expected if iron is given in the preparations and doses stated on p. 472. It is only in the late stages of the disease, when hepatic failure is approaching, that iron therapy begins to fail.

Blood Transfusion is of great value in the treatment of the shock following the severe hæmorrhages which occur in splenic anæmia. By this means we have repeatedly tided patients over emergencies and prolonged life for years. Iron therapy should be started immediately after the transfusion. Blood transfusions should be discontinued only when there is clear evidence that an advanced stage of liver failure has been reached or when hæmorrhages are recurring at short intervals, particularly if grossly enlarged œsophageal varices can be demonstrated by X-rays. At this stage of the disease the patient is living on top of a volcano and the mental misery entailed by the constant fear of another hæmatemesis is of such a degree that it makes it inadvisable to attempt to prolong life.

For the treatment of cirrhosis of the liver, ascites and hæmatemesis, see p. 610.

POLYCYTHÆMIA VERA

Synonyms : Erythræmia ; Splenomegalic polycythæmia ; Vaquez's disease ; Osler's disease.

A rare disease characterized by polycythæmia, increased viscosity and blood volume, and by cyanosis and splenomegaly.

An increase of red cells may be absolute or relative. An example of the latter is the polycythæmia secondary to diminution of the fluid part of the blood, consequent on severe sweating, vomiting, or diarrhœa. Another example is the high red cell count found in individuals with chilblains and Raynaud's disease when blood is taken from an area of local congestion. Capillary stasis causes concentration of the blood in the affected areas. An absolute increase of red cells results from one of two causes : (1) a primary disease of the erythroblastic tissues, analogous to the hyperplasia of the leucoblastic tissues in leukæmia—hence the name "erythræmia"; and (2) a compensatory hyperplasia of the erythron secondary to factors which lead to incomplete oxygenation of the blood. The term "erythrocytosis" should be confined to this type of polycythæmia. The conditions predisposing to erythrocytosis are chronic cardiac and pulmonary disease, either congenital or acquired, living at high altitudes and the toxic effects of various poisons, *e.g.*, carbon monoxide, phosphorus, aniline dyes, etc. A diagnosis of polycythæmia vera should never be made till the more common conditions which cause erythrocytosis have been excluded.

Treatment.—Since the clinical manifestations of polycythæmia vera are directly attributable to increased blood volume and increased blood viscosity, treatment must be directed to the relief of these features by reducing the number of red blood cells in the circulation. For this purpose many different methods have been employed, most of which have proved ineffective. Thus splenectomy is contraindicated. Benzol should not be used because of its excessively toxic and depressant effect on the bone-marrow. Arsenic in large doses (see p. 528) may be of some value and may be tried, should the forms of treatment recommended below fail. The claims regarding the value of splenic extract therapy have not been confirmed. An entirely different type of treatment has been recently suggested, based on the hypothesis that the hyperplasia of the bone-marrow in polycythæmia vera is caused by an excessive production of a hæmopoietic hormone in the stomach, the condition being the antithesis of pernicious anæmia, in which there is a failure in the production of the anti-anæmic factor. Accordingly a diet has been recommended in which articles of food rich in the extrinsic factor of Castle or in the preformed anti-anæmic factor are reduced to the lowest possible quantities. Since polycythæmia vera is a chronic disease lasting for years, such a diet is unphysiological and impracticable. However, a moderate reduction in animal protein and the forbiddance of foods rich in purins (liver, kidney, sweetbread, etc.) are to be recommended in view of the frequency with which a raised blood pressure and its sequels occur in polycythæmia.

The physician has the choice of three main methods of treatment: (1) venesection; (2) irradiation with X-rays or radium; and (3) phenylhydrazine or its derivative acetylphenylhydrazine. A combination of these methods may be used.

Venesection.—To be of any value a large quantity of blood must be withdrawn, since the blood volume is often increased two or three fold. Little relief is likely to follow the withdrawal of less than 40 oz. There can be no doubt that venesection gives more rapid relief from subjective symptoms than any other form of treatment. Its effect is, however, transitory, and it should not be used as the sole method of treatment, both for this reason and because it tends to stimulate the already hyperplastic marrow to increased activity. In an acute exacerbation of subjective symptoms, particularly if they suggest a liability to intracranial hæmorrhage or thrombosis, it is the method of choice.

Technique.—Owing to the greatly increased viscosity of the blood, venesection is unlikely to be successfully accomplished unless certain modifications of the usual methods are employed.

1. A thick-bore French's needle should be used and the rubber connection attached to this and leading to the receptacle for the blood should be as short as is consistent with convenience and thoroughly washed with sodium-citrate solution before use.

2. When the vein has been selected, the needle should be inserted in the direction opposite to that of the blood stream.

3. A vacuum should be maintained in the blood receptacle to hasten the rate of blood flow through the tubing, and so prevent clotting.

Irradiation.—The idea of applying "stimulating" doses of X-rays to the spleen with a view to increasing the activity of the reticulo-endothelial system has now been abandoned in favour of depressant doses applied to the long bones, sternum and ribs. Such treatment to be successful has to be carried out carefully and controlled by repeated blood counts. If the dosage is too small a stimulating effect on the already hyperplastic marrow may be produced, and if too large, aplastic anæmia may result. Irradiation should not be applied to the head, or, in young people, to the pelvic bones, so that alopecia and damage to the gonads respectively may be avoided. Pack and Craver suggest three to six exposures a week until all the long bones have been irradiated. The course may be repeated at intervals of three to six months, depending on the response of the patient. They claim that the general health is improved and life prolonged. It is probable that cases with a high platelet count are particularly suitable for irradiation therapy rather than for phenylhydrazine treatment, since in such cases the tendency to thrombosis, already present, will be increased by treatment with the drug.

Phenylhydrazine Hydrochloride.—The effects of this drug have been carefully investigated by Giffin and Allen, who claim that in thirteen out of fifteen cases fairly good, good or excellent results were obtained. The following features are held to contraindicate treatment with phenylhydrazine: (1) age over sixty; (2) advanced arteriosclerosis; (3) bedridden cases; (4) cases with a history of thrombosis; (5) cases with definite disease of the liver or kidneys. It is essential that the drug should be freshly prepared. In the initial period of treatment, patients should be in hospital so that proper supervision may be carried out, but they should be ambulatory and may, in some cases, receive a course of massage in order to lessen the susceptibility to thrombosis. Dosage: 0·1 gm. in capsule two or three times a day until 3 to 4 gm. are given, or until definite clinical evidence of active hæmolysis (jaundice) occurs, if the amount necessary is less than this. The initial treatment usually lasts from ten to fourteen days. The drug should then be stopped as the effect is cumulative and lasts for seven to ten days after its withdrawal. In cases which prove resistant, one or more courses of treatment with the drug (0·1 gm. b.i.d., for five days) may be given at intervals of ten days. The maintenance treatment should be commenced within a few weeks of the initial course. The amount necessary for maintenance of a blood count at more or less normal levels has to be found by trial and error in each individual case; a dose of from 0·1 to 0·3 gm. on one day of each week is the average amount necessary. Long-continued treatment of this kind may occasionally be followed by a complete remission of the polycythæmic process for long periods. Thrombosis appears to be the main danger, while gastro-intestinal disturbances may cause some difficulty in administering the drug.

Acetylphenylhydrazine.—This has been recommended by Stone, Harris and Bodansky, and by Rosenthal. It is preferred to phenylhydrazine on the following grounds: it is practically as effective, it is less toxic and the dosage is more readily controlled. Dosage: 0·1 gm. once daily in a gelatin capsule, for one or more courses of seven to ten days, during which the red cell count should be carefully watched. For maintenance purposes the dose is approximately 0·1 gm. at intervals of five to seven days. Rosenthal found large amounts necessary in cases with initially high counts (about 10,000,000), *e.g.*, 0·1 gm. daily for three to five weeks.

For an emergency, venesection should be employed. Irradiation appears to be of more general application than treatment with phenylhydrazine, since many cases are not suitable for treatment with the drug. On the other hand, published reports appear to indicate that it is easier to keep the blood level approximately normal for long periods with phenylhydrazine. A combination of phenylhydrazine and irradiation is recommended by Rosenthal for the leukæmoid group of cases.

Symptomatic Treatment.—A patient with polycythæmia may complain of a variety of symptoms which are principally referable to the nervous, gastro-intestinal and cardiovascular systems. Since they are all due to the high blood volume and increased viscosity of the blood, the measures outlined above to correct these conditions are themselves the best form of symptomatic treatment. The administration of sedative drugs to control the insomnia, giddiness and psychic disorders which are so frequently present may, however, be needed (aspirin, phenacetin, bromides, chloral and the barbiturates). For dyspepsia, a light easily digested diet together with alkalis is advised. Constipation should be treated as outlined on p. 467. Purging with salines should be avoided as this will still further concentrate the blood.

The occurrence of hæmorrhage indicates that nature is attempting to relieve the plethora and no treatment should be undertaken to stop it unless excessive quantities of blood are lost. The liability to thrombosis is best reduced by cutting down the intake of foods rich in calcium, such as milk, and by prescribing regular exercise to maintain an active circulation. Some authorities recommend the administration of potassium citrate (30 to 60 gr. q.i.d.), particularly during the time when phenylhydrazine is being administered, because of the increased liability to thrombosis.

ENTEROGENOUS CYANOSIS

Synonyms : Methæmoglobinæmia ; Sulphæmoglobinæmia.

A disease characterized by chronic cyanosis due to the presence of methæmoglobin, or sulphæmoglobin, in the circulating blood.

Treatment.—*Prophylaxis.*—In the great majority of cases the condition is caused by the ingestion of drugs, *e.g.*, phenacetin, acetanilide, nitrates, sulphonal, potassium chlorate and trional, and recently much attention has been drawn to its frequent occurrence during the administration of the sulphanilamide group. The outstanding characteristic of the condition is the presence of cyanosis without accompanying cardiac or pulmonary lesions, and, usually, without respiratory distress. Methæmoglobinæmia is due to a direct chemical action of the of the drugs mentioned on the hæmoglobin of the circulating erythrocytes, and it rapidly disappears after removal of the causative agent. Sulphæmoglobinæmia, which is much more common and persists for several weeks after cessation of the drug, is caused by a sensitization of the red cells which results in a combination between their contained hæmoglobin and hydrogen sulphide absorbed from the intestine. The differentiation between the two conditions is made by spectroscopic examination of the blood. The occurrence of sulphæmoglobinæmia may be prevented in a large proportion of cases by correcting constipation before prescribing any of the drugs mentioned. During their administration, foods with a high sulphur content, especially eggs, should be avoided, and regular bowel evacuations should be produced by liquid paraffin and occasional enemas rather than by laxatives or purgatives, particularly magnesium sulphate, which render the contents of the colon fluid and so increase the formation of hydrogen sulphide.

Curative Treatment.—The alarming appearance of the patient is in striking contrast to the absence of any distress and, usually, no treatment is required other than withdrawal of the causative drug.

In severe cases of methæmoglobinæmia oxygen inhalation (see p. 1098) is indicated, since this procedure very rapidly restores the hæmoglobin to its original state.

Sulphæmoglobinæmia may produce respiratory embarrassment in patients who were severely anæmic before the onset of the condition, and in whom, therefore, the further reduction of hæmoglobin capable of combining with oxygen results in the symptoms of anoxæmia. In such cases blood transfusions should be given at intervals to relieve respiratory distress until reduction of the sulphæmoglobinæmia and increase in the blood level following appropriate anti-anæmia therapy produce a hæmoglobin level sufficient for the needs of the body.

THE PURPURAS

Purpura is a symptom rather than a disease, but the term is used to describe a condition in which extravascular hæmorrhage occurs in the skin and subcutaneous tissues, from the mucous membranes and rarely in serous cavities.

CLASSIFICATION

The purpuras are best divided into two groups :—

- *Primary* or Idiopathic—in which no cause can be found.
- *Secondary* or Symptomatic—where the symptom-complex is due to a recognizable cause.

Both primary and secondary purpuras may be thrombocytopenic or non-thrombocytopenic. Since a search for a cause must be undertaken in every case, the simple classification given below will be found to be of value in helping the practitioner to discover the ætiological factor.

Primary.

(*a*) Idiopathic thrombocytopenic purpura.

(*b*) The anaphylactoid purpuras of Schönlein and Henoch.

Secondary : due to :—

(*a*) *Infections* (usually severe in degree and particularly if a septicæmia is present) with streptococcus hæmolyticus and viridans, bacillus typhosus, diphtheriæ, tuberculosis (especially in miliary forms) and the viruses of typhus fever, measles, smallpox, etc.

(*b*) *Drug Intoxications*, *e.g.*, benzol, organic arsenicals, quinine, aniline dyes, ergot, sedormid, gold, bismuth, mercury, iodides (for industrial hazards connected with these, see p. 495).

(*c*) *Chronic Diseases* of kidneys and liver, malignant disease and rarely, in the terminal stage, of chronic cardiovascular disease.

(*d*) *Exposure to X-rays* or radio-active substances.

(*e*) *The Terminal States of Blood Diseases*—aplastic anæmia, pernicious anæmia, the leukæmias, hæmolytic anæmia, splenic anæmia, Gaucher's disease.

(*f*) *Primary and Secondary Malignant Disease* of bones and bone-marrow, and osteosclerosis.

(*g*) *Avitaminosis*—scurvy.

What has been said on p. 496 regarding the importance of individual idiosyncrasy to toxic agents in the ætiology of secondary aplastic anæmia is equally applicable to the purpuras.

Treatment.—In every case of purpura a search for a possible cause should be made and measures instituted for its removal or neutralization where possible. A study of the list of causal conditions given above will suggest the type of treatment indicated in individual cases. A full blood examination is essential to eliminate the primary blood diseases in which purpura occurs, to assess the degree of anæmia present and to establish whether the purpura is of the thrombocytopenic or non-thrombocytopenic variety.

Splenectomy is of particular value in the control of bleeding in idiopathic thrombocytopenic purpura and should generally not be advised in the group of purpuras secondary to various toxic or infective agents, in which capillary damage is usually the principal defect. In fact, many authorities hold that the operation is contraindicated in the presence of a normal platelet count, because of the real danger of subsequent venous thrombosis.

The treatment prescribed should be based mainly on the severity of the hæmorrhagic state and the cases can generally be classified into three groups :—

1. Where the escape of blood into the skin or from the mucous membranes is small in extent and does not by itself produce incapacity. Thus, a few purpuric spots not infrequently appear during the course of the exanthemata or in children without any obvious cause. This condition is referred to in many textbooks as purpura simplex. On the other hand, a mild degree of purpura may appear in the late stage of very serious diseases such as chronic nephritis, malignant disease and the leukæmias. In both types of case no particular treatment for the purpura itself is required.

2. Where the purpura is sufficiently severe to lead to anæmia and general systemic disturbance. In this group, hæmorrhages from the mucous membranes, particularly nose, gums, alimentary tract and uterus, are of importance.

Treatment is considered under the headings of local and general measures.

Local Measures.—Since hæmorrhagic and septic lesions of the nose and mouth are of frequent occurrence in a variety of diseases, and since the local treatment required is equally applicable to all, this subject will be dealt with in detail in this section and omitted from the sections devoted to the leukæmias, hæmophilia and aplastic anæmia.

The local measures to be described are often successful in the control of hæmorrhage in purpura and hæmophilia during minor or moderate exacerbations of the hæmorrhagic tendency. When bleeding is severe in the above diseases and in the late stages of the leukæmias and aplastic anæmia, local treatment is unlikely to succeed by itself, but it is of definite value in helping to control hæmorrhage, although blood transfusion must also be employed.

Hæmorrhagic lesions and septic processes frequently coexist, but it is convenient to consider the treatment of these two conditions separately.

Hæmorrhagic Lesions

Bleeding from the Gums.—The most effective preparation for the local control of hæmorrhage is Russell's viper venom, which is an extremely powerful coagulant having the additional advantages that it does not injure the tissues and that it acts efficiently even in very low dilutions. It is supplied under the name of stypven, by Messrs Burroughs, Wellcome & Co. Since the efficacy of solutions of the venom decreases rapidly, the venom in dry form and sterile distilled water are supplied in separate ampoules and the solution is prepared by dissolving the powder in the distilled water immediately before use. The site of bleeding should be thoroughly cleaned and all friable clots removed. A gauze dressing soaked in the venom solution is then applied firmly but without undue pressure. Different contrivances according to the site of the bleeding area may be necessary to keep the dressing in position; for example, a well-fitting dental plate may solve this problem admirably and so avoid the repeated application of fresh dressings which is necessary if they are easily displaced by movements of the tongue.

According to Macfarlane, the dressing is more effective if the solution is first heated to 50° C., and, if the bleeding is very intractable, an equal mixture of the venom solution and 1 : 1,000 solution of adrenalin may be tried as a last resort. If stypven is not available, gauze soaked in normal fresh human blood should be applied to the site after it has been properly cleaned. It is important to bear in mind that excessive pressure to the site of hæmorrhage may control the bleeding temporarily, but may cause such devitalisation of the tissues that necrosis and sloughing occur, with hæmorrhage from a larger area than the initial one.

The effects produced by the measures described above are much superior to those obtained by the use of acids, iron salts, collodion, gelatin, the various commercial hæmostatic sera and tissue extracts, and cauterization of the bleeding area by direct heat or diathermy.

Bleeding from Tooth Sockets.—A frequent source of intractable hæmorrhage, particularly in hæmophilics, is the socket left after the extraction of a tooth. The wound should be thoroughly cleaned and a gauze plug soaked in stypven solution inserted. If there is no infection, this treatment is likely to be rapidly successful. Where gross infection of the socket coexists it is obviously undesirable to close the wound completely, and one should be satisfied with light plugging which will allow drainage. In such cases a certain amount of hæmorrhage is unavoidable. When a marked hæmorrhagic tendency is present it is seldom advisable to attempt to reduce hæmorrhage from a tooth socket by the insertion of sutures, since these "cut out" frequently and defeat their purpose by increasing the bleeding area.

Bleeding from the Nose.—Before an attempt is made to stop persistent hæmorrhage from the nose the nasal cavities should first be cleared of all loose blood clots. For this purpose the patient should sniff, through each nostril in turn, salt solution (1 drachm to the pint) at a temperature of approximately 112° F. He should then try to expel any remaining clots by blowing through the nose with the mouth closed while first one side of the nose and then the other is occluded by placing the tip of the thumb against the nostril. If this method does not succeed it may be necessary to remove tough clots by seizing them with forceps or by dislodging them with a small gauze mop held in forceps. The nasal cavities should then be examined in order to determine as accurately as possible the source of the bleeding.

Very frequently Little's or Kieselbach's area on the anterior part of the nasal septum is the site of the hæmorrhage. In such cases it is easily accessible, and the most effective method of treatment is to insert into the nostril a gauze pack, soaked in stypven solution and of sufficient size to ensure firm contact with the bleeding area. If this procedure is not effective the electro-cautery should be applied to the bleeding point.

If the bleeding occurs diffusely from the nasal mucous membrane, anterior packing should first be tried. After all loose clots have been removed, the nasal cavity on both sides is sprayed with 2 per cent. decicain (Bayer Products Ltd.), or a mixture of equal parts of 10 per cent. cocaine and 1 : 1,000 adrenalin solution. The nasal cavities are then packed with strips of ribbon gauze ($\frac{1}{2}$ in. width) soaked in Stypven solution. For this procedure an angular forceps is used, and the packing should commence at the posterior part of the floor of the nose and proceed gradually forwards and upwards until the cavity is filled. At least 1 yd. of gauze is needed to pack each cavity efficiently.

If bleeding continues after these packs have been in position for twelve hours it is probable that hæmorrhage is occurring from the posterior nares, or the upper part of the nasopharynx, or both. In these circumstances the packs should be removed and a combination of post-nasal and anterior packing tried.

After all loose blood clots have been removed the nasal cavities, nasopharynx and soft palate should be anæsthetized by spraying with the solution already mentioned. The tip of a soft rubber catheter (size 8), in which a hole has been bored opposite the eye, is then passed along the floor of the nasal cavity, choosing that side which is of greater capacity or in which the bleeding has been less marked. The catheter is introduced until contact of the tip with the posterior wall of the nasopharynx deflects it downwards and it is seen through the mouth between the faucial pillars. The tip is then seized with suitable forceps (*e.g.*, Luc's) and is pulled for a short distance through the mouth. A roll of gauze about 2 in. in length and 1 in. in diameter, or a bundle of gauze mops (two to three for a child and three to four for an adult) soaked in stypven solution is suspended from the tip of the catheter by thin tape, one end of the tape being passed through the eye and the hole opposite it and tied firmly to the other end. The length of tape between the tip of the catheter and the roll of gauze should be about 1 ft. The end of the catheter lying outside the nose is then gently pulled and, after the pack has passed over the soft palate, it is gradually insinuated into the post-nasal space. By manipulation of the pack through the mouth and by traction on the tape which has now been withdrawn through the nostril, the pack is firmly apposed to the posterior nares. Slight traction is maintained on the tape while that side of the nasal cavity through which it passes is packed with strips of ribbon gauze soaked in stypven solution in the manner already described. The other side is then packed, the tape is cut from the catheter and the two ends are tied tightly over a thin roll of gauze applied to the anterior nares, care being taken that the traction on the tape is sufficient to keep the post-nasal pack firmly in position against the posterior nares.

Nasal and post-nasal packs should not be left *in situ* for more than twenty-four hours without being changed, owing to the danger of pressure necrosis and infection, particularly of the middle ear via the Eustachian tube. This is an important point which must on no account be disregarded.

Oral Sepsis.—Oral sepsis frequently complicates hæmorrhagic lesions of the mouth, especially in the leukæmias. A useful mouth wash for removing sloughs and clearing up oral infection is—

Citric acid	gr. xl
Water	℥i

diluted one part in seven with water before use. Since

spirochætes are almost invariably present in these lesions, good results often follow application of N.A.B. paint (0·9 gm. N.A.B., 9 c.c. glycerin and 9 c.c. water) to the affected areas, or the administration of 0·3 gm. N.A.B. intravenously.

Conclusion.—Although the measures described above are of great value in producing temporary arrest of hæmorrhage and in preventing the development of gross sepsis, it must be clearly realized that the lesions are merely local manifestations of general disease and therefore adequate treatment must embrace control of the causal condition as described in the appropriate sections.

General Measures, by Drugs and Other Procedures.—The multiplicity of remedies recommended for the treatment of purpura is itself an indication that none of them can be held to have consistently a specific action in the control of hæmorrhage.

Adrenalin and Calcium.—Where capillary permeability rather than thrombocytopenia appears to be the particular defect, or where allergy is suggested by clinical examination, *i.e.*, the coexistence with purpura of urticaria, œdema, or arthritis, adrenalin (subcutaneously in 5 to 10 minim doses three times a day) and calcium (calcium lactate 30 gr. four times a day by mouth and/or calcium gluconate 10 c.c. intramuscularly once a day) are indicated.

Vitamin C.—Where a history of dietary deficiency is obtained, with particular reference to fresh fruits and vegetables, and in patients suffering from chronic diseases and infective states both chronic and acute, the administration of vitamin C is worthy of trial, since this vitamin plays a rôle in the maintenance of the integrity of capillary endothelium. For special methods of quantitative estimation of vitamin C deficiency, see Scurvy, p. 410. The quickest way to repair the vitamin C deficiency is by the parenteral administration (subcutaneously, intramuscularly or intravenously) of ascorbic acid. A suitable preparation for this purpose is redoxon forte ampoules (Roche Products Limited), 1 to 2 ampoules being given daily for a week. At the same time, oral treatment should be commenced by ordering 1 to 2 tablets of redoxon, two to three times daily, or the juice of six oranges daily. A failure to obtain results within a week would suggest that the capillary permeability is not conditioned by vitamin C deficiency.

Recent research by Szent-Györgyi and others indicates that the factor concerned with capillary permeability is not vitamin C but another substance called vitamin P, which is found with ascorbic acid in paprika, hips and lemon juice. This substance has been manufactured in the pure state as citrin or hesperidin, a crystalline compound of the flavone group. Although much work still requires to be done before the scope of this new therapeutic agent is clearly defined, there is little doubt that it is of great value in the treatment of those purpuric states in which the essential lesson is an increase in capillary permeability, *e.g.*, Henoch's and Schönlein's purpura and conditions of general vitamin deficiency. Citrin (hesperidin Glaxo) is given by intravenous or intramuscular injection in a daily dose of 50 mg. or orally in doses of 1 gm. daily.

Commercial Liver Extracts have been recommended by various workers. Good results have been claimed for the administration of campolon, 2 to 4 c.c. intramuscularly once daily. In our experience this is of little value except when a megalocytic anæmia is present as well.

Commercial Hæmostatic Preparations.—There are many preparations on the market which are claimed by the manufacturers to have beneficial effects in the control of bleeding. Such claims are invariably backed by testimonials from practitioners who fail to realise that the value of hæmostatic preparations is difficult to assess because spontaneous cessation of hæmorrhage frequently occurs in the secondary forms of purpura. Of such preparations the best known are hæmoplastin and coagulin ciba.

In general our experience suggests that the results obtained from commercial hæmostatic preparations are unsatisfactory.

Snake Venom may be used as a local application by the methods described above or for a general effect on capillary permeability, in which case the moccasin snake venom preparation as originally described by Peck and Rosenthal should be employed. These workers report that a considerable proportion of cases of purpura hæmorrhagica derive symptomatic benefit from this form of treatment. Moccasin snake venom is supplied by Lederle Laboratories Inc., and the initial dose should be 0·1 c.c. of the solution subcutaneously. The injections are given at three-day intervals and the dose is gradually increased up to a maximum dose of 1 c.c. Not infrequently a severe local reaction occurs at the site of injection after the third or fourth dose, due to sensitization of the tissues to the venom or to the protein content of the solution. When this occurs, the patient must be desensitized by a number of small doses (0·1 c.c.) before the larger quantities can be injected. We have had insufficient experience of this type of treatment in the more chronic forms of purpura with capillary damage to express an opinion regarding its value, and a study of the literature shows divergence of opinion. In three cases of idiopathic thrombocytopenic purpura which were fully treated by us with moccasin snake venom no beneficial results accrued.

X-rays to the Spleen.—Mettier and Stone and Hippe and Kochmann claim excellent symptomatic results with concomitant increase in the platelets in cases of idiopathic thrombocytopenic purpura treated by repeated applications of X-rays to the splenic area. We have no experience of this method in the chronic non-thrombocytopenic forms of purpura. In three of our cases of severe thrombocytopenic purpura, however, who received treatment in exact accordance with the methods of the above workers, no beneficial effects were obtained.

Foreign Protein Therapy.—For many years the injection of foreign protein intramuscularly has been held to be of value in the control of purpura. The beneficial effects claimed are presumed to be derived from an alteration in capillary permeability, secondary to the sensitization produced. For this purpose, horse serum, either normal or antitoxic, *e.g.*, diphtheria antitoxin serum, may be employed; 5 to 10 c.c. may be given intramuscularly for several consecutive days. The danger of anaphylaxis must be considered before adopting this method of treatment, and an inquiry should be made into a history of asthma, eczema, hay-fever, etc. If any suspicion exists that a tendency to allergy is present it is advisable to give a test dose of serum (0·1 c.c.) intracutaneously, and one hour later 1 c.c. subcutaneously. If no untoward reactions either local or general occur, the intramuscular injection of 5 to 10 c.c. may safely be given. Probably equally good results, without the danger of anaphylaxis, are obtained if human serum or whole blood is used. The simplest procedure is to aspirate into a sterile syringe, which has been perfused with sterile normal citrate solution, 10 c.c. of blood from the vein of a relative or friend and immediately inject the blood deeply into the patient's gluteal muscles. This may be repeated on several occasions.

Treatment with foreign protein is most likely to be of value in bleeding states associated with prolongation of the coagulation time. Since the coagulation time is normal in purpura, we are not surprised that our experience has shown that this form of treatment has not been successful in the severer types of purpura. Nevertheless the intramuscular injection of 10 c.c. of whole blood is a simple procedure attended by no risk and is worthy of trial.

From what has been said it must be apparent that none of the methods of treatment discussed above can be held to have been proved wholly satisfactory. It is probable that the beneficial effects obtained in many cases can be explained on the basis of a spontaneous remission of the hæmorrhagic state rather than as a direct result of the treatment. Nevertheless, where life is not in danger, one or a combination of the methods described should be advised, together with the local and general measures outlined above. We would, however, earnestly offer this advice, namely, that should the hæmorrhagic state not be controlled within a few days and a progressive deterioration of the patient's health occur, the measures indicated under Group 3 should be instituted at once. Otherwise the tendency to bleed may coincidentally increase with the advancement of anæmia, and the ability to withstand the dangers associated with the measures in Group 3 progressively decrease.

3. In this group are placed the patients whose lives are endangered by severe hæmorrhage, especially from the mucous membranes, which cannot be controlled by the simple measures described above. Such cases are divisible into two groups :—

(*a*) In which the intractable purpura is associated with the terminal stages of certain diseases from which there is no hope of recovery, *e.g.*, aplastic anæmia, leukæmia, chronic nephritis with uræmia, etc. If such a diagnosis is established the patient should be allowed to die.

(*b*) Where the severe bleeding is part of the disease idiopathic thrombocytopenic purpura. If vigorous treatment is immediately instituted on the lines described below, life can be saved and health restored in the great majority of cases. Only two methods need be considered, viz., blood transfusion and splenectomy.

Blood Transfusion.—In many cases a single transfusion of 1 pint of blood (see p. 1079 *et seq.*) may be sufficient to control the hæmorrhage. In others it may be necessary to repeat the transfusion at three to four days' intervals on several occasions. For the subsequent transfusions the amount of blood advised is 250 c.c.

Splenectomy is indicated as an emergency measure in patients who are exsanguinated and in whom the bleeding is not controlled by blood transfusion. The operation should be preceded and if necessary followed by transfusion of blood. The risks of emergency splenectomy are high, the mortality varying from 10 to 30 per cent. in different hands, but the risks from the hæmorrhagic state in these intractable cases of severe purpura hæmorrhagica are even greater. The principal reason why patients are allowed to reach this dangerous stage of shock is the continuation for too long periods of the measures outlined in Group 2. We wish to point out again that splenectomy should never be performed as an emergency operation without first trying the effects of intravenous blood transfusion.

The second group of cases in whom splenectomy should be advised consists of patients with chronic thrombocytopenic purpura whose health and efficiency are being continuously impaired from recurrent hæmorrhage, which is only partly controlled by any of the measures mentioned above. As no emergency exists, the patient can be prepared for operation by the general measures outlined above together with iron and blood transfusions, repeated if necessary to bring the hæmoglobin to a safe level (70 to 80 per cent.) and control the tendency to bleed. The operative mortality in this group lies between 5 and 10 per cent.

Immediately following, or within a few hours of removal of the spleen, capillary oozing in all situations ceases, and with the help of iron the blood level will be restored to normal within two months. Symptomatic cure occurs in at least 80 per cent. of cases, although in some individuals qualitative changes in the blood picture (thrombocytopenia) may still remain.

The Bleeding Tendency in Obstructive Jaundice

There is evidence to suggest that the bleeding tendency commonly seen in cases of obstructive jaundice and chronic biliary fistulæ is due to deficiency of a fat soluble substance called vitamin K, which is not absorbed owing to the failure of adequate fat digestion consequent on the absence of bile in the small intestine. In such cases the prothrombin level of the blood is very low. In all cases of obstructive jaundice if operation is contemplated the prophylactic administration of vitamin K is advised. If bleeding has already developed, the prophylactic dose should be trebled and a transfusion of blood given. Vitamin K may be given as a crude extract of alfalfa (cerophyl, prophylactic dose, one teaspoonful thrice daily) or in the form of an oily solution in capsules (klotogen (Abbott Laboratories) or vitamin K oral (Crookes Laboratories, prophylactic dose, one capsule thrice daily). Bile or bile salts (15 to 30 gr. thrice daily) must always be prescribed when vitamin K is given by mouth. In the near future preparations for parenteral injection will be on the market. These will be of particular value when anorexia and vomiting are present and will do away with the need for the administration of bile salts.

HÆMOPHILIA

Hæmophilia is a hereditary disease characterised by a delay in the coagulation time of the blood and a tendency to recurrent hæmorrhages. Males only are affected, while transmission of the disease is solely through females of hæmophilic stock.

Treatment.—The relative rarity of the disease and the spontaneous fluctuations in the tendency to bleeding which occur make the merits of any therapeutic measures difficult to assess. Treatment may be considered under three headings :—

Preventive.—(*a*) Since the disease is a hereditary one, an effort should be made to control its spread by eugenic measures. Females born of hæmophilic stock should be told that for the sake of posterity child-bearing must not be undertaken ; (*b*) Prophylaxis of attacks of bleeding is obtained by regulating the patient's mode of life and activities so that the chances of trauma are reduced to a minimum. The dangers of trivial injury should be explained to the patient or his parents ; (*c*) Proper preparations for any operative procedure should be undertaken.

Treatment during an Attack of Bleeding—General Treatment.—Energetic measures should be immediately instituted to stop the hæmorrhage, since, if anæmia is allowed to develop, the resulting dilution of the blood which occurs lowers the concentration of the blood-clotting elements. Hence the use of commercial hæmostatic sera and of drugs, such as calcium, adrenalin, ergot, parathyroid extract, œstrogenic substances, etc., cannot be recommended, because there is little evidence that they are of value in altering the course of the disease, and their employment may even be a danger, since their use involves delay in the adoption of measures of proved value. If the site of hæmorrhage is not accessible, or if the bleeding is severe, transfusion of 1 pint of citrated blood should be undertaken. This will control the hæmorrhagic tendency for several days and the transfusion can be then repeated if necessary. In less severe cases the intramuscular injection of 10 to 30 c.c. of whole blood may suffice. In children the intraperitoneal transfusion of blood has been shown to be a satisfactory pre-operative measure.

Local Treatment.—If bleeding takes place from an accessible situation, *e.g.*, nose, tooth socket or a cut, the bleeding area should be gently cleaned and useless clots removed. A dressing soaked in a solution of Russell's viper venom (see p. 510) or normal fresh whole blood or serum should then be applied and kept firmly in position. Special bandages, packs, plates or splints may be required to maintain an effective pressure and reduce movement to a minimum (for details, see p. 510). Hæmatomas and swollen joints should not be opened, and orthopædic treatment should be undertaken by the use of splints, cages, etc., to put the parts at rest until pain and swelling disappear. After the acute symptoms have subsided, heat, gentle massage and passive movements are indicated.

Treatment between Attacks of Bleeding.—(*a*) Induction of Protein Hypersensitivity: The suggestion of Vines, that stimulation of the thrombogenetic functions of the somatic cells may be produced by the induction of a modified form of anaphylactic shock, has received the enthusiastic support of Mills, who claims that so long as a state of hypersensitivity is maintained the coagulation time of the blood is kept low. The method recommended by Mills may be summarized as follows: Sheep or hen serum is used. An intradermal injection is first given to ascertain whether or not the patient is already sensitive. If not, 3 or 4 c.c. are injected intramuscularly and fourteen days later another intradermal injection is given. An urticarial wheal should now appear, indicating that the patient is sensitized. If the coagulation time has not now shortened sufficiently, one should give further intradermal injections at weekly intervals, in different skin areas. This does not tend to reduce the general sensitivity. Thereafter, the coagulation time should be the guide as to the frequency of the intradermal injections. Sensitivity usually lasts for about a year, and at the end of that time it should be renewed by another intramuscular injection of the same or a different protein. Particular care should be taken to avoid injection of the serum subcutaneously while an intradermal injection is being given, as in this way a generalized reaction may be produced which may precipitate the patient into a hæmorrhagic state.

Eley and Clifford treated eight hæmophilic children by the above method, using intradermal injections of horse serum at fortnightly intervals. They confirm Mills' finding that a rapid and marked reduction in the coagulation time of the capillary blood could be obtained and maintained, but the coagulation time of the venous blood was unaltered. The therapy was of convincing benefit in the prevention or control of bleeding from superficial injuries, but was of little value when large vessels were injured, or for the prevention of effusions into joints or of hæmatomas.

(*b*) Placental Extract: A recent study by Eley and his co-workers in Boston has been made of the value of the oral and intramuscular administration of extracts made from human placental tissues. Fifteen hæmophilic children were treated and the data presented clearly show that a marked reduction of both the capillary and venous coagulation time was obtained. The clinical effects appear to be superior to those produced by protein hypersensitivity.

(*c*) Egg White: Timperley, Naish and Clark treated thirteen unselected cases of hæmophilia by intravenous or intramuscular injections of a substance which they have prepared from egg white incubated at 37° C. in the presence of potassium bromide. They claim that the clotting time of the blood was reduced and hæmorrhage was controlled.

In conclusion it would appear that in selected cases some beneficial results may be expected from the forms of treatment detailed above. An extended trial under controlled conditions is obviously desirable in this country and an open mind must be kept until this is done in view of the remarkable variations which spontaneously occur in the hæmophilic state.

(*d*) General Measures, including Diet: The general health should be maintained at as high a level as possible by the administration of a well-balanced diet and by regulated exercise in the fresh air and sunshine. Since there is some evidence to support the view that the coagulability of the blood can be influenced favourably by the absorption of protein from the intestine, a high protein diet has been recommended as a prophylactic measure. In addition to a moderate intake of protein at each of the three main meals, Mills recommends giving a glass of milk or an egg nog between meals and once during the night. If anæmia is present, iron should be prescribed in adequate doses (see p. 472) and treatment continued until a normal hæmoglobin figure is obtained.

(*e*) Removal of Septic Foci: It is well recognized that sepsis can play an important part in lowering the general health, in retarding the response of the hæmopoietic tissues to hæmorrhage, in damaging the endothelial lining of blood vessels and in initiating arthritis or influencing it unfavourably when it has occurred. Accordingly, despite the risks involved, obvious septic foci must be eradicated. The operation should be postponed, if possible, until the disease is in a quiescent state. Transfusion of blood before and after the operation, as well as other measures mentioned above, may be necessary for the control of hæmorrhage.

AGRANULOCYTIC ANGINA

Synonyms : Agranulocytosis ; Granulocytopenia ; Malignant or Primary Neutropenia.

Agranulocytic angina is a rare disease characterized by acute onset, pyrexia, necrotic lesions mainly in the buccal cavity and marked leucopenia with extreme lowering or complete absence of neutrophil polymorph cells. Rarely the course of the disease is chronic with periodic exacerbations. The condition is due to arrest of granular white cell-formation in the bone-marrow.

The term " agranulocytic angina " does not include the severe leucopenias which may occur in septicæmia, acute infectious fevers and aplastic anæmia, or as a terminal event in long-continued debilitating diseases.

Treatment.—*Prophylaxis.*—Recent work has shown that cases of agranulocytic angina may be divided into two groups : (1) in which the cause is unknown, and (2) secondary to the administration of certain drugs, especially amidopyrine (pyramidon), phenacetin, the arsphenamides, certain gold salts, and the sulphanilamides. These drugs possess in common the benzene ring with an attached NH2, or amine group. The most important, because of its very widespread use, is amidopyrine, and it has been estimated that this preparation is the cause of the great majority of cases of agranulocytic angina.

The drugs mentioned above are used with great frequency, but agranulocytic angina rarely develops. This suggests that the disease occurs only in those individuals in whom there is an idiosyncrasy or hypersensitivity to the particular drug employed. This conclusion is supported by the fact that the development of agranulocytic angina bears no relation to the amount of the drug taken, and in patients who have recovered from the disease a minute dose may cause an immediate and profound fall in the number of circulating granulocytes. Unfortunately there is no method whereby the development of such sensitivity may be predicted, and the value of amidopyrine, the organic arsenicals, gold salts, and the sulphanilamide preparations is so great that the serious results which occur in a very small proportion of individuals treated with these drugs cannot be considered as a contraindication to their use in suitable cases. Nevertheless, the possibility of an untoward reaction should be borne in mind and the earliest symptoms of intolerance, namely, drowsiness, weakness, exhaustion and unexplained pyrexia, should immediately raise the suspicion of agranulocytosis, and, if leucopenia is found, the administration of the drug should be stopped at once. In elderly persons and in those debilitated by long-continued illness, it is a wise precaution to perform leucocyte counts every week during treatment by any of the drugs mentioned, and the development of a significant degree of leucopenia should be a signal for the immediate withdrawal of the drug. The ease with which lay persons may purchase proprietary preparations which contain amidopyrine and are sold under trade names giving no information regarding their composition is to be deprecated. Amidopyrine and phenacetin should be available to the public only through the medium of non-renewable prescriptions given by physicians. It is important to realize that although prolonged ingestion of these leucotoxic drugs only rarely produces agranulocytic angina, it causes not infrequently a moderate leucopenia which may markedly reduce resistance to infection.

Curative Treatment.—(1) General Measures : The general nursing and care of a patient with agranulocytic angina are the same as for any acute febrile illness. The application of an ice-bag to the neck may relieve the pain in the throat, and the diet in the acute phase should be of high caloric value, and fluid or semi-solid because of the dysphagia which is frequently a troublesome symptom.

(2) Local Treatment : At least every four hours the mouth should be thoroughly sprayed with $\frac{1}{2}$ to 1 oz. of 1 : 2,000 solution of percaine in glycerin. During the subsequent period of local anæsthesia the patient should be fed and then the gums, tongue, palate and throat should be carefully swabbed, first with 50 per cent. hydrogen peroxide and then with citric acid solution (40 gr. citric acid, 1 oz. water ; diluted one part in seven with water before use).

(3) Treatment of the Agranulocytosis : In every case of agranulocytic angina exhaustive inquiries should be made regarding drugs taken by the patient, and any preparations with leucotoxic properties should, of course, be at once withdrawn. In a proportion of cases recovery then occurs rapidly without further specific treatment. The mortality of agranulocytic angina is so high, however, that in addition, measures to stimulate the leucopoietic tissues in the bone-marrow should be adopted in every case. Leucocyte extracts, parenteral liver therapy and the application of X-rays in stimulating doses have been used for this purpose, and all have proved very disappointing. Blood transfusions are said to be equally ineffective. The most promising form of treatment is the

parenteral administration of the sodium salts of pentose nucleotides prepared from nucleic acid. This product is marketed under the name pentnucleotide and is supplied in the form of a solution in 10 c.c. vials, each containing 0·7 gm. of the salts. Many favourable reports regarding the efficacy of this form of treatment have been published, and some authorities claim that the mortality of agranulocytic angina can be reduced from more than 70 per cent. to approximately 25 per cent. by early and intensive treatment with pentnucleotide. More recent investigations suggest that this optimistic view may have to be modified. However, the balance of evidence at present justifies the early administration of large doses of pentnucleotide in all cases of agranulocytic angina—10 to 20 c.c. should be injected deeply into the gluteal muscles twice daily for the first three days and followed by 10 c.c. once or twice daily for a week. Total white cell and differential counts should be made each day. In favourable cases an increase in the granular leucocytes occurs, usually between the third and fifth days, less often on the first or second day, and this response is accompanied by a fall in temperature and rapid healing of the necrotic lesions.

The introduction of 10 c.c. of fluid into the gluteal muscles frequently causes pain at the site of injection. This may be reduced by vigorous massage and the site of the injections should be varied. General reactions such as rigors, dyspnœa, palpitation and prostration are rare after intramuscular injections of pentnucleotide, but occur with such frequency and severity when the product is given intravenously that this method of administration should be avoided.

When clinical recovery and restoration of the white cells to normal have been achieved, a leucocyte count should be made twice weekly for about three weeks, and another course of pentnucleotide therapy should be instituted at once if a relapse occurs.

It has recently been claimed that oral administration of extracts of yellow bone-marrow produces rapid remission in cases of agranulocytic angina, but the value of this form of treatment must remain in doubt until more experience has been gained.

(4) Prevention of Relapses : All patients with agranulocytic angina due to drugs should be warned against taking the offending preparation in any form in the future.

DISEASES OF THE RETICULO-ENDOTHELIAL SYSTEM

(*a*) Reticulo-endotheliosis.
(*b*) Gaucher's disease.
(*c*) Niemann-Pick disease.
(*d*) Hand-Schüller-Christian disease.

There is no specific treatment for this group of rare diseases. The presence of hypochromic anæmia is an indication for the administration of iron (see p. 472). Some authorities recommend splenectomy in all cases in which the diagnosis of Gaucher's disease has been established, because of the great discomfort caused by the huge splenic tumour in the late stages of this disease. In our opinion the operation is not justified because hepatic enlargement occurs more rapidly after splenectomy. In the Hand-Schüller-Christian syndrome it is claimed that a low fat diet reduces the hypercholesterolæmia and may retard the progress of the disease. Beneficial results may also follow deep X-ray therapy. In this disease, however, there is obvious pituitary dysfunction resulting in diabetes insipidus and retarded growth, etc. The former can be controlled by vasopressin, while the latter may be influenced by anterior pituitary extracts.

THE LEUKÆMIAS

The leukæmias are characterized by qualitative or quantitative changes in the circulating white cells due to an abnormal proliferation of the leucopoietic tissues, the cause of which is unknown. The proliferation affects the lymphoid, myeloid or more rarely the monocyte-forming tissues. In the acute leukæmias the total white-cell count may be little altered and the diagnosis is made by a differential count which shows the presence of an extremely high proportion of stem cells which may be lymphoblasts, myeloblasts or monoblasts. In the chronic leukæmias, on the other hand, the total white-cell count is usually greatly increased, while the stem cells are absent or scanty, and immature cells form only a proportion of the total white-cell count.

The need for accurate diagnosis is apparent when it is realized that the acute forms of leukæmia always terminate fatally within a period of weeks or at the most months, and are materially uninfluenced by any form of treatment, while the chronic forms, although inevitably fatal, can be modified favourably by modern methods of treatment, particularly in regard to improving the well-being of the patient and prolonging economic efficiency.

Treatment of the Chronic Leukæmias.—The treatment of chronic myeloid, lymphoid and monocytic leukæmias is considered together, since the same measures with minor modifications are suitable for all three forms.

General Measures.—The average expectation of life in the chronic leukæmias has been found to be about three years. No matter what form of treatment is employed a fatal termination invariably occurs. Nevertheless, modern treatment with X-rays has considerably increased the period of economic efficiency and prolongs life for a few months. Accordingly, the patient should be advised to continue at his occupation or routine duties for as long as possible. Common-sense measures should be adopted regarding the regulation of the patient's life in regard to overwork, excessive exertion and chilling. Infections produce a marked deterioration in the health of patients with leukæmia. Hence, such patients should avoid close contact with persons suffering from colds in the head, sore throats, influenza, etc., and places where persons are crowded together during epidemics. Should a patient with leukæmia contract a mild infection, he should treat it much more carefully than a normal individual and remain in bed until the condition has completely cleared up.

Careful instructions should be given to the patient that, while exercise in the fresh air, such as walking, golfing and bicycling, is of value in maintaining health, the amount undertaken should always be well within the limit of his tolerance. An ordinary mixed diet should be advised which should contain ample quantities of the foods valuable for blood regeneration (see p. 469), and the total calories should be high in view of the increased basal metabolic rate so frequently present in leukæmia. This can easily be attained by prescribing additional quantities of butter, cream, bacon and the foods rich in carbohydrate. When the appetite begins to fail, bitter tonics may be useful.

Eventually, despite all treatment, emaciation and anæmia develop and the patient will have to give up his occupation and spend more and more time in bed. It is at this stage that blood transfusion is of value in improving the patient's general health and thus allowing the continuation of irradiation therapy.

In the terminal stages, when anæmia is severe and hæmorrhage and sepsis are occurring locally in the nose, mouth, etc., the measures outlined on pp. 510-513 should be taken.

Irradiation Treatment.—Irradiation is the most satisfactory method of treatment available for chronic leukæmia and should be adopted in every case. X-rays or radium are equally effective, but the former is usually employed. The patient should be in hospital for the first course of irradiation, but if for some reason this is impracticable, he may be treated as an out-patient under close supervision. It is not proposed to describe the technique in detail except to say that we have found that repeated application of small graduated doses is a safer and more effective procedure than large doses given at longer intervals. The amount of irradiation required varies widely in different individuals.

In chronic myeloid leukæmia the rays are applied usually to the splenic area and in lymphatic and monocytic leukæmia to the enlarged lymph nodes. If the spleen is markedly enlarged in the latter two conditions it should also be irradiated, although certain authorities are averse to this because severe reactions are stated to follow. The object of treatment is to bring the white-cell count to approximately normal. In practice, this means that treatment should be discontinued when the count is in the neighbourhood of 30,000 per c.mm., because of the liability of a further fall from continuation of the effects of irradiation. The amount of irradiation should be regulated by two factors, namely, the effect on the white and red cell counts and the clinical condition of the patient. Repeated white-cell counts are accordingly essential. If the dosage of X-rays is suitably adjusted, it is usually possible, except in the late stages, to cause a reduction in the white-cell count without any concomitant fall in erythrocytes or hæmoglobin. Should a sudden decrease in the red-cell count occur, this would suggest that the dosage has been excessive. Anæmia itself is not a contraindication to the use of X-rays. On the contrary, since the anæmia is due to a crowding out of erythroblastic tissues by leucoblastic tissue, properly controlled irradiation is generally followed by a rise in hæmoglobin and circulating erythrocytes. Transfusion of blood may be employed in anæmic individuals undergoing irradiation therapy in order to tide them over the period which must elapse before regeneration of red-cell marrow can occur.

When the objects mentioned above have been achieved by the initial course of irradiation, the patient's leucocytes should be counted at least once every three months in order to recognize the early signs of relapse which will inevitably occur.

A single exposure to X-rays may regain control of the situation if given at the beginning of a relapse, while a whole course may have to be repeated if the white-cell count is allowed to approach its former high level.

The effect of subsequent courses of irradiation therapy in reducing the white-cell count decreases markedly even when the dosage is increased. This is due to the fact that fibrosis occurs in the irradiated organs, such as the spleen and lymph glands, and therefore their content of leukæmic cells is much less. Frequently treatment is stopped when only a slight effect is produced by irradiation of these organs. It is possible, however, to obtain a further temporary improvement by careful irradiation of the whole body in a dosage which depresses leucoblastic proliferation but does not materially disturb erythropoiesis. This procedure entails the risk of aplastic anæmia and should therefore be controlled by frequent blood counts.

A time will come when destruction of erythroblastic tissue occurs, with the production of anæmia which cannot be controlled by iron or blood transfusion. When this stage has been reached active treatment should be stopped, and morphia or other symptomatic measures used to keep the patient comfortable.

X-ray Sickness.—The symptoms of general malaise and vomiting which sometimes occur during irradiation therapy are very rarely produced by the small graduated doses of X-rays, which is the method of choice in the treatment of the leukæmias. If the condition develops, however, the course of irradiation should be interrupted and the patient should be confined to bed on a light diet and should be given small doses of a sedative, *e.g.*, $\frac{1}{2}$ gr. phenobarbitone t.i.d., until the symptoms have subsided. Injections of liver extract and the oral administration of glucose have been widely used, but it is very doubtful whether they have any beneficial effect.

Drug Treatment.—Of the numerous drugs referred to in the treatment of leukæmia in the older textbooks of hæmatology, only arsenic, benzol, iodine, iron and liver extract need be mentioned.

Arsenic, like irradiation, is only palliative. Before the advent of irradiation it was the most potent therapeutic agent available. It is mainly in chronic myeloid leukæmia that beneficial effects have been claimed for it. Recently, as a result of the publications of Forkner and Scott, its use has again been recommended. We feel, however, that it is inferior in its action to irradiation and has, in addition, definite disadvantages, particularly the unpleasant symptoms of chronic arsenical poisoning, which no longer entitle it to a prominent place in the treatment of the leukæmias. Hence we do not agree with certain workers that irradiation treatment should not be employed until arsenic has been given a full trial. It is usually stated that arsenic should not be given during treatment by X-rays because of the dangers of secondary radiation, but according to Dr J. E. Blewett, Radiologist to Aberdeen Royal Infirmary, this risk is so slight that it need not be considered. Arsenic will certainly not succeed in cases which have reached the stage of insensitivity to irradiation. Accordingly, we can recommend arsenic only to those patients with leukæmia for whom irradiation therapy is difficult or impossible to procure.

Arsenic is generally given in the form of Fowler's solution (liquor arsenicalis). The initial dose should be 3 minims three times a day, and the dose increased by 1 minim per dose every two days. This is continued until definite toxic symptoms (nausea, vomiting, diarrhœa, tinnitus, and a metallic taste in the mouth) are produced. This amount varies in different individuals from 30 to 60 minims daily. The earliest symptom of toxicity is anorexia, which may appear when the total daily dose is about 20 minims, and it may be necessary to reduce the increments and prolong the intervals between them when this symptom occurs. It should be realized, however, that the patient must take the maximal quantity of arsenic which he can tolerate if results are to be produced.

When full toxic symptoms appear, indicating that the maximal dose has been reached, the drug should be discontinued for two or three days and then started again with about three-quarters of the previous dose. When the limit of tolerance has been reached or the optimal improvement in the blood picture has appeared, the drug is gradually reduced in the manner in which it was increased.

Benzol is a powerful leucocytic poison. It is administered with olive oil in capsules, the initial dose being 0·5 gm. four times a day. The dangers of producing aplastic anæmia are in our opinion so great that they more than counter-balance the fall in the leucocyte count which coincidentally occurs. Accordingly, we recommend that benzol should not be used in the treatment of leukæmia.

Iodine has been recommended in the treatment of leukæmia, especially in the chronic lymphatic form in which a high basal metabolic rate has not infrequently been noted. While it is of some value for the relief of such symptoms as tachycardia, sweating and nervousness, it has little or no effect in the control of the blood picture. Accordingly, it should never be used alone, but only in combination with irradiation therapy. Lugol's iodine in doses of 5 to 10 minims three times a day is the preparation most commonly employed.

Iron.—An iron deficiency anæmia develops sooner or later in every case of chronic leukæmia and requires treatment with dietotherapy and medicinal iron, as described on pp. 469-472.

Liver Extract.—In the acute leukæmias and in the terminal stage of the chronic leukæmias a macrocytic anæmia develops with a high colour index and a red-cell picture resembling pernicious anæmia. The macrocytosis is, however, the result of excessive activity in the remaining portions of erythroblastic marrow, and is not due to a deficiency of the anti-anæmic factor. It is not surprising, therefore, that we have been unable to influence this terminal blood picture by liver or liver extract.

The Acute Leukæmias

Once the diagnosis of acute myeloblastic, lymphoblastic or monoblastic leukæmia is made, it should be realized that a fatal termination will occur within a few weeks. Splenectomy is contraindicated in this as in all forms of leukæmia, and X-rays and radium are generally held to aggravate rather than improve the condition.

Blood transfusion is warranted only if for some specific reason it is desired to prolong life for two or three weeks, or to control severe local hæmorrhage, particularly from the nose and mouth, which is interfering with the comfort of the patient. Accordingly, treatment is purely symptomatic, and sedatives such as morphia should be given in adequate amounts to make the patient comfortable.

Aleukæmic Leukæmia

Definition.—A leukæmia in which the abnormal white cells are found to infiltrate the bone-marrow and many organs of the body although the white-cell count is low or within normal limits. The differential count may be qualitatively normal or abnormal. Diagnosis obviously presents the greatest difficulty unless histological examination of the bone-marrow, obtained by biopsy, is undertaken. Aleukæmic leukæmia may occur in the acute form, clinically indistinguishable from the other acute leukæmias mentioned above, and in such cases treatment is purely symptomatic on the lines already described. In other cases the course is chronic and the question arises whether or not irradiation should be given. The failure of the abnormal cells to enter the peripheral blood makes assessment of the degree of irradiation required extremely difficult. Accordingly, the risks of producing aplastic anæmia are serious, and for this reason some authorities hold that X-rays are contra-indicated. Moreover, there is some evidence to suggest that occasionally irradiation therapy may precipitate an acute phase of the disease. We feel, however, that since the only hope of radically influencing the anæmia lies in the destruction of the leucoblastic tissue which is infiltrating the bone-marrow, irradiation therapy to the spleen or lymph glands should be advised if these organs are enlarged. Obviously, irradiation must be given tentatively in small graduated doses, using the erythrocyte count and the clinical state of the patient to assess its efficacy.

The other measures found to be of value in the chronic leukæmias should also be used in chronic aleukæmic leukæmia.

Hodgkin's Disease

Hodgkin's disease is characterized by progressive enlargement of the lymphoid tissues, commencing in any situation and generally becoming widespread. The histology of the affected tissues justifies consideration of the disease as a specific entity.

Treatment.—Like the leukæmias, Hodgkin's disease is invariably fatal, but the duration of life varies within the very wide limits of a few weeks to about ten years. The general condition of the patient may, for a time, be considerably improved and the progression of the glandular enlargement may be much delayed by irradiation therapy. X-rays are generally to be preferred to radium. All the sites in which there is glandular enlargement, and the spleen if it is enlarged, should be irradiated in turn and a course should consist of small doses at short intervals over a few weeks. The frequency with which the courses should be repeated depends on the condition of the glands, the blood level and the general health of the patient in a manner similar to that described in the section of the leukæmias.

Arsenic is of value in improving the patient's general health, and should be given in the dosage described on p. 528, and iron (see p. 472) should be prescribed in an attempt to correct the hypochromic anæmia which usually accompanies the condition. Lotio phenolis (B.P.C.) and lotio picis carbonis alkalina (B.P.C.) are useful preparations for allaying the pruritus which is occasionally a troublesome symptom.

The general measures which should be adopted are the same as for the leukæmias (see p. 525).

Recently, Gordon has prepared from emulsions of glands a suspension of a virus which he claims to be the infective agent. A few cases have been treated with injections of a vaccine made from the virus with apparently beneficial effects, but sufficient time has not as yet elapsed to enable one to form conclusions regarding the value of this form of therapy.

L. S. P. Davidson.
H. W. Fullerton.

DISEASES OF THE ALIMENTARY CANAL

DISEASES OF THE ŒSOPHAGUS

ŒSOPHAGITIS

INFLAMMATION of the œsophagus may ensue after a foreign body or a corrosive poison has been swallowed. Many *foreign bodies* pass slowly and safely down the œsophagus, and no treatment is required unless breathing is interfered with. A few become arrested, and should only be removed under direct vision through an œsophagoscope. One of the commonest foreign bodies, especially in adults, is a stiff fish-bone, which may penetrate the wall of the gullet and lead to acute mediastinitis. The treatment is surgical, but the mortality is high. Unfortunately, the cause of the perforation is often quite unsuspected. *Corrosive poisons*, swallowed accidentally or with suicidal intent, generally burn the lips, mouth and pharynx, so that immediate diagnosis is easy. Apart from acute œdema of the glottis, which may rarely require tracheotomy, the brunt of the serious damage falls either on the narrow œsophagus or on the mucosa of the stomach. Acute sloughing or perforation of the œsophagus is likely to be rapidly fatal from severe shock. The patient is put to bed, the correct antidote given, if the poison is known, but otherwise nothing whatever is given by mouth. In corrosive poisoning, in contradistinction to other types of poisoning, no attempt to pass a stomach tube must be made. The main immediate treatment is to combat shock, and the agonizing pain demands an immediate injection of morphine.

Simple Stricture.—In patients who survive, stricture is common. The treatment of such cases is difficult, and should only be carried out by experts. The chief difficulty for the physician is to decide the time when gradual dilatation should commence—all acute inflammation must have subsided while dense cicatrization must be forestalled. In most successful cases the primary dilatation must be followed by subsequent courses of treatment, as gradual scarring and contraction may continue for a number of months.

DYSPHAGIA

Difficulty in swallowing is generally the cardinal symptom of œsophageal disease, and when this occurs the first problem to decide is whether the difficulty is due to an organic or functional cause. In one condition, referred to below, the difficulty is in starting the reflex act, but most commonly the fault is in the œsophagus itself. The gullet is, on the whole, firmly fixed in position at its two ends and in its course between them, and the patient can in consequence generally localize the seat of obstruction with great accuracy, pointing to the site with his finger. This is of real help in preliminary diagnosis, since certain conditions affecting the œsophagus are well known to have favourite sites.

Dysphagia arising near the Junction of Œsophagus and Pharynx.—Plummer-Vinson syndrome. Diphtheritic palsy of the soft palate. Dysphagia in certain nervous diseases (*e.g.*, bulbar paralysis). Hysteria.

Dysphagia arising in the Mid-œsophagus.—Carcinoma. Organic stricture following corrosive poisons. Rarely, pressure of an aneurysm, mediastinal tumour, or retrosternal goitre.

Dysphagia arising near the Lower End of the Œsophagus.—Achalasia of the cardia. Carcinoma. Cicatricial stricture. Rarely, peptic ulcer of the œsophagus.

Diverticulum of the Œsophagus is rare, and seldom of importance as a cause of dysphagia.

Diverticulum of the Pharynx just above the œsophagus, and often erroneously believed to arise in it, is more common and of considerable clinical importance. Gradual and progressive enlargement ensues, until finally the sac may retain a large amount of food or fluid. When this occurs, the patient complains of extreme dysphagia and pain on swallowing, the difficulty being referred to the neck and a definite bulge or tumour may be visible. Rapid emaciation always ensues from the difficulty in swallowing. After careful emptying of the sac, a waxed thread is swallowed as a guide for the introduction of a catheter into the stomach. When nutrition has been sufficiently improved by feeding through the catheter, operation may be considered, but the surgical risks are always serious.

Plummer-Vinson Syndrome.—An inco-ordination of the reflex act of swallowing at the pharyngo-œsophageal junction, found almost exclusively in middle-aged women suffering from chronic microcytic (hypochromic) anæmia (see p. 464). The treatment is primarily that of the anæmia, and secondarily similar to achalasia of the cardia. In occasional cases, however, passage of the mercury tube may be impossible owing to the presence of webs or bands. Operative treatment is then required.

Carcinoma of the Œsophagus.—This occurs as a rule at one of the two narrow parts of the œsophagus—at the level of the bifurcation of the trachea (commoner) or at the cardiac end.

Once the diagnosis has been made, only palliative treatment is possible. Radical surgical treatment, up to the present, has been unsuccessful. In the early stages the patient should be encouraged to eat as freely as he can without discomfort, but soon the food must be restricted to semi-solids, and finally only fluids in very limited amounts may reach the stomach. The patient in the later stage is simply starving to death, and the choice must be made between a temporary gastrostomy or the adequate use of morphine. Apart from attempts at radical surgical intervention, efforts have been made to implant radon seeds through an œsophagoscope, and deep X-ray therapy has also been employed without, however, any permanent success. Souttar's spiral coiled metal tube may in certain cases be passed through the constricting tumour and left *in situ* until the end, thus enabling some food to be swallowed. No attempt should ever be made to dilate a carcinomatous stricture.

Achalasia of the Cardia.—This term, coined by Hurst, is used to describe a condition of obstruction at the lower end of the œsophagus, believed to be due to an inability of the cardiac sphincter to relax (achalasia) rather than to muscular spasm. The older term—cardiospasm—is now therefore seldom employed. The condition is chiefly confined to adults of both sexes, and is not uncommon.

Diagnosis is easily made by X-rays following the swallowing of a thin barium meal, and early diagnosis is of great importance, since at that stage permanent cure, or at least permanent amelioration almost amounting to cure, is always possible. If early diagnosis fails, the dilatation of the œsophagus above the obstruction may be enormous, and serious erosion or actual ulceration of the sac may supervene. Passage of any instrument in such cases is difficult and by no means free from danger.

The usual treatment is both simple and effective, and consists in the repeated passage of a single, or, if absolutely necessary, a series of rubber tubes with rounded ends resembling a stomach tube, partly filled with mercury to give weight. The series of tubes recommended by Hurst varies from 24 to 34 gauge, but in practice a single tube of 30 gauge generally suffices. The cost, to a hospital patient, is about 7s. 6d. The patient at first requires encouragement and actual help in passing the tube down the œsophagus and in allowing it, practically by its own weight, to open and pass the obstruction into the stomach. The tube is left in position for fifteen to twenty minutes, after which it is withdrawn and the patient then finds that food can easily be swallowed. Every patient is gradually, but as a rule without much difficulty, taught to pass the tube on himself or herself. At first, even in early cases, the tube may require to be passed before every meal, but eventually its passage is only required daily, weekly, or at irregular intervals. In a few patients it can be dispensed with altogether. In the later stages of treatment the mere passage of the " mercury tube " is sufficient—it may then be withdrawn at once and the meal proceeded with.

In patients in whom the condition is only recognized late, after dilation and elongation of the œsophagus have ensued, treatment is more difficult. The œsophagus should be carefully and repeatedly washed out with normal saline until erosions are healed, and attempts to pass the mercury tube, owing to kinking of the elongated œsophagus, should be undertaken with care. In such patients radiological control is advisable, in association with a thin barium meal. The obstruction is seldom complete, and a fine stream of the barium meal can generally be seen on the X-ray screen demonstrating the course of the channel from œsophagus to stomach.

PEPTIC ULCER OF THE ŒSOPHAGUS

(*Peptic Œsophagitis*)

Peptic ulcer of the œsophagus occurs just above the cardiac sphincter, and is identical with the same ulcer in the stomach, not only in its structure but also in its important complication of hæmorrhage.

Acute Peptic Ulcer of the Œsophagus is a sequel of frequent vomiting, and, most commonly in practice, of post-operative vomiting. Fatal hæmatemesis may occur, especially in children.

Treatment is mainly prophylactic, and depends largely on efficient post-operative nursing. After severe bouts of vomiting a small amount of an alkaline drink should be given. Healing of an acute ulcer is complete in about ten days, and feeding in suspected cases should be confined to citrated milk given in small amounts frequently repeated.

Chronic Peptic Ulcer of the Œsophagus is fortunately uncommon, and is identical with the chronic ulcer of the stomach and duodenum. It also occurs just above the cardiac sphincter, and is believed to depend on the presence of an abnormal area (metaplasia) of oxyntic cells, secreting hydrochloric acid, which should normally be confined to the stomach. Treatment is best undertaken in bed, and should be on exactly analogous lines to those recommended for gastric and duodenal ulcer (p. 542). The chief differences are that food should be taken only when the patient is sitting up and instructions given that he must not lie down for half an hour afterwards. A drink of water is advisable at the end of each meal and olive oil in 2 to 4 drachm doses taken after meals is of particular value for diminishing acid secretion and allaying irritation.

DISEASES OF THE STOMACH

The treatment of disorders of the stomach forms a large part of general medical practice. The disorders belong to two main groups—functional and organic—and although both are of great frequency and importance it must always be remembered that the former exceed the latter in number.

Efficient treatment must always depend on good diagnosis, and this at first may not be easy because of the diversity of symptoms which a patient may refer to his stomach. It is impossible here to enter into the many methods—clinical, clinico-pathological and radiological—which may require to be employed in turn. Before any treatment is commenced after a diagnosis of any form of gastric disorder has been made, a few fundamental points must be kept in mind.

1. The normal functions of the stomach, and the features, so far as they are known, of disturbance of each of them.

   Rational treatment is obviously based on restoration of the deranged function to normal by methods which may be termed, for brevity, "physiological." These methods naturally have particular reference to the functional group, and may only have a partial application in some forms of organic gastric disease.

2. The diathesis or general "make up"—mental and physical—of the patient. The importance of this observation in almost every form of gastric disturbance is universally recognized—one of the chief exceptions being cancer of the stomach.

   Few individuals go through life without experiencing some temporary gastric upset, but in the majority of cases this is without significance. It is well recognized, however, that rather less than one-quarter of the population are of a type which renders them particularly susceptible to gastric disorder, and that this group provides the majority of gastric patients. The group may be enlarged, however, by the addition of normal individuals affected by circumstances which have rendered them prone to gastric disease. A few self-evident examples may be referred to only: faulty habits in food and drink, occupation (with irregular meals or exposure to industrial poisons), persistent business or domestic worry, organic disease of other organs acting reflexly on the gastric secretions and functions. In what may be termed the congenitally susceptible group, always prone to gastric disorder, two types are easily recognized. The first is the hypersthenic, active and often, but by no means always, highly strung type of individual who, on the whole, tends to excess in gastric function and secretion, and whose physiological treatment in consequence must be directed to the inhibition of excessive function. The second is the asthenic, somewhat inactive type of individual, often characterized by a narrow chest, a narrow costal angle and poor muscular development. This type is particularly, but far from exclusively, found in women, many of whose symptoms are ascribed to the concomitant visceroptosis (p. 580). In this second group gastric function and secretion tend to be subnormal, and treatment should be directed to remedying this defect.

The functions of the stomach may now be very briefly summarized, since (except in certain organic diseases of unknown ætiology) it is disturbances of function which we must generally attempt to correct.

The main function of the stomach is its motility, associated with frequent peristaltic waves. This function is quite unknown and unfelt by the normal individual, but gives rise to clamant symptoms in functional and organic disease. Hypermotility of the stomach may be painless, or very painful. The pain is due to tension or to actual organic disease, and both of these may be present together. When the stomach contains food the pain is generally due to overdistension (relieved by eructation or flatulence) or to the pylorus failing to open (due to spasm or organic disease). When for any reason the muscular power of the stomach wall has failed and atonic dilatation has supervened, severe pain is unlikely, except in the presence of actual organic disease.

The secretory function of the stomach comes next in importance, and it may be emphasized at the very outset that as an organ of digestive secretion the stomach falls far behind the pancreas in its potency. The two main secretions of the normal stomach are pepsin and hydrochloric acid, and to this must be added mucus in certain abnormal circumstances. In the treatment of gastric disorders it is remarkable how little importance is attached to pepsin and its action on proteins. We know little about the effects of disturbances in the secretion of pepsin or any symptoms which may in consequence ensue. Protein digestion by the normal pancreas seems always to be adequate for the needs of the body. All our clinical interest in treatment is centred in the secretion of hydrochloric acid—whether it is excessive or diminished or absent altogether, or present at the wrong time in an empty stomach. The effects of abnormalities in the secretion and neutralization of hydrochloric acid are far-reaching in a wide variety of functional and organic gastric diseases, and much of our present therapy is directed to correction of this abnormality of secretion. It must be mentioned, however, that complete gastric health, at least for a time, is apparently quite consistent in some patients with high gastric acidity or with achlorhydria.

Mucus is secreted in the normal stomach in small amount, but in some diseases (*e.g.*, chronic gastritis) is in such excess as to require active therapeutic measures.

Finally, it must be remembered that in recent times we have become aware of another important secretory activity of the stomach—the production of an enzyme (hæmopoietin) which is essential for the complete development of the red cells of the blood and for the health of the central nervous system. This secretion is fully referred to in the section on Pernicious Anæmia (p. 480), as is also the relation of achlorhydria to other forms of anæmia.

When considering the rational treatment of gastric disorders, not only must disturbances of gastric function and structure be considered but also the way in which our remedies may act. Some appear to act directly on the stomach wall, and either are not absorbed, or not until they have left the stomach, *e.g.*, bismuth, olive oil. Some act on the gastric secretion contained in the stomach, *e.g.*, alkalis (to neutralize hydrochloric acid) and dilute hydrochloric acid (to substitute for achlorhydria). Some act during absorption through the wall of the stomach. We have a poor comprehension of the effect of these on an intact mucosa—probably, however, some sedatives act directly on an ulcerated surface. Many drugs used in gastric disorders act only after absorption by their effects on the nervous system—opium, morphine, belladonna, atropine ; or by replacing a necessary hormone—hæmopoietin (as contained in preparations of animal liver and stomach).

The question of dietetics in gastric disorders has been left to the end to emphasize its importance. The main reason for the existence of the stomach, and for its motor and secretory functions, is to receive and deal with the food which is necessary for life. Abuses of food (and drink) have been indicated as causes of gastric disorder. The essential principles of feeding a patient who is suffering from some form of functional or organic gastric disease must be carefully considered, but a few of the most important are indicated here.

The first is that much depends on the duration of the gastric complaint. In general, the dietetic treatment of acute gastric disorders is starvation or partial starvation to rest the functions of the organ which is acutely inflamed. In chronic disorders the nutrition of the body must be maintained—rectal feeding is always a poor and insufficient substitute, and feeding through a duodenal tube only applicable in a few cases and in a few conditions. In gastric diseases, as in other diseases, there has probably been a tendency to think at times too much of the local condition or disease and too little of the importance of adequate general nutrition in combating the effects of prolonged illness.

The giving of food is important for two main reasons : one is to provide for adequate general nutrition, as just mentioned ; the other is that food, when properly given, as described subsequently, forms by far the best way of neutralizing and using up the hydrochloric acid of the gastric juice which is so important in many gastric diseases. It is true that our patients must sleep, during which time feeding is impossible, and thus it is that drugs, particularly for the neutralization of hydrochloric acid, have perhaps their chief value when given at night.

GASTRITIS

Acute Gastritis.—This may result from the swallowing of corrosive poisons, the stomach sharing in the damage done to the œsophagus. Apart from the administration of the antidote, if known, no other treatment is possible.

Acute gastritis of lesser severity (catarrhal gastritis) is exceedingly common, and due to a great variety of causes. Common varieties in practice are the result of indiscretions in food or alcoholic drinks ; but contaminated food, " chill " (especially in the tropics) and scarlet fever in its acute stage may also induce very acute gastric catarrh. In any variety the inflammation may spread downwards to cause acute gastro-enteritis. The cardinal symptom of acute gastritis is vomiting, and when enteritis is superadded, diarrhœa also supervenes.

The treatment of acute catarrhal gastritis is best considered as part of gastro-enteritis, the treatment of which is dealt with under the heading of Diarrhœa (p. 567).

Chronic Gastritis.—This was formerly a common diagnosis. Thereafter came a time when, apart from its recognized existence in habitual alcoholics, the conception of chronic gastritis fell into disrepute, and the use of the term was frowned on in sick reports. Now, again, chiefly as a result of the pathological work of Faber, of Copenhagen, and of developments in radiological and gastroscopic technique, chronic gastritis has come into its own, and is properly regarded, when correctly diagnosed, as an important and by no means infrequent disease. Accurate diagnosis is essential, but, when made, the use of the term is entirely justified.

It is important to treat this disease in as early a stage as possible, not only for the immediate disabilities which arise but still more for the serious consequences, such as carcinoma, which may possibly result from it. Much of the treatment is essentially prophylactic and consists in the removal of such well-known causes as alcoholism, oral sepsis (especially pyorrhœa) and deficient mastication of food (from bad habits or lack of teeth). Excessive use of strong tea, coffee and tobacco have all been blamed as causes, but proof is difficult. The cardinal symptoms of an established case which demand treatment are :—

1. Vomiting, especially in the morning and associated always with an excessive secretion of mucus into the stomach.

2. Diminution or frequently complete absence of hydrochloric acid in the gastric juice. (In the hypertrophic variety of gastritis, hyperacidity occurs.)

The prime causes favouring continuation of the disease having been removed, the first essential in treatment is gastric lavage carried out always before breakfast and in the severer cases at intervals during the day, before meals. In practice either the larger " stomach tube " (with Sanoran's aspirator) or the narrow tube used for fractional test meals (with a large syringe attached) may be used. Patients differ, and as the lavage must be frequently repeated and can finally be entrusted to an individual of moderate intelligence, the easier method should be found and applied. Warm water is in many cases entirely adequate to wash out the stomach and remove the mucus ; but if mucus is present in large amount, 1 to 4 drachms of hydrogen peroxide (10 volumes) is added to 1 pint of warm water. This helps mechanically to " bubble " the mucus away from the gastric mucosa. Treatment by lavage is continued until improvement is manifest, when its use can be gradually discontinued. If lavage is for any reason impossible, the next best substitute is the administration of a teaspoonful or more of sodium bicarbonate in a tumblerful of warm water in the morning, and again before meals throughout the day.

Hydrochloric acid is so commonly greatly diminished or absent in an untreated case of chronic gastritis that this deficiency should be attended to at once, and 1 to 2 drachms of acid. hydrochlor. dil. should be added to a tumblerful of lemonade or orangeade and drunk as a beverage with each main meal. It should be pointed out, however, that the small quantity of dilute hydrochloric acid prescribed cannot be regarded in any sense as " replacement therapy," and we are still in doubt about its mode of action. Further, in some patients pain results and the dosage advised above must be reduced. It is known that after gastric lavage for some weeks the secretion of hydrochloric acid frequently returns in adequate amount.

In the early stages of chronic gastritis, anorexia is common, especially in the morning, while mucus is still in the stomach. Later in the day the appetite generally improves. Alcohol must be entirely forbidden, and smoking restricted to after meals. Meat is digested with difficulty, and should be allowed only once a day. Wholemeal bread, salads, pickles, and the skins and pips of fruit must be avoided, and green vegetables given only when sieved. A bitter tonic containing 5 to 10 minims of tincture of nux vomica and 30 to 60 minims of compound tincture of gentian, taken before meals, may be helpful.

There is no doubt whatever that in patients able to afford it spa treatment is of great assistance for many reasons. Abundance of a mildly aperient spa water corrects the almost invariable constipation and washes out the stomach, while the general spa régime should enable patients to amend their habits. When spa treatment is impossible, bottled spa water may be taken at home, and sodium phosphate, 1 drachm in ½ pint of water, is a substitute for the well-known Carlsbad water.

The patient suffering from chronic gastritis is likely to be irritable, depressed and difficult to handle, and a great deal of common-sense psychological treatment may be required.

GASTRIC AND DUODENAL ULCER

(Syn: Peptic Ulcer)

Chronic peptic ulcer is found (1) on the lesser curvature of the stomach; (2) near the pylorus (pyloric antrum); and (3) in the first inch of the duodenum (duodenal ulcer). Rarely, other parts of the stomach wall are involved, or the ulcers may be multiple.

The treatment of a straightforward case of chronic peptic ulcer is essentially the same, whatever its position. Differences arise in long-standing cases only because each of the varying anatomical positions tends to be associated with special complications. Duodenal ulcer is especially liable to lead to organic pyloric stenosis; ulcer of the lesser curvature to deep penetration into the pancreas or to hour-glass stomach; while ulcer of the pyloric antrum has a well-known tendency, unlike ulcers on other sites, to become malignant. Any chronic peptic ulcer may perforate, when the immediate treatment is surgical.

The difficult problems of ætiology and the great variations in symptomatology of peptic ulcer are not discussed here. All that need be said in introducing rational treatment is that, in the present state of our knowledge, it is believed to be the hydrochloric acid secreted in the gastric juice which continues the existence of chronic gastric and duodenal ulcers, prevents their healing and even breaks down partial healing to produce "recurrences." Many patients suffering from peptic ulcer, especially duodenal ulcer, exhibit great hypersecretion of hydrochloric acid, which, however, in the stomach never exceeds 0·4 per cent. in strength ; others show a more or less normal secretion of acid, but achlorhydria is never found.

It is quite possible that although the presence of hydrochloric acid is the main factor in continuing the active existence of peptic ulcer, this is not the whole truth. Nevertheless, it is by dealing with the hydrochloric acid—by utilization with food, by neutralization with alkalis, and by preventing or diminishing its secretion by drugs and other methods—that we at present obtain our main therapeutic effects.

Utilization of the hydrochloric acid by food—a natural process—constitutes the first and most important line of treatment, and three general points may be made at once :—

1. The food should be smooth and not rough, so as to avoid irritation of the ulcerated surface.
2. It should be given in small amounts at a time, so as to avoid overdistension which might lead to perforation, and also to prevent a great flow of gastric juice.
3. It should be given frequently, so that the total amount is sufficient to sustain adequate nourishment and weight, and to cause continuous neutralization.

Until comparatively recently all that was aimed at in the dietetics of peptic ulcer was to neutralize the hydrochloric acid and to provide sufficient calories. The importance of a balanced diet and of the vitamins in maintaining health apart from mere weight was not fully realized, and a realization of the importance of these matters is rapidly causing changes in our dietetic methods. These changes are referred to in detail subsequently.

The patient suffering from peptic ulcer must sleep, and sleep well, and cannot at the same time be fed. During sleep, however, as a study of the "fasting juice" in a fractional test-meal taken in the morning clearly shows, hydrochloric acid may accumulate in the "empty" stomach, especially if an ulcer near the pylorus has induced spasm or an organic obstruction. It is thus at night, as has already been indicated, that alkalis may be valuable in treatment, although their neutralizing effects must be very incomplete.

With the above general principles in mind, the details of treatment may now be considered. It is presupposed that an accurate diagnosis has been made by the methods now available—clinical, clinico-pathological and radiological.

Initial Management.—The first point to decide, after the diagnosis has been made, is whether treatment should be begun with the patient in bed. This must be regarded as essential, and ambulant treatment at the outset is always unsatisfactory. The ideal time that the patient should remain absolutely at rest in bed is four to six weeks, and as the typical "ulcer patient" is frequently irritable and difficult to manage, the doctor will often require all his patience and resource to insist upon this régime. It has been said that if a patient suffering from peptic ulcer is not entirely relieved of his symptoms after a few days in bed, however inadequate his treatment may be, the diagnosis is probably wrong. This fact must be recognized, and the patient informed that although his discomforts will soon disappear, the ulcer remains quite unhealed.

Two other matters also arise at the very outset of treatment—the problem of smoking and the condition of the mouth and teeth.

Although there is no proof that smoking, even in excess, is a direct ætiological factor in peptic ulcer, there is no doubt that nicotine when swallowed stimulates a flow of gastric juice which, especially in an empty stomach, must be harmful. The advice to be tendered to the patient at the end of treatment for gastric ulcer is dealt with subsequently, but in the earlier stages the writer has no doubt that smoking should be absolutely forbidden.

Many patients suffering from peptic ulcer are found to have defective teeth, either caries, pyorrhœa or an inadequate number of teeth. The front teeth alone may be present, and the molars, so essential for mastication, may have disappeared and may not have been replaced by dentures. It is obviously sound treatment in most cases to begin with a reasonably clean mouth and with provision made for adequate mastication in future.

Dietetic Treatment of Peptic Ulcer.—This section deals with the most important part of our present medical treatment of peptic ulcer, food being the natural way of dealing with the secretion of hydrochloric acid in the stomach. Drugs, such as alkalis, are frequently essential in association with dietetic treatment, but for clearness these are dealt with under a separate heading.

Great care and attention has always been paid in modern medicine to dietetics in peptic ulcer, but since our knowledge is constantly increasing, no finality has been reached, and even at the present time our views are to some extent in process of change. The earlier dietetic treatments were concerned with two things only—efficient utilization of hydrochloric acid and prevention of irritation of the healing ulcer. Proteins and fats entered largely into their constitution. In the acute stages, and particularly after a recent hæmorrhage, it is now realized that too little attention was paid to the provision of adequate calories to maintain weight and strength. In other words, as we now know, in connection with this and other diseases, the disease rather than the patient was chiefly considered. Moreover, the advent of our knowledge of vitamins has altered and amplified our dietetics in many diseases.

Two systems of diet, to be used in the treatment of straightforward cases of peptic ulcer, are still referred to in almost every textbook of medicine—the *Lenhartz diet*, consisting chiefly of milk and eggs, and the *Sippy diet*, made up mainly of milk and cream. Neither of these diets, in their original form, is now used in Britain, but modifications of both of them are still in common use.

Two methods of diet have in recent years attracted attention in Britain. The first is associated with the name of Sir Arthur Hurst, and has already withstood the test of practical experience for many years. The second, recently introduced by Meulengracht, was particularly recommended by him for use after recent hæmorrhage, but is equally applicable to ordinary cases of uncomplicated peptic ulcer. Similar diets have been used independently by others, but the two names mentioned can fairly be used to describe two important modern systems of dietetics in peptic ulcer. Both are arranged to include an adequate caloric intake and a full supply of vitamins. Hurst's régime utilizes a number of drugs in addition to the food; Meulengracht's practically dispenses with drugs. The Hurst régime is given in full in the appendix (p. 557). The Meulengracht diet, as modified by Witts, is referred to again in the section on Hæmatemesis and Melæna, and is also given in the appendix (p. 560).

The chief difficulty of the Hurst régime lies in the fact that it is difficult to carry out in its entirety in private houses, but when circumstances permit of it being undertaken in full, there is no doubt of its great effectiveness. The complete and very elaborate régime described on p. 557 can be modified by the practitioner to suit the circumstances of the case. The Meulengracht type of diet is still on trial, but has already won many supporters; it is naturally greatly preferred by the patients themselves who receive a diet which, although carefully prepared, is of a kind and variety to which they have been accustomed. Time alone can show whether it is as effective for the healing of peptic ulcer as the more complicated Hurst diet.

The dietetic treatment of peptic ulcer is often divided into the " strict ulcer diet " and the " post-ulcer diet " in which greater liberty in choice is allowed.

The healing of a chronic peptic ulcer is a long process, taking many months to complete. We are aware, since the introduction of the direct vision gastroscope, that many ulcers thought to be healed and no longer showing an " ulcer niche " in an X-ray film, are in reality still active although diminished in size. Thus dietetic and other precautions are essential for at least two years, and some restrictions learned by the patient during the active period of treatment must be continued for life.

The problems of alcohol and tobacco arise again in the post-ulcer period. Strong alcoholic drinks of all kinds, and particularly when taken on an empty stomach, should be forbidden, but there is no real objection to more dilute spirits and wines taken along with meals. Smoking on an empty stomach must also be strictly forbidden. Some patients find it possible to adhere to the rule of smoking only after meals and at no other time. Others prefer to give up smoking for life, and as the habit has been stopped during the early stages of treatment, the conditions are not so difficult for the patient.

Drugs in the Treatment of Peptic Ulcer.—*Alkalis* are the most used and probably the most abused remedies in the treatment of real or supposed peptic ulcer. They give immediate symptomatic relief in most forms of " acid dyspepsia," and the amount of alkali powders and tablets of proprietary brands purchased by the public and used without medical advice is incredibly large. When used in excess, or even in moderate amount by susceptible individuals, severe alkalosis (p. 553) may result, and it is extraordinary that this serious complication is comparatively seldom encountered in ordinary practice. When correctly used, alkalis are undoubtedly of the utmost value in the treatment of peptic ulcer under a variety of circumstances, and as an ancillary to correct dietetics.

A number of alkalis are available, which differ somewhat in their action, and this matter requires consideration. Sodium bicarbonate (baking powder) neutralizes hydrochloric acid quickly, but is without prolonged action, induces a marked secondary secretion of acid and produces evolution of gas. This last action may at times be of value in flatulence associated with spasmodic obstruction of the pylorus. Calcium carbonate and magnesium carbonate, on the other hand, neutraliz hydrochloric acid slowly over a long period, and are mildly aperient. Since constipation is frequent in peptic ulcer this is generally an advantage, but if their activity on the bowel is too great, bismuth oxycarbonate may be used in combination with them.

A common type of prescription is as follows :—

℞		
	Calc. Carb.	} āā 1 part
	Mag. Carb. Pond. . . .	
	Bism. Carb.	½ part

Mix and make a powder. Send 10 oz.

Sig.—One teaspoonful or more, in water, as directed.

One of the writers has found tribasic magnesium phosphate (ʒi after each meal and ʒii at night) very useful. If too aperient, this may be combined with tribasic calcium phosphate in varying amount to suit the individual case.

Aluminium hydroxide and magnesium trisilicate have recently been used as antacids in the treatment of peptic ulcer, but are still under trial ; there is no proof that they are more valuable in ordinary medical practice than the alkalis already described, but their use is increasing.

Apart from the alkalis, only two other remedies play any real part in the control of gastric secretion, namely, belladonna (or atropine) and olive oil.

Atropine.—It is claimed that belladonna, or its alkaloid atropine, diminish or even abolish gastric secretion, if given in large enough doses. Many physicians, however, are doubtful whether they can safely be used in adequate amounts for this purpose, although they are undoubtedly valuable for the relief of pylorospasm. Certainly belladonna or atropine should be used with care in ambulant patients, and particularly in those who may drive motor cars. The susceptibility of patients, and the effects on the eyes, vary considerably.

Olive Oil, on the other hand, can do no possible harm, and is frequently given to patients suffering from peptic ulcer with great advantage. When taken on an empty stomach it diminishes the flow of gastric juice, relieves flatulence and is a valuable source of food.

Sedatives. — Bromide, either sodium or potassium, in moderate doses of 10 to 20 gr. thrice daily, or phenobarbitone (luminal), 1 to 2 gr., are often required to assist what may be termed the psychological treatment of patients suffering from peptic ulcer. Many of these patients, as has been stated, are nervous and irritable, and after a short course of bromides they frequently describe themselves as " rested," and regain confidence in themselves. The importance of this side of the treatment cannot be overestimated, but is often forgotten.

Larostidin (histidin) was introduced some years ago for the treatment of peptic ulcer. As a result of thorough clinical trials on controlled series of cases it cannot be recommended and should no longer be used.

Iron.—Anæmia as a result of slow leakage from an ulcer is extremely common, and is treated with iron (p. 471).

Surgical Operation in relation to the treatment of peptic ulcer is discussed under Hæmatemesis and Melæna (see below), Pyloric Stenosis (p. 552) and Hour-glass Stomach (p. 553). The special problems which may follow a primary operation for ulcer are referred to on p. 554.

Treatment of Complications

The complications of peptic ulcer are many, and the treatment required for each must be considered in detail.

Hæmatemesis and Melæna.—Bleeding from the stomach may be followed by vomiting (hæmatemesis) or melæna (bleeding from the bowel), and each has the same significance when the origin of the bleeding is a peptic ulcer. The clinical problems of bleeding from dilated œsophageal veins, in portal cirrhosis and splenic anæmia, have already been referred to (p. 497). In some cases the origin of a sudden hæmatemesis may be impossible to trace, but the immediate treatment at least is the same. A grossly enlarged spleen or obvious signs of portal back pressure should not escape clinical observation.

Hæmorrhage from a peptic ulcer varies greatly in amount, and frequently a poor estimate is made by the patient or his friends. It is best, therefore, to rely chiefly on the clinical features. Moreover, it must be remembered that an initial small hæmorrhage may be followed soon after by a very severe one. A single large hæmorrhage from a peptic ulcer is seldom fatal; the notoriously dangerous cases are those in which bleeding is continued or, more commonly, is repeated in attacks at short intervals within a few days.

Immediate Treatment.—The patient who has just had a severe hæmatemesis is pallid, anxious and in a state of shock. An injection of morphine hydrochloride ($\frac{1}{4}$ to $\frac{1}{2}$ gr.) with atropine sulphate ($\frac{1}{100}$ gr.) should be given at once—the larger dose of morphine is generally preferable—and the patient is made as comfortable as possible wherever he may be. After an hour or two it is generally possible to move the patient into bed. The room is kept quiet and semi-darkened, the patient's head is kept low, and the foot of the bed may be raised. A hot-water bottle, carefully covered, is applied to the feet. The patient is then left undisturbed as far as possible for twelve hours, except that a nurse should watch the pulse-rate. After an initial large hæmorrhage smaller ones are by no means infrequent during the same day, and the chief signs the nurse may observe are increasing restlessness and increase in the pulse-rate, which should be recorded every half-hour at first and every hour later. If restlessness supervenes it may be essential to give a further small dose of morphine and atropine.

During the first twelve hours the physician takes stock of the event, amplifies the history, and lays his plans for eventualities and for subsequent treatment.

Subsequent Treatment.—The chief eventuality the physician faces is the possibility of repetition of bleeding, which may easily end in death. Bleeding from a chronic ulcer may recur up to seven days or thereabouts after the initial attack; thereafter the risk is very greatly lessened. Melæna, which follows every hæmatemesis, gives little help as regards the continuation or repetition of hæmorrhage. It is true that fresh melæna is black, viscid and shiny, but old melæna may persist for many days as black masses mixed with normal fæces.

With the possibility of repeated bleeding in mind the physician must always be prepared. There is a consensus of opinion that when a patient dies from hæmatemesis or melæna, the fatal issue results from diminution in the blood volume rather than from loss of the oxygen-carrying red blood corpuscles. Indeed, if simple hæmoglobin estimations are made, it has been found that a fatal issue may ensue when the hæmoglobin percentage is as high as 60 per cent. or more, the blood volume being diminished and little or no dilution to restore it to normal having taken place. It follows that a diminishing hæmoglobin percentage may even be a good sign, indicative of restoration of the blood volume, rather than a sign of danger or further hæmorrhage.

Blood Transfusion.—The above facts naturally lead up to a consideration of the problem of the desirability or necessity of blood transfusion after severe or repeated hæmatemesis.

Nothing can be urged against the restoration of the blood volume by slow administration of glucose saline by the rectum (after an enema) or by the continuous-drip method intravenously or subcutaneously. The question is whether the intravenous transfusion of blood is better, is at times absolutely life-saving and has no contraindications. Even when full facilities for blood transfusion exist, clinical opinion is at present divided as to its desirability and as to what method and amount should be used. As has been indicated the hæmoglobin percentage may be a fallacious guide, and as blood-volume estimations are quite impossible in ordinary practice, the physician must chiefly rely on his own simple clinical observations and on the carefully taken record of the pulse-rate. A single blood transfusion, even of 800 to 1,000 c.c., supplies many red corpuscles, but not a great volume of fluid. Transfusion of 4,000 c.c. (1 pint=568 c.c.) or more of blood from several donors is only possible in very special circumstances. It had been held by some that blood transfusion, by raising blood pressure, might rather increase the tendency to recurrence of hæmorrhage, but this is quite erroneous. On the contrary the transfusion of fresh blood is likely to enhance the deposition of firm clot in the mouth of the bleeding vessel.

On the whole the present position in general practice with regard to blood transfusion after severe hæmatemesis may be summarized as follows.

Most of the fatalities following severe or repeated hæmorrhage from peptic ulcer result from a greatly diminished blood volume and lack of blood in the cerebral centres rather than from diminution of the red blood corpuscles. Our main immediate object in treatment is to restore the volume of the blood to normal. This may often be satisfactorily done by the administration of glucose-saline solution by various routes but it must be remembered that the main effect is temporary In serious cases, particularly of repeated hæmorrhage, in which both blood volume and red corpuscles are very greatly reduced, transfusion of blood may be essential to save life. Thus to face such an emergency the blood group of the patient should, if possible, always be ascertained, and a suitable donor held in readiness. Should the donor be a near relative cross-matching may, at times, be the simplest test.

The Use of Hæmostatics.—No form of hæmostatic agent either introduced into the stomach itself or parenterally in an attempt to increase blood coagulation, has in practice proved of any real value. Calcium, so often given in the past, is useless.

The Problem of Operation.—The risk of operation to stop severe hæmatemesis is at the best very considerable, even when supported by blood transfusion. If there is no previous gastric history, an acute peptic ulcer may be suspected, and operation should never be attempted. There is no external indication of the site of the ulcer, and even if the stomach is opened no obvious bleeding point may be found. A chronic ulcer is generally easily found by palpation of the stomach wall, and the risks of an emergency operation may at times have to be faced. It is certain that if hæmatemesis recurs at intervals over a period of weeks, operation should be advised. This is particularly necessary in chronic bleeding ulcers near the pylorus, when organic stenosis is commonly found.

Dietetics following Hæmatemesis and Melæna.—The problem of feeding the patient after a hæmatemesis only arises when the immediate shock and the restoration of blood volume have been dealt with. This will vary in cases of differing severity, but the question of food does not as a rule arise for the first twenty-four hours while the patient is under morphine. Thirst, when the patient wakes, is generally intense, and small sips of water may be given without fear, chiefly to moisten the dry mouth and tongue. The sucking of ice has entirely disappeared from modern practice.

In a few cases continued vomiting of "coffee-ground" material may seriously delay the commencement of feeding. If the vomiting continues, it becomes a difficult problem and dangerous to life. Atropine in doses of $\frac{1}{100}$ to $\frac{1}{50}$ gr. has been recommended, but is not very effective. In a serious case the doctor is advised to take the risk of passing a stomach tube, and carefully to empty the stomach, using for the lavage a few ounces of warm water several times repeated. Only the mildest suction should be employed, and the stomach tube should be of the large type. The tube used for a fractional test meal is useless and even dangerous. The risk of dislodging clot from the bleeding vessel is obvious, but the risk may be well worth undertaking.

The methods of feeding a patient after a serious hæmatemesis are at present much under discussion, especially since the publications of Meulengracht.

The usual practice was to wait for two or three days after bleeding had ceased, as shown by general clinical symptoms and a steady fall in the pulse-rate, and then begin feeding by the mouth slowly with albumen water, whey, and soon with citrated milk (2 gr. of sodium citrate to each ounce of milk). The citrated milk is gradually increased until 5 to 7 oz. are being taken every three hours. About this time it becomes essential to clear out the lower bowel of melæna by means of repeated but careful wash-outs of saline. Thereafter the dietetic treatment hitherto employed followed as a rule the Lenhartz, Sippy or Hurst régimes for gastric ulcer.

Meulengracht in 1933 astonished the profession by the

publication of excellent results obtained by feeding a large number of cases of hæmatemesis and melæna, from the very outset or as soon as vomiting had ceased, with an abundant purée or sieved diet of great variety and ample caloric value. He argued that exhausted patients sometimes died after the most scrupulous dietetic precautions, while he noticed that in other patients protracted hæmorrhage at once ceased as soon as they had something to eat. He thereupon began to feed his patients on five more or less natural meals per day, two of them—at 1 P.M. and 6 P.M.—being quite large and very varied. Meulengracht's methods have received widespread support on all sides, and the modification recommended by Witts for patients in Britain has been greatly used. At first, quite rightly, this type of feeding of patients after hæmatemesis was tested in large hospitals, but time has already shown that the mortality rate is even less than with the older methods, and it can now be fully recommended in ordinary practice. Fatalities from hæmatemesis are bound to occur, whatever treatment be adopted, but when a series of cases of this kind is carefully scrutinized in the post-mortem room, it is found that in a number of them the fatal hæmorrhage is not due to peptic ulcer at all but to unrecognized portal cirrhosis of the liver or other causes.

Anœmia following Hœmatemesis and Melœna.—This is inevitable in all cases and, moreover, the hæmoglobin is lost to the body by the hæmorrhage. To enable the bone-marrow to react rapidly, iron must therefore be supplied in full doses as in any other type of hypochromic anæmia (p. 471). There is no reason against the commencement of adequate iron therapy as soon as possible after hæmatemesis has ceased.

Perforation.—This may occur either in an acute or chronic peptic ulcer, but particularly in the duodenal variety. The immediate treatment is surgical, and the success of surgery is remarkable even after perforation has existed for a number of hours. The treatment of perigastric adhesions and abscess are not within the scope of this book. The only aspect of perforation of prolonged interest to the physician is when slow leaking perforation occurs, with strictly localized peritonitis and insufficient general signs to demand immediate operation. Such patients should be given morphine and otherwise treated with the same care as if hæmatemesis had occurred.

Pylorospasm and Organic Pyloric Stenosis.—*Spasm.*—The usual evacuation of the stomach contents may be prevented by spasm of the pylorus, which occurs at some time in almost every case of peptic ulcer situated close to the pylorus, whether on the gastric or duodenal side. It is due to reflex irritation of the ulcer stimulating the pyloric sphincter, but it must be remembered that the same condition occurs in association with many other diseases apart from the stomach, for example, gall-stones and chronic appendicitis. The main effects of pylorospasm are pain and flatulence, and the problems of treatment by belladonna and olive oil have already been discussed.

Stenosis.—Organic pyloric stenosis, due to actual cicatrization of an ulcer, presents an entirely different problem. Even here, however, correct diagnosis may not be easy and a radiological report fallacious, since organic constriction due to scarring may be closely simulated by intense pylorospasm or by a combination of œdema and spasm. The effect of medical treatment of pylorospasm, by belladonna or atropine, should always first be tried. Cases of long standing, with enormous dilatation of the stomach, copious vomiting, and active fermentation of the gastric contents are not often seen nowadays, since diagnosis by X-ray examination is so easy. The clinical evidence of active peristalsis, observed only when the stomach contains food or fluid, is also unmistakable. The treatment is always surgical and gastro-enterostomy is generally performed, a course of gastric lavage preceding the operation. In this condition " gastric tetany " may be observed and call for treatment (p. 427).

Hour-glass Stomach.—This complication occurs as a result of scarring and contraction of a peptic ulcer on the lesser curvature of the stomach. The symptoms are often anomalous, and the diagnosis is generally made by X-rays. There must be few physicians interested in gastric disease who have not confidently diagnosed an organic stenosis when at operation none has been found, the hour-glass contraction being entirely due to spasm. Thus a diagnosis of organic hour-glass stomach should not be made too hastily, but the patient should first be treated carefully as for an ordinary gastric ulcer. When true organic stenosis exists, surgery offers the only relief.

Alkalosis following Alkali Treatment.—This complication has already been briefly referred to, and up to the present too few physicians in general practice are aware of its dangers. As a rule it occurs only when alkalis have been taken in great excess, but in some patients it has followed relatively small amounts. The occurrence of frequent vomiting and the existence of organic renal disease are especially liable to induce alkalosis. The cardinal symptoms are headache, nausea, vomiting and drowsiness, and in severe cases the condition may closely simulate uræmia. This similarity is enhanced by the fact that albumen may be found in the alkaline urine, and the blood urea is always high—even up to 300 mg. per cent. The chloride content of the blood is greatly lowered. The treatment consists in the stoppage of alkalis, and the free administration of normal sodium chloride solution by mouth, rectum, or even intravenously when coma threatens. Ammonium chloride (15 gr.) given by the mouth in capsules three or four times daily is also of value.

Medical Aspects of Surgery in Relation to Peptic Ulcer

Apart from perforation, a number of problems affect the physician in relation to the surgical treatment of peptic ulcer and its complications. Some of these, such as organic pyloric stenosis and hour-glass stomach, have already been discussed.

The physician is fairly often faced with the fact that treatment of a case of peptic ulcer has failed, or recurrence has taken place. Failure may be due to a number of causes concerning the patient, his temperament, his non-adherence to rules of treatment, his occupation, his domestic circumstances and other matters outside the doctor's control. Moreover, failure may be due to unsuspected complications. Surgery is then frequently advised, and the commonest operation at present is gastro-enterostomy. On the other hand, partial gastrectomy in suitable cases and under favourable conditions is being more and more frequently carried out.

The decision to advise operation is sometimes difficult, but the following points are those which should influence the physician in recommending surgery.

1. The age of the patient—the older the patient the greater the surgical risk.
2. The duration of the history of ulcer—the possibility of operating on an acute ulcer must always be excluded.
3. The presence of organic pyloric stenosis, with very persistent delay in emptying the stomach. The difficulties of excluding œdema and pylorospasm have been indicated.
4. Failure to obtain cure after fully adequate and prolonged medical treatment. Many failures and recurrences are undoubtedly due to inadequacy of treatment.

5. Failure (willing or unwilling) on the part of the patient to carry out medical treatment, especially when the patient is the bread-winner.
6. Fear of the onset of early carcinoma in prepyloric gastric ulcer.

The choice between gastro-enterostomy and partial gastrectomy raises certain points for consideration, some of which are beyond the scope of this work. The following matters are, however, of general importance :—

1. The immediate surgical risk.
2. The possibility of complications and sequelæ.
3. The possibility of failure to afford relief.

There is no doubt whatever that the operative mortality from partial gastrectomy is much higher than from posterior gastro-enterostomy. Against this may be set the fact that since hyperchlorhydria is common in peptic ulcer, a partial gastrectomy, whereby part at least of the acid-producing pyloric portion of the stomach is excised, must reduce the acidity, whereas gastro-enterostomy is not so successful in this respect. The chief danger of persisting hyperchlorhydria after the simple short-circuiting operation is jejunal ulceration at the stoma, referred to below. A sequel to be remembered after a successful partial gastrectomy is the occasional development of anæmia. Partial gastrectomy is obviously the correct operation if any suspicion of carcinoma arises.

It is impossible to discuss here the opinions of different surgeons, but it may be said fairly that in most cases the first preference is for simple gastro-enterostomy, with its minimal surgical mortality, partial gastrectomy being reserved for special cases and for those in which jejunal ulcer has followed the simpler operation.

Jejunal or Gastro-jejunal Ulceration.—This sequel to gastro-enterostomy is unfortunately fairly common, occurring generally within a year or two, or even less, after the operation. It is believed to depend on persistence of the same set of circumstances in the stomach as before operation, and especially hyperchlorhydria. The new ulcer, situated at the stoma, in no way differs from the ordinary peptic ulcer of the stomach or duodenum, and must be treated on identical and rigid medical lines. If strict treatment fails, the jejunal ulcer may be excised, the stoma closed and a partial gastrectomy carried out. The operative mortality for this operation is naturally high, but it may require to be faced at a suitable time after the occurrence of the most frequent complication of jejunal ulcer, namely, hæmatemesis and melæna. Partial gastrectomy is easier in these circumstances when the original peptic ulcer is in the duodenum or near the pylorus. The operative difficulties are much greater when a deep penetrating ulcer of the lesser curvature is the primary lesion.

Special Medical Treatment before and after Operation.—Whichever operation is carried out, much can be done to ensure a successful result by careful pre-operative treatment. The stomach is often atonic, or emptying greatly delayed, and persistent vomiting with dehydration may have occurred. Except after recent hæmorrhage, the stomach may be gently washed out with warm water, and food for a few days prior to operation should be given in concentrated form (eggs, junket, jellies) with a minimum of residue. Fluids, such as glucose saline, should be supplied subcutaneously or intravenously. By such measures the risk of post-operative dilatation of the stomach is reduced, and the organ to some extent recovers its tonus.

Following operation, precautions are again essential to re-educate the stomach to an entirely new set of anatomical and physiological circumstances. This is particularly necessary after gastro-enterostomy, since a quite unaccustomed bulk of food is rapidly discharged from the stomach into the jejunum through the stoma. In practice it is best to start with a "strict ulcer" diet, and to develop this in amount and variety very slowly. Although many patients after gastro-enterostomy seem to be able to eat "anything and everything" it is most injudicious to allow them to do so.

Failure after Gastro-enterostomy.—Failure after partial gastrectomy raises no discussion, since nothing further can be done. Failure to cure the peptic ulcer after gastro-enterostomy, or even to relieve symptoms, is unfortunately not infrequent (quite apart from the sequel of jejunal ulcer), and requires discussion. Pylorospasm and flatulence are common, and their treatment has already been discussed. Bilious regurgitation from the duodenum, resulting in vomiting, nausea and inability to eat, is sometimes met with when the pyloric sphincter does not function, or functions abnormally. The exact mechanism in these cases is not fully understood and the results are particularly distressing, since medical treatment is of little value. In such patients the question of "undoing" the gastro-enterostomy and closing the stoma will arise, and this treatment may be successful in spite of the known risks of adhesions and their multiplication.

Hurst's Régime of Treatment in Peptic Ulcer (Details supplied by Sir Arthur Hurst)

Strict Ulcer Treatment

The patient should remain in bed on the strict treatment without alteration until healing is complete. This is shown by the disappearance of a radiological niche and of occult blood from the stools. In no case should the strict treatment be for less than four weeks.

1. Every other hour from 8 A.M. to 10 P.M., 5 oz. of milk. This can be warm or cold and may be flavoured with tea.

2. Every other hour from 9 A.M. to 9 P.M., a 5-oz. feed, which may be made of any of the following:—

   (*a*) Arrowroot, farola, Benger, junket, custard. To any of these red currant, apple or other fruit jelly can be added, and the junket may be flavoured with chocolate.

   (*b*) At least two should consist of a thick soup or semi-solid purée of potato, artichoke, cauliflower or parsnip.

During the night the patient should have citrated milk by his bedside, so that whenever he wakes he can take a feed.

3. A rusk with butter should be eaten with three feeds. A "coddled egg" and some thin bread and butter may be taken once or twice a day by patients who can be relied upon to chew them thoroughly.

4. Small quantities of water may be drunk between feeds. An ounce of strained orange juice should be taken with three or four of the drinks.

5. One ounce of cream should be added to the 11 A.M., 1 P.M. and 5 P.M. feeds, and $\frac{1}{2}$ oz. of olive oil should be taken before the 9 A.M., 2 P.M. and 7 P.M. feeds.

6. Ten grains of sodium citrate in a teaspoonful of water should be added to each milk feed.

7. A teaspoonful of atropine mixture (atropine sulphate, $\frac{1}{150}$ gr. in 1 drachm of water) half an hour before the 8 A.M. and 3 P.M. feeds, and 2 teaspoonfuls before the 10 P.M. feed. The dose should be increased by 10 minims every day until an unpleasant degree of dryness of the mouth or paralysis of accommodation occurs; the dose should then be reduced to that of the previous day.

8. Half a teaspoonful of magnesium trisilicate half-way between feeds and a teaspoonful last thing at night.

9. Wash the mouth out after each feed.

10. No smoking during the strict treatment.

11. If there is any constipation a tablespoonful of liquid paraffin can be taken morning and evening.

The patient should be weighed once a week. If he is too thin and has not gained weight, the feeds should be increased to 6 or 7 oz. If he is too fat and has not lost weight, the feeds should be reduced to 4 or 3 oz.

Ulcer Diet. Stage 2

For two or more weeks between strict diet and post-ulcer diet.

I. 9 *a.m. and* 4 *p.m.*—A tablespoonful of olive oil and a teaspoonful of the atropine mixture a quarter of an hour before the meals.

Weak milky tea.

One or two lightly boiled, poached or scrambled eggs.

Thin bread and butter or toast.

II. 1 *p.m. and* 7 *p.m.*—A tablespoonful of olive oil and a teaspoonful of the atropine mixture a quarter of an hour before the meals.

Fish or chicken with mashed potatoes and other vegetable purées.

Custard and junket, etc.

III. 8 *and* 10.30 *a.m.*, 12, 3, 5.30, 8.30 *and* 10 *p.m.*—Five ounces of citrated creamy milk.

IV. Half a teaspoonful of magnesium trisilicate in water half an hour after each of four meals and again at 9 P.M.

V. A teaspoonful of the atropine mixture at 10 P.M.

VI. The bowels should be kept regular by means of paraffin (1 teaspoonful to 1 tablespoonful once or twice a day) and magnesium hydroxide mixture (B.P.) or milk of magnesia (1 teaspoonful with one or more of the milk feeds).

N.B.—All articles of food allowed in strict diet may also be taken in Stage 2.

Post-ulcer Régime. (*To be followed permanently*)

Avoid alcohol except, if desired later on, a small quantity of light wine or diluted whisky at meals. Avoid effervescing drinks and coffee, except kaffee Hag.

Avoid all pips and skins of fruit (raw, cooked or in jam),

and currants, raisins and lemon-peel in pudding and cake, nuts and all unripe fruit. An orange may be sucked but not eaten. Currants, raisins and figs are particularly undesirable.

Avoid all raw vegetables, whether taken alone (celery, tomatoes, cucumber, water-cress) or in pickles and salad; green vegetables must be passed through a sieve and mixed with butter in the form of a purée. Avoid spinach. Porridge is only allowed if made with the finest oatmeal.

Avoid vinegar, lemon juice, sour fruit; fried fish; pepper, mustard, curry, chutney, excess of salt; new bread; very ripe cheese and cooked cheese; tough meat; pork, made-up and fried dishes, high game, clear and thick meat soup. During the first six months after recovery from an ulcer it is best to avoid meat altogether.

Take plenty of butter and cream and a tablespoonful of olive oil before each meal.

Eat slowly and chew very thoroughly. An adequate time should be allowed for meals; rest for at least a quarter of an hour before and after meals. Meals must be punctual.

Do not smoke excessively; cigarettes should have a plug of wool in the mouth-piece. No smoking at all if any indigestion.

For the first six months: A meal or feed of milk, plain biscuit or plain chocolate should be taken at intervals of not more than two hours from waking till retiring, and again if awake during the night.

After six months of complete freedom from symptoms: A feed should be taken in the middle of the morning, on going to bed, and again if awake during the night, in addition to breakfast, lunch, tea and dinner.

A teaspoonful or 2 crushed tablets of "magsorbent" (magnesium trisilicate—Kaylene Co.) should be taken an hour after meals and also directly the slightest indigestion or heartburn is felt. If the curve of acidity is very high, the atropine mixture should be taken before meals and last thing at night.

The bowels should be kept regular by means of magnesia and liquid paraffin, but no other aperients should be taken.

Have your teeth attended to regularly every six months.

Take no drugs in tablet form.

Special care should be taken to avoid chills. If you get a cold, sore-throat, influenza or other infection, remain in bed on a very light diet until you have completely recovered.

If you have the slightest return of symptoms, go to bed on a strict diet and consult your doctor, and do not wait for the symptoms to get serious.

Dietetic Treatment of Gastro-duodenal Hæmorrhage (Modified from Meulengracht)

Arranged for Two-hourly Feeding

(Witts, *Brit. Med. Jour.* (1937), i., 851)

Feeds by Day.	Food.		Day. 1.	2.	3 and subsequent.
1	Whole milk (fresh or dried)	oz.	5	5	5
	Patent barley or strained porridge	.	Portion	Portion	Portion
2	1 egg beaten up in milk	oz.	5	5	5
	Buttered rusks or cream crackers	.	...	1	2
3	Whole milk (fresh or dried)	oz.	5	5	5
	Marmite to taste	.	...	...	...
	Barley sugar	oz.	1	1	1
	Thin crustless white bread and butter	slices	...	1	2
4	Strained orange or tomato juice	oz.	1	1	1
	Vegetable purée	.	Portion	Portion	Portion
	Pudding	.	,,	,,	,,
	Cream	oz.	1	1	1
	Boiled or steamed fish	.	...	...	Portion
5	1 egg beaten up in milk	oz.	5	5	5
	Barley sugar	oz.	1	1	1
	Butter rusks or cream crackers	.	...	1	2
6	Whole milk (fresh or dried)	oz.	5	5	5
	Fruit purée	.	Portion	Portion	Portion
	Pudding	.	,,	,,	,,
	Cream	oz.	...	1	1
	Thin crustless white bread and butter	slices	...	1	2
7	1 egg beaten up in milk	oz.	5	5	5
	Black treacle or barley sugar	oz.	1	1	1
	Buttered rusks or cream crackers	.	...	1	2
8	Whole milk (fresh or dried)	oz.	5	5	5
	Fruit purée	.	Portion	Portion	Portion
	Pudding	.	,,	,,	,,
Feeds at Night (when awake)	1. Whole milk (fresh or dried)	oz.	5	5	5
	2. 1 egg beaten up in milk	oz.	5	5	5
Between Feeds	Strained orange or tomato juice	oz.	1	1	1
Approximate caloric value			2,545	3,118	3,624

CANCER OF THE STOMACH

The majority of cases of cancer of the stomach are at present unfortunately not recognized until radical operation is impossible, and the physician is only concerned with palliative treatment. Our aim must therefore be, even in the present very uncertain state of our knowledge, to attempt to prevent the occurrence of cancer of the stomach or to recognize its onset at the earliest possible stage.

It is suspected by many that chronic organic gastritis is a frequent precursor of carcinoma, and gastritis should receive adequate treatment.

It is known that cancer of the stomach may be superimposed on chronic peptic ulcer, and especially on the so-called prepyloric ulcer. A chronic peptic ulcer in this dangerous situation should thus receive very special care to ensure permanent cure.

The early diagnosis of cancer of the stomach is not within the scope of this book, but unexplained sudden dyspepsia in men over forty should always be regarded with suspicion, and radiological investigation at once undertaken. In cases of cancer of the stomach recognized sufficiently early, partial gastrectomy does offer a chance—the only chance—of permanent cure. Deep X-ray and radium treatment have been so far unsuccessful. If pyloric stenosis, due to the tumour, is extreme, a palliative gastro-enterostomy may be done, but the operative mortality in such cases is high and life is seldom much prolonged. No operation should ever be attempted if the liver is found to be involved.

The physician is most commonly concerned with palliative treatment, mainly directed towards the relief of gastric discomfort and to procuring adequate sleep. Death usually occurs within six to twelve months after the diagnosis has been made.

The most common site of carcinoma is near the pylorus, and signs of pyloric obstruction quickly appear. The stomach behind the growth becomes dilated and atonic, and hydrochloric acid is absent from the gastric juice. Fermentation of food, delayed greatly in its passage through the pylorus, is inevitable and pus and debris derived from an ulcerating growth add to the patient's discomfort. Lavage of the stomach is therefore frequently required, sometimes several times a day, weak bicarbonate of soda solution (ʒi to 1 pint of warm water) being commonly employed. The diet, when pyloric obstruction is obvious, should be liquid or semi-solid only, but within limits it is often best to let the patient choose what he desires.

36

Odd fancies may emerge, and ice-cream was the only food tolerated and desired by one of the writer's patients.

Sleep may be obtained in the early stages by mild hypnotics such as adalin (carbromol), 10 to 15 gr. at night, but sooner or later opium will be required both for sleep and to alleviate pain and discomfort. Tincture of opium or nepenthe, 20 to 30 minims of either, three times daily, may be given by the mouth, and finally the subcutaneous injection of morphine will be necessary. The usual dose of $\frac{1}{4}$ to $\frac{1}{2}$ gr. may suffice at first, but tolerance soon develops and the dosage should be raised until mental rest from pain is obtained.

Anæmia always develops in carcinoma of the stomach, and may show temporary improvement under treatment with liver extracts and iron.

Various complications, such as jaundice from secondary deposits in the liver, pleural effusion and femoral thrombosis, may all entail alterations or additions in treatment.

One rare variety of cancer of the stomach—leather-bottle stomach—presents many points of difference from the ordinary type. It is very slow in growth—there are proved cases of ten to fifteen years' duration—and pyloric obstruction does not ensue. The stomach, in fact, comes to resemble a long narrow inelastic tube, through which the contents can be seen to hurry during examination by X-rays. Emaciation becomes extreme, being only equalled in carcinoma of the œsophagus, and feeding is unsatisfactory. Milk, eggs, junket and fruit juices are generally acceptable, and alcohol (as spirits or sweet wines) may also be taken. Pain is often considerable in the later stages, and opium by the mouth is generally required. In this very chronic type of carcinoma it may eventually be necessary to administer quantities of opium far in excess of the usual fatal dose.

ANOREXIA NERVOSA

(*Hysterical Anorexia*)

This serious functional disorder is much commoner in females than in males, and occurs especially in adolescence and early adult life. The psychological causes are many, but whatever the origin of the condition the clinical progress is the same. The patient declines to eat, and after a time all desire for food is lost. Emaciation rapidly ensues, and unless treatment is successful death may result simply from starvation. The prognosis depends entirely on the possibility of alleviating the psychological origin of the disorder.

In by far the majority of patients removal from home surroundings is essential and the treatment is psychological. The closest co-operation between the physician and a carefully chosen nurse is required. Every attempt must be made by persuasion to feed the patient frequently, a mouthful at a time, and even when improvement begins the nurse must never leave the sickroom when food is before the patient.

In very severe cases, in which a fatal issue is threatening, glucose must be administered, preferably by the mouth, but otherwise by the rectum or intravenously, and at the same time small doses of insulin (10 to 20 units daily) may be injected with advantage.

SOME COMMON DISORDERS OF DIGESTION

Flatulence.—This has many causes, and is of two varieties—gastric and intestinal—both of which may be present together.

Intestinal flatulence, resulting in the passage of flatus from the bowel, occurs in many organic diseases of the bowel, but also in their absence. The gas results from imperfect digestion of starch, and so starchy foods, especially potatoes, cakes and pastry, should be greatly curtailed. Charcoal, which acts as an absorbent, is useful in doses of 1 to 4 teaspoonfuls in milk three times daily.

Gastric flatulence is of very varying significance, and may be manifested merely by a sensation of fullness and distension or by actual eructations of "wind." Severe distension may at times simulate the pain of angina pectoris.

The causes of gastric flatulence may be functional or organic. By far the commonest functional variety is painless and caused by aerophagy or air swallowing, a habit easily established and difficult to eradicate. In some patients a simple explanation of the facts is sufficient for cure, but others often resent the accusation and strongly deny that they are "air-swallowers." A piece of cork held between the molar teeth or a piece of tape tied quite lightly round the neck just above the larynx will each prevent the occurrence of aerophagy. Flatulence of organic gastric origin occurs in peptic ulcer of all varieties and in carcinoma, and its treatment is discussed elsewhere. The commonest and most persistent gastric flatulence due to organic disease is associated with disease of the gall-bladder, especially gall-stones (p. 619), and its treatment is described under that heading.

Water-brash.—Water-brash consists in the outpouring of

dilute saliva which suddenly fills the mouth. Its exact mechanism is unknown, but it may occur at intervals in almost every form of organic gastric disease. No treatment is possible except for the associated disease.

Hiccup.—This very troublesome symptom is due to sudden spasm of the diaphragm, and again is of very varying significance and importance. It may occur from quickly overfilling the stomach with food or drink, and is then arrested by holding the breath or by inducing sneezing. On the other hand, persistent hiccup, which exhausts the patient, is a sign of many important organic diseases of the bowel and elsewhere, and may be troublesome after operations in the upper abdomen. It occurs in encephalitis lethargica, intestinal obstruction, uræmia, hepatic cirrhosis, carcinoma of the stomach, to name only a few examples. The treatment of persistent hiccup is discussed in the section on Cirrhosis of the Liver (p. 614).

Heartburn.—This term is used to describe a peculiar burning sensation presumed to be in the œsophagus, but its exact situation and ætiology are very obscure. It was formerly thought to be due to regurgitation of acid from the stomach into the œsophagus, but it is now known that it may occur even when achlorhydria is present. A drink of sodium bicarbonate as a rule affords relief.

Nausea.—This symptom, which it is difficult to describe better than "a feeling of sickness unaccompanied by actual vomiting," is also met with in a number of bodily disturbances, quite apart from gastro-intestinal disease. It is complained of frequently in the early months of pregnancy, in migraine, in ocular astigmatism, in fainting, and in diseases of the stomach and gall-bladder. It may be one of the very earliest symptoms of carcinoma of the stomach, and is a constant feature of alcoholic gastritis. The treatment required is concerned with the cause, and no individual therapeutic description is possible.

SOME UNCOMMON DISEASES OF THE STOMACH AND DUODENUM

Syphilis is rare and affects the stomach as a gummatous infiltration resulting in deformity or a mass large enough at times to be mistaken for carcinoma. The resemblance to carcinoma is enhanced, since hydrochloric acid is absent or greatly diminished.

If syphilis is suspected, either from the history or from the evidence of a positive Wassermann reaction, a rapid trial of antisyphilitic treatment (p. 206) should be carried out. There appears to be a consensus of opinion in countries in which gastric syphilis is more common that potassium iodide in full doses is superior to the arsenical remedies. It must always be remembered that a positive Wassermann reaction does not exclude in any way a diagnosis of carcinoma.

Acute dilatation due to sudden atony is met with occasionally after upper abdominal operations, and rarely during the course of acute specific fevers and pneumonia. The characteristic symptom is persistent vomiting of large quantities of dark but not fæcal fluid (" black vomiting "), which may pour out of the mouth unaccompanied by retching. Collapse and dehydration are extreme, and treatment is always urgent. A narrow stomach tube, as used for the fractional test meal, is passed at once, and the stomach kept empty by repeated aspiration. Shock and dehydration are dealt with by the methods described elsewhere. Unless symptoms cease within forty-eight hours, jejunostomy should be carried out, if necessary under local anæsthesia, and the patient fed by this route until the stomach has recovered its tone.

Chronic Duodenal Ileus (or Stasis).—This uncommon condition is believed to be due to visceroptosis, to some congenital malformation or to an anatomical variation in the position of the mesenteric arteries which cross the duodenum. Diagnosis is difficult without confirmation by X-rays, and the symptoms are anomalous. Persistent headache, vomiting and pain simulating duodenal ulcer or cholecystitis are among the most common complaints.

Visceroptosis should be treated as described elsewhere (p. 580), and rest after meals in a position found by experience to give relief should always be advised. In some patients administration of a pint of normal saline on an empty stomach flushes out the duodenum and arrests the symptoms. In severe cases surgical measures such as colopexy and duodeno-jejunostomy have been carried out, but surgery in this condition must still be regarded as in an experimental stage.

DISEASES OF THE INTESTINES

Introduction

It would be convenient to be able to consider treatment under the separate headings of small intestine and colon, but in practical medicine this is generally impossible. In many diseases both the small and large intestine are involved, although in different ways and in differing degrees. Few diseases capable at present of exact definition, interpretation and rational treatment affect the small intestine; many more affect the colon, and are described separately in textbooks.

Chemical Functions.—The small intestine is concerned, over its great length and surface-area with the digestion and absorption of food, the main absorption taking place in the last part of the ileum. So far as treatment is concerned the functions of the small intestine may be upset in two chief ways:—

1. There may be deficiency of absorption of normal essential substances—products of digestion of proteins, carbohydrates and fats, and the necessary vitamins and minerals. Defective absorption may at times be due to undue rapidity of passage through the ileum, thereby affecting the function of the large intestine.
2. There may be absorption of substances injurious to the body—poisons (organic and inorganic), bacterial toxins.

These two conditions obviously involve entirely different lines of rational treatment.

The normal functions of the colon are chiefly concerned with excretion. About 350 gm. of chyme, containing very small amounts of the products of digestion and 90 per cent. of water, normally pass through the ileocæcal valve in a day (Hurst). The average weight of fæces passed daily is 135 gm., containing 75 per cent. of water, and no sugar, coagulable protein or other soluble substances. Thus absorption of much water and of the small amount of nutritive substances which enter the cæcum take place in the proximal colon. The distal colon and rectum merely act as reservoirs, until the important reflex act of defæcation occurs, and this obviously has important bearings on the question of so-called "rectal feeding" and "nutrient enemata."

Intestinal Movements.—The movements of the small intestine are chiefly of two kinds—active and frequent peristalsis causing rapid movement and mixing of chyme, and slower segmentation. The upper part of the small intestine escapes the brunt of many diseases because of the rapidity of passage of its contents, but as the lower ileum is reached, where the main absorption of digestive products takes place, the passage is slower, and this part of the small gut is generally most seriously involved and injured. The rationale for increasing peristalsis and hurrying material through the bowel in certain diseases is thus plainly seen.

The normal movements of the colon are quite different, and have been described as "mass movements." A single powerful peristaltic wave, occurring only at long intervals, pushes along a large mass of material.

The rectum is chiefly concerned with the finely adjusted reflex act of defæcation.

Bacterial Flora.—The bacterial flora of the intestine has important bearings on treatment, quite apart from the problems created by the presence of invading and pathogenic micro-organisms. In the adult, streptococci predominate in the upper part of the small intestine, but in the ileum, with its slower movements, coliform organisms predominate. These facts have been proved in samples taken during surgical operations. In the colon and rectum an enormous number and variety of micro-organisms abound, many of them saprophytic and harmless, but other normal inhabitants, such as streptococci, coliform bacilli, and gas-gangrene bacilli, may become pathogenic. The distribution of the bacterial flora in the whole length of the intestines may be greatly changed in disease, but also, a point of much importance, may be considerably influenced by treatment.

Nervous Mechanism.—The nervous control of the bowel, as it affects not only the ordinary intestinal movements but the reflex act of defæcation, is of the utmost importance in intestinal disease and its treatment. The control is a dual one, both local and central, and rational treatment may be required either to influence the bowel locally or to influence the whole patient through his central nervous system.

DIARRHŒA

Diarrhœa consists essentially in the passage of loose or watery stools. A very rough distinction may be made between diarrhœa arising in the small intestine and that commencing only in the colon; in the former the motions tend to be watery, in the latter only loose and unformed. The stools in diarrhœa may contain excess of fat or starch, blood, pus, excess of mucus, abnormal pigments or deficiency of pigments. The necessity for careful examination, both naked eye and by the microscope, cannot be over-emphasized in order to ensure correct diagnosis and treatment.

Common general varieties of diarrhœa are :—

1. Infective and toxic.
2. Gastrogenous.
3. Nervous and lienteric.
4. So-called carbohydrate dyspepsia.
5. Pancreatic and fatty.
6. Endocrine, *e.g.*, in Graves' Disease.

Infective and Toxic Diarrhœa.—The toxic and infective group is by far the largest, and correct diagnosis is very essential for treatment. The whole range cannot be covered here, but this group includes food poisoning, dysentery, typhoid fever, organic and inorganic poisons, ulcerative colitis, and the toxic diarrhœa of nephritis. Special and specific methods of treatment are found elsewhere, but general principles applicable to most cases (excluding infants and children, p. 283) may be considered in detail.

These general principles are :—

Rest in Bed and Warmth.—This is essential when the diarrhœa is severe and especially if fever is present. Warmth to the abdomen is best applied in these cases by rubber hot-water bottles easily laid aside when the bowels are moved. Poultices and hot wet applications are nowadays no longer required. When fever is absent, and especially in collapse, hot bottles to the feet may also be desirable.

Starvation, but Adequate Supply of Fluid.—In this important aspect of treatment much turns on whether the stomach is also involved in the infective or toxic condition. In such circumstances food of every kind should be strictly withheld in the early stages. Fluids must be given by other routes to combat the rapid dehydration, which may be serious in an adult but still more serious in infancy and childhood. If the effects of a known poison are recognized, or a clear history is obtained, the appropriate antidote is administered and the stomach should be washed out. If the stomach is not seriously involved and vomiting is absent, plain water should be given at frequent intervals by the mouth. Both very hot and very cold drinks are well recognized to increase the symptoms, and should be avoided. When vomiting is present, the fluid must be introduced by intravenous or slow subcutaneous injection (for Technique, see p. 1075). For intravenous use a sterile solution of 0·85 per cent. (*i.e.*, normal) sodium chloride with 6 per cent. glucose added is employed ; for slow "drip" injection normal salt solution alone is required. Occasionally as in bacillary dysentery, it may be valuable treatment to introduce, directly into the stomach, through a fine tube (as used for fractional test meals), a pint of warm normal saline. This is not absorbed, but passes rapidly through the whole length of the intestine, washing out debris and toxins in a watery diarrhœa. The special methods to replace fluids and make up for the great loss of chlorides which occur in cholera are described elsewhere (p. 242).

Diet.—When an exact diagnosis has been made, the problem of feeding the patient at once arises, and the arrangements to be made must differ greatly in, for instance, long diseases such as enteric fever and short illnesses such as the simpler forms of food poisoning. In the latter, when after two or three days the acute symptoms are passing off, the complete rule of starvation must be relaxed, and feeding commenced slowly. Barley water is often used as the first change from water, but the actual feeding is best begun with arrowroot made up with water only, not with milk. Whey may also be acceptable at this stage, or gelatin preparations such as Brand's essence. Later, milk and junket and sweetened fruit juices are commenced, and gradually as the patient improves the full diet is restored.

Drugs. These may be required for three main purposes :—

(*a*) To provide an antidote to a known poison.

(*b*) To exaggerate an acute diarrhœa and quickly rid the bowel of an irritant. This method is particularly suitable in the ordinary simple forms of gastro-enteritis, and castor oil ($\frac{1}{2}$ to 1 oz.) is the most valuable drug and has stood the test of time. It acts by increasing the peristalsis of the whole gastro-intestinal tract, and no part of the oil is absorbed. Saline purgatives (sodium and magnesium sulphate, $\frac{1}{2}$ to 1 oz. in hot water) are much used in bacillary dysentery to wash out the bowel, and the method of introducing 1 pint of normal saline into the stomach in this disease has already been described.

Calomel in small doses ($\frac{1}{12}$ to $\frac{1}{8}$ gr.) given at two-hourly intervals has also many advocates, but is much less used than formerly.

(*c*) To arrest, or partially to arrest, severe and continuing diarrhœa which is weakening the patient by exhaustion, dehydration, pain or sleeplessness.

Opium and its alkaloids, and kaolin are the two important remedies required ; bismuth preparations, tincture of catechu and chalk are useful adjuvants and astringents. Morphine ($\frac{1}{6}$ to $\frac{1}{4}$ gr.) or codeine ($\frac{1}{4}$ gr.) may be injected in adults, and a very well-known mixture for oral administration in adults is as follows :—

℞	Tinct. Opii . . .	♏v to ♏x
	Tinct. Catech. . . .	ʒi
	Mist. Cret. . .	ad ℥i

Sig.—℥i two hourly, or as required.

Kaolin, a china clay, which is a most efficient adsorbent, is particularly useful in chronic diarrhœa, and is often combined with charcoal if much abdominal flatulence and distension is present. Kaolin is not absorbed from the bowel, and large doses may be given, simply mixed with water. An average dose is $\frac{1}{2}$ to 1 oz.

Griping and tenesmus, which exhaust the patient, are best relieved by opium or belladonna and by the application of heat to the abdomen. Suppositories should seldom be employed, and a starch enema (the opium often added is useless) has very limited applications.

When abdominal distension is severe, turpentine stupes applied to the abdomen are very successful, although their mode of action is unknown, as are kaolin and charcoal by the mouth. A turpentine stupe is prepared by wringing out lint or flannel from hot water, and sprinkling the lint with oil of turpentine. This is applied to the abdomen for half to three-quarters of an hour. It should be removed when redness but not vesication has taken place.

(*d*) To treat circulatory collapse. This occurs only in the severest forms of continued diarrhœa, and apart from warmth and large quantities of fluid, which are essential, any of the following drugs may on occasion be required :—

Alcohol (in certain cases only).

Adrenalin (1 to 5 minims of 1 : 1,000 solution intravenously or 5 to 10 minims intramuscularly).

Coramine (Ciba) (1 to 2 c.c. by subcutaneous injection).

(*e*) To change the bacterial flora of the bowel. This method has a very limited application, but in some forms of chronic diarrhœa it may be useful to administer *Bacillus acidophilus*. Spriggs recommends that 4 oz. of a pure culture of *B. acidophilus* should be given daily in a single dose in milk, and care must be taken that the culture is obtained from a reliable source which will guarantee that the organisms are alive and viable. In most samples a minimal bacterial count of 250 millions per c.c. is guaranteed and the directions state the period after preparation within which the culture must be used. Lactose should be taken freely with every meal to provide abundant pabulum for the bacillus —controlled experiments have clearly shown that this is an essential part of the treatment.

Gastrogenous Diarrhœa.—This special variety can only be suspected when no free hydrochloric acid is found to be present in the stomach after a test meal. The treatment is simple and consists in the administration of dilute hydrochloric acid in 1-drachm doses mixed with lemonade or orange juice to be drunk throughout the course of the meals.

Nervous and Lienteric Diarrhœa.—This is more a social trouble than an actual disease, but its occurrence can be devastating to an individual who must attend a public dinner and make a speech, or to a student sitting an important examination. Irritant foods and spices must be avoided beforehand and neither very hot nor ice-cold dishes should be taken. A sedative drug should be employed, and sodium bromide (5 to 10 gr.), luminal ($\frac{1}{2}$ to 1 gr.) and tincture of belladonna (5 to 10 minims) may be tried in turn or in combination, to control the diarrhœa. Closely allied to this form of diarrhœa is the "hair-trigger colon" which often afflicts patients who have suffered from severe enteritis, such as dysentery, it may be several years previously. Such patients are particularly susceptible to chill and whenever they are cold (*e.g.*, after a journey in an open motor car) diarrhœa which is quite uncontrollable may return for a few hours. Such patients learn to avoid chill and should wear for a long period a "cholera belt" (the modern variety of silk and wool is best) around their abdomen.

Intestinal Carbohydrate Dyspepsia.—The diagnosis of this condition is often missed if the stools are not properly examined for starch granules. The essential clinical features are abdominal discomfort and great gaseous distension of the colon, due to fermentation of starch which has passed too rapidly through the small intestine and escaped its proper digestion there. The main point here again is accurate diagnosis, and treatment is very effective. It consists, first, in avoiding or diminishing starchy foods for a time, and using sugars as the main supply of carbohydrates. Taka-diastase (Parke, Davis & Co.), a powerful starch-splitting ferment, is of great value, and enables some starchy foods to be taken. It is available both as a powder or tablet (adult dose, $2\frac{1}{2}$ to 5 gr.), or as a liquid (adult dose, 1 to 2 fluid drachms), taken during or immediately after each meal. Charcoal and kaolin are useful if colonic distension is present. Rarely, at the outset, it may be necessary to use an opium derivative (codein phosphate, $\frac{1}{4}$ gr. or omnopon (Hoffman-La Roche), $\frac{1}{6}$ to $\frac{1}{3}$ gr. to reduce the rapid passage of food through the small intestine With the above treatment the small intestine can generally be retrained to deal with starch quite effectively.

Pancreatic and Fatty Diarrhœa.—See p. 591, “Idiopathi Steatorrhœa.”

Diarrhœa in Graves' Disease.—This may be a particularly troublesome symptom, and may occur either as an early symptom of the disease when the clinical features are no striking, or in the late stages even after an extensive radica operation.

The treatment is difficult and may be long continued, so opium is best avoided. Less powerful intestinal sedatives are often of little avail, and iodine has not had, in the writer' hands, any beneficial result. Two methods are claimed to b successful in a number of cases. Eppinger and van Noorden (1911) introduced the use of rectal injection of adrenalin. An enema is made up of 200 to 300 c.c. of warm water to which 25 to 30 drops of 1 : 1,000 solution of adrenalin is added. Th action is local, and no general effects are observed. Recentl the use of glycerin extracts of suprarenal cortex, such as ar used for Addison's disease and its associated gastro-intestina disturbances, have also been claimed to be effective in th diarrhœa of Graves' disease. (Eschatin (Parke, Davis & Co. cortine (British Organon), dose 5 to 10 c.c. subcutaneously o intramuscularly.)

A large number of cases of chronic diarrhœa sent t hospital because no accurate diagnosis can be made, an because simple treatment is unavailing, prove to be due t some form of partial intestinal obstruction and often to tumou growth in the colon. The diagnosis is generally made b

X-ray examination. If, after complete examination, no signs of tumour are found, the doctor must think of such conditions as ulcerative colitis, uræmia, Addison's disease, tuberculosis of the intestine, amyloid disease, or even chronic arsenical poisoning.

CONSTIPATION

Constipation may be defined as delay in the passage of fæces through the intestine, or delay in their evacuation. Before commencing to treat a case of constipation it is necessary to know that this condition truly exists, and that the patient has not simply "lost confidence in his bowels" (Hutchison). It is therefore generally wise at the outset to stop, for two days at least, all drugs which the patient has generally been taking and watch the result. It must be remembered also that incomplete evacuation of the bowel may constitute constipation just as much as no action at all.

It is essential to have some simple classification on which rational treatment is based. One broad classification may be made at once into organic and functional types. Organic constipation is less common but more serious, and depends generally on some mechanical obstruction or partial obstruction of the lumen of the intestine. The obstruction may be within the bowel—tumour, stricture, foreign body or fæcal impaction—or due to pressure from without—tumour, adhesions, chronic peritonitis. The treatment required is often surgical. Severe abdominal pain, or paralysis of the bowel, may produce the same clinical effects as mechanical obstruction. Functional constipation is exceedingly common, and forms one of the most important chapters in all medical treatment.

Hurst's classification of true or functional constipation is as follows :—

1. Colonic constipation—due to defective movements of the musculature of the colon. The movements may be deficient, or excessive (resulting in spasm—spastic colon).
2. Dyschezia—due to imperfect action of the reflex act of defæcation.
3. Deficiency in bulk of the fæces—due to incorrect feeding, or to unusually complete digestion ("greedy bowel"). In this group the rectum is insufficiently distended to excite the reflex act of defæcation.

Since we may regard the more usual type of constipation which the physician is called on to treat as functional and not organic (this latter type having first been carefully excluded), the following principles must be considered in relation to treatment.

Psychic Factors.—The influence of the mind on the ætiology of constipation (as on some of the problems of diarrhœa) is common knowledge. Some patients simply cannot move their bowels when nervous or worried, in unusual surroundings such as travel, or even at the commencement of a holiday. Workers on alternate day and night shifts are also at a disadvantage, and may be very worried at failure of a previously regular habit. Bodily fatigue is another factor of importance. In all these circumstances the nervous individual may develop great anxiety about his bowels, he begins to take purgatives without advice, and a vicious habit is established.

The general line of treatment is obvious—reassurance that occasional failure of the bowels to act is of no consequence, and that purgatives are quite unnecessary. A sedative mixture alone may be sufficient, along with reassurance, to cure this form of constipation almost at once.

Faulty Habits of Defæcation.—This is certainly one of the worst types of constipation to treat, and is often contracted in childhood and at school. Civilization has brought about many changes in our habits, and defæcation after every meal, still common in savage races, is uncommon with us. Custom has gradually trained most people so that the reflex act of defæcation functions once a day, usually in the morning and most commonly after breakfast. This habit is the result of gradual training. In modern conditions the rush to school, or to catch the morning train may greatly interfere with the habit, unless ample time is allowed ; and the sensation of the "call to stool," once voluntarily suppressed may not easily return again throughout the day. Many schools and offices are very inadequately provided with the necessary conveniences, and there is much room for medical opinion to aid in remedying these matters. Once the habit of regular defæcation is completely broken, the patient becomes constipated and uncomfortable, and as a rule at once takes to cathartic drugs or to enemas and injections. These bad habits and errors in treatment may persist for life, unless training is established and drugs eliminated.

Physical Exercise assists regular bowel movements and improvements in this matter throughout the town-dwelling population have been enormous during the past twenty-five years. Apart from games and the ordinary types of physical activity, adapted as far as possible to the patient's desires and preferences, certain specialized forms of physical exercise are of particular value in constipated patients whose abdominal musculature is weak. These are known as "Swedish exercises," and numerous small books on the methods employed are available. Riding, rowing, skipping and gardening are all valuable for selected patients. When active exercise is impossible, thorough abdominal massage may be essential.

Diet.—Constipation is very frequently the result of faulty diet. The diet may be too dry or too concentrated, and the remedy is to increase the fluid intake. A well-known simple remedy is the early morning drink of a glass of hot water and, as Kantor points out, this remedy is of particular physiological interest. It is only at this time that the stomach and small intestine are empty, and the hot water passes rapidly through to the colon and excites its movements. The diet may be deficient, especially among the poorer citizens, in foods which add the necessary bulk to the fæces to excite the reflex act of defæcation, or slightly irritate the bowel and increase peristalsis. Examples of the first group are vegetables such as lettuce, spinach, cabbage, cauliflower, onions, turnips, and "rough" cereals such as wholemeal and bran. The indigestible skins and seeds of fruits, many of which also contain mild cathartic organic acids, increase peristalsis. Examples are prunes, figs, apples, pears, etc.

An adequate amount of fat, especially butter, is of recognized value, being the normal stimulant for the outflow of bile into the intestine. Olive oil may be used as a medicine for the same purpose, either by itself or as mayonnaise with salads.

Drugs.—Constipation being usually a functional disease, drugs should play a very minor part in its rational treatment. Nevertheless it will be found in practical medicine that the physician must employ them in the earlier stages of treatment, and he must also use them for longer periods, even for life, in certain types of patient. For example :—

1. Patients who fail to respond to general advice, either from carelessness or lack of intelligence. Such patients always have to resort to drugs, and it is best that the physician should advise those which are most suitable.
2. Elderly patients, and chronic invalids suffering from paralysis, heart disease, etc.
3. Patients temporarily bedridden by illness, accident or surgical operations.
4. The residue of cases which for any reason fail to respond to rational treatment without drugs.

The general rules of drug treatment for constipation are :—

1. Avoid all severe purges and cathartics for regular or frequent use, for example, castor oil is a valuable purge, but harmful for regular use.
2. Almost all drugs used for constipation tend to lose, after a time, their original efficiency—the patient's body becomes habituated to them.
3. Drugs used for constipation vary in the period required for their action—the dose must therefore be given at the correct time to ensure a morning evacuation.
4. A suitable dose must be found, which differs greatly in individuals, to give a single soft but not watery motion.

The number of drugs employed for constipation is endless ; only those of proved value, with their special indications, need be mentioned.

Alkaloids which act on nerve endings in the bowel. The alkaloid most commonly used in gastro-intestinal disease is atropine (or belladonna). It is of great value in spastic colon (*q.v.*). Strychnine is a frequent constituent of pills and mixtures, but is probably of little value for increasing peristalsis in the dosage commonly employed.

Vegetable Purgatives and Laxatives, which act either by increasing peristalsis or as mild irritants to the bowel wall. Some of the chief members of this group belong to the anthracene series and include cascara sagrada, senna, aloes, rhubarb and phenolphthalein (a synthetic anthracene). All of these are useful for special purposes, and a most important point common to all is that they have less tendency to lose their efficiency after continuous use than other drugs employed for constipation. Senna and rhubarb are the most drastic, and unless the dose is carefully arranged may act in as short a time as four or five hours. Rhubarb suffers from the disability that constipation follows its use, and it is only suitable, but very valuable, as an occasional purge. Gregory's powder (which contains rhubarb, heavy and light magnesium carbonate and ginger) is well known for its efficiency both as an antacid and as a purgative after an injudicious meal. Senna is best employed as senna pods, which are soaked for several hours at least in cold water. In practice it is advisable to instruct the patient to prepare the next dose at the time the first is taken, and the correct number of pods to ensure one good bowel movement in the morning is quickly found by experience.

Aloes, or its active principle aloin, acts on the colon, and an average dose takes ten or twelve hours to act; it is a common constituent of many pills.

Phenolphthalein is not so much employed alone as formerly, but has the advantage of being almost tasteless.

The anthracene group are by far the most valuable and commonly employed drugs for the treatment of chronic constipation.

Salines.—These are not suitable for habitual use, in spite of wide advertising of their merits as laxatives in small doses; the hot water which dissolves them is really the useful remedy. The mode of action of the purgative doses of the salines has been in some dispute. The commonly accepted view is that they act by extracting water from the bowel wall or by preventing its absorption, but Hurst and others claim that they act on the neuromuscular mechanism of the bowel only after absorption. Sodium sulphate, magnesium sulphate and sodium phosphate are the best examples, and in suitable doses (½ to 1 oz.) act very quickly, especially when dissolved in hot water, and should be taken not long before breakfast to ensure a loose and often watery motion soon after this meal. A disadvantage, even as an occasional purge, is that painful tenesmus may result, and if the whole dose is not evacuated at once frequent small stools may persist throughout the morning. None of the saline purgatives are pleasant to take, and proprietary preparations (*e.g.*, Eno's Fruit Salts) are often preferred by patients.

Mercury Preparations.—Calomel and hydrarg. cum creta are the only mercurial preparations commonly employed for constipation. Calomel decomposes in the intestine, liberating free metallic mercury, which is the active agent in increasing peristalsis of the small intestine. It is far less used nowadays than formerly, and is chiefly applicable as an occasional purge in "biliousness." The usual adult dose is ¼ to 1 gr. at night, followed by a saline purgative in the morning to remove the irritant metal.

Inert Substances Increasing the Bulk of the Fæces.—Careful and suitable dietetics is the best and most rational way of providing for an adequate bulk of fæces, but medicaments may also at times be usefully employed. Liquid paraffin, a mineral and non-absorbable oil, cannot be described as adding bulk, but it acts as a non-irritating lubricant and is often used in combination with other substances with good results.

When liquid paraffin is given alone its great disadvantage is that it frequently leaks from the anus and soils the clothes; this, however, can often be avoided by administration immediately after a meal, so that admixture with the food ensues. The best material to add bulk to the fæces is agar-agar, a dried preparation made from a seaweed, which is not absorbed but takes up a large amount of water. It may be given in shredded form, or as a powder—dose, 1 drachm or much more, according to circumstances. Coreine (Brunet), described as a dried vegetable mucilage, is also useful, the dosage being similar. A large number of emulsions of agar-agar and liquid paraffin are available, but it must clearly be remembered that most of them contain a purgative drug, on which their activity partly depends, and also that in many of these preparations the percentage of agar-agar is relatively small. Emulsio Paraff. Liq. Co. (B.P.C.) contains 50 per cent. of liquid paraffin, 0·75 per cent. agar and 1½ gr. of phenolphthalein per fluid ounce. Dose, 1 to 4 fluid drachms. Agarol (Warner), as sold in this country, is made up of 33 per cent. of liquid paraffin, 16 per cent. of agar jelly and 6 gr. of phenolphthalein per fluid ounce. Agarol without phenolphthalein is not obtainable in Britain. Petrolagar (Petrolagar Co.) contains 66 per cent. of liquid paraffin and 20 per cent. of agar jelly. It can be obtained with or without 1½ gr. of phenolphthalein per fluid ounce. Normacol (Norgine), marketed in Britain by Napp, is described as a desiccated plant mucilage with rhamnaceous glucocides, probably cascara. Treatment with these remedies may be valuable, but in many cases the continued use of phenolphthalein is contraindicated. Agar-agar should be prescribed alone, when the addition of bulk to the fæces is the sole object.

Enemas and Colonic Irrigations.—These have a limited field in the treatment of constipation, but have some important applications in special circumstances. The use of enemata for purposes other than the treatment of intestinal disorders *e.g.*, very concentrated solutions of magnesium sulphate to reduce intracranial pressure, is outside of the scope of thi chapter.

Enemas as used for intestinal diseases are described a high and low. High enemata (colonic lavage, colonic irrigation are given by introducing a soft rubber tube not more tha 2 in. into the rectum and allowing 1, 2 or even more pints o water, warmed to body temperature, to flow slowly into th colon under low pressure sufficient only to ensure the gradua entrance of the fluid. There is no point in using any othe fluid than warm water. Emptying of the colon by the ordinary act of defæcation may occur at once, or an attempt should be made to do so after about fifteen minutes. Low enemata administered as a rule with a Higginson's syringe or a soft tube and funnel may be employed if for any reason the anus and rectum are tender.

Enemata may act mechanically, as chemical irritants, as softeners of hard fæces, or by a combination of these effects. Thermal stimulation is unimportant and an enema introduced at higher temperature than body heat must be avoided.

The enemata in common use are :—

Water or Normal Saline Solution.—These are used for colonic lavage (high enemata) and induce peristalsis merely by mechanical distension of the colon.

Soap and Water Enemata.—The amount commonly employed is 1 pint, and the soap acts as a mild irritant.

Turpentine Enemata.—One ounce of oil of turpentine is emulsified in 1 pint of ordinary starch solution. These are used particularly when there is excessive gas or flatus in the colon, and although their exact mode of action for this purpose is unknown, their efficiency is undoubted.

Olive Oil or Liquid Paraffin Enemata.—Five ounces or more, warmed to body temperature, are introduced slowly at night and are retained if possible until the following morning. A pad of cotton-wool should be placed between the buttocks, to avoid the results of leakage during the night. Olive oil and liquid paraffin, which both act equally well, are used to remove hard dry masses of fæces (scybala) from the rectum. Their power of softening must be slight and only superficial, and their lubricating effect is more important. With their help hard scybala can frequently be evacuated, and as the peristaltic effort of the bowel may be painful and spasmodic, a full dose of tincture of belladonna (10 to 20 minims) or an injection of atropine sulphate ($\frac{1}{100}$ gr.) may be helpful. If this method fails, then evacuation of scybala by the gloved finger is required, and a general anæsthetic may simplify the procedure. It is far safer to use the fingers than the handle of a spoon, as was formerly advised in textbooks, but at times a hard object may be essential to break up concretions.

The chief uses of enemata are in :—

1. Spastic constipation, see p. 585.
2. So-called dyschezia, when for any reason the reflex act of defæcation is lost or impaired.
3. In bedridden, old or paralysed patients.

On the whole enemata should be used sparingly, but they may have great temporary value in suitable cases. Low enemata cannot be described as harmful, but the frequent use of high enemata (colonic lavage) should never be allowed. Colonic lavage is unfortunately fashionable, and may do great harm, not only from irritation of the colon but also because it is so often used in patients whose nervous stability is far from normal.

VISCEROPTOSIS

Visceroptosis from the standpoint of treatment falls into two classes, depending on whether the dropping of the abdominal viscera is due to: (1) fall in intra-abdominal pressure, previously adequate; (2) bodily habitus.

In many persons, both male and female, the abdominal viscera may occupy an unusually low position without any symptom whatever. Thus an X-ray diagnosis alone must always be guarded against, and a diagnosis of visceroptosis rests entirely on the presence of symptoms. The symptomatology in both classes is very complex, and a correct diagnosis may be far from easy. In consequence of this and because the means employed are very time-consuming, visceroptosis is on the whole badly treated, although the patients are often as useless and disabled for work as if they suffered from serious organic disease.

Fall in Intra-abdominal Pressure, Previously Adequate.—This group contains a very great preponderance of females, since its commonest cause is repeated pregnancy followed by inadequate attention to the restoration of abdominal muscle tonus after each confinement. The tendency to visceroptosis is increased when there has been rupture or stretching of the pelvic muscular floor, or unusual stretching of the abdominal wall. In both sexes, abdominal operations, especially if repeated, may bring about the same state of affairs. In this group, the mental factor, which is so prominent from the beginning in the second class, may slowly develop once the condition has become well established.

Bodily Habitus.—It would almost be correct to describe this group as due to "bodily and mental" habitus, by the time the patient reaches the consulting room. The patient starts with a certain type of bodily habitus, consisting of narrow chest, long and narrow costal angle and a tendency to lordosis. This type of body, and the symptoms of visceroptosis which may accompany it, is also most commonly found in women, but is by no means infrequent in males,

To this bodily habitus is added a general state of asthenia, with rapid mental and physical exhaustion. (It must be remembered that asthenia may occasionally be the chief symptom of serious organic disease, such as tuberculosis and gastric ulcer; it may also occur in patients who, because of an accident or otherwise, have been long confined to bed.)

In this type the mental factor is very predominant from the outset, and in addition to general symptoms the patient is constantly conscious of abdominal discomforts which are difficult to explain. In contrast to mucous colitis (p. 585) in which the physical disability is the outcome of a nervous state, here the mental condition must be regarded almost as a sequel to the bodily habitus. Hence it follows in this group that the first line of approach is to treat the physical state, while the mental outlook is strengthened to ensure the co-operation essential for cure.

The treatment necessary for the two groups of patients is different in a few respects, which are mentioned, but on the whole the remedies employed are the same for both.

In the first group the essential treatment is obviously prophylactic, and fortunately the after-care of pregnancy is now greatly improved. Massage and suitable exercises to restore the tonus of the abdominal muscles may be essential, both after pregnancy and at the correct interval of time after abdominal operations. The perineum must be repaired and any tendency to uterine prolapse prevented.

In the second group much could also be done, and perhaps in future will be done, by prophylactic physical training beginning at school. The good effects of physical training, even at a later age, has been plainly shown in recruits for the army found to be under-developed on enlistment.

It will no doubt continue to happen, however, that the physician is first faced with the problems of visceroptosis when both its physical and mental symptoms are well developed, and the general treatment is then as follows :—

Improvement of Nutrition.—Many of these patients are exceedingly thin, and in such cases before any other treatment is contemplated a serious attempt should be made to fatten them, both to improve their general condition and to increase their intra-abdominal supporting fat. This stage of treatment is much more easily carried out in an institution in which full dietetic facilities are available, but if the doctor takes trouble it can be done at home. At the beginning the patient is confined to bed, and a start is made with the best average diet that she will take. Almost invariably these patients have poor appetites, but extra nourishment is added between the ordinary meals which they must be persuaded to take "just like any other medicine." They should be told that as their body improves in condition so they will need more food and their appetite will improve. The best extra food is milk, plain or flavoured with tea, coffee, chocolate or anything else that the patient fancies, or made up in the form of junket, custard, egg-flip or ice-cream. Ice-cream is often of great value in patients who say they "cannot take milk," and many calories may be added in this way. In the rare cases in which there is actual sensitiveness to milk protein, glucose may be used but is not so effective. Butter should be given in as large amounts as possible, and many patients with poor appetites enjoy bread and butter if a little marmite is added to the butter. Provided that the patient is helpful, it is seldom that weight is not gained while in bed, and after two or three weeks the patient may get up and slowly commence remedial exercises while still continuing the enhanced diet and, if possible, increasing it. Remedial exercises should be directed by an expert, in a class of several members to induce competition. A cold rub or cold shower bath, in patients who react, may be helpful.

To obtain a permanent cure by these methods requires great perseverance and patience on the part of both patient and doctor, and when this is remembered it is not to be wondered that at present the failures outnumber the cures. These methods are only likely to be successful in patients who are moderately alert and below the age of forty; if they fail it is necessary to fall back on the palliative treatment of a mechanical support to the abdomen.

Forms of Mechanical Support.—Adhesive strapping is quite unsuitable, except as a temporary or trial expedient, and some form of belt or corset must be employed. These, if a good fit, increase intra-abdominal pressure and undoubtedly to some extent raise and support the abdominal contents.

Certain rules for the purchase and use of all belts and corsets in the treatment of visceroptosis, must be strictly adhered to:—

(*a*) They must always be put on when the patient is lying down, never in the erect posture.

(*b*) Perineal slings and straps are always uncomfortable and should if possible be avoided.

(*c*) The belt or corset should never be taken from "stock," but specially made or specially altered to fit the patient.

(*d*) Some forms of belt or corset suit one patient whilst others do not. All good firms who supply them are therefore willing to lend samples of approximately correct measurement for a few weeks' trial; advantage of this should always be taken, and when the suitable pattern is found a copy should be made to measure.

In Britain, a number of excellent belts or corsets are available, and although only a few are mentioned, this does not exclude other excellent patterns. Of belts perhaps the best known are those of Curtis (London) and Salt (Birmingham). The Curtis belt consists essentially of a thin but strong metal plate, suitably padded, applied (when lying down) to the lower abdomen. It is held firmly in position by two strong but flexible metal arms, united over the vertebral column by a small padded saddle. The belt is comfortable to most patients, never unsightly in any circumstances, and the mobile arms allow the patient to sit down without difficulty. The only difficulty encountered with some patients, especially when they are very thin, is that the pressure of the saddle over the prominent backbone may be intolerable. For this reason, as already stated, a belt of this kind should always be taken on trial. If unsuccessful, a similar metal plate enclosed in a corset may be tried (Curtis, Salt), or a corset alone in which side straps and buckles provide for support in an upward and backward direction. Corsets of this kind made by the "Camp" Corset Company are efficient in less severe cases and are readily obtainable. A point of some importance is that they closely resemble ordinary corsets, and the patient does not feel that she is wearing a surgical instrument. Directions for self-measurement are always supplied by the various makers, and whichever form of belt or corset is finally chosen, it must be given a reasonable trial of several months before any opinion about the result can be given.

Constipation is very common in patients suffering from visceroptosis, and must be treated (p. 573).

Operations of many kinds have been devised for visceroptosis, but all have signally failed and mercifully have all been abandoned. An abdominal operation of any kind is the last thing to be desired in these patients. There are, however, certain individual viscera which, if markedly displaced in the abdomen, may induce symptoms which can only be cured by operation. Chronic duodenal ileus may result from constriction by the mesentery and mesenteric vessels; the symptoms closely simulate those of duodenal ulcer. Extreme ptosis or dislocation of the spleen (so-called wandering spleen) may be followed by torsion of the pedicle or be associated with severe perisplenitis and pain. Removal of the spleen is then indicated. Lastly, severe renal colic (Dietl's crisis) may occasionally arise in nephroptosis. Dropping of the kidneys, if found incidentally during an abdominal examination, should never be mentioned to the patient, as it may simply exaggerate the mental aspects of the case.

Enteritis

The general clinical term "enteritis," although it is not commonly used, except in the form "gastro-enteritis," is useful in that it covers all the organic inflammatory diseases of the intestinal tract.

Inflammation of the intestinal wall may be of many kinds, acute or chronic in its course, catarrhal, ulcerative or gangrenous in its pathology, and due to many causes ranging from bacteria and their toxins, organic and inorganic poisons (mercury, lead, arsenic) and general metabolic disturbances such as uræmia. Most of these forms of enteritis are discussed elsewhere. The clamant general symptoms requiring treatment are diarrhœa (with its associated dehydration and collapse) and toxæmia due to absorption through the inflamed bowel wall. In many cases the exact cause of enteritis can be identified, and special treatment is indicated. In others (*e.g.*, chronic ulcerative colitis) the cause may be unknown or uncertain.

It is important to differentiate a true inflammatory enteritis from a functional disorder such as muco-membranous colic (formerly described as mucous colitis) in which the treatment is essentially different.

CHRONIC REGIONAL ILEITIS

(Syn. : Crohn's disease. Chronic cicatrizing enteritis)

This is an uncommon form of chronic enteritis, affecting the terminal part of the ileum and also spreading into the cæcum. It occurs chiefly in young adult males. The portion of bowel involved becomes thickened and rigid from inflammation, and this is followed by fibrosis, narrowing and ulceration. Tuberculosis has been suspected, because giant cells are often found, but these are probably "foreign body" giant cells associated with necrosis of tissue, and tubercle bacilli have not been found. The symptoms are those of partial intestinal obstruction, a sausage-shaped tumour may be felt, and on

X-ray examination with barium a filling defect (the "string" sign of Cantor) may be evident.

The treatment is essentially surgical. To minimize the operative risk a short circuit of the affected bowel is advised, followed by complete resection at a later stage.

IRRITABLE COLON

(Syn. : Spastic colon)

MUCO-MEMBRANOUS COLIC

(Syn. : Mucous colitis)

Under these headings may be included for convenience what really amounts to a whole group of intestinal disorders, somewhat similar in their ætiology and therefore in the principles of their treatment.

These conditions are not, in the earlier stages at least, to be regarded as a true inflammation or colitis, but as an entirely functional disturbance of the bowel wall and of its secretions. Nevertheless, if the adverse circumstances persist, any one of them may end in a true inflammation.

There are three main factors recognized to be concerned in the ætiology of this group, but there may be others.

1. Nervous and emotional instability.
2. The abuse of cathartics, enemas or colonic irrigations.
3. Disease elsewhere (in the gall-bladder, female pelvic organs, etc.) acting "reflexly" on the bowel. In any individual case only one or a combination of these ætiological factors may be important.

Spastic colon and muco-membranous colic are best regarded simply as differing degrees of severity of the same disorder. The former is very common in both sexes; the latter is comparatively rarely seen nowadays in practice, and is chiefly encountered in women. In both there is tonic spasm of the colon wall, causing hardening and contraction, and the descending colon may be felt through the abdominal wall almost like a bar. Constipation is common, or alternating bouts of constipation and diarrhœa.

In "spastic colon," mucus is generally absent from the stools; in muco-membranous colic shreds of mucus or complete mucous casts of the bowel may be passed. Pain and colic are the chief subjective symptoms. In muco-membranous colic the excessive secretion of mucus is generally described as protective, but another view recently advanced should be mentioned. Not only is mucus in excess, but Charcot-Leyden crystals and eosinophil blood cells are also found in the stools. This has suggested a close analogy with bronchial asthma in which spasm of another bodily tube (the bronchial tree) is also essentially concerned. The influence of nervous instability is well recognized in both affections—are we also now to consider the problem of hypersensitiveness to some foreign protein in relation to the treatment of muco-membranous colic ?

The Nervous Aspect.—After a thorough physical examination, made deliberately in part to impress the patient, assurance must first be given that the condition (as is often suspected) is not cancer. The remainder of the treatment consists essentially in rational psychotherapeutic treatment, and the symptomatic treatment of muscular spasm if this is present. The psychological aspects of every case will differ, and the scope of the examination and treatment cannot be discussed here. The spasm of the colon wall is best treated with tincture of belladonna (10 to 30 minims thrice daily), or with atropine sulphate ($\frac{1}{100}$ gr.) or papaverin (Knoll) ($\frac{5}{8}$-gr. tablet). Morphine must never be used. Occupational therapy and a study of the whole mental and physical health of the patient are both important.

Correction of Abuse of Purgatives.—It will be found that many of these patients, especially those suffering from spastic colon, have treated their constipation by the frequent use of almost every purgative offered to the public. These must be forbidden, and permission only given for olive oil, liquid paraffin or agar-agar. The proprietary preparations which contain phenolphthalein (p. 578) should be avoided in these cases. Colonic lavage not only should never be advised but must often positively be forbidden, as sufferers from an irritable colon are only too prone to consider that it is "the very thing for them." A careful diet which while avoiding coarse residue maintains adequate bulk (see Appendix, p. 596) is a valuable aid to overcoming the purgative habit. Wholemeal breads, unsieved vegetables and fruits containing pips are avoided, but other fruits and vegetable purées should be taken freely.

Reflex Spasm from Disease Elsewhere in the Abdomen.—This is a difficult problem and calls for much care in diagnosis. It is only when disease in some other organ is proved up to the hilt that operation should be recommended in these patients. This is especially true in muco-membranous colic for two good reasons. First, the mental outlook of the patient as a rule makes any operation inadvisable on general grounds. Second, the pain in muco-membranous colic can be made, by the patient at least, to simulate almost any acute intra-abdominal disease. The writer has encountered one male sufferer from muco-membranous colic who in the course of years had five emergency abdominal operations performed in various hospitals. The man himself was convinced, and remains convinced by his colicky symptoms and passage of mucous casts, that there is " something alive " within his bowel, and that some surgeon will ultimately find and remove it.

Irritable or spastic colon is common and a condition for which rational treatment should always effect a cure. Muco-membranous colic, once the complete symptomatology has appeared, always presents a long and exceedingly unsatisfactory therapeutic problem.

CHRONIC ULCERATIVE COLITIS

The treatment of this serious and fairly common disease centres in the first place round the problems of its ætiology. It must be stated that none of the hypotheses so far advanced has yielded anything approaching a uniform, satisfactory or specific line of treatment for the majority of cases.

Most physicians, therefore, continue to treat the disease on general lines, omitting all reference to ætiology. The general treatment will first be discussed and thereafter reference must be made to special methods of therapy for which good results have been claimed.

The disease is almost confined to adults, and it is curious that young children, who are so prone to intestinal diseases, should generally escape.

There is a gradually increasing body of clinical evidence that the disease may appear with great rapidity very soon after some acute mental or psychological disturbance, which suggests some nervous derangement of the mechanism of the bowel. But this view, although manifestly important, has not yet yielded any help in the treatment of the established disease, which even if it appears with great suddenness unfortunately shows little tendency to rapidity of cure. The fact that treatment is bound to be very prolonged, requiring the utmost patience both on the part of patient and physician, is the first thing to realize, once the diagnosis has been made and the common causes of diarrhœa associated with blood, mucus and pus in the stools have been excluded. The course of the average case is a series of ups and downs, and the main general features of the disease for which treatment may be required are fever, toxæmia, anæmia from hæmorrhage, loss of weight in severe cases and exhaustion and dehydration from the frequent stools. Pain is seldom if ever a serious matter in this disease, although abdominal discomfort is always present.

General Treatment.—*Rest in Bed.*—This is the first essential when the diagnosis has been made, and preparations must be made at once for a stay in bed of some months at least and, by no means uncommonly, for a year. A rough rule of value is that the patient must not be allowed up while there is fever, or when the stools number more than two or three in the twenty-four hours.

Dietetics.—This is important in this long-continued weakening disease, for many patients die simply from asthenia. Ulcerative colitis affects the colon alone, and not the small intestine in which all the processes of digestion and assimilation remain, for a time at least, quite unimpaired. The patient may be quite fat and plump at the commencement, and continue so for many months; rapid loss of weight is always a bad sign. A fully adequate diet of high caloric value should be given (see Appendix, p. 598) to mitigate the loss of blood in the stools and the general physical exhaustion. The diet should be free from coarse particles of cellulose, and spices or condiments must be omitted. In patients in whom diarrhœa is extremely severe, great temporary benefit may be obtained by a diet of "pulped apple," although this cannot be continued for more than a few days because the caloric value is so low. This diet, and a modification of it which has proved useful, is given in the Appendix.

Drugs.—Some are required for the control of general symptoms, while others are used for their action on the ulcerated wall of the colon. Sleeplessness is common during the acute phases, when stools may be passed hourly or even half-hourly. Subcutaneous injections of sedatives must be avoided, and codeine ($\frac{1}{2}$ gr.) by the mouth is generally effective, and also helps to diminish the diarrhœa.

Kaolin, kaolin-with-charcoal and other adsorbents have been much employed, but in the writer's own experience have not been effective in controlling the diarrhœa. Charcoal is, however, of real use when there is colicky pain or gaseous distension. Tincture of belladonna, 10 to 30 minims in three equal doses daily, is of value when spasm of the colon is clearly recognized.

Anæmia is always present, and is treated with iron and ammonium citrate, 30 gr. or more, three times daily. If the anæmia becomes severe, blood transfusion should always be carried out. Even when anæmia is mild in degree many physicians believe that small and repeated blood transfusions are the most valuable remedy we possess for combating the asthenia present in this disease.

Local Treatment.—Local treatment of the ulcerated mucous membrane of the colon presents difficult problems, and it is not easy to judge the effects of the various remedies fully. The application of various drugs to the bowel wall by lavage can seldom be carried out successfully unless complete nursing facilities are available. Various drugs have been employed, and in every case it is of advantage not to persist with one of them too long but to change to another. A starch and opium enema (starch, ℥i; tincture of opium, ♏x to ♏xx; water, to ℥ii) may be useful in the early acute phase of ulceration, when there is more tendency to pain and tenesmus. Later, the bowel may be slowly washed out, every second day, with normal saline, flavine (1 : 200,000), argyrol (½ per cent.), or tannic acid in strengths gradually increasing from ½ to 2 gr. to 1 oz. of warm water. Whatever fluid is used about 1 pint should be allowed to run in very slowly under the lowest possible pressure, and the patient should be encouraged to retain the fluid for half an hour. It must be stated that all varieties of irrigation are now much less used than was our former custom.

In serious cases, when the measures outlined above have been unsuccessful, the question of surgical intervention to allow the colon to be washed out from above must arise. Two operations may be performed: (1) *Appendicostomy* or *cæcostomy*, allowing the insertion of a fine rubber tube to carry the irrigating fluid, and (2) *ileostomy*. The latter is the more serious operation in a very ill patient, but has the theoretical advantage of preventing the passage of fæces into the colon so that it can ultimately be thoroughly cleansed. Everyone with much experience must have seen some patients apparently recover as a direct result of one or other operation, but on the other hand almost an equal number die. It is probably the truth that the possibilities of these operations are as a rule only considered too late, when the risk of any surgical intervention is grave. But so far the results have not been sufficiently impressive to indicate early operation as the most hopeful treatment, either to save life or to shorten the disease.

Specific Treatment.—Certain forms of specific treatment, based on views concerning ætiology, must now be discussed.

Antidysenteric Serum.—This method has been recommended especially by Hurst, who believes that the majority of cases of ulcerative colitis are due to a dysentery bacillus, even although the organism cannot be isolated from the stools. He advises, after preliminary desensitization, the intravenous injection of 20, 40, 60, 80 and 100 c.c. of polyvalent anti-dysenteric serum on successive days. It would not be advisable to carry out this treatment, except under hospital or nursing-home conditions, and certainly a supply of adrenalin solution and a suitable syringe should be immediately available in case of sudden anaphylactic collapse. Opinions on the merits of this treatment are divided, remarkable successes having been reported and also many failures. There seems no reason to doubt that a few cases of genuine bacillary dysentery may be followed by extensive ulceration of the whole colon (although the brunt of the infection generally falls on the descending and sigmoid colon), and these may constitute the main successes. It is possible also that the foreign serum-protein may have some non-specific effect. It would be more likely, on pathological grounds alone, for ulcerative colitis to be the result of amœbic dysentery, but this disease must be very rare in Britain. Nevertheless, the writer has himself demonstrated the presence of typical *Entamœba histolytica* in the portal capillaries of a patient who died of "ulcerative colitis" after an illness of six months. This man had never been out of Britain, but worked in contact with men who had been in the East during the Great War. If any suspicions arise from the clinical history it could do no possible harm to try the effects of a course of emetin injections (see Amœbic Dysentery, p. 244).

Bargen's Serum.—Treatment with a serum or vaccine prepared from a micro-organism isolated by Bargen, in America, and believed by him to be the specific cause of the disease, had a transient popularity. The results have, however, been disappointing, and Bargen's serum and vaccine are now rarely used in this country.

It may be emphasized, in conclusion, that the treatment of chronic ulcerative colitis is often disappointing, and the mortality rate, even with the greatest nursing care, is relatively high. Relapses are common, even after apparent cure, but there is no doubt that complete restoration to permanent health may be attained.

In a few cases the disease assumes a really chronic form, and then strictures of the colon and polypoid overgrowth may arise. Both of these conditions are very liable to malignant change, and colectomy may then be the only possible choice in treatment.

After apparent cure, and to guard against the frequent relapses, dietetic precautions should be continued, and a body-belt of silk and wool should always be worn round the abdomen. Purgative drugs must never be employed, but the bowels should be kept regular by suitable diet and the use of liquid paraffin when required.

DIVERTICULOSIS AND DIVERTICULITIS

Diverticulosis.—This is a common condition in adults who have suffered from habitual constipation, or from some acute inflammation of the colon such as dysentery. Its existence is frequently discovered accidentally during an X-ray examination of the bowel for some other purpose. Under such circumstances it is best to tell the patient nothing about it, or to say simply that the colon is not diseased but not quite normal. The early stages of diverticulosis are symptomless. Later, when the pockets or diverticula are fully formed, symptoms may again be entirely absent; but in a certain number of patients the condition leads to complaints of headache, flatulence and colicky pains in the abdomen. Constipation is almost invariable, but occasional attacks of diarrhœa supervene.

Treatment is directed, when symptoms require it, first to the general health of the patient, and second to the almost invariable constipation. Purgative drugs must never be given, but liquid paraffin is always employed. A lacto-vegetarian diet (see p. 599) may also prove of great service for short periods. Other methods of treatment occasionally of value are the rectal administration of a warm douche of normal saline solution, or an enema of warm olive oil run in very slowly at night. Following the latter treatment an absorbent pad must be fixed between the thighs.

Diverticulitis or inflammation of a diverticulum is fortunately comparatively rare, but may be a troublesome problem in diagnosis. The early symptoms are intermittent colicky pain, generally in the left iliac fossa but sometimes elsewhere, with fever, and later an indefinite tender mass is felt. Perforation may occur, requiring urgent surgical intervention, but in by far the majority of cases the inflammation and local peritonitis slowly settle down after expectant treatment and general sedatives.

IDIOPATHIC STEATORRHŒA

(Syn.: Non-tropical sprue. Gee-Thaysen's disease)

This is a condition of unknown ætiology in which there is a disturbance of absorption from the intestine. It is claimed by some that this condition merely represents the adult stage of cœliac disease (p. 285); by others it is held to be a primary disease in the adult.

Fatty stools, due to defective absorption of fat from the bowel, form the most striking clinical feature, but absorption of carbohydrates is also imperfect. Diarrhœa is common, but not invariable. The colon is often dilated. Other metabolic disturbances, particularly of calcium and phosphorus metabolism, are also found, shown clinically by stunted growth, osteoporosis, osteomalacia and tetany. Anæmia is common, and may be either of the microcytic or macrocytic type; indeed, the type of anæmia may change in the same patient during the course of the disease.

The treatment in the first place is dietetic, and a diet high in proteins, low in fat and relatively low in carbohydrates is rational. The symptomatology, however, is so variable that no standardized line of dietetic treatment is applicable for every case. Milk, in spite of its content of fat, is often well borne, and 1,500 c.c. daily may be tried, combined with raw fruit (without pips) or fruit juice. Ripe bananas are useful (as in cœliac disease) because their carbohydrates seem to ferment less readily in the intestines than those from other sources.

On the whole the daily diet for an adult should contain at least 110 to 130 gm. of protein, and, unless diarrhœa is severe, the fats should not be reduced below 50 gm. The amount of carbohydrate allowed depends on the degree of abdominal distension, due to intestinal carbohydrate fermentation. In some patients this is severe, and the carbohydrates should then be confined to ripe bananas; in others a normal or only slightly diminished supply of carbohydrates may be given. Sprulac (Cow & Gate), a dried and defatted milk powder, is often useful. It contains protein 34 per cent., fat 10 per cent., lactose 45 per cent. and mineral salts; 1 oz. is stated to provide 125 calories. Four ounces a day may be given. Achlorhydria is often present, and is treated with dilute hydrochloric acid taken as a beverage with each meal. Anæmia, whether microcytic or macrocytic in type, must be adequately treated (pp. 471, 480). In order to combat osteoporosis and stunted growth, calcium and vitamin D are required. Vitamin D is supplied as radiostol (British Drug Houses), 3 tablets or more three times daily, or as irradiated ergosterol (dose, 3,000 international units per day). Calcium is given by the mouth either as calcium lactate or calcium gluconate, 20 to 30 gr. of either thrice daily. For the treatment of tetany, see p. 426. Marmite (vitamin B) and orange juice (vitamin C) have also proved useful in treatment.

Rest in bed and massage to the muscles are important, and bony deformities may require surgical treatment. Fractures of the bones are not uncommon and special care is required because healing is necessarily slow.

INTESTINAL OBSTRUCTION

The obstruction may be partial or complete, acute or chronic, and may affect any part of the small or large intestine. The causes, as described in textbooks, are commonly divided into those arising in the bowel itself (tumours, malignant and non-malignant, gall-stones, hard fæcal scybala, foreign bodies) and those arising outside of the bowel (herniæ, adhesions and bands, peritonitis). As a rule the obstruction is mechanical, but more rarely is due to paralysis, spasm or peritonitis. Strangulation, volvulus, and intussusception are well-known special varieties of acute intestinal obstruction. Tumour growth is the commonest variety of chronic obstruction in adults.

The diagnosis of obstruction is not difficult, but exact diagnosis both of cause and site is far from easy, although it does not concern us here.

Once the diagnosis of intestinal obstruction has been made, particularly of the acute variety, surgery is almost always indicated, but there are some important medical aspects of treatment.

The higher the acute obstruction in the intestine the greater the danger, and the more intense are the symptoms of vomiting, cramps, shock and dehydration. These, if they persist, are followed by paralysis of the bowel. In spite of much observation on patients, and experiments on animals, the reasons for a fatal issue in acute intestinal obstruction are still far from clear, and because of this our rational therapeutics is limited. It is certain that several factors are at work, including the following :—

1. Overdistension of any hollow viscus is known to produce serious effects.
2. It is known that in a closed loop of bowel in animals, some substance is produced which, on injection, causes splanchnic paralysis.
3. Loss of water and of sodium chloride occur from the vomiting.
4. Loss of blood from the general circulation takes place due to great dilatation of the splanchnic vessels.

The surgeon alone can remedy the first two of these, the third is treated by continuous intravenous injection of normal or hypertonic (p. 1075) saline until chlorides reappear in the urine; the fourth is dealt with by blood transfusion, followed by immediate operation.

In all cases of suspected acute intestinal obstruction, purgatives must never be used, but if the colon is not involved the lower bowel should be cleared with a simple soap and water enema. When the diagnosis of obstruction has been fully made, and preparations for surgery begun, it is legitimate to use morphia for the intense pain. Fæcal vomiting greatly distresses the patient, and the stomach may be washed out with warm water through a small stomach tube.

When the colon is involved, the anaerobic gas-forming bacilli begin at once to play a large part in the issue, and anti-gas-gangrene serum (*B. welchii*) should be administered intramuscularly in doses of 25 c.c. or more.

MEGACOLON

(Syn.: Hirschsprung's disease)

Hirschsprung's disease is the term generally used to describe megacolon in children. In the adult megacolon consists of a uniform dilatation of the rectum and sigmoid colon and at times of the entire colon, unaccompanied by any obstruction. The only certain means of diagnosis is by means of a barium enema, and 5 to 10 pints may easily be allowed to flow in.

The ætiology is believed to be a disturbance of the nervous mechanism of the anal sphincter, congenital in origin.

Constipation is the chief symptom, and scybala may lead to stercoraceous ulceration of the bowel.

When recognized in adult life, it is often remarkable how little the condition interferes with health, and the condition may only be discovered when the patient complains that larger and larger doses of purgatives are required to mitigate the constipation which has troubled them from childhood.

It is frequently stated that purgatives are inadvisable, but the writer has seen several examples of megacolon in which very large doses of simple purgatives enabled the patient to empty the bowel, and good health was maintained. An occasional large enema is often required. Hurst strongly advises the systematic use of a conical rectal bougie to overcome achalasia of the rectal sphincter. The colon is generally greatly elongated in addition to being dilated, and hypertrophy and extreme redundancy of the sigmoid loop occasionally lead to serious complications such as volvulus. Operation is then the only remedy, but the operative risk is considerable.

DIETS FOR INTESTINAL DISEASES

Specimen Diet, and Rules, for Chronic Constipation

Rules—

1. Regular time for meals.
2. Regular, unhurried time for emptying bowels.
3. No cathartics or medicines, unless ordered by physician.
4. Regular exercise, as prescribed.

Breakfast—

Any fruit—fresh, cooked or dried.
Porridge and milk.
Wholemeal bread and butter.
Marmalade, jam or honey.
Coffee, with milk and sugar according to taste.

Lunch—

Soup.
Any fish, meat (with fat) or eggs.
Vegetables—celery, lettuce, spinach, cabbage; or green salads with mayonnaise.
Fresh, preserved or stewed fruits.
Wholemeal bread and butter.

Tea—

Weak tea, milk and sugar.
Wholemeal bread and butter.
Ryvita biscuits.
Treacle scones, treacle gingerbread.

Dinner (as Lunch).

Fluids—in abundance. One tumblerful of hot water on rising, and up to eight tumblerfuls daily. Beer, cider and table waters may all be used.

Avoid—White bread, potatoes and strong tea.

Carbohydrate	321 gm.	approximately.
Protein	87 ,,	
Fat	128 ,,	
Calories	2,784	

Diet Providing Adequate Bulk, but Avoiding Coarse Residue

(Applicable in Spastic Colon and some forms of Constipation)

Early a.m.—

½ pint water flavoured with strained orange, lemon or grapefruit juice.

Breakfast—

Well-strained porridge or cornflakes.

Two eggs, boiled, poached or scrambled ; *or* white fish or smoked haddock ; *or* crisp bacon.

White bread or Hovis bread—not new—crisply toasted.

Butter, honey or golden syrup.

One cup weak tea, with milk and sugar.

11 *a.m.*—

Fruit drink : strained orange juice or grapefruit juice—3½ oz. (100 gm.).

Water to ½ pint.

Lunch or *Dinner* (these may be transposed)—

Cream soup.

White fish, chicken, tripe, sweetbreads, tender liver, fillet steak or chop.

Gravy, or white sauce without parsley.

Creamed potato.

Sieved vegetable.

Curds, custard, jelly, fruit whips, baked apple or soft stewed fruit, without skin or pips.

Cream.

Cheese, water biscuits and butter, if desired.

Tea—

Vita-Weat or Hovis bread (not new).

Tomato pulp or marmite sandwiches.

Plain or Madeira sponge cake.

Butter, jelly or treacle.

One cup freshly made weak tea, with milk and sugar.

Dinner—

Any two courses from lunch. (These two meals may be transposed.)

Carbohydrate	320 gm.	approximately.
Protein	127 ,,	
Fat	145 ,,	
Calories	3,033	

Diet in Continued Diarrhœa

(Schmidt's Test Intestinal Diet)

(Also useful in the early severe stages of ulcerative colitis)

Breakfast—

1 pint milk ; *or* tea or cocoa with much milk.
One buttered roll or bread.
One soft boiled egg.

10 *a.m.*—

One large cupful of strained thick oatmeal soup, with salt or sugar.

Lunch—

One large plateful of thick potato soup.
$\frac{1}{4}$ lb. lean minced or scraped beef, slightly cooked.

4 *p.m.*—

Same as breakfast, without the egg.

Supper—

One plateful thick strained oatmeal soup, with salt.
One or two buttered rolls or bread.
One or two soft boiled or scrambled eggs.

Carbohydrate	242 gm.	approximately.
Protein	127 ,,	
Fat	144 ,,	
Calories	2,772	

Pulped Apple Diet

(In severe diarrhœa and ulcerative colitis)

150 to 175 gm. of peeled, raw, ripe, grated apple pulp seven times daily at intervals of two hours.

First Day—

150 gm. of apple pulp, two-hourly, from 8 A.M. to 8 P.M.
Total, 1,050 gm. Carbohydrate, 158 gm. Calories, 632.

Second Day—

175 gm. of apple pulp as before.
Total, 1,225 gm. Carbohydrate, 183 gm. Calories, 732.

This diet may be continued for three to four days, or the following may be substituted :—

Breakfast, 8 *a.m.*—
Crisp fingers of toast.
Cup of marmite.

10 *a.m.*—
175 gm. apple pulp.

12 *noon*—
Clear broth.
2 oz. lean meat.
crisp toast.

2 *p.m.*—
175 gm. apple pulp.

4 *p.m.*—
2 oz. white fish.
Crisp fingers of toast.

6 *p.m.*—
175 gm. apple pulp.

8 *p.m.*—
Marmite or clear broth to drink.
Crisp toast.

Carbohydrate . . .	125 gm.	approximately.
Protein	35 ,,	
Fat	10 ,,	
Calories	730	

High Vitamin Diet in Chronic Ulcerative Colitis

Directions—
1. Chew all solids slowly and thoroughly.
2. Avoid all hot drinks.

Breakfast—
Sieved porridge and milk.
Two eggs, lightly boiled or poached.
Crisp toast, with butter, honey or marmite.

10 *a.m.*—
Orange juice or glucose lemonade.

Lunch—

Sieved vegetable soup.
Sieved or puréed vegetables—peas, beans, spinach.
If desired, meat, fish or poultry as at dinner (see below).
Boiled rice with butter.
Toast.
Salad of tender lettuce and tomato pulp; olive oil; mayonnaise.

Tea—

Weak tea and milk—not too hot.
Crisp toast and butter, with marmite.

Dinner—

Cream soup.
Meat, fish or chicken—all steamed, not roasted. To begin with, the meat should be minced, and the fish or chicken taken as creams.
Vegetables—as at lunch, sieved and puréed.
Milk puddings—sago, tapioca, custard. Blancmanges, jellies, soft stewed fruit without seeds or skins.

Cod-liver oil, or its equivalent, may be added in certain cases. The raw salad at lunch, if causing irritation, may be discontinued.

Carbohydrate	275 gm.	approximately.
Protein	94 ,,	
Fat	158 ,,	
Calories	2,898	

Lacto-vegetarian Diet in Diverticulosis
(Spriggs)

7 *a.m.*—

½ oz. of paraffin in 2 oz. of warm milk.

8 *a.m.*—

Coffee and milk; 1 tablespoonful of milk sugar.
Wholemeal bread; butter, honey or marmalade.

10.30 *a.m.*—

A glass of buttermilk.
Wholemeal bread and butter.

1 *p.m.*—
Fish (cooked any way); butter sauce.
Salad and dressing.
Compote of fruit.
Cream.
Toast and butter.

4 *p.m.*—
Coffee, with milk or cream.
Marmalade.
Wholemeal bread (toasted if desired) and butter.

7.30 *p.m.*—
Vegetable soup.
Some egg dish (poached, scrambled or omelette) with vegetables or fruit; for instance, may have jam or jelly omelette or *omelette aux fines herbes*.
Cream cheese.
Wholemeal bread.
Butter.

(Modify to suit the individual.)

Light Dry Diet in Flatulent Dyspepsia

On Waking—
Tomato juice—1 oz. in 2 oz. water.

Breakfast—
Egg or white fish.
Rusks or one thin slice crisp toast buttered cold.

11 *a.m.*—
Cup of marmite, preferably made with milk (5 oz.).

Lunch or *Dinner* (these may be transposed)—
Tender steak or lean meat or white fish.
Sieved spinach, carrot.
A very small helping of mashed potato.
Curds or milk jelly.

Mid-afternoon—
3 oz. warm water flavoured with lemon juice.

Tea—
Cream cheese, *e.g.*, St Ivel.
One slice crisp toast buttered cold.
Water biscuit or tea biscuit or small piece plain sponge.

Dinner—
As lunch, but smaller serving of vegetable and potato.

8 *p.m.*—
Milk or milk and cream—5 oz.—to drink.
One tea biscuit.

The following should be avoided :—

N.B.—Drinking with solid food.
Soups, gravies, coffee, strong tea, cocoa.
Pork, duck, goose, sausage, pies, herring, kippers and sardines.
Green vegetables (except sieved spinach and flower of cauliflower), turnip, peas, beans and lentils.
Fruit : at first sugar, glucose, jam, jelly, honey.
Bread (do not eat bread at evening meal).
Porridge, new bread, hot toast, scones, fruit cakes, pastry.
Suet puddings, steamed puddings, milk puddings.

Take Daily—
Milk : ½ to 1 pint should be used daily. Add cream whenever possible.
Butter.
1 oz. tomato juice, lemon juice or 1 oz. orange juice if tolerated.
Ripe banana mashed may be taken, or baked apple pulp.

Carbohydrate . . .	95 gm.	approximately.
Protein	70 ,,	
Fat	75 ,,	
Calories	1,335	

J. W. McNee.
D. Smith.

DISEASES OF THE LIVER, GALL-BLADDER AND BILIARY TRACT, PANCREAS AND PERITONEUM

DISEASES OF THE LIVER

THE liver is absolutely necessary for life, since many of the essential chemical changes in our body included under the term " metabolism " are carried out only by this organ. The greater part of the raw material dealt with by the liver reaches it by the portal vein which drains the intestinal tract ; and the products of digestion which are absorbed into the portal blood stream must pass through the liver. Thus the liver is the main organ concerned with the nutrition of the body. Many of the chemical activities of the liver are quite unknown to us, but it is evident that the breaking-down, storage and re-building of substances essential for the life of every tissue and organ in the body must take place within the polygonal glandular cells of the liver.

In addition to the normal products of digestion other absorbable substances present in the intestine also reach the liver. These may be drugs given by the mouth, or inorganic poisons, or bacterial toxins arising in the intestine in typhoid fever, dysentery, food poisoning and other intestinal infections.

In dealing with these " poisons " (using the word in its widest sense), the liver plays an essential part in the defence of the body, unfortunately hften at the expense of serious damage to itself. This toxiphylactic function of the liver acts in several ways—by destroying, by detoxicating through the formation of harmless derivatives, or by arresting and storing within the liver cells the noxious substances, and so preventing them from entering the general circulation. The resulting damage (hepatitis) may be acute, subacute or chronic, depending on many factors but especially the amount and frequency of the dose.

Apart from the injury to which the hepatic tissues are liable from their important relation to the portal blood, it is obvious that the liver is subject, alike with the rest of the body, to the effects of harmful substances or toxins in the systemic circulation, since the liver has a second blood supply through the hepatic artery. Thus it is that the liver may be damaged in any systemic or generalized disease—acute specific fevers, bacterial septicæmias, syphilis, tuberculosis and many others.

The foregoing short survey of the activities of the liver indicates the directions and the limitations of general rational therapy.

Protection of the Normal Liver against Injury introduced into the body whether therapeutically or otherwise. It is a well-established fact that the liver cells when well filled with glycogen are much less liable to injury than when they are depleted and empty. For this reason an adequate carbohydrate diet, or the administration of glucose, both of which can provide the essential store of glycogen, must be arranged in all circumstances in which a depleted liver might be liable to injury. This applies to the administration of all general anæsthetics, not only the older ones such as chloroform and ether but also to the newer basal anæsthetics. In the arsenical treatment of syphilis similar precautions must be taken, and in industries in which workers may be exposed to liver poisons, whether metals such as arsenic, or carbon derivatives used as commercial solvents, care must be taken that work is not continued for long periods without food.

Treatment of the Damaged Liver.—Here two fundamental points arise and require consideration, since they both modify the results of injury so greatly, and therefore have a profound bearing on all questions of rational treatment.

(*a*) Although the liver is so vulnerable, nature has fortunately provided us with a great excess of hepatic tissue over normal needs. In this way the liver resembles our most important excretory organs, the kidneys. The greater part of the liver may be destroyed by poisons or by tumour growth and yet sufficient remain to carry out perfectly, under normal circumstances and for a considerable time, the requirements of the body.

(*b*) The glandular cells of the liver and the bile-duct system draining them have extraordinary powers of regeneration and repair unsurpassed by any other organ. Thus a liver which has been severely and acutely damaged may later be found to contain large masses of newly formed glandular tissue (nodular hyperplasia), active in function, and with a complete system of bile ducts. It is only when damage has been oft-repeated, as in cirrhosis (*q.v.*), that fibrous tissue seriously interferes with the regenerative powers of the organ.

These two points, the great excess of liver tissue over normal requirements and the extraordinary capacity for regeneration after acute damage, show that the general lines of treatment must lie in protecting the cells that remain undamaged, and in tiding over the time required for repair.

The general lines of treatment are :—

Rest in Bed.—This will help to protect the intact liver cells, since it will diminish the call on the glycogen store of the liver, the body's most easily mobilized source of energy. It will also diminish all the other metabolic activities with which the liver is concerned.

Warmth is provided by rest in bed, and tends to diminish the increased metabolism induced by cold.

Glucose is given in large quantities, either by the mouth or by the subcutaneous and intravenous route, so that the uninjured cells may be protected from any poison which still remains.

Diet should be chiefly carbohydrate in composition, as throwing least strain on the damaged organ. Proteins should be kept down to the minimum bodily requirements, as the metabolism of their derivatives requires hepatic activity. Fats should also be restricted because bile salts, which may be secreted in diminished amount by the damaged liver, are essential for their emulsification and digestion. It has been found in practice that " cooked fats " are a common cause of indigestion and flatulence in hepatic disease. Uncooked fats, such as butter and milk, are less harmful.

Drugs, except the simple saline purgatives, should be used as sparingly as possible in hepatic disease, since most alkaloids are dealt with and finally destroyed by the liver. Restlessness and even delirium may be a serious problem in the most acute forms of hepatic damage (acute necrosis, *q.v.*) and it may then be essential to use powerful hypnotics (both barbitone and opium derivatives). In such case, glucose must be used in large amounts to diminish the primary objections to these drugs.

Avoidance of Known Hepatic Poisons.—The chemical substances known to damage the liver are very numerous, and in the modern developments of industry are increasing every year. Some drugs such as the salvarsan compounds, atophan (phenyl-quinolinic acid; quinolan; cinchophen) must be given, in spite of their known tendency to damage the liver, but atophan especially must be given with care. Gold (as used in tuberculosis and rheumatoid arthritis), phosphorus, santonin and carbon tetrachloride (used for parasitic worms), chloroform, avertin and other basal anæsthetics, trinitrotoluene (used for explosives), tetrachlorethane (used as "dope" for aeroplane wings), and many other "solvents" used in industry are liable to cause severe liver damage. The question of idiosyncracy to liver disturbance is too difficult to discuss and our knowledge too meagre, but certainly anyone known to have suffered from any disease which might injure the liver, such as syphilis, malaria, yellow fever, Weil's disease, gall-stones and chronic alcoholism, should be employed with care in chemical industries, and if occasion arises, treated circumspectly with certain drugs.

Treatment of Disordered Hepatic Function.—We know so little at present about disorders of hepatic function, unassociated with obvious structural change, that our attempts at therapy are rudimentary. Insulin enables us, in diabetes mellitus, to control in some way the storage and mobilization of glycogen in the liver. In pernicious anæmia when the store of the factor (produced in the stomach) necessary for the maturation of the red blood cells is depleted, we can restore this by liver therapy. It is strongly suspected that the liver plays an important part in the manufacture of fibrinogen, and therefore in blood coagulation, but no attempts at hepatic therapy in disorders of blood coagulation are yet possible. In short, there must be very many serious functional disorders of the liver about which we know nothing.

It has been suspected that the liver must produce some internal secretions or enzymes, but the only known secretion of the liver is the bile, which is partly a secretion (bile-salts and cholesterol) and partly an excretion (of a waste product—bile pigment).

Hepatitis

As has been already stated, we know little about functional disturbances of the liver, and the majority (but not all) of hepatic diseases, recognized in textbooks under separate headings, depend on structural changes resulting from injury. These diseases, although clinically and for convenience distinguished by names, can easily, and particularly for purposes of treatment, be included under the one term "hepatitis." They include catarrhal jaundice (acute infective hepatic jaundice), acute necrosis (yellow atrophy) and the acute damage to the liver which occurs in many infective diseases—pneumonia, syphilis, yellow fever, Weil's disease and many others. Moreover the ordinary cirrhosis of the liver is easily and correctly included as chronic interstitial hepatitis, an analogous disease to chronic interstitial nephritis. The general lines of treatment applicable to all varieties of hepatitis have already been given, while the general and specific treatment of certain diseases, such as syphilis, yellow fever, and Weil's disease are dealt with elsewhere. All that remains is to consider the symptomatic or specialized treatment required in some of the common diseases of the liver.

JAUNDICE

Jaundice is a common symptom or sign in many forms of hepatic disease, but although often spoken of almost as such, it is not a disease of itself. It is evidence merely of disturbance of one hepatic function which is concerned with the production and disposal of the bile. Bile, partly a secretory and partly an excretory product of the liver, consists of three essential constituents :—

1. Bile-salts, which are apparently manufactured in the liver alone, and are a true secretion. They have an important function in the digestion of fats.

2. Cholesterol, which exists in the bile as "free" cholesterol, in contrast to the blood-cholesterol, four-fifths of which is bound as cholesterol-ester of higher fatty acids. In passing through the liver the cholesterol-ester appears to be de-esterized, which indicates some activity of the liver apart from mere excretion. The presence of cholesterol in the bile has an important bearing on the formation of gall-stones, but of its function in the body we know very little.

3. Bile-pigment (bilirubin), is a pure excretion which passes out in the fæces and for which the body has no further use. It is the iron-free part of the hæmoglobin molecule, derived from the breaking-down of red-blood corpuscles within cells of the reticulo-endothelial system. Contrary to former beliefs it is now recognized that the liver is not concerned with the manufacture of bile-pigment, but merely with its excretion.

Although presumably the least important constituent of the bile, being merely a waste-product, bile-pigment obtrudes itself strikingly enough in the memory of the clinician, being the cause of the characteristic yellowness of the skin and body tissues in jaundice.

Jaundice may be described as of three varieties :—

1. *Obstructive hepatic jaundice*, arising from obstruction of many kinds to the outflow of bile from the liver. In this variety all three constituents of the bile are retained in the blood, and must be removed from the body in some abnormal way. During excretion by an abnormal route, symptoms may arise and require treatment.

2. *Toxic and infective hepatic jaundice*, which is by far the commonest type, occurs in all forms of hepatitis or damage to the liver. Here again the three constituents of the bile may, for a time at least, be retained in excess in the blood, and give rise to the same problems during their excretion.

3. *Hæmolytic jaundice*, which may occur in conditions of excessive blood destruction, is dealt with under the anæmias (p. 488); and the jaundice of itself involves no problem of treatment.

It is necessary to draw attention here to the fact that mere yellowness of the skin and subcutaneous tissues gives no criterion of the severity and extent of the hepatic damage. The essential feature of jaundice of all varieties is retention of one or all of the constituents of the bile in the blood. The yellow colour in jaundice results from the presence of excess of bile-pigment in the blood (bilirubinæmia), but this may occur before obvious jaundice can be recognized clinically, and may have disappeared long before the yellow staining of the tissues has passed off. Thus only the intensity of bilirubinæmia in the blood may influence prognosis and treatment, and not the colour of the skin.

Catarrhal Jaundice.—This is the commonest disease, associated with jaundice as a symptom, met with in Britain. All recent pathological evidence seems to show that it is essentially a toxic or infective hepatitis, generally of fairly mild degree, and due to an unknown cause. The liver cells are damaged, and the bile ducts also share in the inflammation.

As a rule catarrhal jaundice is not a serious condition, requiring only simple treatment, but no case must be taken too lightly. It must always be remembered that quite suddenly, in an apparently straightforward case, all the signs of the most dreaded form of hepatitis (acute necrosis or yellow atrophy of the liver) may appear.

The treatment of an ordinary case of catarrhal jaundice is on the general lines already described.

1. Rest in bed, and warmth, until it is evident that the hepatic disturbance is not serious, and until bile-pigment, which is at first retained in the blood (resulting in clay-coloured stools) begins to reappear in the fæces.

2. A brisk saline purgative at the outset ; or the well-known Gregory's powder (5 to 15 gr.) may be used and repeated.

3. A light carbohydrate diet, with exclusion of fats.

4. Administration of glucose lemonade (p. 622) to protect the damaged liver cells.

As a rule the ordinary patient who has suffered from catarrhal jaundice may be allowed up in ten days, and is then well, although the yellowness of the skin and tissues may persist for a week or two longer. Occasionally the active phase of catarrhal jaundice is much longer, and intense jaundice with clay-coloured stools may continue for as long as three months. The physician is faced with great difficulty in such prolonged cases, and may rightly fear the occurrence of biliary obstruction from a tumour or other serious cause. Moreover, the liver, from the continued biliary obstruction, becomes greatly enlarged, and is often tender. In such cases, the writer has not hesitated to advise exploratory laparotomy and temporary drainage of the common bile duct. Thick inspissated greenish bile flows from the common bile duct at first, but within a day or two the normal flow of thin brown bile is established, the enlarged liver shrinks, and full recovery gradually takes place.

Itching of the skin (pruritus) is a special therapeutic problem in catarrhal jaundice, but also of many other examples of obstructive and of toxic or infective jaundice. The cause of this symptom, which may be very troublesome and prevent sleep, is not certainly known, although the attempted excretion through the skin of bile salts, retained in the blood, is commonly blamed. The itching may precede clinical jaundice, and continue long after recovery. As a rule, however, in prolonged obstructive jaundice (due, for example, to impacted gall-stone or carcinoma of the head of the pancreas), the itching disappears spontaneously after six weeks or thereabouts. Whatever be the essential cause, the itching (as in other forms of pruritus) is apparently due to irritation of nerve endings in the skin, and local remedies should be used to lessen their sensibility. No general nerve sedatives except bromides appear to have the slightest effect.

Many local sedatives may require to be tried in turn, and as usual it is best to begin with the simplest. Calamine lotion and ordinary household starch can be applied liberally and without restriction. Starch can be used either in a warm bath (4 to 6 tablespoonfuls or more), or a thick starch paste may be "dabbed" on the skin and allowed to dry. Other applications may be tried, but some must be used with care if often repeated. Examples of drugs used are carbolic acid (1 : 60), thymol, camphor, menthol and zinc oxide. Camphor, gr. xx, may be combined with zinc oxide, ℥i, as a dusting powder; or menthol, gr. v, and thymol, gr. x, may be dissolved in 1 oz. of water and used as a paint. Similar amounts of menthol or camphor may usefully be combined with calamine lotion.

Persistent hiccup occasionally occurs in catarrhal jaundice, but is commoner in cirrhosis of the liver, and its treatment is discussed under that heading.

ACUTE (AND SUBACUTE) NECROSIS OF THE LIVER

(Syn.: Acute yellow, acute red atrophy)

The cause of this dreaded, but fortunately uncommon, hepatic disease is often unknown. It may arise in the course of catarrhal jaundice, and during pregnancy, but is occasionally unassociated with any previous change in the body or its functions. Rarely, in certain countries, it has appeared in the form of small epidemics.

It is known, however, to appear after the therapeutic use of certain well-known drugs, of which arsenical compounds and atophan (cinchophen) are the best-known examples. It is by no means unknown in the chemical industry from exposure to a variety of volatile solvents.

When the necrosis of liver cells is very extensive and liver function totally fails, nothing can be done for the patient. The only clinical hope is that sufficient cells may be left intact to allow of regeneration, and glucose administration must be used copiously and continuously, the intravenous route generally being required. Insulin along with the glucose is often recommended, but there is no clear evidence that this is essential. Delirium is often, in the early stages, most violent, and one nurse may be quite unable to control the struggles of the patient. Powerful hypnotics such as morphine, which are in principle contraindicated, may require to be used, but may be without much effect. Later, the patient may sink into coma, and glucose (which it may have been impossible to administer during the height of the delirium) should be freely given intravenously.

CIRRHOSIS OF THE LIVER

(Syn. : Chronic interstitial hepatitis)

This is still one of the commonest chronic hepatic diseases. The essence of the pathology is the effects of oft-repeated damage to the liver cells, which for a time continue to exhibit their remarkable powers of regeneration. Finally, the power of repair is overcome, fibrous tissue fills the gap, and small areas of glandular cells are left isolated amidst the increasing scar tissue. The bile-ducts and portal blood capillaries undergo extreme distorsion and compression in the contracting fibrous tissue, leading to the well-known signs of portal obstruction. Blood continues to be supplied to the liver through the hepatic artery, and the quantity may even be augmented by dilatation of the artery. Finally the functions of the organ totally break down and death results. It must be remembered that when portal obstruction is well-marked, the absorbable products from the intestine which would normally be dealt with in the liver, escape directly into the systemic circulation by collateral veins and lead to some of the disturbances of metabolism common in hepatic cirrhosis.

Once the clinical features of cirrhosis of the liver are fully established, only palliative treatment is possible, but even then much can be done to prolong the life of the patient and relieve some of the most trying symptoms.

The real treatment of cirrhosis is *prophylactic*, or at least recognition of the onset of a chronic hepatitis long before the regenerative powers of the organ have been finally lost. We must aim, in fact, at much earlier diagnosis than has hitherto been made, and this raises at once the problems of ætiology. The writer, from a very considerable experience, has no doubt that in Britain alcohol is still by far the commonest cause of hepatic cirrhosis. Arguments as to how it acts do not concern us here. If diagnosis can be made at the stage sometimes called "pre-cirrhotic hepatitis," then, under a suitable régime of simple treatment and abstinence from alcohol, complete cure can as a rule be promised. The typical case is not a solitary drinker or dipsomaniac, and is not "a martyr to delirium tremens," but an individual who takes too much alcohol because he likes it, and generally accompanies it with too much food and too little exercise. Alcoholic cirrhosis is not confined to the well-to-do, and in our hospital patients an occupation implying easy access to alcohol—barmen and barmaids employees of breweries, etc.—is of great significance. The typical patient in the pre-cirrhotic stage is sallow, has frequent "liver attacks" (of alcoholic gastritis), and complains of headache, irritability and drowsiness. On physical examination the liver is enlarged, often tender, and piles are a common complaint.

Pre-cirrhotic Hepatitis.—The treatment of these patients is simple enough :—

Teetotalism must be enforced for life, and the great probability of complete cure, with the certainty of death if advanced cirrhosis is allowed to supervene, must be stressed to the full.

Rest in bed, warmth, and a restricted diet until all signs of alcoholic gastritis have gone. Gastric lavage may be essential at first to remove the excessive mucous secretion. Milk should be the first diet, and gradually an adequate diet chiefly containing carbohydrates is built up. Glucose lemonade should be the first drink allowed, but later when the patient (who is generally socially inclined) moves about in his business, the writer has been impressed with the value, both as a remedy and for social purposes, of the beverage known as Tonic Water. This ingenious drink contains a large amount of sugar, the sweet taste being concealed by the bitter taste of quinine (see p. 623). It is an excellent and entirely suitable substitute for glucose lemonade in all ambulant cases of liver disease, taken alone and with no alcohol added, and is easily obtainable.

Spa treatment, properly applied, including a correct dietary régime, baths or packs over the enlarged liver, the mild aperient spa water, and not least the discipline and removal from the temptations which have beset him, is often of the utmost value to the well-to-do patient at this early and curative stage of the disease.

Although, as has been mentioned, alcohol is the commonest cause of hepatic cirrhosis in Britain, a number of cases occur in which the effects of alcohol can positively be excluded. A history of typhoid fever or syphilis may sometimes be obtained, but often the ætiology remains obscure, and such patients are generally first seen when the disease is far advanced.

Advanced Cirrhosis.—If cirrhosis of the liver is first seen when the liver is contracted, portal obstruction evident, and jaundice and ascites present, then palliative treatment only is available. There is a fairly common belief that once ascites and jaundice have supervened, death is inevitable within about six months. This is quite erroneous, and with careful handling life and moderate health may be prolonged in a number of cases, but certainly not in all, for five years or more.

The treatment in the late stages is similar to that recommended for the earlier pre-cirrhotic hepatitis, but rest in bed is best avoided until near the end, or until œdema renders walking impossible. It is difficult in many of these patients to stop alcohol altogether, and no rule can be laid down. A patient, treated by the writer, lived and worked very actively for more than five years after ascites had required tapping, while still consuming a bottle of whisky daily.

Tapping of the abdomen should be begun fairly early, before marked œdema of the lower limbs appears, and before breathlessness becomes excessive from the overdistended abdomen. The average amount removed at a sitting from a patient with a moderately full abdomen is 11 to 15 pints. The technique of abdominal tapping is discussed elsewhere (p. 1087), but there are some practical points applicable to cases of hepatic cirrhosis which are worthy of mention. Antiseptics should be applied to the stretched and unhealthy abdominal skin with care, especially tincture of iodine, which in the writer's hands has several times produced marked pustulation. Weak picric acid is generally quite suitable, but a good (although gentle) rubbing with rectified spirits is adequate, and probably the safest of all. A fairly large trocar should be used, simply connected to a fine rubber tube, and the ascitic fluid is allowed to escape by gravity alone into a basin under the bed and invisible to the patient. After novocaine infiltration of the skin and abdominal wall right through to the peritoneum, a short slit made through the skin with a fine scalpel or tenotome allows the large trocar and cannula to be inserted right through the abdominal wall without undue pressure or jerking.

Although the slit made by the scalpel closes and heals far more readily than the rounded hole which the trocar alone would make, a certain amount of leaking after each tapping is to be expected, and may persist for forty-eight hours. Gauze pads and a binder are therefore generally essential, especially if, as happens in suitable employments, the patient is tapped one day and allowed to return to work the next. It has been found by experience that tapping in the flanks is easier for the patient (and the gauze pads are less obvious) than tapping in the middle line. The slit through which the tapping is carried out frequently appears very red and angry after forty-eight hours, and sepsis may be suspected. In practice, however, sepsis very seldom occurs, and there need be no fear, whether the puncture continues to leak or not, of sepsis spreading into the abdomen. The frequency of tapping varies greatly in different cases. At first this small operation may be required once a week, but later (possibly due to adhesions or to peritoneal thickening providing additional collateral vessels) tapping may be needed only at intervals of four to six weeks or more.

The Talma-Morison Operation.—This is carried out by surgeons in different ways, the aim in all operations being to increase the collateral circulation of the blood and relieve portal obstruction. The operation should always be preceded by tapping the abdomen. The peritoneal surfaces covering the liver and diaphragm are rubbed with gauze or scraped to induce adhesive inflammation, and the great omentum (which is rich in veins) may be similarly dealt with, or brought out through an opening to lie beside the rectus abdominalis muscle and securely fixed there.

The results of this operation are difficult to assess, as it has generally been carried out only in the last stages of cirrhosis. The writer has only seen great success in one man, who at the time of the operation was still very obese. In this patient the ascites, greatly complicated by obesity, was checked for two years.

Œdema of the legs and scrotum is a great source of trouble in the late stages of cirrhosis, just as in chronic cardiac failure. Much turns here on the efficiency of excretion by the kidneys, and if this is poor the end is not prolonged. It is well to recollect that œdema of the scrotum and legs must not be regarded as a " stagnant pool " but that even in the worst cases there is a constant but sluggish flow or movement of the fluid. The use of a " cardiac bed," or, failing this, an inclined plane, so that sudden postural alterations of the limbs can be made from time to time, enhances the movement of the fluid and greatly increases the possibility of control of the œdema. The effects of changes of posture are often amplified to a remarkable degree by the use of salyrgan (1 to 2 c.c. intravenously or intramuscularly), which can be injected with safety twice a week in all cases of cirrhosis unless there is also serious renal disease. The results of combined treatment with salyrgan and rapid postural alterations of the limbs are as a rule so satisfactory, that questions of acupuncture or the insertion of Southey's tubes will seldom arise.

Hæmorrhage may occur from various situations—epistaxis, melæna, hæmorrhoids. Bleeding from the rupture of dilated œsophageal veins is fairly common, and may be almost immediately fatal. The treatment is similar to that applicable to any severe hæmorrhage (p. 475).

Anæmia is common in cirrhosis of the liver, especially in

the later stages, and quite apart from active hæmorrhage. Its treatment is dealt with elsewhere (p. 471).

Hiccup is fairly common in a number of hepatic diseases, due to irritation of the diaphragm, and in cirrhosis it may persist without interruption for days, and completely exhaust the patient. The treatment is difficult and various remedies may be tried in turn—bismuth subnitrate (60 gr.), washing out the stomach with water as hot as can be borne, atropine sulphate ($\frac{1}{50}$ gr.), morphine ($\frac{1}{4}$ gr.), and finally cocaine ($\frac{1}{8}$ gr.) by injection.

Coma.—It is seldom justifiable to treat the drowsy toxæmic state which precedes the final coma when the liver totally fails. But one point concerning coma in cirrhosis is of some clinical importance. It happens occasionally that laparotomy is performed on a patient in whom hepatic cirrhosis is never suspected until the abdomen is opened. Such patients, following the operation and the anæsthetic, may rapidly sink into deep coma. Glucose should be administered intravenously at once and the otherwise inevitable fatality may be prevented. It is best to use 20 per cent. glucose in saline, injected very slowly, and as much as 200 to 300 c.c. may safely be given.

SPECIFIC INFECTIONS OF THE LIVER

The treatment of syphilis, malaria, amœbic hepatitis (tropical abscess), hydatids and other infections are all dealt with elsewhere.

SUPPURATIVE PYLEPHLEBITIS
CARCINOMA OF THE LIVER, ETC.

Omitted, as treatment is entirely surgical.

DISEASES OF THE GALL-BLADDER AND BILIARY TRACT

There are two common diseases of the gall-bladder and biliary tract: (1) Cholecystitis or inflammation of the gall-bladder; (2) gall-stones. In the majority of cases, but not in all, the second disease is the sequel of the first.

It is important to consider briefly a few points in ætiology, without a knowledge of which it is impossible to understand rational treatment, both prophylactic and curative.

Microbic infection is the sole cause of cholecystitis, and the essential cause of by far the majority of gall-stones. Much discussion has always arisen as to whether the infecting organisms reach the biliary tract from the blood-stream and are excreted by the liver with the bile, or whether the route of infection is a direct ascent from the duodenum into the common bile duct. We possess no strong evidence in favour of one route as against the other. Typhoid fever is the only specific disease notoriously associated with infection of the biliary tract, but although this is an intestinal disease it is also a septicæmia in its earlier stages. A streptococcus is a common infecting organism in cholecystitis, but there is no proof of its intestinal origin, and indeed its presence has always raised the difficult problem of the influence of focal infection (in teeth, tonsils and elsewhere) in relation to the ætiology of cholecystitis and gall-stones. Coliform organisms (including *B. typhosus*) are also commonly found in inflamed gall-bladders, but other organisms such as staphylococci, gas-forming anaerobic bacilli, and diphtheroid bacilli also are met with.

The precise invading organism is seldom known in the early stages, so that specific prophylactic or curative treatment is impracticable, and only general methods can be applied.

Biliary stasis is universally accepted as an important contributory cause of biliary infection. This occurs in pregnancy, and accounts, in part at least, for the increased frequency of gall-stones in married women. But a sedentary occupation or lack of exercise and obesity are also important in this respect, and require to be remembered in treatment.

Composition of the Bile.—The three normal constituents of the bile—bile-salts, cholesterol and bile pigment—have already been described. When infection occurs, a fourth constituent—calcium—is added, since the inflammatory exudate is rich in lime-salts. Thus the common facetted gall-stones are made up of a mixture of calcium, cholesterol and bile-pigment. The prevention of the addition of calcium to the bile is simply the prevention or cure of the infection. Other alterations in the normal constituents of the bile are also important, not in connection with primary cholecystitis, but with some varieties of gall-stones. Pure pigment stones of bilirubin may occur at an early age in acholuric jaundice (p. 489), and their presence in the gall-bladder is frequently followed by infection and cholecystitis. Cholesterol is increased in the bile in pregnancy, obesity and other conditions, and it is believed that this accounts for the formation of solitary cholesterol gall-stones, which certainly arise in a sterile gall-bladder. Secondary cholecystitis is here again of frequent occurrence. The problem of treating an excess of bile pigment and an excess of cholesterol is discussed later.

The Gall-Bladder.—Both the structure and function of the gall-bladder have important bearings on treatment. The normal gall-bladder wall is thin and almost translucent, but its mucous lining is a complex honeycomb. In chronic cholecystitis the whole wall may become greatly thickened and scarred, and it is claimed by surgeons that the microbic infection lies deep in the wall, and that the presence or absence of micro-organisms, free in the gall-bladder bile, is relatively unimportant. Obviously no medical treatment, probably not even any remedy carried to the thickened gall-bladder wall by the blood stream, can hope to cure this type of infection, and when the gall-bladder wall is thickened and sclerosed surgery is the only therapeutic remedy. If, however, as the writer believes, cholecystitis can be diagnosed early, before permanent changes have occurred in the gall-bladder wall, then medical treatment may effect a cure.

The main function of the gall-bladder is to concentrate the bile, and to empty, or more accurately to empty itself partially, when suitable food enters the duodenum. Advantage is taken of this concentrating power in the diagnostic X-ray method known as cholecystography, and advantage of the ability of the gall-bladder to evacuate its contents is made use of therapeutically.

CHOLECYSTITIS

Acute cholecystitis is of several varieties. Two of these—acute suppurative cholecystitis and acute phlegmonous cholecystitis—are fortunately rare, and fall at once into the realm of surgical emergencies.

Catarrhal cholecystitis is exceedingly common, and is to be regarded as a milder form of infection of the biliary tract, smouldering slowly with the production of definite clinical symptoms, and, unless cured, almost inevitably ending with the sequel of gall-stones.

The treatment of catarrhal cholecystitis is twofold: (1) methods directed to the sterilization of the biliary tract; (2) symptomatic treatment of the flatulent dyspepsia and other clinical features of this disease.

Two methods have been chiefly employed in attempts to eradicate the infecting organisms. The first method presupposes that in the earlier stages of cholecystitis the microbes are still free and accessible in the bile, and not deeply embedded in the wall. Two antiseptics, both excreted by the liver in the bile, have been recommended. Sir Arthur Hurst has strongly supported the claims of hexamine as a biliary antiseptic, when given in large doses. He commences with a mixture containing 80 gr. each of sodium bicarbonate and sodium citrate in 2 oz. of water, given three times daily after meals until the urine has been persistently alkaline for twenty-four hours. Then to each dose of the medicine 100 gr. of hexamine is added, and the patient continues to take 300 gr. of hexamine daily until all symptoms have disappeared. The constant alkalinity of the urine is very important, to prevent irritation of the urinary bladder. Strong claims have been made in favour of this method, but the writer is not at all convinced of its efficacy.

Sodium salicylate, in doses of 30 gr. or more three times daily, has also been recommended, but its activity as a biliary antiseptic is hard to judge.

In the writer's opinion the method now often known as "non-surgical biliary drainage" offers the best chance of cure of a catarrhal cholecystitis. This method takes advantage of the capacity of the gall-bladder to contract suddenly and empty its contents, and arose out of the application of a diagnostic test still commonly employed—biliary drainage after the passage of a duodenal tube. It was found that various substances—irritants such as concentrated solutions of magnesium sulphate and more normal stimulants such as olive oil—when introduced through the duodenal tube, at once excited biliary contraction and a free flow of bile. It was soon realized that here was a therapeutic method by means of which the biliary tract could be emptied at will, and the process repeated when the gall-bladder filled again. An important extension of the method soon appeared, which has made it entirely suitable for ordinary clinical use. It was found that either concentrated solutions of magnesium sulphate or olive oil were quite efficient in inducing gall-bladder contraction when given on an empty stomach, and without the need for a duodenal tube at all.

In practice the method of non-surgical biliary drainage is carried out as follows :—

1. The following prescription is made up :

   Magnesium sulphate, 25 per cent. solution in water.
   Syrup of lemon—just sufficient to flavour.

One teaspoonful or more (the suitable dose varies, but purgation should be avoided) to be taken in a wine glass of water, on an empty stomach, immediately on waking in the morning and at least twenty minutes before breakfast.

2. During the day, advantage is taken of the action of olive oil, and *before* the midday and evening meal a dessert-spoonful of olive oil should be taken to empty the biliary tract. Olive oil acts also in another important way, referred to below. Good olive oil is almost tasteless, but should be bought in small bottles, as it may become rancid.

This method should be carried out daily and systematically for several months, and later, when all symptoms have disappeared, it should be repeated periodically in short courses.

The main symptomatic treatment of catarrhal cholecystitis is concerned with the flatulent dyspepsia which is so common. Dietetics are important, and cooked fat or fried dishes generally aggravate the condition. Olive oil, however, a natural fat, is the most valuable drug we possess for the relief of flatulence, and when taken before meals ($\frac{1}{2}$ to 1 oz.) it greatly diminishes the flow of acid gastric juice. Bismuth and alkalis are also useful in some cases, and are frequently employed.

The question of dietetics in cholecystitis requires consideration for several reasons. First, the problem arises of whether gall-stones can be prevented by diminishing the cholesterol content of the food, since cholesterol is one of the important constituents of biliary calculi. With this end in view egg-yolk, sweetbreads, kidney, liver, cream, suet and other foods rich in cholesterol have been excluded from the diet, but the writer is not convinced that this can alter in any important respect the amount of cholesterol available to the body from many sources.

Cholecystitis (and its common sequel of gall-stones) is very often associated with obesity, and active treatment of this complication cannot be overemphasized (p. 387). Moreover obese patients, who so often state that they eat little, are frequently found on questioning to indulge in just the foods (new bread, hot rolls, pastry) which are particularly liable to induce flatulence even in normal individuals. Other methods directed to the prevention of flatulence have already been mentioned.

Spa treatment is of undoubted value in the treatment of cholecystitis, not only because of the regular dietetic routine followed, away from domestic or business cares, but also because of the effects of the mineral water, best taken hot and always on an empty stomach. The spa water is generally sipped slowly, while walking about, a pint at a time, and is drunk before breakfast and again in the afternoon.

Even in patients who are unable to go to a spa copious drinks of hot water, sipped slowly on an empty stomach, should be taken.

Chronic Cholecystitis.—Chronic cholecystitis may occur either with or without the presence of gall-stones, and the latter condition is dealt with separately.

As has been indicated, when the gall-bladder is chronically inflamed, thickened and sclerosed, and when cholecystography has shown its inability to concentrate bile or loss of its capacity to empty itself, then medical treatment can only be palliative, and in the present state of our resources surgery is the only cure. The palliative methods are the same as those already described.

Gall-stones.—Once gall-stones have formed in an infected gall-bladder there is no known method of dissolving them. Some small ones may pass easily into the intestine, others may block the ducts, and large ones remain in the gall-bladder to set up further inflammation and to be joined by a further collection of stones.

Quacks have for long claimed to dissolve gall-stones, and the method they commonly employ is to administer olive oil in a cachet or enclosed within some form of capsule. As has been indicated, olive oil before meals is our best remedy for the symptomatic treatment of the intense flatulent dyspepsia, and so many of the patients at once experience great relief. The olive oil, given in this way, is saponified into a soap, and to the inexperienced person the masses of soap may bear a fair resemblance to gall-stones, and may be demonstrated to the patient as such. Physicians must be well aware of this error, and able to explain it to their patients whose symptoms soon return when the treatment is stopped.

At present the only certain cure for gall-stones is their surgical removal, and the physician is chiefly concerned with the following therapeutic problems.

Biliary Colic.—As soon as the diagnosis is made this should be treated at once by injection of morphine combined with atropine.

Exacerbations of Cholecystitis in association with Gall-stones.—Such attacks are common, associated with fever, vomiting, intense pain and tenderness over the gall-bladder. The clinical problems of treatment are sometimes difficult, but an attempt must always be made to allow the acute inflam mation to subside before operation is contemplated. Th dangers of waiting are perforation of the gall-bladder an suppuration (empyema of the gall-bladder). Both of thes are fortunately rare, and, if they are excluded, treatment shoul be passive and not active. Pain should be controlled wit morphine and atropine, but no purgative or other drug whic might act on the gall-bladder or biliary tract must be given Diet must be restricted, and indeed starvation is probabl best and most agreeable to the patient until the acut inflammation subsides in a very few days.

Pre-operative Treatment.—Much can be done to increas the safety of an operation for gall-stones. Liver function i always disturbed, and glucose, or fruit drinks, or a combinatio of both, should always be given freely for some days prior t operation.

Obesity is a frequent source of danger, and few surgeon are willing to operate, except in emergency, on very obes patients suffering from gall-stones. For safety the obesit must always be treated by the dietetic and other method described elsewhere (p. 387).

Conservative Treatment of Disease of the Biliary Tract.—I happens fairly frequently that patients who are old and infirm or who suffer from serious disease of other organs (heart, lungs kidneys, diabetes) develop symptoms which point unmistak ably to a disorder of the biliary tract—gall-stones or an acut exacerbation of chronic cholecystitis, or both. Operatior with its grave risks, is imperative immediately only whe empyema of the gall-bladder or perforation are diagnosed, an at a later period when completely obstructive jaundice indicate impaction of a stone in the common bile duct. Otherwis every attempt must be made to avoid operation, and, as ha been indicated, it is remarkable how acute signs and symptom of disease of the gall-bladder may settle down within a fe days, with rest and administration of morphine. The scop of palliative treatment thereafter to be adopted must var with the general condition of the patient, and rigid rules ma be unsuitable. Nevertheless it is often possible to damp dow the biliary troubles of such patients for years, and life ma terminate only by the progress of the other disease. Th writer recollects one old man, suffering also from obesity an auricular fibrillation, in whom many attacks of " intermitten hepatic fever " due to a ball-valve calculus periodicall blocking the cystic duct were treated conservatively an successfully for seven years.

In many of these cases, as in the patient discussed above, it is advisable to carry out at a suitable time the X-ray examination of cholecystography, and there is generally no contraindication to this investigation. The information obtained may be negative or incomplete, but may at times be of great importance to the physician and also to the surgeon if an absolute emergency arises.

Advice Regarding Operations on the Biliary Tract.—When a patient first suffers from biliary colic or from the first obvious attack of acute cholecystitis, the treatment is medical provided the well-known surgical emergencies can be excluded. When, as generally happens, the acute phase passes over, the physician has time to use the appropriate tests for accurate diagnosis, and to consider his patient in respect of age, general health and obesity. Even when gall-stones or chronic cholecystitis have been identified, it may be entirely justifiable to continue medical treatment in the hope of avoiding subsequent attacks, but each case must be judged on its merits.

When operation is strongly advised the physician may be asked to give his reasons, since medical treatment may control the symptoms and since it is well known that gall-stones may be discovered accidentally at necropsy in patients who have never been known to suffer from biliary disease. Further, the physician may often be asked about the possibility of "dissolving" gall-stones, and will be able to explain the secrets of the olive-oil treatment.

When advising operation the rare possibility of cancer of the gall-bladder (p. 622) should not be mentioned, and the writer has generally found it best to allude only in very general terms to the serious acute complications (such as empyema and perforation) that may ensue. The patient may be warned that the presence of gall-stones limits his or her activities "geographically." It may be pointed out that emergency surgery in the upper abdomen is serious even when all the resources of a big city are available, and that in the depths of the country, on holidays abroad or on a sea-voyage the risks of an immediate operation are greatly enhanced. Further, the patient should be told that the liver itself, an essential organ for life, is always injured by the presence of gall-stones and biliary sepsis, and that damage to the heart muscle (myocarditis) is not infrequent.

For these reasons, among others, the patient should be strongly advised to seek operation during a quiescent stage of the disease, after all necessary preparative medical treatment has been carried out.

CARCINOMA OF THE GALL-BLADDER OR BILE DUCTS

Carcinoma of the gall-bladder is almost invariably associated with gall-stones ; but it occurs, however, only in about 4 per cent. of cases. The prophylactic treatment is to remove the gall-stones. Early diagnosis is very difficult, and since the growth rapidly invades the liver, no medical or surgical treatment is usually possible. (It is not unknown to find a very early carcinoma in a gall-bladder removed for gall-stones, and then complete cure may result.)

Carcinoma of the bile-ducts is very unusual, but carcinoma at the ampulla of Vater (whether primary at the end of the common bile duct or in the head of the pancreas does not matter clinically) is exceedingly common ; it is, in fact, the most likely cause of painless obstructive jaundice arising after middle age. Carcinoma involving the head of the pancreas remains at present an almost impossible operative problem for the surgeon, but an important palliative measure must never be forgotten. It is often possible surgically, if the gall-bladder is not diseased or deformed, to join the fundus of the gall-bladder to the duodenum, thus providing free biliary drainage into the intestine and relieving the patient of all the misery of a persistent obstructive jaundice. The writer has had patients who have been able to continue work and enjoy fair health for almost three years after this palliative operation has been performed.

APPENDIX

Intravenous Administration of Glucose

Glucose is used for intravenous injection as a 6 per cent. solution in normal saline, carefully filtered and sterilized. It is often desirable, however, in order to cut down the bulk of the injected fluid, to give glucose intravenously as a 20 per cent. solution in normal saline. There is no danger in this, provided the injection is given slowly.

Glucose Lemonade

$\frac{1}{2}$ lb. powdered glucose or 1 lb. commercial glucose.
1 quart of water.
Thin rind of two lemons.

Add glucose to water and lemon rind ; boil for five minutes, strain, and when cold add juice of two lemons.

Tonic Water

The manufacturers of Schweppes Tonic Water have provided the following details :—

Tonic Water is manufactured from fruit flavourings and essences, finest cane-sugar, and carbonated with pure filtered water. During the process of manufacture and after brief storage practically all the cane-sugar is hydrolyzed or inverted to an equal mixture of glucose and lævulose.

The chief analytical figures for Tonic Water are as follows :—

Specific gravity	1038
Total sugars	9·12 per cent.
Citric acid	0·43 ,,
Quinine hydrochloride . .	0·01 ,,

J. W. McNee.

DISEASES OF THE PANCREAS

Diseases affecting the pancreas give rise to very anomalous clinical and clinico-pathological disturbances. In health the pancreas performs two entirely independent functions.

1. The production of insulin by the islets of Langerhans—internal secretion.
2. The production of pancreatic juice—external secretion.

Disturbances of the internal secretion are discussed in the section on Diabetes Mellitus (p. 323) and only those affecting the external secretion, which are few in number, are discussed here. In some of them glycosuria may be coincidental, but it is rarely severe ; if treatment is required it is the same as in Diabetes Mellitus.

Defects or deficiencies in pancreatic digestion may occur when the pancreatic juice is prevented from reaching the intestine, and from causes which inhibit the secretion or destroy the secreting cells. We do not know whether hypersecretion of pancreatic juice ever occurs, and the physician is only called upon to deal with the deficiencies. Moreover it is only chronic deficiency with which we are concerned, since acute diseases, and especially acute hæmorrhagic pancreatis, are entirely surgical in their treatment. Two chronic diseases—cyst of the pancreas and pancreatic stone—can also be dealt with effectively only by operation.

The diagnosis of chronic pancreatic disease is notoriously difficult and unsatisfactory. Its existence may be suspected when the stools are bulky, pale and frothy, and when the fat content is found to be high—60 to 80 per cent. instead of the normal 15 to 20 per cent. It must be remembered, however, that there are other causes of steatorrhœa, and also that when obstructive jaundice (due to many causes) is present fats may remain undigested from the absence of bile salts rather than from any deficiency of pancreatic secretion. In carcinoma of the head of the pancreas—one of the commonest causes of obstructive jaundice in adults beyond middle age—both the biliary secretion and pancreatic secretion may be deficient in the bowel.

When chronic pancreatic disease has been diagnosed, treatment is carried out in two directions:—

1. A diet is prescribed low in fat but containing an adequate amount of carbohydrate and predigested proteins.
2. An attempt is made to make good the deficiency of pancreatic juice by substitution therapy.

A diet suitable for most patients with pancreatic deficiency is given in the Appendix, and may be modified if the patient is obese, which, however, is unusual.

Substitution therapy has very slowly reached a useful stage of development. Pancreatic juice given by the mouth is valueless, since the enzymes are destroyed in the stomach. All remedies must therefore pass through the stomach unchanged, and several of these containing pancreatic enzymes are now available. Festan (Bayer) is prescribed as tablets (1 tablet or pellet three times daily, with, or immediately after, meals, swallowed without chewing) covered with a protective coating resistant to acid and only soluble on reaching the intestine. It contains all three pancreatic enzymes. Panacoids (Reed and Carnick) is prescribed as tablets "enteric coated," and each contains 2 gr. of desiccated pancreas and 2 gr. of desiccated duodenal substance. Dose, 1 tablet with, or just after, meals.

Pancreatic deficiency is so often only part of the picture of a disease that the physician must at the same time take full stock of other conditions affecting especially the liver, gall-bladder, stomach and duodenum.

DIET IN CHRONIC PANCREATIC DEFICIENCY

Breakfast, 8 *a.m.*—

Peptonized milk or Benger's Food, ½ pint.
Any cereal, with syrup, honey or sugar.
One egg.
Bread, toast, with butter in strict moderation.

Lunch, 1 *p.m.*—

Fish or meat as at dinner.
Vegetables—salad or cooked.
Bread, toast, with butter in strict moderation.
Fruit—raw or stewed; jellies; junket.

Tea—

Cup of weak tea.
Plain tea-bread or cake.

Dinner, 7 *p.m.*—

Light consommé.
Fish, steamed or grilled—serve with white sauce.
Small portion of mutton, lamb, chicken or sweetbread—lightly cooked.
Fruit; custard; trifle.
Weak coffee.

Bedtime—

Peptonized milk, ½ pint.

Water may be partaken of freely throughout the day.

DISEASES OF THE PERITONEUM

There are few diseases of the peritoneum which concern the physician in the first place, except tuberculous peritonitis and ascites, both of which are dealt with elsewhere.

Localized chronic peritonitis or peritoneal adhesions may result from any intra-abdominal operation, no matter how carefully the gut is handled. At times no cause for adhesions can be found. Any subsequent operation merely adds to the number and extent of adhesions, and should never be done after the condition is recognized, except for definite obstruction. The sufferers from abdominal adhesions frequently lapse into a state of chronic invalidism, never being well but never seriously ill, and complaining of many and diverse symptoms of discomfort. The motor and other functions of the intestine are undoubtedly disturbed, but it is not to be wondered at that the symptoms become exaggerated after a time. No cure is possible, but much symptomatic treatment, both physical and psychological, is required. Sedatives should be used with caution, and those of habit-forming type, especially opium, avoided. If a sedative is essential, it is best given in a mixture, the prescription not being shown to the patient. So far as physical symptoms are concerned, constipation and spasm of different parts of the bowel chiefly require treatment. Emuls. Paraff. Liq. Alk. (B.P.C.) is particularly valuable for the former, and tincture of belladonna (5 to 30 minims) is our mainstay for the latter.

J. W. McNee.
D. Smith.

DISEASES OF THE HEART AND CIRCULATION

PRINCIPLES AND LIMITATIONS OF CARDIAC THERAPEUTICS

THE axiom that the first stage in rational therapeutics is accurate diagnosis applies with particular emphasis in diseases of the heart and circulation. Just as a complete and exact diagnosis may safeguard the patient from unnecessary restrictions and ill-chosen remedies, so it must be realized that, with few exceptions, complete restoration of function is not to be anticipated, even with the most energetic measures at our command. Certain defects, by their very nature, are no material handicap and call for no treatment, while for others it must be admitted that remedies, however desirable, are unfortunately unavailing. There is no more important factor in determining appropriate treatment than the ability accurately to assess the degree of circulatory incapacity existing at the moment. It is a well-known fact that many a patient may have definite myocardial or endocardial lesions with striking physical signs and yet be completely free of all symptoms during ordinary activity or even during sustained physical exertion. Of these patients it may be said that their functional capacity is good. They require no treatment for the heart itself, and indeed it is often a question if by any reference to the heart their attention should thus be directed to their circulation. At the other extreme there are those who suffer from all the signs of heart failure even at rest: their functional capacity is minimal, and for them every effort must be made to ease the cardiac burden and relieve their acute discomfort. The first step in treatment, therefore, is the assessment of the degree of circulatory impairment, and this is gauged by the ease with which one or more of the three major cardiac symptoms—pain, dyspnœa or congestion—is induced.

It is important to note that a physical sign in itself, particularly when regarded as the only manifestation of organic damage, seldom warrants active therapeutic measures. A systolic murmur, an irregular pulse, even an enlarged heart, while each demanding careful investigation before its nature can be accurately determined, are not in themselves to be regarded as indications for any particular treatment. It is well known that, in the past, many a patient with a perfectly sound heart has been rested unnecessarily for months at a time on account of an innocent systolic murmur, and all to no purpose. Such a patient was perhaps lucky if he did not receive digitalis in some form or another, though no one has claimed that digitalis has the power to abolish a valvular murmur. Indeed on the contrary, by increasing the force of contractility, or by prolonging diastole, a murmur is often rendered more obvious. Similarly the waxing and waning pulse of sinus arrhythmia has often given rise to difficulty. Here again digitalis, by increasing vagal tone, renders the arrhythmia more striking. This arrhythmia is not a manifestation of disease. An enlarged heart is commonly found in the athlete. As such it demands no treatment. Similarly, in hypertensive heart disease, treatment is to be directed to the patient and not to the blood-pressure level. On the other hand, the detection of an early diastolic aortic murmur during the course of a routine examination in a young or middle-aged adult may be the first sign to suggest a syphilitic aortitis, and thus provide a clue for the early treatment and prevention of future incapacity. There are exceptions to every rule, but it is a good principle which applies with particular emphasis in the therapeutics of heart disease to treat the patient when his symptoms warrant attention, and not his physical signs.

As a further principle it is reasonable to suppose that successful and appropriate treatment depends upon the removal or correction of the provoking cause of the cardiac distress. It has to be admitted, however, that while the ætiological cause of heart disease is often obvious enough, yet unfortunately it is but seldom that treatment can be regarded as successful in eradicating it. The high incidence of rheumatic heart disease in adolescence and early adult life, with all its crippling effects and economic incapacity, make it perhaps the greatest scourge of the white races. We know little about the cause of rheumatic infection, and can do little to eradicate, cure or prevent this important cause of heart disease. Hypertension and arterio-sclerosis are often apparently familial in their distribution. So it is that even those emerging from adolescence may carry with them the defects of past generations, and transmit them to their children. It is common to find both these factors, hypertension and arteriosclerosis, playing an important part in the production of myocardial damage, and all the more regrettable that in the present state of our knowledge we are unable to prevent the ultimate development of grave cardiac and circulatory symptoms by the eradication of the provoking cause. On the other hand, there is every reason for the belief that the rôle of syphilis in the production of heart disease is steadily decreasing, and, when recognized as an ætiological factor, cautious and appropriate treatment may be undertaken with ample justification. Similarly, in that group of cases in which over-activity of the thyroid plays a part, highly skilled surgical measures, appropriately undertaken, may lead ultimately to remarkable recoveries, if not, indeed, complete restoration of cardiac function. Thus it is that in many of the most chronic forms of cardiac disease we are handicapped greatly in the satisfactory treatment of the ætiological factors. On the other hand, there are those cardiac affections secondary to, it may be, acute fevers, nutritional disturbances, chronic alcoholism, or digestive and dyspeptic conditions of one kind or another which may be greatly relieved by appropriate treatment of the exciting cause. In middle life the correction of obesity by dietetic means is of prime importance.

In the relief and treatment of circulatory dysfunctions, without doubt the provision of adequate rest and the regulation of exercise demand a fine discrimination. As pointed out above, the amount of rest to be recommended depends on the circulatory capacity of the individual. In the mildest cases it is only necessary to caution against undue fatigue: actual restriction of activities is unnecessary, and, indeed, should be avoided. There is every reason to suppose that the heart muscle in such people is improved in its tone by appropriate exercise. Unnecessary restriction will only lead to chronic invalidism, and often the production of an anxiety state regarding the integrity of the heart muscle. Much harm can be done by even the best intentions. For those who have dyspnœa or pain more readily induced on slight exertion, then a more sedentary and guarded life should be advised. They should be instructed to live well within their range of activity so that symptoms are kept in abeyance. When distress comes more easily and symptoms begin to appear on slight exertion, then further periods of rest and restricted activities are all the more desirable. Such people benefit from long hours of sleep, perhaps a minimum of nine hours, and many benefit greatly by a short rest after their midday meal. If for economic reasons this is not possible, then perhaps one day in bed each week may suffice to restore the circulation and enable the milder forms of exercise to be undertaken daily without real distress. If early signs of congestive heart failure be present, then more complete rest is urgently required, and a period of days or weeks in bed may be necessary. The amount and degree of rest obtained by lying in bed varies a good deal from individual to individual : it is seldom sufficient merely to order a period of rest in bed without implicit instructions as to the procedure to be adopted. In the more serious cases rest in bed must be absolute, which implies, in addition to the most comfortable and restful position possible for the individual, that arrangements must be made so that he does nothing for himself. He is to be carefully nursed, lifted and helped into different positions as occasion demands : he is to be fed : he is to be denied all but a few visitors. Too often visitors are a tax on the cardiac patient, who is unfit to cope with the presence of even his closest friends. In no system of the body are the beneficial effects of rest as a therapeutic measure better exemplified than in the case of the heart and circulation. It is not an uncommon finding that even in cases of congestive heart failure adequate rest, a suitable diet, and appropriate nursing care may restore to reasonable proportions the inadequate functional capacity, even without the use of cardiac drugs. Such is the importance of rest and activity that each must be gauged in suitable amounts for each individual patient incapacitated by circulatory disease.

Recognizing the remarkable recuperative powers of the circulatory system, it is right to emphasize as a further principle of cardiac therapeutics that the patient must be supported in his illness by an uplifting and encouraging outlook. His progress at first is often slow, and, to allay his fears, ease his suffering and promote peace of mind, the doctor must bring with him to the sickroom a confident and cheerful atmosphere. Heart disease brings with it doubts and fears peculiarly its own, and these can best be countered by a clear statement of facts, tempered with that amount of judicious optimism which the experienced physician will find appropriate for the particular individual's emotional state and mental outlook. The stresses and strains of modern life, the anxieties and doubts which torment the mind of the sick person, throw a burden indirectly on the circulatory system. The doctor in his visit must try to shelter his patient from all the worries attendant upon his illness. A sympathetic understanding of these factors can do much to tide the patient onwards towards recovery.

As a further principle it is desirable to have clearly in mind the indications for the use of those drugs and mechanical procedures commonly employed in cardiac therapeutics. Effective remedies are few, but pharmacopœal and proprietary preparations abound. The discriminating physician will so restrict his therapeutic armamentaria as to be thoroughly familiar with reliable and potent preparations of undisputed activity. The haphazard and indiscriminate use of drugs is at all times to be deprecated, but never more so than in the treatment of circulatory disease in which, with the appropriate use of potent preparations, so much of benefit can be readily accomplished. The intelligent use, for instance, of digitalis may be regarded as one of the triumphs of modern therapeutics, and yet it is probably correct to say that more people suffer from lack of it than are ever poisoned by overdosage. Similarly the use of reliable hypnotics is of prime importance. Long and refreshing hours of sleep demand the use of well-chosen hypnotics, and by their effect appreciably shorten the time spent in confinement to bed. Other symptoms such as cough, pain or excessive dyspnœa in themselves require appropriate treatment to ease the patient's burden. Each step taken is designed to lessen the work demanded of the heart, and by such means much can be accomplished. Dietary regulation has a similar purpose by the reduction of body-weight, and the provision of an adequate supply of vitamins. The restriction of the protein intake, diminishing the specific dynamic action of the protein stimulus to metabolism, serves a similar purpose.

With these broad principles in mind it is desirable to reflect on the limitations of active therapeutic measures. At the outset it will, of course, be realized that complete restoration of function is seldom to be expected, and for the most part structural defects in the muscle, valves and arteries are permanent and irremediable. In consequence a limit is set to what may be attained even by the best régime possible. This must not be permitted to prejudice or discourage the doctor in his endeavour to give adequate symptomatic relief. The fact is that all the measures at our disposal can only alleviate cardiac failure in so far as the myocardium is able to avail itself of the proffered help. A time will surely arise when the futility of whipping the tired horse becomes more and more evident. It has been wisely pointed out that, for the most part, the best that can be accomplished by the intelligent care of chronic cardiac disease is a prolongation of life and relief from suffering, which compares very favourably with all the advantages that can be derived from the early diagnosis and modern treatment of malignant disease (Levine).

Few patients live to suffer from congestive heart failure on more than two or three occasions at most. By assessing the degree and duration of functional incapacity of the circulatory system one may often gauge roughly the extent of the improvement possible from the therapeutic measures to be employed. Fortunately many patients respond more satisfactorily than might be anticipated, provided every provision is made for thorough treatment and careful supervision throughout the illness. In this connection social and economic factors play an important part, for obviously the patient safeguarded in a strong financial position is more likely to reap the benefit of a prolonged rest and change than the labourer whose earning capacity is endangered by many weeks or months of strict medical care, and who in his younger years had no guidance regarding the selection of a suitable occupation in relation to the early cardiac damage. In the particular circumstances the physician must choose a middle course, adapting treatment to the peculiar personal conditions as best he may, and doing all he can to prevent the onset of more serious complications. The skilful use of the procedures of known benefits combined with the full co-operation of the patient, both in an economic and personal sense, will do much to ward off the fatal issue, ease suffering and prolong life.

It is gratifying to record that the intensive study of heart disease during the past twenty-five years has been awarded by a great advance in its therapeutics, thus replacing the blind polypharmacy and inadequate care of the past. Least progress has been made in the treatment of blood-stream infections, but even in this respect there is now more justification than ever for the continued search for effective antiseptic agents. Further gains will be made when the ætiological factors responsible for the ultimate development of myocardial damage can be prevented and adequately treated. Recognizing the limitations and encouraged by the possibility of aiding and guiding the recuperative powers of nature, it is with such broad principles as these that the physician approaches the treatment of heart disease.

A. R. Gilchrist.

THE HEART AND CIRCULATION IN INFECTIONS

RHEUMATIC CARDITIS AND RHEUMATIC FEVER

At the outset it should be stated clearly that treatment of this common and disabling condition is most unsatisfactory. The continued stream of adult cardiac cripples attending our hospitals, the subjects of valvular disease resulting from rheumatic infection in childhood or adolescence, is evidence enough that our treatment of the primary infection is not effective in preventing eventual cardiac damage. Figures such as those of Leonard Findlay ("The Rheumatic Infection in Childhood," Arnold, 1931, p. 158) make melancholy reading. He found that of nearly 700 cases of rheumatic infection in childhood, only one-third escaped cardiac damage, while one-third died within ten years of the first infection, and the remaining third became cardiac cripples, to die in early adult life. If such is the outlook for cases treated with all the resources of a modern hospital, it is apparent that the efficacy of our methods leaves much to be desired. Realization of the limitations of our therapy, however, must not discourage us from treating the victims of this disease as carefully and as intelligently as possible.

Rest.—The two procedures which command universal approval in the management of rheumatic carditis and fever are rest in bed and the administration of salicylate. The child who develops acute or subacute rheumatism should be confined to bed for a prolonged period, during which time he should be at complete rest. Good nursing is essential, and during the presence of active carditis the patient should not be expected or allowed to do anything for himself. The achievement of such complete physical rest in young children who have passed the stage of acute symptoms may present considerable difficulty, but confinement to bed should be maintained even although the child is moving about freely in bed, for to allow such a child up would at once increase greatly the demands made on the heart and circulation. During the period of fever, with its accompanying profuse perspiration, it is usual to keep the patient between blankets, thereby promoting absorption. Careful attention to the toilet of the skin is always necessary, and will lessen the risk of sudaminal rashes. The diet during this period should be fluid and light, as for any other febrile condition. The duration of bed rest is discussed below.

Salicylates.—By general consent, salicylate is regarded as without action on the progress of the cardiac lesions in rheumatism, but exerts a striking and specific effect on the other clinical manifestations, fever and arthritis. Despite misgivings expressed by some authorities, it appears to be without deleterious effect on the heart muscle, and its use, therefore, is not only permissible but imperative in cases with joint involvement. To withhold a remedy that relieves distress so strikingly is to be needlessly cruel; but it should be remembered that it masks the underlying active rheumatic process, and may mislead the unwary into a sense of false security.

To be effective the drug must be given in doses sufficient to produce the symptoms of mild salicylate intoxication: many so-called resistant cases are really due to underdosage. The actual daily dose required to produce saturation with the drug will vary naturally with the age and weight of the patient. The guide to the dose in any individual case is clinical: the abolition of joint pains and of pyrexia, or the development of mild symptoms of salicism, tinnitus, deafness, etc. In general, for an adult, doses of 20 to 30 gr. two or three hourly will be required, a total of 200 gr. per day being commonly sufficient. In children the effective daily dose varies from 60 to 120 gr. per day, according to age. Such doses may produce gastric irritation, and this may be the limiting factor in dosage. Sodium bicarbonate is usually given with the salicylate in doses of 20 to 30 gr. for each 20 gr. of sodium salicylate. This is generally accepted as a measure which reduces the risk of toxic manifestations, though the mode of action is debatable. In cases where sodium salicylate is badly tolerated, acetylsalicylic acid may be substituted. Dosage again has to be pushed so far as the tolerance of the patient permits, or until gastric symptoms prove a bar to further increase. The soluble calcium salicylate, in doses of 15 gr., may be substituted. Though freely soluble this should not be prescribed in a mixture but in powder form with instructions to dissolve one powder in cold water immediately before use. The intravenous administration of salicylate has been advocated by some, but has not been demonstrated to possess appreciable advantages over oral administration. The risk of toxic reactions is much increased, and the method can be said to have little or no place in the treatment of acute rheumatic carditis.

The duration of salicylate therapy on the scale of dosage advocated above is short. Once the fever and pain have subsided, or when symptoms of salicism have appeared, the dosage should be reduced considerably. This can generally be done within a few days at most from the start of treatment.

The drug should not, however, be entirely discontinued, but should be administered in smaller doses so long as the rheumatic process is judged to remain active. The maintenance dose is that which will just suffice to keep pain and fever in abeyance, and for an adult is generally from 100 to 120 gr. per day. Recurrence of acute symptoms is common when the maintenance dose is reduced as low as 60 gr. per day. Should such recurrence occur, the dose must be temporarily increased.

Local treatment for the affected joints should be simple. Wrapping the affected parts in cotton-wool and bandaging to secure rest generally suffice during the few days of acute pain. The application of a liniment of methyl salicylate (B.P.) is in general use, but is of minor importance. Care is essential in those cases where pain lasts more than a very few days, for contrary to general teaching, permanent joint affection may result from rheumatic fever. This rare complication, practically unknown in young children, is seen now and then in adolescent patients. One has seen, for example, a case of acute rheumatic pericarditis in a young adult, with subcutaneous nodules, in which the affected joints included the temporo-mandibular and the small joints of the hands, and where lasting deformity was a sequel. The differentiation of rheumatic fever from " subacute rheumatoid arthritis " in such cases is highly artificial.

In cases where permanent joint changes follow, immobilization during the acute stage leads later to limitation of movement, or even to fibrous ankylosis. It should be a rule, therefore, that passive movement through the maximum range short of causing pain should be performed daily so soon as the most acute symptoms subside, and immobilization during the rest of the day should be in a position optimum for function should fixation occur in spite of attempts to prevent it.

Focal Sepsis.—In many cases of rheumatic fever a focus of streptococcal infection in tonsils or upper respiratory tract remains active throughout the course of the disease. In these cases the question of treatment for the local septic condition arises, and problems requiring great judgment have to be faced. It is a sound rule to confine treatment to conservative lines so long as arthritis or carditis is active, and certainly during the more acute phases. Gargles, sprays and throat paints are of value, while the administration of sulphonamide derivatives may have some influence on the local infection. Radical treatment, by tonsillectomy for example, always demands careful deliberation before it is undertaken for exacerbation of the rheumatic condition, and a severe progressive or even fatal carditis may ensue after an ill-timed operation. In general, no operative interference should be attempted during the period of activity of the rheumatic lesions, and operations such as tonsillectomy should be postponed till convalescence is well established. Where the disease pursues a subacute course, with frequent relapses and continuous low fever, and where gross tonsillar infection is obvious, the question of operative interference at an earlier date must be faced. Operation may have to be undertaken as the only measure which will enable the relapses to be controlled. But in such event, operation must be decided upon only after full consideration of the risks involved weighed against the chances of benefit which may result.

It is convenient to discuss here the advisability of tonsillectomy in rheumatic children who are in a quiescent state. It appears that routine tonsillectomy of healthy children does not protect them against subsequent first attacks of rheumatic fever, and routine tonsillectomy after a first attack does not appreciably lessen the risk of recurrence of the rheumatism. It is probably wise to advise tonsillectomy only when the local condition is such as would demand operation in a non-rheumatic case, and then to choose the time for operation with great care.

Antistreptococcal Serum.—Of recent years the relationship of the hæmolytic streptococcus to the rheumatic infection has attracted increasing attention, and it is now accepted that, if it be not the actual causative agent, this organism at least lays the body open to the rheumatic attack and is closely associated with the infection. Empirically, therefore, attempts have been made to treat rheumatic fever with antistreptococcal serum (Eason *et al*, *Quarterly Journal of Medicine*, 1937, **6,** 93). It seems to be established, and this is borne out by our personal experience, that the administration of such serum has, in some cases, a definite effect on the pyrexia and joint symptoms in cases resistant to salicylate, which are not uncommon. Whether the effects are due to a true attack on the streptococcus, or are entirely non-specific in nature, is open to question. Cases which drag on in subacute fashion over a period of months, with bouts of pyrexia and pain lasting days or weeks, have shown encouraging results with serum treatment. The sponsors of the treatment go so far as to use it in place of salicylate, which they have discarded in view of its admitted inability to affect the cardiac lesions. The effect of serum on the eventual incidence of cardiac lesions cannot be known till a considerable period of years has elapsed. Some cases are resistant to serum and progress, it may be to a fatal issue, in spite of this or any other treatment, but, in our opinion, serum is worthy of trial in otherwise intractable cases. Stock concentrated anti-scarlatinal serum is used, injected intramuscularly in doses of 6 c.c. daily for a week. Severe reactions are unusual during a first course if preliminary tests for serum-sensitivity are carried out. Should, however, a second course be necessary, brisk serum reactions are more common and may be troublesome. They seldom preclude, however, the completion of the planned course of injections.

Duration of Rest.—The question of how long a patient with rheumatic carditis is to be kept in bed is not easily answered. No hard-and-fast time-limit can be laid down, though many clinicians advocate a minimum of three months' bed rest after even a mild attack. There is no doubt that the general tendency is to treat cases of rheumatic fever with insufficient rest. It is distressingly common to encounter cases of established valvular disease who relate a history of previous arthritis treated by a short period of rest followed by a relatively quick return to normal activity. In such cases it is apparent that the doctor had erroneously diagnosed that the heart had escaped damage, and had therefore felt justified in curtailing the period of invalidism. It is wiser to assume that the heart is affected by rheumatism in every case till time has proved one wrong. In all cases with clinical evidence of carditis, bed rest should be prolonged so long as the signs of activity persist, and this may extend over a period of many months. It is not desirable to prolong rest after signs of activity have disappeared. An established quiescent valvular lesion is not benefited by such treatment, and there is evidence that moderate exercise (*e.g.*, games, but no competitive sports) is beneficial for the subjects of early valvular disease.

The criteria for determining quiescence of the endocardial inflammation must therefore be considered. It must be realized that a smouldering inflammation may go on in a valve for many months, and that a process of sufficient intensity to produce eventual gross fibrosis may exist with very little clinical upset. Pulse-rate and temperature may be normal and gross cardiac enlargement absent in the presence of active valvular mischief. Sinus arrhythmia is no longer regarded as a safe indication that the heart has escaped damage, and we have repeatedly confirmed Parkinson's observation that active carditis and sinus arrhythmia may coexist. As is well known, the duration or degree of joint involvement bears no relation to the extent of the cardiac lesions. Subcutaneous nodules when present are indicative of activity, but their absence does not exclude active carditis. The return of the blood sedimentation rate (B.S.R.) to normal is probably as sure a guide as any to the cessation of activity. The B.S.R. is raised in all cases of active carditis, except those with gross congestive failure, but in these cases the failure is easily recognized, and the question of allowing the patient up does not arise. A raised B.S.R. naturally does not necessarily indicate carditis, for many conditions increase it, *e.g.*, tonsillar sepsis, etc. By careful clinical examination the true significance of a raised B.S.R. can usually be assessed. Other criteria of cessation of activity are gain in weight in children (not due to œdema), stabilization of the position of the apex beat and of physical signs in the heart, and a stable pulse-rate, particularly that taken during sleep.

Convalescence.—When the period of complete bed rest is over the return to activity should be very gradual, and should be carefully supervised. Any suspicion of recrudescence of the rheumatic process should be met by a prompt return to complete rest as in the acute attack.

The child who has weathered a rheumatic carditis is frequently sent for a short period to a convalescent home, and then returns to school and to full routine. This is not satisfactory, and is probably responsible for much disability in later life. Convalescence should be protracted, and after the period of hospital treatment the child should be sent for a residence of at least some months, but preferably for a prolonged period (six to eighteen months), to a convalescent home. In some parts of the country special homes have been established by local authorities for such convalescent rheumatic children, where adequate medical attention and supervision are available in healthy surroundings, much on the lines of sanatoria for tuberculosis. The early manifestations of recurrence can thus be recognized and timeous hospital treatment instituted. These homes are not designed for children already the subjects of advanced cardiac disease, for whom unfortunately little can be done, but for the large number of early or incipient cases of cardiac involvement in whom some abatement or arrest of the mischief may be looked for. Provision for the education of the children in such homes is essential.

After-care.—On discharge from such an institution, or after long convalescence at home in areas with no such facilities, the child should return gradually to activity, the limitation of effort being determined by the extent of the cardiac damage. In cases with mild but quiescent cardiac valvular lesions full activity is allowable, with, however, a prohibition on strenuous exertions like competitive sports. Cases with gross damage and marked enlargement must, however, lead quiet, non-strenuous lives. Careful follow-up with periodic assessment of general health and cardiac condition is essential, and any suggestion of renewed rheumatic activity demands prompt measures of rest in bed, etc.

The choice of a future occupation should always be made under the guidance of the doctor. Instances of children or young adults with advanced cardiac lesions engaged in strenuous occupations are all too familiar. One recalls, for example, an undersized lad of fourteen with gross mitral stenosis and auricular fibrillation who was employed as a message boy, cycling with heavy loads in a hilly town. Such cases should not be allowed to occur, and would not if efficient after-care were carried out. In this connection it is well to emphasize that the education of a child should not be neglected during long periods of semi-invalidism. Many rheumatic children leave school at fourteen years with much less than average schooling, and are driven on to the unskilled labour market. Better education means better ability to secure a sedentary occupation, which will not lead so soon to a cardiac breakdown.

TREATMENT OF NON-RHEUMATIC ENDOCARDITIS

Subacute Bacterial Endocarditis.—The fact that probably less than one case in two hundred recovers where this diagnosis has been established is evidence of our therapeutic impotence in this condition. At one time or another practically every new weapon has been tried against the *Streptococcus viridans* in endocarditis lenta, but though an occasional dramatic cure has been claimed, general experience of all suggested methods is depressing. Intravenous antiseptics (eusol, mercurochrome, etc.) had their trial and were found wanting. Blood transfusion and immuno-transfusions (transfusion of blood from a donor previously immunized specifically or non-specifically) are alike disappointing. Of late years sulphonamide preparations have been tried with great hopes, but in our experience without effect. Some drugs of this group (*e.g.*, sulphapyridine) reduce or abolish pyrexia, but do not appear to influence the course of the disease.

In our opinion the less the patient is disturbed by heroic therapy the better. The rôle of the doctor is to put the patient in the best circumstances to fight his battle against the strepto-coccus, to maintain a cheerful outlook and encourage the patient throughout what is often a long and depressing illness, and to treat symptoms as they arise. By the time the diagnosis is reached the patient is usually confined to bed. Good nursing, with attention to skin, diet and bowels, and with due endeavour to provide bright, cheerful surroundings, is essential. Such conditions are more easily attained in hospital than in the average home surroundings, and there is thus a good deal to be said for the removal of such cases to hospital. The patient's comfort is thereby increased and the strain on the relatives somewhat lessened. At the same time it must be remembered that prolonged detention in hospital may not be feasible under existing conditions.

Ulcerative (Acute Bacterial) Endocarditis.—Generally arising as part of a general septicæmia, the existence of this disease is frequently overlooked. Like the subacute variety, it is practically invariably fatal once diagnosed, and treatment is merely palliative. Sera, vaccines, and chemo-therapeutic drugs are generally as ineffective as in the subacute (viridans) form, though possibly sulphonamide derivatives may prove of some use in cases due to the various pyogenic cocci (*Streptococcus hæmolyticus*, staphylococci, etc.). Good nursing and attention to symptoms sum up the treatment of the condition.

THE TREATMENT OF PERICARDITIS

A patient suffering from acute pericarditis, whatever the ætiology, should be nursed at complete rest in bed. In the common variety occurring in the course of an acute rheumati carditis, the general lines of treatment are as described unde that heading. In tuberculous cases the general measures ar those appropriate to tuberculous cases in general. Cases whicl occur in association with pyogenic infections (hæmolyti streptococci, staphylococci, pneumococci, etc.) are treate along lines indicated by the infecting organism, the possibilit of the development of a purulent effusion being kept in mind

The relief of pain may call for treatment, though man cases suffer surprisingly little discomfort even in the presenc of a gross friction rub. Mild analgesics (sodium salicylate, o acetyl-salicylic acid, or codeine in doses of $\frac{1}{4}$ gr.) may suffice but severe pain may necessitate the administration of morphi ($\frac{1}{4}$ gr. hypodermically, with the customary proviso regardin its dangers in young children).

Counter-irritation for the relief of pain has been employe for many years, usually by cantharides blisters. Should suc be employed, the plaster should be applied in one or two sma pieces the size of postage stamps, and large blisters to cover the precordium should never be used. The discomfort produced, the risk of septic skin infection or of toxic absorption from the area, and the interference with subsequent examination of the precordium all render such large blisters most inadvisable. The usual sites for application of small blisters are slightly to the left of the sternum near the base of the heart, or midway between apex and sternal margin. The cantharides is left in position for six to eight hours, or until a blister is raised. The plaster is then carefully removed, the blister snipped with scissors and loose skin removed, and the bare area dressed with an emollient and a sterile dressing held in place by adhesive tape. How far such treatment aids recovery is uncertain. Relief from pain can be more easily attained by simple prescription of analgesics, and, in the case of sensitive children at least, the method has obvious disadvantages which seem to outweigh the claimed benefits. The use of an ice-bag, on the other hand, may give considerable relief from pain without the discomforts attendant on blistering. The ice-bag should be only partially filled with finely chopped ice, to which salt may be added. The bag should be applied to the bare skin of the precordium, and is best suspended from some improvised form of cradle so that the weight of the bag may not cause oppression. It is well recognized from experience in auscultation that pressure over the ribs increases the pain in acute pericarditis.

The development of a large effusion may be associated with symptoms due to embarrassment of the heart's action or to interference with respiration due to partial collapse of the left lung. It is unusual for such symptoms to be severe enough to warrant aspiration of the pericardial effusion, but this rarely may have to be done where cyanosis and dyspnœa are extreme or where the pulse is so far reduced in volume as to be hardly perceptible. Aspiration should be done for diagnostic purposes where there is a question of pus formation in the sac, as in pericarditis developing after pneumonia, or in the course of a septicæmia after osteomyelitis, etc. In these cases the aspiration of a few cubic centimetres of fluid will suffice, while for relief of pressure effects the aspiration of several hundred cubic centimetres may be necessary. Paracentesis may be carried out in various ways. In each case the skin is cleansed and sterilized and then anæsthetized by intradermal and subcutaneous novocain over the area selected for puncture, as in performing a pleural paracentesis. Where pus is suspected, a wide-bore needle (2 mm.) may be necessary, but, in general, a medium bore will suffice (about

1 mm.). The length of needle required depends largely on the site of puncture. The following sites are usually employed: (i) in the fifth left interspace, outside the apex beat but inside the limit of cardiac dullness; (ii) in the fourth left interspace about 1 in. from the sternal margin (far enough from the bone to avoid the internal mammary artery which descends in this region); (iii) in the angle between the ensiform cartilage and the lowest ribs, the needle being directed upwards and backwards to reach the pericardial sac; (iv) from the back, with abducted scapula, in the mid-scapular line in the seventh or eighth intercostal space. Of these, the first two are those most generally used, and appear to be devoid of risk. The penetration of the heart muscle by the needle is of no consequence provided that large coronary vessels be not punctured; this is an unlikely accident from a needle inserted outside the apex beat, or over the area of right ventricle lying 1 in. to the left of the sternum, which is relatively devoid of large vessels. The epigastric and posterior routes are occasionally preferable when a loculated effusion has to be reached; in both these fluid is reached at a deeper level than when an anterior puncture is perforated. When large quantities of fluid are being removed the rate of withdrawal should be slow, to avoid the risk of dangerous pressure changes in the pericardium or heart.

The discovery of pus in the pericardial sac is an indication for surgical intervention. Drainage may be established by open operation, with resection of ribs, or may be achieved by a closed method, by insertion of a tube into the sac through the soft tissue of an interspace and the maintenance of suction. Both methods yield good results, and the decision as to which to employ naturally lies with the surgeon operating.

In non-purulent cases recovery with absorption of the effusion is the rule, except in the cases of terminal acute pericarditis which occur in the last stages of Bright's disease and similar cachectic conditions. Convalescence may be slow and there is no efficient method of hastening the absorption of the fluid. Repeated assessment of the size of the effusion and of the patient's general state will guide the physician in his decision as to management—when to allow the patient to move about in bed, when to allow him up, etc. The general principles for cases of rheumatic carditis are applicable to cases of pericarditis of similar ætiology. Other cases, on recovery from the acute attack, may be allowed fair liberty of exercise, etc., but should be re-examined from time to time during the ensuing years to exclude the development of other lesions or of chronic constrictive pericarditis.

Chronic constrictive pericarditis is a surgical problem, and is dealt with in the section on The Surgery of Cardiac Conditions (p. 713).

THE TREATMENT OF CIRCULATORY FAILURE IN ACUTE INFECTIONS

In the circulatory failure which occurs in acute infections such as lobar pneumonia, two factors are at work: central, due to failure of the poisoned heart muscle, and peripheral, due to failure and dilatation of the poisoned small vessels. Of the two the peripheral failure is generally the more important. This is true even in diphtheria, where many of the deaths are due to peripheral failure, though in some cases the specific action of the toxin on the heart causes sudden (cardiac) death, often many days after the apparent subsidence of the maximum effects of the acute infection.

The treatment of toxæmic circulatory failure really lies in its prevention by early and adequate treatment of the underlying infective condition. In diphtheria, for example, the timeous administration of potent antitoxin reduces greatly the incidence of cases with dangerous circulatory failure. So in lobar pneumonia the giving of the appropriate antiserum at an early stage is of value. In diseases where no specific antiserum exists, or where failure develops during a long illness (*e.g.*, typhoid fever), general measures to reduce toxæmia are employed to the best of our ability.

Once failure has developed, the prospects of successful treatment are not good. It is by then too late for efficient specific therapy, and measures calculated to stimulate the heart or the periphery are disappointing. Of drugs which act on the heart, digitalis is the most widely employed. The use of digitalis in pneumonia, for example, is traditional, though its value is doubtful. It is claimed that in some way the drug improves the efficiency of the heart's action, though even its advocates admit that the heart-rate is not slowed. It is the impression of many clinicians that the use or omission of digitalis makes no difference to mortality rates in lobar pneumonia. This is confirmed statistically by certain recent large-scale observations. The lack of demonstrable effect on mortality holds for cases who were fully digitalized. Cases who receive the drug for the first time near the day of the crisis, and in small doses. manifestly are never digitalized to an extent which would render probable any action on the heart.

Many other drugs which enjoy a reputation as cardiac

stimulants, and which are widely used in conditions of toxæmic circulatory failure, are devoid of direct action on the heart. Strychnine appears to act solely on the central nervous system and the class of " diffusible stimulants " (sp. ætheris nitrosi sp. ammon. aromat.) act reflexly through the same system. None of these is a true cardiac " tonic," increasing the efficiency of the muscle. Adrenaline, it is true, has such an action but it increases the tachycardia which is already a disquieting feature of toxæmic failure, and is known to deplete the glycogen reserve of the heart muscle cells. In short, we do not possess any drug which can whip an exhausted heart to renewed activity or which can render the cells immune to circulating toxins.

Peripheral vascular dilatation, as the principal element in the production of circulatory failure, more frequently demand treatment than the heart condition. Many drugs are available adrenalin, pituitrin, cardiazol, coramine, intravenous hypertoni glucose, etc., and these are discussed in the section on Acut Circulatory Failure (p. 723). The results of their use in toxæmi states are by no means satisfactory. In fact, once such failur has developed, progression to a fatal issue is likely in spite of al therapy, unless the natural body processes succeed in overcomin the toxæmia, as in the crisis phenomenon of lobar pneumonia.

THE TREATMENT OF FOCAL SEPSIS IN RELATION TO HEART DISEASE

The exact rôle of focal septic infection in the productio of heart disease and symptoms is somewhat uncertain. It i recognized that the *Streptococcus viridans* may gain access t the blood from foci, especially in the teeth, tonsils and uppe respiratory tract, and may give rise to a subacute bacteri endocarditis in persons with damaged heart valves. Fo this reason it is advisable to search for, and extirpate, suc foci in all cases of congenital heart disease and in the subjects o rheumatic lesions. Of these latter, it is the cases of aortic diseas or early mitral disease who are liable to develop endocardit lenta; late cases of mitral stenosis are rarely affected.

It is also admitted that foci of sepsis may be of ætiologic importance in cases with heart block of milder grades, and i cases with obstinate extrasystolic irregularities. In such case also, removal of the foci is desirable and generally without ris

The matter is not so simple, however, when symptoms o signs of gall-bladder disease are found in a case presentin clinical evidence of heart disease. It is held by some th many cases of cardiac pain and of congestive failure may ow heir condition to toxic absorption from an infected gall-bladder.)ther clinicians contend that chance association plays a part n the simultaneous occurrence of the two conditions. The ubjects of cholecystitis are of the habitus and age which favour rterial degeneration and its sequelæ of angina and myocardial ailure. The evidence in favour of the so-called "gall-bladder eart" is thus not convincing, and operations for removal f the gall-bladder should only be undertaken when there are lear indications, apart from the cardiac condition, to justify he step. The high mortality which attends this operation in ases with hypertension, obesity and impaired myocardial fficiency should be kept in mind.

I. G. W. Hill.

THE MANAGEMENT OF THE AMBULANT CARDIAC PATIENT

The energetic treatment of heart disease is chiefly concerned ith measures to counteract the more advanced grades of the ifferent types of heart failure, but it is no less important to arn the management of the minor degrees of incapacity in rder that life may be rendered more tolerable, and serious ilure avoided or postponed. The great majority of cardiac atients are able to go about, and, though their activities are stricted, yet with suitable guidance and advice from time to me they can generally lead useful lives of moderate activity. heir appropriate care and supervision depends upon a number factors, of which the more important are the degree of rculatory impairment, the age of the patient, and the tiological cause of the heart disease. The extent of the rdiac damage, the occupation, the environment, the economic rcumstances, the habits and, to some extent, the man's rsonal character and mental outlook influence treatment in widest sense. By this is included the individual's ability to nform to the rules of healthy living, and his willingness to co-erate in the details of therapy as advised by his physician.

It is a recognized fact that, with few exceptions, myocardial mage is an irreversible process, and tends of itself to run a ogressively downward course over the years, ending ulti-ately in one or other type of heart failure, or, it may be, from me relatively sudden complication such as embolism, an ute vascular catastrophe (*e.g.*, rupture of a cardiac or vascular eurysm) or from septicæmia (bacterial endocarditis). Briefly ted, the objects in treatment during the ambulant stage are arrest or retard the downward course by decreasing the cardiac burden, and so to improve the general health of the patient that the liability to infection is reduced. It may thus be said that the patient, however mild his symptoms, has to be taught the principles of healthy living, and treated according to his particular position in relation to his incapacity.

Habits.—It is always worthwhile to review briefly with the patient his habits of life, so that these may be adjusted to conform with physiological principles. Hours of work and hours of sleep are a first consideration. The general health of many people complaining of minor ills of one kind or another is improved by insisting on a minimum of eight hours' sleep each night, and for the great majority of cardiac patients this is certainly a minimum. Nine to ten hours is often preferable and even though all this time may not be spent in actual sleep the mere rest and relaxation is of very definite value, particularly if it become a regular habit. Hours of work vary enormously in different trades and occupations. Certainly in the minor degrees of cardiac embarrassment a maximum of eight hours is as much as most people can accomplish ; if more is attempted, then suitable intervals of rest should be provided. Each individual requires special consideration, but there is no doubt that the avoidance of the rush and tumble of everyday life, and the substitution of regular habits and a quiet and moderate routine, with gentle outdoor exercise from day to day promotes general well-being. Harm results from too sheltered a life, and there is no doubt that muscular exercise up to the point of inducing a healthy degree of fatigue and restful sleep is by its invigorating character of value to the cardiac patient whose response to effort is not greatly impaired. Moderation in food in drink and in tobacco is to be encouraged. The avoidance of infection, particularly infection of the respiratory tract, is of prime importance to the cardiac patient. This is not always easy, but suitable clothing and an abundance of fresh air at all times, with adequate ventilation of the living-rooms at home and in the office and workshop, decreases the risk. In the winter months particularly, when exposed to cold and damp, and when respiratory infections often of minor degree are rife, the cardiac patient is wise to avoid hot, stuffy rooms, crowded places of entertainment and public meetings. Infections of the nose and throat—catarrh and, in particular, bronchitis—throw a considerable burden on the heart and circulation, and may in themselves be responsible in susceptible subjects for a decline in the cardiac reserve, and the actual precipitation of heart failure. It is therefore proper that when an infection becomes manifest, particular care should be taken, and the patient advised to keep to his bed until free of symptoms. Otherwise the cardiac patient must be encouraged to take such exercise as he can up to the limit of his tolerance, provided always that he is ensured a sound and restful sleep each night. His activities are only to be restricted to such a degree that symptoms are avoided. He can take exercise short of producing dyspnœa or undue fatigue.

Exercise.—The amount of exercise suitable for the individual can only be found by actual experiment. Activities are only to be limited when they are sufficient to induce symptoms, undue fatigue, dyspnœa or pain. Thus it is that the degree of circulatory impairment is gauged by a study of the patient's reactions to exercise. The less readily these are induced, the less restriction of activity is required. By living up to the capacity of his tolerance for exercise the more likely is his range of activity to increase. Fatigue or breathlessness decides that his tolerance has been approached or passed, and the rate and amount of work in the future must be reduced to conform with his endurance. Similarly, pain is a signal that the work done has been in excess of that with which the blood supply of the myocardium can cope. Simple restrictions designed so to limit activity that symptoms are kept in abeyance are all that is required in the first instance. Golf, tennis, riding, swimming and even hill walks are permissible, and should be encouraged. Improved tone of the skeletal muscles is associated with an increased capacity for cardiac work. The latitude permitted varies with each individual and the ease with which his physical condition improves.

A further degree of incapacity becomes evident when ordinary activities of a mild nature, such as quiet housework or simple walks on the level, are sufficient to induce fatigue, dyspnœa or discomfort. Social and business activities must be restricted to a greater or less extent. This degree of disability is frequently associated with minor degrees of peripheral œdema noticed about the ankles towards evening. This is a sign of great significance and indicates that more active measures are required if congestive failure is to be avoided. In the mildest cases a few days' rest in bed, with or without the use of digitalis, and the provision of ample sleep are measures designed to enable the restoration of a more satisfactory blood flow. A week or ten days in bed will often enable the circulatory incapacity to right itself, and, thereafter, when activities of a mild degree are resumed, it will usually be necessary to insist on at least one day in bed each week, a rest of an hour or two after the midday meal, and the regular addition of an extra hour in bed each night for some months. Digitalis may be given in small doses of 20 minims of the tincture thrice daily, generally for a week or ten days at a time with three or four days of freedom from the drug.

Focal Sepsis.—In the supervision of the patient in the ambulant stages of heart disease, it is always advisable to have local sepsis, particularly in the mouth and throat, eradicated. The teeth should be overhauled at regular intervals by a competent dentist, the tonsils dealt with if any evidence of local sepsis exists, and appropriate treatment should be undertaken for sinus infection. By removing and correcting infection in these situations much can be done to reduce the tendency to minor respiratory ills, catarrh and infection of the respiratory tract.

Anæmia.—Similarly it is always wise to be on the lookout for even minor degrees of anæmia. Many cardiac patients, especially women, convalescent from rheumatic infection may remain mildly anæmic for months or years after the original infection has died out. Their cardiac symptoms are aggravated by a diminished hæmoglobin content, and their general health can be improved and their fatigue and dyspnœa lessened, by the restoration of a normal hæmoglobin content by the administration of adequate doses of iron for such periods as are necessary. For this purpose ferrous sulphate in doses of 3 gr. four times a day may bring about a striking amelioration of symptoms, particularly with regard to fatigue, and sometimes of pain and præcordial discomfort. Such minor measures as these will do much to maintain the cardiac patient's general health and improve his response to effort, but if with the passage of time a further stage of decompensation is reached and the tendency to congestive failure, nocturnal dyspnœa or anginal discomfort increases, then longer periods of rest are obviously required. The active therapeutic measures for these different types of heart failure are fully discussed on p. 665 *et seq.* In convalescence, after failure has been adequately corrected, drug treatment is almost invariably required, and must be supervised thoroughly from week to week. Digitalis in maintenance doses (p. 679) should be prescribed up to the limit of tolerance when it is indicated, physical activities greatly limited and sound sleep ensured.

Age and Occupation.—The age of the patient is of some importance in determining suitable treatment. In infancy, for instance, the severer grades of congenital heart disease necessitate advice regarding feeding and nursing (p. 663). In childhood and adolescence rheumatic heart disease is prevalent. The rheumatic child, when the active infection has subsided, requires much the same after-care as the tuberculous patient. In this way prolonged semi-convalescent treatment in an institution where the child's education may be continued without the rough and tumble of school life has much to recommend it. In this country the demand for accommodation of this nature is increasing, and various residential homes are available where, under prolonged supervision, with adequate control of the diet, rest, exercise and lessons better progress can be made than in the environment in which the rheumatic infection was originally acquired. Not many of these residential homes are available to the child of middle or better class parents. Where economic circumstances permit, it is justifiable to recommend that these children be taken abroad to tropical or sub-tropical countries where the likelihood of reinfection is diminished, and where, with exposure to sunlight and adequate feeding, nutrition is improved. For this reason the Mediterranean coast, the Canaries and Egypt are often selected for a prolonged convalescence of six or twelve months. Treatment at this stage is directed more to the prevention of infection or its reactivation than to the actual cardiac disease. When the child is ambulant and sufficiently advanced in convalescence to resume even modified school life, continuation of particular care is required so that under-nutrition is prevented, excessive fatigue avoided and exposure to cold and damp minimized, all of which are known to lower resistance and favour reactivation of the carditis. It has already been pointed out that every attempt should be made to educate the rheumatic child so that in later life he may earn his living in a sedentary occupation. In caring for these children the doctor should be prepared to advise the parents regarding the child's employment. In this country an outdoor occupation is inadvisable. Work involving physical strain and sudden or sustained muscular effort is likely to prove detrimental. Employment at a bench, desk or counter is usually preferable. Clerks, book-keepers, typists, telephone operators, cashiers, dressmakers, tailors, all hold sedentary jobs suitable for the young cardiac patient. Similarly there are such skilled trades as electrical mechanics, radio repairers, watch, fountain-pen and jewellery makers to which the youthful rheumatic patient may be suitably apprenticed. Too often it is the journey to or from work which taxes the strength. Greater consideration for the occupational training and employment of the cardiac cripple in suitable industries will be rewarded by happier and longer days for these patients.

In middle age heart disease curbs a man's activities, and when symptoms begin to interfere with the daily routine, a definite modification of his habits and methods of living must be prescribed. Few people are quite so indispensable in their work as is often imagined, and deputies can often be found to share the responsibilities and ease the burden. It depends on circumstances whether restriction should be applied first to the daily occupation or to the hobbies and philanthropic activities. Too many men are allowed to retire from active work without sufficient interests to occupy their minds. The business man in early middle life handicapped by organic heart disease must of necessity be advised to limit his ambitions, lead the quieter life, have longer holidays and rely more and more on his staff for all routine work. At this age period the commoner ætiological factors are hypertensive and syphilitic heart disease, the latter less common than formerly.

ESSENTIAL HYPERTENSION

Hypertension may or may not be associated with generalized arteriosclerotic changes, and in certain instances it is attributable to chronic renal disease, in which case treatment is to be directed to the underlying nephritis. On the other hand there exists a large group of people in whom high blood pressure is the leading physical sign of a condition, the ætiology of which is little understood, and which may persist for years without the production of disagreeable symptoms. This is the state spoken of as "essential hypertension" or "hyperpiesia." After a longer or shorter interval the hypertension is productive of signs of cardiac impairment. The first principle in the treatment of this condition is to endeavour to help the patient to adapt his life to his blood pressure rather than to attempt to direct treatment specifically towards the readings of the sphygmomanometer. The cause of the raised pressure can seldom be attacked at its source, and drugs known to lower blood pressure have at the most only a temporary effect. The reduction in pressure is often itself accompanied by unpleasant symptoms. It is seldom that blood-pressure readings should be communicated to a patient, as this only tends to magnify the condition and focus attention on the least important aspect of his progress. Symptoms are the best guide to treatment, and in general the quiet life recommended for the minor degrees of cardiac incapacity is applicable to the sufferer from this disorder. Long hours of work, business worries, emotional strain and the tension of competitive business are aspects which may be considered with the patient, the doctor advising such restrictions as will allow for a definite routine without the production of further embarrassment. Symptoms are a better guide than millimetres of mercury. Should such measures in themselves prove insufficient to ease the patient, then it is wise that further limitations and restrictions be imposed. If economic circumstances allow, a prolonged rest or leave of absence from work for three to six months is a desirable step. When this has been arranged it is useful to recommend that two to four weeks be spent in more or less complete confinement to bed, the sufferer having previously made such business arrangements as will free him from unnecessary anxieties of one kind or another. The success of this step depends not merely on physical rest, but on the relief which comes from complete mental relaxation. Obviously, during the supervision of such a patient, it is undesirable that he should have his blood pressure recorded at frequent intervals, as this in itself may well become a fixed idea with him, and by concentrating on the systolic level his mental outlook is liable to become distorted and his attitude one of discouragement. After some weeks of rest, outdoor exercise may be cautiously resumed, but if this still continues to be productive of symptoms, then it is probably wise that the man should retire from active participation in the rush and worry of competitive business. Too often retirement is postponed until it becomes synonymous with complete invalidism. On the other hand, there are those who only after many years of raised pressure begin gradually to experience disagreeable symptoms. They are safeguarded by the provision of the restful life, the regular habit of long hours of sleep, the quiet week-end and the protracted holiday. The lesson to be learned is that by adapting the daily routine to the blood pressure, thus keeping symptoms in abeyance, much good can be accomplished over a period of time, provided always that the emotional make-up of the patient is tempered by confidence and reassurance. There is no more important factor in handling these patients than that the fears of high blood pressure should be countered at the earliest opportunity, with the explanation that the condition may exist for years without any serious effects.

Diet.—Dietetic measures have their ardent advocates, but there is no particular food the restriction of which will guarantee a fall in pressure. Many hypertensives tend to over-eat, and if this is associated with obesity, then a clear indication for dietetic treatment does exist. In fact, it may be said that the most successful measure in the treatment of the middle-aged ambulant cardiac patient is the correction of obesity. Even 1 st. in excess of the individual's standard weight for his age and height throws an unnecessary burden on the heart and circulation—a burden which can be readily corrected. The prescription of an exact diet of 1,500, 1,200 or 1,000 calories will do much to ease symptoms without any material difference to the level of the blood-pressure reading (see p. 387). Dietetic treatment can only be successful in so far as the patient is prepared to co-operate wholeheartedly in the measures suggested. In this connection it should be explained to the patient that a loss of 1 to 2 lbs. per week is sufficient. Consequently, according to his excess as compared with the standard for his age and height, many weeks of steady perseverance may be anticipated. He should be instructed to record his weight from week to week so that progress may be accurately gauged, and these figures are certainly worthy of more attention on the part of both doctor and patient than the blood-pressure readings. If he will conscientiously concentrate on his weight loss, the patient will often make reasonable progress, and receive much encouragement. The details of the treatment of obesity are described elsewhere (p. 387). The benefits to be obtained by this method of treatment are so striking that even in those who are not grossly overweight the cultivation of the habit of restricted indulgence is well worth encouraging. A simple diet of 1,500 to 1,600 calories may be prescribed with benefit. There is little to be gained from a total restriction of red meat, at one time so fashionable. The protein intake should be sufficient for the bodily needs. Fresh fruit and abundant vegetables should form a large part of the diet, fluids should be restricted, the minimum amount of salt taken with comfort, and the evening meal should be light and simple. The total restriction of alcohol is unnecessary for those accustomed to take it in moderation, but it is often wise to reduce or discontinue the habit of smoking.

Drugs.—So far as drugs are concerned, a small dose of calomel once or twice a week, and a saline purge, has much to recommend it. When emotional tension runs high and there are obvious nervous influences at work, the prescription of a small dose of bromide or luminal once or twice daily is a useful remedy. Of the former, perhaps 7 to 15 gr. will prove an adequate dose, and of the latter, $\frac{1}{4}$ gr. morning and midday with $\frac{1}{2}$ to 1 gr. at night may be all that is required. The proprietary preparation theominal has some reputation in the control of hypertension, and may be prescribed in the evening in a dose of one to two tablets as such, or the tablet phenobarbitone and theobromine (B.P.C.) may be ordered. This contains a $\frac{1}{2}$ gr. of phenobarbitone combined with 5 gr. of theobromine. Its sedative properties are often of value, particularly about the time of the menopause, when symptoms of hypertension may first become apparent. The symptoms of the climacteric are then mixed with those of hypertension, and occasionally both are benefited by the use of the various follicular hormone preparations now on the market. These would seem to be of particular value in relieving the distressing vasomotor symptoms associated with flushing, headaches and perspiration. Only in exceptional circumstances can thyroid extract be offered as a remedy. It is an uncertain method of weight reduction, as it is so liable, in these patients, to induce tachycardia and occasionally actual anginal pain. When such is the case it must be discontinued immediately. While nitrites have a certain reputation on experimental grounds for the reduction of blood pressure, yet at the best this is only temporary, and no drug is known which has a permanent effect. Attempts to reduce the level of the blood pressure are usually ineffective, and when they do succeed are usually the cause of further embarrassment to the patient. Carefully controlled observations on patients suffering from hypertension treated by the more protracted acting nitrites, such as erythrol tetranitrate, are unconvincing. Nevertheless, from the symptomatic point of view they may be occasionally useful in the relief of morning headache, a trial being made with a tablet of glyceryltrinitrate in a dose of $\frac{1}{400}$ gr. increasing up to $\frac{1}{100}$. If this is unsuccessful, as it often is, then recourse must be made to the more purely symptomatic measures, and for this purpose a full dose of phenacetin, 5 to 15 gr. taken with a cup of hot tea in the early morning, may be helpful. Tablets combining aspirin, caffeine and phenacetin are often more useful.

Surgical Measures.—When symptoms such as giddiness, headache and tinnitus become more pressing, the mechanical relief of the tension is often followed by remarkable comfort, sometimes for weeks on end. In the plethoric individual the withdrawal of 15 to 20 oz. of blood from a vein is a measure often of the greatest value when other methods of treatment prove in themselves insufficient.

In recent years increased attention has been devoted to the possibilities of relief of essential hypertension by surgical means. It is well established that in the earlier stages of the disease, before organic vascular damage has occurred, the chief factor in the perpetuation of the raised blood pressure is almost certainly an abnormal degree of vasoconstriction or increased peripheral arteriolar tonus. On this account various surgical measures have been devised with the intention of easing the peripheral resistance by severing the sympathetic connections between the vasomotor centre and the peripheral arterioles. Bilateral extraperitoneal resection of the splanchnic nerves, the cœliac ganglion and the upper two lumbar sympathetic ganglia is apparently capable of providing some degree of symptomatic relief in the majority of carefully selected patients, and this, strangely enough, without a uniform or substantial reduction of the systolic pressure. In assessing the value of sympathetic surgery, it has been observed that many elderly sufferers from hypertension often receive much relief from their circulatory symptoms by any incidental surgical procedures such as prostatectomy or hysterectomy. The whole subject is therefore still *sub judice*. In younger patients, in whom serious organic vascular damage of a permanent nature has not become firmly established, there would appear to be, at least on theoretical grounds, some justification for surgical intervention. In the later stages of the hypertensive process it is unreasonable to suppose that the relief of peripheral vasoconstriction can accomplish anything of real value. An abrupt fall of blood pressure may well be a source of increased embarrassment when the vascular tree after many years has become firmly adapted to the strain of long-continued hypertension. When further experience makes it possible to select appropriate patients for such surgical procedures, this method of treatment may find a definite place in the therapeutics of hypertension.

In the last stages of the hypertensive process, even before symptoms of cardiac embarrassment become very pronounced and dyspnœa, fatigue and œdema complicate the situation, there should be no hesitation in employing digitalis, as this drug does not raise the blood pressure in the presence of hypertension. The treatment of the final stages, when the heart fails and the blood pressure tends to fall to lower levels, is to all intents and purposes that of congestive, dyspnœic or anginal failure. Treatment of these forms of cardiac distress are fully discussed under the appropriate headings (pp. 665-703).

CARDIOVASCULAR SYPHILIS

It is usual to find that heart disease of syphilitic origin first becomes manifest in middle age. Luetic aortitis is preventable by adequate treatment in the earliest stages of the infection, but when the aorta is damaged, antispecific treatment at the best can only arrest the advance of the disease process.

Powerful remedies in the form of mercury, bismuth and, particularly, organic arsenic, capable of stamping out the infection in the earliest stages, must be used with particular caution in the presence of luetic vascular disease. The rapid resolution of syphilitic tissue with the resulting scarring and fibrosis of the first part of the aorta has led in the past to the so-called therapeutic paradox whereby a rapid improvement in health was followed by as speedy a deterioration. Shrinking and shrivelling of the valve cusps, involvement of the orifices of the coronary arteries in the fibrotic process, with consequent stenosis of their mouths and weakening of the aortic wall, are consequences of ill-judged efforts to eradicate completely all activity in the syphilitic lesions. It is important to temper enthusiasm with a balanced conservatism lest over-zealous attempts to cure should prematurely kill. A treatment too energetic is likely to do more harm than good. The accumulated experience of the past ten or twenty years indicates that the results now obtained are much more encouraging than those attributed to the excessive and ill-judged methods of earlier years. By realizing the dangers and adapting treatment to the special circumstances presented by established vascular syphilis, there is no doubt that the expectation of life may be increased and symptoms eased. Therapy is adjusted to the particular patient after assessment of the extent of the damage, and is *not* directed to his Wassermann reaction. It must be clearly understood that the success of antispecific treatment, so far as the heart and aorta are concerned, is not to be judged by the reversal of the serological reactions, but rather by the relief of the patient's symptoms, the arrest of the pathological process and the avoidance of symptoms of therapeutic shock.

When the aortic lesion is recognized at an early stage, and uncomplicated by a regurgitant leak or frank aneurysmal formation, then treatment may be more intense and thorough than when, for instance, the exact nature of the lesion is only discovered for the first time in the presence of anginal, dyspnœic or congestive failure. The degree of circulatory incapacity is the main factor in determining the intensity of antisyphilitic measures ; the greater the degree of failure, the less intensive must be the treatment of the ætiological agent.

In the absence of congestive failure, or definite anginal symptoms, treatment may be commenced with a preliminary course of either bismuth or mercury intramuscularly, and the simultaneous administration of iodides by the mouth. The usual dose of an insoluble salt of bismuth is 0·05 to 0·1 gm. weekly for four weeks, followed by double this quantity for a further period of eight weeks. The injectio bismuthi (B.P.) 0·5 to 1 c.c., and the injectio hydrargyri (B.P.), 0·3 to 0·6 c.c. are suitable preparations, though various proprietary compounds are popular and in frequent use. Bismuth is to be preferred, but mercury, a less effective alternative, obviates the necessity for repeated injections. Since it can be administered by mouth, a suitable preparation is Hutchinson's pill, which is composed of 1 gr. of grey powder and 1 gr. of Dover's powder. Of this, two or three may be taken daily according to tolerance. During the time that the mercury or bismuth is being administered, iodides are prescribed as a mixture, commencing with a dose of 7½ gr. twice daily and working up cautiously to twice or thrice this amount at the end of a month or two according to tolerance. A careful watch must be kept for symptoms either of iodism or of bismuth or mercury intolerance according to the heavy metal selected. Intolerance is an indication to reduce or discontinue the offending drug. So far as heart cases are concerned, it is probably wiser to prescribe potassium rather than sodium iodide. This is particularly true when congestive failure has threatened, for the sodium ion tends to hold fluid in the tissues (see p. 670).

After three months of preparatory treatment along these lines the use of organic arsenicals may be considered. These should not be used in the presence of true anginal symptoms, nor in dyspnœic or congestive failure, and only with the greatest care if breathlessness is easily provoked on exertion. For intravenous use one of the preparations of neoarsphenamine is used at weekly intervals for a further period of twelve weeks, commencing with a dose of 0·15 gm., increasing cautiously to a maximum of 0·45 gm. at the end of eight weeks. Any unfavourable reaction warrants the discontinuation, or a considerable reduction, of the dosage. It is good practice to advise a period of complete rest in bed during the first month of arsenical treatment. This eases the burden on the heart and circulation, permits of a better adjustment to intensive therapy and prevents overactivity on the part of the patient during a critical phase of treatment.

When the syphilitic damage is judged more extensive, and a free aortic leak is present or definite aneurysmal formation with a mild degree of cardiac incapacity, there may be some hesitation in using neoarsphenamine by the intravenous route, and in these circumstances a preparation less liable to induce therapeutic shock may be used. Acetylarsan, which is dispensed in solution in ampoules ready for intramuscular or subcutaneous injection, is convenient, and very suitable for less intensive treatment. It is given in doses of 1 c.c. (0·05 gm. of arsenic) at weekly intervals, increasing to 3 c.c. over a period of twelve weeks. It is less toxic than neoarsphenamine, and is quite painless on intramuscular injection. Preparations such as sulphostab and kharsulphan are also available for intramuscular injection, but are hardly less toxic than neoarsphenamine. A compound of bismuth with arsenamine sulphonate, known as bismarsen, is popular in the United States, and may be given intramuscularly in doses of 0·1 gm. for six weeks and 0·2 gm. for the following six weeks. In this country acetylarsan and bismuth injections are frequently combined with very satisfactory results.

If no unfavourable effects occur, the arsenical course is completed at the end of the first six months of treatment. A second course of either bismuth or mercury with oral iodides is then repeated for three months, followed by a further course of arsenic. Thereafter it is desirable—if tolerance permits—to repeat annually one course of bismuth or mercury, followed by one course of neoarsphenamine or acetylarsan with bismuth for the rest of the patient's life. Should signs of heart failure ensue, then antispecific treatment is discontinued, and the measures outlined for the treatment of congestive, anginal or dyspnœic failure immediately employed.

Having once suffered from congestive failure, a prolonged course of iodides and mercury is the first essential. Acetylarsan may be used with care and constant observation for signs of intolerance. In the presence of congestive failure, responding to the treatment outlined for this condition (p. 666), antispecific measures are limited to the administration of small doses (7 to 10 gr.) of potassium iodide twice or thrice daily. With further improvement, mercury may be commenced by mouth, but three or four months of steady progress should elapse before a mild course of arsenic is considered advisable.

By such measures as these outlined above, adapted to the individual's particular requirements, much can be done to retard or arrest the advance of the syphilitic process in the first part of the aorta. Well-chosen remedies used with every caution can promote the patient's well-being and prolong life.

The treatment of aneurysms of the aorta or of one of the peripheral arteries is dependent on the cause, which is usually syphilitic. Therapy is based on the principles outlined above. Pressure symptoms demand symptomatic treatment, and for aneurysms in the periphery surgical measures may be considered, rapid or gradual ligation being the procedure usually adopted in accessible situations. The " wiring " of aneurysms, by which is meant the insertion of a fine platinum or silver wire into the aneurysmal sac, in the hope of favouring local thrombosis either by the mere presence of the foreign body or by electrolysis favouring the deposition of a clot, is a procedure often described but seldom practised.

THE SENILE HEART

Past middle life the individual is more than ever at the mercy of his arteries, and in elderly people heart disease, the result of a slow and progressive narrowing of the coronaries takes various forms. Hypertension is often present, and thereby increases the liability to angina or congestive failure Treatment for these states will be found under the appropriate headings. In old age, with generalized arteriosclerosis weakness of the skeletal muscles and diminution in the cardiac reserve advance step by step. The inability to take much in the way of physical exercise eases, to some extent the cardiac burden. Congestive failure comes insidiously often unexpectedly, and runs a short course.

The care of the heart and circulation in the elderly is based on the principles already described, particular attention being directed to physical activity. In such people the risks asso ciated with a prolonged rest in bed are well known, basal congestion, infection and bouts of coughing being the main sources of danger to the heart. Exercise in the open air should be encouraged, sufficient to yield a natural fatigue as distinct from exhaustion and any undue degree of breathlessness Irregular and spasmodic attempts should be avoided, and a definite amount of exercise in the form of short walks should be prescribed according to tolerance, a stated amount being accomplished day by day. In this way blood flow is improved stagnation avoided and muscular tone enhanced. When circumstances permit, especially for those prone to bronchitis and respiratory catarrh, the winter months, being a source of danger, may be spent with profit on the South Coast or abroad in milder climates favoured with more sunshine and warmth and a drier air than is to be found at home.

Diet in the aged presents problems peculiarly its own, but in general the secret of success is to be found in moderation Balfour, acting on the principle that digestive processes are prolonged in the aged, used to insist on a minimum of five hours between meals, no solid food of any kind being taken in the interval. All invalids, and particularly elderly people, should have their principal meal in the middle of the day. It should be as dry as possible, thus diminishing the tendency to flatulence, and safeguarding the circulation from the absorption of bulky amounts of fluid. Salty articles and highly seasoned foods are for similar reasons best avoided. Alcohol has no value as a cardiac stimulant, but, as it increases a sense of well-being and makes for bodily and mental comfort, there is no reason to countermand it in the elderly, who may be accustomed to its use in moderation. Diet will best be light, and adjusted so far as possible to personal idiosyncrasies.

A rest in the afternoon, a light meal in the evening and a long night's rest will often follow naturally. Sleep is to be encouraged. Hot milk or a whisky toddy taken some little time before retiring may be all that is required. Much insomnia and restlessness can be prevented by having the bed alongside a wide-open window. Fresh air as distinct from draughts should be made available in abundance. By such simple rules hypnotics are often unnecessary, but if adequate sleep is difficult to obtain the choice of a suitable drug demands consideration. Paraldehyde, were it not for its objectionable taste when taken by mouth, and its peculiar odour when exhaled, might more frequently be employed on account of its valuable properties. The taste can be disguised to some extent, particularly if dispensed in 20-minim capsules of which three or more make a suitable dose in the first instance, but its excretion is perhaps more embarrassing to the friends of the invalid than to the patient himself. Bromide combined with a small dose of sodium phenobarbitone according to the prescription (p. 669) makes a gentle sedative remedy, and often proves helpful to the elderly patient. Larger doses of a more slow-acting barbiturate such as luminal are also serviceable, but in elderly people tend to be accumulative, and with constant repetition are occasionally responsible after a time for some degree of slight mental confusion. There is a form of sleeplessness not uncommon in the elderly which consists in a period of insomnia occurring for two or three hours in the middle of the night. These people have little difficulty in falling asleep when they first retire to bed, but in the morning are unrefreshed, as their sleep is broken. In the correction of this type of inter-nocturnal insomnia a rapidly acting barbiturate effective for an hour or two is a useful preparation to have available. The proprietary preparation, hebaral-sodium, in 3-gr. capsules, is effective, as it comes into action in the course of fifteen to thirty minutes and the effect wears off in two, three or four hours without any residual "hang-over." This drug can be taken through the night should the occasion demand its use.

Arsenic has some reputation in the treatment of the debility of old age, this being mostly based on the unconvincing evidence provided by the Styrian mountaineers who, having acquired a degree of tolerance to the drug, believe that it enables them to accomplish more work with less fatigue, less effort and less dyspnœa. In therapeutic doses arsenic has no direct effect on the heart or circulation, and any benefits which accrue from its use in the elderly probably result from its "tonic" properties, in improving appetite and relieving weakness and apathy. It may be prescribed as liquor arsenicalis (B.P.) in doses of 2 to 5 minims thrice daily after meals.

When bodily activity declines to such an extent that less and less can be accomplished, and when signs of basal congestion become evident, digitalis is definitely indicated, and may be given in small doses of 15 minims three times a day for a week or ten days at a time according to tolerance. If intermittent courses prove of value, then maintenance doses may be continued as necessary. Tablets of digoxin (0·25 mg.) or Nativelle's digitaline ($\frac{1}{600}$ gr.) are sometimes better tolerated by the elderly person whose digestion is impaired. When frank signs of congestive failure develop, special care must be taken in nursing with a view to the provision of the maximum amount of rest and comfort. The procedures outlined in the section dealing with the treatment of congestive heart failure are then applicable.

HEART DISEASE IN RELATION TO PREGNANCY

Reference has already been made to the question of the selection of a suitable occupation for those afflicted by heart disease in early life. Of all careers maternity may be the most strenuous, particularly in a working-class household, and therefore advice may be sought regarding the suitability of the cardiac patient for the risks and responsibilities of marriage. Just as the contracting parties are unlikely to be dissuaded from their intentions, so it is as a rule unwise and unkind to forbid marriage, but the dangers must be explained to both parties. The probability is that the affected partner will die young. The man suffering from rheumatic heart disease will be debarred from life insurance, and in a short career is less likely to be able to provide adequate support for his dependants after his death. The woman faces peculiar dangers, for the available evidence suggests that even surviving the immediate burdens imposed on her heart by successive pregnancies her days are likewise shortened. It should be realized, however, that the great majority of young women suffering from rheumat heart disease are able, in reasonably good surroundings and with skilled attention during the antenatal period, to bear one or at most two children without serious detriment, after which it may be considered justifiable to advise sterilization.

In no branch of cardiological practice is the ability to assess the degree of circulatory incapacity of greater consequence to the patient. Just as in the healthy woman minor degrees of cardiac embarrassment in the form of slight breathlessness and peripheral œdema often become apparent in the later months, so in the subject of definite cardiac disease a distinct aggravation of symptoms may be confidently anticipated as pregnancy advances. The outstanding danger is the development of congestive heart failure some time before term is reached. Labour under such circumstances is a burden which few will survive, and obstetrical interference undertaken in the presence of heart failure is the straw which breaks the camel's back. Pregnancy must be interrupted either in the earliest months in those likely to develop failure later, or, if it is allowed to proceed, adequate antenatal care and constant supervision must be made available throughout the pregnancy and labour conducted as expeditiously as possible. In determining appropriate treatment, the first duty of the physician is to correlate the degrees of circulatory embarrassment in relation to the period of gestation. Auricular fibrillation adds to the gravity of the situation.

The degree of cardiac impairment is assessed on the ease with which symptoms of circulatory distress are induced. By this means the patient may be graded according to her functional capacity. Group I is composed of those women who have a structural cardiac defect, but who have no associated symptoms. In these women the cardiac lesion is commonly discovered in the course of a routine antenatal examination. Obviously the farther advanced they are in pregnancy with freedom from cardiac symptoms the better is the outlook. As a general rule these women will require no particular treatment, and will be able to accomplish a natural delivery, but they must be kept under observation at intervals of three or four weeks so that their cardiac state may be reassessed from time to time. As the burden of pregnancy increases they will tend naturally to develop symptoms as term approaches, and will thus tend to advance to the next group.

Group II*a* is composed of those who have symptoms of a mild type—breathlessness and fatigue on heavier exertion. This degree of incapacity in the later months is not of serious significance, but up to the fourth or fifth month they likewise must be advised to report regularly for repeated observations.

Treatment consists in the provision of adequate rest with longer hours of sleep. They should be advised to lie down for an hour or two each afternoon, have a long night's rest in bed and avoid fatigue. Such measures as these may be sufficient to check the natural tendency to further signs of distress, as exemplified by the next grade of failure.

Group II*b* is composed of those who have very definite symptoms of breathlessness easily provoked. These women have been forced to decline their heavier household duties, and even with small amounts of exertion they exhibit breathlessness readily, and at night notice some swelling of the feet. This is an indication that particular care is required. Signs such as these occurring in the first three months warrant careful consideration, and usually the advice that the pregnancy be terminated, as by the time the sixth or seventh month is reached congestive heart failure of a more serious grade may be anticipated. Coming under observation about the middle of pregnancy a period of complete rest in bed for three or four weeks is desirable. It is often surprising to find how much good can be accomplished by this measure, particularly if every endeavour is made to ensure adequate sleep. There is probably no more important item in the care of the pregnant woman than the correction of insomnia, and for this purpose the bromide and phenobarbitone mixture (p. 669) recommended in the treatment of heart failure is of the greatest value. At this stage sleep, sound and refreshing, can often accomplish as much or more than digitalis, and at the same time adequate doses of iron to correct the anæmia so common in pregnancy will often help considerably to restore circulatory function. The exhaustion of hyperemesis occasionally aggravates the cardiac state and interferes with drug treatment. Digitalis by the rectal route (p. 681) may then be indicated. The symptoms of Group II*b* in the later months are always a danger signal. These women require rest in view of the natural tendency of the symptoms, if unchecked, to advance to congestive failure. Active measures in the form of enforced rest sleep and digitalis are indicated.

Group III is composed of those who have signs of heart failure at rest. These women, even when confined to bed, are a little dyspnœic, and have a degree of peripheral congestion more or less intense, ranging from a minor pitting œdema of the ankles to extensive anasarca and lumbar œdema. The essentials of treatment are absolute rest, careful nursing, a suitable diet and full doses of digitalis and mercurials. By this means an energetic attempt must be made to rid the patient of congestive heart failure before any obstetrical interference is attempted. With adequate supervision no pregnant woman should be allowed to advance to such a stage of heart failure, as it is of the most serious significance and is only aggravated by obstetrical interference. It is wiser to allow labour to proceed in the presence of congestive failure than to attempt the artificial evacuation of the uterus. In the latter instance she is almost certain to die, whereas with every attempt to support her heart and circulation by medical means she at least stands a chance of weathering the storm. Thorough treatment with a satisfactory response will then permit of Cæsarean section, at which time the opportunity may be taken, with the permission of the patient and her husband, to perform sterilization.

In these patients who have been suitably supervised throughout pregnancy, a successful delivery may be confidently anticipated. They should be admitted to hospital or nursing home a few days—perhaps a week—before term, provided with rest and sleep and, if necessary, digitalized by rapid dosage. During labour a sedative is usually indicated, such as morphia ($\frac{1}{4}$ gr.) and hyoscine ($\frac{1}{150}$ gr.) hypodermically. They should not be denied light anæsthesia. A protracted labour is to be avoided and the timely use of forceps frequently desirable. In the puerperium a longer time in bed will be compensated for by better health in the following months.

CONGENITAL HEART DISEASE

Congenital defects in the architecture of the heart and great vessels vary enormously in the degree of incapacity which they induce. On the one hand there are those individuals advanced in years in whom during the course of a routine examination a hitherto unsuspected congenital abnormality of the heart or aorta is revealed. At the other extreme is the baby surviving perhaps only a few days, cyanosed even to a deep plum colour, dyspnœic and distressed, for whom death is a merciful release. From a clinical point of view, more particularly with regard to prognosis, it is useful to classify congenital heart disease into three broad groups.

In the first group, the most severe, cyanosis is more or less constantly present, and grave structural changes permit of mixing of venous and arterial blood within the heart. Pulmonary stenosis with a large septal defect is an example of such a condition. Here, as a general rule, the course is progressively downwards, and treatment, it must be confessed, can accomplish little. Such cases seldom pass much beyond the age of puberty, and as infants they demand special care in nursing. Nursing difficulties varying in severity are ofte present: the babies become dyspnœic after feeding for only short time. The usual arrangements have to be modified s that they receive small amounts of a high caloric food at mor frequent intervals, thus reducing the difficulties of the actua nursing. As age increases, despite every care regarding die nutrition in many cases fails, and these children are ofte under weight for their age. They are prone to infection Cold, fatigue and exposure should be avoided as predisposin factors, and every attempt should be made to increase resis tance—ultra-violet light, cod-liver oil and malt and th avoidance of crowded places, particularly when infections ar rife, help to decrease the liability to respiratory infection Whooping-cough is a source of particular danger to the chil with a congenital cardiac defect.

The second clinical group is composed of those in whon cyanosis occurs only as a transient or terminal feature. I older children exercise only if taken to excess produce symptoms, or dyspnœa and cyanosis may be temporaril induced by bouts of crying in younger babies. This state o affairs is usually associated with a cardiovascular septal defec such as patency of the ductus arteriosus, or of the foramen oval In the absence of signs of cardiac distress on a reasonable amoun of exertion no particular treatment or restriction of activitie is desirable. It is a matter of adapting activities to the child' capabilities. Every attempt should be made to maintain satisfactory state of general nutrition with freedom fron intercurrent infection. It is probably true that in about hal these cases a long life even of full activity may be enjoye but an equal number of patients often succumb before the ag of twenty is reached, either as a result of congestive failure c the right-sided type or of subacute bacterial infection engrafte on the congenital anomaly. Adequate rest, the avoidance c a strenuous occupation and of unnecessary and unnatura fatigue all help to prolong life and make it more comfortabl Digitalis is indicated when congestive heart failure threaten but so far as the septicæmic state is concerned little can b accomplished therapeutically. Bronchitis and pneumonia are very real source of danger. The majority of these children hav unfortunately to be regarded as invalids all their lives. Like th adult suffering from acquired heart disease they should have long rest in the middle of the day, and slight ailments shoul receive every attention. School is generally out of the questior but some ultimately make better progress than might be antici pated, and after puberty can sometimes undertake light work

In the third or acyanotic group, in which there is no communication between the pulmonary and systemic circulations, the congenital defect may give rise to little or no embarrassment, escape recognition and require no particular treatment. Such instances occasionally come under observation for the first time in adult life. A right-sided aortic arch revealed, for example, by radiological examination may induce in itself no symptoms whatever, and treatment is necessarily out of the question. Similarly coarctation of the aorta, frequently confused with essential hypertension, is not amenable to treatment, and misguided attempts to lower the blood pressure in this condition only result in an aggravation of symptoms. A quieter and more sheltered life may be advised, as by this means such complications as cerebral hæmorrhage or heart failure may be avoided or postponed. The first successful ligation of a patent ductus arteriosus has recently been reported. This gives promise of a real contribution to treatment. Otherwise congenital defects of the heart are outwith the scope of surgery.

A. R. GILCHRIST.

THE TREATMENT OF VARIOUS TYPES OF HEART FAILURE

For clinical and descriptive purposes it is useful to separate the end results of degenerative myocardial disease into three broad groups according to the predominant symptom. Thus it is that we recognize "Congestive Failure" in the presence of peripheral œdema, engorgement of the liver, and distension of the veins. Such a syndrome is frequently accompanied by breathlessness in some degree, but when the dyspnœa is predominant, acute and distressing and the peripheral congestion minimal, the failure is obviously rather different in type. For descriptive purposes it is justifiable to consider this latter form under the general heading of "Dyspnœic Failure." A further group is composed of those in whom pain of cardiac origin is the leading feature, either in the more protracted form associated with coronary thrombosis or in the recurrent paroxysmal type associated with effort. This distressing type of heart disease may be considered under the heading of "Anginal Failure." From a clinical point of view it is of interest to note that, while congestive and dyspnœic failure may be combined in the one individual, it is quite exceptional for congestion to consort with anginal failure, at least in the more acute forms. Dyspnœa, on the other hand, may be in evidence in anginal failure.

CONGESTIVE HEART FAILURE

So far as the immediate treatment of this condition is concerned it matters little whether the patient suffers from valvular or non-valvular disease of the heart. With few modifications the same measures are applicable to the young woman suffering from congestive heart failure secondary to old-standing rheumatic heart disease with valvular defects and aggravated by auricular fibrillation with a fast ventricular rate, as would be applied in the treatment of the same type of failure evident in the man past middle life with no valvular defect, but whose heart has laboured under the burden of a hypertension for many years, and whose peripheral congestion has been of more gradual onset. The fact that the treatment of the congestive failure is similar in each instance does not warrant the conclusion that the ætiological diagnosis for the cause of the condition can be neglected. When the functional capacity of the circulation has been restored and the congestion relieved, further treatment at the ambulant stage may very well depend on this very factor. While we cannot eradicate the cause of rheumatic heart disease, yet a subtotal thyroidectomy may well be indicated for the adequate treatment of congestive failure in the thyro-cardiac, and similarly a suitable course of antiluetic treatment when the ætiological agent is the spirochæta pallida.

There are grades of congestive failure, and it is not difficult to picture on the one hand the young rheumatic subject handicapped by extreme peripheral congestion, greatly swollen legs, ascites, hepatic engorgement and perhaps some hydrothorax, exhausted, cyanosed and breathless on the least exertion. This is an extreme example. On the other hand, in the earliest stages, œdema will only be evident around the ankles towards evening. The first patient will require prolonged and thorough treatment at the earliest opportunity amounting to perhaps four to ten weeks in bed, whereas in the second instance a week's rest followed by advice regarding the restrictions of activity in the future may suffice.

Rest.—Let us consider the more severe grade. At the outset it is wise to explain to the patient that absolute rest will be required, and that this implies confinement to bed for a number of weeks. Many a man will hesitate to submit to this advice on the grounds that he must put his affairs in order, and that he has certain business commitments which demand his personal attention. It is right to explain to him that half-hearted measures have no place in the treatment of cardiac disease, and that more will be accomplished in less time by a strict and complete régime than by temporizing with a serious situation. It can be explained to him that every phase of physical activity increases the work of the heart, and that its burden can only be relieved by the provision of adequate rest. At the same time it must be realized that the full benefit of rest will be denied him if he is forced to retire to his bed with many business problems unsolved and surplus domestic or personal difficulties still preying on his mind. Depending on the circumstances, and guided by the severity of the symptoms, it is often justifiable to permit such a patient to do what he can in the course of a day or two to put his affairs in order, so that he may at once be rewarded by as complete a physical and mental rest as it is humanly possible to attain.

The patient should be put to bed—whether in his own house, a nursing home or hospital depends on many personal factors—and the practitioner familiarizing himself with the particular situation will judge whether adequate nursing care can be provided at home. The rest in bed must be absolute, and everything must be done to render the patient as comfortable as possible by the provision of a suitable number of pillows, support for the arms, a suitable amount of bedclothes and a warm but airy room. Many a patient will beg to be allowed to sit in an arm-chair, saying that his breathing is thereby rendered more free than when he is strictly confined to bed. As a general rule this reflects on the care which has been taken to give him the maximum amount of comfort when in bed. A support for the shoulders, a prop for the feet, a pillow under the knees are all devices which bring comfort, and when this is found the correct position should be maintained. For urination a bottle should be provided, and the only occasion on which he may be permitted to leave his bed is for bowel actions, and for this purpose a bedside commode should be provided. This concession cannot always be permitted, but it is useful to remember that many patients, particularly heavily built and elderly men, expend much mental and physical energy in their unaided gymnastics to master the use of the bed-pan. The provision of a suitable commode at the bedside may result in less expenditure of energy. While there is much to be said for the disciplined routine of the hospital, yet in private practice the experienced nurse will so modify her methods as to avoid disturbing the patient as much as possible, particularly by wakening him in the early morning for washing and bathing. A meal can well be postponed should comfort be found in sleep.

Sleep.—A restful bed is therefore the first essential, but despite this, sleep is seldom as sound or as refreshing as in health unless active steps are taken to provide it. The correction of insomnia is of the utmost importance. Here again half-hearted measures are of little avail. Strangely enough there is often a peculiar reluctance to use opium or one of its derivatives in the presence of heart disease. As a hypnotic there is no drug to compare with it, and time and time again patients will say after an adequate dose that it has provided them with the first night's rest for weeks or even months. In the early evening the patient should be given hypodermically a dose of $\frac{1}{6}$ to $\frac{1}{4}$ gr. of morphine sulphate, and this repeated if necessary in four or six hours. An energetic attempt should be made to ensure a minimum of seven to nine hours' continuous sleep. This is so important that it cannot be over-emphasized, for by this means alone it is often possible to restore in a remarkable way the efficiency of the heart and circulation. Every restless night prolongs the period of confinement to bed, and thus delays recovery. The cardiac patient as a rule tolerates morphia well, though vomiting occurring some hours after its administration is sometimes rightly attributed to the drug. If this be so, then some preparation containing the total alkaloids of opium may be substituted. The proprietary preparations, alopon or omnopon, each adjusted to contain 50 per cent. of morphine, have not the same tendency to induce nausea and vomiting as the single alkaloid—morphia. These drugs are useful and potent preparations. They may be taken in the form of tablets, each $\frac{1}{6}$ gr., by the mouth. When relief from insomnia in cardiac disease is urgently required, it is preferable that a dose of $\frac{1}{3}$ gr. be injected subcutaneously to ensure its rapid absorption. The comfort and peace of mind induced by these opium derivatives is usually profound, and after a few nights of refreshing sleep the dose may be reduced and some other reliable hypnotic gradually substituted. The combination of bromide with chloral is a time-honoured remedy, and is generally effective in heart cases. 20 gr. of potassium bromide and 20 gr. of chloral hydrate prescribed in a mixture may next be employed, the nurse having instructions to repeat the dose in three or four hours should the necessity arise.

In recent years, on account of their reliability and ease of administration, the various barbiturate preparations have shown a tendency to replace the bromide and chloral mixtures of former days in the correction of cardiac insomnia. Luminal (phenobarbitone, B.P.) or its more soluble sodium salt may be given at night in doses up to 2 gr. in tablet form. Ampoules, each 1 c.c. of a 20 per cent. solution (3 gr.), are also available for *intramuscular* injection. This makes a convenient substitute for the subcutaneous injection of morphia, which it may replace after the first few days. At a later stage either a mixture of bromide or one or more tablets of any reliable barbiturate (*e.g.*, soneryl) may be taken by the mouth. Of these there are such a large number that the practitioner will be wise to familiarize himself with the effects of one or two well-selected remedies, or phenobarbitone can be combined with bromide as in the following prescription :—

℞		
	Pot. Brom.	gr. xx
	Phenobarbiton. Sol.	gr. ½
	Liq. Arsen.	♏i
	Syr. Aurant.	♏xx
	Aq. Menth. Pip.	ad ℥ii

Of this mixture 2 drachms in water taken in the evening is often sufficient to induce sleep, and, if necessary, one teaspoonful can be repeated as desired through the night should the occasion arise. In prescribing bromide for the insomnia of congestive heart failure, it is probably wise to avoid the use of the sodium salt, as the sodium ions favour the retention of water in the tissues. The inclusion of a small dose of arsenic is believed to reduce the liability to bromide skin eruptions.

During these first few days the doctor will visit his patient preferably twice in the twenty-four hours, and of these two visits the evening one is the more important, as at this time it is opportune to consider fully the provision of sleep. It is helpful to have the nurse keep a record from day to day of the hours spent asleep. It is worth aiming at a total of ten or twelve in the twenty-four as a minimum, but the drug selected and its dose will be largely determined by the patient's general condition, the amount of sleep obtained during the day and the degree of breathlessness, all of which are of greater importance than any physical sign revealed by examination of the heart.

Diet.—Having made provision for ample rest and for the correction of the insomnia, it is next advisable to draw up a definite dietetic scheme. Too often this is left to chance, and the experience or inexperience of the nurse who, in private practice, may know little of the culinary resources of the household. In hospital practice the routine diet of the ward must be frequently readjusted to suit the special needs of the cardiac patient. In arranging a diet for his patient the doctor will bear in mind the desirability of restricting the total calories in order to reduce metabolism and decrease the work of the heart. On account of portal congestion large meals are badly tolerated ; indeed, anorexia, nausea and vomiting often present special problems of their own. The restriction of protein to 50 or 60 gm. daily, an amount sufficient to compensate for nitrogen loss, reduces its specific dynamic stimulus to metabolism to negligible proportions. Fats as a rule are poorly tolerated, particularly so when jaundice—a fairly frequent accompaniment of the most advanced form of congestive failure—complicates the picture. Carbohydrate furnishes a ready supply of energy and is usually acceptable in an easily assimilable form. It can be given in sufficient quantity to make good the proposed calorie value of the diet. Patients suffering from congestive heart failure commonly complain of thirst, but in the first few days fluid should be restricted to an amount short of producing discomfort : a total fluid intake of 800 to 1,200 c.c. is usually sufficient to quench thirst. As a further principle the diet should be low in salt content, particularly salts of sodium, as clinical experience has taught that the sodium ion is of more importance than the chloride in the retention of tissue fluid. It is undesirable, even were it possible, to exclude entirely the consumption of sodium chloride, but a reduction to 2 or 3 gm. as compared with the usual intake of approximately 10 gm. per day in health is a useful step. Even with such a quantity the diet is apt after a time to become unpalatable, but the salt substitutes on the market are best avoided, as the majority contain sodium. It is as a rule sufficient to advise that salty and spicy articles of food be avoided, that as little salt as possible be used in cooking, and that salt be not served with meals. As a matter of experience, few patients begin to complain about lack of salt until the first week or ten days of treatment has been accomplished, by which time their thirst is usually relieved. Small quantities of salt may again be included in the diet for a few days, returning to the restricted sodium intake as necessary. It is highly desirable that the food should be rich in vitamins, particularly vitamin B_1 and vitamin C, both of which, when administered in deficiency states, have a beneficial effect in the correction of cardiac œdema. Congestive heart failure occurring in the alcoholic, in whom the absorption of vitamins may be defective, often responds in a remarkable way to the parenteral administration of synthetic preparations. Vitamin C itself has a well-marked diuretic effect.

For those adults who do not dislike milk, the Karell diet has much to recommend it, at least for the first few days of treatment. The procedure, which consists in its strictest form in the limitation of nourishment to no more than four glasses of milk, each approximately 7 oz., in the day, thus yielding a total of only 580 calories, is occasionally followed by brilliant results, the venous congestion subsiding, the œdema being relieved by a prompt diuresis, and a distinct amelioration of the patient's distress. There can be no doubt that were such a strict régime applied more often, greater progress might be observed in the first few days of rest in bed. This diet has the virtue that it restricts fluids, keeps the calories low, and reduces the intake of salt, but the frugality of these " meals " cannot be maintained for more than three or four days. In addition many patients dislike milk or find its monotony irksome. Any semi-solid food will therefore be appreciated, and this may take the form of soft boiled eggs, crustless bread with unsalted butter, and fruit drinks flavoured with glucose. A diet of approximately 1,100 calories suitable for the average case and open to modification according to the tastes of the patient is composed as follows :—

Diet for Congestive Failure

Salt Poor. Restricted Fluid.

Early Morning—

Orange or other fruit juice with 1 teaspoonful glucose (total fluid, 3 oz.).

Breakfast—

1 egg—poached, boiled or scrambled.
1 slice crisp toast ; butter ; jelly marmalade.
1 cup milk.

11 *a.m.—*

Orange or other fruit juice with 1 teaspoonful glucose (total fluid, 3 oz.) ; *or*
Small glass of ovaltine or Horlick's (total fluid, 3 oz.).

Dinner—

Small helping pounded fish or sliced chicken or rabbit, or *tender* lean meat—may be served as soufflé or custard.
2 to 3 fingers fairy toast.
Stewed or baked apple or fruit whip, jelly or snow, with sugar.

Tea—

2 plain tea biscuits ; *or*
Finger plain sponge—jelly if desired.
1 cup weak, freshly infused tea with milk and sugar.

Supper (not later than 7 P.M.)—
Stewed or baked apple or fruit whip or custard or curds or jelly with sugar.
2 tea biscuits or Dutch crispies.

9 *p.m.*—
Small glass of Horlick's or ovaltine or plain milk.

Milk daily—$\frac{3}{4}$ pint.
All food should be cooked *without salt*, and no salt served with meals.
Fluid: Fluid content of this diet is approximately 800 c.c.
Calorie Value: Approximately 1,100 calories.
By adding a little cream (3 oz.) to serve with fruit, the calorie value would be increased to approximately 1,300.

The cream and butter of the diet ought to be adjusted according to the weight of the patient, and the fluid limited to 800 c.c. As progress is made the quantities of food may be increased, but the total calories as a rule should not exceed 1,500 while the patient is confined to bed. When convalescence is reached, the diet should be so adjusted as to maintain weight at the correct standard for the patient's age and height. This is of particular importance, as even 1 stone in excess of the correct weight throws a considerable burden on the heart.

The diet outlined above being low in residue has little stimulant action on the bowel, though to some extent this is made good by the inclusion of quantities of fruit or fruit juice which may be increased or varied according to individual requirements. Nevertheless, purgatives will have to be prescribed by the doctor, and in their selection the previous habits of the patient have to be considered, recognizing that brisk purgation is exhausting and does little to relieve congestion. Diarrhœa should be avoided. A daily bowel movement is sufficient. A vegetable pill, perhaps one or more 3-gr. doses of pill aloes (B.P.) at night followed by a saline purge in the morning, may be all that is required. A gentler stimulant which has much to recommend it in those not previously affected by a sluggish bowel is provided by the emulsion of paraffin and agar (B.P.C.) taken in a $\frac{1}{2}$-oz. dose in the evening. A glycerin suppository is in many ways preferable to the saline purge, which is necessarily associated with a large bulk of fluid. One glycerin suppository may be inserted each morning, either a vegetable pill or the emulsion of agar having been taken the previous night. The stool which results is of almost normal consistency, and is unassociated with pain or olic. Many of the proprietary salines in common use contain sodium chloride or other salts of sodium, and though more greeable to take than magnesium sulphate are best avoided. For similar reasons, should an enema be required, 5 to 10 oz. of warm olive oil slowly injected and retained for some hours s preferable to the discomfort associated with liberal quantities of soap and water. Taking into consideration the previous abits of the patient, the urgency of his present symptoms nd the necessity for purgation, the doctor will then decide n the most suitable preparation for immediate use; further neasures will be determined by the response obtained.

It is important to note that acting on the principles outlined bove, remarkable improvement may become evident in the ourse of a few days. This is particularly true of patients dmitted to hospital in varying degrees of congestive failure, vho for one reason or another have been denied adequate upervision in their own homes. It is true that the nursing of he patient may make all the difference between success and ailure, but it would appear that one factor determining rogress which has been poorly assessed in the past is the pro-ision of a better diet. The correction of under-nutrition and vitaminosis may well account for the prompt diuresis which ften appears when the ill-balanced diet of the hospital clientele s corrected more or less automatically on their admission to he wards. Many patients thus treated will respond so satis-actorily that the administration of direct cardiac drugs is nnecessary, and indeed if the use of digitalis is postponed or a few days until progress has been observed, it helps onsiderably in assessing the prognosis. Even a partial diuresis nduced by rest and diet without the use of digitalis betokens favourable response to further treatment.

The Therapeutic Use of Digitalis.—The proper use of igitalis may make all the difference in the treatment of heart lisease. It is not a cardiac panacea, but no other cardiac rug is endowed with such propensities for good. A unique rug having peculiar properties of the utmost value in thera-eutics, its use has to be mastered, and it can never be prescribed n a haphazard or aimless fashion. It is therefore essential to ave a sound working knowledge of the mode of its action, he method of its administration and the results to be expected vhen it is given in adequate dosage for suitable periods at a ime.

In the first instance it is useful to consider when digitalis herapy is indicated. The primary, and by far the most nportant, indication for the administration of this drug is congestive heart failure, however mild or however severe. It is of little or no consequence whether the blood pressure is high or low, whether aortic regurgitation is present or not or whether the heart rate is fast or slow. If congestion is present, then digitalis is indicated beyond a doubt. It is true that when fibrillation is present, particularly if the ventricular rate is high—in the neighbourhood of 150 or thereabouts—a very satisfactory response to digitalis may be anticipated, but a slow, regular pulse, even that of complete heart-block, is not a contraindication to its use when peripheral œdema and venous congestion are present. It is absolutely wrong to suppose that only those patients suffering from auricular fibrillation derive benefit from its use. On the other hand, a regular fast heart, such as occurs in the acute infections, notably pneumonia, or in thyrotoxic states, is not necessarily an indication for its use. Digitalis is also indicated in dyspnœic failure, but yields little or no benefit in the anginal type, and is best avoided. Its administration in the paroxysmal arrhythmias is discussed under this heading. It is occasionally of advantage in the abolition of extrasystoles when these are troublesome to the patient, but they are not in themselves an indication for its use, nor when present do they necessarily contraindicate it.

From what has been said it will be obvious that the milder degrees of cardiac incapacity associated merely with breathlessness on exertion are not an essential indication for digitalis therapy, but it is sometimes difficult to determine the exact stage of cardiac insufficiency which warrants its use. The slightest forms indicated by some degree of breathlessness are usually amenable to restricted activities and longer hours of sleep and rest, and this is equally true of the mildest degrees of congestive failure, when œdema first makes its appearance towards evening. If such measures as rest and sleep in themselves are ineffective, then a certain indication for digitalis therapy may be said to exist. Smaller doses than in the more urgent cases are advisable, and as tolerance to this drug is never acquired its early use does not prejudice full doses should they become imperative at a later date.

It may therefore be said that the primary object in digitalis therapy is to relieve or prevent the characteristic symptoms associated with the two leading syndromes of myocardial insufficiency—congestive and dyspnœic failure. It is in these particular circumstances that real benefit may be anticipated from the use of the drug. If such symptoms of myocardial insufficiency as dyspnœa, œdema, increased venous pressure and congestion of the hepatic, pulmonary or peripheral circulation exist, then digitalis in adequate dosage is likely to be helpful. The use of the drug in the absence of such symptoms finds little or no support in clinical experience. Tachycardia in itself is no certain indication for digitalis. In brief, the object in using digitalis is not to slow the heart-rate, not to counter valvular defects, but to prevent and ease the symptoms of myocardial failure.

It is only natural that as a result of the known efficacy of digitalis a large number of preparations, official and proprietary, should be available for general use, but not all of these are of equal potency or proven efficacy. When digitalis is indicated it is important to use a reliable preparation, and for this purpose there is none better than the tincture of digitalis or the powdered leaf which may be prescribed in pill or tablet form. It is a reassurance to know that in using the latter preparation all the valuable properties of the foxglove are offered to the patient at less expense than the single refined active and inactive bodies prepared by the manufacturing chemists and sold under various trade names. The pill or tablet containing $1\frac{1}{2}$ gr. of the powdered leaf has many advantages. The exact daily amount required is easily regulated, and for a maintenance dose the patient can carry it with him conveniently. The tincture is equally effective, and is the usual source employed in hospital practice, but it is said ultimately to deteriorate on keeping when dispensed in a watery solution. This is no real handicap to its use as relatively small amounts are dispensed at one time and deterioration only takes place in the course of years. The dose should not be counted in drops from a bottle. The size of a drop varies enormously, and it is an inaccurate way of administering the drug. When the pure tincture is in use it is preferable to have a single dose taken each day, say a measured drachm, rather than suffer the vagueness of twenty drops three times a day. Inexact digitalis dosage is fraught with danger to the patient, and confuses the doctor in his management of the case. For these reasons the powdered leaf, at least in private practice, is probably the best preparation to use. In comparing doses of these two preparations, the leaf and the tincture, it is useful to remember that $1\frac{1}{2}$ gr. or 0·1 gm. of the leaf and 15 minims or 1 c.c. of the tincture are all equivalent quantities.

It has been estimated that on the average the body destroys or excretes digitalis at a rate corresponding to $1\frac{1}{2}$ to 2 gr. of the powdered leaf or 15 to 20 minims of the tincture per day. When the daily dose exceeds this amount a proportion accumulates in the tissues, the concentration rising step by step until the excess overflows and the stomach rebels. To obtain maximum beneficial effects it is necessary to saturate the tissues with the drug, and in general the greater the body-weight the more digitalis is required for this purpose. Over-saturation is accompanied by symptoms of digitalis intoxication, but the maximum therapeutic benefit is obtained by a concentration just short of the toxic amount. From what has been said it must be obvious that if small doses are administered daily, say 10 or 15 minims of the tincture, an effective concentration of the drug in the tissues may never be attained, for just as much is eliminated or destroyed each day as is given to the patient. As a general rule seven to nine days will elapse before a daily dose of 60 minims of the tincture produces a concentration sufficient to induce maximum benefit. By doubling this dose the time-lag is reduced to three or four days, as the drug accumulates more rapidly. Thus an effective concentration depends on the rate with which successive doses are administered. The absorption of each dose is virtually completed in the course of six to eight hours, at which time, if auricular fibrillation be present, an effect begins to become evident on the rate of the heart and, if the accumulation is sufficiently great, in the general betterment of the patient.

Recognizing that there are individual variations in the response to drugs, it is nevertheless true that the main factors in determining the amount of digitalis required to produce maximum benefit are the potency of the preparation used and the weight of the patient. Tinctures of digitalis supplied by reliable firms in this country are now sufficiently standardized to correspond on the average with a strength of 1 c.c. to the "cat-unit." Eggleston found that 0·146 c.c. of a standard tincture (1 "cat-unit" per c.c.) per pound body-weight was the average dose required to produce maximum beneficial effect. Theoretically the full digitalizing dose in cubic centimetres of the tincture may therefore be calculated as 0·15 × "cat-unit" value × pounds body-weight. For example, a patient of 140 lbs. will require of a standard tincture 140 × 0·15 × 1 = 21 c.c. of the tincture or 2·10 gm. of the powdered leaf. For clinical purposes 1 c.c. equals 15 minims and 1 gm. equals 15 gr.

It is not suggested that such a large quantity be administered in a single dose, but the total calculated amount may be taken in fractions at intervals of six hours, appropriate doses being approximately half the total (say 10 c.c.) followed by one-quarter (say 5 c.c.) then one-eighth (say 2·5 c.c.), the remainder in smaller doses of perhaps 1·5 c.c. repeated at similar intervals. The first appearance of toxic symptoms is at once an indication for the discontinuation of further doses. *It must be realized that full digitalization by this method of massive doses is inapplicable to any patient who has been taking even small amounts of digitalis or its allied bodies during the previous ten to fourteen days, as obviously, if the tissues are already partially saturated, serious toxic symptoms may be readily induced by the first large dose.* The limitation of the method must be clearly understood before it is applied to any individual, no matter how urgent his symptoms may appear to be.

Various modifications of this method of intensive digitalization have been applied in practice. A suitable one is a single large initial dose calculated on the basis of 1 minim of the tincture to each pound of body-weight. This forms a basis for further therapy. In the first instance a 10-stone patient would therefore receive 140 minims : after six hours 30-minim doses are commenced, and continued at similar intervals until a quantity equal to the original massive dose has been administered. Thus a man of 10 stone would receive in succession at six-hour intervals 140 minims, 30 minims, 30 minims, 30 minims, 30 minims and finally 20 minims to complete the theoretical amount required. Accurate observations on the rate of the heart and a careful supervision are essential during rapid digitalization, as the drug must be stopped on the first appearance of intoxication. The large initial dose in this method has frequently given rise to some hesitation in its employment, and as a result further modifications have been proposed. Thus for a patient whose weight is 10 stone or over, the doses might well be 90 minims, 60 minims and 30 minims at six-hour intervals. In fibrillation an appreciable effect on the heart-rate becomes evident as a rule within six hours and maximum slowing in twenty-four to thirty-six hours. It is misleading to check the effect of the drug by only recording the pulse-rate. With fast ventricular rates diastolic filling is incomplete, and a varying number of beats are in consequence inappreciable at the wrist. The difference between the ventricular-rate and the pulse-rate is spoken of as the pulse-deficit. As accumulation of the drug proceeds the pulse-deficit declines. The pulse-rate may actually increase at first as more beats become effectively transmitted to the periphery. The nurse can quickly learn to record the rate of the ventricles by counting with a stethoscope or by palpation of the apex beat. The pulse-rate in fibrillation may give quite erroneous information.

In cases of auricular fibrillation the control of the ventricular rate frequently coincides with an amelioration of the patient's symptoms. When normal rhythm accompanies congestive failure, the heart-rate may be unchanged or declined by only 10 or 20 beats per minute after full digitalization, and yet symptomatic relief may be just as brilliant. Diuresis commences, dyspnœa lessens, appetite returns and, being more comfortable, the patient is often rewarded by a profound and restful sleep. Digitalis does not cure auricular fibrillation. The ventricular rate is slowed, the rhythm becomes more regular and the efficiency of the heart as a pump is improved, but the fibrillation persists. Digitalis, in fact, tends to perpetuate the abnormal rhythm. In urgent cases of congestive failure, whether fibrillation be present or not, the results obtained by intensive digitalization are generally most gratifying in that distress is promptly relieved. A patient appreciates bold measures when these are based on reason and purposely designed to restore health as rapidly as possible.

Of the pure refined preparations the crystallized glucoside, digoxin, isolated from the leaves of digitalis lanata, has a prompt effect, and is useful for rapid digitalization. In a patient of 140 lbs. or more, a single dose of 1½ mg. (six of the 0·25 mg. tablets in which it is conveniently dispensed), equivalent to 90 minims of digitalis tincture, may be taken by the mouth. In the presence of fibrillation it causes a rapid fall in ventricular rate, reaching a maximum in six to eight hours, at which time, in the absence of toxic effects, dosage may be resumed at a rate of one tablet (0·25 mg.) six-hourly until maximum therapeutic benefit is attained. Digoxin has the advantage that it is probably absorbed more rapidly than a corresponding quantity of digitalis, and as its excretion rate is also more rapid there is less liability to sustained intoxication. On occasion, when symptoms are extremely urgent or when persistent vomiting precludes its oral use (see p. 681), it may be used intravenously.

When the patient's symptoms are less acute and circulatory incapacity more gradual in onset, rapid and intensive digitalization is not so essential. Doses of 30 minims of the tincture thrice daily for three or four days, and subsequently 20 minims for a shorter period of time, may be all that is required, but as a general rule the drug ought to be pushed until symptoms and signs of failure are relieved, or until the mildest symptoms of digitalis intoxication supervene. With few exceptions this is a better guide to adequate dosage than the amount of cardiac slowing recorded. Whatever the method of administration it is usually wise to explain to the patient or his attendant that maximum benefit can only be obtained by an amount just short of that quantity which induces symptoms of intoxication. The dose or doses employed to induce this major effect in the first instance are spoken of as the digitalizing or effective quantity of the drug. This varies for different patients. The dose by which the level of the effect is maintained is spoken of as the "maintenance dose": this quantity requires careful regulation in order to preserve optimum benefit over lengthy periods of time.

Maintenance dosage is commenced a day or two after the effective quantity has been determined. In arranging a maintenance dose in these circumstances, the tissues being already almost fully saturated with the drug, small quantities to counterbalance the excretion rate are all that is required. To avoid the risk of unpleasant symptoms and yet maintain an adequate concentration, the drug should be taken in short courses. The quantity varies for different individuals, and can only be determined by the rough-and-ready clinical method of trial and error. Pills or friable tablets (each 1½ gr.) of the powdered leaf are convenient in regulating the dose, and two or three of these daily (a total of 3 to 4½ gr. or 30 to 45 minims of the tincture) can usually be taken for from four to six consecutive days before mild symptoms of general intoxication appear. An easily remembered rule is to advise the patient to take two pills daily, omitting all medication on Saturday and Sunday of each week. Should symptoms of digitalis poisoning appear before the five days' course is completed, the dose is discontinued for two or three days and recommenced. Some patients will be able to take more than the suggested amount, some less. With a little judicious guidance the intelligent patient will soon learn to regulate his own dosage. He should be encouraged to take as much as his tissues will tolerate. It is probably true that too little attention is given to the regulation of maintenance dosage, and commonly the routine amount taken by the patient tends to be too small rather than too large, with the result that he fails to get full benefit and becomes discouraged. Haphazard administration can accomplish little of value. Overdosage, with its attendant disagreeable effects, dissuades the patient, hinders effective treatment and handicaps his adviser unless confidence can be regained by a full explanation of the effects and uses of the drug.

The toxic effects of digitalis are so uniform in their sequence that the therapeutic dosage can easily be regulated. Particular care must be taken to recognize intoxication at its first appearance. The first unfavourable effect is almost invariably frontal headache, and this is followed by anorexia, nausea and later by vomiting. Loss of appetite is a sign of approaching saturation, and is an indication to reduce or discontinue the maintenance dose. The first appearance of nausea or vomiting is a certain sign that the tissues are over-saturated. Vomiting should be avoided. It distresses the patient unnecessarily.

With a clear understanding of the clinical use of the drug, difficulties in its administration are seldom encountered. It is quite exceptional in hospital practice to meet with a patient in need of digitalis in whom symptoms of general intoxication, nausea or vomiting, are induced by a quantity less than an adequate digitalizing dose, and yet in private practice there are occasionally patients who for one reason or another allege that they are intolerant of the drug. This may result from lack of supervision of the maintenance doses in a prejudiced and bewildered individual, or else it may be a peculiar personal idiosyncrasy. The latter must be rare and well worthy of accurate clinical study. Vomiting, which is the usual symptom of intolerance, may justify the substitution of the tincture for the powdered leaf, or vice versa, or the tincture of strophanthus (2 to 5 minims) or one of the more refined preparations such as tablets of digoxin (0·25 mg.) or Nativelle's digitaline granules ($\frac{1}{240}$ gr.) equivalent to 15 or 20 minims of the tincture, but it must be understood that digitalis or an allied preparation which fails to induce toxic symptoms in appropriate dosage is equally unlikely to be of benefit to the heart.

The nausea and vomiting of portal congestion, a common accompaniment of the advanced degrees of failure, is occasionally confusing in the regulation of digitalis dosage. Vomiting may thus be either a symptom of digitalis lack or of digitalis intoxication. Portal congestion sufficient in itself to induce gastric symptoms is almost invariably accompanied by a swelling of the liver and usually by ascites. Even if the drug is retained by the stomach its absorption is delayed and accumulation takes place more slowly. When congestive failure is present, the ventricular rate high and the auricles fibrillating, it may be taken that digitalis is indicated and that vomiting, if present, is not necessarily an expression of digitalis intoxication. From the point of view of digitalis therapy there are three alternatives. Full doses of digitalis may be continued by the mouth combined with a small dose of tincture of opium (♏x to xx) to act as a gastric sedative, and thus promote retention of the drug, or digitalis may be given by the rectum, or finally an active preparation may be selected for intravenous use.

When vomiting due to congestion of the gastric mucosa precludes the effective oral administration of digitalis, the tincture can be given in doses of 1 to 2 drachms daily by rectal injection. To reduce the tendency to local irritation and promote its absorption, the dose may be added to 2 or 3 oz. of 5 per cent. glucose saline warmed and injected slowly once each day. Rectal administration can be of the greatest value when the nausea and vomiting of a congested alimentary tract handicap the oral use of the drug. It is correct to say from personal experience of severe cases of hyperemesis gravidarum complicated by congestive heart failure, when little or no food could be retained by the stomach, that the rectal administration of digitalis by this method has yielded most gratifying results. The success of the rectal route usually becomes evident in a day or two, by which time the portal congestion subsides, and it is then possible to resume oral administration.

For intravenous use a choice may be made between strophanthin ($\frac{1}{240}$ to $\frac{1}{60}$ gr., B.P.) or digoxin (0·5 to 1·0 mg.) suitably diluted. Intramuscular or subcutaneous injections of either of these preparations is to be avoided on account of intense local irritation and irregular absorption. The former is best given with the usual aseptic precautions diluted in 10 to 20 c.c. of sterile normal saline, and if attempts have been previously made to administer digitalis by the mouth the intravenous dose of strophanthin should not exceed $\frac{1}{150}$ to $\frac{1}{100}$ gr. Thus used, a definite effect on the rate of the heart can usually be obtained within half an hour, and a full action in six hours. If gastric symptoms still persist, then a smaller dose than that formerly administered can be repeated in twelve hours, but great caution is required before a further dose is given, and in any case this should not exceed $\frac{1}{150}$ gr. For intravenous use digoxin is available in convenient ampoules, each containing 0·5 mg. in 1 c.c. of 70 per cent. alcohol. The effective intravenous dose is 0·5 to 1 mg. It must be diluted ten times with sterile saline immediately before use. This is most conveniently done by drawing up the contents of one or two ampoules into a 10 or 20 c.c. syringe, and completing the mixture by filling the syringe with saline to the correct amount. A full dose (1 mg.) will produce a decided effect on the heart-rate within ten minutes, and is maximal in two hours, but it must be borne in mind that a full intravenous dose can only be justified if it is certain that no other digitalis body has been taken by the mouth within the preceding ten days. When the patient is vomiting from time to time as a result of portal congestion, it is often difficult to know how much, if any, of the digitalis previously administered by the mouth has been retained. When intravenous therapy is used it is therefore wise to employ a small dose, say 0·5 mg. digoxin, and repeat this if necessary at intervals of eight or twelve hours, resuming oral administration at the earliest opportunity.

There are other preparations of digitalis and digitalis bodies on the market, some of which are suitable for intravenous use, but it is true that not one of them is superior to a carefully standardized pharmacopœal preparation, and more often than not their activity bears an inverse relation to the volume of advertising matter which accompanies them. Similarly, no benefit ensues from the hypodermic injection of $\frac{1}{100}$ gr. of amorphous digitalin, commonly used by the surgeons in states of circulatory collapse. Refined tinctures, said to be devoid of irritant properties and pure principles ardently advocated by the manufacturing chemists, are, with few exceptions, better avoided. The infusion of digitalis (B.P.) has so many disadvantages that its use has been practically abandoned. It deteriorates on keeping, and has to be given in a dose ten times that of the tincture to obtain the same result. While the whole of the active principles can be extracted in the infusion with special precautions, yet these are not often taken, and it therefore seems that the tincture or powdered leaf are definitely preferable. Tincture of strophanthus has little to commend it for routine use. In full doses its margin of safety is less than digitalis owing to its irregular and slow absorption. The writer has never seen conclusive proof that it was of benefit when digitalis had failed to give relief.

Reference has already been made to the symptoms of digitalis intoxication, which may be grouped under two headings, general and local. It has been pointed out that the first to appear is almost invariably headache which is followed in definite sequence by anorexia, and some six or eight hours later nausea and vomiting if the usual doses are continued. Once induced, digitalis vomiting may persist for twenty-four or forty-eight hours. It is peculiarly distressing to the patient on account of the associated retching, and it is harmful to him by the amount of exhaustion, fatigue and mental depression which accompanies it. Many patients are drowsy for the twenty-four hours or more following rapid digitalization, in spite of adequate sleep on previous nights. Diarrhœa, and in more pronounced cases of intoxication visual disturbances such as difficulty in focusing and the presence of yellow and green vision, may cause anxiety. In elderly men full digitalis dosage may be accompanied by mental confusion, a muttering delirium and hallucinations often taking the form of rectangular figures. The writer has seen these symptoms precede the more common digestive disturbances, and has found them all subside rapidly when the drug was discontinued for a day or two. The central nervous system is more susceptible to digitalis than the gastric mucosa. As regards local symptoms a close watch must be kept on the rhythm of the heart. A heart-rate below 50, the appearance of frequent extrasystoles, especially coupling of the beats, or the appearance of heart-block, either partial or complete, are all danger signals. The irregularity of partial heart-block is easily recognized by auscultation, and from the nature of things is only found when digitalis is administered in cases of normal rhythm. Complete heart-block, on the other hand, may occur either in patients with regular beating auricles or with auricular fibrillation : in the latter instance the heart becomes regular, and when due to digitalis the dissociation usually leads to a ventricular rate higher than that found in complete heart-block of arteriosclerotic origin. The complete heart-block of digitalis is a rare condition, much less frequent than commonly supposed, and when first recognized the ventricular rate is usually about 50 per minute, though higher rates are occasionally observed, particularly if the administration of digitalis is continued, whereas a rate in the neighbourhood of 30 is usual in the arteriosclerotic variety. A more serious and more common indication of digitalis intoxication is the development of a ventricular tachycardia. This occurs as a rule in arteriosclerotic patients, the subjects of advanced myocardial degeneration in whom the response to digitalis has been unsatisfactory with the result that its administration has been pushed to excess in the hope of relieving the congestive failure. It is recognized by the sudden development of an excessively fast ventricular rate usually in the neighbourhood of 150 to 180 per minute. It is accompanied by a marked pulse deficit, so that it may pass undetected unless attention is paid to the rate of the heart. Its persistence for more than a few hours generally leads to an advance in the degree of congestive failure, and the fall in blood pressure which usually accompanies it may be partly responsible for cerebral symptoms ranging from mental confusion to epileptic convulsions. Ventricular tachycardia is a serious sign which usually betokens a fatal issue. The abnormalities of rhythm are more likely to occur before the general manifestations of intoxication in advanced degrees of congestive failure.

There is no specific treatment for digitalis intoxication beyond the obvious necessity of omitting its further administration.

The prescription of a dose of castor oil, with the intention of emptying the alimentary tract and thus avoiding further digitalis absorption, often helps to relieve the patient when the drug has been given by mouth. For excessive intravenous therapy there is no remedy. The intravenous route is, therefore not without danger, particularly if the patient be already even partially digitalized.

To summarize the principles outlined in preceding paragraphs, it will be appreciated that having a clear indication for the use of digitalis it is the duty of the doctor to ensure that the patient receives an adequate amount in as short a time as the urgency of the symptoms demands. Its successful use involves accurate and repeated clinical observation with a close and careful study of the patient, both in regard to the drug's beneficial effects and its peculiar toxic symptoms. Its mastery ripens clinical experience and yields a satisfaction to doctor and patient with which few other drugs can compete The fall in body-weight, the diuresis, the slowing in ventricular rate, the decrease in venous pressure are all obvious effects which can readily be measured and recorded from day to day but the increased bodily comfort and the restoration of a sense of well-being are none the less real, though they defy accurate analysis.

The Use of Diuretics.—Drugs which produce a profuse flow of urine are indicated in the treatment of congestive heart failure when, after a fair trial, the response to digitalis is incomplete or unsatisfactory. From what has been said previously it can be judged that they are only required in a proportion of cases, and that this proportion decreases with the thoroughness with which digitalis is used. If after full digitalization and adequate maintenance dosage for a week or ten days œdema and venous congestion persist, or, as sometimes happens, increase despite the slowing in pulse-rate induced by the drug, then diuretics are to be considered. A large number are available, from which it is not difficult to make the appropriate selection. Clinical experience indicates that of all the diuretics available for use in the treatment of congestive heart failure, there is none to compare with the organic mercurials. In cases of advanced congestive failure it is a waste of time to temporize with the saline diuretics such as potassium citrate and acetate in gr. xv to xx by mouth though highly thought of by the clinicians of fifty years ago when little else was available to them. If diuretics are really required, then it is right and proper to use potent and reliable remedies of known efficacy. For this purpose the injection f mersalyl (B.P.) or the proprietary preparations, salyrgan r neptal, cannot be bettered. These drugs, which are lispensed in a 10 per cent. solution in 1 or 2 c.c. ampoules ontaining a 5 per cent. solution of theophylline, are adminis- ered intramuscularly or intravenously on alternate days. t is usual to commence with a small dose, perhaps 0·5 c.c. y the intramuscular route. In giving the drug, a better effect s obtained when the injection is made into an œdema-free rea, and it is important that the solution be deposited as leeply as possible, and that none escape under the skin, for n the latter situation it may give rise to intense local irritation vhich may pass on to the formation of a sterile abscess, slough- ng of the superficial tissues and local ulceration. A useful ite for the injection is the gluteal region, or if this is œdematous hen the drug may be deposited in the scapular muscles. njections in the region of the deltoid muscle or upper arm are ften painful, and this site is better avoided. When the njection is completed the site ought to be vigorously massaged vith a ball of cotton wool, as this diminishes the local irritation vhich commonly occurs about half an hour after the drug's dministration. Successive doses on alternate days may be radually increased up to a maximum of 2 c.c., and may be ontinued at weekly or bi-weekly intervals, if the occasion lemands it, for many months at a time. On the other hand, f the response to intramuscular injection is judged unsatis- actory, then recourse is made to the intravenous route. For his purpose a vein at the bend of the elbow is usually selected, nd with the customary aseptic precautions the drug is slowly njected diluted in 10 or 20 c.c. of normal saline. Novurit is mercurial compound dispensed in suppositories containing ·5 gm., and in 1-c.c. ampoules (0·1 gm.) with 0·05 gm. heophylline for intramuscular or intravenous use. The uppository is generally an effective, easy and painless method f administering the diuretic, but it may give rise to intense rritation in the presence of local rectal disease. Internal æmorrhoids or fissures may preclude this route of administra- ion on account of acute discomfort usually experienced an our or two after the suppository has been inserted.

The response to these drugs is often so dramatic that there s much justification for the claim that the modern use of ercury in the treatment of congestive heart failure represents he greatest advance since Withering's account of the use of igitalis in 1785. The diuresis induced by any of these pre- arations commences within two hours, reaches a height in ight or twelve hours and is usually completed in the course of twenty-four to thirty-six hours. The actual response depends on a number of factors. It is greater when full digitalization is maintained. and is more abrupt and complete when the

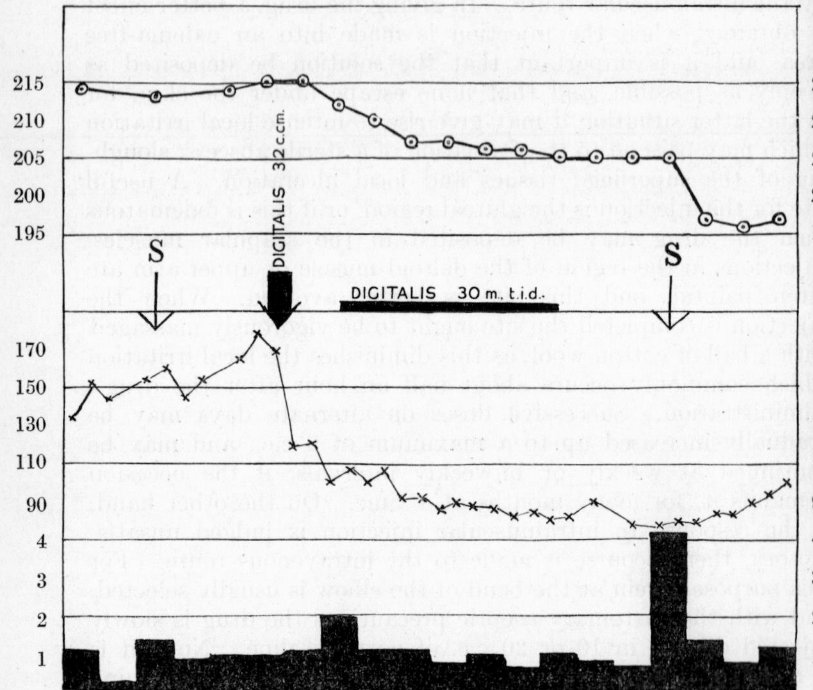

(By courtesy of the "Practitioner.")

Graph showing the effect of massive doses of digitalis tincture in a man, aged forty-six 215 lb. in weight, suffering from congestive heart failure with auricular fibrillation He received successively 15, 8, 5 and 4 c.c. at intervals of six hours on the sixth day of observation without the production of intoxication. He had a remarkabl tolerance for the drug, as two days later 30 minims was begun thrice daily and continued for six days, when nausea was first induced. A fall in body-weigh amounted to 10 lb. It is noteworthy that digitalis potentiates the effect of salyrgan (S). Compare the effect on body-weight and urine output of the dose of 2 c.c. on the third day with that on the seventeenth, when the man had been digitalized

intravenous route is used in preference to the delayed absorption which must result when the drug is deposited into an œdematous area. The volume of urine excreted must also depend on the dose employed and the degree of congestion and œdema existing at the time of its administration. In a digitalized patient in whom an advanced degree of œdema persists, a full dose of salyrgan intravenously may induce an enormous diuresis amounting to 3 to 5 litres in the twenty-four hours following its administration, and the fact that similar doses may be repeated at intervals of two or three days with safety indicates the potency and suitability of these mercurial drugs in the treatment of the more severe grades of congestive failure. They are therefore a useful adjunct to digitalis therapy, not merely in resistant cases but also in those patients who may still have a degree of occult œdema after adequate digitalis therapy. It is not uncommon to find that after all clinical evidence of pitting œdema in the subcutaneous tissues over the sacrum or thigh has disappeared, a single dose of mersalyl may still induce a minor diuresis and corresponding fall in body-weight. The drug may therefore be given to supplement digitalis therapy in any case of congestive heart failure. In the more severe grades it will rid the tissues of excess fluid when repeated at intervals of a week or two during the ambulant stages of treatment. The oral administration of salyrgan in pellets, each containing 0·08 gm., is a procedure at present under trial. Further experience may establish the usefulness of this method as a means of supplementing and maintaining the beneficial effects of intramuscular or intravenous injection.

By its action on the renal cells mersalyl is contraindicated in the presence of parenchymatous nephritis, and when renal function is greatly impaired in the chronic interstitial form of renal disease it can only be used with caution. The assessment of renal damage in the presence of congestive heart failure is always a difficult problem, as albumen and casts in the urine may equally well result from passive congestion of the kidneys as from a true nephritis, but the clinical history, the blood chemistry and particularly in practice the specific gravity of the urine usually help considerably in determining the presence or absence of actual renal disease, a high specific gravity indicating satisfactory renal function.

In virtue of their powers of inducing acidosis, ammonium citrate (gr. v to xx) or ammonium chloride (gr. v to lx) are both mild diuretics which may be used to augment the effect of the mercurial compound when the response to the latter is judged incomplete or unsatisfactory. They are usually unnecessary, but can be prescribed for a week or ten days at a time in doses of 15 to 20 gr. four times a day. Owing to their objectionable flavour these drugs are best prescribed in cachets or enteric-coated tablets, each $7\frac{1}{2}$ gr., but an attempt may be made to disguise their taste in a mixture by including liquid extract of liquorice or syrup of orange, as in the following prescription :—

℞ Ammon. Chlorid. . . . . . gr. xv
Ext. Glycyrrh. Liq. . . . . ♏xxx
Sp. Chlorof. . . . . . ♏x
Aq. . . . . . . ad ℥ss

Sig.—℥ss t.i.d.

If it is thought desirable to use these salts of ammonium they are probably best given for the three or four days preceding the dose of the mercurial. They can then be stopped for two days and repeated in short courses as necessary. Out of consideration for the patient it is always preferable to administer mercurial diuretics in the morning, as if given later in the day the massive diuresis is liable to interfere with sleep.

It is unnecessary to say much regarding the use of the xanthine diuretics, caffeine, theobromine and theophylline (theocine), as these have largely been displaced by the more powerful and efficacious mercurials. Theocine is the most powerful diuretic of the group, and owing to its insolubility is best prescribed in doses of 2½ to 5 gr. in tablets or powders. Theophylline sodium acetate (B.P.), a more soluble salt, may be prescribed in mixtures, but is liable to induce nausea and vomiting. Theobromine sodium salicylate (B.P.), better known under the trade name of diuretin, has also a certain reputation in the treatment of cardiac dropsy, and as it is freely soluble in water it may be prescribed in doses of 10 to 20 gr. in a mixture three or four times in the day. If after a trial of five to seven days these diuretics produce no appreciable benefit, they are best discontinued, but may be resumed again after an interval of a week or thereabouts. Theophylline has been combined with ethylenediamine (as in the proprietary preparation euphyllin) and when given orally in doses of 0·1 to 0·2 gm. thrice daily in tablet form it is occasionally useful on account of its diuretic properties. The natural diuretic urea, in doses of 15 to 30 gm by the mouth, has also been advocated, but is less efficacious in cardiac dropsy than the mercurials or the xanthine compounds.

Recent clinical work has conclusively demonstrated that cardiovascular disturbances are of frequent occurrence in vitamin-deficiency states. These occur commonly in alcoholic subjects, due to defective absorption, and in non-alcoholic as a result of an unbalanced diet or after acute infections when the vitamin requirements are increased by a high metaboli rate. Beriberi in the wet form is the classical example, but it must be understood that minor degrees associated with multiple deficiencies are of common enough occurrence throughout the general population of non-tropical countries. It is for this reason that vitamin concentrates, particularly vitamin B_1 and vitamin C, may be of striking value in the treatment of congestive failure with or without valvular disease. As vitamin B_1 deficiencies are frequently associated with gastro-intestinal and hepatic disorders, it is advisable to administer the synthetic substance parenterally in doses of from 5 to 20 mg. twice or thrice daily. This dose is open to modification, because as yet there is insufficient information on the daily requirement of this vitamin, its storage and its utilization. Its administration is usually associated with diuresis, slowing of the pulse and elevation in the arterial pressure. Vitamin C has diuretic properties even in health, and, administered to patients with congestive failure in tablet form as ascorbic acid (B.P.), each 50 mg., three or four times a day, is capable of inducing and maintaining a profuse diuresis even when other therapeutic measures have failed. Vitamin C deficiencies are more common than formerly supposed, and when present usually respond promptly to full doses by the mouth, or the synthetic preparation may be given parenterally in doses of 100 to 500 mg. It may actually induce a diuresis in excess of that produced by digitalis, though not with the same degree of clinical improvement nor with reduction in the ventricular rate. When the response to digitalis is incomplete the probability of the presence of a vitamin deficiency should be borne in mind, as it may be readily corrected by full doses of ascorbic acid or vitamin B_1, and the patient can be maintained in good health by adequate vitamin intake readily provided by the consumption daily of fresh food rich in vitamins.

Mechanical Procedures.—Of mechanical methods of treatment one of the most important is the old remedy of venesection, which so often produces even within a few minutes striking benefit to the cardiac patient. Its use has tended to be neglected in recent years, with the result that the precise indications for its employment are difficult to determine. It is certainly true that most benefit is likely to accrue from this method when both the arterial and venous blood pressures are raised, though there are exceptions even to this rule as striking benefit may result in the acute forms of left-sided failure with pulmonary œdema when there is little or no engorgement of the neck veins. It is contraindicated in the presence of anæmia or a low arterial blood pressure. When the liver is acutely engorged, painful or pulsating, and there is much cyanosis and pulmonary œdema, the procedure may generally be used with considerable benefit, and this increases the more rapidly the blood is withdrawn. In urgent cases it is only necessary to incise an engorged vein at the region of the elbow and allow the blood to spurt. A needle of as large a bore as can be inserted into a vein may be used as an alternative, a tourniquet being lightly applied round the upper arm. By this means 300 to 600 c.c. of blood may be rapidly withdrawn. It is a method of treatment which opens a wide field for further investigation as regards its beneficial effects, the indications for its use and the development of an improved technique such as might be accomplished by the adaptation of suction methods to increase the rate of blood loss, either by a modification of the Potain aspirator or by a foot pump. The sudden withdrawal of blood eases the burden on the right side of the heart, diminishes pulmonary and hepatic congestion and often appears to permit an improved response to digitalis therapy. The method is certainly less efficacious in long-standing cases of heart failure when, after months or years, cirrhotic changes have occurred in the liver and other organs.

Hydrothorax or ascites seldom warrant mechanical interference until a fair trial has been made with other methods of treatment. Fluid at the base of the right lung is a common occurrence in congestive failure, and may on occasions be bilateral. If it is resistant to treatment and the chest more than half full, then a two-way syringe is a convenient method of withdrawing it. At the conclusion of the paracentesis the injection into the peritoneal or pleural cavity of 1 to 2 c.c. mersalyl suitably diluted is a procedure which has been practised, but has little to recommend it, as the mercurial is probably not absorbed any more freely from either cavity than after its intramuscular injection. The mechanical removal of large quantities of fluid from either the thorax or peritoneum often appears to expedite recovery.

As a last resort it is sometimes justifiable to insert three or four Southey's tubes subcutaneously into the swollen legs usually in the neighbourhood of the ankle. If this procedure is adopted a more satisfactory drainage results if the legs are kept pendent, the excess tissue fluid being thus displaced to the periphery by the force of gravity. Large quantities of œdema fluid can be removed by this method, or through multiple incisions made in the skin, due precautions against sepsis being taken. Copious absorbent dressings are necessary. The danger of sepsis has probably been over-emphasized, but the method is one more adapted to hospital than private practice. As a general rule only temporary benefit results.

Symptomatic Treatment.—The measures already described are in themselves usually sufficient to ease the patient's discomfort, but from time to time other symptoms arise for which relief is sought. Amongst these, cough, attributable to the pulmonary congestion, is often trying to the patient, particularly when it occurs in repeated paroxysms, and tends to interfere with sleep. As congestion subsides under the influence of digitalis and diuretics, bouts of coughing as a rule become less frequent, but should they in themselves place a burden on the heart and fatigue the patient a gentle sedative cough mixture may be prescribed. For this purpose 2 to 4 drachms of the Brompton mixture,[1] repeated if necessary, is a suitable remedy. On the other hand, chronic bronchitis with an asthmatic element occasionally complicates congestive heart failure, and in these circumstances a cough mixture of a more stimulating type incorporating a small dose of ephedrine hydrochloride is often helpful. On account of its stimulating properties to the sympathetic system ephedrine, however, is best avoided until a satisfactory response has been recorded, and even then is only to be used with caution. Pulmonary embolism or thrombosis may give rise to considerable pain if there be an associated pleurisy, and the hæmoptysis which commonly accompanies the infarct may cause a good deal of mental anxiety. From both points of view, morphia is the best drug to employ in the first instance : later the pain may be soothed by hot applications in the form of fomentations or antiphlogistine poultices.

Oxygen therapy has as a rule only a limited application in the treatment of circulatory disease. It will do nothing to correct cyanosis which results from circulatory stasis in the periphery. On the other hand, pulmonary congestion and œdema of the alveolar walls may interfere with the normal oxygenation of hæmoglobin in the lung capillaries. This lends itself to treatment if it is possible to increase the partial pressure of oxygen in the lung alveoli. It can be realized that both factors, pulmonary congestion and peripheral stasis, frequently coexist. The final test of the value of oxygen is the effect of its administration to the patient. If the cyanosis promptly disappears when oxygen is inhaled in sufficient quantity, then its use should be continued, usually with benefit.

[1] Brompton mixture :—

℞	Liq. Morph. Hydrochlor.	ʒjss
	Acid Hydrocyan Dil.	ʒss
	Syr. Tolut.	ʒj
	Inf. Ros. Acid. Rec. . . . . . . ad	ʒvj

Few patients will tolerate an oxygen mask for long, and in private practice in the absence of a suitable oxygen tent a nasal catheter smeared with a little 1 per cent. cocaine ointment is probably the method of choice. The flow of oxygen should be regulated at such a rate as to control the cyanosis, or at least reduce its intensity to as great a degree as circumstances permit. This usually implies a flow of 2 to 4 litres per minute. A tube and funnel has no place in oxygen therapy, as by this means it is impossible to increase the oxygen content of the alveolar air to an extent sufficient to benefit the patient. It is only worth while persevering with oxygen therapy if the patient derives real benefit and can comfortably tolerate the method of administration. Dyspnœa is often apparently lessened by its use.

Convalescent Care.—When peripheral œdema has subsided, and it is obvious that the patient has regained strength and is sleeping comfortably at night, he may be allowed to leave his bed and sit in a chair for gradually lengthening periods. Twenty minutes or half an hour is usually sufficient in the first instance. This period may be increased by fifteen minutes daily, provided it is unaccompanied by any undue fatigue or a return of peripheral congestion. After ten days or a fortnight he may be permitted to walk short distances in his room, and later, depending on economic circumstances, a resumption of duty may be considered. It is almost invariably necessary that a patient who has suffered from congestive heart failure should have his activities greatly curtailed. For many months it is a wise rule to insist that the week-end should be spent resting, if not entirely in bed, and that at the most only half a day's work should be attempted. Those in a more secure financial position should be advised to retire from active business. The details of drug treatment depend on circumstances, and these are discussed under the heading of the Care of the Ambulant Cardiac Patient (p. 645).

A. R. Gilchrist.

ANGINAL HEART FAILURE

Treatment of an Attack of Coronary Thrombosis.—The immediate treatment of a case of coronary thrombosis consists in securing absolute rest in bed and the relief of pain by administration of morphia in full doses. Should the attack occur when the patient is at work or away from home, he should be given morphia ($\frac{1}{4}$ or $\frac{1}{3}$ gr. hypodermically) immediately on diagnosis, and should be sent home or to hospital or nursing home by car or ambulance. He must be assisted with his undressing, and should from the outset be debarred from all avoidable exertion. He must not rise to the toilet, and should not even sit up on the bed-pan. He will require to be lifted in bed for attention to bowels and for changing of linen, and even for change of position, so that the services of two strong nurses, trained or untrained, are desirable. It is unwise to allow a woman to undertake single-handed the nursing of a relative or other patient with this disorder, for the day and night nursing and the lifting involved impose too great a strain, and the temptation for the patient to ease the burden by doing things for himself is too great. It is wiser to send the patient to hospital at the outset than to move him some days later when his condition may be even more precarious.

The amount of morphia required to relieve pain is variable. The initial dose of $\frac{1}{4}$ to $\frac{1}{3}$ gr. should be repeated unhesitatingly in an hour should pain be unrelieved, and further repeated doses are likely to be required during the first twenty-four to forty-eight hours. For the later doses oral administration of the $\frac{1}{4}$-gr. tablets at the hands of the attendant, under medical direction, is satisfactory. A limit is set to dosage only by the development of general toxic symptoms, for the drug exerts no deleterious effect on the heart. The relief of pain and the rest for mind, body and heart obtained by adequate doses render the drug invaluable.

Nitrites and other vasodilators are useless in coronary thrombosis, and should not be administered, particularly as shock is usually marked and the blood pressure already greatly lowered. The administration of digitalis during the first week, and especially during the first few days, is inadvisable. The risk is due to the drug heightening the excitability of the ventricular muscle, and thereby favouring the onset of ventricular fibrillation, to which the coronary lesion predisposes. The use of digitalis in cases showing gross congestive failure is dealt with below. Quinidine sulphate, as a cardiac depressant, may lessen the risk of ventricular fibrillation, and in cases where there seems to be likelihood of this developing (cases with bursts of extrasystoles, or with ventricular paroxysmal tachycardia) it may be given in small doses (3 gr. thrice daily in cachet).

Shock should be treated on symptomatic lines by warmth, etc., but such drugs as adrenalin, ephedrine or pituitrin should not be given on account of their cardiac actions (for which see p. 730). Coramine and cardiazol may be given, but should be reserved for desperate cases who appear in imminent danger of death. They are not required or desirable in the average case.

The diet of the patient during the first few days should be one demanding the minimum of effort in ingestion, and easily assimilated. The type of diet recommended for cases of severe congestive failure (see p. 671) will prove generally suitable.

Purgation should be avoided. The instillation of a few ounces of olive oil into the rectum, followed by a saline enema in the morning, is a safe and effective method of opening the bowels.

Various complications may arise during the first few days or weeks, and may demand treatment. Of these, progressive congestive failure should be treated along the usual lines. It may be necessary to give digitalis, especially if auricular fibrillation is present, but the drug should be given during the first few days only after a consideration of the risks run by its respective administration or omission. Diuretics such as the organic mercurials (salyrgan, neptal, novurit, etc.), or the purines (theobromine sodium salicylate, theocin sodium acetate) are of value, and venesection may afford relief in cases with great venous engorgement. Troublesome dyspnœa, interfering with sleep, can be treated by administration of euphyllin (0·1 gm.) by the mouth, or as a suppository per rectum (0·36 gm.) repeated two or three times a day. Cyanosis is an indication for oxygen therapy, by tent if available, or by nasal catheter. Should the procedure cause great distress or restlessness it should be discontinued. The development of progressive congestive failure after infarction is a very unfavourable sign, and the mortality of such cases is likely to be high despite treatment.

The occurrence of embolism is an ever-present risk, and cannot be foreseen. It is favoured by exertion on the part of the patient, but the risk cannot be eliminated entirely even by most careful nursing and attention. The treatment of cases where embolism has occurred is on symptomatic lines, and absolute rest is secured by morphia. From the nature of the cases surgical intervention is not generally practicable where arterial embolism of main limb vessels has occurred.

Recurrence of pain may occur at any time, and even slight persistent pain recurring over a period of days is disquieting. The treatment of such cases is renewed administration of opiates and prolongation of the period of rest in bed.

The actual duration of confinement to bed can be taken as six weeks in an average uncomplicated case. There are definite risks to life throughout the first few weeks after a coronary accident (recurrence, embolism, rupture of the softened area of muscle, failure), and these are increased by exertion. After six weeks or so these risks are greatly reduced, and a gradual return to activity can be permitted. The patient is first allowed to wash and feed himself, to sit up in bed for meals and later to rise to the toilet. Eventually, some eight weeks after the infarct, he should be up and walking about in his room for a few hours daily. The question of his future activities must then be considered.

Difficulty will often be experienced in persuading a patient to stay in bed for the prescribed period, particularly if, as often happens, he feels perfectly well a few days after the attack. The difficulty is naturally greatest in mild cases, or in those who have had no pain. It is advisable, however, to insist on a full period of recumbency even in cases with relatively minor symptoms. Explanation that the heart has been damaged, and that it takes about six weeks to heal properly, will usually render the patient amenable to discipline. But one must be careful not to induce a state of undue apprehension of the hazards to be run, for much dispeace of mind may result, and more harm than good be done. The attitude of the doctor towards his patient is, in fact, worthy of some comment. The patient is generally aware from his own sensations of the seriousness of his condition. An attitude of unrelieved gloom on the part of the attending physician is not only inhuman but is not justifiable in view of the fact that two out of every three cases recover who survive long enough to be seen by a doctor. The risks to be run during convalescence must be kept in mind by the doctor, but must not be used as a bogey to frighten a patient into submission. And it should be realized that not the least of the patient's risks is that of developing an eventual cardiac neurosis which may be much more crippling than his true organic lesion.

Cases who have suffered an attack of coronary thrombosis, whether or not residual effort angina persists, should in their after-care be treated on the same lines as the subjects of effort angina (see p. 697).

Treatment of Attacks of Angina of Effort.—It is unusual for a patient to be seen by his doctor while actually suffering in an attack of effort angina. The attacks are of short duration and occur while the patient is about his daily business, and even if a medical man is summoned the pain is likely to have abated spontaneously before he reaches the patient. A patient whose pain has lasted without intermission for half an hour or more in spite of resting should probably be regarded as a case of coronary thrombosis and treated as such.

The patient who is habitually seized with precordial pain while walking generally realizes that continued effort aggravates his discomfort, and soon learns that he must stand still when pain comes on. In many cases this alone is sufficient to secure subsidence of the pain within a few minutes, and no medication is required. In more severe or resistant cases one or other of the quickly acting nitrites can usually be relied on to afford speedy relief, and patients, the subjects of effort angina, frequently carry such preparations in readiness for emergency use. The preparation most widely used is amyl nitrite, carried in small ampoules or "perles" containing 3 to 5 minims. These are individually encased in fabric covers, permitting them to be broken in the fingers without fear of cuts from broken glass. The broken ampoule is held to the mouth, and a few deep breaths taken with the mouth open. The action is speedy and relief from pain is frequently achieved. The vasodilator action produces flushing and often headache or giddiness, and the patient may hesitate to use the drug on that account, for such discomforts are to many harder to bear than a mild attack of pain. In severe attacks, of course, the benefits from nitrite far outweigh the unpleasant side-actions. Amyl nitrite fails to afford relief in a considerable number of cases, and the manner of its administration render the user conspicuous in public. Dosage also is difficult to gauge. For these reasons the drug has been largely replaced by another, nitroglycerin, which is more reliable and, being taken orally, is less liable to cause embarrassment. Nitroglycerin is dispensed in tablets, frequently chocolate-coated, containing the desired dose together with milk-sugar to make up a convenient weight. The dose required to abort an attack is variable in different cases, but it is convenient to prescribe the B.P. tablets of Tab. Glycerylis Trinitratis containing $\frac{1}{100}$ gr., and to adjust the number of tablets taken to secure the appropriate dose. While relief may follow the taking of as little as $\frac{1}{200}$ gr., $\frac{1}{100}$ gr. is usually required and sometimes $\frac{1}{50}$ gr. or even exceptionally $\frac{1}{25}$ gr. may be necessary. It is important to instruct the patient to chew and suck the tablets and not to swallow them, as absorption has been proved to be most rapid from the buccal mucous membrane. Another point of importance is that this substance deteriorates when kept in contact with air for long periods, and therefore only small quantities of tablets should be prescribed at a time. Tablets stored in bulk should be kept in full bottles sealed with paraffin wax.

If nitrites are not available and the attack is severe and

prolonged, alcohol, as whisky or brandy, may afford relief. But the use of alcohol even occasionally is not to be recommended, in view of the obvious danger of habit formation. Morphia likewise, which relieves the pain, is very undesirable in cases with chronic recurrent pain, from the risk of addiction.

After subsidence of the pain in an attack, many patients are able to resume walking or other activity where they left off, but should be warned that a slower pace than that which provoked the pain is to be adopted.

The Management of Cases of Angina of Effort and of Convalescent Coronary Thrombosis.—The treatment of actual attacks of pain should be looked upon as a very minor part of the treatment of a case of coronary disease. Reduction in the number of attacks is of vastly greater importance, and a great deal can be done by wise management to achieve this end. Much more will be achieved by regulation of the mode of life at work and at play, of habits regarding meals and the use of alcohol and tobacco, and by advice on other mundane matters than by the administration of drugs. It is a travesty of our therapeutic knowledge to diagnose a case as one of effort angina and to send him away merely with a box of amyl nitrite "perles" and instructions to take one when the pain is felt.

A large proportion of cases are of the overweight, thick-set type, and in these reduction in weight is probably our most potent therapeutic agent. The loss of one or two stones of superfluous weight greatly eases the burden imposed on the heart, and in our experience has repeatedly led to striking improvement in the exercise tolerance without the use of any drugs. The sufferer from angina should be encouraged to attain a weight slightly under that which is average for the height, age and sex. This can be achieved by simple dietetic restrictions, provided the co-operation of the patient is secured. Thyroid extract as a weight-reducing agent is not to be recommended in angina cases, in view of the increased cardiac load it imposes. Should its use be considered in an obstinate case the effect on the heart must be most carefully observed, and it is wiser to discard it entirely in cases of cardiac pain. A further dietetic point hinges on the well-known tendency of attacks to occur when exercise is taken soon after a meal. Heavy meals are to be avoided, and a rest or short sleep after lunch or dinner may greatly reduce the frequency of attacks in some patients.

The family physician, from his knowledge of the patient's habits and mode of life, is best qualified to instruct him as to what to do and what to avoid in his daily routine. A large proportion of cases occur in the active type of business man around fifty years of age, and in these a careful consideration of the case will reveal what steps can be taken to reduce the demands that are made on the circulation. The avoidance of business worries, relegation of as much work as feasible to juniors, the giving up of committee work involving responsibility or the strain of meetings, etc., are all points requiring consideration. Physical effort can be reduced considerably by taking a little thought—securing offices or bedroom on the ground-floor where there is no lift; going late to the office and leaving early, and thereby avoiding the bustle and rush inevitable when the usual morning and evening train or bus is taken between suburb and city; cutting down the week-end golf from two strenuous days to a pleasant easygoing round, and so on. In cases occurring in men who are employed in heavy manual labour, or in vocations demanding physical effort (postmen, rent collectors, shopkeepers, etc.), it may be difficult to reduce exertion at work without jeopardising the man's livelihood. In certain cases it may be necessary to change the occupation, where feasible, or to recommend retiral. Each case demands careful assessment, and great judgment in weighing the risk involved by continued work against the financial worry and hardship that will follow invalidism. Certain occupations should never be permitted to the subjects of severe angina, because of the risk not only to themselves but to others—*e.g.*, drivers of locomotives, buses, etc.

In any case, whatever other measures are taken to spare the heart, it is always possible to arrange that the patient can have at least eight hours' sleep each night, with the additional rest of Saturday afternoon and Sunday in bed if required. At the outset of treatment in severe cases considerable betterment is frequently to be obtained by an initial period of two to three weeks absolute rest in bed. The relief from attacks so attained may persist after return to activity, usually as an increase in the amount of work required to provoke an attack. Periodic spells of bed-rest of this type are of value in many cases who otherwise have difficulty in securing enough rest.

The use of drugs is of minor importance, but nitroglycerin has recently been proved to be valuable in preventing, as well as in cutting short, attacks of pain. A patient who habitually gets pain on doing a specific act may prevent such attacks by taking $\frac{1}{100}$ or $\frac{1}{50}$ gr. of nitroglycerin a few minutes before performing the exertion. Attacks produced regularly by climbing a flight of stairs may thus be prevented, or the strain of an important business meeting may be undertaken without liscomfort. Many tablets can be taken daily over long periods vith no apparent untoward results. For example, in cases of *ngina decubitus* who are attacked by pain on turning in bed, or sitting up for a meal, or straining at stool, anything from en to twenty tablets may be necessary to keep the patient free rom pain throughout the day. The ambulant case who is ising nitroglycerin to prevent attacks must be warned that hey are intended to allow him to pursue his essential daily ousiness at a very low level of energy expenditure, and are not o be taken with the object of allowing him to return to a more trenuous mode of life.

The widely advertised vasodilators of tissue origin (muscle ind pancreatic extracts, etc.) are of little or no value in the reatment of angina, and should be avoided. Drugs of the affeine group (theobromine and theophyllin or theocin) have ome reputation as coronary vasodilators, but their action is light. A combination of theobromine (5 gr.) and phenobarbitone ($\frac{1}{2}$ gr.) taken as a powder or tablet twice a day is ometimes useful; its action is probably mainly due to its edative barbiturate content. A combination of theophyllin ind ethylene diamine, sold as "euphyllin," is probably more efficient as a coronary vasodilator than the simple purines, hough opinions differ as to its efficacy in practice. It is worthy of trial should nitrites fail, and can be given as a tablet by nouth in doses of 0·1 gm. or as a suppository (0·36 gm.), epeated in either case twice or thrice daily.

The place of surgery in the treatment of angina is discussed on p. 713.

I. G. W. Hill.

DYSPNŒIC HEART FAILURE

Occurring in acute forms this type of failure is usually an expression of left ventricular strain. The typical breathless ttacks occur at night when the patient, about to fall off to leep, wakens in distress, acutely uncomfortable, sits up in oed, struggles for air, and literally fights for his breath and or his life. The severer attacks of so-called cardiac asthma or paroxysmal nocturnal dyspnœa tend to pass on to acute pulnonary œdema, suffocation and death. The milder forms are requently heralded by periodic breathing of the Cheyne-Stokes ype.

The minor degrees of distress are eased to some extent by he resumption of the upright position, and as much fresh air s can be obtained from the wide open window. A support o the back and shoulders, often supplied by a table across the bed on which the arms may be rested, eases the burden, bu the real relief comes from morphia, which should be given liberally as early as possible in the attack. A quarter of a grain is usually sufficient to relieve the situation appreciably, but i may be repeated if necessary. As a rule within a few minute apprehension is decreased, and the breathlessness checked in some measure. There is no completely adequate explanation for the mechanism of the onset of these attacks in which pulmonary congestion and broncho-spasm seem to play so large a part. The mode of recovery is equally mysterious. Morphia probably damps out abnormal reflexes and decreases the venous return to the heart by the mere reduction in muscular effort.

Digitalis takes second place in the treatment of the acute phases. That it is useful there is no question. To be effective it or an allied drug must be given in a large dose, preferably intravenously, but only then if the patient has not had one of the digitalis bodies in the previous ten days. For intra venous use digoxin (1 mg. or more for heavily built, plethori individuals) is exceedingly useful. Digifoline is a proprietary preparation of digitalis bodies suitable for intravenous use in a dose ranging from 2 to 6 c.c. It has a clinical reputation in the treatment of this condition, but as with all digitalis bodie required urgently in large doses particular care must be taken to ensure that it may be administered with safety.

In from ten to twenty minutes after these drugs have been administered a definite easing of the respiratory embarrassmen should be evident. The patient should not be left unattended until it is obvious that the dyspnœa is well under control that the cough has ceased and that sleep is bringing comfort Unyielding cardiac asthma tends to advance a stage furthe to acute pulmonary œdema, a treacherous condition. It onset is heralded by an irritating spasmodic cough, and late by the production of pink, frothy sputum at first scanty in amount and later becoming copious. In the earliest stage atropine, $\frac{1}{100}$ gr. hypodermically, repeated intravenously i necessary, is well worth using, but as a general rule with th appearance of the characteristic sputum a venesection will be required. This is best done by taking a scalpel and making a short longitudinal slit through the skin into an engorged vein at the bend of the elbow. The blood is allowed to spurt After 10 to 15 oz. have been withdrawn, thus unloading the right side of the heart, a simple dressing and firm bandage applied with the arm elevated will rapidly arrest the bleeding.

There is often some hesitation in deciding under condition of emergency such as these whether the use of adrenalin i varranted in the acute respiratory difficulties of left ventricular ailure. Adrenalin is a powerful myocardial stimulant, and s contraindicated in both congestive and anginal failure. It ncreases cardiac work, but in small doses the element of roncho-spasm in the production of cardiac asthma may be ased by its use, and possibly the tendency to acute pulmonary edema diminished. When it is judged that despite all his listress the patient is not passing into a state of collapse, vhen the pulse is of good volume, and particularly when the hysical examination yields evidence of broncho-spasm in the orm of sibilant rhonchi, inspiratory fixation of the chest wall nd inspiratory retraction of the interspaces, then, contrary o general custom and belief, adrenalin may be used with enefit in small doses up to a maximum of 0·25 c.c. of the in 1,000 solution. Just as adrenalin can relieve the distress f true bronchial asthma so in dyspnœic failure it may play minor but helpful part, bronchial relaxation reducing the orced muscular efforts of breathing. Adrenalin, however, is n itself unlikely to abort an attack of cardiac asthma, as there re other factors than the mere broncho-spasm, but used in he small doses recommended in association with morphia or ligitalis it does appear to be of value under certain conditions nd in certain people.

The intravenous administration of 0·24 to 0·48 gm. of uphyllin (theophyllin with ethylendiamine) has also been ecommended, but hardly seems as effective as morphia. For his purpose it is obtainable in ampoules containing 0·24 gm. lissolved in 10 c.c. of sterilized distilled water. The injection nust be made slowly at a rate not in excess of 2 c.c. per minute. t may be combined with intravenous digitalis medication. f, despite the measures already suggested, the attack continues hen the administration of oxygen should certainly be commenced by nasal catheter if a tent or oxygen chamber is not eadily available.

Such a critical state as cardiac asthma or acute pulmonary edema demands careful investigation for any exciting cause. Ioreover, the recurrence of attacks is rendered less likely if the riginal be treated by a sufficiently long period of rest in bed. t is often the case that even by the following day the patient eels, though perhaps tired, almost fully restored to health. 'his is misleading, and absolute rest in bed for at least three veeks should be insisted upon. In cases attributable to an cute coronary thrombosis a longer period of rest in bed is esirable. During the period of convalescence from the acute ttack every endeavour should be made to ensure complete relaxation and adequate sleep. Simple dietetic measures ma be commenced, particularly with a view to the reduction o excess weight, and as a rule it is worth while commencin maintenance courses of digitalis such as two $1\frac{1}{2}$-gr. pills of th powdered leaf for five or six days at a time, depending on th patient's tolerance, omitting two to three days at the conclusio of each course as necessary. Despite such measures, bout of nocturnal dyspnœa may continue, necessitating repeate emergency injections of morphia. To some extent this ca often be countered by the administration of small repeate doses of opium during the afternoon or evening. Tincture o opium may be prescribed in a mixture in a strength of 5 t 10 minims to the drachm, and of this 1 drachm taken at 2 P.M. two drachms at 4 or 6 P.M. and repeated at 8 or 10 P.M. ma succeed in preventing the more acute disturbance through th night. Euphyllin in tablets of 0·1 gm., of which one or tw may be taken three times a day, is sometimes helpful. Thi drug is capable of checking Cheyne-Stokes breathing whe given intravenously, and is always worthy of trial. A quiete life and shorter hours of work are certainly desirable for man months after the acute phase of the illness is past. Digitali usually requires to be continued indefinitely.

Pulmonary Disease in Relation to Dyspnœic Failure.—Acut dyspnœa often associated with retrosternal discomfort may b a manifestation of pulmonary embolism or extensive thrombosi in the branches of the pulmonary artery. Such a state o affairs places an enormous burden on the right side of th heart, and is usually associated with some degree of shoc which tends to advance. Morphine, oxygen and coramine ar indicated.

Chronic lung disease, particularly in the form of emphysema throws a gradually increasing load on the circulatory system chiefly on the right side of the heart. Dyspnœa, bouts o coughing and repeated infections in the form of bronchitis lea to increasing cardiac difficulties. It has been pointed out tha congestive heart failure of the right-sided type is more ofte attributable to an acute exacerbation of the bronchitis than t an actual advance in the degree of emphysema. Treatment i these cases is therefore directed towards the chronic bronchiti and the prevention of acute attacks. Emphysema is incurabl but dyspnœa may be lessened by a well-fitting abdominal be to raise the level of the diaphragm and better health promote by a change in climate and appropriate expectorant mixture (see p. 849). In the treatment of congestive failure, suitab sedative or stimulant expectorant mixtures must be continue dyspnœa and distress relieved if necessary by the steam kettle and oxygen administered from time to time to decrease the cyanosis, which in this type of failure is usually intense. Digitalis is prescribed and diuretics used as outlined in the treatment of congestive heart failure.

A. R. GILCHRIST.

DISORDERS OF RHYTHM AND INDICATIONS FOR THEIR TREATMENT

The presence of a cardiac arrhythmia is an indication for reatment only when the abnormal rhythm interferes with he efficiency of the heart's action. Sinus arrhythmia is a ıormal mechanism and requires no treatment. Occasional extrasystoles, or even short bouts of paroxysmal tachycardia, nay occur in healthy hearts with no effect on cardiac efficiency. Minor degrees of heart block and auricular fibrillation with a slow ventricular rate are indications of cardiac damage, out do not in themselves necessarily limit the capacity for effort. In treating all arrhythmias attention should be directed primarily to the maintenance of ventricular efficiency, and in some auricular disorders, *e.g.*, fibrillation, this can be done vithout fundamental change in the abnormal rhythm.

AURICULAR FIBRILLATION

Treatment has here to be considered under two heads: *a*) That of the disordered ventricular action resulting from he auricular disturbance; and (*b*) that of the disturbance of he auricular contractions, the fibrillation *per se*. Of these, the ormer is usually by far the more important, and as in most ases it alone demands attention, it will be considered first.

When auricular fibrillation supervenes in a person whose ıeart is otherwise relatively healthy (as in cases of toxic goitre, nany rheumatic cases and cases of paroxysmal fibrillation) he ventricles beat irregularly at a high rate—over 120 and ven as high as 180 per minute. The high rate, and the nefficiency conditioned by the total irregularity, usually deterıine the speedy onset of symptoms of congestive failure, and elief of those symptoms will follow reduction in the ventricular ate by suitable treatment. For this purpose bodies of the igitalis series are unrivalled.

On the other hand, patients whose heart muscle is exensively fibrosed (old arteriosclerotic and hypertensive cases) equently have slow, though irregular, ventricular rates in ıe presence of auricular fibrillation, owing to inability of a damaged *a-v* bundle to transmit as many impulses as a healthy bundle. In such cases auricular fibrillation may exist witl an apex or pulse rate of 60 or 70 per minute ; symptoms o failure due to high rate alone are absent, and digitalis lose its dramatic effect.

In a case of auricular fibrillation accompanied by tachy cardia and congestive failure, the patient should be at rest ir bed and nursed as a case of failure, with the customary restriction of diet and fluids, etc. Sleep is secured in many cases by simple measures, such as the barbiturates, but there need be no hesitation in giving morphia ($\frac{1}{6}$ or $\frac{1}{4}$ gr.). Thi drug is relatively safe even in desperately ill patients, anc often affords striking relief from sleeplessness due to dyspnœa It is worthy of emphasis that the widespread mistrust o morphia in cardiac patients is baseless, and that the drug is o great value.

The patient should be fully digitalized without delay. Th administration of digitalis is along the lines laid down on pp 673-684. The choice of preparation and mode of administratio will depend on the urgency of symptoms and the need for speedy action. Whatever method of administration is employed an whatever preparation is used the patient should be kept unde observation during the period of digitalization. Palpation o the pulse is no real guide to the heart-rate, in view of the puls deficit in such cases, and the apex-beat should be auscultate daily during this period. In hospitals the senior nurses shoul chart the apex-rate as ascertained by auscultation, as well a the pulse-rate. The reduction of the apex-rate to 80 pe minute is desirable ; reduction to 70 or even 60 per minute i of itself harmless, but gives an indication that dosage must b reduced. The development of pronounced bradycardia (unde 60), of coupled rhythm, due to ventricular extrasystole following each normal beat, or of any of the other clinica manifestations of digitalis intoxication, are all urgent indica tions for temporary cessation of administration. It is usuall safe to start again after twenty-four hours remission, givin smaller (maintenance) doses of about 15 to 20 minims o tincture per day, or its equivalent. In cases of gross over dosage, forty-eight hours or even longer may have to elaps before the drug is restarted. It is important to realize tha individual variation in susceptibility to digitalis is considerabl and no fixed amount can be stated as that required fo digitalization. In general a total of 300 minims is enough, bu a few patients require much less and some, notably hyper thyroids and febrile cases, much more.

Once the apex-rate has been reduced to the chosen level (70 to 80) an endeavour is made to hold it there by small maintenance doses of digitalis. For this purpose a daily dose of 15 to 20 minims usually suffices, but the exact dosage has to be worked out for each individual patient. In the writer's opinion it is more convenient to use a pill of the powdered leaf than the tincture for maintenance dosage—the risks of error in dosage are reduced, the stability of the drug is certain, and the solid form is more convenient, especially for patients who are travelling. Any dose of tincture can be calculated as powdered leaf very simply, 1 gr. of the solid form being equivalent to 10 minims of the tincture. The pellets of digitaline marketed by Nativelle are also very potent and reliable, and equally convenient. The equivalents in tincture are roughly 15 to 20 minims for the $\frac{1}{240}$-gr. pill, and 7 minims for the $\frac{1}{600}$-gr. pill.

The duration of digitalis treatment is generally for life. All cases on digitalis should be seen every few days after initial digitalization till the apex rate has been stabilized, and thereafter should be examined at least once weekly for some time. Patients who have been taking digitalis for months or years should occasionally be examined : instances are frequent in our experience where a patient has taken digitalis for long periods without adequate supervision, and where clinical examination reveals quite inadequate control of the heart-rate, with consequent limitation of the exercise tolerance or even congestive failure. Underdosage rather than overdosage is the rule in these neglected cases, and in general one may say that failures of digitalis in practice are frequent, and are almost always due to inadequate dosage. The only method of assessing dosage correctly is by frequent examination of the patient.

One point deserves to be mentioned with regard to digitalis in cases of paroxysmal fibrillation. From animal research it is known that vagal stimulation increases the ease with which auricular fibrillation can be evoked, and prolongs the duration of induced paroxysms. Digitalis, by its action as a vagal stimulant, has a similar action, and the drug is therefore contraindicated in the treatment of short recurring paroxysms in man. It has to be given should failure develop in such an attack, but the possibility of converting paroxysmal attacks to established fibrillation should be kept in mind.

In cases with a low ventricular rate in the untreated state, digitalis is not indicated in the absence of congestive failure. Should failure be present, the drug may be given with due caution lest untoward bradycardia result. Some benefit results in many cases, but the results are less likely to be dramatic than in the usual cases with high ventricular rate.

Treatment of the auricular disorder may be considered once the apex-rate is suitably controlled. It is well recognized that a proportion of cases of auricular fibrillation can be restored to normal rhythm by quinine derivatives, particularly quinidine sulphate. The prospect of success and the duration of the restored normal rhythm in any given case vary with a number of factors, and the use of the drug is not without risk ; a full understanding of these points is essential before the treatment be embarked upon.

The drug is of most value in cases of auricular fibrillation of comparatively recent onset, without grave signs of muscle damage (enlargement, etc.) and particularly when the exciting cause of the arrhythmia has been traced and removed—for example, in cases of auricular fibrillation in hyperthyroid cases after operation. It is of some value, too, in cases of rheumatic origin of fairly recent onset, though here the prospects of lasting restoration of normal rhythm are less. It is of little value in cases of fibrillation of several or many years' duration, or in patients with grossly enlarged hearts and congestive failure. Should normal rhythm be restored in such cases, it is likely to be of short duration, and the benefits obtained are not commensurate with the definite risk involved in the treatment. Cases, too, with a previous history of embolism are unsuitable for quinidine, embolism from an auricular clot being a known risk of quinidine therapy, and the risk being increased by similar embolic accidents in the past.

In justice it must be admitted that, while from the foregoing it is evident that in our opinion quinidine is greatly limited in its value, in other centres the drug is much more freely used. It is argued that even a few additional weeks or months of normal rhythm is a considerable gain for a patient who is progressing toward the usual terminal phase of, say mitral disease. Against this, one could quote cases of mitral disease who, when fibrillating with a well-controlled ventricular rate, were less dyspnœic and able for more effort than when normal rhythm was present.

Should quinidine therapy be decided upon after due consideration, the drug should only be given after careful preliminary digitalis treatment. The ventricular rate should be well controlled, and congestive failure should have been abolished. The use of quinidine without these precautions is dangerous. A test dose of 0·2 gm. (3 gr.) quinidine sulphate in cachet is first given: some—a very few—patients show idiosyncrasy in the form of nausea, vomiting, tinnitus, or even collapse. Should no toxic symptoms develop, the drug is given in doses of 0·3 gm. (5 gr.) four-hourly throughout the twenty-four hours, with one dose omitted during the night to allow of eight hours' sleep; this dosage is kept up for several days or even a week. Electrocardiographic control is desirable, and careful clinical observation, preferably in hospital, essential. Should the fibrillation persist after this course it is repeated after an interval of a week, during which digitalization is maintained. The proportion of cases that returns to normal rhythm varies with the type of case selected for treatment, but averages about one-third. In post-operative cases of thyrotoxicosis, practically all cases can be restored to normal rhythm—in fact, spontaneous reversion is common and may occur up to three weeks after thyroidectomy. The actual risk to life (from embolism, etc.) in well selected cases though real, is low, and has probably been exaggerated.

In our opinion quinidine is a drug requiring considerable judgment in selection of cases, and skilled observation and care during its administration. It is a drug that for the treatment of auricular fibrillation has little place in general practice.

AURICULAR FLUTTER

Unlike auricular fibrillation, the disordered auricular mechanism in this condition is influenced considerably by digitalis. In doses sufficient to produce ventricular slowing as in auricular fibrillation, this drug also causes conversion of auricular flutter to fibrillation in a considerable proportion of cases. The cessation of all digitalis medication in such a case, once fibrillation has developed, is followed in about one-third of the cases by return to normal rhythm; in another one-third of the cases the rhythm reverts to flutter, in the remaining one-third fibrillation persists as an established condition. In the former case, a second attempt with digitalis may succeed in establishing normal rhythm, or quinidine may be tried. In the latter case, the fibrillation is treated in the usual way, and again quinidine may be tried. In any case, the restoration of normal rhythm has the same prospects of duration as it has in cases of auricular fibrillation, and there is a similar risk of embolism.

In the treatment of a case with digitalis, the drug is given as in comparable cases of auricular fibrillation, and careful observation of the patient (especially his apex rate) is essential. Whenever marked slowing occurs together with total irregularity at the apex, fibrillation may be assumed to have developed. This has occurred in our experience after a single intravenous dose of strophanthin, but it is more usual to induce it by oral administration of the tincture of digitalis over a period of some days. Electrocardiographic control is useful, but hardly essential. When fibrillation supervenes, all digitalis is stopped for a few days, and a return to normal rhythm awaited.

An alternative method is to use quinidine. After preliminary digitalisation, to secure a slow ventricular rate and abolition of congestive failure, quinidine is given in similar dosage and method as for auricular fibrillation. Quinidine slows the rate of the auricular contractions, so that an auricular rate originally between 250 and 300 per minute falls gradually—it may be below 200 per minute. At this stage there is a danger that the ventricles may follow the full auricular rhythm (1 : 1 flutter) instead of responding to every second, third or fourth auricular cycle as at the beginning of treatment. Should this occur a dangerous ventricular tachycardia at 180 to 200 per minute may arise. This accident, however, is very rare. The slowing of the auricular rhythm to 200 or thereabouts is frequently followed by abrupt resumption of normal rhythm. Large doses of the drug are then stopped, and after twenty-four hours small doses (3 gr. once or twice a day) are restarted and maintained for a few weeks.

It is our practice to use digitalis for flutter cases in the first instance. Quinidine is reserved for those which fail to respond to digitalis. In either case should normal rhythm be restored, its duration depends on the same factors as in case of fibrillation treated with quinidine. Recurrence of flutter or fibrillation at an early date is likely in cases with grossly enlarged hearts or old-standing disorders of rhythm, and in those where a toxic factor (hyperthyroidism), is still operative.

PAROXYSMAL TACHYCARDIA

Supraventricular Paroxysmal Tachycardia occurs frequently in people with no other discoverable abnormality in their cardiovascular systems, but also in various pathological conditions—rheumatic heart disease, toxic goitre, etc. In cases with an exciting cause, such as the last named, efforts should be made to remove it.

During attacks various measures may be employed to cut short a paroxysm. Any one of a number of procedures may result in the abrupt cessation of the attack, and many patients soon learn how to treat their own symptoms. The particula method which meets with success varies in individual cases, but frequently remains fairly constant for any particular individual. Bending the head low between the knees when seated on a chair, holding the breath, attempting forced inspiration or expiration with nose held and mouth closed, pressure over the abdomen, and vomiting, are all examples of procedures that patients may find useful in cutting short the attacks. The physician may stimulate the vagus reflexly and strongly by pressure over the carotid sinus on one or other side, and this frequently arrests the paroxysm. If this is attempted the patient should lie on a couch, and pressure with the finger tips of one hand should be gently exercised over a point level with the lower border of the thyroid cartilage at the anterior border of the sterno-mastoid. The heart should be auscultated the while, and abrupt slowing or cessation of the sounds is the signal for immediate release of pressure. In some instances a first attempt is ineffective, but success may follow repeated attempts or stimulation of the sinus on the other side. Cases resistant to such sinus stimulation may yield to reflex vagal stimulation through the fifth nerve, from pressure on the eyeballs. Again recumbent, the patient is told to close his eyes firmly. Pressure with the finger-tips on both eyeballs sufficient in degree to cause slight pain may produce cessation of the paroxysm. Ocular pressure, however, is unpleasant and painful, and is now seldom employed.

If all such attempts prove ineffectual, the induction of vomiting by emetics, or the production of nausea by subemetic doses of tinct. ipecac., may cut short the attack. A tight abdominal binder is often effective, especially in children.

In cases where these simple measures are ineffectual, attacks may sometimes be brought to an end by full digitalization. Quinidine sulphate is, however, more generally useful, and in doses of 0·3 gm. (5 gr.) three or four times a day by mouth, will usually bring the attack to an end. Hypodermic administration of $\frac{1}{4}$ to $\frac{1}{3}$ gr. morphia may secure needed rest for an anxious and exhausted patient.

With the development of symptoms and signs of congestive failure or of pain, indicating exhaustion of the heart muscle, the arrest of the paroxysm becomes more urgent. Prompt arrest may be brought about by intravenous administration of quinine preparations, either quinine hydrochloride, or quinidine sulphate, 0·3 gm. (5 gr.) in 10 c.c. saline. Dramatic arrest may likewise be achieved by the intravenous injection of a drug of the parasympatho-mimetic group, *e.g.*, Mecholin or Doryl. These are allies of acetylcholine, a substance which recent physiological research has shown to be released at their terminations when parasympathetic nerves are stimulated, and which produces the characteristic parasympathetic effects on various organs. Acetylcholine is broken down too readily in the body to be of value in therapeutics, but other more stable esters of choline share some of its properties. Of these, acetyl-β-methyl-choline (the chloride of which is marketed as Mecholin) and carbaminoyl-choline (which is marketed also as a chloride as Doryl) may be given intravenously to refractory cases of paroxysmal tachycardia. Fraser ("Croonian Lectures," 1938) advocated Mecholin as preferable for this purpose. A usual dose is 25 mg. intravenously, though from 10 to 60 mg. may be required. The effect is produced within a few minutes, and abrupt return to normal rhythm occurs in a high percentage of cases. Doryl is given in smaller doses (0·05 to 0·12 mg.), and is also effective. It has been noted, however, to produce auricular fibrillation in some cases. With either of these drugs other symptoms of excessive vagal stimulation may occur—nausea, vomiting or diarrhœa.

It should be remembered that the attacks tend to cease spontaneously and are generally of short duration—minutes or hours. Every day that passes in a resistant case renders the spontaneous arrest more likely to occur within a short time and whatever medicament is being used will probably be given the credit of the cure.

Ventricular Paroxysmal Tachycardia is less common than the other form, and generally occurs in patients with grave myocardial disease, *e.g.*, after recent coronary infarction, etc. It may also occur from gross overdosage with digitalis. One form, however, is innocent and occurs in relation to exercise in apparently healthy people. In general, vagal stimulation is useless in treating these cases. Mecholin, doryl and allied drugs are of no value in this form of tachycardia and treatment by quinidine or digitalis is usually required. Quinidine is given as for supraventricular cases, and is very effective: the rate during the paroxysm may fall gradually under quinidine before normal rhythm is abruptly restored. Digitalis, though it can produce paroxysms of ventricular origin as a toxic effect, is paradoxically of value in arresting those of other origin. It is risky, however, in cases of recent coronary infarction, and in our experience inferior to quinidine. Treatment in cases of ventricular tachycardia with grave cardiac disease and gross failure is a more urgent matter than in the average case of supraventricular origin, and intravenous quinine hydrochloride (5 gr. in 10 c.c. saline, given slowly) may be calle for. Such drastic methods are, however, generally unsuitable for use in general practice, and are best reserved for hospital use with electrocardiographic control where practicable.

Patients who have recently had an attack of paroxysmal tachycardia or who are liable to repeated attacks, are generally benefited by a maintenance dose of quinidine sulphate (3 to 5 gr. per day) over a period of weeks. Any obvious exciting factor (excess of tobacco or alcohol; thyrotoxicosis; septic foci in teeth or tonsils, etc.) should be attended to. Many cases are resistant and attacks recur at intervals over long periods of years without serious effects on the general health.

HEART-BLOCK

The treatment of minor grades of heart-block is directed towards elimination of the cause. Little can be done by drugs to improve the conductivity of a damaged *a-v* bundle. Many cases are due to excessive dosage of digitalis, and clear up when the drug is withheld. Others are due to an intercurrent streptococcal throat infection, and subside as this clears up. Many occur in cases of active rheumatic carditis, and for these there is no specific treatment beyond the usual régime of rest and salicylate. A few cases are due to reflex inhibition of the bundle through vagal stimulation, and in these atropine in full doses ($\frac{1}{50}$ to $\frac{1}{30}$ gr. intravenously, or full doses of tincture by mouth) may prove useful. In the minority of cases which are of syphilitic origin, potassium iodide may be of benefit, but it should be realized that actual gummata of the bundle are very rare. In that very large group of cases which occur as part of an ischæmia of heart muscle brought about through arterial degeneration, we have no specific drug of any proved value, and iodide has not in our hands deserved its time-honoured reputation. It is to be realized that simple prolongation of the *a-v* conduction time, or the occurrence of "dropped beats" is of no moment as regards the mechanical efficiency of the heart. Longstanding cases of 2 : 1 heart-block may have little or no limitation of effort, and demand no special treatment. It is to be emphasized, too, that digitalis is not advisable in cases of partial heart-block as the drug may depress the bundle further and aggravate the condition.

Established complete heart-block is likewise not amenable to therapy. Such cases are usually due to scarring in the bundle region, and from the nature of things are irreparable. The management of such a case, however, is important: the patient should be warned to live within his reserve, and cautioned as to the risks involved by strenuous exertion, such as running upstairs, lifting heavy articles, etc. Unduly strenuous acts produce in such cases sudden syncopal attacks, since the heart is unable to accelerate to meet the demands for increase blood-flow to the tissues, and the cerebral circulation suffers accordingly.

High-grade heart-block in an unstable state is manifested clinically in many cases by recurrent classical Stokes-Adams attacks, to relieve which therapy may be of some value. The treatment of such cases is dealt with under Cardiac Syncope on p. 725.

EXTRA-SYSTOLES

Extra-systoles occurring in young people with no other cardiovascular abnormality do not require treatment, and as a rule are very resistant to any medication. The patient should be reassured as to the innocent nature of his abnormality, should he be aware of it, and should not be allowed to permit the arrhythmia to interfere in any way with his normal activities. We are familiar with cases of persistent extra-systolic irregularity in healthy young athletes, and in men who, having had the disorder for many years, have reached the allotted span without mishap.

Patients who are greatly troubled by abnormal sensations due to extra-systoles may require a sedative, such as bromide (10 gr.) or phenobarbitone (½ to 1 gr.). There is some evidence that the barbiturates may also diminish the frequency of extra-systoles in some cases (Brow, Long and Beattie).

Extra-systoles developing *de novo* in a patient demand careful overhaul to exclude organic cardiac disease, and also a search for possible exciting factors, of which examples are: heavy meals before retiring to bed; flatulence; tobacco in excess; septic foci in teeth or elsewhere; and digitalis overdosage.

Multiple extra-systoles may cause a pulse irregularity so great as to simulate auricular fibrillation. If one is certain that digitalis has not played a part in their genesis this drug in full doses is most useful in treating the condition. To be effective, digitalization must be thorough, and its administration does not differ from that in cases of auricular fibrillation. The continued administration of digitalis to a patient already intoxicated by it, is, of course, highly dangerous, and may lead to ventricular tachycardia and sudden death. Hence the necessity of making certain that digitalis is not responsible for the condition before starting treatment. Extra-systoles appearing in a patient receiving digitalis in any but the smallest doses should be assumed to be due to the drug till proved of other origin by their persistence for several days after cessation of digitalis therapy. Quinidine sulphate (3 to 5 gr. twice or thrice daily) is useful in some cases, and is relatively safer than digitalis in the first week after a coronary thrombosis.

Coupled rhythm, or *pulsus bigeminus*, though not always due to digitalis, very frequently is and should always be regarded as such in a new patient till proof is available that the drug has not been exhibited. Keeping this rule will avoid accidents from digitalis overdosage.

SINO-AURICULAR BLOCK, NODAL RHYTHM, ETC.

There is no indication for medication in cases of sino-auricular block, or in the other rare disorders such as interference-dissociation. Some of these are prone to occur under digitalis therapy, and should such a cause be suspected the drug should be temporarily withheld.

SURGERY IN THE TREATMENT OF CARDIAC DISEASE

For certain cardiac conditions relief may be obtained by surgical intervention on structures not anatomically connected with the heart itself, as, for instance, by sympathetic nerve section in cases of angina pectoris, or by thyroidectomy in cases of heart disease caused by thyrotoxicosis. The perfection of technique in surgery and in anæsthesia, particularly in respect of intra-thoracic operations, have, however, brought operations on the heart itself within the range of the possible. Direct attacks have been made on the stenosed orifice in cases of mitral stenosis, and the constricting bands have been removed in some cases of chronic adhesive pericarditis. Such operations, however, are emphatically outwith the scope of the average general surgeon, competent though he may be to deal in an emergency with such conditions as wounds of the muscle or hæmorrhage into the pericardium. Deliberate operations on the heart should be left for those who are specially interested in this field of surgery, in whose hands alone can such operations be undertaken with reasonable safety. No attempt will be made here to enter into details of technique. It is enough to indicate which types of case may be submitted to operation, with the prospects of relief which may be attained.

Mitral Stenosis.—Operations for the relief of this valvular lesion have been performed sporadically for a number of years. In the early attempts the constricted orifice was stretched by the fingers of the operator : later, an instrument (valvulotome) was designed to punch out a portion of the thickened cusps, converting the stenosed valve into an incompetent one. The mortality of such operations is extremely high, even in the hands of the few specialist surgeons who undertake them. The after-results are by general consent unsatisfactory. In our opinion the operation as at present performed is not one to which we should advise any patient to submit.

Pericardial Disease.—Surgical operation is imperative in cases of purulent pericarditis, the establishment of free drainage by open or closed methods being as essential as in cases of pleural empyæma (see under Pericarditis).

In cases of chronic adhesive pericarditis operation may sometimes be usefully undertaken. In the type of case where the thickened pericardium is bound firmly to adjacent structures (ribs, sternum) a great deal of useless work is done by the heart muscle at each systole. In such cases it suffices after reflection of the pectoral muscle and soft tissues to resect the ribs and divide adhesions to sternum, etc. Very striking improvement in the cardiac condition may result, and there are many records of patients with severe congestive failure who, after such operations, have returned to practically normal life. The operation on this type of case appears to be relatively simple and to carry a low mortality. In the other type of case, where adhesions to outside structures are absent, but the two layers of pericardium are matted together, possibly extensively calcified and where constricting bands around the orifices of the venæ cavæ are common, the operation is considerably more difficult and dangerous. The amount of interference required will vary from case to case, but a very extensive "decortication" of the heart may be necessary, stripping from the surface of the muscle the mass of scar tissue and calcium salts which impedes its movements. In many cases bands of scar tissue constrict the openings of the great veins, and these have to be divided. It is readily realized how great the technical difficulties may be, and in practice the surgeon must often rest content with partial operations. The results of such operations though the initial mortality is rather high, are very satisfactory.

In contradistinction to operations for the relief of mitral stenosis, these operations on the pericardium offer such good prospects of relief with such a moderate mortality that all cases where adhesive constrictive pericardial disease has been diagnosed should be referred to a competent surgeon for advice. This is especially desirable in cases with congestive failure which fail to respond to medical treatment.

Operations for the Relief of Cardiac Pain.—A great variety of operative procedures for the relief of pain in angina pectoris have been tried at one time or another, but those at present in use may be divided into the following groups: Operations on the sympathetic ganglia (resection or injection with alcohol); thyroidectomy; and operations for establishment of a collateral circulation. The last group, which is still in the experimental stage, may be dismissed briefly. While other methods aim at merely symptomatic relief, operations of this group aim at revascularization of the ischæmic area of muscle. Various methods have been employed, such as the use of grafts from the adjacent pectoral muscle or from the omentum. In each case the surface of the epicardium is stripped, and the graft (pectoral muscle or omentum) with its blood supply intact is stitched to the raw surface. The mortality appears to be surprisingly low, and good results are claimed. The operations are, however, at the moment carried out by only a very few surgeons, and the method has still to win general acceptance. On *a priori* grounds operations of this type would seem most likely to yield lasting results in cases where progressive disease of the natural nutrient vessels has rendered the myocardium ischæmic.

Thyroidectomy in cases of angina pectoris has been widely employed, with at least initial success. The original operation was a complete excision of the gland, designed to produce myxœdema, similar to that performed for the relief of congestive failure. Investigation has shown, however, that relief from pain is immediate, and is not dependent on the fall in basal metabolic rate which takes place in the weeks following operation. Some cases after operation have had their basal metabolic rate raised to normal by administration of thyroid extract, without return of pain. This paradox has led some authorities to suggest that the operation is effective because it involves the section of some nervous pain-pathway running over the anterior surface of the thyroid gland, and for which no other anatomical or clinical evidence exists. Those who believe this to be the case have modified the original operation to a seven-eighths partial thyroidectomy such as is performed in cases of thyrotoxicosis. The exact mode of action of the operation is therefore by no means clear, but there is no question that a considerable percentage of patients are very markedly improved after operation. The operative mortality appears to be low (3 per cent. in a series of sixty-seven cases in Boston hospitals, quoted by Means). The indications for operation will be discussed, together with those for sympathectomy, below.

It is well established that the sensory pain paths from the heart run in the sympathetic fibres and ganglia of the cervical and upper dorsal chain, principally on the left side, though occasionally in cases with right-sided pain the right chain appears to carry the sensation. These nervous paths may be interrupted by resection of the stellate and upper dorsal ganglia, or by injection of the ganglia with a sclerosing fluid (alcohol). Preference for one or other of these methods varies with individual surgeons; in skilled hands either method yields good results. The injection is relatively a minor procedure, performed under local anæsthesia, and very effective when skilfully performed. In some cases an obstinate intercostal neuritis results from implication of posterior roots in the resulting scars. Sympathectomy demands open operation, and, as a rule, general anæsthesia. The operative mortality, however, is surprisingly low, and many of the possible pitfalls of the blind injection operation are avoided. In our experience a mild neuritis may follow the operation, but this has rarely been persistent or severe.

Cases of *angina decubitus* of extreme severity have been restored to a fair degree of activity and have been able to take up such duties as those of caretakers, etc. One case of angina of such severity that pain was induced by any exertion, however slight, is now so far improved as to return (without medical sanction !) to work underground in a coal-mine. Absolute relief from pain cannot be promised in any individual case, but is usually achieved. The objection raised by Mackenzie, that operation by relieving pain abolished the "red light" that signalled danger in over-exertion, appears to have been exaggerated. We have not met any instance where the abolition of pain has led to unfortunate results. The tenure of life in cases of coronary disease is notoriously uncertain, and an occasional unforeseen death in a case which has been operated upon should not rashly be attributed to the operation. We have noted further that many of the patients, though free from actual pain after operation, are still conscious of a vague sense of oppression on exertion, which indicates to them that the limit has been reached and acts as the warning against strenuous activity.

The question when to advise operation (thyroidectomy or sympathectomy) in a case of angina pectoris is one of considerable difficulty. The general attitude in this country is conservative, and in common with others we comparatively rarely send cases for surgical treatment. Probably only 4 or 5 per cent. of cases are suitable for operation by present-day standards. We advise it where pain is very severe and frequent, particularly in the type of case where, despite the maintenance of complete rest in bed, pain is relieved only by repeated administration of nitroglycerine. In such cases the relief obtained is generally so striking and untoward effects are so rare that operation will probably be resorted to more frequently in the future. Operation is also worthy of consideration in cases where pain severely limits exertion and where the heart, as judged by clinical, radiological and electro-cardiographic examination, is relatively little damaged. Operation on this type of case is by comparison rare, and its advisability is a matter of debate.

Thyroidectomy for Congestive Heart Failure.—Complete extirpation of the thyroid gland has been advocated as a measure in treatment of severe congestive failure, the rationale being that with a lowered basal metabolic rate the demands made on the heart to sustain a circulation adequate for the body at rest will be diminished. While some encouraging results were obtained, the general concensus of opinion now is that the operation has little place in the therapeutics of cardiac failure. The proportion of cases showing improvement, and the degree of betterment secured, seem inadequate to justify this major operation on critically ill patients.

Subtotal Thyroidectomy in Cases of Thyrotoxicosis.—This subject is discussed fully in the section on Diseases of the Thyroid Gland. It is sufficient here to emphasize two points. First, that serious cardiac decompensation with auricular fibrillation is of itself no contraindication to operation in cases of thyrotoxicosis. Naturally, the cardiac failure should first be treated as a pre-operative measure, but the presence of severe cardiac decompensation, far from militating against operation, is an absolute indication that operation should be undertaken. No matter how late the case, how advanced the cardiac damage, there is no doubt that only harm can result from continued thyroid toxæmia. If the patient can be brought into a reasonable state, and the extreme congestion reduced, then operative removal of seven-eighths of the gland holds out a prospect of considerable amelioration, if not of cure, of the cardiac condition. Secondly, there is little doubt that many cases of thyrotoxic heart disease escape recognition. In cases of unexplained congestive failure in the middle-aged, especially with auricular fibrillation, and even in the absence of overt ocular or nervous signs of thyroid disease, the possibility of thyrotoxicosis as the cause of the myocardial failure should be kept in mind. Careful search for signs of hyperthyroidism such as loss of weight, sweating, glycosuria, etc., and a full examination of the thyroid gland may reveal the true cause of the heart symptoms. Paroxysmal auricular fibrillation in apparently healthy people should likewise suggest careful examination to rule out hyperthyroidism.

I. G. W. Hill.

THE CARDIAC NEUROSES

The conception of the heart as the organ of emotion dates from the earliest times. Avicenna, the ancient Arabian physician, who classified falling in love amongst the mental diseases, claimed that by a study of the pulse—its rate and rhythm—it was possible under particular circumstances to identify the person loved and to base on this knowledge an appropriate treatment. Such phrases as "broken-hearted" and "half-hearted" are remnants of the pre-Harveian notions of the circulation, notions which contain more than a nucleus of truth. There is every justification for the view that the circulatory system is a sensitive index of the individual's emotional state existing at the moment. In health, blood flow, both local and general, heart-rate and rhythm, blood pressure and vasomotor tone are all attuned by passing thoughts and ideas, even, it may be, of a most trifling nature. These reactions may well be intensified a hundredfold in the face of major emotional experiences. Sudden grief, joy, anger, shame. fear and such-like may each impose a burden on the circulatory system, with the production of acute symptoms ranging from perhaps no more than blushing or palpitation to giddiness, syncope, precordial discomfort, profound collapse or even sudden death. As a general rule the physiological reaction of the circulatory system to emotion is as short-lived as that experienced after physical exertion, but individuals vary as much in their mental balance, sensitivity to pain, whether it be bodily or mental anguish, and in their emotional make-up as in their general physique.

In this normal reaction of the heart to emotional stimuli we have the basis of an understanding of the altered mechanism of the cardiovascular system in those varied conditions which are roughly classified for descriptive purposes as functional circulatory states. Imaginary heart disease, neurocirculatory asthenia (the effort syndrome), "angina innocens," and the cardiac neuroses form a group of different but related conditions associated with much distress, disability and economic incapacity. Often they are entities in themselves unrelated to any structural defect in the heart or circulation. This is not the place to review in detail the symptomatology of these various functional states, but as a general rule they are the products of conscious or unconscious emotional trends, anxiety for the future and lack of confidence in the present being firmly rooted ideas. It is equally true that an individual may constantly complain of disagreeable sensations identical with those produced by a passing emotion in a healthy individual without being aware at the moment of any exciting cause. In other words an emotion can act without awareness in consciousness and from the point of view of treatment be less easy to detect and eradicate. The psychiatrist may divide such individuals into groups composed of anxiety states, obsessional neuroses and conversion hysterias. Quite commonly there may be a true psychosis, sometimes associated with an anatomical basis as in cerebral arteriosclerosis or in hypertension.

It is important to realize that not infrequently a functional nervous state consorts with an organic lesion, and treatment is therefore all the more complex. True angina pectoris is an outstanding example of an organic disease in which violent attacks may be induced by transient emotional disturbances recognized by the patient as anger, fear or worry. Similarly in rheumatic heart disease, long-continued anxiety, doubts and fears for the future may be the means of inducing a succession of symptoms mimicking serious disease. This is not uncommon in mitral stenosis—symptoms being partly organic, such as dyspnœa and fatigue, and partly functional as submammary pain and giddiness. The knowledge, or even the suspicion, that the heart is the site of a morbid process is sufficient in the mind of most people to induce a train of symptoms based on fear, and culminating ultimately in an anxiety neurosis if unchecked at their beginnings. It is true that the mental reaction to doubt is apparently more intense in the case of the heart than in any other organ of the body. In the mind of the layman heart disease spells, if not sudden death, something incurable and irremediable. Only in the last stages of heart disease can it be said that there is a decreased response to emotion. It is remarkable that so often individuals in the final stages of congestive heart failure are naturally sanguine and retain, despite all their discomforts, an optimistic outlook. They are brave patients.

The term "imaginary heart disease" is best applied to those conditions which give rise to signs or symptoms simulating those of true organic disease, but in which the heart is not the seat of any structural defect. Innocent murmurs, precordial aches and simple syncopal attacks often suggest organic disease to the mind of the individual, a doubt which is intensified by an inadequate diagnosis and a faulty explanation of the mechanism of the production of the symptoms. It has been well said that the diagnosis of a " weak heart " or a " strained heart " under such circumstances reflects more on the doctor, who is weak and whose diagnosis is strained, rather than on the patient's heart. These are terms to avoid. It is always a mistake to offer a half-hearted diagnosis, particularly when the integrity of the heart is in doubt, without a thorough and complete examination. Only then is it possible to assess the relevant facts. Such a diagnosis as a " weak " or " tired " heart may sow the seed of a protracted cardiac neurosis on very fertile ground. A hasty remark, a look or a nod, even an expression of doubt on the face of the examiner, may bring in its trail fears of crippling disability. With the universal knowledge regarding the vital function of the heart, symptoms are easily magnified, and unless checked in the most thorough way possible at the earliest opportunity, doubts accumulate and become more and more difficult to dispel.

Faced with such an individual the first step in treatment is the most thorough and careful examination possible, having first of all gained his confidence by encouraging the patient to give as full and as detailed an account of his symptoms as he may. The electrocardiograph and the X-ray have their therapeutic as well as their diagnostic uses. The examiner being satisfied in his own mind as to the nature of the disturbance, further treatment depends on winning the patient's co-operation by an intelligent discussion of the means whereby symptoms of a cardiac nature are produced. This is not always easy, nor is it always immediately fruitful in its results, as much must depend on the intelligence, education and co-operation of the patient. The physician must be prepared to justify his diagnosis and take as firm a stand as all the circumstances will permit. If the heart is judged sound then it is a contradiction in terms to prohibit activities or to prescribe cardiac tonics.

In other instances it must be admitted that the basis of the circulatory neurosis is more deep-seated and repressed, so that only the special measures of the trained psychiatrist are likely to be fruitful. The family doctor, who is prepared to devote time and care to his patient, and has the opportunity to study him as an individual, knowing his upbringing, his personal traits and frailties, can do much to help and guide the neurotic. An earnest endeavour to analyse the particular situation and oot out the source, origin and nature of the conflicts by frank liscussion will accomplish far more in the long run than is o be attained by hasty and injudicious instructions to take a est at a spa or a sea voyage in the tropics. The congregation f neurotics at health resorts often accentuates an individual's lifficulties and widens the scope of his symptoms. Genuine motional disturbances, reflected in circulatory symptoms, nay result from all kinds of stresses and strains in modern ivilization. Domestic worries, difficult economic circum-tances, thwarted ambitions, private jealousies, sexual excesses, hameful dealings are all factors which, when frankly discussed nd analysed, are often found to be in some measure correctable. Vhen their true significance is appreciated, confidence gained nd the facts faced in their true perspective the individual nay realize that his difficulties are often less embarrassing han might at first sight be imagined. In this way the family octor can often ease the burden and reduce the emotional ension responsible for the individual's lack of adaptation. 'irculatory symptoms can thus be eased and in time righted vith perseverance, encouragement and reassurance. Simple xplanations of the effects of pent-up emotions on the heart nd circulation gradually come to be appreciated and understood s confidence is regained. Drugs are usually not required, but nsomnia must be corrected as adequate sleep is a first essential. epeated examination of the heart and daily or weekly records f blood pressure are to be avoided, as thereby attention ontinues to be fixed on the circulation. Treatment is neces-arily protracted, recovery is slow and only by perseverance is elapse prevented. Ross has shown that a large number of atients affected by the common neuroses, who are treated by frank discussion of their symptoms, will become well and keep ell. By demonstrating how their symptoms arise as emotional eactions, and by proving how they are retained because they re misinterpreted and by persuading the individual to appre-ate their real value, much can be done to restore him to veryday activities. It is in short a method of restoration f confidence combined with the banishment of fear (Ross). nxiety produces mental and physical exhaustion, and when is is adequately corrected by a short rest and the provision sleep, it is right that these people should be encouraged to ke as much exercise as they can endure. Constant encourage-ent, persuasion and a judicious optimism will rescue many om lives of incapacity. It is useless to offer to the con-rmed neurotic the bald statement, even after a thorough amination, "Your heart is sound: go and forget about it."

An encouraging clap on the back serves only to increase hi discomfort. To him his symptoms are genuine and he ha had no explanation for them. He distrusts more than ever The neurosis is accentuated.

The effort syndrome or neurocirculatory asthenia is worth of more detailed study in view of its intractable nature. Here as in the simpler neuroses, it is our first endeavour to offer a explanation for the symptoms, reassuring as far as is justifiabl and explaining the nature of the nervous and circulatory upset The eradication of sepsis is important, but the most successfu measures are those directed to simple outdoor exercise governe again by the patient's endurance, so that confidence is regained The neurasthenic must be made to do more than he thinks h can. Light walks, gradually increasing in range and in rat for half an hour or so morning and afternoon, are of grea benefit, associated later with a gentle outdoor occupatio These patients must be well fed, and have ample hours of slee Drugs are of little or no value, and digitalis, as in all th neuroses, should not be prescribed, as by increasing the forc of contractility it is liable to make the patient more awa of his heart. In any case it does nothing to improve th circulation in health. The occurrence of this syndrome in th convalescent period after such acute illnesses as influenz pneumonia or even tonsillitis, particularly in young adult makes for special care in selecting an appropriate time f return to work. A hasty convalescence predisposes to th form of functional cardiac instability.

Treatment is rendered more complex when functional stat and organic disease co-exist. It requires a fine discriminati to steer a middle course, combining reassurance and encourag ment with such physical limitations and drugs as the hea itself demands. In particular, in coronary disease associat with angina and hypertension, there is almost invariably a undercurrent of emotional tension, the correction of which ca only be approached by a frank discussion regarding simp rules of behaviour, and the demonstration that fear is oft unfounded. For this reason it is usually as unwise as it unkind to offer the information to a patient that he suffe from angina, though actually the prognosis in such a conditi may run to ten or twenty years, for such a statement prejudic his progress and increases his anxiety. A simple explanati of his symptoms is all that an intelligent patient or his frien will desire.

THE TREATMENT OF ACUTE CIRCULATORY FAILURE

In preceding sections attention has been chiefly directed o the treatment of those chronic forms of heart disease which ıltimately lead to one or other of the common types of cardiac ailure. Congestive, dyspnœic and anginal failure are for the nost part the end results of chronic degenerative lesions within he heart itself, and though each is liable to acute exacerbations hese forms of chronic failure must be sharply differentiated rom the various syndromes attributable to acute circulatory nsufficiency. Heart failure and circulatory failure are ıot synonymous, for they differ in their exciting cause, nechanism of production and hence also in their rational reatment.

The term "acute circulatory failure" includes a wide ariety of related conditions ranging from the mildest forms of imple syncope to the most profound degree of collapse, shock, oma and sudden death. The failure of the circulation in these tates is more often attributable to a disordered regulation of he peripheral circulation than to any essential or intrinsic efect in the heart itself. A sudden decrease in the volume of lood in active circulation is the fundamental mechanism in he production of these circulatory syndromes. Thus it is hat the symptoms associated with a profuse hæmorrhage differ nly quantitatively from those of a simple syncopal attack. n the first instance blood is suddenly lost to the exterior, nd the circulating blood volume is correspondingly reduced. n the second, the privation is none the less real as the amount f blood in active circulation is depleted by the stagnation of ırge quantities in the arterial and venous reservoirs. Peri- heral dilatation as an acute disorganization of the vasomotor ıechanism leads to pooling of the blood in stagnant areas with consequent reduction in the venous return to the heart, a ecreased output per beat, low peripheral pressure and more r less profound symptoms attributable to acute starvation f the central nervous system. Syncope, shock and collapse iffer from each other only quantitatively (Weiss). Initially, arious factors determine the onset and development of these ndromes, and treatment is determined by the correction of ıe exciting cause and the restoration of an adequate blood olume in *active* circulation to the vital centres.

SIMPLE SYNCOPE

Cerebral anæmia in an acute form has many causes, and no the least frequent are those which operate through the nervou pathways. Disturbances of the autonomic nervous syste leading to hypotension and transient cardiac inhibition ar often reflex in origin, originating either from the highes cerebral centres or along the afferent pathways provided b the peripheral sensory nerves. Acute emotional distress hypersensitivity of the carotid sinus, stimulation of the pleur or other sensory nerve endings may each reflexly precipitat syncope. Hence attacks may be prevented by such differen measures as the avoidance of emotional strain, the correctio of psychological conflicts, the stripping of the coats of th carotid artery on the side of the more sensitive sinus, or b the adequate employment of local anæsthesia when surgica measures are contemplated (Weiss). All these are method of prevention appropriate for particular cases. In postura hypotension, which is often attributable to syphilis of th central nervous system, but which also occurs in a milde form in the severer anæmias, attempts to prevent the peculia repeated seizures ought to be directed to the ætiological cause When this is irremediable and permanent, symptomatic relie may follow the use of ephedrine ($\frac{1}{8}$ to $\frac{1}{2}$ gr.) three or four time a day. Similarly mechanical support to the splanchnic are in the form of a suitably padded elastic belt and the develop ment of increased muscular tone by a course of abdomina exercises are measures which may be employed to supplemen drug therapy. The force of gravity constantly puts a burde upon the fine adjustments of the circulatory mechanism Individuals prone to faint discover this fact for themselves When attacks threaten they frequently lie down or adopt sitting posture with the trunk flexed and the head throw forward between the knees. Hot stuffy rooms, long hours i the erect posture without food or exposure to cold and damp ar factors which predispose to syncope in susceptible persons.

The loss of tone in the voluntary muscles which accompani the act of fainting serves the purpose of immediately correctin the cerebral anæmia by facilitating the return of blood to th heart and the vital centres. Treatment of the actual attac consists in loosening the clothing about the neck and ches and in placing the patient prone, or an even better effect ma be obtained by the adoption of a modified Trendelenbu position. By laying the victim on his back and elevating th feet some inches from the ground, venous return is facilitate lassage from the periphery towards the heart has a similar ffect. Pronounced bradycardia and hypotension of reflex rigin in severer cases may be corrected by the subcutaneous dministration of adrenalin solution (0·25 to 0·5 c.c.) or tropine sulphate ($\frac{1}{100}$ to $\frac{1}{50}$ gr.). When consciousness is egained alcohol has little to recommend it, but hot drinks of trong tea or coffee are often serviceable.

CARDIAC SYNCOPE

Syncope of cardiac origin is attributable to an intrinsic isorder of the heart beat. The symptoms may closely resemble simple faint or may proceed to convulsive seizures and actual pileptiform attacks. The attack is usually transient and esults from either extreme bradycardia, ventricular arrest or entricular fibrillation on the one hand, or from an excessive entricular rate as in the paroxysmal arrhythmias on the other. n either instance the symptoms are similar, and are due to erebral anoxæmia. The prevention and treatment of the aroxysmal tachycardias, a potent cause of syncope in elderly eople, have already been discussed (p. 708).

Stokes-Adams seizures are syncopal attacks associated ith a defect, transient or permanent, in the conducting echanism of the heart-beat. In the majority of instances ey can be prevented by the regular administration of ephedrine ydrochloride in doses sufficient to increase by a few beats er minute the slow idioventricular rate. For this purpose a ose of half a grain of ephedrine by mouth in tablet form at ther four or eight hour intervals may be sufficient. Larger oses may cause over-stimulation and exhaustion of the entricular centre. While ephedrine is the most reliable drug use for this purpose it is not effective in every case, probably r the reason that the mechanism responsible for ventricular rest varies in different individuals. Barium chloride in oses of $\frac{1}{2}$ to 1 gr. by mouth in a mixture thrice daily has an perimental justification for its use in the treatment of heart-ock in that it increases ventricular excitability, but clinical sts in patients liable to Stokes-Adams attacks have not lly substantiated this claim. If ephedrine alone fails to event seizures, barium may be prescribed in addition. ropine is not of great value, but may be tried if ephedrine d barium fail.

Recovery from the actual Stokes-Adams attack usually curs before any particular treatment can be prescribed. e ventricles resume their rhythm spontaneously. In the more severe attacks, as the circulation is in abeyance, sub-cutaneous or intravenous injections or inhalations are valueless as the drugs are not transported to the heart. Therefore, in desperate cases recourse must be made to an intracardia injection. Adrenalin is the remedy of choice. A fine needl about 3 in. long attached to a syringe charged with 0·25 c.c adrenalin (1 : 1,000 solution) is inserted into the fourth lef intercostal space about one finger-breadth from the sterna border. This site avoids the internal mammary artery an diminishes the likelihood of puncture of an underlying branc of a coronary artery or vein. The needle-point is inserted t a depth of 2 in. or more, and if the ventricular cavity i reached blood may be withdrawn into the syringe. Th injection is then made, but actually it is of little consequenc if the adrenalin is deposited either in the myocardium o within the cavity of the ventricle. The resumption of ventri-cular contractions is as a rule so immediate that it is questionabl if the restoration of rhythm is attributable to the drug or t the local irritation of the needle in the myocardium. Ventri-cular systole is accompanied by an oscillation of the syring and needle, and in a few seconds, if respiratory failure has nc also ensued, by the rush of oxygenated blood through the ski of the face and neck. This method is life-saving, not merel in Stokes-Adams seizures, but also in the cardiac arrest c anæsthesia, electrocution and in anaphylactic shock. There also every justification for its employment in asphyxia neona-torum, and in apparent death from the asphyxia of drownin It must be obvious that the intracardiac injection of adrenali is an emergency measure not without danger. Only the urgenc of the situation justifies its use for which, fortunately, there now ample experimental and clinical support.

It occasionally happens that Stokes-Adams seizures follo each other in rapid succession, the patient regaining consciou ness only to lapse back again into coma every few minute perhaps twenty or thirty attacks occurring in the course an hour. The milder seizures may amount to no more than transient giddiness, but others proceed to profound coma an clonic convulsions. Here, again, adrenalin is the drug to us Within fifteen minutes of a subcutaneous injection successi seizures may be arrested. When these are severe and rapid recurring, it may be judged advisable to give the drug intr venously, and for this purpose 0·5 c.c. of a 1 : 10,000 solutic is ample. This dosage is easily accomplished by drawi 0·5 c.c. of the standard 1 in 1,000 solution into a syringe, ar rediluting it by the addition of 4·5 c.c. normal sterile salin

After mixture 4·5 c.c. of the solution are discarded and the remaining 0·5 c.c. slowly injected into a vein at the elbow. Its total bulk may be augmented by further dilution, thus decreasing the risk of ventricular fibrillation.

Very occasionally Stokes-Adams seizures are due to this arrhythmia. Ventricular fibrillation is not necessarily a fatal condition, but if co-ordinate contraction of the ventricle is not quickly restored, death soon follows in a matter of minutes. The condition can only be recognized by the electrocardiograph, and when Stokes-Adams attacks are due to this abnormal mechanism it may well be justifiable to use quinidine sulphate in their prevention. Doses of 0·2 gm. in cachets three or four times a day are then worthy of trial.

COLLAPSE AND SHOCK

These terms, which are virtually interchangeable, are employed to denote an advanced degree of acute circulatory insufficiency, more gradual in its onset, more protracted in its course and of much more serious significance than the simple syncopes. The student will have to turn to textbooks of surgery for a description of their symptomatology, though, in fact, there is no fundamental difference between " medical " collapse and " surgical " shock. The underlying mechanism, provoked by numerous agents, is similar in all three—syncope, collapse and shock. The amount of blood in active circulation is strikingly reduced. Shock and collapse may occur relatively suddenly in the acute infections, notably lobar pneumonia ; in acute sepsis as in peritonitis ; in the course of acute intoxications, particularly delirium tremens ; after spinal anæsthesia ; as a result of mutilating trauma and profuse hæmorrhage ; accompanying thrombosis and infarction, notably in the heart, lungs and brain ; after an instrumental labour and in the post-operative period particularly in middle-aged people with or without organic vascular disease. The peripheral circulation is disorganized as a result, it is believed, of dilatation of the smallest venules with either an associated dilatation or constriction of the arterioles. It is associated with capillary paresis and in the later stages with an alteration in the permeability of the walls of the finest vessels (Weiss). Compensatory adjustments are impaired by the associated anæmia of the central nervous system. Clinically the ashen-grey colour, the impaired mental acuity, the shallow respirations, the thready pulse, the cold perspiration and the fall in blood pressure make a fairly characteristic syndrome.

As regards treatment, posture is of the first importance. A

horizontal or sitting posture may have to be maintained in certain instances, but whenever possible pillows should be withdrawn from beneath the head, and the foot of the bed raised on blocks to a height of 2 ft. or more. By this means alone the blood supply to the heart and brain is considerably facilitated. Cooling of the skin surface increases shock, and this must be countered by the application of a generous amount of warmth, either in the form of numerous hot tins, or by the application of a "shock cage" in which heat is maintained by electric bulbs. Heat may be employed internally as well as externally by the provision of hot drinks either in the form of normal saline or as salty soup by the mouth, and by a hot solution of glucose, 5 per cent., in normal saline by the bowel if need be. The correction of dehydration relative or absolute is particularly valuable in the acute circulatory failure of fever and in post-operative collapse, but considerable judgment is required regarding its use, in view of the danger of overloading the right side of the heart and increasing the transudation of fluid through the weakened capillary walls as occurs in the most advanced degrees of shock. If it is judged that the collapse is relatively mild, early in its onset and the heart fundamentally sound, then the restoration of a satisfactory volume of blood in active circulation can be brought about by transfusion of a $\frac{1}{2}$ to 1 pint of blood or by a continuous intravenous saline drip. By this means 3,000 to 8,000 c.c. of fluid may be added to the circulation in the course of twenty-four hours. To the normal saline thus used various substances of value in the treatment of shock may be added—glucose, insulin, coramine and eucortone all may serve a useful purpose. The latter, an aqueous solution of the active principles of the suprarenal cortex, is believed to regulate the volume of the circulating fluid within the vascular system and is worthy of a more extended clinical trial in the treatment of shock and collapse than it has received to date. It may be given in doses of 2 c.c. every hour subcutaneously for an adult, or if added to the transfusion fluid then 2 c.c. of eucortone to each litre, if run at a rate of 400 to 500 c.c. of saline per hour, would appear to be adequate dosage. After two or three hours, if progress be made, the rate of flow may be reduced to half this quantity.

Anoxæmia has a detrimental effect on the central nervous system and aggravates all the features of shock. Oxygen therapy will be of value in those forms of anoxæmia in which œdema of the lung alveoli interferes with the absorption of oxygen. Pulmonary infarction and œdema, commonly associated with shock in the early stages, and the basal congestion which may rapidly follow an acute coronary thrombosis are examples of conditions in which oxygen therapy may be of value. In an emergency a nasal catheter is the best method of administration if an oxygen tent is not available.

Pain is a potent cause in the perpetuation of those reflexes disorganizing the peripheral circulation and promoting symptoms of shock. A fine discrimination is required to assess the appropriate dose of morphia to relieve the pain without augmenting the disordered peripheral circulation. It will be recalled that morphia itself in full doses acts through the parasympathetic system. As a general rule morphia is well tolerated in the early stages of shock and may be given in full doses if pain is at all severe. After some hours when the collapse is more advanced and the patient's general condition has deteriorated, then small doses are justifiable. It must be borne in mind that the detrimental effect of severe pain is to be dreaded more than the reaction of the peripheral circulation to the drug.

When the symptoms and signs suggest that the major factor in the production of the acute circulatory failure is a depression of the vasomotor centre, there are a number of useful drugs which may be employed with benefit. One of the best is strychnine, which is perhaps not so fashionable now as formerly. Clinical experience, particularly in the collapse of lobar pneumonia, indicates that this drug is of distinct benefit when given at hourly or even two-hourly intervals in doses of $\frac{1}{30}$ gr. or more. It increases the tone of the peripheral muscles, and may thus help the return of blood to the heart. It facilitates reflex action and there is evidence to suggest that it augments the tone of the vasomotor centres. It has no effect on the heart. There is no justification for the employment of digitalis in shock or collapse. The probability is that drugs of the digitalis group accentuate the degree of shock by inducing a further diminution in the volume-output of the heart. While the subcutaneous injection of camphor in oil in doses of 3 gr. or more is ineffective owing to its slow absorption and insolubility, other synthetic organic compounds such as coramine (pyridine carbonate of diethylamide) or cardiazol (pentamethylenetetrazol) appear to be useful and effective remedies when given parenterally in sufficient dosage. The former is supplied in a 25 per cent. solution in 1 c.c. ampoules, and the latter in a 10 per cent. solution also in similar ampoules. In circulatory collapse of vasomotor origin either of these drugs may be administered intramuscularly in doses of 1 c.c. or more at hourly or two-hourly intervals. It is doubtful if they are really active by the mouth, and in circulatory collapse they can only be given intravenously with considerable caution and well diluted. In actual practice their intravenous use is perhaps limited to the collapse of barbiturate, morphine or carbonmonoxide poisoning. They are probably less effective in the presence of organic heart disease, but may be used to counteract the minor degree of peripheral collapse when morphia is indicated, *e.g.*, in the profound shock of coronary thrombosis. On account of its cardiac stimulation and its power to constrict the peripheral arterioles, there is little justification for the use of adrenalin in profound collapse or shock, and pituitrin, for the reason that it decreases cardiac output, is not without danger. The fact is that the ideal drug for the treatment of peripheral circulatory failure has not yet been found. Weiss has suggested that a chemical substance which exerts a constricting effect solely on the venules will be of particular benefit, whereas a substance which simultaneously induces constriction of the arterioles as well may further impair the blood supply to the tissues. A drug with such selective properties has yet to be demonstrated. Until further clinical research has differentiated more sharply the different varieties of shock and collapse appropriate treatment must be based on rough and ready principles, the practitioner assessing the situation as best he may. Obviously all the methods outlined above are not desirable in every instance, but a selection may be made as the clinical state appears to indicate.

A. Rae Gilchrist.

DISEASES OF THE BLOOD VESSELS OF THE LIMBS

THE diseases to be considered in this chapter call for treatment because they diminish the supply of blood to a limb or limbs. The resulting nutritional changes are determined by the duration and the intensity of the ischæmia, and vary in severity from dryness and glazing of the skin when the impairment of blood flow is slight to massive gangrene when it is severe. The management of cases of this nature is the more satisfactory the earlier the presence of impairment of blood flow is discovered, and the more accurately the underlying pathological process is identified. Therefore we consider it advantageous to deviate from the general plan of this book and to include in this chapter brief descriptions of the normal control of blood flow to the limbs, of tests of its efficiency and of the pathological processes which may reduce it. The clarification of many of these problems is of comparatively recent date, and owes much to the researches of Lewis and his collaborators.

NORMAL PERIPHERAL BLOOD FLOW

The amount of blood which reaches the tissues of the limbs depends on the calibre of the arterial tree, which in turn depends on the tonus of the smooth musculature of the arterial blood vessels. Arterial tonus is controlled (1) partly by the activity of vasoconstrictor fibres belonging to the sympathetic nervous system, which are ultimately distributed to the vessels by way of the somatic nerves of the limbs, and (2) partly by the influence of chemical substances, either manufactured locally (products of muscular activity, which cause vasodilatation) or conveyed by the blood stream (adrenalin, which causes vasoconstriction). The arterial vessels may be grouped in two sets: those supplying the muscles, which are controlled exclusively by the mediation of chemical substances, and those supplying the skin and subcutaneous tissues, in the control of which the sympathetic nervous system plays much the most important part. The latter set of vessels takes part in the general vascular reactions which help to maintain the body at a constant temperature. When the temperature of the environment changes, that of the blood tends to follow the changes. The autonomic centres in the brain are sensitive to changes in the temperature of the blood which reaches them. When it is increased, the response is a generalized complete inhibition of vasoconstrictor tonus, so that a rapid flow of blood results, with a correspondingly increased loss of bodily heat. When it is decreased, generalized vasoconstriction of the superficial vessels is the response, which results in conservation of bodily heat. Adaptation to low environmental temperatures might be expected to be most difficult in the hands and feet, which provide the end-stages of the peripheral circulation, and which might not be warmly clad ; the supply of heat to these parts by the circulation is greatly facilitated by the presence of special shunts (arteriolo-venous anastomoses) between the subcutaneous arterioles and veins. When these anastomoses are relaxed by their controlling nervous mechanism, the resulting rapid increase in blood flow quickly warms the extremities.

For the development by the tissues of an adequate response to trauma and to bacterial infection, it is essential that both the peripheral vessels and the mechanisms for controlling the flow of blood in them should be normal.

PATHOLOGICAL PROCESSES WHICH REDUCE BLOOD FLOW

The processes which reduce the amount of blood flowing through arterial vessels may be classified into two groups :—

Group I.—An Organic Change is Present from the First in the Lumen or Wall of the Affected Vessels

A. Thickening of the wall of arteries : In arteriosclerosis and syphilis.

B. Embolism : The embolus may (1) originate in the heart (auricular fibrillation, infarction, bacterial endocarditis), or (2) be detached from an atheromatous patch in an artery.

C. Thrombosis : (1) In arteriosclerosis (elderly patients of both sexes, especially diabetics) ; (2) in thrombo-angiitis obliterans (young or middle-aged males) ; (3) in syphilitic arteritis ; (4) in polycythæmia vera, and leucæmia ; (5) as a result of external pressure (tumours, cervical rib); (6) after debilitating diseases (pneumonia, typhoid); (7) without any apparent cause.

GROUP II.—THE OBSTRUCTION TO BLOOD FLOW IS OFFERED BY SPASM OF THE VESSEL, AND ORGANIC CHANGES ARE (AT LEAST AT FIRST) ABSENT.

A. As a result of trauma: A rare cause in large arteries; particularly after bullet wounds in their vicinity.

B. As a result of local hypersensitivity to cold: This is encountered in the small arteries of the hands and feet. Intermittent spasm of these vessels gives rise to the Raynaud phenomenon. The common type is the bilateral and symmetrical form met with in young women, and the phenomenon may also appear in the hands of those who work with vibrating tools. In both these types organic changes in the walls of the vessels may ultimately be superimposed on the original spasm. These tend to increase and to perpetuate the obstruction to blood-flow.

A. SUDDEN OBSTRUCTION OF LARGER ARTERIES

When a main artery is obstructed by an embolus, the patient experiences numbness or pain in the limb and the skin becomes at first blanched and later cyanosed. Pulsation is absent beyond the site of lodgment of the clot. The temperature of the skin falls slowly to that of the environment. Loss of sensation and of power appear, and progress from the distal parts towards the proximal. The area involved in these changes depends on the availability of the collateral vessels, which are at first narrowed by reflex vasoconstriction. If they are inadequate, a sharp line of demarcation forms at a level which varies with that of the arterial block. Distal to this line the limb becomes gangrenous.

Since such an obstruction is likely to be permanent and progressive, the clot should be removed surgically (1) when it is aseptic, (2) when the general condition of the patient warrants such interference, and (3) when operation can be carried out within ten or twelve hours. The lodgment of a septic clot (as in bacterial endocarditis) is a fatal complication. In other cases unsuitable for operation, the development of a collateral circulation must be encouraged by warming the unaffected area of the body to about 45° C. (113° F.) by means of an electric cage, electric lamps, or hot-water bottles under sufficient coverings. When the area which will become gangrenous has been demarcated, it must be kept scrupulously clean and dry by the application of spirit followed by a sterile dusting powder,[1] and enveloped in a sterile, dry dressing. If the patient survives, it may be amputated later.

B. GRADUAL OBSTRUCTION OF THE ARTERIAL VESSELS

In practice this is a very common condition. As a rule, the morbid process affects both the superficial vessels and those of the muscles; but not infrequently the clinical features may direct attention particularly to one set, and they will be described from this aspect.

1. The Superficial Vessels

The patient may complain :—

(*a*) *Of Cold Feet.*—This is usually accompanied by changes in colour. Cyanosis is frequently present, and always indicates a slow circulation; if present in warm surroundings it must be regarded as abnormal. In the most severe cases the skin has a pale, waxy appearance. Blanching of the distal parts of the limb when it is elevated above the horizontal is frequently present, particularly in thrombo-angiitis obliterans. If the temperature of the environment is constant and the surface of the skin dry, surface temperature varies directly with the amount of subcutaneous blood flow; therefore the temperature of the skin provides an index of the efficiency of the superficial circulation. For accurate observations, special skin-thermometers of the thermo-electric type are necessary; in clinical examination a satisfactory estimation may be made by first palpating the skin of the suspected area with the dorsal surfaces of the middle phalanges of the fingers and then palpating the skin where the circulation is adequate (*e.g.*, feet, forehead). Moreover, if both arms, or both legs, be exposed to a warm environment (23° C., 73° F.), then any difference in skin temperature is due to reduced blood flow on the less warm side.

(*b*) *Of Nutritional Changes.*—The growth of the nails may be greatly retarded, and perspiration diminished or absent. Any breach of the epithelium heals very slowly or not at all, and there is a tendency for the development of indolent ulcers,

[1] A suitable powder is a mixture of boric acid, 1 part; zinc oxide, 2 parts; and powdered starch, 3 parts.

especially on the heel and in the interdigital clefts of the toes. As the vascular occlusion progresses, areas of dry gangrene may develop, and this is often precipitated by careless nail-cutting or corn-paring (p. 737). Such an area may ultimately include a phalanx or an entire digit. In the final stages the foot, or the foot and leg, may become gangrenous. Both ulcerative and gangrenous processes are, as a rule, extremely painful.

2. The Deep and Superficial Vessels

The patient may complain of *pain*. The cardinal symptom of inadequate blood flow to the muscles is *intermittent claudication*, a cramp-like pain in the calves and fronts of the legs which restricts exercise. This appears most rapidly if the patient walks uphill or fast, and in its most severe form it may force him to halt after he has walked as little as fifty yards. Claudication disappears if the patient rests.

Very inadequate blood flow in both superficial and muscular vessels is sometimes associated with severe pain which occurs during rest, especially at night; this is usually felt in the heel and/or in the sole of the foot.

In every case in which the history or physical signs are suggestive of vascular insufficiency, the pulses of the limbs must be carefully examined (Figs. A, B, C, D); this should be done when the subject is warm, because pulsations are then maximal. This examination does not supply complete proof of absence of blood flow, because (1) vessels may pursue an abnormal course, (2) additional abnormal vessels may be present, (3) a partial obstruction proximally situated may diminish pulsation without seriously reducing blood flow (*cf.* coarctation of the aorta), and (4) although the walls of a vessel may be too rigid to pulsate it may be transmitting a fair quantity of blood. The inexperienced observer may mistake the twitchings of adjacent tendons for arterial pulsation, particularly of the dorsalis pedis and posterior tibial arteries.

(*a*) **General Treatment.**—This will include advice as to diet; since no individual food factor is known to be of ætiological importance, the patient should be allowed a reasonable latitude in arranging his daily menu. Patients must be warned not to put on weight, because the increasing inability to take exercise naturally tends to lead to obesity; the heavier the patient the greater the strain on his feet and legs (for anti-obesity diet see p. 389). Alcohol is best limited to whisky and water at bed time. Glycosuria, if present, should be corrected, because it may be of ætiological importance and because it predisposes to septic complications. In thrombo-angiitis obliterans smoking must be stopped completely. Rest pain is usually relieved by placing the legs in a dependent position, and the patient may be able to sleep in a chair. It is a wise plan to arrange for the patient to have a succession of good nights at the beginning of treatment, by giving a mild hypnotic-analgesic (*e.g.* soluble barbitone gr. v with acetylsalicylic acid gr. v, phenobarbitone

Fig. A.—Pulses in the Arm.

The Brachial Artery corresponds to a line drawn from the outer wall of the axilla at the junction of its anterior and middle third to the mid-point of the elbow.

The Radial Artery is palpated to the radial side of the tendon of the flexor carpi radialis.

The Ulnar Artery, which is not always palpable, lies to the radial side of the tendon of the flexor carpi ulnaris.

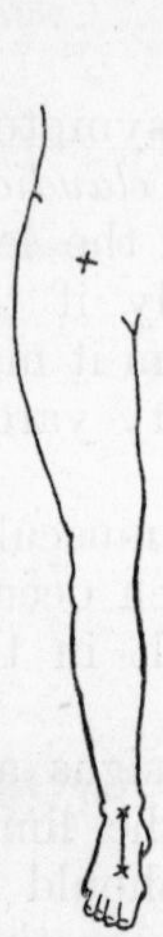

Fig. B.

The Femoral Artery is palpated at a point midway between the anterior superior iliac spine and the symphysis pubis.

The Dorsalis Pedis runs from a point midway between the two malleoli to the base of the first interosseous space.

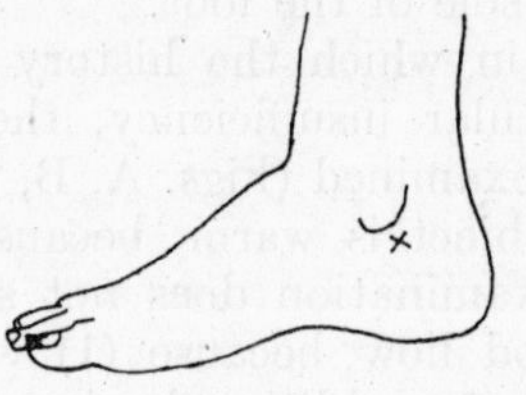

Fig. D.

The Posterior Tibial Artery is palpated at the mid-point between the posterior border of the internal malleolus and the inner border of the os calcis. In the average adult this is $\frac{3}{4}$ in. behind the malleolus.

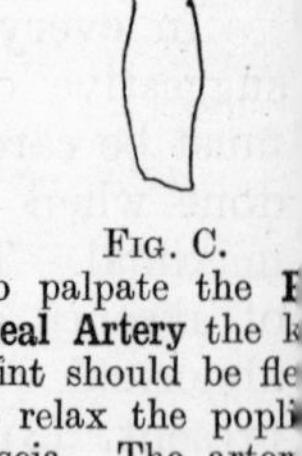

Fig. C.

To palpate the P liteal Artery the k joint should be fle to relax the popli fascia. The arter felt at the mid-p of the popliteal sp

gr. iss with acetylsalicylic acid gr. x, or one of the proprietary preparations such as Empyrin or Veganin). Lack of sleep makes these old people (and often their households) irritable and unco-operative; after a good sleep they are different people, and the doctor will have the household with him. Clothing should be warm and not constricting. Woollen underclothes should reach the wrists and ankles, and bed socks must be worn.

(*b*) **Care of Threatened Areas.**—For the prevention or postponement of nutritional lesions the care of the threatened areas, especially of the feet, is of supreme importance. Patients should be given definite written or typewritten instructions;

these should be carefully explained to the patient and the importance of close attention to the carrying out of every detail strongly emphasized. It is quite true to point out that neglect of these instructions may mean the loss of a leg.

The feet and legs must be washed daily with *tepid* water and soap, dried carefully (especially between the toes) with a soft towel, and powdered with a dusting powder. Clothing must not compress them; thus socks should be woollen, seamless and of a good fit; boots and shoes must be roomy without being loose, without irregularities which might press on the soles of the feet (nails), and either soled with rubber or with an extra rubber sole. Prolonged standing is harmful; prolonged walking must be forbidden, the patient being instructed to stop within his known "claudication-distance." The feet must be protected from even the slightest trauma; thus nails should be cut straight and well away from the quick; corns should be pared only superficially, and never treated with destructive applications (*e.g.*, salicylic acid). Those who can obtain the services of a skilled chiropodist should avail themselves of these, and the patient's doctor should be willing to act as chiropodist if required. The patient must avoid crowds, in which his feet may be trampled on with disastrous results. And finally, the feet and legs must never be exposed to cold, particularly to cold water (gangrene has followed incautious "paddling" in the sea).

(*c*) **Care of Nutritional Lesions.**—The appearance of any breach of surface, however trifling, is of such potentially grave moment that the patient must rest in bed until healing has taken place. *Abrasions* should be gently cleansed with surgical spirit, and protected by a dry dressing of gauze or lint, held in position by a small strip of adhesive plaster (which must never completely encircle a digit) or by a light bandage. *Ulcers* about the toes or on the heel are as a rule very painful, especially when dressed; for this reason a suitable local application is an anæsthetic ointment.[1] If the ulcer is not painful, balsam of Peru or 4 per cent. thymol in liquid paraffin are alternative applications. *Small areas of dry gangrene*, *e.g.*, up to a digit, must be kept aseptic and dry by the application of spirit two or three times a day, and are best exposed to the air, under a cage or box, without any dressing, in order to promote drying. Mechanical attempts to hasten the separation of the slough should never be made. The local application of heat is not good practice, for this raises the metabolic rate locally and increases the demand on an already

[1] Unguentum cocainæ; "Anæsthesin" ointment (Bayer Products Ltd.).

deficient blood flow. Local removal, *e.g.*, of a digit, should never be considered until a clear line of demarcation has formed; even then the decision to amputate locally is a matter of some judgment. In arteriosclerosis local removal may be considered if the tissues appear to be reacting well on the proximal side of the gangrenous toe; the incision should follow the line of demarcation, and the skin proximal to this must not be handled with forceps. The wound should be left open, or at most one loose stitch inserted. In thrombo-angiitis obliterans local removal of a digit is hardly ever worth while, as pain is likely to persist after this type of amputation. Local anæsthesia must not be employed to remove gangrenous digits, because it produces local tension; nitrous oxide or nitrous oxide and oxygen are the anæsthetics of choice. Sometimes an angry reddening of the skin is seen about the base of a gangrenous digit, perhaps associated with lymphangiitis of the foot and leg. This often heralds extension of the gangrenous process, but occasionally it is due to retention of pus by the hard skin of the gangrenous area; before more extensive measures are tried search should be made, particularly in the sole and interdigital clefts, and any small abscess drained by raising the dry black skin.

In diabetes the problems are a little different. If the patient is young, even a small area of gangrene, especially if it becomes infected, should be regarded as an urgent surgical condition of great gravity, and one requiring care in hospital[1]; whereas in older patients the gangrene is more often of the dry type and does not call for so urgent or so extensive treatment.

It must be emphasized again that if a small gangrenous area such as a digit is left to separate almost of itself, which is often the wisest plan, pain must be controlled, especially at night; but only as a last resort should morphine or one of its derivatives be employed for this purpose.

A major amputation is required (1) when gangrene is massive from the first, (2) when it involves more than the digits, (3) when it is associated with spreading septic infection and (4) when it gives rise to intolerable pain. At least the relatives, and often the patient, should understand that the pathological process is bilateral and that the other leg may be affected at a later date.

(*d*) **Measures Designed to Improve Blood Supply.**—1. *By Drugs.*—Numerous attempts have been made to improve blood flow by the administration of acetylcholine and its

[1] Since it is likely to be more of an infective than of ischæmic type.

derivatives. The action of these substances is transitory, because they are rapidly destroyed in the body by a specific esterase. Their use is not recommended.

2. *By Operation.*—When the obstructive process is segmental, and parts of the arterial tree unaffected (a condition of affairs which may be found in thrombo-angiitis obliterans), an attempt may be made to improve the total blood flow in the limb by operation. The result of such an attempt depends on the availability of collateral channels, and/or their capacity to dilate. This can be determined by tests, which must be carried out in a hospital properly equipped to do so (see p. 741). If the test is satisfactory, two procedures are available. The first is *arterectomy*, in which the obstructed segment of artery is first determined by radiography after the injection of an opaque fluid and then resected. The diseased segment of the artery is said to act as an irritant, which produces reflex vasoconstriction of the remainder of the arterial tree. The second is *sympathectomy*, in which the vasoconstrictor nerves to the limb are divided, so that vasodilatation results. Sympathectomy is *never* indicated in arteriosclerosis, and arterectomy but rarely. In thrombo-angiitis obliterans neither operation should be undertaken except after very careful preliminary study, and it must be emphasized that *claudication is not relieved* by sympathectomy, because the control of muscular vessels is predominantly chemical.

3. *By Buerger's Exercises.*—The patient lies on his back, in bed or on a couch. A leg is elevated to from 60 to 90 degrees above the horizontal, and retained in this position by resting the heel on a support for from one-half to three minutes, the period required being that necessary to produce blanching. As soon as this is established the foot is allowed to hang over the edge of the bed until reactionary hyperæmia or rubor appears, and kept dependent for one minute longer ; the total length in this position is from two to five minutes. The leg is then placed in the horizontal position for three minutes. The placing of the limb in these three successive positions constitutes one cycle, and each leg should be exercised in this way for six cycles three times a day. To be effective, the treatment must be faithfully carried out ; if instituted early, its beneficial results are beyond doubt.

4. *By the Induction of Intermittent Reactive Hyperæmia.*—This is a most useful method of dilating the vessels in obstructive arterial disease. It is accomplished by the application of a pneumatic cuff to the thigh (or arm), which is alternately inflated to a pressure of 30 to 70 mm. of mercury for two

minutes, and deflated for two minutes, the cycle being maintained by an apparatus driven from the domestic electric mains,[1] or by a cheaper but rather cumbersome apparatus regulated by the domestic water supply.[2] One of the most beneficial results of this treatment is the relief of the severe rest-pain of thrombo-angiitis obliterans, frequently within an hour or two of the application of the cuff. The distance which the patient can walk before claudication appears is steadily increased. In cases of this type from six to ten hours' treatment is necessary in each day, at a pressure of from 40 to 60 mm. Hg.; as patients readily accustom themselves to sleep while treatment is being applied, the hours of sleep can be utilized. After four to eight weeks of intensive treatment, each patient will discover the duration of his daily "maintenance" period of treatment for himself. When nutritional lesions dominate the clinical picture, the duration of treatments should be thirty to sixty minutes three times a day, and the pressure 30 to 35 mm. of mercury. The improvement to be expected, although less striking than in the former type of case, is often valuable. A contraindication to treatment is existing thrombo-phlebitis, or the possibility of its appearance (*e.g.*, the migratory phlebitis of thrombo-angiitis obliterans).

C. INTERMITTENT OBSTRUCTION OF ARTERIAL VESSELS

This group includes the cases in which the Raynaud phenomenon is the presenting physical finding. The essential feature of the commonest type, which is met with in young women, consists of attacks characterized by the sudden arrest of the inflow to the fingers, and possibly to a less extent to the toes. Usually an attack is precipitated by exposure to cold. The general physical findings are similar to those described in Section A. At first nutritional changes are absent, but in severe cases of long standing, areas of superficial gangrene may occur at the tips of the fingers, as the result of the appearance of organic changes in the walls of the digital arteries.

1. **General Treatment.**—By far the most important principle in the treatment of this condition is avoidance of cold. Although local climatic conditions may make this difficult, at the least the patient must avoid cold in its most provocative form—cold water. Those who can afford it should winter in a warm,

[1] The Chalmers-Edina Engineering Company, Leith.
[2] Messrs Baird & Tatlock (London).

dry climate. Much can be done to reduce the frequency and severity of attacks by the adoption of proper clothing. The trunk should be warmly clad in order to minimize the amount of vasoconstrictor tonus imposed on the peripheral vessels. The limbs should be warmly clad from the root of the limb (clavicle, groin) to the hands and ankles ; this keeps the blood warm on its way to the digits. For the hands, warm, loose-fitting gauntlet gloves are essential ; for the feet stout boots or shoes, allowing room for two pairs of stockings, and with additional rubber soles. The patient should sleep in a warm bed, with arms and hands under the bedclothes, so as to ensure at least eight hours each day of inhibition of vasoconstrictor tonus. Unfortunately for their comfort, most of these suggestions are as a rule rejected by young women, sometimes with scorn and often with hilarity.

When the condition follows the use of vibrating tools, the workman must find some other employment.

2. **Operative Treatment.**—When the patient has placed herself under the best possible conditions, and the attacks continue to be a source of economic or social disability, operation may be considered. This takes the form of division of the sympathetic vasoconstrictor fibres to the limb, and, if the point of section is properly chosen, permanent vasodilatation of the superficial vessels follows. Of necessity, sweating is also abolished, and the dryness which results may be troublesome in the hands.[1] Before operation is undertaken it is essential that the capacity of the vessels to dilate be already demonstrated. This is a matter for the hospital clinic, where it is assessed by observing the rise in the surface temperature of the affected limbs when vasoconstrictor tonus is inhibited by heating a sufficient area of another part of the body. In practice the hands are most commonly tested ; and the heat is applied by placing the feet and legs in water at 45° C. (113° F.). After a certain interval the temperature of the hands may rise to as high as 36° C. (97° F.), and must reach 30° C. (86° F.) before operation is justifiable.

Sympathectomy operations are not dangerous, and the period of disability is short (two to three weeks). No serious undesirable after-effects follow a well-planned operation.

ERYTHRO-CYANOSIS

This is the term which Lewis employs to describe a condition which occurs almost exclusively in adolescent and young adult females. It is characterized by areas of defective circulation

[1] It may be minimized by the use of an emollient (cold cream) or glycerin.

situated on the legs, particularly on the antero-lateral aspect, just above the external malleolus. Such areas are bluish-red in colour, and the skin is atrophic. The patients suffer in addition from cold feet, and burning pain is commonly felt when the blue areas are warmed. The condition is, as a rule, present only during the cold season, and disappears more or less completely during summer. In advanced cases the skin may actually break, with the formation of indolent ulcers. Some œdema of the ankles and feet is commonly associated.

Patients should be advised to wear woollen stockings, advice which, owing to the dictates of fashion, is rarely followed. In advanced cases, with severe ulceration recurring each winter, lumbar sympathectomy is indicated.

J. R. Learmonth.
W. M. Arnott.

DISEASES OF THE NOSE, THROAT AND EAR

THE NOSE

Introduction

CONSIDERATION is given in this section to the treatment of the commoner affections of the nose and the nasal accessory air sinuses. Surgery plays its own part in connection with these affections, but as such it receives no present attention.

Similarly, lesions of the nose, throat and ear, caused by syphilis, tuberculosis and malignant disease are not dealt with; they are more appropriately discussed in the sections set apart for that purpose.

Physiology of the Nose and Nasal Accessory Sinuses in Relation to Treatment

Some knowledge of the physiology of the mucous membrane of the nose and that of the nasal accessory sinuses is essential to the intelligent treatment of diseases of these structures. The chief symptoms are, for the most part, the result of derangement of nasal physiology and, therefore, treatment is, in the main, an attempt to restore physiology to normal. The variation from normal may be in any one of the different elements of the nasal mechanism. Mucous membrane, of columnar ciliated type, is the structure upon which function is based. There are slight variations in the membrane in the different parts of the nose, as the more important functions are localized to certain areas. The mucous membrane is rich in glands which secrete the mucus which is essential to the life of the cilia. Under the basement layer of the epithelium is connective tissue stroma, containing blood vessels and spaces which contain blood. These spaces form the erectile tissue of the nose, and are capable of engorgement with blood or of retraction, according to the functions of the nose in the supply of moisture and warm air to the lung. This erectile tissue is located chiefly in those parts of the nose upon which the air stream impinges—the anterior end of the inferior turbinate, its lower edge and the anterior end of the middle turbinate. This tissue is under the control of the sympathetic nervous system, and derangement of this is responsible for a great many symptoms of nasal disease which call for treatment. Mucus is secreted by the glands of the nose, and this has functions of its own. As has already been mentioned, it provides a medium in which the cilia of the columnar cells may live and work, and in order that they may carry out their function properly the mucus must be of the correct consistency. The mucus also has the function of protecting the membrane which lines the nose, and its absence or removal is immediately followed by changes in the mucous membrane and by symptoms of nasal discomfort. Particles of foreign material and bacteria inhaled into the nose are caught in the mucus, and are eventually eliminated through the alimentary canal.

Principles of Treatment

The main requirements for comfort in the nose and for normal physiology are adequate drainage, adequate aeration and ciliary activity ; and it is towards the restoration of these that treatment is directed.

Common Nasal Remedies.—These consist of douches, sprays, drops, inhalations, powders and salves of various types. In accordance with the physiological principles which we have enunciated, no remedy which interferes with ciliary function is to be permitted. Therefore any remedy containing drugs in sufficient strength to paralyse or interfere with ciliary activity, as, for example, strong solutions of ephedrine, cocaine or irritants, must be avoided. Ointments or other applications which remain in a thick state within the nose will clog the mucous membrane, and thus prevent ciliary movement. Powders act as irritants and are not recommended. Douches, when used, must be isotonic, because water tends to paralyse ciliary activity. The main function of a nasal douche is to remove accumulated secretions which coat the mucous membrane and the nasal passages and prevent proper aeration and drainage. By removal of this accumulation the ciliary membrane is given an opportunity to recover, but it must be remembered that, as the function of mucus is to protect the membrane, the repeated and continued use of the nasal douche, by depriving the membrane of its protection, will tend to defeat its own end. Therefore, when a douche is used to cleanse the mucous membrane, the membrane should be protected with some solution which will prevent excessive drying. A spray of light oil is used for this purpose after a douche, to replace the mucus which has been washed out.

Oily Sprays.—These should be of light oil, of a non-clogging type and, if medicated, must not contain harmful preparations of drugs.

Drops.—These are not as effective as oil used from an atomiser, as it is difficult to obtain an adequate and even spread of the solution throughout the nasal cavity. They have the merit, however, that they are simpler to use, require less apparatus, and in many cases are all that is required for comfort. Oil should never be used as drops or sprays in young children or infants, owing to the danger of inhalation of the oil and the production of lung complications. Saline and ephedrine solution is used very frequently as a decongestive, in the form of drops or spray. The solution should be isotonic and should not contain more than 2 per cent. of ephedrine.

Inhalations.—Inhalations of steam, medicated with menthol, camphor, eucalyptus, oil of pine or other substance, are frequently used in cases of nasal congestion. They are often of considerable benefit to those suffering from acute congestion of the nose, and the steam forms a convenient vehicle for the application of small quantities of soothing drugs to the mucous membrane. Prescriptions containing these remedies will be found in the Appendix (see p. 773).

Other Forms of Treatment.—Certain of these call for mention since, although outside the scope of medical treatment, they cannot be classified under a surgical heading. They are the galvano-cautery, the use of caustics and sclerosing solutions, ionisation and various forms of radiation therapy. These have as their object the reduction of the bulk of the mucous membrane of the nose to provide aeration, or the correction of the sensitiveness of the mucous membrane to particular irritants.

INJURIES OF THE NOSE

Treatment will vary according to the nature of the injury and the problems which it presents. Generally speaking, the conditions calling for attention fall roughly into three categories :—

1. Fractures.
2. Hæmatomata.
3. Epistaxis.

Fractures of the Nose.—Simple fractures are treated by replacement of the displaced bones. If seen immediately afte injury, an attempt may be made to correct the deformity If, however, there is considerable swelling of the soft parts o the nose, it is wiser to allow this to subside, in order tc ascertain the extent of the deformity before replacement i attempted. The commonest deformity is a depression of one nasal bone with deviation of the nose to the opposite side Before this deviation can be corrected, the depressed lateral nasal bone must be elevated. This can be done with any flat instrument from within the nose and replacement is then a simple matter. An anæsthetic, as a rule, is required for this manipulation.

In compound fractures of the nose it is wiser to allow the lacerations to heal before attempting any manipulation of the bones. Needless to say, only the simplest forms of injury can be treated in this fashion. Where deformity or displace ment is considerable, a plastic operation is desirable. This also applies to all cases when more than five or six weeks have elapsed since the injury.

Hæmatoma consists of effusion of blood between the layers of the septum. If the symptoms are not urgent the hæmatoma should be left alone, as it will disappear after a period of about a week ; but if very large and causing trouble it may be aspirated after cocainizing a small area of mucou membrane on one side or the other. Suppuration in the hæmatoma is always a possibility, and when this occurs the hæmatoma should be opened and drained. With loca anæsthesia, a small incision is made on one side of the swelling and the pus is evacuated. A small drain is inserte into the wound and the abscess may require to be reopene daily for some days.

Epistaxis.—In such cases two areas of the nose may require treatment. The first and commonest area is Little' area. This is the name given to the part supporting th aggregation of veins found at the anterior end of the nasa septum. The other area is the ethmoidal, in the upper par of the nose, which may also be the site of bleeding due to othe conditions. The treatment of bleeding from the nose varie according to the area from which the bleeding is coming. I some instances it is unwise to treat the epistaxis immediately because, if the loss is not severe or profuse, it may act as relief to the patient as, for example, in cases of high bloo pressure. On the other hand, when bleeding becomes profus and troublesome to the patient, it will require to be controllec f the bleeding must be stopped, there are two methods vailable. The bleeding may be controlled by pressure, hat is by packing, or the actual bleeding point may be bliterated.

The Control of Bleeding by Packing.—If the nose is full f clot, an attempt should be made to get rid of this by louching. A solution of equal parts of peroxide of hydrogen nd water, used cold, is an excellent solution for syringing the ose. After the nose has been douched, it should be packed ightly with gauze wrung out with 5 per cent. cocaine solution ontaining adrenalin (5 minims to 1 drachm of cocaine). This acking should be left in for a few minutes and, when removed, he nose will be found to be comparatively insensitive and the vork of packing the nose will be rendered very much less npleasant for the patient. The doctor is able to carry out he packing more thoroughly when the nose reacts to the ocaine; also the mucous membrane will swell later, and by ripping the pack, will increase its efficiency. The packing is arried out with 1-in. ribbon gauze soaked in solution of ydrogen peroxide (10 volumes). The floor of the nose is rst packed. Six inches of the pack having being doubled, ith a pair of angled forceps it is passed right back along the nferior meatus. From the floor of the nose the pack is built p towards the roof, being firmly pushed into all crevices of he nasal cavity. In the vast majority of cases this is sufficient control the bleeding, but if insufficient, a post-nasal plug ill be required. To form the post-nasal plug, a piece of gauze folded until it is of a size which will fit tightly into the asopharynx of the patient. On an average, the gauze should e about the thickness of the thumb and perhaps not quite long. It is tied round the middle with tape. This tape is assed through the nose on the side which it is proposed to ack, and by it the pack is firmly anchored in the nasopharynx. he insertion of the pack, unless carried out with some degree f skill, is an unpleasant experience for the patient. To inimise the patient's discomfort, it is wiser to cocainize not nly the floor of the nose but also to spray the palate and the asopharynx with a little cocaine. A catheter is passed through e nose into the pharynx, where it is grasped by a pair f forceps and drawn out of the mouth. The end of the tape tied to the catheter, which is drawn back through the ose bringing the tape with it. By depressing the tongue, the ack can be slipped into the back of the throat, from which sition it can easily be pushed into the nasopharynx, this ing assisted by traction on the tape. The tape should be anchored to the face by means of strapping. The packing then carried out as detailed before, using the post-nasal pac as a base. In this way severe hæmorrhage can be controlled.

Control of hæmorrhage may also be accomplished by mea of a pneumatic plug. A large-sized finger cot is tied to fine gum-elastic catheter which is passed back into the nos The bag can then be inflated, filling the nasal cavity. A plu or clamp closes the catheter and the bag remains inflated.

The Control of Epistaxis by Obliteration of the Bleedin point.—Cases in which the bleeding is from Little's area len themselves to treatment by this method. The bleeding-poi should first be identified and the front part of the no packed with local anæsthetic, for example, cocaine solutio (5 per cent.) with adrenalin. When this has been left in for few minutes, the bleeding will be found in all probability to b very much less, and the bleeding veins will be seen to stan out clearly in the mucous membrane of the nose. Obliteratic can be carried out either with the actual cautery or with chromic acid bead. The electro-cautery is used at a dull re heat, and each vein in turn is obliterated with the point of th cautery, the cauterizing being made as superficial as possib consistent with the stoppage of the bleeding.

To control bleeding by chromic acid, a chromic bead mu be made. To make this, a probe is heated gently in a spi flame and some crystals of chromic acid are picked up on th point of the probe. The flame is then applied to the probe short distance above the crystals. After a moment or two th crystals melt, and will run down to form a drop on the poi of the probe. As soon as the crystals melt, the probe withdrawn from the flame and, by rotating the probe gentl a drop will adhere to the point of the probe until it cools. Th point of cooling is marked by the change from a bright, shinin black bead to one of a dull coke-like appearance. The bea is then used in a similar fashion to the cautery, but it mu be used sparingly and the excess of acid must be wiped aw immediately after each application.

General Treatment.—Brisk nasal hæmorrhage is frequent an alarming experience for a patient, and it is very oft wise before commencing treatment to give the patient injection of morphia or other sedative. This will help in ma cases to control the bleeding by keeping the patient qui and will make subsequent manipulations very much easier f the doctor. It is not proposed to deal here with nas hæmorrhage as the result of blood disease or other system conditions, as the treatment of epistaxis in these cases, apa 'om the purely local measures detailed above, belongs properly) the sections in which these diseases are found.

AFFECTIONS OF THE NOSE

Rhinitis.—*Acute Rhinitis.* (See Coryza.)

Purulent Rhinitis.—This form of infection is most fre- uently seen in conjunction with the exanthemata, and gnifies a virulent infection in the mucous membrane of the ose. Locally, it is treated with douches and ordinary cleanli- ess in conjunction with the general measures of the diseases uring the course of which the condition occurs.

Membranous Rhinitis.—As this condition is most frequently ue to the Klebs Löffler bacillus, the treatment is the same as cases of diphtheria. Other forms of membranous rhinitis e found in patients suffering from marked debility, and in ich cases they may be treated with mild alkaline douches, istillations of drops, such as argyrol (10 per cent.), protargol 0 per cent.), and other non-irritant applications. (For rescriptions, see Appendix.)

Chronic Rhinitis.—The treatment of chronic rhinitis depends a considerable extent upon the stage to which the chronic ondition has advanced. In the earliest stage the return of omfort to the patient depends upon the restoration of ciliary tion and, as this is prevented by the want of proper aeration the nose and the clogging of the mucous membrane with ickened secretions, treatment should be directed towards the lief of this condition, and alkaline douches are indicated. halations of menthol will help to decongest the mucous embrane. Menthol must not be used, however, in very oung children. A spray containing 0·5 to 1 per cent. of hedrine in normal saline or liquid paraffin is useful for a ort period, but should not be prescribed for prolonged use.

Where the rhinitis has progressed to the hypertrophic rm, which means the laying down of fibrous tissue within e mucous membrane, then treatment must be directed in e first place to the removal of the non-functioning fibrous ucous membrane, and this, therefore, will entail operative rocedures.

Atrophic Rhinitis.—In atrophic rhinitis there is such ktensive damage to the mucous membrane, and sometimes the underlying tissues and structures, that treatment alone ffers little hope of restoration of function. Treatment there- re resolves itself into the problem of providing the maximum omfort for the patient under the circumstances. This means that the accumulation of secretions which, owing to the lacl of ciliary function, dry and form crusts within the nasal cavity has to be removed, otherwise the patient would suffer fron chronic obstruction of the nose. A certain amount can b done to moisten the thin and dry nasal mucous membrane but, except in the *earliest stages*, the condition cannot be cure and even then can only be checked.

The removal of the crusts is best carried out by means o douching, with or without the preliminary softening of th crusts within the nose. If the crusting is heavy, the patien should be instructed on rising in the morning to plug botl nostrils with cotton-wool to moisten the crusts. After abou half an hour, he should douche the nose with a weak salin solution, *e.g.*, 1 teaspoonful of salt to a pint of warm water Where the crusting is not so heavy and the condition is in th earlier stages, the nose should be douched with mild alkalin solution (see Appendix, p. 773).

The nose can be douched morning and night ; but, i douching once daily is sufficient, the cleansing should b confined to this one occasion. Excessive douching is apt t lead to irritation and further discomfort. After douching, th nose should be sprayed with an oily solution. A light oil i best for this purpose and may contain some essential oil t render the odour pleasant. This helps to protect the mucou membrane, and also tends to delay the formation of crusts.

Other forms of treatment may be tried, as, for instance plugging the nose for one or two hours daily with gauze o wool soaked in glucose solution. Recently an oily spray o Oestrin has been found to be of value.

Ozœna.—This affection is usually looked upon as a separat entity, but it closely resembles atrophic rhinitis, the onl additional feature which has to be combated being the fœto which is characteristic. This condition should be treated in similar manner to the above, the nose being plugged on risin and then douched with a weak saline solution once or twic daily. Efficient cleansing of the nose will ensure the dis appearance of the disagreeable odour, and will at least permi the patient to mix with other persons. If the cleansing i done properly and is persisted in for a sufficiently long time the tendency to crust-formation and the fœtid odour wi disappear and the patient will be left with a rather dry nose but most of the unpleasant symptoms will have disappeared.

Nasal Polypi.—The treatment of nasal polypi is symp tomatic only, in so far as this section is concerned. A carefu search must first be made for the underlying cause, and th reatment will depend upon what is discovered. Treatment nay be instituted, for example, on account of an allergic asis for the polypus formation, or investigation may necessitate he treatment of an underlying affection of the sinuses. Local reatment of the polypi consists in their removal by forceps nd wire snare. Occasionally, it is found that polypi disappear pontaneously, but delay in treatment should never be allowed n the hope that this may occur.

Syphilis and Tuberculosis.—These conditions are fully dealt vith elsewhere and need not be mentioned here (see pp. 206, 92).

Nasal Allergy.—The question of allergy is also considered n another section. Local treatment, however, may be called or in the nose. Ephedrine is the most useful drug in such ases. Ephedrine is applied either as drops or a spray (0·5 or per cent.) in normal saline solution or a light oil.

Other treatments, such as radiation of various types, may e used ; infra-red rays are sometimes of value when directed o the mucous membrane. Ultra-violet rays do not appear o have as great value as infra-red.

Radium has become popular in certain quarters and has een used mostly where there has been polypus formation vithout underlying sinusitis, but as the danger of necrosis nd perforation of the septum is considerable, this form of reatment must be used with extreme care and only under xpert guidance. Zinc ionization will in many cases give omplete comfort to the sufferers from nasal allergy. This reatment involves the packing of both nasal cavities with auze or wool soaked in 2 per cent. zinc sulphate solution hrough which an electric current is passed. This has the ffect upon the nasal mucous membrane of restricting the pasmodic discharge and the irritability which are characteristic f the condition. It has been used to a great extent in cases f specific nasal allergy, as, for example, hay-fever, but is lso of value in the non-specific types of sensitivity.

Foreign Bodies in the Nose.—Removal is the only treatment or foreign bodies in the nose. If a foreign body is close to he nasal vestibule anteriorly, it is usually easily removed, rovided a suitable pair of forceps is at hand and adequate ssistance is available to control the patient. If the patient s old enough to co-operate, it will be found of considerable dvantage to shrink the nose with 10 per cent. solution of ocaine containing adrenalin (1 : 1,000)—5 drops of adrenalin o the ounce of cocaine solution. This will facilitate manipulaion and, by the shrinkage of the nose, will render the removal f the foreign body a comparatively simple matter. In the case of a small child, the patient must be controlled by another person, preferably not the mother, and it is useless to attempt the removal of the foreign body unless the assistant is capable of holding the child perfectly still. It may be necessary, in cases of doubt, to give an anæsthetic in order to make a complete examination of the nasal cavity. An anæsthetic in such cases should never be given without adequate preparation, for the child is frequently frightened and resistive, and, as such, may make an extremely bad subject for anæsthesia. When it is decided to give an anæsthetic, a finger should be inserted into the nasopharynx and placed in the choana of the nostril which is being examined, as it is possible to push the foreign body backwards into the nasopharynx whence it may be either inhaled or swallowed. The finger in the nasopharynx will prevent such an accident and will also assist, in certain cases, in gripping the foreign body. If it is thought that the foreign body is radio-opaque, such manipulation should be preceded by an X-ray of the skull. Occasionally, if a foreign body has remained in the nostril for some time, it will form the core of a concretion. These concretions may be very large, and it may be found advisable to break them up before removing them.

SINUSITIS

In the treatment of sinusitis the aims are similar to those in affections of the nose, namely, the relief of pain and the restoration of function. The loss of ciliary function for a prolonged period may render treatment unavailing. If, therefore, surgical treatment is to be avoided, the early stages of the physiological derangement must not be neglected. As pain is so frequently the result of obstruction to drainage, the relief of pain in many cases becomes the problem of securing the release of contents obstructed within the sinus. As the sinus can only drain through the small ostium into the nasal cavity, treatment is primarily directed towards restoring the patency of the ostium. Agents are used which have the function of shrinking the mucous membrane of the nose. Of these, the simplest are steam inhalations containing menthol which not only help to shrink the mucous membrane but also have an analgesic action and will relieve the accompanying discomfort. Ephedrine (1 per cent.) in isotonic saline solution or oil may also be instilled into the nose. This will help to shrink the turbinates and will open up the œdematous middle meatus. These drops can be repeated at frequent intervals as required, and may be sufficient to promote a flow of secretion from the sinuses. In certain cases where the turbinates show very marked engorgement, a pledget of wool soaked in cocaine (10 per cent.) can be inserted into the upper part of the nose against the middle turbinate. This causes a very marked retraction of the turbinate and will frequently be successful in relieving an obstruction. It may have to be repeated, however, at frequent intervals, and it must be remembered that cocaine has a reaction which may defeat the original purpose of its application. Rest is of the utmost importance in the treatment of sinusitis, and a patient should always be advised to refrain from business or other activity, since return to health will be delayed if he insists on carrying on with his daily work. Another essential is that the patient should remain in the same temperature as far as possible, to prevent changes in the tension in the nasal mucous membrane. Accordingly, rest in bed is generally advisable, as this provides the easiest method of controlling the patient's activity ; and should there be any constitutional disturbance, this must be insisted upon. For the pain itself, apart from measures which aim at the relief of tension within the sinuses, the application of heat in various forms is the most valuable way of relieving the patient. Radiant-heat baths will frequently cause an immediate diminution in the congested condition of the sinuses and relieve the patient. On the other hand, they may possibly increase the patient's discomfort ; in such cases the radiant-heat baths should be immediately discontinued. Short-wave diathermy is also of value, though in the very acute stages this may cause even greater pain and is best reserved for the subacute stage when the sinusitis is commencing to clear up. Heat may be applied as fomentations over the affected sinuses, or, if available, electric pads may be used instead.

In the purulent stage of the infection, where there is considerable constitutional disturbance, the object of treatment should be to avoid operative interference if that be possible. Surgical measures should be reserved until the acute stage has passed. It may happen, however, that increasing severity of symptoms, such as swelling or increase of pain, may render it necessary to undertake some operative measure for the relief of the patient. In the maxillary sinus the simple process of proof-puncture may be sufficient to give the patient relief. Proof-puncture, however, in the stage of acute inflammation may be extremely painful, so that the question of anæsthesia, local or general, must receive careful consideration. This procedure has its greatest value where the sinus is filled with purulent fluid. In many cases of the most acute type, however, there is no cavity within the sinus, the whole space being occupied with œdematous mucous membrane. In which case proof-puncture will accomplish nothing and will merely give the patient added pain. Where proof-puncture is found to be of value, it may be repeated on three or four occasions. Each case must be judged by the individual reaction to the procedure, but as a rule it should not be repeated within two or three days' time, and if after three or four punctures sufficient improvement is not obtained, it is obvious that proof-puncture is inadequate and further operative interference must be considered.

Chronic Sinusitis.—In chronic sinusitis it is frequently worth while to attempt to clear up the infection before having recourse to surgical means, for sometimes the symptoms are referable to a slight and intermittent degree of obstruction to drainage. Full investigation of these cases should be undertaken before treatment is finally decided upon. Where gross infection is shown by radiography, and where there is obviously polypus formation within the sinus, then conservative measures are not likely to achieve cure and recourse must be had to surgery. Where, however, the infection is not severe, proof-puncture and lavage with saline solution may be sufficient to allow the cilia to recover function.

The displacement method of introducing agents within the sinuses is a useful one. It consists of applying suction to the nose in such a way that when the head is placed in a suitable position the ostia of the sinuses are submerged in the solution which is being introduced. The air is drawn out of the sinus by the suction, and the drug allowed thereby to find its way in. Ephedrine in saline (½ per cent.) is frequently used in this way; by its gradual elimination it gives a prolonged action and keeps the ostium shrunk, thus allowing drainage over a considerable period. Short-wave diathermy, by causing a certain degree of hyperæmia within the sinus, may be effective in clearing up an infection which has not been too long established.

Complications of Chronic Sinusitis.—The chief complications of sinusitis which require treatment are osteomyelitis, abscess formation without the sinuses, such changes in the eyes as are induced by pressure either upon the orbit or upon the optic nerve, and meningitis. This last is a late complication due to extension of the disease.

The treatment of these complications of sinusitis is mainly palliative, pending the arrival of surgical assistance. Osteomyelitis of the bones of the face, that is, of the maxilla and the frontal bone, when established, calls for immediate surgical treatment. In the early stages, however, there may be a degree of hyperæmia of the bone which can be held in check by local measures such as fomentations and the application of heat. The accompanying septicæmia may be treated by those alive to the possibility of its presence before surgical aid has arrived. For the detailed treatment of septicæmia the reader is referred to the appropriate section. Localized abscess formation around the sinuses in the earlier stages calls for palliative treatment by fomentations and the application of heat to relieve pain. The use of poultices or blisters is to be deprecated, as in so many of these cases subsequent surgical treatment is demanded and the result is that incision may have to be made through blistered and damaged skin. Such conditions greatly increase the difficulty of surgical treatment and also the likelihood of widespread infection of the skin and soft tissues. An obviously fluctuating swelling, where radical treatment cannot be undertaken, may be incised ; this may be all that is required for the immediate relief of symptoms. Occasionally, the diagnosis of the presence of pus offers difficulty to the inexperienced, and in such cases a fairly large bore-needle and a record-syringe may be used to aspirate the suspicious swelling in order to locate the pus. In this way unnecessary incisions on the face may be avoided. Where meningitis is established, the treatment is along general lines after the primary focus has been adequately dealt with (see p. 980).

THE PHARYNX

TONSILLITIS

Acute Tonsillitis.—The treatment of this affection depends upon the stage to which the illness has progressed. In the earliest stages, where there is merely a hyperæmia of the tonsillar region, simple precautions may be sufficient to abort the disease. But it must be firmly impressed upon the reader that this condition must never be treated as of small consequence, and fairly stringent regulations of the patient's activity at the beginning of the illness may save him from great trouble at a later date. As a working rule, one may say that if there is any general disturbance, such as rise of pulse-rate or temperature, a feeling of illness, malaise, or shivering, then the patient should be put to bed. Regulation of the bowels is a first consideration, but unnecessary purging should be avoided. Owing to his sore throat, the patient will, in all probability, limit his intake of fluid, and it is therefore unwise to increase fluid loss by excessive purging. Where there is rise of temperature, antifebrile drugs may be used, such as the salicylates. The local treatment consists chiefly of gargles and paints, which should be of a mild nature. There should be no nipping or burning with any of the drugs used. The mucous membrane is in an inflamed condition and requires soothing and not irritation. A gargle of carbolic acid, sodium sulphocarbolate, sodium bicarbonate and glycerin (see Appendix) may be used.

Boroglycerin is a good paint in early acute cases. There may be, even in the earliest stages, a marked glandular involvement. The glands of the submaxillary and upper cervical region may be tender and swollen, limiting thereby the movements of the neck. These conditions may be met by hot fomentations of boracic, poultices of linseed, or applications such as kaolin. These give relief and also reduce swelling.

In the follicular stage of tonsillitis, in which the tonsils are found to be spotted, treatment is frequently simpler, as at such a stage the patient is usually quite willing to retire to bed. The symptoms are rise of temperature and of pulse-rate, with associated pain and difficulty in swallowing. This may be so severe as to determine the nature of the patient's diet, confining it to fluids such as tea, barley water, glucose and orange juice, strained soup and porridge. Locally, gargles and paints are again required, and treatment of the glands of the neck should they be enlarged and tender.

In the membranous form of tonsillitis there is an extension of the infection from the above stage, and treatment has to be correspondingly energetic. The patient's general condition, as a rule, is weaker and his fluid intake is usually considerably limited owing to the extreme pain in swallowing. In such cases, if the patient does not seem to be taking sufficient liquid by the mouth it must be given in other ways. This may take the form of a rectal saline, but the best method is the administration of glucose (5 per cent.) in normal saline by the continuous-drip system. In this stage of the infection, gargles are frequently ineffective, as the patient may lack the strength to use them. The membrane also frequently covers parts of the throat to which the gargle does not reach. Under these circumstances an antiseptic spray may be the best means of cleansing the infected parts. The spray may consist of hydrogen peroxide and water, in equal parts, or a solution of glycerin of thymol (see Appendix, p. 774). Soothing paints, also, are excellent, because they help to ease the local condition and stimulate swallowing and the flow of saliva. Inhalations may be required because the inflammation is seldom localized and there is frequently hyperæmia of the larynx. A useful inhalation consists of 15 to 20 drops of tinct. benzoini co. in 1 pint of hot water.

It is important to maintain as much movement as possible in the throat and to keep the surfaces constantly cleansed. It is for this reason that sprays are of such value, for, even if the saliva is deficient, they induce swallowing movements or the coughing up of infected material. In children, especially, the spray is useful when the throat becomes really sore. A child sometimes refuses to gargle or drink, and it is in these cases that the greatest danger occurs from dehydration. Further, the throat is held completely quiet so that the infection becomes severe and there is little or no cleansing of the parts locally. In order to spray the throat, a certain amount of force may be required to control the child properly, and, as it is unlikely that the mother will be able to carry out this treatment adequately, it is usually best to have these cases under the charge of a nurse or to place them in hospital. An excess of affection has before now been responsible for tragedy in the case of a child.

Complications.—Of the complications of tonsillitis, peritonsillar abscess or quinsy is the most frequent. In the early stages, in which the tonsillar region is slightly swollen and the soft palate is showing only a little sign of œdema, palliatives are indicated, such as frequent hot gargles and fomentations to the glands. Sleep is usually interfered with, and it is an excellent thing to give a sedative at night in order to conserve the patient's strength. The question frequently arises as to when is the correct time for surgical assistance. It may be said that when the soft palate has a distinct bulge on one side and the tonsil is pushed towards the mid-line, then an attempt may be made to locate pus behind the tonsil. Many cases are seen only when there is an obvious bulge in some part or other of the swollen soft palate. In such cases it is a simple matter to push a pair of blunt forceps into the soft swelling and evacuate the pus. Where, however, no point of softening exists, the peritonsillar abscess is best opened from the superior tonsillar crypt. A long pair of blunt-pointed forceps is used. If desired, the throat may be sprayed with cocaine (10 per cent.), or an anæsthetic lozenge may be given to the patient to suck. This rarely has the effect of lessening the pain of the opening of the abscess, but it frequently diminishes the amount of trismus present and helps to give the patient confidence. The forceps are inserted into the superior tonsillar crypt and pushed sharply upwards and outwards through the capsule into the abscess cavity, and widely opened. This is followed by a gush of pus and the patient experiences a very great sense of relief. Hot gargles are given and treatment continued as before until the swelling has disappeared from the side of the throat.

Abscesses may occur in other parts of the throat as the result of tonsillar infection. These are more frequent in young children. They occur either in the nasopharynx or in the hypopharynx, and their treatment demands evacuation at an early stage of the infection. Correct treatment is of the utmost importance, and the possibility of this affection being present should never be lost sight of in unexplained illnesses in young children, where there is difficulty in breathing or swallowing. In all cases of acute tonsillitis and its complications, when general infection is marked, the use of sulphanilamide is of the greatest value in reducing the toxæmia accompanying the infection.

Chronic Tonsillitis.—Chronic tonsillar infection occurs with comparative frequency in adults, but many are unaware of their disability. These patients are symptom-free, because they have acquired immunity to their infection, and it is not until some general infection, or lowering of resistance, causes a break down of the immunity, that symptoms appear which demand attention. The use of palliative treatment in such a case is to enable the immunity to be built up again. Therefore, although it may not be necessary to remove tonsils at all times when they are found to be infected, the problem of treatment is that of the patient's ability to sustain the operation without injury to body or mind.

Palliative treatment may consist of painting the tonsils in cases of chronic tonsillitis such paints are of a faintly irritating character, the commonest of these being Mandl's paint. Gargles may be recommended, as they serve the purpose of exercising the pharyngeal muscles and ensuring an adequate blood supply to the parts concerned. In such cases, also, suction is recommended as likely to remove the debris and infected material from the tonsil and, no doubt, as far as the surface is concerned, it will do so. But a consideration of the anatomy of the tonsil will suggest very strongly that the tortuous channels of small size which constitute the crypts are not likely to be adequately evacuated by any method of surface suction. Radiation of various kinds has been used in tonsillitis ultra-violet and infra-red may be applied directly to the tonsil by means of the Kromayer or other lamp with special applicators. These produce hyperæmia within the tonsil, and the increased blood supply may reasonably be expected to deal with some of the earlier forms of infection. Where, however, infection has been established over a prolonged period, with the usual fibrous tissue formation and replacement of columnar epithelium with other forms, such treatment cannot reverse the established pathological changes. Gamma radiation has been recommended for treatment in inflamed tonsils, and there is no doubt that radiation will remove tonsillar tissue, if used in sufficiently large doses. But it is equally evident that if used in sufficient dosage to destroy the tonsil, the side-effects are such that the treatment does not justify the expenditure of the time and money required. Either the reactions are severe—very much more so than with a simple tonsillectomy—or the treatment is so prolonged that the expense will be a very serious consideration.

The technique of removal of the tonsils does not fall within the scope of this section, but the practitioner may have to make the decision as to when the tonsils should be removed, and to know the appropriate method. Operations for tonsillectomy are many and the details vary according to the ideas of the surgeon concerned, but they all aim at the complete removal of the tonsil and its surrounding capsule. The tonsil may be dissected out from its bed or may be removed completely by diathermy coagulation. The coagulation technique has received prominence of recent years and considerable claims have been made for it. The complete removal of the tonsil by coagulation involves some half a dozen sittings and occupies a considerable period of time.

There is practical unanimity of opinion that removal by surgical dissection is the quickest and most satisfactory method. The disadvantages of the operation are that the patient is confined to bed for some days and has to cease work during that time. He is subject to a certain amount of operative risk, possibly to an anæsthetic and to the psychological upset inseparable from the idea of an operation. The advantage of the coagulation method is that the patient need not necessarily be off work, that the treatment can be carried out in the consulting room or office, and, though frequently painful, is not so incapacitating as operation and can be applied in cases where the physical state of the patient contraindicates surgical measures. The outstanding disadvantage of the method is that it is impossible to guarantee complete removal of the tonsil in every case. Diathermy coagulation has no selective action upon the tonsillar tissue, and if complete coagulation of the tonsil is guaranteed, it is impossible to ensure that the deeper structures of the throat are left unharmed. The treatment tends to be lengthy and is frequently more painful than those carrying it out are wont to admit.

PHARYNGITIS

The treatment of pharyngitis is a twofold problem. In the vast majority of cases of pharyngitis, we are concerned with a remote cause which is having a local effect. It is essential in the first instance to inquire with care into the patient's habits, surroundings and type of work. Habits, particularly with regard to smoking and alcohol, require investigation. The presence or absence of gastric trouble, rheumatism and like diseases may modify the attitude towards treatment. Excessive dust or a special type of atmosphere may be found to be of ætiological importance. For instance, the presence of ammonia fumes or other forms of irritant may require to be eliminated before treatment can be successful. Inflammation or suppuration in other parts of the upper air passages may be causing the pharyngitis. One of the commonest of these causes is a sinusitis, and the sinusitis will require treatment before any improvement can be expected in the pharynx. Treatment of chronic tonsillitis may be necessary, though it should be noted in this connection that the removal of tonsils for the cure of pharyngitis should not be undertaken, except after most careful consideration, as in most cases the tonsillectomy will tend to aggravate the chronic pharyngitis rather than to improve it.

The local treatment of pharyngitis depends upon whether the condition is acute or chronic. In the acute stage palliatives only should be considered, and soothing applications to the pharynx must be made until the acute symptoms have subsided. Gargles are rarely of value in a pharyngitis, apart from helping the flow of saliva and assisting in the lubrication of the mucous membrane. Sprays and paints of boroglycerin or glycerin and tannin are of real value. Steam inhalations are soothing in the more severe types of case. These may be medicated, as, for instance, with friars' balsam. Lozenges containing menthol or other drugs are soothing to the patient. In the chronic stage, treatment is more of the nature of counter-irritation, and such applications may be made to the pharynx locally as will help to stimulate the resolution of the inflamed mucous membrane. Paints, such as Mandl's paint, or the careful touching of the inflamed portions of membrane with iodine or with silver nitrate (10 per cent.), will help to reduce the irritation. The cautery or diathermy, also, may be used to destroy the red lymphoid nodes in the pharyngeal wall. These measures, however, must be employed with the greatest care. If the cautery is employed the throat should be painted with 10 per cent. cocaine, after which the fine cautery point may be used very sparingly on the enlarged lymph nodes.

Retro-pharyngeal Abscess.—The difficulties caused by retro-pharyngeal abscess are chiefly those of diagnosis; but where obstruction of the nasopharynx or larynx is being caused by abscess formation, the relief of the obstruction is the treatment immediately required. The abscess, if causing obstruction, must be opened, and this may be done by the oral route, except in the case of abscesses which have their origin in tuberculous cervical caries.

NEUROSES OF PHARYNX

Sensory Neurosis.—Paræsthesia, or the underlying cause of paræsthesia, may be found to be some degree of pharyngitis or enlargement of lingual tonsil and, in such cases, removal of these is the first step in treatment. The majority of patients who appear for treatment for this unpleasant sensation in the pharynx are cancer-phobes, and in such cases one of the most important parts of the treatment is the suggestion to the patient that there is no underlying disease and that a little local treatment is probably all that is required.

Anæsthesia of the Pharynx.—This condition usually accompanies lesions of the base of the brain, and therefore is not amenable to treatment.

Glosso-pharyngeal Tic.—The treatment of glosso-pharyngeal tic falls into the category of surgical treatment and consists of nerve resection.

PATERSON-KELLY SYNDROME (PLUMMER-VINSON)

The local treatment of this obstruction consists in the stretching of the stricture through a laryngoscope or the œsophagoscope. The blind intubation of these cases is to be deprecated, and, in the first instance, treatment should be carried out under direct vision by those experienced in such procedures.

THE EAR

DISEASES OF THE EXTERNAL EAR

The Auricle.—*Injuries.*—Hæmatoma of the auricle calls for treatment on account of its unsightliness and the possibility of subsequent infection with destruction of the cartilage. Where large, it is best treated by aspiration of the swelling, with proper aseptic precautions. The ear should be cleaned with spirit and a hypodermic syringe and needle should be inserted into the auricle and blood-stained fluid withdrawn. This should be repeated if necessary. The ear should then be bandaged firmly, or, if inflamed, should be covered with an ichthyol and glycerin soak (10 per cent.).

Perichondritis.—When inflammation has supervened, treatment consists in the application of soothing remedies. Ichthyol and glycerin (10 per cent.) or boric fomentations should be applied ; and if pus forms, it should be evacuated.

Skin Affections.—*Furunculosis,* or hair-follicle infection, calls for soothing treatment in the first stages. The ear should be packed with gauze soaked with ichthyol and glycerin and heat applied outside the ear in the form of boric fomentations or a thermal pad. Ultra-violet radiation has been tried in the effort to abort the abscess or to cause it to develop quickly. Short-wave diathermy may be used for the same purpose. It is better to avoid incision as far as possible, but where the furuncle is very large and pus has obviously formed, then incision may be undertaken.

Otitis Externa.—The treatment of otitis externa varies according to the stage of the disease and its particular type. In many of these cases the ear is filled with discharge and debris : it may therefore be essential to cleanse it by syringing. If possible this course should be avoided, and if syringing has to be resorted to, the ear should be carefully dried afterwards.

In the very acutely inflamed type, where there is some perichondritis, the treatment should be the same as that outlined for furunculosis. When the most acute stage has passed, then the ear should be packed with strips of gauze soaked in aluminium acetate solution (8 per cent.). The same solution is used for the drier and more scaly types of infection: it soothes and quickly dries up the skin. To cause the condition to clear up finally, a useful application is $2\frac{1}{2}$ per cent. alcoholic solution of gentian violet. The external meatus should be swabbed with this solution, and the solution should be dried in the meatus by a blower.

Wax in the Ear.—Wax in the ear is removed by syringing. Where the wax is very hard, before syringing it should first be softened by the instillation of drops of saturated solution of bicarbonate of soda. Half a dozen drops of this should be instilled four or five times for one to two days preceding the syringing. The syringing of the ear may be carried out either with an ear-syringe, which should have finger-rings, or, in default of this, with a Higginson's syringe. The temperature of the syringing fluid is of importance and the optimum temperature is blood heat, for by the use of such a temperature, unpleasant effects upon the internal ear are avoided. Warm water, preferably boiled, is quite effective, or tap water with a few drops of antiseptic added may be used. The patient should be instructed to hold the basin or kidney-dish underneath the ear to catch the waste water, and a trough which fits around the ear will be found of great advantage in avoiding splashing. Unless the person carrying out the treatment is experienced, a sharp nozzle should not be used upon the syringe as this is liable to damage the meatal wall. The stream of water should be directed against the posterior superior aspect of the meatal wall. By doing so the plug of wax is loosened and the water passing behind the wax tends to force the plug outwards. Great force must not be used, and if considerable difficulty is being experienced, it will assist if the posterior edge of the wax plug be elevated from the meatal wall to make a point of entry for the stream of water. During the syringing frequent inspection of the meatus should be made in order to ascertain the progress of the removal.

After the plug of wax has been removed the ear should be dried of excess fluid. If, as sometimes happens, some epithelium is removed along with the wax and a raw place is left on the meatal wall, it is wise to pack the ear with a strip of gauze soaked in aluminium acetate solution (8 per cent.) for twelve hours to prevent the possibility of infection. Where there is known to be a perforation in the drum, wax should not be removed by syringing, but preferably by being picked out if necessary after softening. Where there is a perforation of the drum there is a possibility of the water passing through into the middle-ear cleft and setting up an acute inflammation.

Keratosis Obturans.—This condition consists of the impaction of a very large plug of wax in the inner part of the external meatus with subsequent epithelial destruction by pressure. The hardness of the plug may be such that a general anæsthetic may be required to accomplish its removal.

Foreign Bodies in the Ear.—From the point of view of treatment, foreign bodies in the ear may be divided into three classes—vegetable, mineral and animal.

Vegetable foreign bodies, *e.g.*, a pea, should not be removed by syringing. If the initial syringing is unsuccessful, the foreign body will swell with the water and give the patient excruciating pain, and also render the subsequent removal extremely difficult. Mineral foreign bodies, such as glass beads, are most easily removed by syringing. If this fails, a proper equipment of ear-forceps, hooks, etc., is required for their safe removal. Insects and such animal foreign bodies should be killed first by the instillation of spirit drops or chloroform vapour, and then syringed out. In small children, anæsthesia is frequently required for the safe removal of the foreign body. It is useless to attempt to remove a foreign body from the ear of a kicking, struggling child. In such cases the proper preparation should be made for the anæsthetic. A lengthy administration may be necessary since some foreign bodies may tax the ingenuity and the patience of the operator if they are to be removed without damage to the drum.

AFFECTIONS OF THE DRUM

Rupture of the Drum.—Whether this occurs as a result of a concussion, for example from a blow or gun-fire, or from a fracture of the skull, the main principle of treatment is masterly inactivity. In cases where rupture has taken place and suppuration, as may frequently happen, sets in, then the treatment is the same as that of conservative treatment for acute otitis media, to which the reader is referred.

Myringitis Bullosa.—Very large hæmorrhagic blisters may occasionally be opened, but as long as the hearing is good and the constitutional disturbance is slight, soothing drops—for instance, carbolic (4 per cent.) in glycerin—should be instilled.

Herpes.—Herpes of the auricle and meatus may occur as part of herpes zoster oticus (Hunt's disease). The local condition is treated as in otitis externa, the chief symptom requiring attention being pain.

DISEASES OF THE MIDDLE EAR

Acute Otitis Media.—In acute otitis media treatment is required on account of pain, deafness, discharge from the ear and constitutional disturbance. The condition, from the point of view of treatment, falls naturally into two groups: firstly, treatment of acute otitis media before discharge appears in the ear; and, secondly, after discharge has made its appearance.

Acute Otitis Media before Discharge.—Pain is here the chief complaint. As this pain is due to irritation of nerve-endings in the acutely inflamed and tightly stretched drum membrane, direct application to the inflamed membrane may be made by means of anæsthetic drops. One of the most useful forms of application is carbolic acid in glycerin (4 per cent.); to this may be added cocaine (20 per cent.). Heat is a favoured form of application, and warm drops of oil have been used traditionally as a soothing application to the ear. This, however, is not a good method of treatment, as the ear is liable to be damaged by such instillations. Heat applied, as a fomentation of boric lint wrung out of hot water or a saturated solution of magnesium sulphate, outside the ear, is equally effective.

Constitutional symptoms also call for treatment. The rise of temperature and pulse-rate with a general feeling of illness may be met by confining the patient to bed. In cases of constipation, treatment should begin with a purge, though violent purging should be avoided. Fluids should be given freely; starvation is not indicated, and the patient should be given a good sustaining diet. Drug treatment should not include antifebrile drugs. The administration of such drugs as aspirin, antipyrin, etc., may bring the temperature down, but at the same time they so obscure the clinical picture that it is difficult to form an accurate estimate of the progress of the infection. If the pain is severe, it may be relieved by sedatives. Sulphanilamide may be given from the beginning of the illness, as the constitutional symptoms in this case are signs of toxæmia. The dosage may be 6 to 8 tablets daily for an adult, and up to 6 for a child of seven years.

Treatment after the Discharge Appears.—The chief principle in treatment at this stage is the encouragement of the free flow of discharge. In addition to promoting the flow through either the perforation or the paracentesis opening, an endeavour must be made to promote the reopening of the natural drainage channel—the Eustachian tube. Once discharge is established, nature must be assisted in drying up the secretions.

There are two principal methods of treatment of this type of affection, and there are two distinct schools of thought regarding the proper method of management. These methods are referred to as the dry method and the wet method. The dry method aims at introducing nothing into the area which is likely to convey sepsis into the middle ear. The wet method consists in cleansing the ear with the simplest form of apparatus, namely, the syringe, and then adopting measures as in the dry method which will help nature to dry up the discharge. The dry method entails a considerable amount of attention. The ear has to be cleansed carefully under direct vision at frequent intervals. In one of the most successful methods a wick of wool or gauze is inserted into the meatus, close to the perforation, so that it acts by capillary attraction in withdrawing fluid rapidly from the middle ear. The ear may then be mopped dry at intervals and drying drops instilled, *e.g.*, of boric acid and rectified spirits.

In the dry method, nothing is gained by mere wiping of the outer part of the ear. The ear must be dried right to the drum and all excess of secretions and debris must be removed so that a completely clear channel is left for the discharge. In addition, the external meatus must be wiped with antiseptic before mopping the ear, so that sepsis is not transferred from the outer part to the inside of the ear.

The wet method of treatment consists of instilling into the ear drops of peroxide of hydrogen which by their action tend to loosen the discharge which accumulates in the ear. This discharge is then syringed out with an antiseptic lotion. This may consist of boric lotion, lysol (1 teaspoonful to a pint of water) or other weak antiseptic. After syringing, the ear is mopped dry as far as possible and, if desired, drying drops are instilled into the ear.

The relative value of these methods is worth consideration on account of statements having been made that it is almost a malpractice to syringe the ear when it is the seat of an acute otitis media. Theoretically speaking, the dry method is the best for dealing with an ear suppuration, but it presupposes a knowledge and a skill which is not to be expected or demanded from the average nurse. In cases where treatment is carried out at home or has to be done by an overworked district nurse, the wet method has a distinct advantage and is widely used in certain clinics, notably in Scotland, where the distressing results assumed by certain writers have never been observed.

Besides the methods detailed above for improving the condition of the ear, other means may be used for withdrawing discharge from the middle ear. When available, suction is of use in skilled hands. The ear may be cleared to some extent of discharge by catheterizing the Eustachian tube and blowing air through the middle ear. This should not be done in the earlier stages of the disease, but is useful for helping to empty the middle ear when the disease is beginning to resolve.

nflation of the Eustachian tube must always be done at the nd of treatment. After the ear is dry, the hearing in the najority of cases is subnormal and inflation of the Eustachian ube will do a considerable amount towards restoring it to ormal and, in many cases, will prevent permanent deafness. This inflation should always form the last step in the treatment, nd must never be neglected.

Indications for Paracentesis.—Although paracentesis is a urgical procedure, it must sometimes be undertaken by those vho are at a considerable distance from hospital service, and t is therefore essential that the medical practitioner underaking the treatment of acute otitis media should have a clear dea of the conditions which demand this procedure. One of he first effects of an acute infection on an ear-drum is the roduction of pain, owing to the irritation of the nerve endings y the inflammation and the tension; if the pain becomes xcessive, relief may be obtained by paracentesis. Secondly, f there is increasing toxæmia with obvious middle-ear infection nd the tympanic membrane is bulging, relief may be expected y the release of the contents of the middle ear. Again, if a lrum is evidently upon the point of perforation, indicated by yellowish area appearing at the most prominent part, mmediate relief by paracentesis may obviate the sloughing f the drum membrane; a surgical cut so made will heal apidly, causing less permanent damage to the drum structure han if a portion of the membrane is allowed to slough out. Vhere deafness is becoming more marked, owing to increasing ension in the middle ear, paracentesis may afford the most ertain method of ensuring rapid and complete return of earing.

In the treatment of these cases of acute middle-ear nfection, one principle must always be observed, viz., that reatment is to be directed towards the prevention of deafness: e can do little or nothing for a patient once the hearing has een lost for a period. In this case above all others, prevention s better than cure.

An adequate source of light is required to carry out aracentesis. This may be obtained either from an electric amp, the light from which may be focused upon the ear by neans of a head-mirror, or it may be obtained from an electric uriscope. Before carrying out a paracentesis the ear must e cleansed thoroughly and completely so that a clear view f the drum-membrane is obtained. General anæsthesia is dvisable in all cases. When the patient has been properly næsthetized, a paracentesis knife is introduced and the drum is incised in the posterior half in the form of a J, the upright portion commencing a little below the posterior horizontal fold of the drum and the incision being brought round in the lower part to finish just below the handle of the malleus. This procedure must, of course, be carried out with proper aseptic precautions, and the after-treatment is that for discharging ear.

Complications of Acute Otitis Media.—Treatment of complications of acute otitis media is almost entirely a surgical problem. Although questions of treatment of such conditions as septicæmia and meningitis may arise, they should always be preceded by adequate surgical measures, and their treatment is fully dealt with elsewhere.

Chronic Otitis Media.—Treatment of this condition depends to a great extent upon the type of suppuration, the part of the ear cavity which is affected, the duration of the condition and the presence or absence of bone disease. It is obvious, therefore, that an adequate knowledge of the state of affairs in the middle ear is essential for the proper planning of the treatment. In the consideration of such a case the circumstances of the individual must not be overlooked, and treatment should be selected with regard to these circumstances, as, for instance, the patient's means and the conditions of his work, as well as from considerations demanded by the nature of the suppuration.

The treatment of chronic otitis media has three chief aims of which the first and most important is the assurance of safety to the patient. The preservation of hearing is next in importance, for hearing is usually the equivalent of earning power. Lastly, provided the first two conditions are satisfied treatment should reduce to a minimum the loss of working time. Both surgical and conservative treatment play a part in the cure of chronic otitis media. Surgical treatment is essential in the presence of certain complications, such as brain-abscess, labyrinthitis, necrosis of bone and extensive cholesteatoma formation. Conditions such as these do not admit of any other treatment than surgical operation. The selection of the type of operation will fall upon the surgeon who will make his decision in view of the conditions present and in keeping with the principles which have just been laid down.

Conservative Treatment.—This must be regarded as the method of choice. If a polypus is present in the ear, this may be removed, and granulations may be scraped or touched with silver nitrate or chromic acid. The object in view in the treatment of chronic otitis media is to dry up the discharge. To do this, the ear must first be cleansed of accumulated debris, wax, etc.; secondly, drying agents are instilled into the ear; and, thirdly, special forms of treatment may be used. To cleanse the ear, peroxide of hydrogen drops can be instilled in order to loosen any accumulated debris. This should then be syringed out with boric lotion or other mild antiseptic. In cases of very copious discharge, this may be done morning and evening, but in most cases, once daily will be found sufficient. Syringing is sometimes carried out in special ways: where the chief infection is located in the attic, a cannula may be introduced into the attic region which is then syringed out. In the same way, syringing may be carried out through perforations. Drops, instilled into the ear, have for their objects antisepsis and the drying up of the discharge. The simplest method is the introduction of spirit. This may be rectified spirit or industrial spirit. It is usually combined with a small quantity of boric acid. About 5 to 6 drops are allowed to run into the ear from a warm teaspoon or dropped in from a fountain-pen filler. This should be done once or twice daily, according to the amount of discharge, and where syringing is being carried out, should form the last stage of the treatment. In certain cases attempts have been made to introduce agents via the Eustachian tube, such as argyrol, protargol and oils of various kinds. In addition, powders are used, with the object of drying up the ear. The simplest powder for this purpose is boracic acid powder. This is blown into the ear from a powder-blower. The use of boric acid powder with 0·75 per cent. of iodine is an improvement upon plain boracic acid. The principle of this treatment is that the boracic acid dissolves in the discharge of the ear and liberates nascent iodine, which exercises a powerful antiseptic action and assists materially in drying up the discharge. These powders should not be used in the early stages of treatment because, if there is a great deal of discharge, they will merely block the ear; they are most useful during the later stages of treatment, when the ear is almost but not quite dry. A large quantity of powder should not be used, but only sufficient to produce a light coating.

Special forms of treatment are sometimes used, as, for instance, ionization. In some hands this treatment gives beneficial results. It consists in passing an electric current through the ear, using zinc as the positive pole in the ear. The application of the zinc is carried out by filling the ear with zinc sulphate solution, 2 to 4 per cent., and placing in the zinc sulphate solution the positive zinc pole. Before carrying out this treatment the ear must be cleansed with the utmost care, and dried. Where there is a perforation, special precautions must be taken to make sure that the middle ear is completely filled with zinc sulphate solution. This is done either by massaging the solution into the ear, to exclude air bubbles, or in certain cases where a perforation exists, a cannula is used to introduce the solution into the middle ear. Current to the extent of 5 ma. is used for ten to twenty minutes. Three or more applications may be required to obtain a good result. This treatment is particularly useful in young people, such as school children, but is quite useless where extensive disease exists, in particular bone disease or granulation formation.

Progressive Middle-ear Deafness.—*Otosclerosis.*—Treatment in the case of otosclerosis is unsatisfactory. Where chronic catarrh in the nose exists, Eustachian inflation may give some benefit, but if catarrh and the frequency of colds is very marked, it may be justifiable in certain cases to do some operation on the nose to ensure freedom from obstruction.

Chronic Adhesive Process.—This condition gives very much the same symptoms as otosclerosis, and treatment is equally unsatisfactory.

Deaf Aids

While we are unable to prescribe treatment which will cure patients of these forms of deafness, we can do something to assist them to hear, and the practitioner is often asked for advice regarding artificial aids to hearing. A knowledge of such instruments is therefore essential to every practitioner.

There are two chief classes of aid—the mechanical and the electrical. The first group includes the familiar ear-trumpet, auricles and artificial drums. The second includes non-valve electrical instruments and valve instruments. The advantage of the mechanical instrument lies in its lightness and portability and the fact that there is no upkeep. Its disadvantage is, however, that it is comparatively limited in its scope, and while such things as auricles may be concealed in the ear, the old-fashioned trumpet, although for many cases the most satisfactory form of hearing-aid, is so conspicuous that many patients refuse to use it. The auricle is, in effect, a miniature trumpet or shell which collects the sound and transfers it to the ear. Artificial drums may consist of small pledgets of wool soaked in glycerin or paraffin, etc., or they may be small discs of oil-silk which are introduced into an ear in which there is a perforation of the drum, in order to close up the deficiency in the drum-membrane. In certain instances they do excellent service.

Of the electrical aids, from the point of view of performance, the valve instrument is very much superior to the non-valve type. The non-valve type has, as a rule, a carbon microphone which may be single or multiple, and is, from its portability, suitable for people who are engaged in hard work and who require the use of both their hands. It can therefore be used by manual labourers. The valve instrument is considerably more bulky than the non-valve type of aid. It may consist of one to three valves, and as scientific instruments these have reached a high pitch of perfection. They give powerful amplification, and the electric circuits can be so adjusted that a particular part of the hearing range can be amplified to correspond with the greatest deficiency in the patient's hearing. The disadvantages of these aids are their expense and their bulk. Modern development, however, is helping to produce aids which are very much smaller than formerly ; some can be divided into portions which may be carried in the pockets about the person. They require a considerable amount of battery renewal, but the batteries are of a type readily procurable in any part of the country. The type of patient likely to benefit from a hearing aid is the young person who finds it essential to work for a living and whose deafness is beginning to make this difficult. It is these people who are likely to take the small amount of trouble which is necessary to understand these instruments and to get the best out of them. Those suffering from middle-ear deafness are particularly favourable cases for the use of electric hearing aids. Elderly people suffering from nerve deafness are not generally successful in using these instruments. They are sensitive in regard to their appearance, and as a rule do not take the trouble to understand them well enough to obtain good results. The majority of these people are past the necessity for earning their living and regard their hearing more in the light of a social amenity than as a means of livelihood.

THE LARYNX

LARYNGITIS

Acute Laryngitis.—This condition is usually part of a general infection of the upper air passages, and treatment of laryngitis in a great many cases must include the treatment of the upper respiratory infection also. The first principle of treatment of laryngitis is rest of the larynx. Resting the larynx involves not only the avoidance of vocal function, but also the avoidance of muscular effort. As a considerable muscular effort is required from the larynx every time the thorax is braced or the arms used vigorously, quite obviously movement will frequently cause effort in the larynx and this must be prevented. For this reason the patient is best nursed in bed, even although constitutional symptoms may not seem sufficiently severe to demand this treatment. This has the further advantage that the patient is kept in an even temperature, which is a most important point in treatment.

General febrile conditions will be met by antifebrile measures, laxatives, etc., as for coryza. Locally the inflamed larynx must be soothed. This may be done by steam inhalations, sprays and direct applications. Steam inhalations may be medicated, and if so, with soothing and not with irritating agents. Tinct. benz. co. is one of the most useful of these: 15 to 20 drops should be placed in half a jug of boiling water and the steam inhaled for fifteen minutes at a time.

Sprays may be of light oils and may contain essential oils to make them pleasanter to the larynx and trachea. Oily solutions may be applied directly to the larynx by means of a dressed probe.

Frequently there is acute pain in the neck, and applications of heat—kaolin poultices, linseed poultice, thermal pads, etc. —give comfort and relief.

Chronic Laryngitis.—The first step in the treatment of a chronic laryngitis consists in an intensive search for the exciting agent. The removal of the cause of the irritation is essential. If it is impossible to identify any one cause, then all sources of irritation must be eliminated, such as tobacco, alcohol, the presence of fumes, frequent contact with dust, etc. The voice should be put at rest for a period, provided the patient's economic condition will permit. Inhalations of tinct. benz. co should be prescribed to be used at night-time only, and a soothing spray can be used frequently throughout the day.

Locally the larynx can be painted with mild preparations and in very chronic and resistant cases a weak solution of silver nitrate ($2\frac{1}{2}$ per cent.) or zinc sulphate (5 to 10 per cent.) may be tried. This, however, must be used with the utmost care. Complete examination of the upper respiratory passages must always form part of the preliminaries to treatment, as a sinusitis or other infection may be found which will require treatment before any improvement can be expected in the laryngeal condition.

If it is possible to change the patient's environment, this is frequently a valuable measure, and in such circumstances warm, south-westerly exposures should be chosen.

APPENDIX

Nose

℞	Sodii bibor.	ʒii
	Sodii bicarb.	ʒii
	Sodii chlor.	ʒii

Sig.—One teaspoonful to a pint of warm water.

℞	Menthol.	0·5 per cent.
	Ol. Limon (B.P.) . . .	0·5 per cent.
	Paraff. Liq.	℥i

Sig.—Use in an atomiser.

Ear

℞	Sol. Aluminii acetatis, 8 per cent. .	℥j

Sig.—Soak ½ in. ribbon gauze in solution and pack into the ear once daily.

℞	Ichthyol in glycerin, 10 per cent. .	℥i

Sig.—Soak ½ in. ribbon gauze in solution and pack into the ear once daily.

℞	Iodi resublimati . . .	0·75 per cent.
	Pulv. Acid. Boric. . . ad	℥i

Sig.—Use in a powder blower as directed.

℞	Acid. Boric.	gr. xv
	Sp. Rectificati	℥i

Sig.—Ear drops.

Scarlet Red Drops

℞	Scarlet red	gr. xxv
	Sp. Rectificati	℥i

Sig.—Ten to fifteen drops to be instilled into the ear as directed.

Larynx

℞ Tinct. Benzoin. Co. . . . . . ℥i

Sig.—Fifteen to thirty drops in a jug of hot water, for an inhalation.

Pharynx

℞ Sod. Bicarb. . . . . . . gr. xlv
Liq. Thymol. Co. (B.P.C.) . . . ℥i
Glycer. . . . . ℥i

Dilute eight times with water.

Sig.—The throat spray or gargle, to be used as directed.

℞ Phenol.
Sod. Sulphocarbolatis . . āā ʒss
Sod. Bicarb. . . . . . . ʒss
Glycer. . . . . ʒv
Liq. Carmin. (B.P.C.). . . . . ♏v
Aq. Aurant. Flor. . . . . . ℥iv

Sig.—Dilute with an equal quantity of water and use as a gargle.

Mandl's Paint

℞ Iod. . . . . gr. v
Pot. Iod. . . . . gr. xxv
Ol. Menth. Pip. . . . . . ♏v
Glycer. . . . . . . ad ℥i

Sig.—Use as a paint in chronic pharyngitis.

I. S. Hall.

DISEASES OF THE RESPIRATORY SYSTEM

THE PREVENTION OF ACUTE RESPIRATORY DISEASES

(Coryza, Acute Bronchitis and Broncho-pneumonia)

THE commonest predisposing cause of the more severe respiratory diseases, such as bronchitis and pneumonia, is coryza and influenza. This is particularly the case when infection occurs in individuals whose resistance is lowered from any cause. It is for this reason that we believe that in the field of prevention, education of the individual sufferer from the common cold in regard to his social obligations is of prime importance. It would constitute a definite advance in prophylaxis if infected individuals, particularly during the first twenty-four to forty-eight hours of the disease, would isolate themselves in their homes, or, failing this, refrain from entering places of public entertainment such as cinemas and theatres, etc., where people are crowded together. They should keep as far apart as possible from non-infected persons and should cough and sneeze into a handkerchief with the head averted from neighbours, who should not be submitted to the direct line of fire of infected droplets.

It should be explained to persons in the acute stage of coryza that isolation at home is not merely a social obligation required for the prevention of infection of others, but that rest in a constant temperature is the best means of obtaining a rapid cure and limiting the liability to more serious disease from extension of the inflammation.

During epidemics of acute coryza and influenza, it is particularly important for certain individuals to reduce their chances of infection to a minimum by not entering places where persons are crowded together. This advice applies to elderly and debilitated people in general, sufferers from cardiac and pulmonary disease and, in particular, those with chronic bronchitis, asthma, bronchiectasis and tuberculosis.

In view of the grave complications which may occur in infants and young children, every effort should be made to limit the risks of exposure to infection. Doctors, dentists and nurses have a grave responsibility when suffering from sore throats or colds in the head, and should take particular care to avoid infecting their patients, especially infants and debilitated persons.

Lastly, we would stress the desirability of the early removal to hospitals of infants and young children with measles and whooping-cough. Good nursing and general care, which are not available in many working-class homes, reduce the pulmonary complications which are the principal cause of the mortality.

As conditions exist to-day, the average individual can scarcely hope to avoid infection at some time during the winter months. Every effort should be made to build up the constitution and raise the general resistance of persons who are peculiarly susceptible, or those with chronic organic disease, by giving common-sense advice on the following points :—

1. The avoidance of excessive mental or physical fatigue.

2. The avoidance of undue exposure to wet and cold, by staying indoors when the weather is unseasonable, particularly if cold is combined with fog or mist. This does not mean that fresh air and exercise are harmful—on the contrary, regular open-air exercise, when the weather is suitable, so long as it is within the limits of the patient's tolerance, is one of the most important factors in building up the natural resistance. The beneficial effects of fresh air can be continued at night by insisting that bedroom windows are kept open. In addition, in schools and institutions where the dormitory system is in existence, the beds should be spaced at least 7 ft. apart, and during times of epidemics every alternate bed should be reversed.

3. The wearing of heavy clothing in the house leads to an unhealthy condition of the skin, an organ which plays a most important part in allowing the patient to adjust himself to changes of temperature and pressure. Light clothes should be worn indoors, with, for outdoor use, an overcoat of a thickness to suit the climatic conditions. The fact is well recognized that although females muffle themselves up much less than males, they are noticeably less susceptible to colds. Wet and therefore cold feet, especially if endured for hours in the office or factory, are a potent factor in lowering the vitality,

often with serious consequences. The obvious preventive measure is the use of stout footwear. Health as well as comfort may be dependent on having a dry pair of shoes and stockings available at the place of work.

4. Since chronic irritation of the air passages predisposes to infection, attention should be directed to the irritation produced by an atmosphere of cigarette smoke. In certain cases it may be necessary to prohibit or at least curtail smoking. The individual's occupation should be ascertained. Should it involve exposure to excessive amounts of dust or chemical fumes in the atmosphere, a change of occupation may be necessary. It may be sufficient, however, to abate the nuisance by means of respirators, fans and ventilators. In parenthesis, we would draw attention to the difficulty of getting workmen to use respirators, even after considerable care has been taken to explain the need for this precaution.

Local Measures.—The nose and throat should be examined for abnormalities which impair the free entry of air and lead to mouth breathing, *e.g.*, deflected septum, polypi, enlarged tonsils and adenoids. Chronic infection of the air sinuses and tonsils, if present, should receive attention, since this may cause a lowering of resistance to the viruses of the common cold and influenza.

Practical experience does not encourage the wearing of masks by healthy individuals as a safeguard against infection. A mask is more likely to be effective in preventing the spread of infection if worn by persons actually suffering from the disease.

Gargles and spraying with mild antiseptics night and morning are believed by many to be of value as a preventive measure. Listerine, hydrogen peroxide, glycerin thymol co., etc., are commonly used for this purpose. An atomiser is required when oily solutions are advised. Mild antiseptic solutions, or normal saline, may also be used as a nasal douche. We would remind the reader not to use any forcible measures for the introduction of fluids into the nose (see p. 780). Douching is more effective if reserved for the later stage of coryza, when it will remove any thick secretion obstructing the airway. In our experience, the preventive value of local applications to the nose and throat has been exaggerated.

Diet and Tonics.—In poorly nourished or debilitated patients, dietetic measures are important in building up the resistance. It is seldom that a diet is deficient in a quantitative sense, since calories can be purchased very cheaply in the form of carbohydrates such as bread and potatoes. The qualitative deficiencies present in the diet of the working classes are mainly in animal proteins, minerals and vitamins. This can very easily be corrected by the ingestion of an extra pint of milk a day and some fresh fruit and green vegetables. Iron, when anæmia is present, and cod-liver oil to increase the intake of vitamins A and D should be prescribed. On the other hand, obesity is a potent factor in lowering the resistance, particularly if the patient is taking a diet deficient in animal proteins, vitamins and minerals. Accordingly, the caloric intake in such individuals must be reduced (see p. 389), while the so-called protective foods must be given in adequate amounts.

Faulty Posture and Breathing.—Proper ventilation of the lungs requires efficient and full movements of the diaphragm. This not only empties the lungs of air lying dormant at the bases, but corrects the tendency of the blood to stagnate in the large abdominal veins. Faulty breathing is frequently accompanied by faulty posture, for the correction of which an understanding of the principles of body mechanics, as enunciated by Goldthwaite and Swaim of Boston, is necessary. Drugs are useless for this purpose, and reliance must be placed on special exercises carried out regularly every day. Reference to the section on rheumatic diseases (p. 952) will indicate the great importance of correcting these abnormalities as a means of raising the general resistance.

Vaccine Therapy.—No more controversial question exists in medicine than the value of vaccines in the prophylaxis and treatment of disease. In our experience vaccines are rarely useful, and are often harmful when given in the acute stage of any disease. With regard to the prophylaxis of such a condition as the common cold, it is extremely difficult to assess the merits of vaccine therapy because of the wide variation in susceptibility and resistance in different individuals, and in the same individual at different periods. Since it is now established that the infective agent of a common cold is a filterable virus, it seems unlikely that the manifold claims made in the medical press during the past twenty years regarding the value of prophylactic anticatarrhal vaccines can now be maintained. Since the more serious complications such as sinusitis, tracheitis and bronchitis are due to secondary invaders which can be incorporated in a vaccine, the possibility exists, and there is some evidence to support it, that vaccines may prevent or reduce the severity of such complications. For this purpose, the mixed catarrhal vaccine, as sold by the British Drug Houses and other firms, may be given subcutaneously on three or four occasions at weekly intervals in the late summer or early autumn to individuals susceptible to coryza and its complications. In view of the short period of immunity conferred, the course should be repeated in January or February. The dosage recommended is 0·25, 0·5 and 1 c.c., and 1 c.c. at weekly intervals. If anything more than a mild degree of local or general reaction follows an injection, the dose should not be increased at the next injection, and may possibly have to be reduced. Prophylactic immunization should not be undertaken if coryza is already present, in view of the danger of a serious reaction.

For the prevention or amelioration of recurrent winter cough which so frequently occurs in chronic bronchitis, a mixed catarrhal stock vaccine is frequently employed. Some authorities stress the importance of having the organisms in the patient's sputum identified and an autogenous vaccine made. There is more to be said for this procedure if a single organism is present in almost pure culture. Whether a stock or autogenous vaccine is employed, it is essential to proceed with great care in regard to the dosage. It is generally agreed that the maximal dose of vaccine should be less than the amount which will produce any general reaction. In view of the great variation in individuals the dosage can be found only by trial and error. Accordingly, it is wise to start with a very small quantity of vaccine, *e.g.*, 0·1 c.c., containing from 1 to 5 million organisms. The subsequent doses should be given at weekly intervals and progressively increased, but always with care to avoid general reactions. By this means the patient's immunity mechanism is believed to be steadily stimulated. Reactions, on the other hand, may induce a state of increased sensitivity to bacterial antigen, and, if severe, may precipitate an acute illness.

ACUTE CORYZA

Synonym : Acute rhinitis (" cold in the head ").

Definition : A catarrhal inflammation of the nasopharynx due to a filterable virus ; a secondary infection with pyogenic organisms usually follows.

Treatment will be considered under two heads, (1) measures to abort the infection in the early stages and (2) treatment of the established condition.

Measures to Abort the Infection in the Early Stages.—When an individual comes home from work with a slight soreness of the throat and stuffiness of the nose, it is sometimes possible to abort the incipient coryza by one or more of the following measures.

He should take a hot bath, followed by a hot drink of lemon or black-currant juice sweetened with sugar, to which 1 oz. of whisky may be added should the patient desire it. Five to ten grains of aspirin and the same quantity of Dover's powder will secure a good night's rest. Such traditional remedies as a teaspoonful of ammoniated tincture of quinine, or 5 minims of oil of cinnamon in hot milk, are widely valued by public opinion.

Local treatment to the nose with lubricants or astringents may be tried. Glegg recommends the instillation of 1 to 2 drachms of a mixture of paraffinum molle 1 part and paraffinum liquidum 3 parts into each nostril in turn while the patient lies on his back. This procedure should be repeated several times during the day.

For the purpose of shrinking the congested mucous membranes, a 1 per cent. solution of ephedrine in saline, or an oily solution containing some of the essential oils (with or without ephedrine) may be sprayed into the nose through an atomiser (for prescriptions, see p. 848). "Endrine" can be used in an atomiser or 1 to 2 drops can be run into the nose by means of a pipette. "Benzedrine" produces a rapid shrinkage of the mucous membranes and can be purchased in a convenient form of inhaler. Local astringents, since they shrink swollen mucous membranes and thereby clear the exits of the air sinuses, are held to be of value in reducing the risks of sinusitis. Though the claims made by the manufacturers regarding the efficacy of their preparations in aborting the common cold are often exaggerated, there is little doubt that a temporary symptomatic improvement does occur. It is necessary, however, to utter a warning against the excessive use of preparations of this type. If used too frequently the secondary reaction which follows the vasoconstriction may cause a turgescence of the mucous membranes greater than before, and may lead to an increase of inflammation or even necrosis of the epithelium. Accordingly, local vasoconstriction should not be attempted more than three or four times in the twenty-four hours.

Douching with warm normal saline assists in freeing the airway by removing secretions and organisms, although it does not produce such dramatic effects as obtained from vasoconstrictor drugs. It is advisable to run the saline into the nose gently from a pipette, stopping at once if any tendency to swallowing or retching occurs. The nose should not be blown for at least a quarter of an hour after the operation. These instructions are given in order to avoid forcing infected material into the Eustachian tube.

Treatment of the Established Condition.—If the measures already described fail to abort the condition and the patient has reached the acute stage of coryza with profuse rhinorrhœa, the most important question to be decided is whether he should be allowed to go to work or be confined to the house. If fever is present, or if the patient is old or debilitated, or has any coexisting serious organic disease, there can be no doubt about the advisability of remaining in bed. Personally, we advise all sufferers from acute coryza to stay at home, if possible, since we believe that by far the most effective way of obtaining a rapid cure is to remain indoors in an even temperature in a well-ventilated but warm room for twenty-four to forty-eight hours. By this means the liability to the serious sequelæ from extension of the inflammation to the nasal sinuses and the bronchial tree is reduced to a minimum.

Individuals with acute coryza should realize that they are suffering from an infectious disease which they may pass on to others with results which may be disastrous. Hence they have a moral obligation to isolate themselves during the acute infective stage, *i.e.*, during the first twenty-four to forty-eight hours.

It is a time-honoured custom to start the treatment of any acute disease with a purge. Since this question will arise in all the acute respiratory diseases, we propose to discuss it fully now in order to save repetition.

Our own feeling is that the routine administration of calomel or castor oil at the beginning of an illness is to be deprecated, since purging is invariably followed by an upset of the normal rhythm of evacuation, and, if carried too far, has a debilitating effect. Accordingly, if the patient has had a regular daily evacuation of the bowels up to the onset of the illness, we do not advise the administration of an initial purge. If, however, the patient has been constipated for the preceding day or two, an aperient will have to be given. Two to three grains of calomel followed by Epsom salts in the morning has been shown by long clinical experience to achieve a satisfactory evacuation. Calomel, however, does not suit everyone, and it is wise to enquire of the patient which laxative he has found to be most satisfactory. This preparation will cause the least disturbance to the patient, and a double dose will ensure a satisfactory evacuation. Should constipation persist, it is better to rely on small doses of a mild laxative such as senna, milk of magnesia or cascara at night, followed next morning by an enema. A single evacuation from an enema is less exhausting to a debilitated patient than a series of watery motions resulting from a purgative.

Since acute coryza in the vast majority of cases is a self-limiting disease of short duration, no question arises of supplying a diet which will meet the maintenance caloric requirements. A light, easily digested diet, of the type used in fevers (see p. 4), whose constituents should, within reason, meet with the patient's approval, is all that is required. Fluids should be taken in abundance. The patient should drink daily at least 4 to 6 pints of water, fruit drinks, tea, etc.

Drugs.—Provided there are no complications, the only drugs required are aspirin (10 gr.), which may be taken three or four times a day, and Dover's powder (pulv. ipecac. et opii) (5 to 10 gr.), taken at night with a hot drink.

Local Treatment.—In our experience the most suitable form of local treatment is the inhalation of steam impregnated with friars' balsam, menthol or eucalyptus. Special vessels are sold for inhalation purposes, but simpler and as effective is the use of a jug which will hold approximately 2 pints of water. The jug should be half-filled with water from a kettle that has been " off the boil " for a few minutes, thus reducing the risk of scalding the patient's face or cracking the jug. One teaspoonful of friars' balsam is added to the hot water for its sedative effect, while the addition of a small crystal of menthol or 5 to 6 drops of oil of eucalyptus will stimulate a freer flow of secretion. The jug is surrounded by a towel whose ends are gathered together to form a funnel through which the patient inhales the vapour. It is advisable to keep the eyes outside the funnel in order to avoid irritation from the medicated steam. When sinusitis is present, the exits from the sinuses may be enlarged and drainage facilitated by shrinking the nasal mucous membrane by the local application of astringents (see p. 780) before the inhalation of steam. If the nares are blocked by thick viscid secretion, gentle douching with warm normal saline is recommended and should be carried out after the steam inhalation.

Complications.—For the treatment of sinusitis, tonsillitis, tracheitis, etc., the reader is referred to the appropriate sections.

ACUTE BRONCHITIS AND BRONCHO-PNEUMONIA

Acute bronchitis is an acute inflammation of the mucous membrane of the bronchi, which may be mild or intense and may affect the trachea, bronchi or terminal bronchioles. The further down the bronchial tree the inflammation spreads the more serious will be the systemic manifestations. No sharp dividing line exists between tracheitis, bronchitis, capillary bronchitis and broncho-pneumonia.

A primary form of broncho-pneumonia is described in infancy and early childhood, but in the great majority of cases it is secondary to an inflammation of the terminal bronchioles. When this extends into the air vesicles, it leads to small lobular areas of consolidation and collapse, scattered mainly throughout the bases of the lungs. The conditions leading to bronchitis and broncho-pneumonia have already been discussed in the sections dealing with the prevention of acute respiratory diseases.

Treatment must vary in every case depending on the severity of the infection and the resistance of the individual.

In mild cases of tracheo-bronchitis in healthy persons, confinement in a warm well-ventilated room at an even temperature for a few days and the administration of a simple expectorant cough mixture may be all that is required. At the other extreme, some patients with acute bronchitis and broncho-pneumonia may be so seriously ill that they will need the best of nursing and medical treatment if a successful issue is to be obtained.

General Measures

The patient must be confined to bed in a warm room at a constant temperature of 65° F. It is so essential to conserve the strength of those patients who are seriously ill that they must be relieved of every effort. Skilled nursing, accordingly, is always necessary. Unless this can be afforded, hospital treatment is indicated.

The patient's night-wear should consist of a light woollen vest, a flannel bed-jacket and pyjama trousers. The common mistake of allowing the patient to be covered with several layers of thick heavy clothing is an important factor in inducing restlessness and discomfort, so preventing sleep. Tepid sponging of the whole body, avoiding undue exposure, morning and evening, and of the face and hands on other occasions when the patient feels feverish is very comforting. If the patient is not debilitated and little or no fever is present, a hot bath may be ordered provided the bathroom is close to the bedroom and the patient returns immediately to bed. The night-wear should be changed at frequent intervals if sweating is present.

Diet.—A light, easily digested fluid or semi-solid diet should be ordered (see p. 4). It should be given in small amounts at two-hourly intervals along with a plentiful supply of fluids in the form of weak tea, barley water, fruit juice in water sweetened with glucose, etc. One tumblerful of fluid should be taken at least every two hours during the day.

To prevent intestinal distension, bulk and roughage in the diet should be avoided. A choice should be made from the following articles : milk (which may be citrated by the addition of 2 gr. of sodium citrate to each ounce), milky foods (Bengers, Allenburys, Ovaltine, etc.), milk puddings, ice-cream, custards, jellies, eggs, broth, gruel and vegetable purées.

In old and debilitated persons the nurse should alter the patient's position in bed from time to time, to prevent him from slipping down into a flat position, since this may increase the difficulty in breathing and the liability to hypostatic congestion. The patient should be permitted to assume the position in bed which he finds most comfortable. In general, this is the inclined position, the patient's back being supported by pillows or a bed rest and his knees by a bolster placed beneath them. If available, beds specially constructed for the nursing of cardiac and respiratory cases are convenient.

Symptomatic Treatment

Insomnia and Restlessness.—When the small tubes are affected and the patient is in a weak, toxic condition, it is essential to ensure sufficient sleep. Before resorting to hypnotics, the following measures should be tried. Sponging with tepid water, placing the patient in a comfortable position, rearranging the bedclothes, getting the patient to pass water and giving 10 gr. of aspirin and a hot lemon drink with or without the addition of whisky are simple measures, which, when given by a skilled nurse, are often sufficient.

The commonest cause of sleeplessness in bronchitis is a distressing, painful cough, in which case the best hypnotic is a sedative cough mixture (see p. 850). When insomnia is due to the restlessness caused by fever and toxæmia, potassium bromide (15 to 30 gr.) and chloral hydrate (10 to 20 gr.) are two excellent preparations which may be given singly or in combination. Should these be unsuccessful the barbiturates may be tried, veronal and medinal (5 to 10 gr.), dial ($1\frac{1}{2}$ to 3 gr.), prescribed in tablet form. Paraldehyde (2 to 4 drachms by mouth or 4 to 6 drachms emulsified in 2 oz. of saline per rectum) is a safe and good hypnotic. The unpleasant taste may be disguised by taking it with an equal quantity of whisky flavoured with syrup of orange. Unfortunately, whether given by mouth or by rectum, a nauseating smell in the breath may persist for several days. Opium or its alkaloids should be used only if sleep is being prevented by a hacking cough or severe pain in the chest. Its use in full doses is dangerous, if there is much secretion in the lungs or if marked cyanosis is present. This warning is given lest by the stoppage of the cough reflex the bases of the lungs become water-logged with the danger of death from asphyxia. If there is much secretion it is advisable to give $\frac{1}{100}$ gr. of atropine sulphate along with not more than $\frac{1}{6}$ gr. of morphine or $\frac{1}{12}$ gr. of heroin.

Delirium.—A mild degree of delirium is frequently present in pneumonia, the patient suffering from hallucinations and mild confusion. Marked delirium is one of the most serious complications and indicates intense toxæmia and anoxæmia. Treatment of these severe cases is unsatisfactory because the amount of sedative required to control the delirium may produce a fatal issue from depression of the respiratory centre. Oxygen is obviously indicated, although the mask or nasal catheter or even the oxygen tent is often badly tolerated. The patient must be restrained if necessary by strapping the limbs to the bed. A warm, wet pack at 100° F. is sometimes helpful. In general, however, reliance has to be placed on hypnotics despite their danger. Morphia is contraindicated. Chloral hydrate (30 gr.), potassium bromide (30 gr.) or one of the barbiturates, dial (3 gr.), medinal (10 gr.), may be tried if the patient can be induced to swallow. Otherwise, per rectal or parenteral treatment must be employed. Five to eight drachms of paraldehyde emulsified in 2 oz. of normal saline or avertin in a dose of 0·06 gm. per kilogram body-weight may be given per rectum.

Cyanosis.—The removal of 10 to 20 oz. of blood from a vein (see p. 1074) is recommended when cyanosis develops or when the veins of the neck are distended. Venesection is particularly effective in plethoric individuals, with whom, indeed, it may be useful even before the appearance of cyanosis.

The early administration of oxygen in adequate quantities is essential in all persons suffering from capillary bronchitis and broncho-pneumonia with cyanosis (for details, see p. 1098).

Circulatory Failure.—In patients seriously ill with evidence of a failing circulation, the question of cardio-respiratory stimulants will invariably arise.

Their routine administration is to be deprecated, and the

choice of drug must be decided according to the circumstances of each individual case.

Alcohol.—Alcohol is used much less frequently to-day than it was thirty years ago. This is certainly due to the fact that in the past it was the practice to starve feverish patients, whereas to-day every effort is made to keep them in caloric equilibrium. As Hutchison says, "We have swung, in fact, from a regimen of starvation mitigated by tippling to one of mild stuffing modified by total abstinence. There can be no doubt that the change is, on the whole, wise, though perhaps it has gone too far."

Brandy or whisky may be used. Good whisky is better than bad brandy. Half to one ounce of spirits three or four times in the twenty-four hours is generally sufficient.

Whisky and brandy are usually considered as stimulants, though, in fact, they are sedatives. Nevertheless, for the following reasons, alcohol is of value, particularly in elderly persons or those accustomed to taking it regularly :—

1. It promotes rest and sleep, and lessens apprehension.
2. It dilates the peripheral blood vessels, inducing diaphoresis and augmenting heat loss.
3. It is a source of energy, easily absorbed and metabolised.

Digitalis.—The routine administration of digitalis in capillary bronchitis and pneumonia is a matter on which acute controversy exists. In febrile conditions accompanied by heart failure and auricular fibrillation, no one doubts its value, but it is certain that in febrile states digitalis will not slow a rapid pulse whose rhythm is regular. Those who prescribe digitalis where the rhythm is regular maintain that it improves the tone of the cardiac muscle and lessens the tendency to cardiac dilatation. Whether it has such an action is disputed both by pharmacologists and physicians. Nevertheless, many experienced physicians believe that elderly people or patients with chronic heart disease benefit from the onset of the illness by the administration of 10 to 15 minims of tincture of digitalis three times a day. We do not prescribe digitalis as a general routine, but only when the earliest signs of cardiac failure appear, when we prefer to rely on the rapid effect of the intravenous injection of 0·5 mg. digoxin (B., W. & Co.), followed by 0·25 mg. by mouth every six hours. The full effect of the drug can be obtained in a few hours by this method.

Other stimulants which require mention are coramine, cardiazol, pituitrin, adrenalin, strychnine and caffeine. In acute heart failure we believe that coramine given in doses of

2 to 4 c.c., intramuscularly or intravenously, is a valuable drug. The dose can be repeated four-hourly if required. When the failure is more peripheral than central, 1 c.c. of pituitrin or 5 to 10 minims of adrenalin may be given subcutaneously. The beneficial effects as estimated by the rise in blood pressure are of short duration, lasting less than an hour. It is our practice in critical cases, where the circulation is failing, to give alternate injections of coramine and either pituitrin or adrenalin at two-hourly intervals. Strychnine is probably employed more often than any other drug for the treatment of cardiac failure in acute respiratory disease. Strychnine is essentially a respiratory stimulant, and any beneficial effects it can have on the heart must be secondary to an improvement of pulmonary ventilation. In the usual dosage of $\frac{1}{100}$ gr. subcutaneously, it is of no value at all. When strychnine is considered desirable, $\frac{1}{60}$ to $\frac{1}{30}$ gr. must be given before any result can be expected. The dose may be repeated in four to six hours. Caffeine is widely used and safe, and may be given in the form of caffeine and sodium benzoate (B.P.), 2 to 5 gr. subcutaneously every four to six hours.

The stimulants mentioned above are in everyday use for the treatment of circulatory failure, but it appears to us that much of the benefit claimed from them is exaggerated, being based on uncritical clinical observation. The circulation fails because of anoxæmia, dehydration and toxæmia. The rational procedure is the prevention or limitation of circulatory failure by the use of oxygen, infusion of glucose saline (200 c.c. of 25 per cent. glucose) and the administration of sulphapyridine. or serum, if it is available for the particular causative organism. These must, of course, be given sufficiently early and in adequate amounts.

Dehydration.—Dehydration is indicated by dryness of the tongue and skin, a low urinary output and a low blood pressure. If the patient is unable to take sufficient liquid by the mouth to restore the tissue fluids, 1 or more litres of 5 per cent. glucose in normal saline should be given intravenously by the drip method (see p. 1075). By this means the patient will receive an addition of sodium chloride to maintain the electrolyte balance as well as 50 to 100 gm. of glucose to restore the depleted glycogen reserves in the liver. The intravenous infusion of isotonic fluids is strongly contraindicated in the presence of pulmonary œdema.

Tympanites.—Minor degrees of meteorism may occur from the ingestion of excessive quantities or unsuitable articles of food. It is desirable, therefore, to examine the motions for the purpose of correcting the diet. If thick curds are being passed per rectum, the quantity of milk should be reduced, diluted with water and citrated or peptonized. Marked abdominal distension is usually the result of paralysis of the intestinal muscle consequent on toxæmia. For its prevention, early diagnosis is of first importance along with the use in adequate quantities of oxygen, serum if possible, and intravenous infusions of glucose saline.

For its treatment the following measures should be tried. An enema containing either ox bile, magnesium sulphate (1 oz. to ½ pint of water) or 1 per cent. sodium bicarbonate should be given and thereafter a soft rubber catheter (rectal tube) should be passed and left in position. An ox bile enema is prepared by adding 1 oz. of fresh ox bile to 2 oz. of warm water.

To induce peristalsis and so expel the gaseous contents of the bowel, turpentine stupes may be applied every half-hour to the abdomen. These are prepared by sprinkling 1 to 2 drachms of turpentine on a piece of flannel wrung out of boiling water.

Should these simple measures fail, 1 c.c. of pituitrin may be injected subcutaneously, the same quantity being repeated one hour later if necessary. Occasionally, meteorism may be relieved by small doses of calomel ($\frac{1}{8}$ gr.) every hour, or, alternatively, castor oil (ʒi) every three hours until the bowels move.

Cough, Spit and Pain in the Chest.—In the early stages the patient has an irritating non-productive cough, accompanied by pain under the sternum. The objects of treatment are to loosen the sputum, lessen the cough and relieve the discomfort. For these purposes the following measures are indicated :—

External Measures.—The room should be well ventilated and a constant temperature maintained around 65° F. A fœtid stuffy atmosphere is itself a potent factor in maintaining an irritating cough. Moistening the air by steam from a steaming kettle at a distance of several feet from the patient is comforting. The steam may be medicated by the addition to the water of a few drops of oil of eucalyptus or terebene. The steam tent may be used instead or the steam may be inhaled directly, as already described under the treatment of acute coryza.

For the retrosternal soreness, local applications of heat to the chest are of value. A light linseed poultice may be employed, but it should be removed before it is cold. In patients severely ill with marked dyspnœa a poultice is contraindicated because of its weight. Antiphlogistine or cataplasm kaolin (B.P.), heated and spread in a thin layer on lint, is light and comforting and retains its heat for a longer time. Should the patient object to poultices, relief may be obtained by applying a mustard leaf or plaster, or a rubefacient liniment, such as lin. terebinth. acet. or lin. camphor.

A mustard plaster may be made in the home by mixing equal parts of household mustard and wheat flour into a paste with warm water and spreading it between two layers of muslin. The plaster should be left in position over the sternum until the skin becomes red, when the preparation should be removed. This usually occurs within twenty to thirty minutes.

Internal Measures.—To loosen the secretion an expectorant mixture should be prescribed, containing potassium citrate (30 gr.) and liq. ammon. acetatis (2 to 4 drachms) as a basis, to which may be added one or more of the following drugs: potassium iodide (1 to 3 gr.), tinct. ipecac. (10 minims) or syr. tolu. (30 to 60 minims).

Such a prescription, while loosening the secretion, may not be efficient in relieving the pain accompanying the cough. For this reason, tinct. opii camphorat. is frequently added to the prescription in doses of 10 to 20 minims. It may appear contradictory to prescribe drugs which check the cough and dry up the secretion with others which loosen the spit. Nevertheless clinical experience has shown that such a combination may in practice be beneficial. Personally, we prefer to keep the opiate separate from the loosening mixture and give it in a single dose of sufficient strength to control the cough for several hours and thus ensure a proper rest. This is particularly desirable at night. For this purpose a linctus will be found to be satisfactory, such as elixir diamorph. et terpin. (B.P.C.), or linctus scillæ co. (B.P.C.) ($\frac{1}{2}$ to 1 drachm) or syrup codein phosphate (B.P.C.) (1 to 2 drachms). Alternatively, heroin hydrochloride in doses of $\frac{1}{20}$ to $\frac{1}{10}$ gr. or codein phosphate ($\frac{1}{4}$ to $\frac{1}{2}$ gr.) may be prescribed.

The beneficial effects of hot drinks in relieving painful spasm and loosening secretion are not fully realized, and the action of the expectorant mixture should be augmented by sipping a hot lemon drink after each dose.

High-pitched rhonchi and prolonged expiration are evidence of spasm of the bronchioles. The drugs to use are the antispasmodics, *e.g.*, ephedrine sulphate ($\frac{1}{2}$ gr.), tinct. stramonii (15 minims) or tinct. lobeliæ ætheris (15 minims) (see Appendix).

When the secretion becomes loose and copious, stimulating expectorants should be added to the mixture, and for this purpose ammonium carbonate (5 gr.) or ammonium chloride (10 gr.) may be prescribed in combination with syrup scillæ ($\frac{1}{2}$ to 1 drachm), tinct. ipecac. (10 minims) or syrup tolu. ($\frac{1}{2}$ to 1 drachm).

The expectoration of a foul-smelling spit rarely occurs in bronchitis or broncho-pneumonia, being usually an indication of abscess formation or gangrene of the lung. For its treatment, see pp. 815, 818.

Another rare type is plastic bronchitis (acute fibrinous bronchitis) in which casts of the bronchi are coughed up. The measures outlined under acute bronchitis are required to loosen the spit. The intense dyspnœa accompanied by physical signs suggestive of asthma usually fails to respond to the injection of adrenalin. Treatment consists of the administration of intranasal oxygen and a linctus of heroin combined with apomorphine (elixir diamorph. et terpin cum apomorph. (B.P.C.) ($\frac{1}{2}$ to 1 fluid drachm)).

Pulmonary Œdema.—Rarely a condition of bronchorrhœa occurs, as indicated by a profuse expectoration and the presence of bubbling râles scattered throughout the lungs. In severe cases pulmonary œdema may develop, in which case the prognosis is very bad. Pulmonary œdema is a medical emergency requiring prompt treatment. Atropine ($\frac{1}{25}$ to $\frac{1}{50}$ gr.) should be injected subcutaneously at once and repeated if necessary at two-hourly intervals. Venesection (10 to 20 oz.) should be carried out and oxygen given continuously by the intranasal route.

Pulmonary œdema occurring in lungs, the seat of inflammation, responds less favourably to the injection of atropine sulphate than when the primary cause is left-ventricular heart failure. It is doubtful whether morphia should be given for pulmonary œdema associated with severe respiratory diseases because of its depressant effect on the respiratory centre. If, however, restlessness is marked, morphia ($\frac{1}{6}$ gr.) may be justified. According to Bullowa, treatment should consist of the administration of oxygen under pressure by means of a Haldane mask, which relieves the anoxæmia by increasing the depth of respiration through the Hering-Breuer reflexes and by breaking up the foam obstructing the atria. The increased pressure is obtained either by means of an obstruction in the expiratory exit of the mask or by a high oxygen feed. In addition, he recommends the intravenous injection of 100 c.c. of 50 per cent. sucrose with the object of abstracting fluid from the tissue spaces. Sucrose is stated to be better than glucose because its effect is more lasting. The beneficial effects should appear within an hour.

Dry cupping may also be tried as this reflexly stimulates the capillaries to absorb fluid.

Serum Therapy and Chemotherapy

Serum therapy is of real value in broncho-pneumonia if the infecting organism is a pneumococcus of a type for which serum is available (see p. 798). Unfortunately the infection is usually a mixed one or the pneumococcus isolated will be found to belong to Group IV (see p. 799).

The sulphonamide group of drugs is of real value in broncho-pneumonia. For details of dosage and administration, see pp. 806-808.

Convalescence

After an acute attack of bronchitis or broncho-pneumonia, it is most desirable that the patient should have a holiday of at least two to four weeks before returning to work, to ensure complete resolution of the diseased process in the lungs. If possible, convalescence should be spent in surroundings where the patient can get sunshine, change of air and scenery and good nourishing food, including plenty of milk. Most hospitals have a convalescent home which is suitable in these respects, while for better-off patients a holiday at the seaside should be ordered. In this country, however, a sheltered inland resort may be more beneficial in winter-time. Care should be taken not to send the patient to a holiday resort at a long distance from his home until he is physically fit for the journey. While no artificial measures are so valuable as exercise in the fresh air along with good food, nevertheless, ultra-violet radiation and tonics (cod-liver oil and vitamin preparations such as adexolin and yeast), while supplemental, should not be omitted. Breathing exercises should be undertaken for from five to ten minutes night and morning in all cases in which incomplete resolution is suspected from the presence of poor air entry or residual crepitations at the bases of the lungs. Should an irritating non-productive cough continue, as is not infrequently the case, it must be controlled by the use of a sedative linctus.

Pulmonary Fibrosis.—Post-pneumonic fibrosis usually manifests itself by recurrent attacks of bronchitis, and has been named by some writers " chronic pulmonary catarrh." Bronchiectasis should be excluded in all doubtful cases by means of radiograms after the introduction of lipiodol. The most important single measure in the prevention and treatment of this condition is prolonged convalescence at a bracing inland or seaside resort. It is a common mistake to send such patients to a convalescent home for two or three weeks. The practitioner should insist on at least two months of convalescent treatment, which should include good food, cod-liver oil and regular breathing exercises.

If resolution has not occurred as judged by clinical and radiological examinations, treatment on the above lines must be resolutely continued for at least another six months, since it is only by this means that permanent fibrosis and bronchiectasis can be avoided.

For the treatment of fibrosis of the lung in tuberculosis, pneumoconiosis, etc., see appropriate sections.

CHRONIC BRONCHITIS AND EMPHYSEMA

Treatment will be considered under three headings: (1) correction of factors of ætiological importance; (2) general measures; and (3) local measures.

Correction of Factors of Ætiological Importance.—Chronic bronchitis sometimes follows previous attacks of the acute form, sometimes it appears insidiously as a concomitant of organic disease. In elderly patients it may develop without recognizable cause in the form of a chronic cough, worse in winter.

The treatment of chronic bronchitis does not merely consist of prescribing a cough mixture, but entails in the first instance the study of factors which may be of importance in its causation. For example, in a case where it is associated with obesity and cardiac disease, the prescription of a rational diet along with digitalis and the regulation of the patient's activities, mental as well as physical, will prove more useful than any cough mixtures.

The patient's occupation should be ascertained, since it may be maintaining or at least aggravating the cough. Each individual case calls for a separate decision. For instance, working in a dust-laden atmosphere may be very deleterious. The remedy may lie in the use of a respirator, or better ventilation in the factory or workshop. Possibly no remedy will be really effective short of a complete change of occupation.

The nose and throat should be carefully examined for abnormalities which by obstructing the airway encourage mouth breathing, and for infected tonsils or accessory sinuses whose secretions may be draining into the bronchial tubes.

Lastly, we would recall the danger of overlooking chronic fibroid phthisis which not infrequently masquerades as chronic bronchitis.

General Measures.—These aim at increasing the patient's own power of resistance. Diet is important here, but it must be adjusted to the needs of the individual. In debilitated persons, for example, abundance of butter, cream, milk and bacon will increase the calorific value of the diet, while the overweight person with cardio-renal disease needs the weight-reducing measures as outlined on p. 387.

Regular exercise in the fresh air should be prescribed, always within the limits of the patient's tolerance, but during fog and damp weather he should stay indoors. Those who can afford it will derive much benefit from a winter spent at a resort suitably situated with regard to warmth and sunshine. Unfortunately, the French and Italian Rivieras can have spells of unpleasant weather in the winter, when they offer no more advantages beyond more accessible resorts. To be assured of warm weather and sunshine, it may be necessary to go as far as Egypt or the north coast of Africa. The cost of a long journey with its attendant risks may easily outweigh the benefit obtained, unless the patient is prepared to stay for at least six weeks in the place selected. If the patient cannot stay for more than two or three weeks at the resort, the family doctor should consider carefully the choice of a place nearer home.

A tepid or warm bath, followed by vigorous friction with a rough towel, is an excellent measure for stimulating the skin. This should be followed by breathing exercises (see p. 843). Common-sense advice should be given regarding the deleterious effects of wearing excessively heavy and thick clothes. Footwear should be sufficiently strong in construction to prevent wet feet.

We are satisfied that smoking is a factor of importance in maintaining and augmenting chronic bronchitis, and we have seen much benefit arising in individuals who have taken our advice and given it up. In general, however, this advice will not be accepted *in toto*, in which case the patient may be persuaded to limit himself to a pipe after each meal. The inhalation of cigarette smoke is particularly harmful.

It is unnecessary to draw attention to the effects of excessive quantities of alcohol on the general resistance, but little harm will be done if it is taken in moderate amounts.

Vaccines, either stock or autogenous, are beneficial in a proportion of cases. Great care must be taken in regulating the dosage to avoid reactions which are undoubtedly harmful. The reader is referred to p. 778, where vaccine therapy is discussed in detail.

Local Measures.—The general principles described under the treatment of acute bronchitis in regard to expectorant drugs are applicable to chronic bronchitis. In particular, we would again draw attention to the need for studying in every case the quantity and character of the sputum and any associated symptoms such as cough, pain, dyspnœa and bronchial spasm.

When the cough is irritating and the spit tenacious, a mixture for loosening the cough should be prescribed. For this purpose alkalis, potassium iodide and ammonium chloride are of value. The addition to the mixture of one or more antispasmodic drugs (tincture of strammonium, tincture of lobelia ætheria (10 to 15 minims) or ephedrine hydrochloride (½ gr.)) is indicated if bronchial spasm is present. When the secretion is profuse the stimulating expectorants (ammonium carbonate, ipecacuanha, the balsams of tolu and peru, and squills) are recommended.

For the irritating non-productive cough, tinct. opii camph., or the sedative linctuses (linctus scillæ co. (B.P.C.), linctus diamorphin et scillæ (B.P.C.) and syrup codein phosphat.) or sedative lozenges (troch. glycyrrhizæ (B.P.C.)) should be recommended.

We are in favour of prescribing sedative drugs separately from those used for the purpose of loosening or stimulating the expectoration. By this means the total amount of opiate given in the twenty-four hours can be reduced, since the sedative drugs are only employed as the occasion demands.

Inhalations of medicated steam, as already described, are comforting and should not be forgotten.

When the spit is fœtid, creosote (3 minims) in capsules or perles, or five drops of terebine on a lump of sugar several times a day, are of value.

Suitable prescriptions for the above drugs can be found in the Appendix.

Emphysema.—Emphysema is a concomitant of chronic bronchitis in a greater or less degree. The condition is incurable, and treatment consists of stopping or limiting the process by treating the bronchitis. Common-sense advice must be given to the patient in regard to regulating his life within the limits of his tolerance to effort. Breathing exercises may be tried, but in general will not be found to be so useful as in asthma. They should be combined with a course of massage to the muscles of respiration with the object of increasing their efficiency. In the late stages of emphysema cardiac failure may supervene. Suitable measures for its treatment will be found in the section devoted to diseases of the heart.

LOBAR PNEUMONIA

Although the specific treatment of lobar pneumonia by means of chemotherapy and antipneumococcal serum constitutes a major advance, good nursing under the best conditions still plays an extremely important part in bringing the disease to a successful conclusion. Unless the financial situation permits the employment of day and night nurses and the use of a bedroom with plenty of fresh air and freedom from disturbance by other members of the household, hospitalization should be recommended. Removal to an institution should take place in the early stage of the disease, as after the fifth day the risks involved by the journey are so serious that they more than counterbalance the subsequent advantages. It is our experience that the family doctor is apt to hesitate until a sudden turn for the worse makes him order an ambulance. At least half of our cases are admitted on the fourth or fifth day of illness. In consequence the patient is less able to stand the journey, while the best results from serum therapy cannot be obtained. Practitioners tell us that they are unwilling to remove patients to hospital until unequivocal signs such as dullness on percussion and bronchial breathing have developed. Transfer to hospital could be recommended at a much earlier stage if more reliance were placed on the classical symptoms of rigor, pain in the chest, fever, dyspnœa and cough occurring suddenly in a previously healthy individual. If it is decided to hospitalize a patient with pneumonia, under no condition must he be allowed to walk a single step as this may induce a collapse. A stretcher and ambulance must be employed.

General measures with regard to *nursing*, *fresh air*, *position of the patient in bed*, *diet*, *care of the bowels*, etc., and the symptomatic treatment of *circulatory failure*, *pulmonary œdema*, *cyanosis*, *cough*, *tympanites*, *insomnia*, *restlessness*, *delirium*, etc., have been fully described in the section devoted to acute bronchitis and broncho-pneumonia (p. 784). These are equally applicable in lobar pneumonia, and hence it is only necessary to refer briefly to certain additional points before dealing in detail with specific serum therapy.

Lobar pneumonia is a sharp intense infection, from which the patient generally dies or recovers within ten days. Accordingly, it is unnecessary to attempt by dietetic measures to maintain the patient in metabolic equilibrium, as is so important in long-continuing fevers. Nevertheless, the daily caloric requirements may be as high as 3,000 to 4,000 calories when the temperature continues around 104° F. It is considered helpful to conserve the patient's strength and prevent dehydration by ensuring an intake of at least 2,000 calories daily. This can be done by the use of small two-hourly feeds of the articles mentioned on p. 784, with intervening drinks of water or fruit juice sweetened with glucose or lactose. Sleep is of such value to the patient with pneumonia that it should never be broken for the purpose of giving feeds or drinks, making examinations or undertaking procedures such as changing the linen, washing the patient, etc. Visitors should be excluded or severely limited, although due consideration should be given to individual circumstances. For instance, during the first three days of the illness it may be advisable on occasions to let the patient discuss business or family affairs which may be worrying him, with the object of removing causes of apprehension and anxiety before the critical stage of the disease has been reached.

Reference must be made to the usefulness of expectorant cough mixtures in lobar pneumonia. For several years we employed, routinely, a mixture containing ammonium carbonate, potassium iodide, tinct. ipecac., but were never satisfied that it was effective in loosening the viscid spit. The sister in charge of the pneumonia wards was emphatic that it failed in this object and, in addition, caused gastric upset in many persons. The exudate in the alveoli is liquefied by a process of autolysis and is largely excreted by the kidneys after absorption into the blood stream. If our views are correct, expectorant cough mixtures can play little part in the treatment of lobar pneumonia. Accordingly, we have stopped the routine prescription of such expectorant mixtures as tend to upset digestion, and give instead a simple alkaline mixture containing potassium citrate (20 to 30 gr.), sodium bicarbonate (20 to 30 gr.), liq. ammon. acetatis (2 to 4 drachms) t.i.d. This mixture encourages diuresis and diaphoresis, corrects the tendency to acidosis, soothes the gastric catarrh and is quite as efficacious as any other combination of drugs in helping the liquefaction of the sputum. We have had no reason to be dissatisfied with the change.

Pain and Restlessness.—1. *Morphia.*—Severe pain from pleurisy is present in the majority of cases of pneumonia at the beginning of the illness. It leads to much distress, restlessness and insomnia and to shallow breathing which increases the liability to anoxæmia. In our opinion, if relief is not obtained by the local application of heat (see p. 788), or strapping on the chest (see below), or sedative drugs such as potassium bromide, chloral hydrate or aspirin, then morphia is indicated. We consider morphia is of great value in obtaining some hours of rest and sleep, and we routinely use it during the first three to five days of the illness. One-sixth of a grain should be given subcutaneously in the evening, and the dose may be repeated in two hours if necessary. Some physicians prefer $\frac{1}{12}$ gr. of heroin hydrochloride in the belief that it is a less potent respiratory depressant and tends to cause less intestinal distension. In the later stages of the disease morphia has to be given with great caution. It is contraindicated if marked cyanosis or much secretion in the lungs is present. The last twenty years have seen a considerable change of opinion in favour of the use of morphia in pneumonia. A study of the recent writings of the English authorities leads us to believe that the views expressed above are generally accepted.

2. *Strapping.*—Fixation of the hemithorax with strips of adhesive tape relieves pain by diminishing movement of the inflamed pleural surfaces on each other. If strapping is to be effective, careful attention must be given to the following details. The tape should be 3 in. wide and should extend to the unaffected side at least 4 in. beyond the middle line, both in front and behind. While a single strip over the lower ribs may be sufficient to relieve pain in some cases, in others three pieces may be required. The upper two strips cross in the axilla, passing above and below the breast, while the remaining strip is used to fix the free margin of the ribs. If hair is present it should be removed by shaving. The strips of plaster should be placed in position during full expiration. Strapping the chest on the lines indicated above does not interfere with physical examination or counter-irritation, should this be considered necessary.

Artificial Pneumothorax.—Artificial pneumothorax has been advocated in America for the treatment of pneumonia. One of us has been privileged to examine a series of patients treated with this method. Proof is still lacking that pneumothorax can compare with chemotherapy in reducing the mortality in pneumonia, and we do not think that it will ever become a routine therapeutic procedure. For the relief of pain, however, the separation of the two inflamed pleural membranes by the introduction of 400 to 500 c.c. of air into the pleural cavity is extremely effective. The procedure may have to be repeated if pain returns. Artificial pneumothorax is particularly indicated for the relief of pain which is not controlled by strapping, counter-irritation and mild analgesics, and when the administration of morphia is contraindicated by the presence of marked cyanosis or excessive secretion in the lungs.

Quinine.—Quinine has been claimed by certain authorities to be of specific value in the treatment of pneumonia. This claim is based largely on experimental work on animals, which has shown that even traces of quinine in solution can protect mice injected intraperitoneally with pneumococci. Accordingly, the preparation "optochin" (4 gr. six-hourly) has been advocated for the specific treatment of the pneumonias. Its failure to control pneumonia in human beings, together with its inherent danger of causing blindness, led the workers at the Rockefeller Institute to abandon its use.

Another preparation which has frequently been employed is a combination of quinine and urea hydrochloride. It is given by the intramuscular route every four hours in doses of 15 gr. Some twenty years ago one of the writers tested this preparation in a series of cases of pneumonia. Although a fall in temperature could regularly be obtained following each injection, the effect was transitory and not necessarily accompanied by clinical improvement. We are not aware of any properly controlled series of cases which, on statistical analysis, has shown that any quinine preparation is effective in reducing the mortality of pneumonia. Nor do we believe that reduction of temperature by antipyretic drugs is indicated except when hyperpyrexia is present. As pyrexia constitutes one of the body's defence mechanisms, to lower it artificially by drugs would appear to us to reduce rather than increase resistance, and may, in fact, tend to induce a state of collapse. Since pyrexia and the other manifestations of fever are the direct result of the toxic action of the invading organisms, neutralization of the infection by specific immune serum or chemotherapy is more rational than the employment of antipyretic drugs.

Serum Therapy

Treatment of the pneumonias with type specific antipneumococcal serum has been practised in America on a large scale for more than ten years. Ample evidence of a controlled nature and confirmed by statistical analysis is available to show that serum therapy can markedly reduce both the mortality and the morbidity of the disease. Our experience during the past eight years in Aberdeen fully confirms the views expressed by our American colleagues. It may be asked, why is it, if this is the case, that serum is used so little in this country. There are several possible explanations. First, the cost of treatment is so high as to be prohibitive except to the rich or to the poor treated in hospital. On an average the cost of serum is £10 per patient. Second, technical difficulties connected with the repeated intravenous injections of serum make it unsuitable for the family doctor attending patients in their homes, particularly if they are unable to afford the attention of a private nurse. Third, the special laboratory facilities which are required for typing the pneumococcus in the patient's sputum are available in only a limited number of places. For these reasons, serum treatment can never be widely used unless the public health authorities in each area make themselves responsible for the provision of the hospital accommodation and the laboratory services required. This has been done in Aberdeen, and we believe that the results have fully justified the work and expense entailed.

The pneumococci have been shown by agglutination reactions to belong to several types. Originally, they were separated into Types 1, 2 and 3, and Group IV. Group IV has recently been divided into many types, viz., 5, 6, 7, etc. Serum is available for pneumococcal infections due to Type 1 and 2, and more recently for Types 5, 7, 8 and 14. While the most striking results have been obtained from Type 1 serum, a considerable reduction in the mortality has been shown to follow serum treatment in Types 2, 5, 7, 8 and 14. No satisfactory serum is available for Type 3. To obtain the best results, serum must be given early and in adequate dosage, as is revealed by statistical analysis of the results obtained when serum is given in the first three days of the disease as compared with the fifth day or later. Serum is sometimes of value in cases treated from the fifth day onwards, but the general opinion is that after this date the results attained do not warrant its administration as a routine procedure because of the high costs involved. The low mortality rate from pneumonia in persons between the ages of five and twenty suggests that in this age group it is rarely necessary to use serum. This has been our practice for the past three years in Aberdeen, provided the blood culture is negative and there are no unfavourable factors present, *e.g.*, serious cardiac or renal disease. Nevertheless, it must be emphasized that no one can predict the course of any individual case of pneumonia, and even in mild cases there may be a sudden transition from a condition of apparent safety to one of the utmost gravity. Serum is of particular value in two classes of patients. First, in people of forty years of age and over, as the mortality rate is more than doubled as compared with those of twenty-five and under. Second, in individuals with an infection of the blood, the presence of bacteræmia denotes a severe infection with a high death-rate and indicates the need for large quantities of serum to sterilize the blood.

Recently, a therapeutic serum has been developed which is derived from rabbits. It has been shown that the rabbit produces antibodies to the pneumococcus more rapidly and in greater quantities than does the horse. In addition, the antibodies are believed to have greater diffusibility in the body owing to the smaller size of the rabbit globulin molecule. While encouraging results have already been reported, sufficient time has not yet elapsed for the final evaluation of rabbit serum.

It now seems certain that this country will not suffer for its tardiness in organizing a national compaign against pneumonia by serum treatment, since recent work on sulphapyridine (M. & B. 693) clearly indicates that chemotherapy, because of its cheapness, ease of administration, rapidity of action, lack of serious toxic reactions and effectiveness against pneumococci of all types will supplant serum therapy.

Reactions.—It is essential that physicians who are to give serum parenterally should realize that reactions are liable to occur, which, if not promptly and effectively treated, may result in the death of the patient. This danger should, however, in no way influence the doctor against utilizing serum where it is indicated, and it seems to us that general practitioners are on the whole unnecessarily scared of this procedure. With the refined and concentrated antipneumococcal serum made by the Felton process and sold by the Lederle Manufacturing Company, we have had no deaths due to anaphylaxis among hundreds of cases of pneumonia treated during the past eight years, and severe serum reactions have rarely been encountered. Bullowa puts the chance of a serious reaction at 1 in 300 and the chance of death from pneumonia without serum at 1 in 4.

The reactions which may occur can be divided into two main groups :—

1. Due to acquired or inborn sensitivity of the patient to foreign protein.
2. Due to causes other than allergy.

Reactions due to Serum Sensitivity.—The reactions may occur within seconds or minutes of the intravenous injection of serum or may not appear for one or two hours. When they occur in close proximity to the time of injection they are called anaphylactic reactions, but when they occur some days later (usually about the seventh day) they are called serum sickness.

Anaphylactic reactions may usually be recognized as belonging to one of two types. In some cases the principal feature is the appearance of a severe asthmatic attack due to bronchial spasm, whereas, in others, gastro-intestinal symptoms such as nausea, vomiting and defæcation may appear. These latter symptoms are believed to be associated with spasm of the capillaries of the liver.

Tests for Sensitivity.—Before serum is administered parenterally, it is advisable to test for sensitivity. This is done by making certain inquiries and carrying out certain tests. A careful history should be obtained from the patient in regard to (1) previous attacks of asthma, hay fever, eczema, urticaria, etc., and, in particular, if such symptoms were related in any way to sensitivity to horse serum, horse hair, horse dander and rabbit fur, since the horse and the rabbit are the two animals commonly used for the production of antipneumococcal serum; (2) previous injections of, and reactions to, immune serum, *e.g.*, diphtheria or tetanus antitoxic serum.

There are three tests commonly employed in testing for sensitivity.

1. *The Ophthalmic Test.*—Into the outer canthus of the conjunctival sac of one eye, one drop of a 1 in 10 dilution of normal horse serum is dropped. Normal horse serum, if not available, may be replaced by one drop of a 1 in 10 solution of the serum to be used. Material for the ophthalmic test is usually supplied by the manufacturers, along with the packet of immune serum. The other eye acts as a control. In from five to ten minutes, if the patient is sensitive, itching, watering and reddening of the eye appear. In general, the degree of local conjunctivitis runs parallel with the degree of general sensitivity. The test may be difficult to interpret if previous conjunctivitis is present, while a false negative reaction may occur if the serum is washed away by excessive lachrymation.

2. *The Intradermal Test.*—0·2 c.c. of normal saline is injected into the skin of the volar surface of the forearm. If the control injection of normal saline is done first, the same syringe and needle can be used for introducing intradermally 0·2 c.c. of a 1 in 100 dilution of normal horse serum, 2 in. distant from the control. A positive reaction is recognized by the appearance in from five to twenty minutes of a wheal

of at least 10 mm. in diameter surrounded by a zone of redness. This test is more difficult to interpret than the ophthalmic test, and less reliance can be placed upon it unless the wheal and flare are well marked, and extension of the wheal in the form of pseudopodia is present.

3. *The Blood-pressure Test.*—Recently, workers of the Rockefeller Institute have shown that serum removed from rabbits immunized with pneumococci is of high therapeutic potency. Since rabbit serum produces a positive intradermal reaction in the majority of normal persons, a new test for sensitivity had to be devised. The Rockefeller workers claim that if, after an intravenous injection of 0·1 c.c. of serum diluted with 5 c.c. of normal saline, the fall in blood pressure does not exceed 15 mm. Hg., and no symptoms of shock appear within five minutes, then the patient may be considered to be non-sensitive and the injection of rabbit serum may be proceeded with.

The Value of Tests for Sensitivity.—Due caution is required in the assessment of the value of the tests for sensitivity. We have had patients with negative tests for sensitivity who have had reactions and others who have had no reactions despite the presence of positive tests. In general, however, it may be said that a history of previous allergic manifestations and sensitivity tests are both of value, because the liability to, and the intensity of, reactions is usually greater in those who give positive results than in those who do not. Thus, Bullowa had 36 patients with anaphylactic reactions among 79 showing positive skin tests, as against 58 with reactions among 197 with negative skin tests. On the other hand, the same worker states that among 3,250 patients treated with serum during the past eight years, 8 deaths (0·2 per cent.) occurred in such close proximity to the intravenous injection of serum as to suggest that they were anaphylactic in origin. In all 8 cases, both inquiry for previous allergic manifestations and tests for sensitivity were negative. It is clear, therefore, that even in the presence of a negative history and tests, the greatest care should be taken to administer immune serum extremely slowly as described below, and to have in readiness a syringe filled with potent adrenalin. Adrenalin should be contained in tightly stoppered bottles or glass ampoules, as it is rapidly oxidized if exposed to air.

Serum should not be given to patients from whom a clear history is obtained of asthma caused by emanations from horses, or if the eye test is positive, or if the intradermal test is strongly positive.

Serum may be given to patients with a history of other types of asthma, hay fever, etc., or who have had a previous administration of horse serum, if the tests for sensitivity to horse serum are negative, provided the risks involved are recognized and the precautions described below are undertaken.

In general, these rules should not be departed from unless a careful consideration of the factors influencing prognosis, *e.g.*, age, bacteræmia, etc., suggests that the risks of anaphylaxis are more than counterbalanced by the benefits which may be expected from serum therapy. In this case, an injection of 7 to 10 minims of a 1 in 1,000 solution of adrenalin should be given six minutes by the clock, before the introduction of the serum, which should be injected into the vein extremely slowly (see below). Should a reaction occur, the administration must be stopped and another injection of adrenalin given. By this means it may be possible, although at considerable risk, to continue the serum treatment some minutes later during the period of refractoriness (anti-anaphylaxis). In general, severe reactions, whether allergic or thermal, indicate the discontinuance of the administration of serum. Attempts to desensitize the patient by means of small, gradually increasing doses of serum have been found by Bullowa to be unsatisfactory, and, in addition, may lead in bacteræmic cases to a fatal delay in administering sufficient serum.

Treatment of Anaphylaxis and Serum Sickness.—*Anaphylaxis.*—At the first sign of anaphylaxis 0·5 c.c. of a 1 in 1,000 solution of adrenalin hydrochloride should be given intramuscularly. Massage at the site of injection increases the rate of absorption. The injection should be repeated in a few minutes if relief is not obtained. The shock in severe cases demands immediate treatment by lowering the head, administering stimulants, *e.g.*, sp. ammon. aromat. (1 drachm in water), brandy or whisky (4 drachms in water) or coramine (1 to 2 c.c. intramuscularly), surrounding the patient with hot bottles or the electric cage and administering oxygen through a nasal catheter. Artificial respiration may have to be started. If the blood pressure has fallen greatly, a transfusion of 500 to 1,000 c.c. of gum saline or blood may be given.

Serum Sickness.—Serum sickness is recognized by one or more of the following manifestations—malaise, rise in temperature, pains in the muscles and joints, urticaria and eosinophilia. It may commence at any time between the first and the twelfth day after the injection of serum. The commonest day for the occurrence of arthralgia is the seventh. The symptoms may be mild or severe. In our experience they occur in about 25 per cent. of cases, but produce major discomfort to the patient in only 10 per cent. of cases.

In the majority of cases the myalgia and the arthralgia last only thirty-six hours, and can be controlled by analgesic drugs. Nothing is better than a powder containing aspirin (10 gr.), phenacetin (5 gr.) and codein (¼ gr.), which can be given every four hours until the pain is relieved. Putting the joints at rest by splints is of great value when pain and swelling are marked. For the urticaria a subcutaneous injection of 5 minims of adrenalin is indicated. The injection can be repeated several times in the twenty-four hours. The application of calamine lotion to the skin is comforting to the patient. At the same time ½ gr. of ephedrine sulphate thrice daily should be prescribed because of its prolonged adrenalin-like action. Calcium lactate (30 gr. four-hourly by mouth) and calcium gluconate (10 c.c. of a 10 per cent. solution by the intramuscular or the intravenous route) is of undoubted value in severe cases. We have found little benefit from calcium or adrenalin in the control of arthralgia and use these preparations mainly for the treatment of the urticarial rash.

Reactions not due to Allergy.—*Vasovagal Attacks.*—Very rarely the patient may collapse when the needle is introduced into the skin. The patient is suffering from a "faint" or vasovagal attack, as recognized by the pallor of the face, bradycardia, weak pulse and low blood pressure. Treatment consists of lowering the patient's head to improve the circulation to the medulla and the administration of diffusible stimulants. Occasionally, it may be necessary to inject adrenalin and to carry out the other measures described for the treatment of shock.

Thermal Reactions.—These reactions occur within thirty to ninety minutes of the injection of serum, and can be recognized by the presence of chill (rigor or shivering), rise in the temperature, malaise and sometimes nausea and vomiting. The rigor is followed by sweating. Thermal reactions occur in about 20 per cent. of patients receiving serum.

The chances of a thermal reaction are greatly reduced (1) if scrupulous attention is paid to the preparation of rubber tubing, syringes, needles, etc., used for the injection of the serum, and if refined and concentrated serum is employed which past experience has shown to be free from thermogenic substances; (2) if serum is administered very slowly. We have had little serious trouble in this direction with the Felton pneumococcal serum.

During the stage of chill the patient should be kept warm with hot blankets and hot bottles, hot fluids should be given along with 15 gr. of aspirin, repeated, if necessary, in one hour. If the temperature rises unduly high, the patient should be cooled down by placing on his forehead, wrists and ankles towels wrung out of iced water. Ephedrine is of no value. According to Bullowa, adrenalin increases and prolongs the rigor and hence is contraindicated, while amyl nitrite shortens the reaction.

Serum Administration.—Since approximately 60 per cent. of all cases of lobar pneumonia are either Type 1 or Type 2, a duovalent serum has often been given during the twenty-four hours which used to elapse before the bacteriologists' report was available. With the modern Neufeld method, the type of pneumococcus can be identified within an hour. Where facilities exist for the use of this method, the use of duovalent serum is unnecessary as well as uneconomical.

It is most essential that the bacteriologist should receive sputum which has recently been coughed up by the patient, and that the sample should represent the exudate from the lungs and not merely contain the salivary secretion from the mouth. When no spit is being brought up, swabbing the larynx may enable the organism to be identified. Another method used in some clinics is to puncture the consolidated area of the lung with a fine needle and aspirate some blood-stained material, which is then injected into the peritoneal cavity of a mouse. When the type of pneumococcus has been identified, the appropriate serum can be obtained.

If serum has been kept in the refrigerator, it can be brought to room temperature (65° to 70° F.) by leaving it exposed to the air, by warming it in the hand or by immersion in warm water. Hot water, *i.e.*, above blood heat, must not be used, since overheated serum tends to produce thermal reactions. The slowness with which the serum must be administered does away with the need for keeping it at blood heat. Serum should always be given intravenously, as by this route it is more effective. It is introduced into a vein in the forearm from a needle attached to a 20-c.c. syringe. When the vein cannot be felt or seen in a collapsed or obese individual, it may be necessary to cut down. In this case it may be advisable to give a drip transfusion of glucose saline, to which the serum has been added. The rate of flow should be about 4 c.c. a minute.

Dosage.—Concentrated and refined serum, as sold by the Lederle Company, contains 10,000 units in approximately 5 c.c.

of serum. A unit of antibody is the amount which will protect a mouse from 1,000,000 fatal doses of pneumococci.

The first dose of serum should not exceed 5 c.c. and must be given extremely slowly. This is the most important point in reducing the incidence and severity of reactions. At least three minutes should be taken to introduce the first cubic centimetre, while the remaining quantity can be given at the rate of 1 c.c. per minute. If there is no reaction within two hours, the speed at which the serum is introduced at the subsequent injection may be more rapid, but in our opinion never faster than 2 c.c. every minute. An interval of two hours should elapse between the first and the second, and the second and the third doses. Subsequent doses should be given at four to six hourly intervals. For the second and subsequent injections the dose of serum should be 40,000 units, *i.e.*, 20 c.c. of serum. The object to be achieved is to get a high concentration of immune bodies in the patient's blood as quickly as possible. In general, it may be said that the initial amount of serum given in divided doses should be at least 60,000 units for Type 1 and 100,000 units for Type 2 pneumonias. The total dose of serum required in a case of Type 1 pneumonia of average severity is approximately 100,000 units, while in Type 2 pneumonia the amount approaches 200,000 units. A mild case treated early with 60,000 units may be expected to have a crisis within twenty-four hours, while a severe case with bacteræmia may need 2, 3 or 400,000 units. The assessment of the dosage is largely based on the response of the patient. A fall in temperature, a slowing of the pulse and a feeling of well-being suggests that an adequate dose has been given. If the temperature rises and the pulse accelerates again, a further dose should be given at once. In the special pneumonia services established in America, repeated estimations of the antibodies (agglutinins) in the blood are routinely performed. It is held that the persistent presence of excess of antibodies indicates that additional serum is unnecessary.

Chemotherapy

Chemothrapy received a great impetus with the advent of sulphanilamide. The effect of this drug on the control of diseases due to hæmolytic streptococci was so dramatic as to stimulate research into allied compounds which would be equally efficacious against other micro-organisms. Of the many preparations tested, 2-sulphanilyl-aminopyridine[1] (first prepared in the research laboratories of May & Baker Ltd.,

[1] Now generally described as sulphapyridine.

and marketed under the trade name, M. & B. 693) deserves special mention because of its remarkable property of controlling pneumococcal infections. In a recent paper, Evans and Gaisford (July 1938) report the results obtained from treatment of 100 cases of lobar pneumonia with this drug. The case mortality rate was 8 per cent. as compared with 27 per cent. in a controlled series observed at the same time. Apart from some degree of cyanosis which appeared in a quarter of the patients, no tendency to the development of toxic effects was noted. The authors have also treated forty cases of broncho-pneumonia in children. Only two deaths occurred. There was no difficulty in getting the babies to take the tablets, which were crushed and suspended in glucose saline. No toxic manifestations were observed. This work has received ample confirmation by other clinicians as well as by the writers.[1]

Sulphapyridine is a white powder with a slightly bitter taste, and is soluble in water to the extent of 1 part in 1,000. Experiments on animals and on human volunteers show that the drug is rapidly absorbed from the alimentary tract and rapidly excreted in the urine. The concentration of the drug in the blood stream and cerebrospinal fluid of animals reaches a maximum within three hours and falls to half this figure in the fifth hour. Upon this evidence is based the treatment of human beings by four-hourly doses, the concentration of the drug in the blood being thus maintained continuously at a high level. Sulphapyridine has been shown to possess a toxicity for laboratory animals of approximately one-fourth that of sulphanilamide, and clinical experience suggests that it is also less toxic to human beings than other allied drugs. *In vitro* tests, as well as experiments designed to show its curative value in experimental infections in animals, indicate that sulphapyridine is much superior to sulphanilamide in pneumococcal infection and quite as efficient in streptococcal and meningococcal infections. The drug approaches the ideal chemotherapeutic agent in that it is possible to maintain a concentration in the blood stream which causes, by a bacteriocidal action, direct changes in the pneumococci and, by a bacteriostatic action, a prevention of their multiplication. As a result the invading organisms can be destroyed by the leucocytes, which are themselves not adversely affected by the drug.

[1] During the past year records have been published of approximately 2,000 cases of lobar pneumonia treated with sulphapyridine in different countries. The average mortality was approximately 5 per cent. in contrast to the usual figure of 20 to 30 per cent.

Dosage in Pneumonia and Other Respiratory Diseases due to Pneumococci or Streptococci.—Sulphapyridine is supplied in the form of compressed tablets for oral administration, each tablet containing 7½ gr. (0·5 gm.) of the active substance. For parenteral administration ampoules are available containing 1·0 gm. of the sodium salt in solution in water. Parenteral treatment is only advised when vomiting is a serious feature of the case. The tablets may be chewed and swallowed with a drink of water, or suspended in the form of a powder in milk or glucose saline. The aim of treatment is to obtain as rapidly as possible, and to maintain, a high concentration of the drug in the blood stream. Severely ill patients should receive an initial dose of four tablets (2 gm.), and the same dose should be repeated in four hours Thereafter. two tablets should be given every four hours for the next two days except during sleep. By this time marked clinical improvement can be expected. During the third day the dose is reduced to one tablet four-hourly, which is decreased to one tablet eight-hourly during the fourth and fifth days. A total of between forty to fifty tablets (approximately 20 to 25 gm.) on a decreasing scale during five days are thus given. The manufacturers suggest the following doses for lobar or broncho-pneumonia in children :—

Age . .	One to three months	Six months to two years	Three years	Five years.
Dose in tablets	¼, four-hourly	½, four-hourly	¾, four-hourly	1, four-hourly.

In very severe cases the initial dose may be doubled.

Toxic Reactions.—With the exception of nausea and sometimes vomiting, serious toxic reactions are relatively rare. Occasionally a complaint of dizziness or general malaise is made, and, more rarely still, a rash, fever or cyanosis may appear. The administration of alkalis (*e.g.*, 10 to 20 gr. of sodium bicarbonate in water fifteen minutes before the drug is swallowed) is believed to be of value in overcoming or reducing nausea or vomiting. Aperients should be given sparingly or should be replaced by enemata when required. The saline and sulphur-containing drugs must be avoided and preference be given to liquid paraffin or one of the vegetable laxatives (see p. 86).

PLEURISY

(See p. 136)

ACUTE EMPYEMA

Empyema may complicate any type of pneumonia and at any age. When it is suspected an exploratory puncture should be carried out in order to ascertain the character of the pus, which should be examined bacteriologically. In addition, an X-ray film should be taken in bed as it provides valuable information concerning the position and size of the effusion.

The appropriate time for, and the method of treatment of empyema is governed by such important considerations as the age and general condition of the patient, the extent of the empyema and the infecting agent.

The ordinary (pneumococcal) type of empyema in *adults* usually develops after the crisis of lobar pneumonia, when the respiratory reserve has increased. The pus is thick and is usually localised to the lower and posterior part of the pleural cavity, and the lung surrounding the empyema is often adherent to the chest wall. Therefore, there is no risk in performing open drainage, which is more effective and certain than other methods. Drainage should be done under local anæsthesia by rib resection at the most dependent part of the cavity. Large coagula should be removed. The drainage tube should be of wide bore and, for convenience of dressing, may be attached to a bottle containing antiseptic beneath the bed.

The streptococcal type of empyema may not differ materially from the pneumococcal and may be treated on the same principles. But when, as is common in broncho-pneumonia, the effusion develops in great bulk while the patient is still ill with cyanosis and dyspnœa, open drainage would—in the absence of pleural adhesions—reduce the respiratory reserve still further and prove hazardous. Therefore the toxæmia and the pressure within the thorax should be relieved either by repeated aspiration or closed (*i.e.*, air) drainage.

Aspiration carried out daily is exhausting to the patient, does not reduce toxæmia completely and may lead to cellulitis of the chest wall. Closed drainage, with a catheter through an intercostal space, is to be preferred as it keeps the pleural cavity empty, diminishes toxæmia more promptly and allows the lung to re-expand. Sometimes, though it must not be relied upon, no further operation is required. Usually when the patient's condition has improved sufficiently and the lung has secured adhesion to the chest wall, open drainage should be carried out on the same lines as for pneumococcal empyema.

With very large effusions—either of the pneumococcal or streptococcal type—which cause marked displacement of the mediastinum, immediate open drainage may be dangerous. In such cases aspiration of approximately 20 oz. of pus should be carried out two or three days before drainage is performed; alternatively, temporary intercostal drainage by a catheter may be performed to serve as a means of gradual decompression.

Empyema in Children.—In children over five years the treatment of empyema need not differ in its essentials from that in adults. Very frequently closed drainage suffices, but in a proportion of cases it fails and open drainage is ultimately required. Open drainage should never be employed in infants and children under three. It has a much higher death-rate than closed drainage. Closed drainage is almost always sufficient. It should be performed under local anæsthesia.

Post-operative Management of Empyema.—It is an advantage to irrigate the pleural cavity regularly after the patient has recovered sufficient strength to tolerate the procedure. Warm saline should be used at first, later an antiseptic solution—such as weak eusol (half eusol, half water)—is preferable, as it helps to dissolve fibrin. The solution should be kept from strong light in a dark bottle. The patient should be so placed that the opening in the chest is uppermost and the cavity is completely filled so that all surfaces are cleansed.

Recovery is accelerated if the patient is nursed in the open air. Breathing exercises should be started as soon as possible in order to promote expansion of the lung. Active inspiratory exercises—known as M'Mahon's—are of the greatest value; they require the supervision of a trained masseuse.

The progress of lung expansion and diminution in size of the empyema cavity should be estimated periodically by radiograms, perferably taken anteroposteriorly and laterally. In no circumstances should the drainage tube be removed so long as any significant cavity remains; failure to observe this rule is very common and is the usual cause of recurrence of infection and chronicity of the empyema.

SPONTANEOUS PNEUMOTHORAX

Pulmonary tuberculosis is the most common cause of spontaneous pneumothorax, and routine radiological examination suggests that lesser degrees of the condition are not infrequent and that it often passes unnoticed. In rare instances it is the first evidence of pulmonary tuberculosis.

Till recent times tuberculosis was considered the almost invariable cause of spontaneous pneumothorax. It is now recognized, however, that when spontaneous pneumothorax occurs in an apparently healthy person it is more often due to some non-tuberculous defect in the alveoli or the pleura, such as an emphysematous bulla, or a direct tear of the pleura from traction by adhesions. Sometimes the pneumothorax recurs at varying intervals, and in some instances is bilateral or alternating. It is so seldom complicated by effusion that a simple origin may be inferred.

The escape of air into the pleural cavity may result from softening of superficial tuberculous foci, rupture of a cavity or the dragging effect of adhesions. If the opening in the pleura is oblique or valvular, a serious rise of intrapleural pressure may occur (tension pneumothorax). The escape of infective material usually results in pyopneumothorax (see below).

In a well-marked case of spontaneous pneumothorax there is usually sudden and severe pain in the chest and urgent dyspnœa and cyanosis. In the more severe cases hasty relief is necessary if fatal asphyxia is to be averted.

An X-ray examination should be carried out in order to ascertain the degree of pneumothorax and the presence of such complicating features as effusion and mediastinal displacement. Spontaneous pneumothorax may create considerable shock, alarm and anxiety, and morphia ($\frac{1}{4}$ gr.) is required for the control of these symptoms.

In many cases the lung quickly re-expands, and this should be awaited if there is only slight distress. If there is urgent dyspnœa and, especially if the heart is much displaced, the intrapleural tension should be relieved immediately. In an emergency the insertion of an aspirating needle into the pleural cavity is sufficient for decompression. If the opening in the lung is valvular and/or symptoms recur, the needle should be left in place and connected by rubber tubing to a bottle of antiseptic beneath the bed. This improvized water valve allows air to escape from, but not to re-enter, the chest. Later, if necessary, further air can be withdrawn by means of an artificial pneumothorax apparatus.

A very full and careful examination should be carried out to exclude the possibility of pulmonary tuberculosis. The milder cases should be treated by expectant measures. Urgent cases should be treated on the lines laid down above.

When the pneumothorax recurs at frequent intervals, and especially if it is incapacitating the patient, an attempt may be made to induce adhesions of the visceral or parietal pleura. *Oleothorax*—using olive oil—may succeed. Alternatively, the injection into the pneumothorax cavity of tincture of iodine ($2\frac{1}{2}$ per cent.), 1 to 10 c.c. at intervals of three or four days may create sufficient inflammatory reaction to bring about the requisite degree of adhesion.

Pyopneumothorax.—Following spontaneous pneumothorax of tuberculous origin an effusion develops in a large proportion of cases. At first the fluid is clear and tubercle bacilli are few in number, but there is a special tendency for the infection to progress so that the effusion becomes purulent—pyopneumothorax. Not infrequently a superadded pyogenic infection occurs or, still more serious, the pus may reach the surface or rupture into the large bronchi via a fistula.

The prognosis is always bad, more especially if the infection occurs during the advanced stages of the disease. If the pyopneumothorax complicates early disease of the lung, and especially if the other lung is healthy, active measures should be adopted before toxæmia undermines the patient's strength. The aim of treatment is to cleanse the pleura, to promote expansion of the lung and to allow the chest wall to shrink to its maximum amount before any drastic operation is performed. Sometimes repeated aspiration alone succeeds. If toxæmia persists, there need be no hesitation in carrying out "closed" suction drainage, which will allow of more thorough cleansing of the pleura by irrigation. In favourable cases, when the maximum degree of natural shrinkage of the chest has occurred, usually after several months, thoracoplasty—done in several stages—may lead to a successful issue.

BRONCHIECTASIS

There are wide variations in the clinical picture of bronchiectasis. The patient may complain only of recurrent cough, or repeated hæmoptysis (bronchiectasis hæmorrhagica sicca) or the classical picture of chronic ill-health, toxæmia, fœtid sputum and clubbing of the fingers may be present. There is, in addition, a large intermediate group in which health is not impaired for a great many years despite the expectoration of large amounts of sputum. The type, stage and localization of the disease, as well as the age, social circumstances and general health of the patient are factors which must be taken into consideration in determining the most suitable method of treatment.

Prophylaxis

A history of one or more attacks of capillary bronchitis or broncho-pneumonia, usually in childhood, is of such frequent occurrence as to suggest that a failure to obtain complete resolution of the inflammatory process is a factor of great ætiological importance in bronchiectasis. Accordingly, the family doctor should realize the essential need for thorough treatment in the acute stage of broncho-pneumonia by the measures outlined on p. 783, and the need for preventing the child from resuming its ordinary activities until every method has been tried to promote complete resolution. Such measures include a good diet, fresh air, a holiday at a convalescent home and breathing exercises carried out regularly two or three times a day. If atelectasis is present and fails to respond to the above measures, the use of a bronchoscope may be necessary to remove inspissated mucus or pus causing bronchial obstruction.

The bronchoscope should also be employed for the treatment of lobar collapse due to obstruction of a bronchus by a foreign body. The latter should be removed as soon as possible because of the liability of the bronchial tree to infection and dilatation.

Medical Treatment

Although the disease is a slowly progressive one, and medical treatment is only palliative, it can do much for the improvement of the general health, the reduction of toxæmia if present, the promotion of effective drainage of the bronchiectatic cavities and the reduction of the fœtor of the sputum. Even in cases selected for surgical treatment, a pre-operative course of treatment on medical lines is always indicated.

General Health.—The measures for the raising of the general resistance advocated for the prophylaxis of acute respiratory disease (p. 776) and the treatment of chronic bronchitis (p. 793) are equally applicable in bronchiectasis since patients suffering from this disease are particularly liable to attacks of acute respiratory infection. Fresh air and exercise are the best tonics, but attention should be paid to climate, good food, suitable clothing, etc. Tonics to stimulate the appetite may be given, and cod-liver oil may be prescribed during the winter. Iron is indicated if anæmia is present (see p. 471). Every case should be examined for chronic infection of the nasal sinuses, a frequent concomitant of bronchiectasis. Infected tonsils and adenoids and septic teeth should be removed. Patients with pyrexia will require rest in bed, and if possible should be nursed in the open air under sanatorium conditions.

Postural Drainage.—The most important medical measure for improving the general health and reducing the quantity and fœtor of the sputum is the emptying of the dilated bronchi and cavities by postural drainage. If regularly and efficiently carried out, the sputum may be reduced from several ounces to a trace in a few weeks. The resulting improvement in the general health is often remarkable.

Intermittent Postural Drainage.—This is carried out by instructing the patient to lean over the edge of the bed. The head should be well below the level of the body, which is supported by placing the hands on the floor so that the bases of the lungs are uppermost. A basin is placed on the floor to catch the expectoration and the vomit should this occur. This posture should be adopted two or three times a day before meals for a period of ten to fifteen minutes. We would again emphasize the fact that to obtain satisfactory results from postural drainage, it must be carried out persistently and with attention to detail.

Continuous Postural Drainage.—In patients with excessive expectoration, particularly if toxic manifestations are present, who fail to respond to intermittent postural drainage, it is advisable to arrange for continuous postural drainage. This means that the patient must be kept in bed for several weeks until the quantity of sputum expectorated has been reduced to a minimum. The position the patient should adopt will depend on the site of the pulmonary lesions. The posterior bronchi of the lower lobes are most frequently affected in bronchiectasis, and when the disease is situated in this region, the patient should lie prone (*i.e.*, face downward) with the head supported by one pillow and the foot of the bed raised to a height of about 12 in. A special postural drainage bed may be used in which the frame is hinged across the middle so that the centre of the bed can be raised to varying heights. Such a bed may be improvised by the use of a Bradford frame, the most suitable angle of inclination being between 20 and 30 degrees. When the disease is localized in other sites, appropriate postures should be adopted (see above). At the beginning of postural treatment an increase in the amount of sputum usually results, but once drainage is established a gradual diminution occurs. Many patients at first will be unable to tolerate more than five or ten minutes three times a day in the appropriate position. After a few days, drainage may be maintained for a large part of the day and night. During the first few days a slight rise in temperature, along with an increase in toxæmia may occur. The liability to hæmoptysis is slightly increased, but large hæmorrhages sufficient to endanger life are very rare. Severe reactions or hæmorrhage necessitate the cessation of postural drainage, which may be started again cautiously a few days later. The strain of coughing is very exhausting to patients acutely ill or debilitated by fever and toxæmia. In such cases, postural treatment should be discontinued, if the exhaustion produced more than counterbalances the effects of the removal of sputum. When the sputum has been reduced to a constant minimum quantity continuous drainage should be replaced by intermittent postural drainage.

Bronchoscopic Drainage.—In certain cases, when there is thick and tenacious purulent material in the cavities, or obstruction caused by swelling of the mucous membrane of the bronchi, aspiration through a bronchoscope often results in the establishment of free drainage. The procedure may have to be repeated several times, but should be abandoned as soon as adequate drainage can be secured. Bronchoscopic drainage immediately prior to the operation of lobectomy is invaluable and should be performed in all cases where there is purulent expectoration. Repeated lavage of the infected cavities through a bronchoscope with normal saline and mild antiseptics has not been of much value.

Drugs.—The intratracheal injection through a laryngeal cannula of oily solutions containing mild antiseptics such as gomenol, 5 per cent., or menthol, 5 per cent., in olive oil, has been advocated for the purposes of disinfecting the bronchial tree, but the results have been disappointing. To aid the removal of pus an expectorant mixture followed by a hot drink will be found useful (see p. 849). Inhalations of steam medicated with tinct. benzoin. co. (1 fluid drachm to 1 pint of hot water) are also helpful. In general, opiates are dangerous and contraindicated. If the cough is exhausting the patient, the use of a sedative linctus may be unavoidable, but if possible it should be reserved for securing sleep at night.

Fœtid Sputum.—When the sputum is foul smelling, an examination should always be made for spirochætes and fusiform bacilli, and if these are present arsenic should be administered. The intravenous injection of N.A.B., 0·3 gm. or the intramuscular injection of sulpharsphenamine, 0·3 gm., should be given once every four or five days for a few weeks.

In advanced cases the fœtor of the sputum is often exceedingly disagreeable to the patient and his friends. Life to him may be unbearable and ordinary social intercourse impossible. For the purpose of reducing the fœtor, the administration of garlic, 30 gr. in a capsule, has been recommended, but the best deodorant is creosote, which may be given in capsules containing 3 minims, three times a day.

Inhalations of creosote are recommended in every textbook. The patient sits or lies in a room specially set aside for the purpose, and a quantity of creosote is volatilized in an iron container. The vapour is very irritating, and the patient must wear close-fitting goggles to protect the eyes. The fumes are inhaled for a short period every day. At first the patient may be unable to tolerate more than a few minutes in the chamber, but the duration of exposure should be gradually increased to a maximum of half an hour. The coughing brought about by the irritating fumes encourages expectoration and after prolonged treatment a considerable reduction may occur in the amount of sputum along with the disappearance of the fœtor. Our experience leads us to believe that the creosote chamber is employed much less frequently to-day than in the past. Probably the beneficial effects obtained were largely the result of emptying the cavities of pus consequent on the paroxysms of coughing induced by the irritating fumes. If this explanation is correct, efficient postural drainage is to be preferred to the creosote chamber, since it is more convenient and less irritating to the patient.

Hæmoptysis.—Hæmoptysis is a fairly common symptom in bronchiectasis. The hæmorrhages are usually small and of little significance ; large hæmorrhages, so profuse as to endanger life, are rare. The symptomatic treatment is similar to that adopted in hæmoptysis from other causes such as tuberculosis (see p. 132). In bronchiectasis, however, when the bleeding is a possible source of danger to life, operative treatment may be indicated if the case fulfils the criteria discussed below.

Vaccines.—The question of vaccine therapy in chronic respiratory diseases has already been dealt with (p. 778). In early cases the administration of an autogenous vaccine may be of benefit. In advanced cases, however, vaccines should not be used, both because of their failure to produce good results and because of their tendency to induce severe reactions.

Surgical Measures

Lobectomy.—Lobectomy is the only operation which offers complete cure in bronchiectasis, but it is not an operation which should be undertaken lightly. A decision to advise lobectomy calls for sound clinical judgment, the co-operation of physician and surgeon, and the consideration of a number of factors. The services of a surgeon specially trained in surgery of the chest is essential, since in inexperienced hands the operation carries with it a high mortality. Unfortunately, the prolonged training required by the thoracic surgeon has led to the supply falling short of the demand. The exact site and extent of the disease should be carefully determined by lipiodol examination.

In general, only cases in which the disease is entirely or mainly confined to one lobe are suitable for lobectomy. Elderly people do not stand the operation well, and one should hesitate to advise lobectomy if the patient is over the age of forty. Children, on the other hand, are much better risks than adults. The general condition of the patient, as shown by the degree of toxæmia and the amount of sputum, is a factor which demands careful consideration. The risks of operation vary directly with the amount of sepsis present. Chronic ill-health with marked toxæmia usually indicates the presence of numerous adhesions, which add considerably to the technical difficulties of the operation. In such cases the operative mortality may be as high as 40 per cent. On the other hand, in young adults and children suffering either from dry hæmorrhagic bronchiectasis or bronchiectasis with expectoration but with no toxæmia, the operative mortality varies from 2 to 17 per cent. in different hands.

It must be remembered, however, that persons who suffer from bronchiectasis may remain in good health and live as normal members of society for many years. Lobectomy should only be considered if the disease is extending, sputum increasing or the general health deteriorating in spite of efficient medical treatment. No hard-and-fast rules can be laid down, and each case should be considered on its own merits. For instance, one would have more hesitation in advising lobectomy in the case of the breadwinner of a large family than in a young unmarried woman in whom the constant expectoration of foul pus makes her a social outcast, or in whom life becomes unbearable because of the mental anxiety resulting from repeated hæmorrhages. The social circumstances are frequently of paramount importance in influencing the decision in favour of operation.

Pre-operative Measures.—The operative risks can be reduced considerably if efficient medical treatment is carried out prior to the operation. This includes improvement of the general health, eradication of septic foci in the upper respiratory tract and reduction of the amount of sputum by postural treatment and bronchoscopic drainage.

Other Operative Measures.—*Thoracoplasty.*—The results of thoracoplasty are far from satisfactory. An extensive resection is required, the operation carries a high mortality rate and there is no guarantee that the cavities will be completely collapsed.

Phrenic Evulsion.—Paralysis of the diaphragm is not recommended. It seldom causes collapse of the cavities, while the expulsive power of the diaphragm is lost with resultant interference with drainage.

52

Artificial Pneumothorax.—The cavities in bronchiectasis are so thick-walled that a collapse of any therapeutic value is rarely produced. In addition, collapse of the lung is often prevented by the presence of pleural adhesions. For severe hæmorrhage which fails to respond to medical treatment, artificial pneumothorax may have to be considered.

ABSCESS AND GANGRENE OF THE LUNG

Abscess of the lung may arise without apparent cause, may complicate pneumonia or bronchial carcinoma, or may follow surgical operation or the inhalation of a foreign body, etc.

From the point of view of prophylaxis, the prevention and treatment of post-operative complications are of importance (see p. 820). It is not sufficiently realized that every patient, who is about to undergo a major surgical operation under general anæsthesia, should first have any sepsis in the mouth and throat treated. Since abscess of the lung may follow dental extraction, the removal at one operation of a large number of septic teeth under general anæsthesia is to be deprecated.

In the early stages medical treatment is indicated, since complete spontaneous cure frequently occurs by rupture of the abscess into a bronchus with expectoration of the pus. The treatment of abscess of the lung in each individual case varies with the cause and duration of the abscess, the site and extent of the lesion, whether rupture into a bronchus has occurred and the general condition of the patient.

The exact site of the abscess should be determined at the earliest possible moment by means of antero-posterior and lateral radiograms, and if necessary by the introduction of lipiodol. Exploratory puncture of the chest with a needle in order to locate the abscess should not be attempted on account of the risks of infecting the pleural cavity.

Medical Measures.—Measures should be taken to improve the general health by diet, tonics and good nursing (see p. 776). It is of advantage to nurse the patient in the open air if the weather is good and the patient is not too enfeebled. Every effort should be made to promote effective expectoration of the pus, since this is the fundamental principle of medical treatment. For this purpose *continuous postural drainage* carried out on the lines described on p. 814 should be instituted. When the abscess is situated in the upper zone the patient should be supported in the sitting position by pillows. When the abscess is situated in the middle zones the patient should be treated lying supine on his side, or prone, according to the position of the lesion as demonstrated by a lateral radiogram of the chest. For a lesion in the lower zone, the foot of the bed is raised about 12 in., and the patient lies supine in the lateral position, or prone, depending on whether the abscess occupies the anterior, lateral or posterior region of the lower lobe.

Inhalations of medicated steam are soothing, and will often help to loosen viscid sputum. Stimulating expectorants may also be prescribed (see p. 849). The cough is often very irritating and exhausting, especially in debilitated patients. As far as possible the use of opiates should be avoided, but the practitioner may be forced to prescribe a sedative linctus (see p. 850) to secure rest and sleep.

Bronchoscopy.—If the presence of a foreign body or bronchial carcinoma is suspected, bronchoscopy should be performed as soon as possible. Bronchoscopy is indicated in all cases which are not responding to postural drainage, or in which the general condition is deteriorating, or where radiograms reveal progressive enlargement of the cavity. Where poor drainage is due to the obstruction caused by granulation tissue, swollen mucosa or inspissated pus, aspiration through a bronchoscope may result in the establishment of free drainage. But, if the abscess is draining freely into a bronchus, bronchoscopy is unlikely to give better results than efficient postural drainage.

The presence of a foul sputum, containing large numbers of Vincent's organisms (spirochætes and fusiform bacilli) demands the employment of arsenical compounds such as N.A.B. 0·3 gm. intravenously or sulpharsphenamine 0·3 gm. intramuscularly.

Surgical Measures.—Surgical measures are chiefly reserved for cases in which the abscess is single and situated near the periphery of the lung. They should only be advised when, after at least six to eight weeks of adequate medical treatment, effective drainage has not been secured, and the patient is losing ground as evidenced by intractable cough, loss of weight, and toxæmia, or if the radiograms show an extension of the abscess cavity. No hard-and-fast rules can be laid down, and the decision, if and when to advise operation, is often exceedingly difficult. The operation usually indicated is thoracotomy, which consists in the majority of cases of a two-stage procedure, the first to cause adherence of the two layers of the pleura by the introduction between them of a sterile gauze swab, the second consisting of rib resection and a wide incision to establish external drainage.

Pneumonectomy and lobectomy are serious operations, and are seldom advisable.

Thoracoplasty has not justified the expectations of those who have advocated it, and cannot be recommended.

POST-OPERATIVE PULMONARY COMPLICATIONS

The treatment of such complications as bronchitis, pneumonia, abscess of the lung and empyema have been dealt with elsewhere. Sulphrenic abscess calls for surgical measures.

Atelectasis

Atelectasis is one of the commonest post-operative pulmonary complications. It may be patchy or lobular, or may involve an entire lobe (massive collapse). The onset is usually sudden and occurs within the first twenty-four to forty-eight hours after the operation, particularly an abdominal one. The immediate cause of the collapse is obstruction of a bronchus by inspissated mucus or purulent secretion. Numerous factors predispose to retention of bronchial secretions, but if steps are taken to correct these beforehand, the liability to post-operative collapse will be greatly reduced.

Prophylaxis.—*Before Operation.*—When respiratory infection, *e.g.*, bronchitis, is present, the risk of atelectasis is increased, and major operations should be postponed if possible. Heavy smokers are particularly liable to post-operative pulmonary complications. Accordingly, it may be advisable to stop or reduce smoking for one or two weeks prior to operation.

If postponement is possible for a month or longer individuals with deformities of the chest or faulty methods of breathing should be given a course of remedial exercises before operation.

Secretions are apt to stagnate in the bronchi of elderly patients particularly if they are obese and flabby. Before operating on these patients measures should be taken to reduce their weight (see p. 387), and gas and oxygen anæsthesia are to be preferred to ether at operation.

After Operation.—CO_2 is the natural stimulant of the respiratory centre. For increasing the depth of respiration in individuals who breathe weakly after severe operations the inhalation through a nasal catheter of 5 per cent. CO_2 in oxygen has been found of great value. It may be given for half-hour periods every two or three hours for the first twenty-four to forty-eight hours after the operation.

After all major operations the position of the patient should be changed three or four times during the day. The nurse should remove the pillows, place the patient on his side, and, while supporting the abdomen with the hand, encourage him to cough. Constricting bandages around the lower part of the chest and abdomen interfere with expansion of the lower lobes and should never be allowed. Flatulent distension has a similar effect and should be corrected. The suppression of the cough, for example, by pain in the wound, is a potent factor in the production of atelectasis. Small doses of morphine, not more than $\frac{1}{6}$ gr., will relieve the pain sufficiently to enable the patient to breathe more freely and to cough without discomfort. Large doses of morphine are contraindicated since they stop the cough reflex. Atropine should not be used after operation as it tends to increase the tenacity of the mucus in the bronchial tubes, thus rendering its expectoration more difficult.

Treatment.—At the onset of a severe case of atelectasis, the usual remedies for shock will be necessary (see p. 727). If cyanosis and dyspnœa are present, oxygen should be given continuously through a nasal catheter.

Many patients will respond to simple measures, such as encouragement to cough, frequent changes in position, and the administration of an expectorant mixture containing potassium iodide and ephedrine if bronchial spasm is present (see Appendix).

Morphine (in small doses, $\frac{1}{6}$ gr.) should be used only if the patient is suffering from severe pain, which cannot be relieved by the milder sedative drugs such as aspirin, phenacetin and codeine, and by the local application of heat (see p. 788).

Oxygen with 5 per cent. carbon dioxide will promote deep breathing and may help to dislodge the obstructions in the bronchi.

If the above measures fail and collapse of the lung still persists at the end of a week, bronchoscopy should be seriously considered with a view to removing the obstructing secretions.

Pulmonary Embolism and Infarction

The symptoms vary with the size of the infarct. If a large vessel is occluded death usually occurs with dramatic suddenness. In less severe cases, collapse, pleuritic pain in the chest and hæmoptysis are the prominent features. The pain usually preceeds the hæmoptysis by some hours. The fear occasioned by the spitting of blood may be minimized by forewarning the patient of its probable occurrence and by giving him appropriate reassurance.

Prophylaxis.—Thrombo-phlebitis, a common cause of pulmonary embolism, should be treated by immobilization of the limb until such time as organization of the clot has taken place. On an average this means absolute rest for a period of six weeks.

Treatment.—An injection of $\frac{1}{6}$ to $\frac{1}{4}$ gr. of morphine may be given if pain is severe, and measures for treating shock instituted (see p. 727). The patient should be kept warm by the use of hot bottles or the electric cage. To improve the cerebral circulation the head should be lowered by raising the foot of the bed on blocks. Diffusible stimulants such as spiritus ammon. aromat., 1 fluid drachm, or $\frac{1}{2}$ oz. of whisky or brandy may be given.

When the patient has recovered from the state of shock, the recumbent position may be resumed. Twenty-four hours later the patient should be supported by pillows in a sitting position so as to prevent hypostatic congestion and broncho-pneumonia. These not infrequently cause a fatal result one or two weeks after the infarction.

INTRATHORACIC NEW GROWTHS

Malignant Tumours

Bronchial Carcinoma.—The radical cure of cancer of the lung by the complete extirpation of the affected lobe is rarely possible, since by the time the patient presents himself for examination, metastasis to the bronchial glands and elsewhere has nearly always occurred. With improved methods of diagnosis, and of surgical technique, it is reasonable to hope that there will be an increase in the number of cases suitable for operation.

The great majority of cases will have to be treated on medical lines. Radium needles or radon seeds introduced directly into the growth through a bronchoscope have given disappointing results. Deep X-ray therapy may cause shrinkage of the growth, and may be useful in the later stages of the disease in alleviating distressing symptoms, such as pain, stridor and œdema. Prolongation of life, however, can only be expected in a very small proportion of cases.

Sooner or later measures will have to be taken for the relief of breathlessness, pain and cough. Increasing doses of liquor morphin. hydrochlor. should be given three or four times a day. In the late stages, morphine should be given freely by hypodermic injection. Heroin is preferred by some, and the combination of morphine and cocaine (of each $\frac{1}{4}$ gr.) has been recommended.

Lymphosarcoma and Hodgkin's Disease, affecting the mediastinal glands, often respond in a remarkable manner to deep X-ray therapy. Life may be prolonged for one or two years, but unfortunately these tumours always recur, and the disease is sooner or later fatal. For the general treatment of these diseases, see p. 530.

Non-malignant Tumours

The prognosis in innocent tumours and cysts of the lung and mediastinum is better than in malignant cases. Provided the patient survives the operation, complete cure may be expected. The decision to recommend operation may be very difficult. If the tumour is discovered accidentally, it is advisable to watch the rate of growth by means of serial radiograms. Operation should be performed only if the tumour is increasing in size, or if pressure signs develop. In the majority of cases, however, when the patient consults his doctor signs of pressure are manifest. In such cases, operation should be carried out, if, after careful consideration of the size and position of the tumour and the general condition of the patient, reasonable prospects of success may be expected. Otherwise treatment must be on symptomatic lines. It may be possible to remove such tumours as adenomata and fibromata of the larger bronchi by means of the bronchoscope.

SPECIFIC NON-TUBERCULOUS INFECTION OF THE LUNG

Pulmonary lesions may be produced by syphilis, fungus infections (actinomycosis, aspergillosis, etc.) and hydatid disease. For their treatment, see appropriate sections.

ACUTE ŒDEMA OF THE LUNGS

In Pneumonia, see p. 790. In Cardiac Disease, see p. 699.

ASTHMA

Definition. A spasmodic contraction of the bronchial muscles causing paroxysmal dyspnœa which is chiefly expiratory in character.

Treatment will be considered under two headings: (1) treatment of the acute attack; (2) the management of the asthmatic state.

TREATMENT OF THE ACUTE ATTACK

If the attack of asthma is of sufficient severity to require the attendance of a doctor, the following measures should be instituted. The patient should be sent to bed and propped up in the position which he finds most comfortable. The most effective way of relieving bronchial spasm is to stimulate the sympathetic nervous system. For this purpose a subcutaneous injection of adrenalin hydrochloride, 1 : 1,000 solution, should be employed. Adrenalin loses its potency with keeping, particularly if exposed to the air or to sunlight. It should therefore be kept in tinted rubber-capped bottles in the dark and even then should be renewed every three months. The earlier in the attack that adrenalin is given, the more effective will be its action. Thus, a small dose such as 3 to 5 minims, if given at the onset of wheezing, may completely abort the attack, while twice this quantity may be unsuccessful in bringing relief to a patient in whom the paroxysm has lasted for an hour or two. It is for this reason that we believe that patients whose paroxysms are not controlled by the measures described in the section devoted to the management of the asthmatic state, should be instructed how to inject themselves with adrenalin. Should the initial dose fail to control the attack, the dose may be repeated at half-hour intervals. There is no evidence, as far as we know, that any harmful effects result from the frequent injection of small amounts of adrenalin, even when asthma and hypertension coexist. In some cases, however, when many daily injections are given over a period of weeks, the individual appears to acquire a partial tolerance to the drug as shown by the poor effects produced even when large doses are given. Adrenalin should always be injected very slowly by the subcutaneous route. After introducing the needle under the skin and before injecting the drug, the piston of the syringe should be slightly withdrawn to make sure that the needle is not in a small vein, since the intravenous injection of adrenalin causes unpleasant reactions, *e.g.*, tremor, bursting headache, faintness, palpitation or even collapse.

Counter-irritation to the chest is soothing to the patient and in some cases undoubtedly helps to relieve bronchial spasm. For this purpose one or other of the following may be tried—a linseed poultice, with or without the addition of mustard, a kaolin poultice, dry cupping the back of the chest, the application of hot turpentine stupes or a mustard leaf to the sternum.

Should three or four injections of adrenalin at half-hourly intervals fail to control the paroxysm of asthma, pituitrin either alone or combined with adrenalin (asthmolysin) in a dose of $\frac{1}{2}$ to 1 c.c., should be given subcutaneously. Some cases which have failed to respond to adrenalin will respond to the above combination.

In a very small proportion of cases of great severity the measures already described fail to bring relief. The patient may be described as being in "status asthmaticus." To break this state, it will be necessary to introduce antispasmodic drugs under the skin every one to two minutes. A 1 c.c. syringe filled with adrenalin should be strapped to the skin of the forearm after introducing the needle under the skin. One minim should be injected every minute until relief has been obtained. As much as 100 minims may be required in a severe case. Thereafter, to prevent a relapse, it is advisable to give 1 to 2 minims every quarter of an hour for the next hour, twice in the second hour, and once an hour for another two or three hours. This method will be found to be effective in controlling the majority of cases of "status asthmaticus."

Should no result be produced, however, by the end of an hour, it will be necessary to use in addition one or other of the following narcotic drugs: (1) morphia should be given in a dose of $\frac{1}{6}$ gr. and should not be repeated for at least four hours. Morphine is in general contraindicated in asthma because of the liability to habit formation. In addition there is the danger of asphyxia because the large amounts of mucus which may be secreted after the spasm has been relieved will not be removed if the cough reflex has been abolished; (2) $\frac{1}{2}$ oz. of ether mixed with $\frac{1}{2}$ oz. of olive oil for every 20 lbs. of body-weight should be administered per rectum.

When the paroxysm has been relieved by one or other of these measures, the patient should be given an antispasmodic mixture (see Appendix) and $\frac{1}{2}$ gr. of ephedrine hydrochloride every six hours. If the attack has been severe and prolonged the patient will be exhausted and should be advised to stay in bed for twenty-four hours or longer. He should take a light easily digested diet in small quantities at two-hourly intervals, and large amounts of fluid of which fruit juice sweetened with glucose should form a part.

THE MANAGEMENT OF THE ASTHMATIC STATE

"Many physicians feel their responsibility ended after the control of the acute paroxysm" (Coca).

This attitude cannot be too strongly deprecated to-day in view of the advance of knowledge in regard to the factors which underlie the asthmatic constitution. Every effort must be made (1) to ascertain the immediate exciting cause of the paroxysm; (2) to determine the ætiological factors; (3) to institute therapeutic measures to prevent recurrence or, if this is impossible, to diminish the number and severity of the attacks.

The management of the asthmatic state does not consist in giving an antispasmodic mixture, but entails the taking of a careful clinical history and the making of a complete investigation of all systems. Apart from certain general measures, treatment therefore varies in every case since it will depend on the recognition of the causative factors and the assessment of their relative importance. Hence it can be understood why the claims of certain enthusiasts, that their own particular remedy is a cure for all cases of asthma, are totally unconvincing. Asthma resembles the chronic rheumatic diseases since in both there exists a constitutional basis which can be affected by a wide variety of exciting agents.

While for clearness of description the ætiological factors must be separately considered, in practice they frequently occur in combination. Hence treatment is often unsuccessful because one factor has received exclusive attention. The importance of the combination of factors is well exemplified by the story of Trousseau. He found that oat and stable dust was only able to induce him to have a very mild form of asthma. Likewise, when he was out driving with his coachman and got into a passion, no asthma resulted. If, however, he lost his temper with his coachman in the stable where he was in contact with dust, an extremely severe paroxysm of asthma occurred.

The Psychological Factor

In our experience the most important single factor in asthma is the psychological one. The typical asthmatic is a highly strung, over-anxious, emotional and intelligent person, whose broncho-constrictor centre in the medulla is in a peculiarly irritable condition, being easily influenced by many types of minor stimuli. If we accept the constitutional basis of asthma as being of great importance, we can understand the danger of using the word "cure," since the removal of some abnormality in the nose or the correction of some dietary indiscretion may temporarily relieve the asthma but will leave unchanged the underlying constitutional basis. It is not surprising, therefore, that asthma may again occur when the broncho-constrictor centre is irritated by other stimuli.

It should be noted that the broncho-constrictor centre, which for constitutional reasons is excessively irritable, will react to psychological stimuli of a degree insufficient to have any effect on normal individuals.

It is only within the last few years that the real importance of the psychological factor in asthma has been fully realised. It is the influence of this elusive factor which makes it so difficult to assess the value of any one therapeutic measure. It has long been known that the majority of cases of asthma cease having attacks on entering a hospital ward and often promptly relapse on returning home. The enthusiastic believers in allergy would suggest that the results depend on the removal of the patient from contact with some sensitizing allergen. We believe that in the majority of cases the results are effected by the psychological influence of white-coated doctors and efficient sisters, which gives the patient a hope that something definite is going to be done to improve his condition. In addition, he is transferred to a tranquil environment from one which may be keeping him in a state of nervous tension. The patient's skin reactions may have been positive to dust, feathers, etc., before he entered hospital and will continue to be positive while he is free from asthma in the hospital ward, even though he is sleeping peacefully on a feather pillow. Any treatment involving injections or special manipulations is calculated to inspire confidence in the patient. We, like others, have obtained excellent results in the management of the asthmatic state by injections of distilled water. Since 50 to 60 per cent. of all asthmatics can be improved by a simple antispasmodic mixture and cheerful encouragement by the family doctor, it follows that the claims made for many forms of treatment commonly employed to-day must be accepted with due reserve.

The following case histories are given with the object of illustrating the psychological factor in asthma :—

Case 1. Mrs A., an asthmatic of long standing, had severe attacks periodically. She had lived in the same house for many years. No evidence of allergy was obtained from the clinical history or from skin tests. Her married life had always been unhappy owing to her belief in her inferior social status to her husband. Her sexual life had also been unsatisfactory, although she was the mother of two healthy daughters. A careful analysis of her asthmatic attacks indicated a close association between them and her fear and loathing of her husband. During his absence abroad her asthma quietened down to a mild chronic condition, but anything which brought his presence back to her mind would start a paroxysm, *e.g.*, a conversation with a friend, or reading in a newspaper about his career. The receipt of any letter from him, particularly if it contained any suggestion that he would be coming home on leave, was sufficient to induce a severe attack of asthma, which lasted for several days despite the repeated injection of adrenalin. All efforts at curing the patient have failed as she will neither accept the situation nor agree to a divorce. Possibly if the psychological aspect had been treated many years previously, results would have been different.

Case 2. A boy aged sixteen, the son of brilliant parents, had had periodic attacks of severe asthma since the age of six. He had eczema in infancy and there was a family history of asthma on his father's side. Skin tests were positive to horse and cat hair, dust and pollen, but negative to all ingestants tested. He had received many kinds of treatment including non-specific desensitization. His feather pillow had been replaced by one of sorbo rubber. Periodic attacks of asthma continued just the same. Our analysis of the events immediately preceding his attacks made it clear that anything which induced a state of nervous tension would precipitate an attack. Recently the boy's mother telephoned one of us that he had severe asthma. Inquiry elicited the information that he had been sitting examinations for the preceding three days. An assurance that the attack would immediately subside without any treatment when the results of the examinations were announced, particularly if he had done well, was justified by its immediate cessation on the following day, when the boy was given first-class honours. It is difficult to know to what degree the conscious or unconscious mind was responsible for the attack. The state of nervous tension induced by the examinations could not be avoided by this brilliant youth. On the other hand, the occurrence of asthma at the time of the examinations would be a good excuse if he failed to do well, while if he were successful the accomplishment would be all the more creditable, in view of his physical incapacity. Some two weeks after the examination, when the boy was entirely free from asthma, we repeated his skin tests and found them triple positive to the above-mentioned inhalants.

At the same time, tests performed on his three brothers and sisters who were non-asthmatics were negative. The clinical history of eczema and the family history of asthma, together with the positive skin tests, suggest an undoubted allergic factor. Nevertheless, the boy is free from asthma for months on end, despite the presence of cats in the house, or even when he is sleeping on feather pillows. If an allergic factor in this case is the cause of the asthma, it would appear to operate only or chiefly when a state of nervous tension is induced by psychological causes. Concentration on treatment of the allergic factor without correcting the underlying psychological factor is in our experience the principle reason why disappointing results are so frequently obtained in the treatment of asthma.

Case 3. A boy of ten had had asthma for several years. Skin tests were strongly positive to dust, horse hair and feathers. A history of eczema during infancy was obtained. His father wished to know if asthma was an infectious disease, because his other son, aged eight, suddenly started to have asthma. No evidence of an allergic basis was found in the younger child, and inquiry suggested that the asthma was induced in order to receive the favours (sweets, petting by the mother and leave from school) which the elder brother obtained when he had asthma. The position was explained to the child, and suitable advice given to the parents. The child ceased having attacks, and has remained well ever since.

Assessment of the Psychological Factor.—For the assessment of the importance of the psychological factor, information regarding the following points must be obtained : (1) personal relations with family and friends ; (2) occupation and relations with employer ; (3) financial circumstances ; and (4) the patient's opinion regarding his state of health, *e.g.*, the fear of disease.

Strauss suggests that help may be obtained by attempting to get an answer to the following ten questions :—

1. Does the patient volunteer the information that he is, generally speaking, " nervy " apart from his asthma ?
2. Does he state that excitement or emotion of any kind precipitates an attack ?
3. Does he habitually live under conditions involving excessive worry or emotional strain and stress ?
4. Is he temperamentally a person who finds it difficult to adapt to his social environment ?
5. Is his libidinal life reasonably and legitimately satisfied or satisfiable—judging by superficial standards only ?

6. Was he considered to be nervous as a child ?
7. Are there any obvious pointers to determinant " complexes " in the psychoanalytical sense ?
8. Is a crudely purposive (unconscious) factor detectable and probably a link in the causal chain ?
9. Does the patient superficially impress the investigator as being " neurotic " or well-balanced ?
10. Is the family history " neuropathic " ?

Lastly, we agree with Halliday that it is highly important for the doctor to make full inquiries into the following three points :—

1. What kind of person is this ? Is he over-aggressive, emotionally unstable, shy and seclusive, etc. ?
2. Why did he take ill when he did ? Inquiries should be made with regard to the mode of behaviour and psychological factors operating at or before the time of the *first* attack of asthma.
3. What is the person getting at ?—*i.e.*, for what end or purpose is this behaviour ? An attack of asthma may enable a person to attain what he desires or to avoid something which is unpleasant.

Should the above investigations reveal a psychological element of importance, much can be done by the intelligent practitioner to improve matters. This is particularly the case in children.

Children.—The situation must be explained to the mother, so that her natural desire to protect the child may not defeat its own object by inducing a state of nervous tension. Often the mother herself is in a state of nervous tension over some personal problem which is unconsciously transmitted to the child. This aspect is often not realized, and successful results may not be obtained in the treatment of the child if the psychological factor in the parents is neglected. Over-anxiety of the mother leads to pampering the child and making him wear excessive clothing. This must be corrected. There must be no suggestion that he is a delicate child and different from other children, and he must be induced to play with them in order to gain confidence. He must not be withdrawn from school for mild attacks so that he does not use his asthma as a means of avoiding his responsibilities. If the father has adopted a domineering attitude, this must cease. It is important to get the school-teacher to co-operate in these efforts.

Should the family doctor fail to obtain satisfactory results either because of his lack of experience or personality, or because of his inability to obtain the parents' co-operation, the child should be referred to a child-guidance clinic where expert psychological treatment will be available and where organized play therapy is being regularly carried out.

Adults.—A different method must be adopted for treating the psychological element in adults.

Careful questioning will frequently reveal that a state of mental conflict or anxiety in the patient, consequent on unhappy relations between husband and wife, parents and children, employers and employees, etc. Any cause of anxiety, however, may start an asthmatic attack. For instance one of our patients, who had been instructed to inject himself with adrenalin, told us that on one occasion he was unable to lay hands on his syringe. The terror induced by the mere thought that he had lost his syringe was sufficient to induce a paroxysm of asthma. In other cases, the attack of asthma is used by the patient as a means of escape from performing duties which he finds to be unpleasant, or for the acquisition of sympathy. The family doctor, by the use of explanation and persuasion, can play an important part in relieving the mental conflict or the anxiety states. The mere unburdening of the patient's troubles, followed by a kindly and simple explanation by the doctor of their effect in the production of asthma, is not infrequently sufficient to relieve nervous tension and to produce improvement. In some cases, however, the psychological factor is so complex and so deeply ingrained that it is necessary to refer the patient to a psychologist.

The Allergic Factor

A state of inherited hypersensitiveness to foreign substances is commonly present in asthma. The sensitizing agent is usually a protein, although occasionally it may be a drug, *e.g.*, aspirin. The assessment of this factor may be difficult, since sensitivity to a substance may vary from time to time for reasons not clearly understood.

In investigating the allergic factor it is essential to obtain a careful history of how and when the original attack of asthma commenced. In general, it may be said, that the earlier in life asthma commences the more likely will an allergic factor be found. This probability is increased by the coexistence of eczema, urticaria, prurigo, hay fever or migraine, or a family history of allergy.

The allergen may be absorbed by ingestion or inhalation. The alimentary route is of particular importance in infancy. The commonest foods causing asthma in order of frequency are wheat, egg, milk, chocolate, beans, potatoes, pig products and beef.

In childhood and early adult life, inhalants are of great ætiological importance. The chief inhalants are animal emanations, such as horse dander and feathers, house dust, moulds, pollens and orris root, which is so frequently used in face powders. In middle age and late life a history of a lung infection so frequently precedes the original asthmatic attack as to suggest bacterial allergy.

Although the taking of a careful history regarding an allergic factor is of the utmost importance, we would utter a warning against the doctor accepting the patient's statement too easily. Again and again we have had patients who claimed that certain articles of food or some animal emanation produced an asthmatic attack and yet, when the supposedly offending article was brought into contact with the patient in a disguised form, no asthma resulted. Such experiences suggest that the patient's deductions are often at fault in assessing the part played by any factor in starting an asthmatic attack. In other cases the asthma results from psychological causes, as exemplified by the story of the patient who believed that her asthma was due to emanations from roses and immediately had an asthmatic attack at the sight of an artificial rose.

Despite these experiences, if the history and skin tests are positive, we recommend that contact with the causative allergen should be avoided or reduced to a minimum, because, although it may not induce an attack in hospital, it may do so in the patient's home if accompanied by a state of nervous tension or anxiety. In addition to taking a careful history it will be necessary to make certain tests for ascertaining sensitivity. For this purpose, solutions of the common inhalants and ingestants can be obtained from leading manufacturers, such as Bencards.

Intradermal Test.—The most satisfactory test is made by introducing 0·01 c.c. of the solutions of extracts to be tested into the skin of the volar surface of the forearm. A control injection of carbol-saline is also made. A positive reaction is recognized by the appearance within ten to fifteen minutes of a wheal of at least 5 mm. in diameter. Pseudopodial extensions from the wheal indicate definite sensitivity.

Scratch Test.—Another method of skin testing is to place the solution of the extract on the skin, which is scarified through the drop with a needle.

Interpretation of Skin Tests.—The interpretation and the clinical significance of the skin tests is far from easy. Thus a patient may give a history of allergy to a certain substance and the skin test may be negative, or more frequently a positive test may be found in the absence of a suggestive clinical history. Again, in our experience, multiple sensitivity is present rather than sensitivity to a single allergen. Lastly, a positive skin test to a solution of house dust is so commonly present in asthmatics that its significance is difficult to assess, particularly since a similar reaction not infrequently occurs in normal persons without asthma. From what has been said, it is clear that the results obtained from skin testing are often unsatisfactory and many physicians have accordingly given them up. We believe, however, that they are of value in a proportion of cases both for the purpose of recognizing and confirming sensitivity and for helping to eliminate the allergic factor in cases which we believe to be purely psychological. Some of our most intractable cases of asthma belong to this category and have negative skin tests.

Avoidance of the Offending Substance.—When the clinical history and skin tests suggest that the sensitizing agent is an ingestant or an inhalant, measures should be instituted which will enable the patient, if possible, to avoid contact with it.

Ingestants.—If the allergen is some uncommon foodstuff such as strawberries, pork or shell-fish, its recognition is usually easy and its elimination from the diet may produce dramatic results. If, on the other hand, the allergen is a common foodstuff such as wheat, egg or milk, both recognition and avoidance will be difficult because these articles appear on the table in various disguises. To identify the offending substance elimination diets must be used. The bowels are emptied by calomel and Epsom salts, and the patient is placed on a simple basic diet. This diet should consist of one or two articles of food to which the patient is not sensitive. For this purpose orange juice or a milk diet (provided the patient is not sensitive to milk) will be found satisfactory. The patient remains on this basic diet for three days. Thereafter another article of food is added to the diet on each successive day until the offending foodstuff is discovered by the occurrence of asthma, or reactions resembling the symptoms of the disease under investigation. The offending article can then be eliminated from the diet. When complete elimination is not practicable, marked reduction in the quantity of the allergen in the diet may be sufficient to produce an improvement.

Inhalants.—If feathers or horse dander have been definitely inculpated from the clinical history and from the presence of strongly positive skin tests, feathers in pillows and quilts should be replaced by the best Java kapok. Horse-hair mattresses should be covered with rubber sheeting or replaced by the sorbo rubber mattress as supplied by the Dunlop Rubber Company. Chairs and sofas stuffed with horse hair should be replaced by articles of furniture stuffed with kapok. Owing to the expense involved these changes should only be advised if the asthma is not controlled by the other measures described for the management of the asthmatic state, nor should a too optimistic attitude be adopted since in our experience the results are not infrequently disappointing.

A dusty atmosphere undoubtedly predisposes to attacks of asthma, but whether this is due to a specific sensitivity to the dust, or to mechanical irritation of the asthmagenic area in the nose, we are not prepared to say. In either case, the less the patient comes in contact with a dusty atmosphere the better. Accordingly, the minimum of furniture should be kept in the bedroom and a vacuum cleaner should be used for removing dust from the floor, crevices and ledges.

If the patient is sensitive to orris root then face powders must be prohibited or special preparations free from orris root used. These may be obtained from any chemist (Queen products).

Lastly, sensitization may occur to inhalants with which the patient comes in contact during his work, *e.g.*, in mills, breweries or stables. If desensitization with the particular allergen fails to produce benefit, a change of occupation must be advised.

Specific Desensitization.—Should the patient find it impossible to avoid the offending allergen, desensitization may be attempted. In the case of ingestants two methods are available. A solution of the offending article may be injected subcutaneously in increasing doses. Alternatively, minute quantities of the food itself may be added to the patient's diet and the amount gradually increased. Desensitization is much more frequently employed against inhalants. When sensitivity is multiple it is advisable to use a solution containing a mixture of the commoner inhalants, *e.g.*, feathers, dust, animal hair and orris root. A mixed inhalant solution with full directions, may be obtained from C. L. Bencard, Endersleigh Gardens, Hendon, London. In general, it is advisable to start with the subcutaneous injection of 0·1 c.c. of the weakest solution and cautiously to increase this dose at intervals of from five to seven days according to the local reaction. The occurrence of a general reaction such as an asthmatic attack necessitates the reduction of the dose at the next injection. In order to minimize the risk of general reactions, 2 or 3 minims of adrenalin should be injected simultaneously. Specific desensitization is most successful where only one allergen is concerned. It has certain risks, fortunately rare, and should not be practised by those unfamiliar with the technique.

Before embarking on a course of desensitizing injections the patient should be told that the process involves frequent injections over many weeks. The idea that beneficial effects can be obtained from two or three injections is fallacious. In our experience the benefits claimed to result from specific desensitization have been greatly exaggerated. Any improvement which may result is seldom lasting. We have already drawn attention to the great importance of the psychological factor in the treatment of asthma, which is particularly apparent when parenteral methods of treatment are employed by an enthusiast. Nevertheless, specific desensitization is believed to be of value by many authorities, and details of the technique have accordingly been given.

Non-specific Desensitization.—For this purpose many substances have been used, such as peptone, tuberculin, milk, T.A.B. vaccine, sulphur, etc. We do not intend to discuss these preparations in detail because we feel that their exponents have in general taken an unduly optimistic view of their value, and we suspect that the psychological effects of injections have been overlooked. While it is true that 60 to 70 per cent. of cases of asthma may obtain benefit by non-specific desensitization, in our experience the improvement is seldom lasting. Nevertheless, it is worthy of trial when other measures have failed. Occasionally, dramatic success is attained, while in others cases temporary relief occurs which enables the patient to regain his confidence.

Peptone.—Armour's peptone No. 2 (5 per cent. solution), is chiefly employed and can be given intravenously or intramuscularly, the latter route being considerably safer. Starting with 0·3 c.c. (5 minims), the dose is slowly increased every four or five days until a maximum of 2 to 3 c.c. is given, after which the dose is gradually reduced.

Tuberculin.—This method is contraindicated in the presence of active tuberculosis. The initial dose should be 0·1 c.c. of 1 : 1,000,000 Koch's old tuberculin. The dose is given subcutaneously and should be gradually increased at weekly intervals, due care being taken to keep below a dose which produces general reactions.

Milk.—Whole milk which has first been boiled may be injected subcutaneously or intramuscularly at intervals of five to seven days, starting with an intitial dose of 1 c.c. and gradually increasing to a maximum dose of 10 c.c. The proprietary preparation " xifal milk " is extensively used for this purpose.

Sulphur.—Sulphur in colloidal form in 1 and 2 c.c. ampoules in 0·1 and 0·5 per cent. solution is marketed by British Drug Houses Ltd. and Crooke's Laboratories. It is given intramuscularly or intravenously at weekly intervals.

T.A.B. Vaccine.—The initial dose is 25 million organisms injected intravenously, which is increased by 25 to 50 million at weekly intervals up to a maximum of 500 million. The severe reactions which may occur indicate great caution in this form of treatment.

Auto-hæmotherapy.—Five to ten cubic centimetres of blood are withdrawn into a syringe from a vein in the patient's arm and immediately injected into the muscles of the buttock. A course consists of six to ten injections at weekly intervals.

The Infective Factor

Acute infections of the upper respiratory tract will precipitate an attack of asthma in the majority of sufferers. Accordingly, the measures already described for the prevention and treatment of acute respiratory infections are particularly required in asthmatics (see p. 775 *et seq.*).

Vaccines.—Vaccines are recommended for the treatment of asthma : (1) if there is a history of asthma starting directly after severe respiratory infections ; (2) if there is expectoration of a purulent sputum ; (3) if there is evidence of lung damage as shown by clinical or radiological examination.

The question whether autogenous or stock vaccines should be employed, with details regarding dosage and technique, have been fully discussed on pp. 778, 793, and this information is equally relevant to the treatment of asthma. Many authorities believe that the vaccine treatment of asthma is extremely useful, but their investigations are seldom properly controlled. We believe that the anticatarrhal vaccines usually employed act in a non-specific rather than in a specific manner. Nevertheless, vaccine treatment is worthy of trial in cases of asthma with lung damage, who have failed to respond to other forms of treatment. It is again necessary to recall that vaccines should be given cautiously and in amounts which fail to produce general reactions.

The Nasal Factor

A nasal factor is commonly present in asthma and is frequently of importance. There are two ways in which it may operate : (1) if the asthmagenic area in the nose is in an abnormally sensitive condition it will readily be irritated by dust, cold air, purulent material, etc., thus inducing through a reflex mechanism an asthmatic attack ; and (2) organic diseases, such as polypi, deflected septum, hypertrophy of the turbinate bones and infections of the nasal sinuses, all tend to cause asthma, both by interfering with free ventilation and by increasing the liability to infections of the nose and throat.

In taking a careful history it is important to record the occurrence of sneezing, watering and itching of the nose prior to the asthmatic attack, whether the symptoms occur at any particular season of the year, and the effects, if any, produced on the patient by a dusty atmosphere. A positive history in these respects favours an allergic basis. Owing to the similarity of the symptoms of allergic rhinitis and rhinitis due to a vasomotor neurosis, skin tests may be required for their differentiation.

To determine whether organic disease is present an examination of the nose and throat should be made. A pale boggy colour of the mucous membrane of the nose suggests an allergic factor, while redness and congestion indicate infection. These appearances are deceptive where, as often happens, infection occurs in a mucous membrane already allergic. The presence of eosinophilia in the nasal secretion is a valuable indication of the importance of the allergic factor.

Experience has shown that the surgical treatment of nasal abnormalities in asthma is disappointing. It is true that relief is often obtained for a period of weeks or even months, but the majority of cases relapse. This suggests that many nasal abnormalities are not the cause of the asthma but its result. Accordingly, a conservative attitude should be adopted towards nasal surgery.

The asthma should be treated on the general lines indicated while local measures should be employed to reduce the œdema and swelling of the mucous membrane of the nose. Freer ventilation will be secured along with better drainage of the accessory sinuses and lowered irritability of the asthmagenic area. This may be achieved by local application of the cautery, or of astringent and anæsthetic drugs, or zinc ionization (for details, see Paroxysmal Rhinorrhœa). Infected antra should be treated by proof puncture and lavage, rather than by open operation.

If the measures described fail to bring relief, the question of the correction of the nasal factor by surgical measures must be considered. The principle which we advocate is that radical surgical treatment should be advised only if the abnormalities present are such that even if the patient had not asthma, surgical measures would be necessary. The position should be explained to the patient without undue optimism.

The Gastro-intestinal Factor

The gastro-intestinal factor may cause asthma either because the patient's digestion is upset by some article of food or for reflex reasons consequent on flatulent dyspepsia or constipation.

In general, it will be found that asthmatics do best if they take a good breakfast and lunch, and a light evening meal. It is particularly important that they should take no food within an hour and a half of going to bed. While considerable latitude should be allowed the patient with regard to the composition of his diet, obviously he should avoid any food to which he is sensitive, and anything likely to cause dyspepsia and flatulence. Large meals should be prohibited, two or three courses being sufficient. Flatulent dyspepsia and constipation should be treated as outlined on pp. 563, 573.

In about one case in four an atonic dyspepsia accompanied by achlorhydria is present. In such cases benefit will be obtained from hydrochloric acid and pepsin (see p. 467). We are unwilling to accept the statement by several authors that the routine administration of hydrochloric acid or nitro-hydrochloric acid is of curative value in a high proportion of cases of asthma. Any benefit derived from giving 30 to 60 minims three times a day of hydrochloric acid to a patient whose stomach is already secreting hundreds of cubic centimetres of acid in the twenty-four hours can only be explained on psychological basis.

Drugs

Sedative Drugs.—Many asthmatic patients, particularly those in whom the psychological factor is prominent, live in a state of constant nervous tension. For such persons potassium bromide (15 gr. b.i.d.) or small doses of phenobarbitone ($\frac{1}{2}$ gr.) are of value.

Antispasmodic Drugs.—Chronic asthmatics, who have failed to respond to the various forms of treatment outlined above, should be instructed to inject themselves with adrenalin, the most useful drug available for the treatment of asthma. By this means many patients, who would otherwise be semi-invalids, can be enabled to live a practically normal life. A dose as small as 2 minims, if given at the onset, may be sufficient to abort the attack. The patient should discover for himself the smallest effective dose. In general, however, some degree of tolerance develops and it will be necessary, as time goes on, to increase the dose gradually. In addition, the knowledge that severe attacks may be prevented restores confidence, which so many asthmatics have lost.

Although drug treatment is only palliative, the anti-spasmodic drugs are of value in the treatment of asthma. A mixture, if persistently used for several months, will often lessen the frequency and severity of the attacks. The drugs commonly employed are lobelia, stramonium or belladonna in the form of a tincture in doses of 10 to 15 minims. Sir Arthur Hurst informs us that from personal experience he has found lobelia and belladonna of little value, but that stramonium in doses of at least 30 minims of the tincture, given at night for short periods, is worthy of trial. Iodide of potassium is generally added to the mixture to liquefy the tenacious mucus (see Appendix). Ephedrine sulphate and hydrochloride are valuable antispasmodics. While not so rapid or constant in its action as adrenalin, ephedrine has the advantages that it can be taken by mouth and has more lasting effects. The dose is $\frac{1}{2}$ gr. two or three times a day for an adult, $\frac{1}{4}$ gr. for a child over the age of seven, $\frac{1}{8}$ gr. for an infant.

Ephedrine may be added to the mixture of antispasmodic drugs described above, but we prefer to give it separately in tablet form so that it can be omitted from the evening dose should it lead to sleeplessness. Some persons are unable to take ephedrine because of the occurrence of unpleasant symptoms, such as nausea, palpitation, sweating and occasionally dysuria. These reactions may be prevented or at least reduced if ephedrine is prescribed with one of the following: luminal, $\frac{1}{2}$ gr.; phenazone (ephazone tablets); sodium amytal, 1 gr.

Synthetic ephedrine (pseudo-ephedrine) is sold by leading manufacturing firms, *e.g.*, tabloid pseudo-ephedrine hydrochlor. (B. W. & Co.) and ephetonin (Napp). It is cheaper and produces unpleasant reactions less frequently than ephedrine. On the other hand, it is doubtful whether it is as efficacious as natural ephedrine in relieving bronchial spasm.

When asthma occurs principally at night a dose of a strong sedative linctus should be taken half an hour before going to bed. It may prevent the onset of coughing, which not infrequently occurs when the patient leaves the warm living-room and enters the cold bedroom. Antispasmodic drugs are included in the prescription. A single dose at night will often prevent the early morning bronchial spasm. The sedative drugs usually employed are tinct. opii camph. in doses of 30 minims or syr. codein phosphate, B.P.C., 1 drachm (see Appendix).

Inhalations.—Adrenalin, ephedrine and cocaine in oily and watery solutions may be used singly or in combination in the form of inhalations. The solution should be sprayed into the nose by means of a simple atomizer or by a pump worked by hand or driven by an electric motor or volatilized by oxygen. We recommend a hand atomizer, as it is equally efficient, more portable and much less expensive than the instruments worked by mechanical means. A high-grade atomizer should be used in order to deliver the finest possible spray. The original cost of the atomizer will soon be recovered by the less wasteful use of expensive drugs. The combination of ephedrine 1 per cent. and cocaine 1 per cent. in equal parts is generally satisfactory. Ephedrine is preferable to adrenalin since its local effect is more prolonged and the secondary reaction less marked. Cocaine is an excellent astringent and local anæsthetic, while with a 1 per cent. solution there is practically no danger of habit formation.

Many patients prefer the inhalation to the injection of adrenalin, even though the effects are not so dramatic or prolonged. Moreover, the mere knowledge that they can readily avert an incipient attack of asthma gives considerable confidence, and relieves anxiety and tension.

Inhalations of smoke from burning powders or cigarettes containing potassium nitrate with stramonium and lobelia leaves are commonly employed by asthmatics. In general they cannot be recommended because the temporary relief obtained is more than offset by the irritant effects on the bronchial mucous membrane.

Morphia.—The use of morphia in the management of the asthmatic state is contraindicated because of the dangers of habit formation, and of pulmonary atelectasis.

Glucose.—The administration of glucose is useful in children, particularly if they are nervous or poorly nourished. It may be given in 1 or 2 drachm doses after meals, or as honey or barley sugar.

Calcium.—Calcium has been employed in many forms in the treatment of asthma, but there can be no doubt that it is of little value.

Caffeine.—Caffeine may be of value in all types of asthma, and particularly in elderly patients with some degree of cardiac weakness. Two to four tablets containing 2 gr. of caffeine citrate may be taken before attempting an effort which tends to make the patient unduly breathless. Caffeine should be avoided in the evening as it induces insomnia.

General Measures

Apart from the investigation and treatment of the special factors already described, the family doctor can always give valuable help by his common-sense advice on general health measures. Physical fatigue and nervous strain are potent factors in the production of asthma, and these must be counteracted by reorganization of the patient's life, both in regard to work and play. This entails careful investigation of the family, social and business relations of the patient, and, of course, each individual case must be treated on its own merits.

Artificial sunlight treatment is a valuable tonic in raising the general health and may be recommended for debilitated children, particularly in winter. For the same reason cod-liver oil, iron and yeast may be given.

Climate.—Climatic conditions are believed to play an important part in asthma. In general, it may be said that a cool dry climate without marked variations in humidity and temperature is the most suitable. Many asthmatics feel much better when living in the mountains at an altitude of 3,000 ft. It has been suggested that high altitudes produce beneficial biochemical changes in the blood or that the pure air is free from allergens and mechanically irritating particles. Nevertheless it is impossible to say what climate is suitable for each individual case of asthma. We have had patients who tell us that they keep free from attacks in Glasgow in spite of the fog and smoke, while others have come from Glasgow to Aberdeen to find relief in the cool, bracing air. This suggests to us that some at least of the benefits credited to a change of climate are in reality due to a psychological factor, since the climatic change is generally accompanied by the removal of disturbing influences which have kept the broncho-constrictor centre constantly irritated.

This aspect is well brought out by the following case

history. Miss A. had to be removed from school in Aberdeen at the age of sixteen because of asthma. Her doctor ordered this on the grounds that the climate was the essential ætiological factor.

She went to her home in the country some forty miles away, where she remained free from asthma. At the age of eighteen she went to the University of Glasgow, where she was very happy, took part in many social activities and had no asthma. Having taken her degree, she returned home, and within six months asthma started again. She then took a post in Aberdeen as under-manageress of an hotel, and remained in this situation for three years, during which time she had only an occasional attack of mild asthma.

Our analysis of the psychological aspects of this case is as follows: While at school in Aberdeen she was unhappy and objected to the discipline. She reacted to this state of nervous tension by having asthma, which obtained for her sympathy and preferential treatment and finally enabled her to leave her unhappy surroundings. On returning to her home in the country, she was free from the restrictions which were imposed on her at school, and so she kept well. Her reaction to home life in the country was different on her return from Glasgow. The absence of cinemas, theatres and dances made existence in the country seem dull and monotonous, and home life now appeared to offer many restrictions compared to the freedom which she enjoyed in lodgings in Glasgow. Again she reacted to these psychological factors by having asthma. These in turn disappeared when she accepted a position in Aberdeen which gave her her freedom and satisfied her social desires. If our deductions are correct, climatic conditions had nothing to do with the onset or disappearance of the asthma, for it will be noted that at different periods of her life she had asthma and was also free from asthma in the same district.

Spa Treatment.—Enthusiastic spa physicians claim remarkable beneficial effects from the waters of their individual spas, whether administered internally, externally or by inhalation. Temporary beneficial effects are certainly frequent, but we have little hesitation in saying that they are largely due to the improvement in the patient's health and mental outlook, which result from a holiday under pleasant conditions, and from the unintentional psycho-therapy of the enthusiastic spa physician.

Prevention of Upper Respiratory Infections.—In the majority of sufferers the occurrence of any respiratory tract infection will precipitate an asthmatic attack. It is of the utmost importance, therefore, that every care should be exercised in their prophylaxis and treatment. Preventive measures have been fully described on p. 775.

Postural and Breathing Exercises.—Long-continued asthma leads to over-expansion of the lungs and changes in the thorax, which assumes the so-called barrel-shape with hypertrophy of the accessory muscles of respiration. In addition, the pulmonary distension leads to a state of emphysema, which, as Hurst has rightly pointed out, is for a long time functional rather than organic in origin. Lastly, the respiration of the chronic asthmatic becomes of the upper thoracic type through his failure to use the diaphragm and abdominal muscles. In consequence a considerable proportion of the air contained in the lower lobes becomes stagnant. For the treatment of these conditions postural and breathing exercises are of paramount importance. A large proportion of chronic asthmatics will derive marked benefit by undertaking a course of remedial exercises. This necessitates the help of a qualified physio-therapeutist, not only to give instruction in the physical exercises but to loosen the stiff thoracic muscles by applying massage. The book published by the Asthma Research Council, entitled "Physical Exercises for Asthma," fully describes suitable exercises in detail (obtainable for 1s. post free from the Secretary, King's College, Strand, London, W.C.2.).

HAY FEVER

Hay fever occurs in individuals who are hypersensitive to the pollen of grasses and is characterized by itching and watering of the eyes, sneezing and running at the nose, and a hacking cough.

The hay-fever season usually starts in the south of England about the middle of May and continues throughout June and July. In Scotland, the season is two or three weeks later. In America allergic symptoms to the pollen of ragweed are common in the autumn, usually from August to October.

Symptomatic Treatment.—When the grasses are pollinating the sufferer from hay fever should avoid country districts where the air is heavily laden with pollen, but pollen is so widely disseminated that severe symptoms may occur in the middle of a large city. In a severe case it may be necessary for the individual to remain indoors with the windows closed, only venturing out during damp and rainy weather. A long sea voyage may be recommended in the case of a wealthy patient. Special pollen filters can be purchased in the form of masks which the patient wears during the day. Such appliances, however, are cumbersome and seldom tolerated.

Conjunctivitis may be very distressing and painful. For its prevention and treatment close-fitting dark glasses should be worn. Immediate relief can be obtained by the instillation of 1 or 2 drops of the following solution into each eye :—

Liq. adrenalin hydrochlorid. 1 : 1,000	.	1 drachm.
Cocaine hydrochlorid. . . .	.	$1\frac{1}{2}$ gr.
Saturated solution boric acid .	ad	1 oz.

Ephedrine is an excellent substitute for adrenalin and may be instilled into the eye in a strength of 2 to 3 gr. to the ounce of saturated boric solution.

The troublesome sneezing and irritation of the nose may be temporarily relieved by the instillation of nasal drops containing ephedrine in 1 to 3 per cent. solution in distilled water or liquid paraffin. A useful spray consists of 1 per cent. ephedrine sulphate and 1 per cent. cocaine in liquid paraffin.

For the relief of the hacking cough a sedative linctus should be administered (see Appendix).

It is beneficial to prescribe ephedrine by mouth in doses of $\frac{1}{2}$ gr. night and morning. It may be combined with $\frac{1}{2}$ gr. luminal or $\frac{3}{4}$ gr. sodium amytal if any untoward effects are experienced.

Since many sufferers from hay fever are nervous individuals, it is well to prescribe small doses of a mild sedative throughout the season.

Pre-seasonal Specific Desensitization.—Pre-seasonal specific desensitization entails the subcutaneous injection of pollen extract in increasing quantities before the onset of the hay fever season. Suitable extracts may be obtained from leading manufacturing firms (Parke, Davis & Co., Bencards, Duncan & Flockhart, etc.) The solution is supplied in rubber capped bottles containing so many units of pollen per cubic centimetre. The results of pre-seasonal desensitization have varied in the hands of different writers, but it may be said that the practitioner can expect complete relief or marked improvement in the majority of cases. A very small number may be completely cured by one course of injections, but the majority of patients will require desensitization during successive years. After a number of courses, many patients will be able to enjoy considerable comfort for the next year or two. The majority, however, return to their former condition, requiring further desensitization.

Treatment must be commenced at least ten weeks before

the beginning of the pollen season, *i.e.*, about the end of February or in the first week of March.

Intradermal skin tests should first be carried out to determine the degree of sensitivity. Very sensitive cases may not tolerate more than five units of pollen extract for an initial dose, while the least sensitive cases can receive 500 units. The extract is given subcutaneously at intervals of four to seven days, and the dose should be gradually increased until a maximum of 100,000 units is reached before the onset of the hay fever season. This dose should be repeated weekly for three to four weeks after the season commences. After the needle of the syringe has been inserted it is important to withdraw the piston to ensure that the point of the needle is not in a small vein. The intravenous injection of pollen extract may give rise to a severe general reaction. To each injection, 2 minims of adrenalin (1 : 1,000 solution) should be added in order to slow the rate of absorption and lessen the risk of a general reaction. After the injection the patient must be kept under observation for half an hour in case any local or general reaction occurs.

General Reactions are fortunately rare, but may be alarming and even fatal. Prompt measures must be adopted as soon as the first symptoms appear. Itching of the palms of the hands and conjunctivæ are indications that a general reaction is commencing. An immediate injection of $\frac{1}{2}$ c.c. of adrenalin should be given subcutaneously. To prevent further quantities of pollen extract reaching the circulation a tourniquet should be applied to the arm proximal to the site of injection. If more severe symptoms such as urticaria, swelling of the neck and face, asthma or collapse occur, a further injection of 1 c.c. of adrenalin must be given. If the patient is in a state of collapse artificial respiration must be started at once and 2 c.c. of coramine injected intramuscularly. The occurrence of a general reaction calls for a reduction of the next dose of extract to one quarter and this should be combined with 5 minims of adrenalin. Subsequent doses must be increased cautiously.

Local Reactions are more frequent and are evidenced by redness, swelling and itching at the site of injection. The schedule of dosage need not be interrupted for a mild local reaction, but if it is large and painful the subsequent injection should be repeated instead of being increased.

Desensitization by " rush inoculation " as advocated by Freeman may be used if sufficient time is not available for the full pre-seasonal course of injections. This method is not without danger and should only be practised by those with experience in the treatment of allergy. The course, which consists of subcutaneous injections of pollen extract every one and a half to two hours, may be completed in from two to four days.

Perennial Desensitization.—The perennial method has given good results in some hands and poor results in others. Monthly injections are given throughout the year, the dose being the highest dose attained at the end of the first pre-seasonal course. This method obviates the necessity of frequent visits to the practitioner.

Seasonal Desensitization.—Desensitization may still be attempted even when the patient presents himself after the symptoms of hay fever have appeared. The initial dose is calculated from the degree of the patient's sensitivity to pollen extract as determined by intradermal skin tests. It varies from 5 to 500 units and is given daily for three to five days. The dose is then increased cautiously and the intervals between injections lengthened. The danger of serious reactions and the uncertainty of success obtained make it doubtful if desensitization should be attempted when the patient is actually suffering from hay fever.

Zinc Ionization.—Zinc ionization as described for the treatment of paroxysmal rhinorrhœa has given good results in hay fever. It should be carried out at the commencement of the hay fever season and in most cases will have to be repeated on two or three occasions during the season.

Conclusions.—Pre-seasonal specific desensitization is advised as the method of choice.

Desensitization by the oral route or by the local application of pollen ointment cannot be recommended because of the disappointing results obtained.

Seasonal desensitization should not be undertaken by the general practitioner because of the dangers involved. If the patient presents himself for treatment while suffering from hay fever, reliance should be placed on symptomatic treatment together with zinc ionization if this is available.

PAROXYSMAL RHINORRHŒA

(*Vasomotor Rhinitis*)

Paroxysmal rhinorrhœa is a condition characterized by paroxysms of sneezing and watery discharge from the nose. In many cases it is allergic in nature, being often found in association with asthma. The allergens responsible are usually inhalants such as pollens, horse dander, dust, orris root and flour. Foods (wheat, egg, fish) are rare causes, and drugs, especially aspirin, are occasionally responsible for allergic nasal symptoms.

Sensitivity to one or more allergens may be revealed by a detailed history combined with intradermal skin tests (see p. 832), which should always be performed. In many cases, however, no evidence of allergy can be found. In these a hypersensitivity to bacterial proteins may be present, or more frequently a state of "primary vasomotor disturbance" is present for which no satisfactory explanation may be available.

The first step is to exclude from the patient's environment all allergens to which he shows hypersensitiveness (see p. 831). If this is impossible, or if the condition does not improve, specific desensitization should be carried out. This entails weekly subcutaneous injections of extracts of the offending allergen or allergens in increasing concentration. It is usual to start treatment with a weak extract, the initial dose of which is 0·1 c.c. The solutions may be obtained from Messrs Bencard.

The general health should be maintained by the usual measures and care should be taken to avoid fatigue, worry and cold, which are important precipitating factors. Varnish, smoke and perfumes often act as mechanical irritants and are liable to produce an attack. If the patient's work entails spending many hours in a dust-laden atmosphere, a change of occupation may be desirable.

Striking relief may be obtained during a paroxysm by the application of astringent drugs to the nasal mucous membrane. Ephedrine is extensively used and may be applied to the nose as an ointment (5 gr. to 1 oz. of soft paraffin). "Ephregel" is a convenient preparation. Probably better results are obtained by the use of an oily or aqueous solution containing 0·5 to 1 per cent. of ephedrine. Nebula ephedrine co. (B.P.C.) or "endrine" may be dropped into the nose or may be used in an atomizer. If the preparation is being used over a long period, the use of an atomizer is much more economical. "Benzedrine" which is supplied in inhalers is also useful. These preparations should not be used more than four or five times a day. Ephedrine by mouth in doses of ½ gr. night and morning is also helpful in preventing and relieving attacks.

Zinc ionization of the nose is widely used, but results seem to show that it is most successful in cases in which no specific allergen can be found. The method consists in impregnating the cells of the mucous membrane of the nose with zinc ions. After spraying the nose with a solution of equal parts of decicain (2 per cent.) and adrenalin (1 : 1,000), both sides are packed with ribbon gauze saturated with a 1 per cent. solution of zinc sulphate. The positive electrode is then inserted while the patient grasps the negative pole. A current of from 7 to 10 ma. is then passed for fifteen minutes. The procedure should be repeated for three or four sittings at ten to fourteen day intervals, depending on the reaction in the nose. Complete relief may be obtained for several months.

Many cases can temporarily be relieved by cauterization to the inferior turbinates, using either a saturated solution of trichloracetic acid or chromic acid (40 per cent.) or a fused bead of silver nitrate. The electro-cautery, heated to a cherry-red heat, is also effective and may be applied to Francis' area or tubercle of the septum.

It is generally agreed that no operation, however trivial, should be undertaken until the allergic symptoms have subsided or have been brought under control. Operative procedures on the nose and throat frequently fail to cure paroxysmal rhinorrhœa. Accordingly, surgical treatment is contraindicated except for the correction of pathological conditions irrespective of the presence of paroxysmal rhinorrhœa. The aim of surgical treatment should be restoration of function and the elimination of infection. Infected adenoids and tonsils, sinusitis, polypi and deflected septum, should be treated on the usual lines.

Radium has its advocates and good results have been claimed, especially if used after the removal of nasal polypi.

APPENDIX

Oily Solutions of Essential Oils with or without Ephedrine

Nebula menthol. et thymol co., B.P.C.

Contains approximately—

Menthol.	gr. ix
Thymol.	gr. i
Camph.	gr. ix
Phenol.	gr. ix
Paraff. Liq. . . . . . to	℥i

Nebula ephedrinæ co., B.P.C.

Contains approximately—

Ephed. Hydrochlor.		gr. iv
Menthol.		gr. ix
Camph.		gr. ix
Oil of thyme.		♏x
Paraff. Liq.	to	℥i

Nebula eucalyptol co., B.P.C.

Contains approximately—

Eucalyp.		♏xl
Camph.		gr. ix
Menthol.		gr. ix
Thymol.		gr. ½
Paraff. Liq.	to	℥i

Antispasmodic Cough Mixture

℞	Pot. Iod.		gr. v
	Tinct. Bellad.		♏x
	Tinct. Stramon.		♏xv-xx
	Ext. Glycyrrh. Liq		♏xv
	Aq.	ad	℥ss

Sedative Antispasmodic Mixture

℞	Ephed. Hydrochlor.		gr. ½
	Tinct. Stramon.		♏xv
	Syr. Codein. Phos.	ad	ʒi

Expectorant Cough Mixtures

℞	Ammon. Carb.		gr. v
	Pot. Iod.		gr. iii
	Tinct. Ipecac.		♏x
	Ext. Glycyrrh. Liq.		♏xv
	Aq.	ad	℥ss

℞	Ammon. Chlorid.		gr. x
	Tinct. Scill.		♏x
	Sp. Chlorof.		♏x
	Syr. Tolu.		♏xxx
	Aq.	ad	℥ss

Alkaline Cough Mixture

℞	Sod. Bicarb.		gr. xx
	Pot. Citrat.		gr. xxx
	Liq. Ammon. Acet. Dil. . .		ʒii-iv
	Aq. Chlorof.	ad	℥ss

Sedative Linctuses

1. Linctus scillæ co., B.P.C.

   Contains—

Tinct. Opii Camph. . .	Equal parts.
Oxymel scill. . . .	
Syr. Tolu.	

   Dose—½ to 1 fluid drachm.

2. Linctus diamorphin. et scillæ, B.P.C.

   Contains—

   Diamorphine hydrochloride . gr. $\frac{1}{40}$ in each fluid drachm.

   Dose—½ to 1 fluid drachm.

3. Syr. Codein. Phosph., B.P.C.

   Contains—

   Codein. Phosph. . . . gr. ¼ in each fluid drachm.

   Dose—½ to 2 fluid drachms.

4. Elixir diamorphin. et terpin., B.P.C.

   Contains—

   Diamorphine hydrochloride . gr. $\frac{1}{18}$ in each fluid drachm.

L. S. P. Davidson.
I. Gordon.

RENAL DISEASES

NEPHRITIS

Introduction

ALTHOUGH the classification of nephritis has been obscured by the over-elaboration and subdivision of most workers, the treatment fortunately remains fairly clear. That this is so is mainly due to the fact that its basis rests upon no pathological classification but is almost wholly symptomatic, being regulated by the nature and the degree of the renal upset. It is therefore necessary to preface the treatment of nephritis with a short discussion of the changes which are present in the kidney at the various stages of the disease. The acute stage develops in most cases seven to twenty-one days after a streptococcal condition in some other part of the body, most commonly the throat. This may have been so slight as to have been forgotten or never noticed by the patient. With the onset of nephritis the glomeruli are rendered ischæmic for a brief period, which is yet sufficiently long to cause damage to the glomerular membrane and the tubule. As a result the permeability of the glomerular membrane is increased, while the concentrating power of the tubule is diminished. Consequent upon the glomerular ischæmia and its sequelæ are the characteristic findings of acute nephritis, namely, oliguria, blood, albumin and tube casts (blood and epithelial) in the urine, impairment of concentrating power, increase in the nitrogenous constituents of the blood, raised blood pressure and œdema. As initial improvement occurs, blood diminishes in the urine, while the output increases; œdema diminishes; blood pressure falls and nitrogen retention disappears. Later the œdema disappears while the albuminuria diminishes and still later, in most cases, clears up entirely. The concentrating power of the kidney, however, takes longer to be restored. In most cases the restoration of normal concentrating power is the final proof of recovery. The treatment of acute nephritis is determined by the stage present as detailed above.

Complete recovery occurs in the majority of cases where treatment is patiently persevered with. Failing this complete recovery, the condition may pass on to the second stage of glomerulonephritis characterized by the persistence of increased glomerular permeability but little or no impairment of the concentrating power of the tubule. At this stage, therefore, albuminuria is the predominant sign, being present for long periods without associated œdema, which, however, develops eventually in most cases. The characteristic blood chemistry findings are a lowered plasma albumin content and an increased concentration of cholesterol. There is no nitrogenous retention, impairment of renal function or hypertension with its associated cardiac changes.

The third stage of glomerulonephritis is marked by sclerosis of the affected glomeruli and consequent upon the withdrawal of blood from these the albuminuria disappears. Because of the reduction in the number of functioning kidney units, impaired concentrating power associated with the occurrence of azotæmia develops. Chemical analysis of the blood shows an increased nitrogenous content, and later there may be found a decreased calcium content and lowered CO_2 combining power. Hypertension with its associated cardiovascular and retinal changes is also present.

It has to be understood that the above simple clear-cut division into the three stages of nephritis is seldom encountered clinically. Gradations from the one stage to the other are commonly found so that treatment may be necessary in cases which feature mixed symptoms of two stages.

"Uræmia" may occur both in the acute and in the third stages of the disease. The condition found during the acute stage is due more to cerebral œdema than to true uræmia, this latter being regarded as a symptom complex consequent upon failure of the kidney to excrete toxic substances. The true uræmic condition is found in the third stage. The symptoms of the two types of "uræmia" and their treatment vary as do their causes.

Acute Nephritis

Treatment is based upon a consideration of the characteristics of the typical case and the normal course followed towards recovery. At the onset of the condition the aim should be to avoid irritation of the damaged organ and to give it functional rest, imposing upon it no avoidable strain until complete recovery has been obtained. The treatment therefore must run parallel with the functional ability of the kidney. Due regard must, however, be paid to the general condition of the patient, this being maintained at the highest possible level so that the desired renal recovery may be facilitated.

Rest.—Rest in bed is essential from the moment of diagnosis. It has been customary to place the patient in blankets and clothe him in flannel, but, now that sweating is not so frequently resorted to in treatment, these procedures may be modified provided the patient is always kept warm and free from draughts. The duration of rest in bed should be much longer than is generally advised. Too often the disappearance of albuminuria is regarded as the index of cure ; impairment of concentrating power is present in the majority of cases long after the urine is free of albumin ; no case should be allowed out of bed until complete recovery has taken place, *i.e.*, until the urine, blood pressure and blood chemistry are normal and the concentrating power has been fully restored. This may even entail complete rest in bed for months. As long as there are indications of improvement this treatment should be continued ; when the condition becomes stationary, the advisability of allowing the patient up has to be admitted and future treatment must follow along the lines indicated later for the chronic stages.

Diet.—*Protein and Fluid.*—The dietetic treatment most generally followed at the onset of the condition is the complete elimination of all protein, glucose and fruit juices being the sole sources of food. The fluid intake is restricted until the signs of acute damage are waning. For this purpose 1 to 1½ pints of fluid only are permitted until the hæmaturia has diminished and diuresis has occurred. Volhard goes even further and advises complete withdrawal of fluid and food. Supporters of this line of treatment suggest that they are thereby lessening the burden on the kidney by providing it with no extra water and no exogenous nitrogen for excretion. It has to be borne in mind, however, that endogenous nitrogen is constantly being produced from tissue breakdown and consequently, even on a protein-free diet, a certain amount has to be excreted by the kidney or retained in the blood. Further, tissue breakdown without tissue replacement means deterioration of the general condition and decreased resistance to infection. Formerly milk was permitted in the acute stage, the diet consisting of milk in amounts up to 3 pints per day. Such a diet contains 1,680 c.c. of water, 60 gm. of protein and 3 gm. of sodium chloride. Admittedly this amount of protein is in excess of the requirements for the tissue needs of a resting individual. It has to be remembered that in caseinogen all the essential amino acids except cystine are present and that this is found in lactalbumin. Further, with a strictly limited administration of essential protein the nitrogen excretion is no greater than when protein has been wholly withheld. Up to 20 oz. of milk can be given without increasing the daily excretion of urea. It has accordingly been the writer's custom to compromise between the above two methods in the treatment of the initial stage, giving alternate two-hourly feeds of citrated milk (see p. 551) and glucose fruit-juice solution, the total amount of fluid over twenty-four hours being restricted to not more than 2 pints (see p. 863, Diet I). The protein in this quantity of milk has been shown to cause no rise above the endogenous level in the nitrogenous content of the urine of a normal individual, and is not likely to do so in any but the severest cases of acute nephritis characterized by almost complete anuria. The citrate added to the milk not only helps to make it more digestible but assists the kidney to secrete a more bland, neutral or mildly alkaline urine. Following the appearance of diuresis and the lessening of the hæmaturia, the caloric intake is increased by the addition of further carbohydrates and fat, as bread, cereals, fruit, butter and cream. By this means the dietetic intake is raised to 1,500 calories per day, and this is continued until the hæmaturia has disappeared. At this stage it is advisable to carry out a renal function test to determine the concentrating power of the kidney because this gives a guide as to the protein intake to be allowed. The writer is in the habit of employing Calvert's urea concentration range, details of which are given below.[1] For those unable to carry out a urea concentration test, valuable information can be obtained from estimating the specific gravity of the first specimen of urine passed in the morning, provided a heavy albuminuria is not present. The specific gravity of this specimen in a normal individual should be 1,020 to 1,025 ; the lower the specific gravity, the less the protein that can be given with safety. As the patient on Diet I (see p. 863) is not in

[1] *Urea Concentration Range.*—Fluid intake is restricted from noon. At 10 P.M. patient is given 15 gm. urea in 100 c.c. of water flavoured with orange. Bladder is emptied at 11 P.M. and urine discarded. Any urine passed before 7 A.M. is kept (specimen 1) and bladder emptied at 7 A.M. (specimen 2). Two pints of fluid are given at 7 A.M. ; urine voided and discarded at 8 A.M. ; and bladder emptied and specimen 3 kept at 9 A.M. Specimen 1 or 2 contains the maximum urea concentration and specimen 3 the minimum concentration.

A normal kidney shows a maximum power of 3·5 per cent. or over and a minimum of 0·4 per cent. or less. Early inefficiency is shown by fall in the maximum. As inefficiency advances, the maximum continues to fall while the minimum rises. In extreme inefficiency the maximum and minimum approximate (maximum under 1·5 per cent., minimum up to or over 1 per cent.).

nitrogen balance, the daily protein intake must be increased to 50 gm. within a fortnight. Care must be taken that the additional protein is of high biological value (*i.e.*, protein of meat, fish, milk, cheese or eggs). Thereafter a renal function test is reapplied at regular intervals, and as the concentrating power of the kidney improves or the specific gravity of the urine increases, the protein content of the diet is raised. When a maximum concentration of up to 2·5 per cent., or specific gravity of 1,018, is reached, a protein intake of 75 gm. may be given: a rise in the maximum to 3 per cent. or over (specific gravity 1,020+) permits the giving of a normal diet with 100 gm. or over. A suitable dietetic scheme of treatment throughout all phases of this condition is given in Diets I to IV (pp. 863, 865). The presence of albuminuria is not regarded as an indication for altering these dietetic measures. The above protein intakes are within the limits of the kidneys' ability to deal with urea; the allowance of this full amount of protein ensures the maximum restoration of the general condition which deteriorates with too low protein intakes. Further, the writer wishes to emphasize the need for allowing the maximum protein intake consistent with the renal power present at any particular phase. It is now becoming increasingly accepted that such a procedure stimulates the return of kidney function and gives an earlier restoration of power than the previously adopted course which aimed at sparing the kidney.

Salt.—The part played by sodium chloride in the occurrence of œdema is still debated, but it would appear that of the two ions sodium is the more important. It is necessary, therefore, to limit the intake of sodium, but the food need not be made unpalatable by the withdrawal of chloride which can be administered in sufficient amount for savouring purposes by the use of potassium chloride. Selarom (Bayer) is a suitable preparation for this purpose.

Vitamins.—The vitamin content of the diet should be maintained throughout in view of the influence of these factors on infective processes (vitamins A and D) and capillary permeability (vitamin C). The value and rôle of vitamins K and P have not yet been fully established and so their use cannot be discussed in the treatment of the hæmorrhage of acute nephritis. Vitamins A and D can be given as adexolin or similar preparation. Sufficient vitamin C should be provided in fresh juice of citrus fruits, vegetables and milk.

Focal Sepsis.—In the majority of cases the streptococcal infection preceding the acute nephritis requires no treatment by the time the kidney is affected. Unfortunately no certain prophylaxis can be adopted to prevent nephritis following on such an infection. Nevertheless it may be that the lesion is present along with the nephritis, and any of the sulphonamide preparations may be used in full doses without detriment to the renal state (see p. 83). After the nephritis has cleared up a search for foci of sepsis should be made and any found should be eradicated. Unless tonsils are definitely septic, however, they should not be removed. Nephritis should not be added to the list of diseases, already far too large, which immediately suggest tonsillectomy. Where, however, hæmolytic streptococcal pus is present in the tonsils, tonsillectomy is necessary, but it should be delayed if at all possible until complete renal recovery has taken place. When recovery becomes markedly retarded, and especially when hæmaturia persists, it is unwise to delay removal of septic foci any longer. A temporary increase in hæmaturia may occur, but this is usually followed by a more rapid improvement. An excessively conservative attitude in regard to the removal of septic foci is as unjustifiable as undue haste.

Drugs.—*Alkalis.*—The administration of drugs is of little service in the treatment of acute nephritis. Alkalis are of value in rendering the urine more bland and for this purpose potassium citrate and potassium bicarbonate should be given in sufficient doses to keep the urine alkaline to litmus. Twenty to thirty grains of each at four-hourly intervals may be required initially, but later this dose can be decreased. Alkalis can be administered conveniently along with the milk.

Diuretics.—Potassium citrate is the only diuretic that is permissible. The purine group (caffeine, theobromine and theophylline) act as kidney irritants ; urea may already be present in the blood above the normal amount ; the mercurial preparations, though excellent in cardiac failure even in the presence of albuminuria, are strongly contraindicated in acute nephritis. As the acute state passes off, diuresis will occur naturally. It cannot be urged too strongly that this natural diuresis be awaited patiently.

Purgatives.—The use of massive doses of jalap, salts and other drastic cathartics is fortunately now generally discontinued. The improvement (if any) which followed the fluid removal which they achieved was heavily outbalanced by the strain which they occasioned the patient. An easy motion once daily, achieved, if need be, by the aid of a mild aperient (cascara, senna, etc.) is all that is necessary. Mercurial purgatives are contraindicated on account of their possible irritant action on the kidney.

Diaphoretics.—Diaphoretic measures are now fairly generally abandoned. Except, possibly, in incipient "acute uræmia" the drastic sweating by hot packs, hot baths and pilocarpine cannot be recommended. Even in incipient "uræmia" its value lies in the elimination of water, not of nitrogenous products as previously stated, and the withdrawal of water from the tissues can be more efficiently and easily secured by the means detailed below.

Symptomatic Treatment.—The measures discussed above are sufficient in the vast majority of cases, but in a few the appearance of certain special symptoms and signs calls for further treatment. Of these anuria, excessive œdema and "acute uræmia" are the chief.

Anuria.—Oliguria naturally relieved by diuresis in the course of a few days occasions no alarm or need for treatment other than the above: complete suppression necessitates an attempt to force kidney action. The most suitable method is the intravenous administration of a solution of 4·285 per cent. sodium sulphate and 10 per cent. glucose in normal (0·9 per cent.) saline. Magnesium sulphate (1 per cent.) is frequently added where signs of tetany are present. The solution can be administered in quantities of 500 c.c. doses, this being preferred to the continuous-drip method. The treatment of anuria by decapsulation of the kidneys has been carried out with very doubtful success. It certainly is not recommended, except in acute cortical necrosis.

Œdema.—Œdema seldom fails to yield to the dietetic and general measures detailed above. In a few cases, however, persistent excessive œdema, ascites and hydrothorax are encountered and these have to be treated by mechanical means. (For technique, see pp. 1087, 1088). The impaired renal function contraindicates the high protein diet and urea administration recommended for removal of œdema in chronic glomerulonephritis (second stage). The necessity for the avoidance of drastic diuretics and the inefficacy of cathartic and diaphoretic measures have already been sufficiently stressed.

Acute Uræmia.—The "uræmia" encountered in acute nephritis is an œdema of the brain rather than true uræmia, the resulting symptoms of headache, amaurosis, coma and convulsions being all due to increased intracranial pressure, possibly associated with high blood pressure. The gastro-intestinal symptoms found in true uræmia are usually absent. Venesection, with removal of 10 to 20 oz. of blood according to age and general condition, and lumbar puncture removing

30 to 40 c.c. of cerebrospinal fluid, may yield dramatic results. After lumbar puncture care must be taken to keep the head low lest a pressure cone develop. The administration of hypertonic solutions (especially magnesium sulphate) can be recommended strongly ; rectally 8 oz. of 25 per cent. magnesium sulphate ; intramuscularly 6 to 10 c.c. 25 per cent. magnesium sulphate ; and intravenously 10 to 20 c.c. 10 per cent. magnesium sulphate, or 40 c.c. 30 per cent. sodium chloride, or 200 c.c. 50 per cent. glucose, or 50 per cent. sucrose are all measures which may be adopted to lower the intracranial pressure. If intravenous administration is adopted, a preceding venesection will add to the value of the therapy. Of the above alternative procedures intravenous magnesium sulphate and sucrose administration are the most successful.

After complete recovery from acute nephritis, no dietetic restrictions are necessary. This point requires stressing as too frequently restriction of protein is unnecessarily imposed. The patient should, however, be warned about the danger of exposure to chills and wettings. He should be advised to treat all future infections, particularly those of the throat region, with special care. Instruction should be given in regard to the wearing of warm clothing and thick footwear in winter weather, and to the need for changing the shoes and socks if they are wet.

Second Stage of Glomerulonephritis and Nephrosis

(*Chronic Parenchymatous Nephritis, Nephrotic Syndrome, Hydræmic Syndrome, Chronic Nephritis with Œdema, Hydropigenous Nephritis*)

It is customary to regard this stage as being characterized by the presence of a heavy albuminuria, but by the absence of azotæmic and hypertensive changes. The drain upon the plasma albumin by the heavy albuminuria results in a lowering of the protein osmotic tension of the blood. An important factor, secondary to this hypoproteinæmia and resultant œdema, is the passage in excess of sodium from blood to tissues. The absence of azotæmia is associated with a normal renal efficiency as demonstrated by renal function tests.

In *chronic nephrosis* a very similar clinical picture is present. There is heavy albuminuria, œdema and a normal renal concentrating power. The changes in blood chemistry are characterized by lowered plasma albumin, markedly increased cholesterol and a normal nitrogen content.

It is not fully realized that for long periods a patient may remain œdema-free despite constant albuminuria and that it is not until the plasma albumin concentration falls below 3 gm. per cent. (normal albumin being 4 to 6 gm. per cent.) that œdema occurs. Further, it has to be remembered that the general condition has to be maintained at all costs as patients with this disease show a greatly increased tendency to septic diseases. In the treatment of this condition one should concentrate on raising the lowered plasma albumin content and on improving the general condition of the patient, largely ignoring the albuminuria which is a permanent feature. For this purpose a high protein diet is necessary: 120 gm. per day is the minimum, but up to 200 gm. per day may be given. With such a protein intake ample potential replenishment of plasma albumin is made and the urinary loss thereby compensated for, while at the same time the general condition of the patient is maintained. At this stage of the disease the kidney has no difficulty in eliminating the end products of protein metabolism, hence no objection can be taken to such a régime on the basis of the increased urea production which it entails. Indeed, the increased urea excretion aids in eliminating œdema by promoting diuresis. Further, as there is no hypertension, the possible pressor action of protein need not be considered. A suitable high protein diet is given in Diet V (p. 866). The salt intake should be limited, especially when the plasma albumin is falling towards the level at which œdema occurs. A safe rule at all times is to allow no salt to be added at table. Unless œdema is present, however, no objection may be taken to its use in cooking. The rôles of the Na and Cl ions have been discussed under acute nephritis. Many of the nephritic diets are barely adequate in iron for the increased needs of the nephritic patient, and consequently iron in any of the usual forms may be necessary (see p. 471). The vitamin content is also commonly deficient and will require supplementing. The rôle of Vitamin P in the control of capillary permeability would suggest its usefulness in this stage of the condition as the albuminuria is entirely consequent upon the increased glomerular permeability. In the few cases, however, where the writer has had the opportunity of using it, he has seen no change in the amount of albuminuria. Septic foci must be searched for and, if present, eradicated. When the patient is free of œdema, it is unnecessary to restrict the fluid intake, this being guided by the patient's own desire. If the fluid intake is unduly restricted, it adds to the kidney's difficulty in excreting the large amount of nitrogenous waste products resulting from the high protein intake. On the other hand, it is unnecessary to force fluids upon the patient at this stage of the disease. As long as œdema is absent the patient should be allowed to be up and to perform his usual occupations. He must, however, be guarded against chills and intercurrent infections which are likely to accelerate his downhill progress. When œdema develops he must be put to bed and a more drastic régime instituted, including a high protein salt-poor diet. In addition, diuretic measures have to be considered. Attempts to raise the osmotic tension of the plasma by the intravenous administration of 15 to 30 per cent. solution of acacia (1 gm. of acacia per kilogram body-weight) are reported to have been helpful, but in the writer's experience this procedure has not proved efficacious. Osman recommends massive doses of alkali, giving sufficient citrate and bicarbonate to maintain the *p*H of the urine constantly at or above 8. Again, the writer has not found this method of treatment helpful. The administration of diuretics also holds out little hope of success. Diuretics are unlikely to be successful unless the hypoproteinæmia is corrected. Of the diuretics urea may be given in doses of 100 to 250 gr. t.i.d., this amount being easily excreted by the normally functioning kidney in addition to that produced from the high protein intake. The mercurial diuretics are of great value provided there are no signs of acute renal damage. It is usually advisable, however, to start with a small test dose of ½ c.c. only of the mercurial used. (See treatment of cardiac œdema for full details, p. 684.) Premedication with ammonium chloride or other acid salt can be given, as at this stage of chronic nephritis acidosis and uræmia do not occur. Frequently, the removal of fluid by mechanical means is followed by rapid improvement. Paracentesis abdominis and thoracis are commonly followed by diuresis and lessening of the œdema. Subcutaneous tapping is less often successful. The technique of these procedures is given on p. 1087. The inadvisability of drastic purgation and diaphoresis has already been noted (p. 856). Epstein recommends thyroid administration in the treatment of nephrosis. It has been noted that patients with nephrosis frequently tolerate large doses of thyroid. The writer has not found this of value. Nor does the administration of suprarenal cortical extract in large doses intravenously prove any more successful. This latter attempt at endocrine therapy is based upon the supposed controlling influence of the suprarenal cortex upon cholesterol metabolism which is presumably grossly disturbed in nephrosis.

Third Stage of Glomerulonephritis

(*Chronic Interstitial Nephritis, Azotæmic Nephritis*)

When the condition reaches this stage, the affected glomeruli become sclerosed, blood flow through them is thereby prevented, and consequently albuminuria and œdema diminish or disappear. The reduction in nephrons, however, leads to impairment of concentrating power and other renal functions. This eventually gives rise to the characteristic changes in the blood chemistry of which the increased nitrogen content is the most frequently noted. At the same time hypertension develops and following upon this hypertrophic changes take place in the heart.

In the stage of azotæmia the diet can no longer be maintained at a high protein level, but has to be based upon the power of the kidney to excrete nitrogenous waste products. Too often in the past, however, protein intake has been drastically curtailed with resultant damage to the general health. *It may safely be said that more damage can be done at this stage by protein starvation than by protein excess.* The degree of renal function should be determined by renal efficiency tests and by estimation of the blood nitrogen. These estimations should be repeated at intervals to ascertain the progress of the condition, the diet being regulated by the result. The diets given in Diets II to IV under Acute Nephritis can again be employed, starting with Diet IV (p. 865) where only a mild degree of functional impairment is present, and then descending the diet scale as the impairment increases. As the tendency at this stage is towards acidosis, an alkaline ash diet is commonly advised. In our experience equally good results can be obtained by the administration of 30 to 60 gr. of potassium citrate t.i.d. Fluid intake can no longer be restricted as a greater excretion of water is necessary to compensate for the lessened power of concentration, otherwise blood nitrogen retention and uræmia must follow. As hypertension is a feature of this stage of the disease, care must be taken to restrict food rich in purines, such as liver, sweetbreads and kidneys, as these are believed to have a pressor action. It is usually best to allow the patient to follow his normal activities as far as possible, due regard being given to the state of his heart and general health (see p. 650). The end is inevitable and no point is served by withdrawing him from congenial employment until the condition forces it upon him. Any œdema present at this stage will be largely of cardiac origin and should be treated accordingly (p. 665). The mercurial diuretics must be used with caution.

Uræmia is the natural termination in about a third of cases. While its onset may be inevitable, it frequently occurs earlier than need be owing to the presence of some other condition such as heart failure, prostatism, infections, gastro-intestinal disturbance or a superadded acute nephritis. A search for such precipitant causes should constantly be made, and if discovered, prompt treatment instituted. In most of them pre-renal loss of fluid into the tissues or by vomiting and diarrhœa leads to an insufficient circulation of fluid through the kidney, with resultant retention of products which would otherwise have been excreted. Eventually, however, no method succeeds in compensating for the impaired concentrating power and true uræmia arises. Gastro-intestinal symptoms develop insidiously and later nervous symptoms ensue associated with gradual onset of drowsiness and coma. Tetany may also occur as the result of the low calcium and raised phosphorus content of the blood.

The treatment of this type of uræmia is much less successful than that of the form occurring in the acute stage and is mainly of a symptomatic nature. Venesection and lumbar puncture may give transient benefit when headache, fits and other cerebral signs are present. The beneficial results of these procedures are much less evident than in pseudo-uræmia. The intravenous administration of hypertonic solutions is of no service in chronic uræmia. Acidosis, as indicated by uræmic asthma, may be counteracted to some extent by the intravenous administration of alkali. The alkalis should be given along with saline when, as commonly occurs, the chloride content of the blood is also low. For this purpose 30 to 50 c.c. of 8 per cent. solution of sodium bicarbonate should be given along with 500 c.c. of normal saline. Where latent or active tetany is present, calcium gluconate (10 c.c. 10 per cent. sol.) intramuscularly may be given two or three times a day. The administration of 500 c.c. of a 1 per cent. solution of magnesium sulphate intravenously is also helpful. The gastro-intestinal symptoms are frequently most distressing, ulceration of the mouth, anorexia, vomiting, diarrhœa and constipation being the commonest. The vomiting and diarrhœa increase the pre-renal deviation of fluid, decrease the chloride content of the blood and increase the acidosis. They thus call for further intravenous administration of saline and alkali, and to these a weak glucose solution may be added (5 per cent.) to prevent the tendency to ketosis. Sedatives will be called for in all such cases : any may be given, even the morphine group. The danger of morphine in chronic kidney disease has been over-emphasized. It is now known that morphine has no detrimental effect on renal function. Since, however, excretion is seriously impaired, due care must be taken to guard against over-dosage.

Diet I

Milk, Glucose and Fruit-juice Diet for the Initial Stage of Acute Nephritis

(Protein content, 20 gm.)

(The glucose fruit-juice mixture is a 30 per cent. solution of glucose in water with the juice of 1 or 2 oranges or lemons added to each pint for flavouring purposes.)

8 *a.m.*—5 oz. citrated milk.
10 *a.m.*—5 oz. glucose fruit-juice mixture.
12 *noon*—5 oz. citrated milk.
2 *p.m.*—5 oz. glucose fruit-juice mixture.
4 *p.m.*—5 oz. citrated milk.
6 *p.m.*—5 oz. glucose fruit-juice mixture.
8 *p.m.*—5 oz. citrated milk.

During Night—5 oz. glucose fruit-juice mixture.

With improvement in the renal condition the milk can be wholly or partly replaced by a milk and cream mixture, while bread and butter, Benger's food, arrowroot or other light cereals may be added.

When urea range lies between a maximum 1·5 to 2 per cent. (specific gravity below 1,018), place on Diet II. When the urea range shows a maximum concentration of 2·5 per cent. (specific gravity 1,018), Diet III is given. With a maximum rise to 3 per cent. (specific gravity 1,020+), Diet IV is used.

Diet II

(Approximately 50 gm. protein)

Breakfast—
Grapefruit or orange with sugar.
2 oz. bread.
Butter and marmalade.
Tea with milk and sugar.

Forenoon—

1 apple or orange, if desired.

Dinner—

2 oz. meat or $2\frac{1}{2}$ oz. fish.
Large helping of vegetable (except peas or beans).
Average helping of potato.
Cereal pudding with milk from ration.
Stewed, tinned or fresh fruit.

Tea—

$1\frac{1}{2}$ oz. bread.
Tomato, cress, lettuce, cucumber, if desired.
Butter and honey or jam.
Tea with milk and sugar.

Supper—

2 oz. bread.
Butter.
Glass of milk from ration.

Daily Rations—

2 oz. meat.
$\frac{3}{4}$ pint milk.
$5\frac{1}{2}$ oz. bread.

Two tea biscuits may be taken in place of $\frac{1}{2}$ oz. bread, as far as their protein content is concerned.

DIET III

(Approximately 75 gm. protein)

Breakfast—

6 tablespoonfuls porridge with milk from ration.
$1\frac{1}{2}$ oz. bread.
Butter.
Marmalade.
Tea with milk and sugar.

Forenoon—

1 apple or orange, if desired.

Dinner—
3 oz. meat or 4 oz. fish.
Large helping of vegetables (except peas and beans).
Average helping potato.
Cereal pudding with milk from ration.
Stewed, tinned or fresh fruit.

Tea—
2 oz. bread. Tomato, lettuce, cress, cucumber, if desired.
Butter and honey or jam.
Tea with milk and sugar.

Supper—
1 egg or $\frac{3}{4}$ oz. cheese ; *or*, omitting 1 oz. meat at dinner, 2 oz. meat or $2\frac{1}{2}$ oz. fish.
2 oz. bread.
Butter.
Glass of milk from ration.
Fresh fruit if desired.

Daily Rations—
3 oz. meat.
1 egg.
$5\frac{1}{2}$ oz. bread.
1 pint milk.
6 tablespoonfuls porridge.

One and a half ounces bacon, *or* 1 egg+1 oz. milk, may be substituted for 6 tablespoonfuls porridge.

Two tea biscuits, *or* $\frac{1}{2}$ oz. spongecake, may be substituted for $\frac{1}{2}$ oz. bread.

Diet IV

(Approximately 96 gm. protein)

Breakfast—
6 tablespoonfuls porridge with milk from ration.
1 egg.
$1\frac{1}{2}$ oz. bread.
Butter.
Marmalade.
Tea with milk and sugar.

Forenoon—
1 apple or orange, if desired.

Dinner—

$2\frac{1}{2}$ oz. meat or 3 oz. fish.
Large helping vegetables (except peas and beans).
Average helping of potato.
Cereal pudding with milk from ration.
Stewed, tinned or fresh fruit.

Tea—

2 oz. bread.
Tomato, lettuce, cress or cucumber, if desired.
Butter and honey or jam.
Tea with milk and sugar.

Supper—

2 oz. meat or $2\frac{1}{2}$ oz. fish.
2 oz. bread.
Butter.
Glass of milk from ration.
Fresh fruit, if desired.

Daily Rations—

$4\frac{1}{2}$ oz. meat.
1 egg.
$5\frac{1}{2}$ oz. bread.
$1\frac{1}{2}$ pints milk.
6 tablespoonfuls porridge.

One and a half ounces bacon, *or* 1 egg+1 oz. milk, may be substituted for 6 tablespoonfuls porridge.

Two tea biscuits, *or* $\frac{1}{2}$ oz. spongecake, may be substituted for $\frac{1}{2}$ oz. bread.

DIET V

FOR CHRONIC NEPHRITIS WITH ŒDEMA

(Approximately 130 gm. protein, low salt)

Breakfast—

2 eggs or 2 oz. fish (unsalted).
2 oz. bread.
Unsalted butter.
Marmalade.
Tea with milk and sugar.

Forenoon—

Glass of milk from daily ration.

Dinner—

4 oz. meat or 5 oz. fish (unsalted).
Average helping vegetables (except peas and beans).
Average helping of potato.
Cereal pudding with milk from ration.
Stewed, tinned or fresh fruit.

Tea—

2 oz. bread.
Salad now or at supper, with 1 hard-boiled egg, *or* egg may be used in cooking, *i.e.*, in cereal pudding.
Unsalted butter and honey or jam.
Tea with milk and sugar.

Supper—

4 oz. meat or 5 oz. fish—unsalted.
2 oz. bread.
Unsalted butter.
Glass of milk from daily ration.
Fresh fruit, if desired.

Daily Rations—

8 oz. meat.
3 eggs.
$1\frac{1}{2}$ pints milk.
6 oz. bread.

All food to be prepared without salt.
No salt allowed with meals.

J. D. S. CAMERON.

HYDRONEPHROSIS

In hydronephrosis there is dilatation of the renal pelvis and calyces with non-infected urine. If the urine becomes infected the condition of pyonephrosis is established.

Hydronephrosis may be congenital or acquired. The congenital form arises in connection with various developmental anomalies affecting not only the kidney but also the lower parts of the urinary tract. It sometimes arises without any anatomical abnormality being visible, and it is presumed in such cases to be due to a neuromuscular inco-ordination of the same type that gives rise to megacolon and hypertrophic pyloric stenosis.

The acquired forms of hydronephrosis arise as a result of obstruction to the urinary flow and may be unilateral or bilateral. The chief causes are blocking of the urinary tract by stone, neoplasm or inflammatory products (*e.g.*, renal tuberculosis ; ureteric stricture ; pressure on the ureter from without by tumours, inflammatory masses or adhesions ; torsion of the ureter when the kidney is abnormally movable). These conditions usually give rise to a unilateral hydronephrosis, but may affect both kidneys. Bilateral hydronephrosis is, however, more commonly due to obstruction to or occlusion of the lower parts of the urinary tract (*e.g.*, neoplastic or inflammatory masses in the bony pelvis, urethral stricture, prostatic hypertrophy, phimosis or the presence of some mass such as a calculus in the bladder). If the obstruction to the urinary flow is intermittent, the conditions are favourable for a progressive increase in the degree of hydronephrosis, while a permanent obstruction leads to a more rapid destruction of renal tissue from pressure, so that the hydronephrosis tends to become stationary.

Minor degrees of hydronephrosis, such as occur in cases of generalized visceroptosis, may give rise to no symptoms and require no special treatment except when periods of exacerbation due to kinking of the ureter (Dietl's crises) cause pain and sometimes also vomiting and collapse.

Large or progressively enlarging dilatations of the renal pelvis may require surgical interference to remove the cause of the obstruction, and in every case where hydronephrosis is diagnosed or suspected a thorough urological examination should be made in order to determine (*a*) the cause and (*b*) whether the obstruction is unilateral or bilateral. The operative treatment of hydronephrosis is beyond the scope of this work, but it may be emphasized that surgical exploration is to be preferred to making an attempt to reduce the distension by aspiration. Where no cause for the hydronephrosis is found that can be dealt with by operation, certain palliative measures may be employed. An intermittent hydronephrosis that is not giving rise to any serious symptoms can be left alone, but the patient should be kept under careful observation. A hydronephrosis that is associated with generalized visceroptosis may sometimes be prevented from developing acute obstructive phases by controlling it with a surgical belt, but the fitting of these appliances in women of the nervous type, who are usually the subjects of visceroptosis, is often a matter of difficulty. A simple arrangement of pad and binder may be more comfortable than one of the more elaborate and rigid forms of belt. Patients of an introspective type seem to find relief from wearing a support even when there are no acute symptoms. The measures described for the treatment of visceroptosis (see p. 580) are applicable to these cases. When a Dietl's crisis threatens or develops the patient should be put to bed, heat should be applied to the loins and a sedative such as potassium bromide (15 gr. thrice daily) should be given in conjunction with belladonna (10 to 20 minims of the tincture thrice daily) to diminish any tendency to spasm and achalasia of the ureteric sphincters. If pain is severe, however, morphia may be necessary. In hydronephrosis associated with visceroptosis or "floating kidney," operative treatment should be avoided.

When there is an obstruction to the urinary flow that for any reason cannot be dealt with by operation, it is sometimes possible to relieve the pressure on the kidney tissue by ureteric catheterization, but this procedure should not be adopted without careful consideration of the nature and extent of the obstruction. If there is likely to be any risk of carrying infection into the renal pelvis from the lower parts of the tract the procedure should be avoided. Rest and the administration of belladonna in the doses indicated may be sufficient to relieve an exacerbation of the hydronephrosis by diminishing spasm. Prolonged pressure on the renal parenchyma by the retained fluid will ultimately lead to loss of function in the glomerular apparatus so that renal insufficiency results. This must be treated on the lines indicated for the treatment of chronic nephritis with renal failure (see p. 861). When infection occurs in a hydronephrosis a much more serious condition arises. It is important, therefore, to avoid instrumental interference as far as possible and to treat promptly any slight bacilluria or pyuria that may arise (see below).

It should scarcely be necessary to mention the need for testing the efficiency of each kidney separately if nephrotomy or nephrectomy is contemplated.

INFECTIONS OF THE URINARY TRACT

The management of a case of infection of the urinary tract depends not only on the particular part most affected but also on the age of the patient and the type of infecting organism. There are, however, certain principles which are of general application. The term "pyelitis" is frequently used in a broad sense to include not only suppurative inflammation of the renal pelvis but also the associated inflammation of the ureter and bladder. It must not be forgotten that there may also be an extension of the inflammatory process into the tubular system of the kidney so that a pyelonephritis is produced.

Pyelitis may be acute, subacute or chronic. It may develop insidiously or come on suddenly without prodromal symptoms. In many cases the infection attacks a previously healthy urinary tract, but in others its development is favoured and its duration prolonged by the presence of some abnormality, such as calculus, tumour or tuberculosis.

Apart from local abnormalities in the genito-urinary organs there are many general conditions which predispose to the occurrence of urinary infection. Common causes of this type are influenza, the state of lowered resistance that follows the exanthemata, the cachexia of chronic renal or cardiac disease, malignant disease or tuberculosis. Chronic constipation, colitis, diverticulitis, anal fissure and infected hæmorrhoids are frequently factors in the development of urinary infections—particularly with organisms of the coliform group. In all cases of urinary infection with *Bacillus coli*, therefore, a careful examination should be made to exclude such pathological conditions in the large bowel, which should receive appropriate treatment if found to be present.

Pyelitis is common in pregnancy, and in this state there are mechanical factors with dilatation of the ureter and achalasia of the ureteric sphincters which are favourable to the growth of organisms on account of the stagnation of the urinary flow to which they give rise. In young persons, and in middle-aged adults who have no pre-existing disease of the urinary tract, the infection usually gives rise to a pyelitis with only a moderate inflammatory reaction in the kidney and in the lower part of the urinary tract. In elderly subjects the bladder infection is often the most troublesome feature, and is most resistant to treatment. The deformed bladder of the elderly man with prostatic hypertrophy forms a favourable site for the continued activity of the infecting organisms which grow in the residual urine that is left behind after the incomplete evacuation of the bladder. Similar factors favour the continued growth of organisms in the bladders of women with uterine prolapse and cystocele.

In the acute form of pyelitis there is often a very severe general disturbance from toxic absorption. In the early stages the febrile reaction and its accompanying symptoms may be so prominent that the existence of an infection of the urinary tract may be overlooked if the examination of the urine is not properly carried out. In severe cases there is high fever with rigors, headache, lumbar pain and general prostration. Signs of bladder irritation, though often present, may be so indefinite as to be overlooked. This is particularly likely to occur in children who are unable to describe their symptoms accurately.

The essential point in the diagnosis of infections of the urinary tract is the demonstration of pus and organisms in the urine. Pus may be so abundant as to be obvious on casual inspection of the urine, but is frequently scanty in amount, and its presence can then be detected only by microscopic examination. The old-fashioned test with liquor potassiæ ("ropiness" when the reagent is added to the urine) is of little value. When it is positive, the amount of pus present is usually sufficient to be visible to the naked eye. Absence of "ropiness" on the other hand is no indication of the absence of pus or bacilluria. It must be emphasized, therefore, that the only reliable way of ascertaining whether pus and organisms are present in the urine is by microscopic examination. If there is any question of contamination of the urine, as, for example, by the vaginal discharges, it is necessary to obtain a catheter specimen. Even where this is not considered necessary it is well to allow the first part of the bladder contents to be evacuated before the specimen for examination is collected. In this way confusion will be avoided between a true pyuria or bacilluria and contamination of the urine with pus from the urethra or genital passages.

If any appreciable amount of pus is present it will be seen in a fresh wet preparation of the urine examined under a low or medium power lens. If the urine is examined after centrifugalization it must be remembered that a normal urine may show a few leucocytes in the deposit and that this must be taken into account in interpreting the results and correlating it with the clinical findings. As a criterion of the results of treatment, culture of the urine is commonly made, and it is frequently found that after a successful course of medication the urine has become sterile. This does not necessarily indicate, however, that there is no residual nidus of infection which may again become active when the antibacterial action of the drug is withdrawn.

A great variety of organisms may be found in urinary infections, but the commonest is the group of coliform bacilli. *B. coli* may occur as a pure infection or as part of a mixed infection along with enterococci or streptococci. *B. proteus* is an important infective agent on account of its strong urea-splitting action which gives rise to an alkaline ammoniacal urine and necessitates special precautions in treatment. Certain of the coccal infections (streptococcal and staphylococcal) involve the same difficulty, though in less marked degree than *B. proteus*. Urea-splitting with ammonia formation does not occur to any extent with *B. coli* and the paratyphoid group, so that control of urinary reaction in these infections is simplified.

Care should be taken that an underlying infection with *B. tuberculosis* is not overlooked. If there is any reason to suspect its presence the appropriate methods of searching for it should be applied, and it should not be assumed that because there is a heavy infection with a coliform or coccal organism the whole bacteriological picture has been established. Since non-pathogenic organisms, particularly coliform bacilli, may multiply at room temperature in a specimen of urine, the true cause of a urinary infection may be missed if there is delay in examining the specimen.

In the investigation of a case of infection of the urinary tract it must be remembered that the fundamental cause of the condition may be some abnormality or disease outside the genito-urinary system. It is necessary, therefore, if a satisfactory course of treatment is to be laid down, that a full general examination of the patient should be made. In many cases it is futile to attempt to overcome the infection by giving urinary antiseptics without also dealing with the following factors should they be present: (1) malnutrition, due to an insufficient or improperly balanced diet; (2) lowered resistance, due to some metabolic disorder such as diabetes mellitus; (3) chronic intoxication from a diseased appendix or from some lesion of the gastro-intestinal tract such as colitis, diverticulitis, inflamed hæmorrhoids, fistula or carcinoma; (4) anæmia, whether it be nutritional, post-hæmorrhagic or dyshæmapoietic in type; and (5) mechanical or nervous causes leading to interference with the regular or complete emptying of any part of the urinary tract.

General Management of the Patient.—Having diagnosed the presence of infection of the urinary tract, the first point to decide is whether the patient may be treated as an ambulatory case or must be confined to bed. In all cases where the infection is acute, and in most cases where it is subacute, rest in bed is essential. The need for this is clear in severe cases with general febrile and toxic manifestations, but it may not be so obvious to the patient when the infection is only subacute. It should be explained to him that his recovery is likely to be much quicker if he submits to a period of complete rest. After the fever has settled and the toxæmia has subsided, the patient may be allowed up for short periods as this helps to promote drainage, but he must not be allowed to expose himself to chill and should avoid exertion until convalescence is well established.

Diet.—During the acute febrile stages of pyelitis, the diet should be restricted to water, glucose, fruit juices and diluted milk. As soon as the toxæmia shows signs of clearing, light farinaceous foods, bread and butter, toast, or plain biscuits may be added to the diet. With further improvement, egg and fish dishes and vegetable purée may be added to the diet. When the method of treatment adopted does not necessitate the restriction of fluid, large quantities of milk may be allowed, either fresh milk, buttermilk, or milk shakes (that is, milk flavoured with fruit syrup). The quantities of food may be gradually increased, but until convalescence is definitely established, these dietary restrictions should be continued. Reference is made below to certain forms of treatment which necessitate a restriction of the fluid intake, and to others in which the amount of fluid must be increased above the normal. The dietary management of the patient must be modified according to which of these methods is chosen.

Regulation of the bowels is important, as in many cases chronic constipation is present. If the patient's physical condition permits, 4 to 8 drachms of castor oil is a suitable preliminary treatment. Otherwise a soap and water enema (1 oz. of green soft soap to each pint of warm water) should be given and may be repeated daily. In some cases an olive oil enema may be required to dislodge inspissated fæces (10 oz. of warmed olive oil run in, under gravity, through a rubber catheter). It is undesirable to give cathartics as their action may tend to encourage the passage of coliform organisms from the gut, but the regular evacuation of the bowels should be secured by giving small doses of cascara and belladonna. The former improves the tone of the muscular wall of the gut, while the latter minimizes any tendency to spasm, not only in the gut but also in the urinary tract. Hyoscyamus may be added for the same reason, and the following mixture three times a day after food will be found effective.

Extr. Casc. Sagr. Liq. . .	♏x
Tinct. Bellad.	♏v
Tinct. Hyoscy.	♏v
Syrup Zingib.	ʒi
Aq. . . . . . to	ʒiv

Sig.—One tablespoonful three times a day after food.

It is seldom that the administration of this mixture fails to produce a normal evacuation of the bowels once or twice in the twenty-four hours, but occasionally an additional dose of liquid extract of cascara (1 to 2 drachms) may be required each evening for the first few days.

Control of Pain in Pyrexia.—Apart from irritation in the bladder and urethra, severe pain is not usually a prominent feature in pyelitis, but there is often a good deal of dull aching and discomfort in the abdomen and in the lumbar region. This pain may respond to the local application of heat by means of rubber hot-water bottles, a hot compress or an electrically heated pad. It may also be alleviated by a simple analgesic such as the following:—

Acid. Acetylsalicyl.	gr. v
Phenacet.	gr. iii
Codein. Phosph.	gr. $\frac{1}{6}$

In some cases it is necessary to control pain with an opium preparation, such as $\frac{1}{6}$ gr. morphine sulphate and $\frac{1}{100}$ gr. atropine sulphate hypodermically. Irritability of the bladder and dysuria may be lessened by giving 10 minims of tincture of hyoscyamus in $\frac{1}{2}$ oz. of water thrice daily.

Pyrexia is best controlled by tepid sponging, but care should be taken to avoid chilling the patient by exposing large areas of the body surface. If the analgesic mixture of aspirin, phenacetin and codeine referred to above is being used, it will tend to lessen the fever.

Alkalis.—The reaction of the urine in pyelitis may be either acid or alkaline. In the common form of infection with coliform organisms, the urine is acid unless it has been lying in the bladder for a sufficient time to allow of decomposition. A great deal may be done to inhibit the growth of organisms in the urinary tract by altering the reaction of the urine so that it is unfavourable to them. Artificially induced changes in the reaction in the urine slow down the rate of growth of organisms. These changes in reaction can be brought about very easily if the dosage of the drugs used is properly adjusted, but if the amounts given are inadequate they will fail to produce any improvement. In the common form of urinary tract infection, with a highly acid urine, the aim is to produce a sudden change to alkalinity. This can be done by giving sufficient amounts of sodium citrate, sodium acetate or sodium bicarbonate. If it is desired to change an alkaline urine to an acid one, the most suitable drugs to employ are ammonium chloride or sodium acid phosphate. Reference is made below to the use of these acidifying drugs in connection with mandelates and hexamine. The alkaline diuretic treatment, in addition to inhibiting the growth of many of the common types of organisms, has a beneficial effect in other ways, because it produces a large amount of dilute non-irritating urine which minimizes local irritation and mechanically flushes out the urinary passages. In many cases the administration of alkalis alone will be followed by an arrest of the infective process, but it is desirable to combine it with sulphapyridine (see below). Failure to obtain good results with the alkaline method is generally due to inadequate dosage or to failure of the patient to co-operate. The first essential is to make sure that the patient is taking large amounts of fluid. A minimum of 5 pints of water—alone or combined with barley water, fruit drinks, tea, or diluted milk—should be insisted upon. The intake should be spread as evenly as possible over the twenty-four hours, so that at no time does the urine become highly concentrated. The output of urine following this intake should be somewhere in the region of 100 oz., and if the diuretic response is unsatisfactory the fluid intake may be further increased. Failure to obtain a sufficient output of urine is generally due to the patient not having carried out the instructions with regard to fluid intake.

The amount of alkali to be given depends to some extent on the response of the patient. As a preliminary, 30 gr. each of sodium citrate and sodium bicarbonate with $\frac{1}{2}$ oz. of liquor ammonii acetatis may be given in water every two hours for the first day or two. The reaction of the urine to litmus must be taken each time the bladder is emptied, and as soon as the urine becomes frankly alkaline the dosage may be cut down by giving the mixture only once every four hours. Some patients are very resistant and require larger doses for a longer period. There is sometimes a better response if sodium bicarbonate (30 gr.) is added to each dose for a day or so, but on the whole, citrates and acetates are less upsetting to the digestion. Another very simple method of securing alkalinization of the urine is to prescribe sodium citrate alone, in solid forms, and to instruct the patient to take a teaspoonful (approximately 60 gr.) every two hours until the litmus turns blue, and thereafter every four hours. Should he subsequently find the litmus failing to turn blue he should resume the two-hourly doses until the reaction is again adjusted. Occasionally patients object to the insipid taste of sodium citrate. This may be overcome by giving 6 minims of concentrated infusion of gentian in $\frac{1}{2}$ oz. of water with each dose of citrate. It is useless to attempt to treat infection of the urinary tract by this method if the urine does not become alkaline. To prevent hypochloræmia from the free diuresis, 1 to 2 drachms of sodium chloride should be included in each day's diet.

If the alkaline diuretic treatment is carried out in the manner described, pyuria may be expected to diminish within a few days and may even clear up completely, but the duration of the treatment is lessened and the cure is more effective if this régime is combined with the administration of sulphanilamide (see below).

Urinary Antiseptics.—*The Sulphonamides.*—The introduction of the sulphonamide group of drugs has given us a new and potent weapon for use in the treatment of infections of the urinary tract. The different types of sulphonamide preparations with their relative advantages and disadvantages have been discussed in detail on pp. 83-86. It is as yet premature to say dogmatically which of these drugs will prove to be the most effective in dealing with the varying infections which may occur in the urinary tract. Recent work, however, suggests most strongly that sulphapyridine (M. & B. 693 or Dagenan) is the drug of choice in all types of urinary infection.

The sulphonamide preparations have been used alone, but there is evidence that they are more effective if combined with the alkaline diuretic treatment described above. In the writer's experience this combination has much to commend it and, particularly in infections with *bacillus proteus*, it has given very encouraging results. The beneficial effects of diuresis and of alkalinization of the urine need not be sacrificed, while the additional antibacterial action of the sulphonamide helps to reduce the time required for the sterilization of the urine. Sulphapyridine is given orally in doses of 7½ gr. four times a day in addition to the alkaline diuretic régime described above. With this combined treatment there is a rapid diminution in fever and toxæmia, and it is common to find that not only does the pus disappear from the urine within a week or ten days but that the urine becomes sterile on culture. In using these sulphonamide preparations it is necessary to avoid the administration of any drug containing sulphur, *e.g.*, magnesium sulphate, and the ingestion of any articles of diet which are rich in sulphur, *e.g.*, eggs. Further reference to the dosage of sulphanilamide preparations will be found in another section (see p. 83).

Mandelic Acid.—About 1931 there was introduced a method

of treating pyelitis by inducing a ketosis. The patient was given a "ketogenic" diet in which the normal balance of carbohydrate and fat was upset by restricting the former and increasing the latter until ketonuria was produced. The method was troublesome to use and uncertain in action but seemed to contain a principle of some value. Investigation showed that B-hydroxy-butyric acid has a powerful action in preventing the growth of organisms if the urine is sufficiently acid (*p*H 5·3). Hydroxy-butyric acid cannot be given orally because it is destroyed in the upper part of the alimentary tract, but mandelic acid was shown by Rosenheim to be an effective substitute for it. The use of mandelic acid in infections of the urinary tract marks a very striking advance, and with modifications has become established as a standard method of treatment. On account of the necessity for giving some additional drug to alter the reaction of the urine, and also because of the unpleasant and irritating effects of mandelic acid in the stomach, it is now customary to use one of the salts, such as sodium, ammonium or calcium mandelate.

In giving mandelic acid or one of its salts the reaction of the urine must be kept at or below *p*H 5·3. If the acidity should become less than this the antibacterial action of the mandelic acid is lost. When the fluid intake is restricted this degree of acidity may develop spontaneously, but if it does not, ammonium chloride must be given in addition. The common method of acidifying the urine for this purpose is to give 15 gr. (1 gm.) of ammonium chloride four times a day. In some cases this is insufficient to render the urine highly acid and multiples of this dose up to as much as 6 or 8 gm. may have to be used. Treatment with these large doses cannot be continued for long on account of the irritating effects of the ammonium chloride, and in some patients even the smaller doses are not tolerated. The newer preparations such as calcium mandelate and ammonium mandelate are on the whole less irritating and less nauseating. Though slightly more expensive, they are preferable to ammonium chloride and mandelic acid. It should be emphasized that unless the urine reaches the proper degree of acidity it is useless to attempt to continue the treatment with mandelates.

The usual basic dose of mandelic acid is 45 gr. (3 gm.) four times a day. The equivalent of this in the form of sodium mandelate is 50 gr. (3·43 gm.). If it is desired to use a non-proprietary preparation, the following mixtures are effective :—

No. 1.—Ammonium Chloride Mixture

Ammon. Chlorid.		℥ss
Extr. Glycyrrh. Liq. . . .		ʒiv
Aq.	to	℥viii

Sig.—One tablespoonful four times a day before food.

(*Note.*—Ammonium chloride may be given dry in cachets if preferred.)

No. 2.—Sodium Mandelate Mixture

Sod. Mandelate . . .		℥iss
Syr. Aurant. . . .		℥iss
Aq.	to	℥viii

Sig.—One tablespoonful four times a day after food.

The reaction of the urine must be tested regularly by adding 5 drops of a buffered solution of methyl-red to $\frac{1}{2}$ in. of urine in a test-tube. At *p*H 5·3 the colour is bright pink, but above this the colour is orange or yellow indicating that the urine is alkaline or not sufficiently acid. This indicator solution can be purchased ready for use. A number of drug manufacturers supply preparations of ammonium or calcium mandelate under proprietary names. These are more palatable and quite reliable, but are necessarily slightly more expensive than non-proprietary mixtures. Examples of these preparations are :—

Mandelix.—Dose, 2 drachms four times a day. Supplied by British Drug Houses Ltd.

Mandecal.—Dose, 4 to 5 gm. (1 level dessertspoonful four times a day). Supplied by British Drug Houses Ltd.

Ammoket.—Dose, 4 drachms four times a day. Supplied by Boots Pure Drug Co. Ltd.

Neoket (mandelic acid, sodium bicarbonate and sodium acid phosphate without ammonium chloride).—Dose, 2 drachms four times a day. Supplied by Boots Pure Drug Co.

When one of these preparations is given the reaction of the urine usually reaches the proper degree of acidity, but if there is failure to get a *p*H 5·3, doses of 10 gr. of ammonium chloride may be given three or four times a day until the reaction is corrected. There are exceptionally resistant cases, but usually, if the mandelic acid treatment is carried out carefully, the urine becomes sterile within seven to ten days unless there is some anatomical abnormality such as a deformed bladder or a renal calculus. An undesirable point about the treatment with mandelic acid and its derivatives is the necessity for some restriction of the fluid intake, and in cases where there is renal disease the drug may produce irritation of the kidneys. If signs of such irritation should appear, *e.g.*, hæmaturia, gross albuminuria, or a heavy deposit of casts, the drug should be stopped and one of the other methods of treatment substituted. On account of its tendency to irritation, and because of the necessity of restricting the fluid intake, it is undesirable to use mandelic acid in the initial stages of acute pyelitis. When the patient is febrile and toxic, the alkaline diuretic method should be used until the acute phase has passed off.

It would be premature to make a final assessment of the relative values of mandelate and sulphapyridine, but experience up to the present with these two methods of treatment indicates that mandelate is as effective when there is little or no urea-splitting (particularly in pure infections with *B. coli*) while sulphapyridine is more effective in those cases where urea-splitting takes place freely as in infections with *B. proteus*, streptococci and in mixed coccal and bacterial infections.

Hexamine (Hexamina) "British Pharmacopœia," 1932 (Hexamethylene tetramine).—Hexamine is also sold under various names of which the best known is "urotropine." In prescribing it the official pharmacopœial name "hexamine" should be used. Five to fifteen grains are given orally as a single dose, 40 to 60 gr. being commonly used in the twenty-four hours. The bactericidal action of hexamine depends upon its breaking down in an acid medium with the liberation of formaldehyde. In using hexamine the urine must be acid, and it is customary to give 20 to 30 gr. of sodium acid phosphate, 5 to 30 gr. of sodium benzoate, or 5 to 20 gr. of ammonium chloride three times a day to acidify the urine. If the fluid intake is restricted during the administration of hexamine there is a liability to irritation of the kidneys. If large amounts of fluid are given this tendency is overcome, but the concentration of formaldehyde in the urine tends to become so low that it has little or no bactericidal action. While it would appear that the continued presence of quite low concentrations of formaldehyde in the urine has some effect in inhibiting the growth of organisms, particularly in chronic infections of the urinary tract, the difficulty of giving really large doses of hexamine limits its usefulness in the treatment of the more acute forms of infection. If hexamine is used it is important to watch the reaction of the urine and also to give the maximum amount of the drug that the patient can tolerate. The chief use of hexamine and of the various proprietary preparations containing it is in the treatment of cases of chronic catarrhal infection of the urinary tract, and particularly of the bladder. In all acute and many subacute cases of urinary tract infections, however, hexamine is contra-indicated. Even in chronic infection it is inferior to sulpha-pyridine and mandelates.

Pyridine.—Several dyes of the pyridine series are used as urinary antiseptics. Two of the best known are phenyl-azo-alpha-alpha-diamino-pyridine hydrochloride (trade mark, " Pyridium "—Menley & James Ltd.) and butyloxy-diamino-azo-pyridine (trade mark, " Neotropin "—Schering-Kahlbaum A.G.). Both are dispensed in coated dragées containing $1\frac{1}{2}$ gr. (0·1 gm.) of the dye. Two or three of these dragées are given thrice daily by the mouth. The dye is excreted in the urine in high concentration if the fluid intake is restricted. Many favourable results have been reported, but in my experience the action is uncertain. The cost of these preparations is relatively high, and patients often object to them on account of the staining of underwear and bed-linen which is apt to occur.

Hexyl-resorcinol 1 in 3 dihydroxy-4-hexylbenzol is sold under the trade name " Caprokol " (British Drug Houses and Sharp & Dohme Ltd.). It acts in either an acid or an alkaline urine, and has a powerful antibacterial action in suitable concentration. It is believed to act mainly by lowering surface tension, and when it is given the fluid intake must be restricted. It cannot be given along with sodium bicarbonate. It is dispensed in gelatin capsules containing 0·15 gm. in olive oil, and is also obtainable as a 2·5 per cent. solution in olive oil The dosage is two to four capsules thrice daily immediately after food, or 3 to 6 drachms of the solution. Each drachm contains 0·1 gm. of the drug. In the writer's experience hexyl-resorcinol is inferior to alkaline diuresis or mandelic acid in acute cases, but it is useful in subacute cases, particularly where cystitis is causing bladder irritation. If given over a long period the expense of this proprietary preparation must be taken into account.

Drainage of the Ureter.—In some cases of pyelitis, particularly in those associated with pregnancy, there is difficulty in maintaining satisfactory drainage of pus from the renal pelvis. One factor interfering with drainage is achalasia of the ureter and this may to some extent be overcome by giving atropine (5 to 10 minims of tincture of belladonna in water three times a day). It is sometimes impossible, however, to overcome the tendency to stagnation of urine and accumulation of pus in the ureter and renal pelvis in spite of free diuresis. If this natural process of lavage is insufficient to clear the tract it is occasionally necessary to catheterize the ureters and wash out the renal pelves. For this purpose acriflavine (1 in 5,000) or silver nitrate (1 in 5,000) may be used. The procedure requires special technique and experience and should only be carried out by a urologist. I have sometimes seen striking improvement after such lavage when the ureteric catheters were left in position for twenty-four hours to establish drainage. These periods of recurrent blocking of the ureter are usually associated with an increase in toxæmia and hyperpyrexia, and the fact that the hold-up may cause a temporary diminution of the pus in the urine may lead to difficulty in diagnosis. Lavage of the bladder is sometimes the most effective way of dealing with the residual cystitis which is found particularly in elderly people who have had an acute infection of the urinary tract or an acute or subacute exacerbation of a chronic infection. Bladder lavage may be carried out daily, or on alternate days, for one to two weeks and after that at longer intervals. A non-irritating fluid should be used such as normal saline, boracic lotion, 1 in 5,000 acriflavine or 1 in 10,000 silver nitrate. After the bladder has been washed out and emptied, 10 c.c. of 10 per cent. argyrol may be injected into it just before the catheter is withdrawn.

Summary

In the initial stages of acute pyelitis when there is fever and general toxæmia, the most satisfactory treatment is the diuretic alkaline régime. Sulphapyridine may be given in suitable doses in combination with this. Until all signs of general disturbance have settled down the patient must be kept at rest in bed in an even temperature, and his activities should be restricted for some time thereafter. In the majority of uncomplicated cases pus will have disappeared and the urine will have become sterile on culture within ten days. If the infection persists one of the mandelate preparations should be used unless there is some contraindication such as active renal disease. Hexamine, hexyl-resorcinol and pyridine dyes may all be found useful in chronic cases, but are on the whole less likely to arrest the infection than either mandelic acid or sulphapyridine in combination with alkali. It is only rarely that drainage and lavage of the renal pelvis is required, but bladder lavage is frequently useful in overcoming a residual cystitis.

It cannot be emphasized too strongly that in the application of these methods of treatment the regulation of the reaction of the urine is of the first importance. Unless attention is paid to this point the results are likely to be unsatisfactory and the course of the illness unduly prolonged. Further, it is of paramount importance to make sure that no obstructive lesion, stone or underlying tuberculous disease is present in the urinary tract, and to treat any pathological condition which may be present in the colon.

RENAL CALCULUS

While the radical treatment of renal calculus is a surgical matter, there are many points in the management of the patient that are the concern of the physician. In cases where there is an excess of those constituents of the urine that tend to form calculi, certain dietary and medical measures may lessen the formation of crystalline deposits and so minimize the risk of calculus formation. Again, renal colic, hæmaturia, anuria and the infection of the urinary tract that so frequently accompanies renal calculus are all amenable to medical treatment.

Any patient who is threatened with renal calculus, whether he has signs of actual calculus or has merely been passing gravel or crystalline accumulations, must be given large quantities of fluid. In many cases it will be found that he has been habitually taking less fluid than his normal requirements, but whether this is the case or not he should be instructed to take a definite volume of fluid every day. Water, barley water, lemon drinks such as potus imperialis may be prescribed, or one of the natural mineral waters such as Vichy, Evian or Contrexéville may be ordered. It does not matter very much which is used so long as the volume of fluid is adequate, that is, 4 to 5 pints in the day. If there is an abnormal concentration of urates, uric acid or oxalates in the urine alkali should be given in moderate doses. The large doses used in the treatment of pyelitis are not required, but 20 to 30 gr. of potassium citrate three times a day should be prescribed, and should be continued for months at a time. If the urine is kept strongly alkaline there may be a tendency to the deposition of phosphates round an oxalate or uric acid stone, so that care should be taken to keep the reaction of the urine just on the alkaline side by suitable regulation of the dosage of citrate. If there is any tendency to colic or irritation, 10 minims of tincture of belladonna should be given three or four times a day for two or three days. This short course may be repeated from time to time as required. In such cases it is particularly important to make sure that the patient is taking a large amount of fluid so as to keep the urine dilute and non-irritating. Incidentally, the administration of belladonna and the production of a free diuresis may be followed by the passage of small calculi which would otherwise have remained impacted in the urinary tract.

Since phosphatic deposits occur in an alkaline medium, care should be taken to keep the urine faintly acid if there is known to be a tendency to the formation of phosphatic calculi. The fluid intake must be liberal, as in dealing with the other forms of calculi, and small doses of sodium acid phosphate (10 gr. four-hourly) may be given if necessary to control the reaction of the urine.

Regulation of the diet is necessary if there is any tendency to the excretion of excessive amounts of uric acid or urates in the urine. The amount of meat, eggs and other sources of animal protein should be cut down and the patient should be instructed to take a liberal amount of fruit and vegetables. All substances rich in nucleo-proteins (*e.g.*, kidney, liver, sweetbreads and beef) and also such purin-rich beverages as tea and coffee must be eliminated from the diet or reduced to a minimum. In general, the dietary restrictions are those necessary in the treatment of gout (*q.v.* p. 962).

The modifications of the diet that are necessary when there is a tendency to the formation of oxalate calculi are described below in connection with oxaluria (see p. 885), while those necessary for the prevention of the formation of phosphatic calculi are described in connection with the treatment of phosphaturia (see p. 884).

When the patient's circumstances permit, a course of treatment at a spa is often an effective prophylactic measure, but if the patient is willing to co-operate fully in the treatment there is no real advantage in putting him to the trouble and expense of giving up his ordinary duties and leaving home.

Renal Colic.—Renal colic occurs when a calculus enters the ureter or when the ureter is attempting to pass it into the bladder. Severe pain may also arise after a calculus has entered the bladder or while it is passing along the urethra. The pain or renal colic is of such a commanding nature that prompt measures are necessary for its relief. The most effective drug for this purpose is morphine. A $\frac{1}{4}$ gr. should be given in combination with atropine sulphate ($\frac{1}{100}$ gr.), and this injection of morphine and atropine may be repeated at intervals of three or four hours until the severity of the pain is controlled. In some cases it may be necessary to give inhalations of chloroform to obtain relief from the agonizing pain until the morphine has had time to act.

After the attack of colic has passed off the patient should be kept in bed for a few days and the urine should be examined daily for blood and pus. Even if no pus is found it is well to give a course of urinary antiseptic treatment as a prophylactic. If there is reason to suspect that the calculus is of the type that forms in acid media, citrate should be given in the doses indicated above, while in the other type of case with a tendency to phosphatic deposits the urine should be kept acid and hexamine given in doses of 10 gr. four times a day.

In the majority of cases where there is a calculus of considerable size, surgical treatment will be necessary sooner or later, but the management of the patient before and after the operation should be along the lines indicated. Particular care must be taken to diminish the risk of infection of the urinary tract, and if it does develop it should be treated in one of the ways described in the section devoted to that subject.

PHOSPHATURIA

The normal urine contains large amounts of phosphate, and the formation of a deposit of phosphates when the urine is amphoteric or alkaline is not an indication of disease.

Certain individuals, however, tend to excrete an unusual amount of phosphate. These are usually people who are taking large amounts of fruit and vegetables in their diet. Phosphaturia is also found in patients with hyperchlorhydria and in nervous and debilitated people with muscular wasting. This excessive concentration of phosphates in the urine can be dissipated by diminishing calcium-rich foodstuffs such as milk, eggs and vegetables and increasing the amount of meat, cereals and potatoes. The administration of 30 minims of dilute hydrochloric acid three or four times a day is also useful in such cases. The acid can be given at meal times, well diluted and flavoured with 1 or 2 drachms of syrup of lemon. Phosphaturia occurs also in association with cystitis when there has been ammoniacal decomposition of the urine. This is seen commonly in the common form of cystitis that accompanies prostatic hypertrophy. It usually clears up when the cystitis is treated by one of the methods described in the section on infections of the urinary tract.

OXALURIA

Oxaluria is a condition in which crystals of calcium oxalate appear as a deposit in the urine. The oxalates are derived usually from foodstuffs rich in these salts. These are mainly such vegetables or fruits as spinach, rhubarb, tomatoes and strawberries. Oxaluria may occur when such articles of diet are taken in large amounts, and it is believed that individuals with a highly acid gastric secretion are particularly prone to develop oxaluria when these forms of fruit or vegetable food are taken in excess. The oxalate crystals may cause irritation and pain and there may even be some degree of hæmaturia. Sometimes signs of general disturbance are found, such as headache, dyspepsia and lassitude. Oxalate calculi may form—the so-called "mulberry stone." These give rise to the usual symptoms of renal or ureteric calculus.

The main point in the treatment of oxaluria is the restriction of all articles of diet that are rich in oxalates. In addition to the fruits and vegetables mentioned above, it is necessary to forbid or restrict the use of tea and cocoa, since these contain oxalate. Milk, eggs, sugar, butter, wheatmeal and rice may all be allowed with safety as they are the foodstuffs least likely to lead to a persistence of oxaluria. Peas, which are rich in magnesia, may be allowed in large quantities, and magnesia can be given daily in the form of magnesium sulphate or carbonate.

J. N. Cruickshank.

CHRONIC RHEUMATIC DISEASES

INTRODUCTION

THE rheumatic diseases, both acute and chronic, are, for the most part, diseases of temperate climates. In countries enjoying this mixed blessing they constitute a serious menace to the health and well-being of the community. Only within recent years have statistics been compiled which indicate the magnitude of the problem. It is officially admitted that one-sixth of the total annual invalidity of insured persons in Great Britain is due to rheumatic disease in one or other of its forms. In Scotland, with a population of approximately 5 millions, 50,000 insured persons are totally incapacitated annually, for an average period of sixty days. Investigations carried out by the writers indicate that at least 300,000 new cases of rheumatic disease requiring medical treatment occur annually in Scotland, of which about 75 per cent. belong to the group of fibrositic diseases affecting muscles, nerves and tendons. Such figures give some indication of the enormous economic loss resulting from the ravages of this group of diseases, and of the vast amount of pain and misery entailed. They are the greatest scourge of modern civilization and have amply earned the title "Public Health Enemy No. 1."

When the section on treatment has been perused, it will become clear that many of the complex and specialized measures required for diagnosis and treatment are outside the scope of general medical practice, and it is officially admitted that there is an urgent need for the provision of special facilities for the treatment of the more chronic forms of rheumatic disease. It is for these reasons that we advocate most strongly the establishment of a national scheme for the control and treatment of the chronic rheumatic diseases, the essential feature of which would be the provision by local authorities in selected areas throughout the country of clinics in charge of physicians who have received special post-graduate training, and who would decide whether patients suffering from chronic rheumatic disease should be treated by the family physician at home, at the treatment centre as out-patients or in hospital. Only by accurate diagnosis in the early stages of the more severe forms, and by the immediate institution of the proper lines of treatment, can the regrettably common legacy of permanent incapacity be reduced or avoided. The problem of ætiology is so complex, that for its elucidation the physician must have at his disposal the help of a team of specialists in all branches of medicine, by whose concerted efforts the problem of each individual case can be unravelled.

The Governments of Sweden, Russia and other Continental countries have accepted the fact that the chronic rheumatic diseases constitute the major cause of invalidity and have put into operation plans for the control of this scourge. It is to be regretted that this country is lagging far behind many of her Continental neighbours in this respect.

Before any scheme of treatment is adopted for an individual case, it must again be emphasized that accurate diagnosis of the type of rheumatic disease present is vitally important. To label a patient rheumatism and prescribe analgesics is no longer justifiable in view of the great advances in treatment which have been made during recent years. When a diagnosis has been reached, the next step is to estimate the degree of activity of the disease process. This is especially applicable to the rheumatoid or chronic infective type, where the disease may be encountered for the first time in the acute, subacute or chronic stage. Accurate knowledge as to the activity or otherwise of the disease processes is essential if treatment is to be applied in a rational manner. The measures adopted during the acute or active phase differ radically from those employed in the subacute or chronic state, and the use of over-strenuous measures at the wrong time may lead to disaster. To estimate the degree of activity on clinical grounds alone may present considerable difficulty. The local and general condition must be carefully considered. Determination of the sedimentation rate of the red blood cells should be carried out in every case of arthritis. The technique of this test is simple and should be undertaken by every family doctor who wishes to treat the more severe forms of chronic rheumatic disease. Accordingly the technique of the test is described in the appendix. Often, in an apparently quiescent case, the test will reveal a marked degree of activity indicating the possibility of a relapse, especially if too radical forms of treatment are employed. Repeated determinations of the sedimentation rate at weekly intervals throughout treatment serve as a useful index of the progress of the case. As the disease process is overcome the reading will gradually return to normal. It must be borne in mind, however, that this return lags considerably behind clinical improvement, and in the presence of an obvious change for the better in the patient's condition the importance of a rapid rate must not be overstressed as long as the tendency is for it to fall and not to rise.

When the physician has reached a correct diagnosis and has assessed the degree of activity present, the next step, before embarking on a scheme of treatment, is to institute a thorough search for ætiological factors, and it is at this stage that the aid of specialists, in the various systems where focal sepsis is prone to occur, must be invoked. Expert opinion is essential before the patient is condemned to lose his teeth, have his tonsils removed or sinuses drained, to quote one or two examples.

Many factors are believed to play a part in the ætiology of the different forms of chronic rheumatic disease—infection, environment, constitution, occupation, the anatomic type of the patient, impairment of the body mechanics, etc. In a particular case one factor may appear to dominate the picture. For example, a thorough soaking may precipitate an attack of lumbago, but the underlying cause may be a low-grade infection, or a metabolic disturbance secondary to faulty dietetic habits. The physician should remember that a healthy body has, until its vitality is impaired, a remarkable capacity for withstanding isolated insults offered to it by its environment externally and its owner internally. Accordingly, although the amelioration of pain is the first consideration both of the patient and his physician, the latter will not have fulfilled his obligations until he has made an effort to discover and remove the underlying cause and has thus restored to the body its ability to withstand the insults with which it will inevitably be faced.

The first consideration in the treatment of chronic rheumatic disease is to secure the co-operation of the patient. Chronicity is an essential feature of the more severe forms of the disease, and unless the patient has full confidence in his physician's understanding of his trouble, and in his ability to treat it effectively, little or no progress is likely to be made. It should be explained that dramatic results must not be expected and that reliance should be placed on the judicious application, not of one form of treatment but of a combination of methods which have been carefully thought out. His confidence won, his co-operation secured and the fundamental principles underlying correct treatment observed, a prospect of progressive improvement lies before the patient. Treated early and adequately, the outlook in the severe forms of chronic rheumatic disease is far from being as gloomy as has been formerly held by the laity and the profession. A return to the enjoyment of useful citizenship can be attained in a surprisingly high proportion of cases.

There are three fundamental principles which govern the treatment of all forms of chronic rheumatic disease :—

1. The improvement of the general health of the patient.
2. The elimination or correction of ætiological factors.
3. Treatment of the local manifestation of the disease.

CLASSIFICATION

It has been thought advisable to adopt as simple a classification as possible, using the nomenclature in common use among general practitioners rather than the more recent terminology based on ætiological concepts over which opinion is still sharply divided. From the point of view of treatment, the chronic rheumatic diseases can be divided into three main groups :—

1. Rheumatoid arthritis.
2. Osteo-arthritis.
3. Non-articular rheumatic diseases.

In a recent paper Osgood has given an excellent definition and comparative classification of the two main groups of chronic rheumatic arthritis, which we quote verbatim :—

" The first, which affects females more often than males, is of more common occurrence in the asthenic individual and has its greatest age incidence in the earlier decades, is called *rheumatoid* arthritis or *atrophic* arthritis or *proliferative* arthritis or *ankylosing* arthritis : ' Rheumatoid ' because it is not rheumatic fever but presents a somewhat similar articular picture (in the British Isles this is the synonym most commonly employed) : ' Atrophic ' because very early in its course we may appreciate characteristic atrophy (halisteresis) or erosion of bone structure and soon accompanying atrophy of the musculature ; ' Proliferative ' because Nichols and Richardson (1909) showed that an early change, perhaps the very earliest, is a proliferation of the synovial membrane of the affected joints, which becomes thickened (pannus) with the formation of synovial tabs or villi ; ' Ankylosing ' because, in an unchecked disease, the joints may eventually become ankylosed, at first by fibrous adhesions and later by true bony fusion.

"In this first great type we include Still's disease in children and, at least for the present, the 'Marie-Strümpell' syndrome, or 'spondylose rhizomélique,' the main ankylosing lesions of which usually appear first in the sacro-iliac joints and spine. The so-called root joints, *i.e.*, the shoulders and hips, frequently are also affected."

There has been much controversy whether rheumatoid arthritis occurs in two forms: (1) the so-called classical or primary type, where a focus of infection is not demonstrable, and (2) the secondary or focal type in which infection is believed to play a definite part. From the point of view of treatment, differentiation between these two forms is unnecessary except in so far as sepsis has to be dealt with in one form and not in the other. In parenthesis, the writers do not wish it to be understood that they agree with the subdivision of arthritis of the rheumatoid type into the two forms mentioned above.

Osgood's definition of group 2 is as follows:—

"The second great type, in which there is no striking difference in sex incidence, although the sthenic body type exhibits it most frequently, and in which subjective symptoms do not usually appear before the age of forty years, is called *osteoarthritis* (or arthrosis), or *hypertrophic* arthritis, or *degenerative* arthritis, or *non-ankylosing* arthritis: 'Osteo-arthritis' (or arthrosis) (the usual British term) because the bony changes are evident early in the disease; 'Hypertrophic' for the same reason, the articular bone-end changes representing overgrowth or hypertrophy in the form of chondro-osseous spicules or ridges; 'Degenerative' because, as Nichols and Richardson (1909) also demonstrated, the initial changes seem to appear in the articular cartilage in the form of fibrillation and degeneration; 'Non-ankylosing' because neither fibrous nor true bony ankylosis of the joints of the extremities occurs even as an end result of an unchecked disease. One spinal exostosis or spur may fuse with an impinging spur, but the articular bone ends, even after the degenerated cartilage has been completely absorbed, become eburnated (often actually polished), but do not fuse."—"A Survey of Chronic Rheumatic Diseases," pp. 227-278. Oxford University Press, 1938.

We have followed the committee appointed by the British Medical Association in 1933 in excluding from the chronic rheumatic diseases arthritis occurring in the following conditions:—

1. Acute or subacute rheumatic fever.

2. Specific infections : Gonococcal, dysenteric, tuberculous, syphilitic, pyogenic.
3. Metabolic and blood diseases : Gout, hæmophilia.
4. Organic nervous disease : Charcot's joints in tabes and syringomyelia.

The reader is referred to the appropriate sections for the treatment of the primary condition in this group, while the general principles enunciated in the section on chronic rheumatic diseases are in general applicable to the joint manifestations.

PROPHYLAXIS OF THE CHRONIC RHEUMATIC DISEASES

The importance of diagnosis and treatment in the early stages of disease has been recognized for many years. More recently this principle has been extended to include the preventive aspect of medicine which implies (*a*) the recognition and treatment of individuals whose anatomical and physiological make-up differs in certain respects from the normal, and whom clinical experience has shown to be peculiarly liable to develop certain diseases, and (*b*) a study of the effects of external factors in producing disease in normal persons and in those rendered more susceptible by inherent constitutional abnormalities. These principles have been recognized for some time as of fundamental importance in tuberculosis, but in our opinion they are equally applicable to the rheumatic diseases. Accordingly, it appears to us desirable to describe briefly the anatomical and physiological deviations from the normal which occur frequently in individuals who eventually develop chronic rheumatic disease, and also the various external factors of ætiological significance.

Although chronic arthritis does not respect age, sex, social position or anatomic type, clinical experience has shown that (1) a considerable proportion of cases of rheumatoid arthritis are of the asthenic, visceroptotic type, easily fatigued and emotionally unstable ; (2) the proportion of females to males is about 3 to 1 ; (3) the age incidence lies chiefly between puberty and forty-five years of age ; (4) the victims, prior to the onset of arthritis, have often a sluggish deficient peripheral circulation, indicated by their clammy, chilly extremities and inability to tolerate exposure to changes in temperature. In contrast to this group, the majority of sufferers from osteoarthritis are either of normal build or are of the sthenic, stocky type, with a tendency to obesity and have usually a placid or cheerful outlook. They are often active, energetic people, both mentally and physically. The chief incidence of the disease falls in the latter half of life. It should be pointed out that individuals of the asthenic type are candidates not only for rheumatoid arthritis but for many other forms of chronic disease.

Prophylaxis will be considered under two headings : (1) the improvement of the "soil" by measures directed towards raising the general resistance, and (2) the eradication or reduction of other factors of ætiological importance.

Prophylaxis of Rheumatoid Arthritis

Measures for Raising General Resistance.—The general physique can be improved by breathing and postural exercises, details of which will be found in the appendix. Exercise such as walking, cycling, golfing, etc., in the fresh air should be advised in amounts short of producing fatigue. Should the individual wish to join a gymnastic class organized under the physical fitness campaign, care should be taken that the exercises prescribed are well within his capacity, otherwise more harm than good will result. Attempts to improve the circulation should be made by the use of tepid or warm baths every day followed by a brisk rub down with a rough towel. Bathing in cold water is generally contraindicated in this class of person. A short annual course of treatment at a spa, if financial circumstances permit, is, we believe, of great value as a preventive measure. Clothing should be light but warm, and the avoidance of wetting and chilling of the feet by the use of suitable footwear is to be recommended. Because of the asthenia and the tendency to become easily fatigued, the family doctor can give useful advice on how to conserve energy, by orderly arrangement of work. For the same reason the doctor should see that adequate rest is obtained, by warning against late hours and by suggesting an hour's rest in the afternoon, if necessary. Mental fatigue is as important as physical fatigue, and the doctor must play his part by adjusting, by simple psychological means, the minor worries and troubles which beset all of us. Since candidates for rheumatoid arthritis are generally spare individuals below their normal body-weight, common sense advice regarding the quantitative and qualitative characters of the diet should be given, stress being particularly laid on the value of fruits, vegetables and the dairy products—milk, eggs and cheese. Any tendency towards constipation should be corrected by the measures outlined on p. 573. The anæmia which is so frequently present in women in the pre-arthritic stage should be treated with iron (see p. 471). Cod-liver oil is valuable.

By adoption of the régime described, the general resistance will be raised and the liability to infection, believed to be of importance in the ætiology of rheumatoid arthritis, will be lowered. Should, however, any type of infection develop, it should be treated in the asthenic individual with more than the usual care and a longer period of convalescence advised than would be the case in a normal person. When focal sepsis is found to be present which the body resistance cannot overcome after being raised as high as possible by the measures outlined above, eradication should not be delayed in view of the known importance of focal sepsis as an ætiological factor in arthritis.

Prophylaxis of Osteo-arthritis

Osteo-arthritis is more an arthrosis than an arthritis, being a degenerative condition and an accompaniment of the ageing process. It is probable that the most important factor is a constitutional defect in the patient's articular cartilage, which is therefore unable to withstand repeated micro-traumata as satisfactorily as the cartilage of more fortunate individuals. The constitutional factor is analogous to that conditioning the incidence of arteriosclerosis and hypertension. French workers believe that minor congenital abnormalities of the joints are also predisposing factors which are more important than has hitherto been believed. Certain factors, however, can cause or accelerate the process and these may be partly or wholly remediable. They are gross injuries leading to dislocations of joints, fractures of bones which involve the articular surfaces, and excessive or long continued strains. Accordingly, a short discussion of some of these is appropriate. When a bone is fractured a secondary osteo-arthritis will result in adjacent joints unless proper alignment of the fragments is procured. When a fall or injury occurs, producing trauma of the joint structures and contusion of the overlying tissues, proper treatment by rest followed by heat, massage and movement may delay and minimize the effect of the trauma in conditioning the occurrence of osteo-arthritis. Long-continued trauma from occupational strains is a common cause of osteo-arthritis. It is well recognized that individual trades produce arthritis in particular sites. For example, stone-masons commonly suffer from osteo-arthritis of the wrist, elbow or shoulder, and in agricultural labourers the spine and hips are usually affected. The question arises, when early signs of osteo-arthritis are noted by the doctor, whether a change of occupation should be advised before the affected joints become hopelessly crippled. The decision in such a case will depend on the circumstances, but the advice to change one's occupation in middle age can seldom be taken for economic reasons.

More hopeful fields for the reduction of arthritis and fibrositis in industry lie in the province of public health administration. Improvement of working conditions in factories, workshops, mines, etc., on the following lines would go far to lower the incidence of the rheumatic diseases in industry: (1) the elimination of exposure to draughts, excessive heat and cold; (2) the provision of rest shelters; (3) the installation of hot baths with the opportunity of changing wet clothes; (4) the adoption of mechanical appliances which would reduce the strain on workers to a minimum by performing weight-lifting operations; (5) the selection of individuals for certain occupations on the basis of physical suitability, and especially the exclusion of people past middle age from occupations throwing excessive strain on the joints.

Another factor which leads to continuous joint strain and undue pressure on the articular surfaces is obesity. Its correction by diet, exercise and endocrine therapy (discussed on p. 387) is a preventive measure of great importance in many conditions other than osteo-arthritis.

Postural defects produce osteo-arthritis for the same reason as does obesity, and their correction by special exercises or orthopædic measures is as important in its prevention as in that of rheumatoid arthritis. The commonest faults are lumbar lordosis and scoliosis, genu varus or valgus, pes planus.

Focal sepsis is believed to be of much less ætiological importance in osteo-arthritis than in rheumatoid arthritis, but nevertheless, obvious foci should be eradicated when present, as the chronic toxæmia resulting therefrom may be a factor in impairing the general health and thus accelerating the degenerative processes.

TREATMENT OF RHEUMATOID ARTHRITIS

The treatment of rheumatoid arthritis is governed by the stage of the disease and the degree of activity present when the patient is first seen by the medical practitioner. We have arbitrarily divided the diseases into three stages, although in practice no sharp dividing line exists.

Treatment of the Acute Stage of Rheumatoid Arthritis

In order that the objects of treatment may be better understood, a brief description of the main clinical features in the acute stage will be given. Although the joint symptoms are predominant, there is also general systemic disturbance. The patient complains of lassitude even when at rest and of excessive fatigue on the slightest effort. There has been a progressive loss of weight and the appetite is poor. The extremities are cold and clammy, and the body sweat has a peculiarly rank odour. A moderate fever ranging from 99° to 101° F. may be present. Blood examination shows a moderate or even marked degree of hypochromic anæmia, often a slight polymorphonuclear leucocytosis and a marked increase in the sedimentation rate of the red blood corpuscles. Many joints are swollen and painful, the small joints of the hands and feet usually being the first to be affected. The lesions are mainly peri-articular at this stage, only rarefaction of the bone ends being seen on X-ray examination. Muscular wasting is an early and prominent feature of the disease. The treatment of such a patient embodies two fundamental principles :—

1. General treatment which includes measures (*a*) to promote the patient's vitality and increase his resistance to infection, and (*b*) the eradication or correction of ætiological factors.
2. Local treatment of the joints.

General Treatment.—The principles applicable to other forms of infection, particularly tuberculosis, are of fundamental importance in rheumatoid arthritis and must be carried out with scrupulous attention to detail if the best results are to be obtained.

As already stated, the *psychological aspect* is of particular importance in all diseases which tend to run a prolonged course. Accordingly the physician must secure the intelligent co-operation of the patient by taking him into his confidence, by explaining in simple language the nature of the disease and the principles on which the treatment to be adopted is founded, and by assuming an optimistic attitude regarding the results to be expected.

Rest, both physical and mental, is the first object to be achieved. In the acute stage rest must be complete, and this means that the patient must stay in bed for weeks or even months if necessary until the active phase is past. The desirability of this rest period being undertaken under the best conditions is as important in rheumatoid arthritis as in tuberculosis. Fresh air, sunshine, cheerful surroundings, good nursing and nourishing diet are all factors of importance in improving the physical and psychological state of the patient. It is advisable to explain to the patient that the prescription of rest must be considered as only the first step in an organized scheme of treatment. Recumbency affords the opportunity of correcting faulty posture and, as Goldthwait says, " enables the physician to remodel the body no longer handicapped by the unfavourable influences of gravity." Lastly, rest in bed enables the nutrition of the patient to be more rapidly improved by dietetic treatment. An important factor in securing rest is the control of pain, which impairs appetite, causes insomnia and increases physical and mental fatigue. For this purpose analgesic drugs must be prescribed in adequate quantities (see p. 899). The practitioner must realize that the analgesic drugs are prescribed solely for the purpose of obtaining rest and thus allowing the other aspects of the therapeutic scheme to be brought into operation, and not because they possess any specific curative properties.

After a week or two of complete rest, when the more active symptoms such as pyrexia may have abated, other measures of value in raising the general resistance will be employed. A short exposure to *ultra-violet rays*, given on alternate days, acts as a stimulant to the skin and a tonic to the mind. On the other days light *massage* (*effleurage*) to the body, but excluding the joints, improves the circulation, allays spasm and acts as a general sedative. *The care of the skin* is an important feature in the treatment, because of the defective peripheral circulation and the marked tendency for these patients to sweat a great deal. Accordingly, tepid sponging of the whole body, followed by gentle rubbing with a soft towel, should be carried out at least once a day. Night-wear should be of woollen material, and care should be taken to change the garment as often as required to avoid having damp material next the skin. Even at this early stage *exercises* should be prescribed for the purpose of improving the circulation and correcting faulty posture. They are carried out in the recumbent position, and their frequency and amount graduated to suit each individual case in accordance with the degree of asthenia present. Breathing exercises are designed to teach the patient to use his diaphragm and abdominal muscles more efficiently, as by this means the ventilation of the lungs is increased, the oxygenation of the blood improved and the accumulation of blood in the dilated splanchnic vessels mobilized, with concomitant improvement in the general circulation. Postural exercises are given for improving the tone of the spinal and gluteal muscles. We are satisfied, from daily experience of these measures, that the claims made by Goldthwait and Swaim regarding the beneficial effects produced are justified, and we strongly recommend their adoption in every case of rheumatoid arthritis. Details of the exercises for use in the acute stage are given in the appendix.

The Removal of Septic Foci.—Since it is generally agreed that an infective factor is of particular importance in rheumatoid arthritis, the problem of focal sepsis requires careful consideration. In some cases the history and clinical manifestations show that an infection has occurred of such virulence as to warrant the deduction that it is the prime ætiological factor. In many cases, however, the evidences of infection are more uncertain, and in others the most careful clinical investigation leads to negative results. It is possible, however, that in the last group infection may have played a part, although evidence of its occurrence can no longer be found or alternatively it may be present but cannot be located by available methods of investigation. From this it may be argued that the response of the body to infection is frequently of equal importance in causing the disease as the infection itself. Accordingly, it is not surprising that the results obtained by the eradication of focal sepsis are frequently unsatisfactory if it constitutes the only therapeutic procedure. If a focus of infection exists, which is not removed, it will seriously mitigate the chances of recovery, even when all other forms of treatment have been applied. The discovery of focal infection and the assessment of its ætiological importance may offer the greatest difficulties, since it is recognized that focal sepsis may occur as the result of the lowered vitality of the individual, consequent on the disease. It follows from this that when doubt exists a conservative policy should be adopted until sufficient time has elapsed to evaluate the effects of the measures for raising general resistance. If improvement occurs, conservative treatment should be continued until its maximum effects have been obtained, and the patient's condition is such that eradication of the focus will entail the least danger of precipitating a relapse, should the focus still show signs of activity. If, on the other hand, no benefit accrues from conservative treatment, it is probable that the focus of infection is responsible for the continued activity of the disease, and its removal should be undertaken.

Septic foci are of two types, those which are easily accessible for investigation, *e.g.*, teeth, tonsils, etc., and those which are not, *e.g.*, gall-bladder, appendix, etc. We do not intend to describe the symptoms and signs on which the diagnosis of infection in any individual organ is made, or to give in detail the methods of treatment required, but will merely enumerate in order of importance the sites in which foci of infection in rheumatoid arthritis are likely to occur :—

1. First in frequency and importance is tonsillar sepsis. The younger the individual the more frequently will this be found.

2. Dental sepsis. In our experience apical abscesses are more important as sources of infection than pyorrhœa alveolaris. In the more elderly patients dental sepsis is as important as tonsillar sepsis.

3. The accessory air sinuses, particularly the maxillary antrum.

4. Sepsis of the urogenital tract. In males, where no obvious sepsis of the mouth or throat can be found, the prostate should always be palpated and its secretion examined under the microscope for organisms and pus cells. Gonococci are seldom demonstrated in the smears, the original invasion having been succeeded by a low-grade infection, usually streptococcal or staphylococcal in origin. The latter organisms are held by some authorities to be primary infective agents in many cases. If prostatitis is present, drainage of the organ must be assisted by prostatic massage, which at first must be done very gently and gradually increased in vigour, otherwise severe local pain and constitutional disturbances may result. Vaccine treatment of chronic prostatitis is believed by some observers to be of particular value. In women, pelvic sepsis, with the exception of chronic salpingitis, is not of the same ætiological importance as it is in men. We have had under our care cases of rheumatoid arthritis with multiple and widespread lesions which failed to respond to all forms of treatment until tubal infection was discovered and eradicated. Some physicians, however, believe that chronic cervicitis is a frequent source of toxæmia in rheumatoid arthritis and claim excellent results from the use of pelvic diathermy.

5. Chronic cholecystitis and appendicitis may be sources of infection. In view of the deleterious effects which major operations may have on severely debilitated individuals, unequivocal signs of infection must be present before laparotomy is advised.

Since the family doctor cannot be expected to have specialized knowledge of all the organs of the body, the need for team work is obvious in the investigation of a case of rheumatoid arthritis, and the physician in charge of the patient should have at his disposal the services of a laryngologist, dentist, radiologist, etc.

In conclusion, we would again stress the difficulty of recognizing and assessing the importance of septic foci and the need for wide experience and sound judgment in deciding what measures should be adopted in each individual case.

Drug Treatment.—Of the hundreds of remedies used in the treatment of the chronic rheumatic diseases the majority are useless, some may be harmful and only a limited number are of proved value. Pemberton and Osgood put the position clearly when they state "That commercial firms should endeavor to exploit this field is not surprising ; that physicians should continue to believe the claims made by some firms for their products is disappointing and reveals not a little the unfamiliarity of the profession with the disease." Although no drug, with the possible exception of the gold salts, can be held to have a specific curative action in rheumatoid arthritis, this does not mean that drugs have no place in the treatment. Intelligently used, they play a definite part in helping the patient along the road to recovery. For simplicity, the drugs used can be classified under two main headings :—

1. Drugs used for their known pharmacological effects.
2. Drugs used empirically.

Drugs used for their Pharmacological Effects.—The most important drugs in this group are the analgesics and hypnotics. For the control of pain in rheumatoid arthritis, the salicylates have stood the test of time. It is now generally agreed that acetylsalicylic acid (aspirin) is superior to sodium salicylate in this respect. Apart from their analgesic action, the salicylates are of value because they promote a better blood flow by dilating the capillaries and influence metabolism as evidenced by an increased excretion of uric acid. When pain is severe, especially in the acute stage, it is essential that it should be controlled and aspirin in doses of 10 to 15 gr. should be given every four hours. In fevered patients this may lead to excessive sweating, but the analgesic effect should be maintained by reducing the amount of aspirin to 8 to 10 gr. and combining it with 5 gr. of phenacetin and 2 gr. of caffeine or $\frac{1}{4}$ gr. of codeine. In the acute stage it is a common mistake to give insufficient amounts of analgesic drugs. Aspirin is insoluble in water, but soluble in a solution of potassium citrate. Calcium acetylsalicylate has the advantage of being soluble in water and is believed by some to cause less digestive disturbance. Other drugs of great value in the control of pain are phenazone (antipyrin), dose 5 to 10 gr., and amidopyrine (pyramidon), dose 5 to 10 gr. The latter may be used in conjunction with the barbiturates, as in "allonal" (dose, one 2½-gr. tablet) and "veramon" (dose, one 6-gr. tablet). Amidopyrin should be used with great care, if at all, in elderly persons with marked debility, because of the danger which occasionally arises from its leucotoxic effect (see p. 521). Insomnia is frequently the result of pain and disappears with its relief, in which case the analgesic drugs may also act as hypnotics. In some cases, however, their action must be reinforced by hypnotics, and for this purpose a mixture containing 10 to 15 gr. of potassium bromide and 10 to 15 gr. of chloral hydrate, with or without the addition of 10 to 15 minims of tincture of opium, should be used as a sleeping draught. The barbiturates may be employed as alternatives. Phenobarbitone (dose, ½ to 2 gr.), medinal (dose, 5 to 10 gr.) and dial (dose, 1½ to 3 gr.) are useful preparations for this purpose. The injection of morphine or heroin is contraindicated because of the danger of habit formation.

For the correction of the hypochromic anæmia, so commonly found in cases of rheumatoid arthritis, iron should be prescribed in the doses detailed on p. 471.

In view of the generalized decalcification of the skeleton almost invariably present in the more severe cases of rheumatoid arthritis, many physicians believe in the administration of calcium by mouth in the form of calcium lactate (dose, 15 to 30 gr. t.d.s.) or intravenously as calcium gluconate or lævulinate (doses, 5 c.c. daily or 10 c.c. two or three times a week). To ensure its absorption when given by mouth, vitamin D in the form of cod-liver oil or one of its concentrates (ostelin, adexolin) should be prescribed in addition.

Tonics are of value for improving the appetite and general tone. Easton's syrup (syr. ferri, phos. cum quinine et strychnin B.P.) is one of the best known preparations used for this purpose, the dose being one teaspoonful three times a day. Strychnine combined with iron and arsenic is available as pil. ferri carb. cum arsenic et strychnine B.P. (dose, one thrice daily). When the patient is very nervous the best tonic may be a sedative, such as the bromides or barbiturates. Cod-liver oil and preparations such as yeast tablets and marmite in our experience are valuable preparations for raising the patient's lowered vitality.

Thyroid extract is seldom indicated in rheumatoid arthritis, although its value is well recognized in stout individuals who are suffering from osteo-arthritis and fibrositis, particularly at the menopause.

Drugs used for their action on the gastro-intestinal tract are discussed in the appropriate section.

Cinchophen (atophan) and colchicum, the specific action of which is to increase the excretion of uric acid, are contra-indicated in rheumatoid arthritis. Cinchophen in particular should not be prescribed in the acute stage because of the known dangers of its toxic action. Alkalis, however, particularly potassium citrate, may be employed, especially in combination with the salicylates because they reduce the liability to gastric irritation and because they act as mild diuretics. The mineral waters obtained at spas have a similar effect.

Drugs Used Empirically.—Mention must be made of drugs which are commonly prescribed in the chronic rheumatic diseases and which appear, not infrequently, to have beneficial effects, although no satisfactory explanation of a scientific nature is available with regard to their mode of action.

Arsenic is claimed by Pemberton and Osgood to be one of the most useful drugs in the treatment of arthritis because of its influence on blood formation and on metabolism. It should be pointed out that few modern hæmatologists would agree that arsenic is a hæmatinic and proof of any specific effect on metabolism is wanting. If arsenic is to be given it should be prescribed in small doses over a prolonged period. The preparations most commonly used are liq. arsenicalis B.P. (Fowler's solution), starting with a dose of 1 to 2 minims three times a day and gradually increasing up to 5 minims three times a day, or cacodylate of soda, $\frac{1}{4}$ gr. three times a day.

Iodine is probably more frequently employed in the chronic rheumatic diseases than any other drug, but its use is largely empirical and its mode of action obscure. Like arsenic, it should be given in small doses over long periods. Potassium iodide is the cheapest form of iodine available and is best prescribed in small doses of 1 to 3 gr. two or three times a day. It is more fashionable, however, to use Lugol's solution (liq. iodi. aquosis B.P.) in doses of 5 minims twice or thrice daily, or the French tincture (liq. iodi. simplex B.P.) in the same doses. The irritant effect of iodine on the stomach is reduced if the preparation is taken in milk.

Ortho-iodoxy benzoic acid originated in America where it was hailed with enthusiasm as a valuable drug in the treatment of rheumatoid arthritis. When given by mouth it causes much gastric upset, and after absorption, sweating, fever and a leucocytosis occur. These effects suggest that its action is on the lines of non-specific protein shock therapy. The fact that ortho-iodoxybenzoic acid has been omitted from the list of "New and Non-official Remedies" of the American Medical Association suggests that the original claims were grossly exaggerated, and in view of its toxic action we believe that it is of little value in the treatment of rheumatoid arthritis, and certainly not in the acute stage.

Histamine and bee venom and the thiosinamine group of drugs are not suitable for use in the acute stage and will be dealt with in the section devoted to the subacute and chronic stages of rheumatoid arthritis.

Although the hair and nails of patients with rheumatoid arthritis have been shown to have a low sulphur content, there is no satisfactory proof that defective sulphur metabolism occurs in this disease. Nevertheless, many experienced physicians believe that sulphur is of undoubted value in the treatment of the chronic rheumatic diseases. Spa waters containing sulphur enjoy a considerable reputation, but the good effects produced are more likely to be due to the régime of spa treatment and the benefit which is derived from the laxative properties of the drug. Sulphur is available combined with guaiacol in the form of Chelsea Pensioner (Confectio Guaiaci Co. B.P.C.), dose 1 to 2 drachms, or as confection of sulphur (B.P.), dose 1 to 2 drachms. For those who wish to give the drug in the colloidal state, collosol sulphur (Crookes) 1 to 2 drachms thrice daily in water after food can be recommended.

Sulphur by injection is used for the production of pyrexia, and thus employed its action is entirely non-specific. The reaction produced is relatively mild and less exhausting to debilitated patients than that produced by the intravenous injection of T.A.B. vaccines. It is available combined with milk in the preparation Pyrolactin D (Research Products, London), the initial dose being 2 c.c. intramuscularly. Sulphur in oil or aqueous collosal sulphur may be used. Colsul (British Colloids) is a 1 per cent. solution of sulphur in olive oil and the initial dose is ½ c.c., which is increased at each injection by ½ c.c. to a maximum of 5 c.c., or until a sufficient degree of pyrexia has been produced. An increase in stiffness and pain for twelve hours after the injection is claimed to be a desirable symptom. The injections should be given at weekly intervals. The type of case where this treatment is indicated is discussed on p. 908.

Sulphonamide.—Little work has been done up to the present on the treatment of rheumatoid arthritis with the new sulphonamide preparations, and what information is available does not suggest that good results are to be expected. In view of the part played by the hæmolytic streptococcus in the ætiology of many cases, further research on this problem is required.

Radio-active Compounds.—The authors have no personal experience of the employment of radio-active compounds by injection in the treatment of rheumatoid arthritis, but Mathieu-Pierre Weil claims good results from their use. In view of the dangers of late untoward effects, this form of treatment should be left in the hands of those with a thorough knowledge of the technique involved.

Gold Therapy.—The most important advance in the drug treatment of rheumatoid arthritis was the introduction of gold salts by Forestier nearly ten years ago. British and Continental workers are agreed that beneficial results can be expected in about 70 per cent. of cases, and that this improvement warrants the exhibition of gold salts despite the attendant risks. Further time must elapse before final judgment can be passed in regard to the best preparations, dosage and the ultimate effects produced, but it is already clear that chrysotherapy should be considered as merely a unit in the general scheme of treatment, which includes the removal of ætiological factors and the raising of the patient's general resistance by every means available. The failure to recognize this principle, and the indiscriminate use of gold in unsuitable cases of chronic arthritis, is already beginning to bring into disrepute what we believe to be a valuable method of treatment. The reactions which not infrequently follow chrysotherapy are sometimes due to excessive dosage, and sometimes due to an individual idiosyncrasy to the drug which cannot be predicted at present by any known method.

For the prevention of gold salt reactions, many substances have been advocated. Among these are calcium gluconate, sodium thiosulphate, liver extract, glucose and vitamin concentrates. Opinion is divided as to whether any of these substances is effective. We use none of them, and during the past three years have never had any severe reactions. This may be partly due to good fortune, but we believe that it is mainly the result of the care taken in watching for the first sign of intolerance and in limiting the total amount of gold given over a course of ten weeks to 1 gm.

There does not appear to be any contraindication to the

exhibition of gold during the acute stage of rheumatoid arthritis, but in our opinion it is perhaps better to withhold the drug until any septic foci have been dealt with and the patient has had a few weeks' complete rest, both mental and physical, and is better able to respond to what, in the present state of our knowledge, must be regarded as a non-specific stimulus to the disease-fighting mechanism.

Chrysotherapy is contraindicated both in the acute and chronic stages of rheumatoid arthritis if organic disease of the heart, kidneys, liver or hæmopoietic tissues is present, and it is not advisable to use gold in the presence of any form of skin disease with the possible exception of psoriasis, in view of the danger of causing an exfoliative dermatitis.

The oil-soluble and the water-soluble salts appear to be equally effective, provided the dosage of the gold salt is the same. We personally use the preparation, Myocrisin, which is a 50 per cent. solution of sodium aurothiomalate in water. Injections should be given by the intramuscular route, and the first should not contain more than 0·01 gm. The interval between injections should be at least five days, and the dose should be increased to 0·05 at the second and 0·1 gm. at the third injection, providing no untoward reactions have occurred. Thereafter, injections of 0·1 gm. are given. The total dosage of a course should not exceed 1·5 gm., or better still, 1 gm. The occurrence of any of the following manifestations indicates the need for the immediate cessation of gold therapy :—

1. Generalized erythema of the skin, or vesicular or macular eruptions. Continuation of the treatment may lead to a severe exfoliative dermatitis.

2. Albumin, casts and red blood cells in the urine. Slight albuminuria is not in itself a danger signal and it occurs with relative frequency during the administration of gold, but should casts and blood cells accompany it the drug must be stopped at once, otherwise a toxic nephritis may result. The urine should be examined regularly before each injection.

3. The appearance of jaundice is a sign of toxic hepatitis, and although often mild and transitory, should be regarded as a contraindication to the further use of gold for some months.

4. Purpura of the skin or mucous membranes. This is a sign of grave significance, as it indicates that damage to the hæmopoietic tissues has occurred.

5. Leucopenia. Fatal agranulocytic angina may result from the administration of gold salts.

Less serious complications of gold therapy are stomatitis, diarrhœa, proctitis and general malaise. Their appearance is a sign for the reduction of the dose, less frequent injections or, if the symptoms persist, cessation of the treatment for some weeks.

The first course should be followed by a second after an interval of at least ten weeks, and in the majority of cases a third, or even a fourth, course may be required before the full benefits of chrysotherapy are obtained. If no improvement results from the first course of treatment, a second should be given before this method of treatment is discarded. When improvement does occur, the gain should always be consolidated by further courses.

To obtain the best results from chrysotherapy, it should be instituted as early in the course of the disease as possible. Gold has the effect of temporarily increasing the sedimentation rate, which should begin to fall within two or three months from the commencement of treatment. The maintenance of a high sedimentation rate after this period indicates continued activity of the disease and suggests re-examination of the patient in regard to factors of ætiological importance.

Vaccines.—The use of vaccines in the treatment of disease has always been the subject of much controversy, and opinion is still divided over their value in rheumatoid arthritis. A survey of the literature indicates that while vaccine therapy is no longer enjoying the widespread vogue of a few years ago, there are still physicians of experience who firmly believe that it has a definite place in the treatment of rheumatoid arthritis. Equally good results are claimed by those who use vaccines, by those who do not and also by others using non-specific forms of protein therapy. Published reports suggest that there is little to choose between the results obtained by stock and autogenous vaccines, and the variety of organisms used in their manufacture—streptococci, staphylococci, *B. coli*, etc., appears to indicate that any benefit obtained must be of a non-specific character. The reader is referred to a critical review by C. C. Okell, late Professor of Bacteriology, University College Hospital, London, published by the British Committee on Chronic Rheumatic Diseases in the third volume of their Reports (1937), in which he states : "We are asked to believe that by injecting dead bacteria, a method apparently without any curative value in any human or animal disease, we can benefit a disease whose ætiology is entirely unknown and which for all we know may not be a microbic disease at all."

The writers believe that vaccine therapy should never be used as the sole form of treatment. Moreover, if it is decided to use vaccines the course should be delayed until the scheme of treatment outlined in this section has been carefully carried out for some months. If progress has become stationary, vaccine therapy may be justified, although we personally prefer to rely on gold salts. It is a matter of personal opinion whether stock vaccines or autogenous vaccines made from organisms isolated from a septic focus believed to have been of ætiological significance should be employed. It is generally agreed that a vaccine should be given over a prolonged period, in small doses, with the careful avoidance of significant reactions. The production of a constitutional disturbance may have a serious deleterious effect on the patient's health and on the local manifestations of the disease in the joints. This is particularly liable to occur in the active stage of the disease when fever is present. Accordingly, we feel that vaccine therapy is contra-indicated except in the subacute or chronic stages. Although some authorities claim that the best results are obtained from the intravenous injections of vaccines, this is disputed by others, and since the technical difficulties are greater and the chances of serious reactions higher, we advise the practitioner to continue using the subcutaneous route. The intervals between injections should be about a week and the initial dose should be sufficiently small to ensure that no general reaction results. Usually, an amount of vaccine containing approximately one million organisms will fulfil this requirement. Some authorities believe that even a smaller initial dose is indicated. For subsequent injections, the dose is gradually increased until a feeling of slight malaise or an increase of pain in the joints occurs. This reaction is usually accompanied by a small rise in temperature, the recognition of which is of importance in assessing the subsequent dose of vaccines. It is advisable, therefore, to take temperature readings night and morning, or better still, at four-hourly intervals during the twenty-four hours after the injection. Even a mild reaction is an indication that the dose of vaccine should not be increased at the next injection. Should a similar reaction occur with the same dose, a decrease to the amount which fails to provoke a reaction is indicated, and this dose should be continued for two or three injections, after which an attempt may again be made to increase it. The course should be continued as long as improvement is occurring. Should no benefit accrue within from two to three months of the institution of the course, injections should be stopped. On the day of injection and for twenty-four hours thereafter, all forms of active physiotherapy should be withheld, since they tend to increase the reaction to the parenteral administration of foreign protein. The one undoubted benefit which the weekly injection of any substance including vaccines has to offer is, that it enables the physician to see his patient at regular intervals, and gives him the opportunity of reviewing the progress of the case and of making adjustments to the therapeutic programme when necessary. In addition, parenteral treatment appears to have a more beneficial psychological effect on patients in general than peroral treatment, and anything which helps the patient to keep up his courage is of value in all forms of chronic debilitating disease.

Non-specific Protein Therapy.—This form of treatment is employed much less frequently to-day than fifteen years ago, thus indicating that the original claims regarding its beneficial action were undoubtedly exaggerated. The parenteral injection of a foreign protein results in a rise in temperature accompanied by an increased blood flow, leucocytosis, a heightened metabolism and changes in the permeability of cell membranes. Similar effects can be produced by raising the body temperature by the use of hot-air cabinets, short-wave machines or general diathermy. Although we have no experience of these latter methods we understand from our American colleagues that the effects produced and the results obtained are of a similar nature to those resulting from protein shock therapy. Accordingly, the opinions expressed below are equally applicable to fever therapy in rheumatoid arthritis. The degree of the reaction accompanying protein shock therapy depends on several factors, the chief of which are the type and amount of material introduced, the route used for injection and the patient's individual sensitivity. The most marked effects result from the injection of foreign protein by the intravenous route. A temperature of 103° or higher, with marked malaise and local joint pain, may result from the intravenous injection of a vaccine containing 100 million typhoid and paratyphoid organisms. Although occasionally a dramatic improvement of a permanent nature occurs, more frequently, any increased range of movement and decreased swelling which results are only of a temporary nature, and the patient's general health may be adversely affected.

A course consists of a series of intravenous injections of T.A.B. vaccine given at intervals of five to seven days. Fifty million organisms are given on the first occasion, the dose being doubled at each subsequent injection, due consideration being given to the degree of reaction previously obtained. Owing to the exhaustion produced, a course should rarely consist of more than six injections.

In the acute stage of rheumatoid arthritis, particularly if

the patient is severely debilitated, this method of treatment is definitely contraindicated as it may endanger life. Under these conditions, should it be decided to use non-specific therapy, the intramuscular injection of milk or sulphur should be employed, since the constitutional reaction produced is very much less.

Preparations used for this purpose are given at weekly intervals in increasing amounts, a course lasting from six to ten weeks. The following are some of the preparations used and their initial doses :—

Boiled milk	5 c.c.
Peptone solution (Allen & Hanbury)	0·3 c.c.
Xifal-milk	2 c.c.
Yatren-Casein	½ to 1 c.c. of the weak solution.
Pyrolactin D	2 c.c.

Our own feeling is that vaccines and non-specific protein therapy have only a limited value in the treatment of rheumatoid arthritis and should be reserved for the subacute and chronic stages of the disease, when the general lines of treatment described by us have been carefully applied and a stage has been reached where further progress is not being made.

We would impress on our readers that their indiscriminate use in unsuitable amounts in debilitated sufferers from rheumatoid arthritis may lead to harmful results.

Diet.—We wish to state categorically that no one particular diet can be held to have a specific curative action in rheumatoid arthritis, nor can dietary deficiency be considered as an important ætiological factor, except in so far as under-nutrition leads to a lowering of the general resistance. Patients suffering from this disease are usually considerably under weight, therefore a diet should be prescribed to correct this state. During the acute stage the patient may be unable to take a diet of high caloric value, because of lack of appetite and digestive disturbances which result from the hypotonia of the gastro-intestinal tract so commonly present. Pemberton records excellent results in patients who are afebrile and who are not excessively under-nourished, by insisting on a marked reduction in the food intake for a few days. For the first two days nothing but orange juice and water is permitted, and thereafter the protein and fat content of the diet is gradually increased by the addition of milk, eggs and butter. An ample supply of fruit and vegetables, particularly in the raw state, is then allowed, but the rich carbohydrate foods are strictly limited. On this régime he claims that the digestive powers of the patient may be regained more rapidly than if a larger diet is given from the start, and that swelling of the joints may be markedly reduced. A diet should be aimed at which contains sufficient calories to raise the patient's body-weight and to maintain it at an approximately normal figure. Each meal should be small, and intermediate feeds of patent milky foods may be required. Stress must be laid on the importance of varying the articles of food, serving them in as dainty a form as possible and complying in reason with the patient's likes and dislikes. The tendency of many doctors to prohibit animal protein such as beef, mutton, chicken, etc., in the chronic rheumatic diseases has no justification in rheumatoid arthritis, since an adequate supply of protein is required for the building up of wasted muscles. The patient should be encouraged to eat liberal amounts of fatty foods because of their high caloric content. Milk, cream, butter and bacon are valuable in this respect, particularly the first which is rich in calcium, phosphorus and vitamins A and D. At least 2 pints of milk should be taken daily in some form or another. Ample fresh fruit and vegetables are indicated. The idea that fruit is harmful in chronic rheumatic disease because of its acidity is entirely fallacious, since the acids are absorbed in the form of citrates, tartrates and malates, and actually tend to alter the hydrogen-ion concentration of the blood towards the alkaline side. In the early stages it may be advisable to give fruit in the form of juices or jellies, and vegetables in the form of purées. The foods rich in carbohydrate, such as bread, cereals and potatoes should generally be limited. We make a practice of ensuring that the diet is high in vitamin B by giving concentrates such as yeast tablets ii t.i.d., or bemax or marmite 1 to 2 drachms daily in the form of a hot drink or spread on bread and butter in the form of a sandwich, because we believe that vitamin B plays an important part in maintaining the health of the nervous system and the tone of the gastro-intestinal tract. If adequate fresh fruit is given, the vitamin C content of the diet will in general be sufficient. Because of the decalcification of the skeleton we attempt to procure the best absorption possible of the calcium and phosphorus in the diet by supplying, in addition, vitamin D in the form of cod-liver oil or one of its concentrates such as radiostoleum or adexolin. In emaciated individuals who fail to gain weight because of their lack of appetite, insulin given before lunch and dinner may be of definite value. The initial dose should be 5 units half an hour before meals, and this should be slowly increased to 15 to 20 units twice daily. It is advisable to ensure that adequate carbohydrate is taken in the meal following the insulin, and for this purpose orange juice sweetened with 1 oz. of glucose will suffice.

Gastro-intestinal Tract.—It has long been recognized that patients with rheumatoid arthritis have a poor appetite and frequently suffer from digestive disorders. Since radiographic studies indicate a general hypotonia of the stomach and intestines, the latter showing elongation, dilatation and ptosis, with markedly reduced haustration, it is not surprising that stasis of the intestinal contents is present. Accordingly, the supporters of the theory of auto-intoxication hold that the bowel must be considered as an important site of focal sepsis in rheumatoid arthritis. We feel, however, that the gastro-intestinal abnormalities are more likely to be the result rather than the cause of the disease. Such a view does not imply, however, that their treatment should be neglected. For this purpose dietetic measures are of particular importance, for it has been shown by Fletcher of Toronto that in such cases it is possible to restore partially or entirely the normal tone of the bowel.

The dietetic treatment of rheumatoid arthritis has already been described, and the need for supplying a high vitamin diet and the addition of vitamin B concentrates in particular has been stressed. Additional measures are the avoidance of purgatives and the use of liquid paraffin in small doses two or three times a day, supplemented, if necessary, by mild laxatives such as salines, senna or cascara. Postural and breathing exercises (see p. 952) and abdominal massage are also helpful. Colonic lavage does not appear to us to be a physiological method of treating constipation. If used at all it should be given on alternate days on three or four occasions, with the object of emptying a heavily laden colon, as a preliminary to the institution of the régime already described. For further details regarding the treatment of constipation see p. 573.

For the flatulent dyspepsia associated with the achlorhydria, present in about 20 per cent. of cases, 30 to 60 minims of dilute hydrochloric acid is of value (see p. 467).

Intestinal antiseptics, such as salol or guaiacol, are frequently prescribed, but there is little scientific evidence to justify their use. Sulphur is also advised both because of its supposed intestinal antiseptic qualities and because of the somewhat doubtful evidence of abnormal metabolism of sulphur in rheumatoid arthritis.

Local Treatment.—During the acute stage of rheumatoid

arthritis the affected joints are swollen and exquisitely tender. The slightest movement is accompanied by severe pain and the muscles moving the joints are continuously in spasm. The patient soon discovers the position of greatest ease for the throbbing joints, and is often aided by sympathetic relatives, who little realize that by placing the joints in the flexed positions of the patient's choice they are preparing the way for the establishment of the dreadful deformities which are only too commonly the permanent legacy of rheumatoid arthritis. Such a patient lies with flexed knees, flexed hips, flexed elbows. The forearms and hands are laid on the chest, the wrists in a position of palmar flexion, and the feet are allowed to remain plantar flexed for lengthy periods. As the disease progresses, peri-articular and intra-articular adhesions form and movement becomes progressively more limited.

There are two fundamental principles underlying local treatment during the active stage of the disease. The first is the prevention of deformity and the second is the maintenance of function. The spasm of the surrounding muscles is Nature's attempt to immobilize the inflamed joints and is largely responsible for the wasting which is such a prominent feature of the disease. As a result of the long-maintained position of flexion, the flexor groups of muscles undergo compensatory shortening and thus still further limit the range of movements. Pain, therefore, must be relieved at all costs. It has already been emphasized that analgesics in adequate dosage are essential, but this alone will not suffice. The affected joints must be completely immobilized in order to avoid stretching of the inflamed structures, and this is most satisfactorily obtained by application of properly fitting splints. The relief obtained by fixation in such splints is of great therapeutic value, as it allows the patient to sleep without the large doses of sedatives previously required, with consequent improvement in the mental outlook. The muscles, relieved of their burden by the splint, relax and wasting is reduced to a minimum. Thus, the fundamental principle of rest must be applied locally to each affected joint if the patient is to enjoy the mental and physical rest so essential to his well-being.

Light, easily removable, perfectly fitting splints can be made quickly and simply with muslin bandages impregnated with plaster of Paris. The technical details for their manufacture are given in the Appendix. Whenever possible the splints should be skin-tight, as this ensures complete immobilization of the joints, since the slightest movement within the splint will induce the return of pain and spasm. In very thin patients it may be necessary to pad the bony prominences. This is best done by means of small pieces of chiropodist's felt, which are easily cut to shape and adhere to the skin. Before applying the plaster the skin should be oiled or the limb encased in stockinet, which forms an effective lining to the splint. Since in some of the more severe cases ankylosis may take place in spite of treatment, the splint should hold the joint in the position which will produce the best functional result, should this occur. For example, the wrist should be put up in slight dorsiflexion, the foot midway between dorsi and plantar flexion.

Although we believe that splints made by the plaster technique are ideal, their application requires some degree of technical skill, and other materials may be found more convenient. Aluminium can readily be cut and shaped to form a splint for any joint, and can be purchased in sheets of the correct thickness for this purpose. Poroplast when soaked in hot water becomes pliable and can be moulded to any shape required. When dry it forms a light and rigid splint.

The use of properly fitting splints is probably the most important recent advance in the treatment of the joints in rheumatoid arthritis. By this means swelling is reduced more quickly and pain relieved more effectively than by any other method. Whatever material is used, the splint should be easily removable in order that the second principle underlying treatment may be observed. Function is maintained in the inflamed joints during the acute phase of the disease by passive movement. The splints are removed once daily and each affected joint is gently moved. The movements should be well within the patient's limit of tolerance, and if any increase in pain or stiffness results it is an indication that this has been exceeded. A single movement daily is sufficient to prevent the occurrence of ankylosis. Any effort to force the inflamed joints through their full range of movement will result in increased disability. A full dose of an analgesic, such as codeine and aspirin, or veramon given 1 to 2 hours previously, will reduce pain to a minimum. Passive movement should be preceded by heat in some form, because of its effect in diminishing pain and spasm and improving the local circulation. The particular form of heat employed is not of great importance, provided that the joints are thoroughly warmed. Radiant heat, or infra-red lamps which are portable and can be plugged into any lighting circuit, are admirable sources of heat for this purpose. Moist heat, in the form of mud packs, peat packs or cataplasma kaolin, are also of great value as a preliminary to passive movement. Perhaps one of the best methods of applying local heat is by means of paraffin wax baths. Full details regarding the use of mud and wax are given in the Appendix. The nutrition and tone of the muscles are maintained by light massage (*effleurage*), but the joints themselves are avoided as no useful purpose, but rather the reverse, is served by massage applied over a swollen and inflamed joint. The patient must also be taught to contract the muscles without moving the joints (static contraction), since voluntary contraction is the physiological method of maintaining the health of muscles. In the early stages, especially when marked wasting is present, faradic stimulation may be necessary, but should be replaced by active contractions as soon as possible. As the activity of the disease begins to subside and the patient's general condition starts to improve, active movements of the joints are instituted, assisted at first in order to throw a minimum strain on the articular structures. Later, simple exercises are prescribed (see Appendix), but weight-bearing must be avoided until the active phase of the disease has passed. External applications of ointments, such as wintergreen (ungt. methyl. sal. B.P.), iodex with methyl sal., Scott's dressing, Bengue's balsam, unguentum capsici B.P., or the proprietary preparation rheumogen, are useful as rubefacients and counter-irritants, but are only of limited value in the acute stage of the disease when the skin over the joints is atrophic and easily irritated.

The more active forms of local treatment are not applicable during this phase of the disease, when they do more harm than good. They will be fully discussed in the treatment of subacute and chronic stages.

Subacute Stage of Rheumatoid Arthritis

The patient may reach the subacute stage after weeks or months of treatment in the acute stage. Alternatively the disease may commence insidiously and the patient presents himself for treatment in the subacute stage. Characteristically one or more of the joints is swollen and painful, a considerable degree of asthenia and muscular wasting is generally present, fever is absent, but the sedimentation rate is raised to a figure of 30 to 50 mm. in one hour. In such cases the investigations described and the measures advised for the raising of the general resistance and the eradication of factors of ætiological importance must be undertaken with the same attention to detail as in the acute stage. This includes the search for septic foci and their eradication, the provision of adequate mental and physical rest, attention to the gastro-intestinal tract, the prescription of a nourishing diet, the instruction of the patient in breathing and postural exercises, the administration of drugs, including the gold salts, and the application of local measures for the relief of pain, prevention of deformity and maintenance of function. In cases which have passed into the subacute from the acute stage, the transition from recumbency to active movements and weight-bearing must be made gradually.

It is essential to bear in mind the fact that rheumatoid arthritis is a general disease, and that even if the weight-bearing joints are not or only slightly involved, this in no way invalidates the need for general bodily rest for considerable periods in the day in order to counteract the general fatigue invariably present. The failure to obtain adequate rest in women of the working classes treated at home is an important factor in mitigating against the production of good results from treatment of these cases. The benefit derived from resting the swollen and painful joints in splints is as great in the subacute stage as in the acute, but the number of hours per day during which the joints are immobilized becomes less and varies according to the degree of activity still present. Thus, in some cases, splints fitted to the wrists may be worn only at night, while in more active cases they may have to remain in position throughout the day except at meals.

In the subacute stage physiotherapy plays a more important part in the treatment than it does in the acute stage. The measures for the application of heat locally, *e.g.*, radiant heat, wax baths, mud packs, etc., are as useful in this stage as they are in the acute. In addition, hydrotherapy may be extremely valuable as a means of improving the function of the skin as well as for its effect of causing absorption of effusions and helping to restore movements to stiff joints. Accordingly, it is only in the subacute and chronic stages of the disease that it is advisable to send patients to spas for treatment, and this should be done before irreparable structural damage to joints has occurred if the best results are to be obtained. Ætiological factors such as focal sepsis should be corrected first. The family doctor in making his selection of the spa should be guided by certain considerations, such as the weather, which may be expected at the time of his patient's visit, the nature of the water, the type of treatment desired and the general amenities available. For elderly, feeble patients there is an obvious advantage in choosing the spa nearest the patient's home, while in other cases the further the patient is removed from the influence of home and relatives the better. A reliable guide for the choice of a spa is now available to the medical profession in the official handbook of the British Health Resorts Association. A full report of the patient should be sent by the family doctor to the spa physician. The main cost of spa treatment is that of board and lodging, which may vary from three guineas a week upwards, depending on whether the patient is in a boarding-house or in a luxury hotel, while the cost of actual treatment averages about a guinea a week. The average duration of a " cure " is about three weeks.

Physiotherapy.—We have already discussed the part played by hydrology as a preventive measure in frigi-sensitive individuals who are peculiarly liable to develop the chronic rheumatic diseases, in re-educating the skin to respond more normally to the effect of cold and damp. Hydrology also plays an important part in the treatment of chronic rheumatism. The use of hyperthermal waters is of particular value. Aldred-Brown has recently summarized the results that may be looked for as follows :—

" There are many types of baths that may be used and they may be given at varying temperatures. The triad of heat, moisture and movement are again the important means to this end.

" The results that may be looked for are as follows :

" (*a*) The relief of pain. The action of hot water is unfailing : its physiological action may be brought about in two ways : (1) by dilatation of the superficial capillaries thus relieving the congestion of enlarged blood-vessels—pressure pain is thus diminished at the site of an inflammation ; (2) as a counter stimulus inhibiting the pain stimulus.

" (*b*) The relaxation of spasm of the muscles.

" (*c*) Improved nutrition of all the structures of the body by redistribution of the blood circulation.

" (*d*) Reabsorption of effusions in joints.

" (*e*) The prevention and correction of deformities which is made possible by the above changes.

" Although every properly equipped hydrological establishment possesses, rightly, a large variety of different types of baths, it is certain that the duration and temperature of the bath for each individual case is far more important than the type of bath. For the therapeutic application of hydrology to chronic rheumatism and gout there are, in my opinion, three baths that can fulfil all requirements. These are the Deep Bath with undercurrent douche, the Subaqueous Massage Douche, and the Hot Pool Bath with active and passive movements."

In the deep bath the patient can stand or sit in water at a temperature of from 95° to 100° F. The bath is of a sufficient size to allow of free movement of all the joints, and of sufficient depth to reduce the action of gravity to a minimum. Controlled percussive massage is applied by an undercurrent douche of water ejected from a 2-in. hose-pipe at a temperature 5° to 10° hotter than the bath (subaqueous massage). The massage douche may be of the Vichy type, where general massage of the muscles is given to the patient lying in a shallow trough under a fine spray of hot water. Finally, each joint is put through its possible range of movement, without the use of force. In the Aix type of massage douche the patient may be sitting on a stool or reclining on a table. General massage is given, while a jet of hot water, emerging from a hose carried over the operator's shoulder, is played on the part being treated. The usual temperature of the water used is 100° to 105° F., and the treatment lasts for twenty minutes. The hot pool is a small swimming bath with parallel bars running across it to enable the patients to support themselves while taking exercise. Undercurrent douches may also be provided. Patients who are unable to walk may be lowered into the bath on a canvas stretcher or a chair operated from a gantry. The hot pool bath is of particular value in enabling the operator to manipulate the joints and in aiding the patient to move his joints actively without weight-bearing.

Following any form of hydrotherapy it is important that the patient should be placed in hot wraps in order to achieve free sweating and to maintain it for fifteen to twenty minutes after the bath. The patient should then be allowed to cool down slowly in a warm room, at least one hour's rest being prescribed. Immersion baths cause considerable exhaustion to debilitated patients. They should not exceed ten minutes in duration, and in general should not be given more than three times in a week. Particular care must be observed in prescribing immersion baths in cases of rheumatoid arthritis, as more harm than good may result if excessive fatigue is produced. (There is real need for issuing a warning regarding the dangers of overtreatment in asthenic individuals suffering from arthritis.) On alternate days the joints should be treated by local applications of heat in the form of mud packs, wax baths, kaolin poultices, radiant heat, etc.

Electrical treatment may also be of service, and the continuous or galvanic current, diathermy and short-wave treatment are valuable for their sedative effect. The interrupted current (Faradism) is used to improve the condition of wasted muscles in the neighbourhood of arthritic joints. Ionization with sodium salicylate, potassium iodide or histamine is of value both in relieving pain and dispersing effusions.

Massage plays an important part in the treatment of all rheumatic diseases. It should be applied to the muscles surrounding the joints. If massage is to be applied to the joints the disease process must be quiescent, and it should be of the light stroking type (*effleurage*).

Movements, active and passive, and re-educational exercises are of the greatest value in the restoration of function. In the subacute stage movements of the joints under water is particularly beneficial. Re-educational exercises, under the guidance of a properly trained technician and devised according to the individual patient's needs, play an important part in the prevention and correction of deformity and the restoration of function.

Much can be done at home for individuals who, for financial or other reasons, are unable to visit a spa. The various methods for the production of local heat already described are available everywhere, and electrical treatment can be given in all general hospitals and modern nursing homes. Hydrotherapy may be provided in the patient's home by using the household bath, which should be filled with 30 to 40 gals. of water at a temperature of 98° to 105° F. The addition of 3 to 6 lbs. of common salt will make a brine bath with a saline content equivalent to that of sea water. Epsom salts (1 to 2 lbs.) or washing soda ($\frac{1}{2}$ to 1 lb.) can also be used. A mustard bath is another excellent means of raising body temperature and causing a rubefacient effect. Half an ounce of mustard is made into a smooth paste with cold water before being added to the bath. This method is contraindicated in the presence of any skin disease and should not be used in patients with rheumatoid arthritis and psoriasis. The patient is completely immersed in the bath for a period of from five to fifteen minutes, depending on the general condition. Thereafter he should be well wrapped in hot towels and remain in bed for at least an hour. For more debilitated persons partial immersion baths should be employed, since they are much less exhausting. The patient sits in a hip bath half filled with water at 100° F., with his feet in a foot bath containing water at a temperature of 100° to 105° F. The duration of the bath should be from ten to twenty minutes, and it should be followed by a similar rest period as already described. Complete or partial immersion baths should not be given on more than three days a week.

Drugs.—In addition to those mentioned in the section devoted to the acute stage, the following drugs have been claimed to be of value in the subacute and chronic stages and will therefore be discussed briefly.

The use of bee venom has been advocated by some in the treatment of rheumatoid arthritis, on the basis of the freedom of bee-keepers from rheumatic diseases. Its main action appears to be counter irritant. It is applied in the form of an ointment (forapin) or by intradermal injection (apicosan, apicur) over the affected joints. Instructions as regards dosage are supplied by the makers of the individual preparations. Histamine is another drug used both for its local effect in causing vaso-dilatation and for its general effect in producing diffuse flushing, decrease of stiffness and alleviation of pain. It can be administered in ointment form by inunction, in solution by subcutaneous injection or by ionization. The dosage by injection is 0·1 mg., increasing daily by 0·05 mg. until it reaches 0·5 mg., and this dose is repeated two or three times a week. The patient should lie down for an hour after the injection to avoid headache and dizziness. The thiosinamine group of drugs (fibrolysin, iodolysin, cicatricine) are claimed to have the property of resolving pathological fibrous tissue. Their administration is followed by a general reaction with fever and malaise, and is not without danger. In view of the uncertainty regarding their mode of action, and their toxic effects, they are perhaps better avoided in the treatment of rheumatoid arthritis.

The claims made on behalf of all the drugs mentioned above have probably been exaggerated. They are certainly contra-indicated in the acute stage of the disease, where the principles of rest and relief from pain are of paramount importance.

Chronic Stage of Rheumatoid Arthritis

If all cases of rheumatoid arthritis were correctly treated in the acute and subacute stages, deformities would be met with much less frequently. However, much can now be done to improve the lot of those patients in whom the active phase of the disease has passed, but in whom marked deformities have arisen in the joints.

In addition to the physiotherapeutic methods already described, special procedures are required for the correction of deformities and restoration of function, which are wholly orthopœdic in nature and may include surgical intervention in a small proportion of cases (see Surgery in Arthritis, p. 942).

Correction of Deformities.—The commonest deformities are fixed flexion of the hips, knees and elbows, limitation of abduction and rotation in the shoulders, limitation of movement or ankylosis of the wrists in palmar flexion and of the ankles in plantar flexion, subluxation of the metacarpophalangeal joints with ulnar deviation of the fingers, subluxation of the interphalangeal joints, flat foot and hallux valgus. The joints usually become fixed in the position which is most comfortable to the patient during the acute stage, as has been previously mentioned. The maintenance of the joints in these positions for long periods leads to the formation of intra- and extra-articular adhesions, destruction of the cartilage becomes complete and in the more progressive cases bony ankylosis ensues.

A brief description of some of the methods used for the correction of the more common deformities will be given, but for full information on this subject the reader is referred to the works of those orthopœdic surgeons who have made a special study of the chronic rheumatic diseases (R. B. Osgood, A. G. Timbrell Fisher and H. Platt).

Flexion of the Hips and Knees.—There are several methods in use for the correction of this deformity. Except in very severe cases the hip joints are rarely seriously involved in rheumatoid arthritis, but they are maintained in flexion by the deformity of the knees. In cases of long duration, shortening and fibrosis of the quadriceps and other muscles may occur and give rise to a secondary flexion deformity of the hips.

Weight Extension.—The limb is placed in a modified Thomas' splint and about 10 to 15 lbs. extension applied in the usual way. If a Balkan beam is available the limb in the splint is slung from this. This method does nothing to allay muscular spasm and the patient may experience considerable pain. The weight is removed once daily for the passive movements of the joint and the application of massage and faradism to the muscles.

Serial Plasters.—One of the most important advances in the technique of correction of deformities is the use of serial plasters (see Appendix). It is of particular value for the correction of flexion deformities of the knees, but can be used in any joint which is accessible to the application of plaster. In the case of the knees, a complete plaster is applied to the limb and bivalved when dry to allow of movement of the joint and massage to the muscles. After three to six days complete rest in the plaster, it is found that the knee is now capable of an extra few degrees of extension. This gain is consolidated by the application of a new plaster. After four to six plasters have been applied, complete extension will frequently have been attained. In more resistant cases manipulation under a general anæsthetic may be required before a full range of movement can be restored to the joint. The advantages of serial plasters are that no strain is thrown on the articular structures, the muscles are put at rest, spasm is overcome and pain is relieved.

Wedge Plasters.—This is a modification of the serial plaster method. A rather heavier plaster is applied with an anterior slab over the knee to act as a hinge. Twenty-four hours after application the plaster is sawn through three-quarters way round at the knee, leaving the anterior slab intact. Every two to three days, wedges are inserted behind the knee. Great care must be taken not to put too great a strain on the joint by forcing in too large wedges. The wedges merely "take up the slack," *i.e.*, maintain the extension gained by passive relaxation of spasm and stretching of adhesions. The wedge plaster, therefore, simply takes the place of a number of serial plasters, the advantage being that only one or two plasters are required. Some obstinate cases which do not respond to serial plasters, do well with this method. The great disadvantage is that the treatment of the muscles is impossible while the plaster is in position.

Manipulation.—Manipulation under a general anæsthetic is of value in properly selected cases of rheumatoid arthritis. Certain criteria must be observed. The first and most important is that the active phase of the disease must be past. X-ray films of the joints must be studied carefully and bony ankylosis excluded. Subluxation is also a contraindication in most cases. Although a joint cavity may still be present in the knee, the patella may be firmly ankylosed to the lower end of the femur, and unless this can be mobilized little functional gain will be obtained from manipulation of the joint. Great care must be exercised if the bones are markedly decalcified, otherwise a fracture may result. Certain joints react well to manipulation—knees, hips and shoulders. Results are less certain in the wrists and ankles and good seldom comes of manipulation of the elbows. The presence of severe cartilaginous damage may not preclude some return of movement, but the after-treatment must be prolonged and weight-bearing avoided for some weeks.

When minor degrees of pain and disability are present, local infiltration of the peri-articular structures, on one or more occasions, with $\frac{1}{2}$ per cent. solution of novocain according to the technique described for the treatment of fibrositis (see p. 937), followed by heat and movements, may be sufficient to banish pain and restore full function.

In cases where abduction has become limited in the shoulder but where the degree of activity precludes manipulation under an anæsthetic, full movement may be restored by the use of an aeroplane splint (see Fig. 1). When first applied it is adjusted so as to hold the arm in the position of maximum

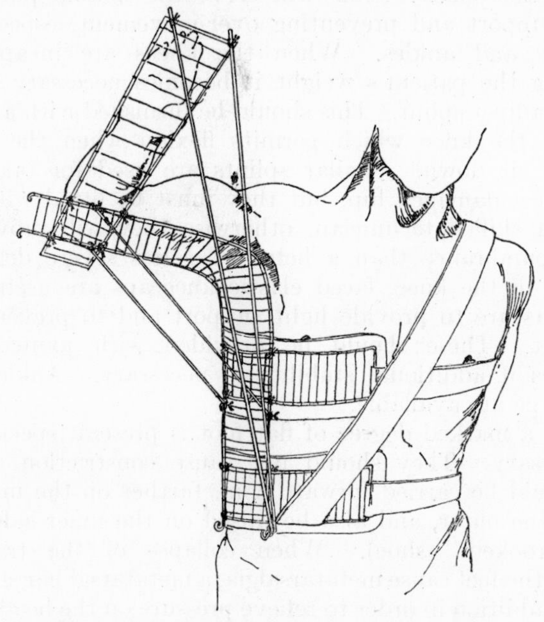

FIG. 1.—Aeroplane Splint in Position. Padding on the arm-piece has been omitted for the sake of clearness. This type of splint is readily constructed from lengths of wire splinting as shown.

abduction compatible with comfort. The arm is bandaged firmly to the splint, which must be well padded. The rest obtained will relax spasm and in a few days more abduction becomes possible. The splint is now adjusted to hold the arm in the new position. This process is continued until full abduction has been restored. The underlying principle is exactly similar to that of the serial plaster method. Heat and movement to the joint and massage and exercise for the muscles are employed daily.

In more severe cases the damage to certain joints may be of such a degree that appliances are necessary to supplement the impaired function before the patient can regain the power to walk. The simplest of these is crutches, which serve a useful purpose in the transitional stage between recumbency and unaided weight-bearing. It is important that they should be of the correct length for each individual case, otherwise they may be the cause of further deformity, especially of the spine and hips. Another simple method of supporting an unstable joint is the application of a firm bandage, preferably crêpe or elastoplast. This will serve the double purpose of lending support and preventing over-movement, especially in the knees and ankles. When the knees are incapable of supporting the patient's weight it becomes necessary to fit a walking calliper splint. This should be furnished with a locking device at the knee which permits flexion when the patient wishes to sit down. Similar splints are used for taking the weight off a damaged hip, but they must be fitted with great care by a skilled technician, otherwise they will prove more of an encumbrance than a help. For less severe degrees of disability in the knee, laced elastic kneecaps are useful when the objects are to provide light support and to prevent over-movement. These should be provided with jointed metal side-pieces if additional stability is necessary. Anklets of a similar type are available.

When a marked degree of flat foot is present, special shoes are necessary. They should not cause constriction and the heels should be carried forward ½ in. further on the inner side than on the outer, and also be raised on the inner side of the sole ("crooked" shoe). When collapse of the transverse arches of the feet cause metatarsalgia, a metatarsal bar should be fitted in addition in order to relieve pressure on the heads of the metatarsal bones. Considerable relief from pain may also result from the use of small pads of chiropodist's felt over the metatarsal heads plus the application of adhesive plaster round the foot, immediately proximal to the heads of the metatarsals.

In the very rare cases of rheumatoid arthritis in which the spine becomes involved, or where the posture is very bad, it may be necessary to fit a spinal brace. Here, again, expert opinion is required regarding the particular type of brace suitable for each individual case.

In the chronic stage of rheumatoid arthritis it is of paramount importance to prescribe a carefully thought-out scheme of exercises, both for the correction of faulty body mechanics and for the restoration of function after deformity has been corrected. Details of exercises of value for these purposes will be found in the Appendix.

OSTEO-ARTHRITIS

For the definition and prophylaxis of osteo-arthritis see pp. 890, 893.

Treatment of the established disease is in the main palliative, since it would be unreasonable to expect that degenerated cartilage or bony outgrowths can be repaired or removed by drugs, vaccines or physiotherapy. Treatment may be divided into (1) general, which includes the removal or correction of ætiological factors ; and (2) local.

General Treatment.—If the patient is suffering severe pain in a weight-bearing joint such as the hip or the knee, the best method of taking the strain off the joint and relieving the pain is to confine the patient to bed for a week or two. During this period the joint should daily be put through the full range of movement of which it is capable, without force being used. Patients with severe arthritic pain have frequently reached this state by accepting the advice of their friends or medical attendant, that the best treatment is to "walk it off" otherwise the joint will become stiff. Not only is this advice unwise, but it is also inaccurate, since ankylosis does not occur in osteo-arthritis. For patients with less severe pain, modified rest should be ordered to meet the individual requirements of the case. If the patient is unable to accept this advice because of his occupation, the mechanical devices discussed below may be of value in relieving the strain of weight-bearing in an individual joint. The occupational factor, as has already been mentioned, is of great ætiological importance in all chronic rheumatic diseases including osteo-arthritis, and the doctor must discuss with his patient the question of whether it is possible to change or modify his occupation, should it be unsuitable. Similar advice may have to be given regarding hobbies or pastimes, such as golf, fishing and shooting, which may throw an undue strain on the affected joints.

Obesity is commonly present in individuals with osteo-arthritis, and reduction of weight by suitable dietotherapy is of great importance (see p. 387). If the obesity affects the abdomen particularly, the patient tends to assume a posture which throws still greater strain on the weight-bearing joints, and exercises for the correction of bad posture (see Appendix) should be carried out regularly.

If clinical evidence of thyroid deficiency is also present, as is not infrequently the case in women at the menopause, thyroid extract should be prescribed in suitable doses.

A regular motion of the bowels should be ensured by an adequate fluid intake and the use of ample fresh fruit and vegetables in the diet, assisted when necessary by a small dose of salts in the morning.

A conservative attitude should be adopted towards septic foci and their eradication, as osteo-arthritis is not believed to be the result of infection. Nevertheless, obvious septic foci should be removed, both on the grounds of general health and because of the possibility of their accelerating the degenerative processes in the joints (see p. 894).

Drugs play only a small part in the treatment of osteo-arthritis. Analgesics (see p. 899) are prescribed when necessary for the relief of pain. Potassium iodide, arsenic, guaicum and sulphur (p. 901) may be tried individually or in combination, and appear to be of some value in a proportion of cases, although their mode of action is not any clearer in osteo-arthritis than in the other chronic rheumatic diseases (see p. 901). Buckley states that the injection of 1 to 2 c.c. of lipiodol every three weeks, or at longer intervals, into the muscles in the neighbourhood of the affected joints produces relief from pain and stiffness in many instances. Gold salts which are of use in rheumatoid arthritis are valueless in osteo-arthritis and fibrositis, and are therefore contraindicated for this reason and because of the associated dangers of toxic reactions. Vaccines, and non-specific protein shock therapy play no part in the treatment of osteo-arthritis.

Local Treatment.—Physiotherapy and not drug therapy is the essential feature of the treatment of osteo-arthritis. By this means, muscular spasm can best be relaxed, pain relieved and the circulation of blood and lymph in the neighbourhood of affected joints improved, with the hope that the degenerative processes may be retarded. Physiotherapy enables movements of the joints to be undertaken more freely, with concomitant improvement of function. If a single joint is affected, such as the knee, considerable relief may be obtained from the local application of heat. Any of the methods already described on p. 912 may be used, but mud packs are of particular value. In deep-seated joints such as the hips or spine, the analgesic effects of heat may be best attained by means of diathermy or short-wave therapy. Recently, Kahlmeter has published a paper embodying the results obtained in a large series of patients treated by deep X-ray therapy, and claims beneficial results in a high proportion of cases. In our more limited experience definite symptomatic improvement resulted in about 50 to 60 per cent. of cases in a carefully controlled series. Accordingly, we believe that deep X-ray therapy is worthy of a trial in cases which have resisted the simpler and less expensive methods.

In joints more superficially situated, ionization with potassium iodide, sodium salicylate, or histamine is sometimes useful. Counter-irritation is another simple measure which should be tried. This may be obtained by the use of rubefacient ointments (see p. 913), mustard leaves, blistering fluid (liq. epipasticus, B.P.) or by means of the electro-cautery.

Massage should be given to the muscles surrounding the joint with a view to improving the local circulation and dispersing fibrositic lesions which are frequently present. It is inadvisable, however, to attempt to apply heavy massage over the painful bony exostoses in the neighbourhood of the joints.

Hydrotherapy (see p. 915) is of the greatest value in osteoarthritis, particularly the deep-pool bath in which the patient can move his limbs under warm water, which relaxes spasm and eliminates the effect of gravity, thus enabling movements to be carried out with the minimum of pain. The undercurrent douche should be applied at the same time.

For those unable to visit a spa, a hot bath at home, medicated or otherwise (see p. 917), is a useful substitute in enabling the patient to obtain the benefits of heat and movement.

Orthopædic Procedures. — Manipulation under a general anæsthetic may be a valuable procedure, but it must be employed with great caution and only in selected cases where there is considerable pain and limitation of movement with only moderate bony changes. In such a case, peri-articular adhesions and capsular thickening are believed to be largely responsible for the disability which is present and much benefit may be obtained from manipulating the joint in a gentle manner under full surgical anæsthesia. This must be followed by daily movement of the joint preceded by heat.

In the case of the hip, when marked spasm and shortening of the adductor muscles is present, in addition to manipulation it may be necessary to perform a tenotomy of the adductor tendons.

Mechanical appliances for the relief of weight-bearing joints may be necessary if the measures already outlined fail to give relief. The indications for surgical treatment are discussed on p. 942.

CHRONIC MENOPAUSAL ARTHRITIS

(*Chronic Villous Arthritis*, *Climacteric Arthritis*)

There is a form of arthritis which occurs commonly in women about the time of the menopause. Those affected have, as a rule, been considerably overweight for some years and show signs of the subthyroid state. The joints principally affected are the knees, but minor changes are usually present in the hands. In the early stages of the disease the affected joints are swollen and painful owing to thickening of the peri-articular structures, hypertrophy of the synovial membrane or less commonly to the presence of fluid in the joint cavity. The condition is a proliferative synovitis rather than an arthritis, since X-rays reveal little or no bony change. In untreated cases the disease slowly progresses until typical signs of osteo-arthritis occur.

Various factors appear to play a part in the ætiology of this disease, but the most important from the point of view of treatment is obesity. Menopausal endocrine deficiencies may influence the onset directly by giving rise to premature senility and the early appearance of degenerative changes in the joints, or indirectly by leading to obesity.

The condition is one which is peculiarly amenable to treatment in the early stages. The first step must be to reduce the strain thrown upon the knees by excessive weight. If this object is attained by careful regulation of the diet, and, where necessary, by the administration of thyroid, combined with suitable general and local treatment, the appearance of the cartilaginous and bony changes of osteo-arthritis may be indefinitely delayed. A suitable diet of low calorific value is prescribed, and the patient must be impressed with the importance of adhering to it strictly. For details of a suitable diet, see p. 389. A small dose of thyroid (thyroideum, B.P., $\frac{1}{4}$ to $\frac{1}{2}$ gr. twice a day) should be administered with the object of correcting any endocrine deficiency and to augment the effect of the reducing diet. The dose must be adjusted to suit the requirements of each individual case. Few drugs have been found to have much beneficial effect in chronic menopausal arthritis, with the exception of the analgesics, but many physicians believe that iodine, in the doses detailed on p. 901, is of value. The peripheral circulation is often sluggish, and the skin is tacked down to the subcutaneous tissues. Tender fibrositic areas are commonly present around the joints and in the scapular region. Hydrotherapy and the other methods of applying local heat followed by massage, as already described on p. 924, do much to improve the circulation, disperse the fibrositic thickenings and restore the function of the joints. Adequate rest to the joints themselves must be insisted on, walking being reduced to a minimum for some weeks, until the swelling and pain have greatly subsided and a substantial reduction in weight has been secured. Crêpe bandages or elastoplast should be applied to the knee in order to maintain an even pressure, which will aid the reabsorption of effusion and provide support during weight-bearing. These should be retained when the patient returns to active life and until the quadriceps muscles have regained their normal tone. Faradic stimulation and static contractions should be used during the time when the patient's activities are restricted. Spa treatment is particularly suitable for patients with menopausal arthritis as the physiotherapeutic and hydrological facilities available are of the utmost value. When very marked synovial proliferation is present, resulting in nipping of fringes between the articular surfaces, surgical intervention may become necessary (see p. 942).

Excellent results are to be expected from the use of deep X-ray therapy in this disease. If the treatment is employed in the early stage, before radiological evidence of osteo-arthritis has appeared, complete cure follows in a proportion of cases. In more advanced cases the progress of the disease may be arrested and relief of symptoms may result. As a rule more than one course of treatment is required. The prescription of dosage and the length of the course should be in the hands of a radiologist skilled in the use of deep X-ray therapy and familiar with its application to diseases of the joints.

When the disease is treated early, the prognosis is good. If osteo-arthritic changes are established when the patient is first seen, the treatment is the same as already described for that disease on p. 923.

SPONDYLITIS

Arthritis affecting the spine occurs in two main forms—spondylitis osteo-arthritica (spondylosis deformans) and ankylosing spondylitis (spondylose rhizomélique, spondylitis ankylopœtica).

The ætiology and pathology of osteo-arthritis affecting the spinal articulations are identical with those of osteo-arthritis arising in any other joint. It occurs in those whose occupation has thrown a strain on the back over a period of years. It is a slowly progressive condition, and marked degenerative changes may be present before symptoms appear. It is often discovered in people past middle life during the course of a routine examination. Trauma, obesity, occupation and postural defects may all play a part in conditioning the onset of symptoms, and these factors should receive attention in the early stages of the disease.

When symptoms arise they are due to pressure of osteophytes on nerve roots or to reactionary fibrositis in the surrounding muscles and ligaments. Pain may be severe but is often absent, and in more advanced cases muscular wasting and disturbances of sensation may manifest themselves owing to pressure on nerve roots.

The methods of treatment already described for osteo-arthritis in other joints are equally applicable when the spine is affected. Local heat and massage do much to allay the pain arising from the muscular spasm commonly present. Diathermy, short-wave therapy and the various forms of baths may afford considerable relief. Repeated courses of deep X-ray therapy are beneficial in a considerable proportion of cases. Ætiological factors must be corrected, and in the cases where the nerve roots are being subjected to pressure by osteophytes surgical intervention may occasionally become necessary.

Ankylosing Spondylitis is a disease mainly of early adult life, and is much more common in males. Its incidence is relatively small, but when it arises it is an extremely serious condition which completely incapacitates the sufferer and may even endanger life. The pathology is that of infective or atrophic arthritis, and it has been called rheumatoid arthritis of the spine, although in the opinion of a number of observers it is an entirely different disease. The onset of symptoms referable to the spine is preceded by a period during which the patient complains of vague pain in his muscles and joints. The estimation of the sedimentation rate at this time may suggest the presence of some infective process, and X-rays of the spine and pelvis may show the early changes of ankylosing spondylitis. The disease affects particularly males in the early twenties, well developed and of an active mode of life. In the majority of cases the first joints to show radiological changes are the sacro-iliacs, which become ankylosed very early in the course of the disease. As the disease progresses the intervertebral and costovertebral joints are involved, the spine becomes rigid and the thoracic cage immobile. If the disease remains unchecked it spreads centrifugally to involve the hips, knees, shoulders, elbows, and may in severe cases affect the hands and feet. The joint changes are accompanied by generalized muscular wasting. In the early stages, patients are usually ambulatory, with the result that, owing to decalcification and softening of the vertebral bodies, the spine assumes a kyphotic position, and unless treatment is instituted early, this deformity will become permanent owing to the deposition of calcium in the ligaments and capsules of the joints. The calcification and later ossification of the joint capsules is a characteristic feature.

General Treatment.—The disease is believed to be infective in origin, and a scheme of treatment exactly similar to that described in the section on rheumatoid arthritis must be adopted (see p. 895) including rest in bed in the active stage to overcome fatigue and prevent deformities, and the application of all the measures already detailed to raise the general resistance and improve the health of the patient. A careful search should be made for septic foci in the teeth, tonsils, etc. At one time the view was widely held, especially in France, that the gonococcus was the causative organism in ankylosing spondylitis, but the negative history and the absence of bacteriological evidence in many cases do not uphold this view.

The value of vaccines, gold and protein shock therapy is as much a controversial subject in ankylosing spondylitis as it is in rheumatoid arthritis. Gold must certainly be given with great care as sufferers from this disease are often particularly sensitive to the drug. Buckley is of the opinion that beneficial effects may result from the use of Ponndorf's vaccine, which contains antigens of streptococci, staphylococci, pneumococci, gonococci, *B. tuberculosis* and *B. Pfeiffer*. It appears to act as a desensitizing agent. The vaccine is put up in tubes. A quarter of a tube is the initial dose and it is applied to a scarified area of the skin. A local reaction follows, varying from a slight redness to the formation of a scab. A general reaction may occur and is considered a favourable sign. The dose and area of scarification are increased slowly, until a whole tube is being used. The interval between applications is two to three weeks at first, increasing to two or three months towards the end of the course, which should consist of twelve to fifteen applications. Absence of reaction after two or three doses have been applied should be regarded as a contraindication to the continuation of the treatment.

Drugs should be used with discretion as in rheumatoid arthritis, analgesics again being the most valuable.

Local Treatment.—In the early stages of the disease, when no deformity of the spine has yet arisen, its occurrence may be prevented by the use of a spinal shell. This is made from plaster of Paris while the patient is lying face down with the spine in the optimum position. The back is oiled and the plaster applied "skin-tight" in order to ensure perfect fit, and the shell extends from occiput to sacrum. When dry the shell forms a light, comfortable splint in which the patient lies both day and night during the active stage of the disease. When the subacute stage is reached the patient is fitted with a spinal brace, which he wears throughout the day, his nights being spent in the plaster shell.

The costo-vertebral joints become involved early in the course of the disease, and unless their mobility is maintained by special breathing exercises the thoracic cage becomes fixed, often in the position of expiration. Breathing exercises should be commenced as soon as the patient comes under medical care, and should be continued daily for the rest of his life. (For details of the exercises, see p. 952).

The large joints, hips, shoulders and knees must be put through their full range of movement every day. Should they become involved by the disease process, they are treated along the same lines as the joints in rheumatoid arthritis.

If kyphosis has already become established it can be wholly or partly corrected by the use of serial plaster shells. While the plaster is still wet it is manipulated so that it becomes a little straighter than the patient's spine. After about one to two weeks spent in this shell the patient will have settled into it and his spine will be in contact with the splint. This procedure is repeated until the deformity has been corrected as much as the changes already present will allow. At the same time, mobility is restored to the ribs by the exercises already mentioned. After the acute stage is passed the physiotherapeutic measures already described are utilized for allaying pain and restoring function. Heat in all its forms, massage, exercises for the correction of postural defects and hydrotherapy all play their part. Opinion differs regarding the value of deep X-ray therapy in this disease, and final judgment must be deferred until further experience has been acquired. It is, however, worthy of trial where pain has not been relieved by the measures described above.

Ankylosing spondylitis is in the majority of cases a steadily progressive disease and no method of treatment has yet been found to stay its advance. The rôle of the physician is to prevent deformity and maintain function to the best of his ability. A rigid spine is not in itself a crippling deformity if good position has been insured by early and adequate treatment. Forcible manipulation with or without an anæsthetic should never be used in ankylosing spondylitis at any stage, as more harm than good will result.

STILL'S DISEASE

A rheumatoid type of arthritis occurs occasionally in children between the ages of three and ten. It is accompanied by fever, glandular enlargement and splenomegaly. There is a tendency for the infantile proportions of the limbs to persist, probably due to interference with normal growth by the disease processes. The findings in the joints do not appear to be specific for the disease, but common to all types of chronic infective arthritis. The disease tends to run a prolonged course, although dramatic remissions have been recorded occasionally following the eradication of a septic focus or the use of gold therapy.

The treatment is that of rheumatoid arthritis (see p. 894).

FIBROSITIS

Definition.—Fibrositis may be defined as a non-suppurative inflammatory reaction of the fibrous supporting tissue of the body. The inflammation may involve the capsules of joints (capsulitis), the sheaths of nerves (neuritis), the subcutaneous connective tissue (panniculitis) or the aponeuroses, tendons and interstitial fibrous tissue of muscles (tendinitis, myositis). The specialized connective tissue of bursæ and synovial membranes may also be involved by a similar process (bursitis, synovitis), and care must be taken to distinguish these conditions from a true arthritis, in which cartilaginous or bony changes are present.

Since the measures for the prevention and successful treatment of fibrositis are based essentially on a knowledge of the ætiological factors involved, it is considered desirable to deal with this aspect first.

Ætiology.—Although the ætiology of fibrositis is still unsettled, several factors are recognized as being of particular importance. More than one may be at work, and until all are adequately dealt with treatment may fail to accomplish a cure of an isolated attack of fibrositis or may produce only a temporary alleviation of symptoms, to be followed by relapse when the patient resumes an unsuitable occupation or returns to an uncongenial environment. In some cases focal sepsis seems to be the underlying cause, while in others a metabolic defect is the principle factor at fault. Some authorities believe that the defect in metabolism is conditioned by the liver being unable to complete the metabolism of purine bodies. Others hold that a failure of digestion with consequent absorption of toxic products is responsible. In a small proportion of cases, the underlying cause of fibrositis is true gout, and this should be borne in mind in the investigation of the more chronic cases. In many instances the patients appear to lack the ability to accommodate themselves to changes in temperature and barometric pressure, and it is for this reason that so many fibrositic subjects can forecast a change in the weather by reason of an exacerbation of their pain or stiffness. The skin is the principal organ which enables human beings to adapt themselves to changes in their environment, and all investigators of the group of chronic rheumatic diseases are agreed on the frequency with which abnormalities of the skin and its underlying capillaries are found. Damp and cold act by depressing the local or general circulation, and lead to accumulation of the end products of metabolism in the muscles. Lastly, the importance of the occupational factor in the chronic rheumatic diseases, especially fibrositis, must never be forgotten. Statistics clearly indicate the high incidence of all forms of rheumatic disease in occupations involving exposure to damp, cold and excessive strain, and particularly if work is undertaken in postures which throw excessive and prolonged strain on one group of muscles and joints. The importance of fatigue as an ætiological factor has long been recognized.

The practitioner would be well advised in each case of fibrositis to search for and evaluate the importance of the following factors :—

1. Sepsis.
2. Diet.
3. Metabolic defects.
4. Trauma and occupation.
5. Climate.

Treatment will be considered under three headings :—

I. Removal or correction of factors of ætiological importance.
II. Treatment of the general condition.
III. Treatment of the local condition.

Removal or Correction of Factors of Ætiological Importance. —The measures to be outlined are necessary both for prophylaxis in subjects who are constitutionally predisposed to fibrositis and for the prevention of recurrences in established cases. They are in the main applicable to all forms of chronic rheumatism, and only a brief reference need be made to those already discussed under Rheumatoid Arthritis. This applies particularly to the eradication of focal sepsis, because the same considerations govern this problem in fibrositis (see p. 891).

In every case a careful inquiry should be made into the patient's dietetic habits, and articles of food and drink which the history suggests are of ætiological importance should be forbidden. In general, individuals with chronic fibrositis are better if the intake of purines and proteins is restricted. This is particularly true of the fibrositis of gouty origin. In patients who are overweight, especially females at the menopause, much benefit can be obtained from a reduction of the total calories in the diet, with the addition of a small dose of thyroid extract if some degree of thyroid deficiency is present, as is quite frequently the case (see p. 396).

The measures for improving the function of the skin consist of advice on clothing, regular exercise in the fresh air and hydrotherapy at home or in a spa. These have already been discussed on p. 915.

It is seldom possible to secure a change from an unsuitable environment or occupation, but common-sense advice (see p. 891) on the observation of the fundamental rules of health and the avoidance of fatigue may go far towards reducing the liability to recurrences.

Treatment in the Acute Stage

General.—During an acute attack of fibrositis, the patient should be put to bed in order to secure complete rest to the affected part. This is especially necessary if the back or lower limbs are involved. In milder cases with no constitutional disturbance, where the disease affects only the arms or shoulders, a sling may provide adequate rest. The patient's bowels should be opened with calomel (2 to 3 gr.) given at night, followed next morning with ½ oz. of Epsom salts. In elderly people the laxative to which they are accustomed may be ordered in double the usual dose. A light diet should be prescribed, preferably lacto-vegetarian in type, and the patient should be instructed to drink large quantities of fluids. At least six to eight glasses of water should be taken daily. Alkaline spa waters such as Vichy water are excellent, failing which the following alkaline mixture should be taken three or four times a day after meals :—

℞		
	Pot. Cit.	gr. xxx
	Liq. Ammon. Acet. Dil. . . .	ʒii
	Aq. Menth. Pip. Dest. . . ad	℥ss

For the control of pain analgesics in sufficient amounts are necessary. Aspirin in doses of 10 to 15 gr. three or four times a day will be adequate in most cases, but may sometimes require to be reinforced with a stronger analgesic such as codeine (see p. 899). During the acute stage in the severest forms of sciatica, morphia may be the only drug which gives relief. When aspirin is not well tolerated calcium aspirin or the salicylates may be tried. Sodium salicylates (20 to 30 gr.) with an equal amount of sodium bicarbonate should be given three or four times a day. Where there is evidence of a gouty basis, 15 minims of the wine of colchicum should be added to the mixture during the acute stage. Numerous other drugs have been recommended for fibrositis, but they are of little value during the acute stage, and should be reserved for the more chronic forms of the disease (see p. 937).

In view of the sluggish peripheral circulation so commonly found in sufferers from fibrositis the application of general heat in the form of a bath, if the patient's condition permits, or by means of a radiant heat cabinet in bed, is a useful form of treatment. Free sweating should be encouraged, but care must be taken with elderly patients and those who perspire only with difficulty, or undue exhaustion and discomfort may result. During the application of general heat, copious draughts of plain water or barley water help to promote diaphoresis. The addition of Epsom salts, mustard or washing soda (see p. 917) to the bath water serves as an additional stimulus to the skin. After such a bath the patient should be dried, wrapped in towels and returned to bed as quickly as possible to avoid chilling. These principles of general treatment are applicable whatever part of the body is affected by the disease.

Local Treatment.—The most important principle in local treatment during the acute stage of the disease is to secure absolute rest of the affected part. When the muscles or peri-articular structures of the shoulder girdle or arm are involved, a sling should be applied. In intercostal fibrositis (pleurodynia) the effected side of the chest should be immobilized in the position of maximum expiration by the application of broad strips of adhesive plaster. The plaster should extend well across the mid-line. In lumbago, in addition to rest in bed, the affected spinal muscles are immobilized in a similar fashion by strapping or by the application of a belladonna plaster, which acts as an efficient support and keeps the part warm. During the acute stage of sciatica the pain may be so severe that the patient will not tolerate any form of fixation of the affected limb. He will insist on being allowed to move it at frequent intervals, as only by doing so can he make the pain tolerable. In milder cases a splint or light weight extension may be applied with benefit. The comforting effects of heat will be confirmed by all who have suffered from fibrositis. The various methods of applying heat and counter-irritation locally have been discussed on p. 912 and in the Appendix. They include portable radiant heat and infra-red lamps, hot bottles, bags of hot salt, linseed and kaolin poultices, mud packs and the use of a hot iron applied to a towel over the affected part. The method used in any one case will depend on the material available and the part of the body affected. Massage is usually contraindicated during the acute stage because of the pain it produces and its inefficiency on account of muscular spasm. In less severe cases very light friction, with the application of a counter-irritant, may bring relief.

Subacute and Chronic Stage

Within a few days the acute condition has, as a rule, subsided, and more active physiotherapeutic measures must be employed, the chief of which is massage which should be preceded for at least fifteen to twenty minutes by heat. This will induce a relaxation of spasm and relief of pain. As a result, the masseuse is more easily able to disperse the products of the inflammatory reaction deep in the muscles, and thus prevent the deposition of pathological fibrous tissue in the form of nodules and bands, which so frequently cause the condition to become chronic. Benefit may be derived from the use of counter-irritants, and these should be rubbed into the skin over the affected muscles. As the condition of the patient improves, the massage should become firmer and deeper, and any nodules present should receive special attention.

Deep massage for the removal of chronic fibrous nodules is likely to cause pain, and this cannot be avoided if the pathological lesions are to be resolved. Poor results are often due to the desire of the masseuse to avoid hurting the patient. At this stage massage should be followed by gentle passive movements to stretch the affected tissues and prevent shortening. This is particularly important when the peri-articular structures of a joint are involved. If neglected fibrous contractures may develop, and manipulation under general anæsthesia may be required to restore full movement. Finally, active exercises should be prescribed in order to overcome residual stiffness and correct any postural defects which have arisen.

Under this régime 80 to 90 per cent. of patients suffering from acute fibrositis will be completely relieved in one to two weeks, and provided the underlying cause has been found and dealt with (see ætiology), no recurrence need be expected. In more intractable cases, or in those who have developed fibrous thickenings as a result of previous attacks, a course of hydrotherapy at a spa is of particular value. Immersion baths with undercurrent douches, followed by vigorous massage, have a markedly beneficial effect in improving the tone of the circulation and dispersing fibrous nodules in muscles. Turkish (hot air) and Russian (vapour) baths are available in many cities and are also useful, but should not be prescribed more than once or twice a week because of their exhausting effect if taken too frequently. It is to be hoped that the interest now being taken in the rheumatic diseases will lead to the establishment by municipal authorities of rheumatism treatment centres with hydrotherapeutic facilities in every industrial area.

Diet.—No dietetic restrictions may be required for the patient who has an isolated attack of fibrositis conditioned by a single factor which disappears by itself or can be removed, *e.g.*, trauma, infection, excessive exposure to wet or cold. On the other hand, where repeated acute attacks of fibrositis occur or where a state of chronic fibrositis persists, despite attempts to correct or remove underlying ætiological factors, a full investigation should be made into the following factors: (1) Idiosyncrasy to any particular food or drink; (2) any digestive disturbances with particular reference to dyspepsia associated with achlorhydria or with defective carbohydrate digestion; (3) the presence of constipation; (4) signs of sluggish liver function; (5) clinical or chemical evidence favouring a gouty basis.

In general it will be found advisable to reduce the rich starchy foods, such as bread, pastry, suet puddings, etc. This will help to correct defective carbohydrate digestion and will at the same time reduce the overweight patient. Next the protein, and particularly the purine part of the diet, should be reduced or modified. This is especially necessary if a gouty basis is suspected. Liver, sweetbreads, kidney and rich soups are best avoided, and the patient should limit himself to a small helping of meat or bird once daily. There is little evidence to suggest that beef or mutton in equivalent quantities are more harmful than chicken or game. In short, a modified lacto-vegetarian diet will frequently be found to be of service to many patients suffering from chronic fibrositis. The diet should be constructed from the dairy products (milk, eggs, cheese and butter), plenty of fruit and vegetables, both cooked and raw, milk puddings, custard and junket. Rhubarb and strawberries should be forbidden if oxaluria is present. Plenty of fluids should be taken between meals ; the alkali spa waters are valuable. Alcohol should be forbidden or greatly reduced in quantity. Beer and sweet wines are particularly harmful to some sufferers from fibrositis. If it is considered necessary to allow alcohol, it should be in the form of spirits, preferably whisky well diluted with water.

A modified lacto-vegetarian diet with plenty of fruit and vegetables, assisted where necessary with liquid paraffin, is the best treatment for constipation.

Drugs.—Numerous drugs have been recommended for fibrositis, those most commonly employed being iodine, arsenic and sulphur (for details of administration and dosage, see p. 901). While we do not deny the value of aspirin and other analgesic drugs as symptomatic remedies, we believe that the beneficial effects obtained from iodine, arsenic and sulphur have been exaggerated. The practitioner is entitled to prescribe one or other of these drugs should he wish to, provided he realizes that in fibrositis reliance should be placed on physiotherapy rather than drug therapy. Mention has already been made of the value of thyroid extract in overweight patients suffering from mild degrees of hypothyroidism. Where a gouty basis exists atophan should be given a trial (see p. 964), with due regard to the possibility of toxic effects on the liver. Some authorities recommend the use of bee venom (see p. 918) in the more chronic cases of fibrositis ; if no benefit results after four to six doses have been given, the method should be abandoned. Vaccines have been used in cases believed to have an infective basis, but the results are no more satisfactory than in other forms of chronic rheumatic disease, and this line of treatment is not to be recommended. A mild form of protein shock may be of benefit in resistant cases, and Buckley has found the preparation Pyrolactin D, which contains milk and sulphur, to be of value for this purpose (see p. 908).

Local Infiltration.—Infiltration of the affected area with a solution of ½ per cent. novocaine in normal saline is a very valuable method of treatment in three types of cases: (1) Localized persistently painful areas situated in muscles or at their tendinous attachments ; (2) fibrositis involving the capsules and ligaments of joints ; (3) neuritis due to involvement of the nerve sheath or interstitial fibrous tissue.

In the first type of case, having located the painful area,

20 to 40 c.c. of the novocaine solution are injected into and around the part, the skin having first been anæsthetized by an intradermal wheal. To obtain the maximum benefit the affected muscles are then firmly kneaded and passively stretched in order to break down and disperse fibrous deposits. The anæsthesia produced is sufficient to allow of this being done without undue discomfort to the patient. The bulk of fluid injected exerts a mechanical effect in softening and disrupting pathological fibrous tissue. The patient is then given a course of heat, massage and exercise.

When the capsule and ligaments of a joint are involved, these structures are thoroughly infiltrated and the joint put through its maximum range of movement without undue force being used. Adhesions will often be felt giving way and the operator should be satisfied with a moderate gain in movement. No attempt should be made to put the joint through its full range by force. The procedure can be repeated on two or three occasions, when a full range of movement will be restored in many cases. Heat, passive movements, active movements and graduated exercises will complete the cure.

In fibrositis of the gluteal muscles the trunk of the sciatic nerve may be involved as it emerges from the pelvis. Rapid relief from pain may follow the injection of 40 to 60 c.c. of novocaine solution around the sciatic notch, the bony points of which can be readily palpated. It is unnecessary to inject the solution into the nerve itself. The injection is followed by heat and massage to the gluteal region.

We have been greatly impressed by the value of novocaine infiltration in cases which have failed to respond to heat and massage applied for weeks or even months. There is no object in using stronger solutions of novocaine than $\frac{1}{2}$ per cent. as this induces adequate local anæsthesia, and the liability to reactions in those sensitive to novocaine is correspondingly reduced. We have used this method successfully for the treatment of painful lesions in the occipital, scapular, lumbar and gluteal regions. The amount of solution injected varies with the site of the lesion. From 3 to 5 c.c. may be effective in the occipital region, while 20 to 40 c.c. may be required for the lumbar and gluteal regions. To infiltrate the capsule and periarticular structures of a large joint, such as the shoulder or the knee, 60 to 80 c.c. may be necessary.

Manipulation.—In more advanced cases of fibrositis involving the capsules and periarticular structures of joints, in cases of low-back pain due to lumbosacral and sacro-iliac strain and in cases of sciatica due to involvement by fibrous tissue of the nerve roots at their exit from the spinal canal, the simple measures outlined may be insufficient to effect a cure. In these cases manipulation under a general anæsthetic may be indicated, but as this should be done only by an individual with a special training in orthopædics, we do not propose to discuss the technique employed.

It is now proposed to discuss briefly fibrositis in various sites where it may present difficulty in diagnosis or where special forms of treatment should be employed.

Cervical Spine and Occipital Region.—Fibrositis of the occipital aponeurosis is a common cause of persistent headache, variable in intensity but usually worse in the morning. Isolated nodules may be present along the occipital ridge, tender on pressure, or there may be a diffuse tenderness of the whole scalp. The fibrositic process not infrequently involves the trapezius muscles on one or both sides, giving rise to recurring attacks of "stiff neck." Should the general and local measures already described fail to relieve the symptoms, a manipulation of the cervical spine will frequently effect a cure. This can be carried out by an experienced operator without a general anæsthetic. It may be necessary to repeat the procedure on several occasions. Heat and massage following the manipulation play an important part in the treatment. When acutely tender nodules are present in the occipital region, the injection of 2 to 3 c.c. of $\frac{1}{2}$ per cent. novocaine into each tender spot is often of value.

Shoulder.—Fibrositis, when it involves the capsule and periarticular structures of the shoulder, may give rise to serious disability in the form of pain and limitation of movement. These cases are frequently diagnosed as arthritis, but a careful study of the X-ray picture will reveal no change in the joint itself. The onset of the condition may be insidious following some minor trauma, and the patient may not seek medical advice until considerable limitation of movement has developed. Treatment in the first place should consist of heat followed by gentle stretching of the contracted capsule. This should be carried out daily and continued so long as increased range of movement results. Should the condition resist this line of treatment, infiltration of the periarticular structures with $\frac{1}{2}$ per cent. novocaine should be tried. The needle is introduced through the deltoid, beneath the tip of the acromion process, and the solution deposited in front, behind and above the joint, which is then gently manipulated. In long-standing cases manipulation under a general anæsthetic may become necessary.

Subacromial Bursitis.—The subacromial bursa situated under the acromial process is not infrequently the site of inflammation. During the acute stage pain is felt on all movements of the shoulder, but is most severe on abduction. With the arm by the side, pressure over the head of the humerus is painful. This tenderness disappears if the arm can be abducted more than 90 degrees. During the acute stage, this range of movement is frequently rendered impossible by pain and spasm of the muscles moving the joint. Treatment at first consists of rest in an arm-sling, heat and a gently daily movement to prevent the formation of adhesions. Most cases will recover in three to four weeks under this treatment, but should adhesions form, infiltration or manipulation may become necessary.

Lumbago.—Pain in the lumbar region may arise from many causes. In the majority of cases the history of sudden onset of pain and stiffness in the lower back, following a chill or unaccustomed exercise, will make the diagnosis clear, *i.e.*, acute fibrositis of the lumbar muscles. In such cases the adoption of the general measures outlined and the elimination of factors of ætiological importance will lead to cure and reduce the possibility of recurrences to a minimum. In more chronic and persistent cases a careful search for the cause must be undertaken, which should include an X-ray picture of the lumbar spine in order to eliminate secondary carcinoma of the spine, sacralization of the fifth lumbar vertebra, caries, osteomyelitis, old injuries to the vertebral bodies or their processes, spondylitis, etc. In women with persistent backache a pelvic examination should always be made, as the presence of a gynæcological abnormality may be responsible for the pain. It should be remembered, however, that minor abnormalities may be found which are not necessarily responsible for the low-back pain. Many gynæcological operations have been performed for this purpose quite unnecessarily. In men the prostate should be examined and malignant growths of the rectum excluded. Bad posture due to obesity, knock knees, flat feet or occupational causes may give rise to persistent pain in the lumbar region, and the patient should be examined in the erect posture in a good light. Correction of postural abnormalities by re-educational exercises (see p. 952) will often banish troublesome backache of years' duration.

In chronic cases where tender areas are present in the lumbar muscles or their tendinous insertions, infiltration with novocaine, followed by heat, massage and exercise is indicated. For chronic fibrositis of the lumbar muscles which fails to respond to conservative treatment, or where pain is due to lumbosacral or sacro-iliac strain, manipulation of the spine under a general anæsthetic should be carried out.

Sciatica

Pain over the distribution of the sciatic nerve can arise from a number of causes, and successful treatment depends upon arriving at an accurate diagnosis of the underlying condition. The first step is to exclude pathological conditions in the spine or pelvic organs by X-ray and pelvic examination. In the majority of cases these structures will be found to be normal. It must then be decided whether the sciatica pain is due (1) to direct involvement of the nerve or its roots by a fibrositic process or (2) whether it is a referred pain. It is the opinion of certain authorities that pain in the distribution of the sciatic nerve, where objective signs of neuritis are absent, is not due to involvement of the sciatic nerve or its roots, but is of the nature of a referred pain conditioned by pathological lesions involving sensory nerves which enter the cord at the same segmental level as that from which the sciatic nerve arises. In the first type of case examination will reveal objective signs in the shape of diminished or absent ankle jerk, exaggerated knee jerk (due to hypotonia of the ham strings), muscular weakness, and in severe cases some degree of wasting. Lasegue's sign (extension of the leg with the thigh flexed) will be positive. The patient will complain of tingling and numbness as well as pain, and the foot on the affected side will be cold. In root sciatica the patient tends to lean away from the affected side. In the second group of cases the complaint is of pain alone, and examination will reveal no alteration in reflexes and no muscular wasting. Lasegue's sign may be positive or negative. Scoliosis of the lumbar spine is frequently present, and the convexity may be towards or away from the affected side. Pain referred to the distribution of the sciatic nerve may arise from pathological conditions in the sacro-iliac and lumbosacral regions, *i.e.*, fibrositis involving the lumbosacral and sacro-iliac ligaments, strain of the sacro-iliac joint arising from trauma or defective posture. Fibrositic lesions in the gluteal and lumbar muscles, which do not involve the nerve or its roots, may give rise to referred pain in the distribution of the sciatic nerve.

In the acute phase of all types of cases treatment is the same and consists of the general measures outlined, including analgesic drugs, rest in bed and heat in the form of mud packs, kaolin poultices, radiant heat, immersion baths, etc. In cases which do not recover under this treatment in a reasonable time, other measures may become necessary. When the nerve or its roots are involved, infiltration of the tender areas in the lumbar muscles or the gluteal region may give relief (see p. 938). In deep-seated lesions, involving the nerve roots emerging from the spine, manipulation of the spine combined with epidural injection (see p. 1096) should be carried out.

In the second group of cases, where the pain is referred in nature, spinal manipulation followed by exercises to correct faulty posture will usually be necessary. Hydrotherapy, physiotherapy and exercise play an important part in the treatment of the more chronic type of case, and a visit to a spa will often materially reduce the period of disability.

Convalescence.—After a severe attack of fibrositis, which has required prolonged physiotherapy for its cure, a holiday of at least a fortnight in a bracing place at the seaside, or in a convalescent home for those less fortunately situated, should be advised, and a tonic containing iron, strychnine and quinine prescribed (see p. 900). Exercises should be prescribed to be undertaken daily in order to keep the muscles of the affected area supple.

THE RÔLE OF SURGERY IN THE CHRONIC RHEUMATIC DISEASES

Before discussing the part played by surgery in the chronic rheumatic diseases, it must again be emphasized that early and adequate treatment will, in the vast majority of cases, obviate the necessity for surgical procedures. Surgery has no place in the treatment of the acute or subacute stages of rheumatoid arthritis, but offers to an arthritic derelict who has failed to respond to physiotherapeutic measures the only hope of regaining some degree of useful function.

Before surgical measures are considered in the treatment of rheumatoid arthritis, certain criteria must be observed. These have been clearly defined by Pemberton and Osgood as follows :—

1. Arrest or quiescence of the disease.
2. Preliminary treatment to improve the patient's general condition as much as possible.
3. Correct appraisal of the patient as an operative risk.
4. A knowledge of the patient's psychology and a belief in his ability to maintain morale.

5. An accurate estimate of the number and nature of the operations which will be required to attain the functional objective.
6. Provision for carrying through the entire operative campaign. This includes (*a*) special hospital facilities and optimistic, experienced nursing; (*b*) consideration of the patient's financial resources in relation to after-treatment, especially physical therapy and prolonged "follow-up."
7. Thorough training in joint surgery, good judgment and meticulous technique on the part of the surgeon.

In rheumatoid arthritis deformities requiring surgical correction may be present both in arms and legs. When this is the case the arms, as a rule, should be dealt with first, as the psychological effect on the patient of being able to feed herself and attend to her toilet is valuable in fortifying her for the more serious and time-consuming procedures required for the restoration of the ability to walk.

It is not proposed to give details of the various operations, but merely to mention the object of each and the type of case on which they can most profitably be performed.

Synovectomy.—This type of operation is indicated in cases of rheumatoid arthritis and occasionally in cases of menopausal arthritis, where other forms of treatment have failed to reduce swelling and disability, and recurrent effusion and pain result from the nipping of tags of proliferated synovial membrane between the articular surfaces. The operation consists of the removal of as much as possible of the hypertrophied synovial membrane in the affected joint.

Capsulotomy.—This operation consists of the division of contracted ligaments and joint capsules which are causing flexion deformities, but where a free range of movement exists up to the position of deformity. It is particularly applicable to the knee-joints, but may be used in other joints such as the hip and elbow.

Arthrotomy.—In rheumatoid arthritis an isolated mass of proliferated synovial membrane may give rise to disability, as a result of being pinched between the articular surfaces during movement of the joint. In osteo-arthritis individual chrondo-osseous spurs may limit motion, or loose bodies may be present in the joint cavity. In these conditions arthrotomy may be required for their removal. The existence of extensive articular damage is, in general, a contraindication to the operation, because permanent relief of the arthritis is unlikely to result.

Osteotomy.—Osteotomy is employed for restoration of the normal alignment of joint surfaces when a useful range of movement is still present in the joint, or for the correction of mal-alignment in a joint which has already become ankylosed. For example, osteotomy may serve a useful purpose in correcting the flexion and adduction deformities which are common in more advanced cases of osteo-arthritis of the hip joint.

Drilling of the Head of the Femur (Forage).—In osteo-arthritis it has been claimed that relief from pain and increased range of movement may result from drilling the head of the femur. This procedure is based on the belief that the circulation to the head of the bone is thereby improved. The operation is simple and without risk, but sufficient time has not elapsed to come to a conclusion regarding its permanent value.

Acetabuloplasty.—In this operation the upper and anterior parts of the acetabular margin are removed on the basis that pain may occur in osteo-arthritis due to the contact between the neck of the femur and the hypertrophied rim of the acetabulum on abduction. The operation is also of too recent origin for its value to be estimated.

Arthrodesing Operations.—When a joint has become unstable and useless from a functional point of view, considerable benefit may be derived from a procedure which deprives it of all motion but renders it stable. A joint may still be capable of a limited range of movement, but be so painful that from the patient's point of view the movement can be put to no useful purpose. Here, again, artificially produced ankylosis may banish pain and enable the patient to use the limb. In view of the fact that ankylosis occurs in the course of the disease in many cases, the operation has only a limited application in rheumatoid arthritis, but in osteo-arthritis this never occurs, and arthrodesis of the hip, and less frequently of the knee, may be recommended in selected cases.

Reconstruction Operations.—Many procedures have been devised by Sir Robert Jones, Whitman, Bracket, Lorenz and others for the reconstruction of joints affected by chronic arthritis. Their objects are to retain motion, relieve pain and render the joint stable, and they are mainly used in osteo-arthritis.

Arthroplasty.—In this operation the joint is completely exposed, the bone-ends remodelled and a piece of fascia interposed to prevent ankylosis and allow free smooth motion. In osteo-arthritis the operation is mainly applied to the hips.

In carefully selected patients with rheumatoid arthritis whose general condition is good and who will co-operate willingly in the long post-operative period required to secure a functionally good result, this operation is believed to have a wider application than was hitherto thought. A high degree of surgical skill is essential, and infinite patience on the part of both the surgeon and the patient is required. Weight-bearing must be delayed for at least two months, and for several weeks longer it must be aided by crutches and a stabilizing apparatus applied to the joint. The best results are obtained in the elbow, knee and hip.

Sympathectomy.—In certain cases of rheumatoid arthritis the limbs are cold and clammy. A cervical sympathectomy in the case of the hands and a lumbar sympathectomy in the case of the feet will have the effect of rendering them warm and dry. In early cases, some relief of pain and improvement in function may result, but operations on the sympathetic system have a very limited application in rheumatoid arthritis.

This brief survey of the rôle of surgery in chronic arthritis may help to indicate that the outlook, even in the arthritic derelict, may not be so hopeless as has been previously thought. Success depends upon the close co-operation of physicians and surgeons who have made a special study of the problems presented by the chronic rheumatic diseases.

APPENDIX

METHODS OF APPLYING LOCAL HEAT

Dry Heat.—Salt or sand retains heat for a considerable period and may be used when other methods of applying dry heat are not available. The amount required varies with the part to be treated. Enough must be used to completely cover or enclose the group of muscles or joint affected by the disease. The substance is heated in a metal container over a fire or in an oven, and is applied directly to the part or filled into sand-bags which are then packed around it. Hot-water bottles of the rubber-bag variety can be applied to a painful area or moulded to a joint and are available in the majority of homes. They should be held firmly in place by a bandage or a flannel binder. Electrically heated pads which can be plugged into any electric-light socket can be purchased cheaply and are very handy. The pad is applied over the part to be treated and the controlling switch turned to full. When the temperature begins to cause discomfort the current is reduced. These pads can be kept in position for two to three hours. The old-fashioned method of applying local heat by means of a hot iron over a towel or brown paper may afford relief in cases of fibrositis of the spinal and gluteal muscles. Radiant heat and infra-red lamps form clean and efficient sources of heat. Such lamps cost approximately 30s. and last for many years. An electric radiator or gas fire can be used if the patient cannot afford a portable lamp, and are satisfactory but not so handy. Exposure to radiant heat or infra-red rays should not exceed fifteen to twenty minutes at a distance of 2 ft. The time of exposure will vary in each individual case, depending on personal sensitivity, and care should be taken particularly with the first two or three exposures to avoid over-exposure, which may cause burns.

Moist Heat.—A simple method of applying moist heat is by means of a mud-pack. Pistany mud can be bought in the form of dried cubes or in a compress ready for use. Boiling water is added to the dried mud and the temperature adjusted to 110° to 115° F. The mud is then applied directly to the painful muscles or joints and covered with a waterproof sheet and a blanket. The pack remains in position for one to two hours. In the case of the mud compress it is dipped into hot water (temperature 120° F.), shaken and applied in the same way as the dried mud. The initial cost is twenty-one shillings for the compress and twelve shillings per cube, but the mud or compress can be used repeatedly. Packs made from powdered Fuller's earth form a cheap and effective substitute for spa mud. The earth can be purchased in bulk for a few pence a pound. It is mixed with hot water, spread on calico or linen and applied as described above. Peat is also employed for this purpose and can be bought in convenient packages for home use. Another convenient method for applying local moist heat is the use of cataplasma kaolin or antiphlogistine poultices. The material is packed in tins and is heated by placing the tin and contents in a pan of boiling water. When thoroughly hot the contents are spread on calico or linen and applied as already described to the affected joint or muscle. It should be left in position for two to three hours.

Paraffin-wax Baths.—One of the best methods of applying local heat is by means of paraffin-wax baths. The wax can be obtained in bulk from oil merchants or through any chemist. A double boiler or steamer is used to melt the wax, the melting-point of which is around 110° F. The receptacle should be of sufficient size to permit the immersion of a hand or foot. When the limb has been immersed the patient should be instructed to keep it perfectly still for a few seconds or the sensation of heat may become unbearable. It is withdrawn and immersed repeatedly, the wax being allowed to solidify on the limb after each immersion, until five or six coats of wax have been applied. The part is then wrapped up in jaconette and cotton wool for twenty to thirty minutes. The skin perspires freely beneath the wax and a local vapour bath is formed. At the end of the treatment the wax is easily peeled off and leaves an intense erythema of the skin which lasts for some time. The wax can be used again and again. This method is very valuable in the treatment of hands and feet of those affected by rheumatoid arthritis. Pain is eased and movement of the joints is improved. When the affected joint cannot be immersed in the wax (knee, shoulder, etc.), several coats of hot wax are applied by means of a large paint brush, jaconette and cotton wool being used to retain the heat as before.

Glove Bath.—A method devised by Ray for the local application of heat to the hands or feet has been found to be of service. The hand or foot is covered by a rubber glove or rubber sock several sizes too large, and then immersed in water at a temperature of about 110° F. for fifteen to twenty minutes. The skin perspires freely within the rubber covering, pain is relieved and movement improved. The effect of this form of treatment can be enhanced by the application to the limb, before it is covered with the rubber, of oil of wintergreen or iodine.

All the methods outlined can be used in the home and are comparatively cheap. More elaborate procedures are available in the hydrological establishments at the spas, but those described above are equally efficient and the average patient or his friends can readily be taught to use them effectively.

MANUFACTURE OF PLASTER SPLINTS

Wrist Splint.—Soak a plaster-of-Paris bandage 3 yds. long and 4 in. wide in lukewarm water, to which a little salt has been added (ʒi to ʒii to a basin of water). On a smooth surface (a sheet of thick plate-glass is perhaps the best) make a slab 14 to 16 in. long by rolling the bandage backwards and forwards upon itself. As each successive layer of bandage is added it is rubbed smooth with the palm of the hand in order to get rid of air bubbles. When the slab is complete it is grasped firmly with the finger and thumb about 6 in. from one end and compressed into a bar (see Fig. 2), which is then placed between the first finger and thumb of the patient's hand, the shorter end of the slab being on the palmar aspect. This end is moulded across the patient's palm just proximal to the metacarpophalangeal joints, and round on to the dorsal aspect of the hand and wrist.

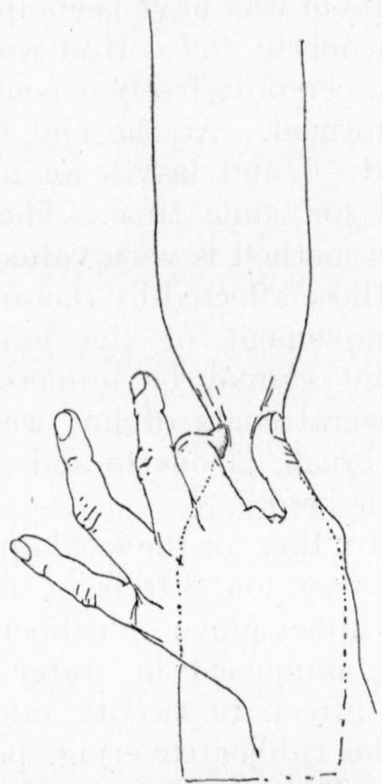

Fig. 2.—Showing how Plaster Slab is Compressed to Form a Bar by the Forefinger and Thumb.

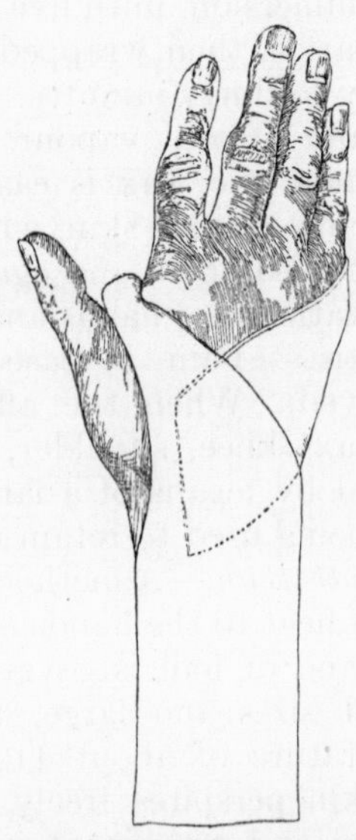

Fig. 3.—Showing the Slab Moulded into Position, short end across the palm and over the dorsum of the hand, long end over dorsum of the hand and up the forearm.

The other end of the slab is moulded across the dorsum of the hand and up the forearm (see Fig. 3). A plaster bandage is now applied to the forearm and wrist, which is held slightly in dorsiflexion and the transverse palmar arch maintained by pressure of the operator's thumb (see Fig. 4) until the plaster has firmly set. The plaster on the anterior aspect of the forearm and wrist is now cut away (see Fig. 4) and the splint slipped off. The splint is allowed to dry for twelve hours, after which it can be readily slipped on and off and when in use kept in place by a bandage (preferably crêpe) applied to

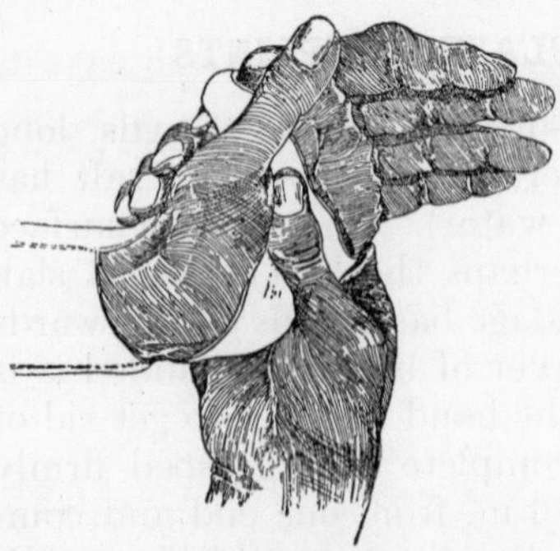

Fig. 4.—Showing how the Splint is Moulded to hold the Wrist in Dorsiflexion. Dotted lines on the anterior aspect of the wrist indicate where plaster is to be cut.

the forearm. This type of splint is used when the wrist alone is involved. In the acute stage its function is to prevent deformity and secure absolute rest to the joint. In the subacute and chronic stages, where flexion deformity of the wrist already exists, a series of these plasters may be used for its correction, according to the technique already described for the knee (see p. 950).

Hand and Wrist Splint.—Make a short slab of plaster bandage 3 to 4 in. wide and 6 to 8 in. long, consisting of six thicknesses of bandage. It is moulded around the fingers and hand. Make a second slab 10 to 12 in. long and 4 in. wide, consisting of six to eight thicknesses of bandage. Apply it along the forearm, hand and fingers, overlapping the first slab (see Fig. 5). The two slabs are now fixed together with a plaster bandage. While the plaster is still soft, ulnar deviation is corrected, the wrist dorsiflexed and the palmar arch restored. When the plaster is firm, the splint is slipped off and trimmed in order to ensure its easy application and removal. When in use it is held in place by a forearm bandage, as shown in Figs. 5 and 6. The splint is used for rest in the acute stage, and correction of ulnar deviation and flexion deformity of the wrist in the subacute and chronic stages.

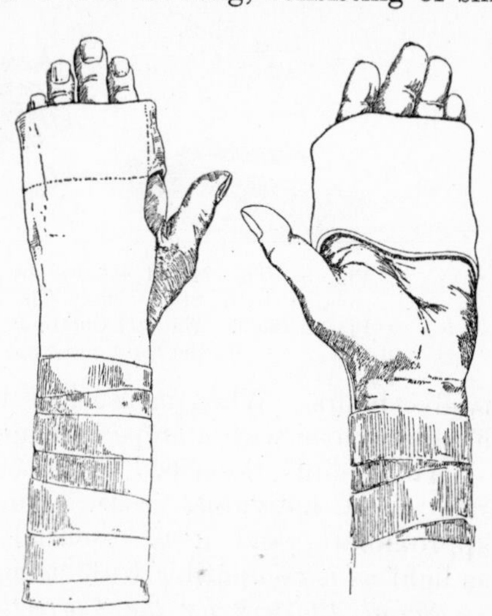

Fig. 5.—Hand and Wrist Splint—Posterior Aspect.

Fig. 6.—Hand and Wrist Splint—Anterior Aspect.

Rest Splint for Use in the Acute Stage of Rheumatoid Arthritis.—For the manufacture of this type of splint a mould is required, consisting of a length of aluminium 4 in. wide and about 18 in. long. It is bent at one end so as to form an eminence upon which the hand rests (see Fig. 7).

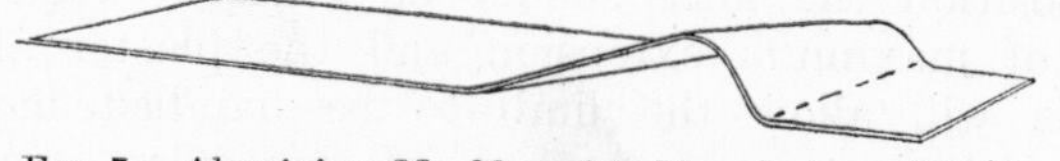

Fig. 7.—Aluminium Mould used in Manufacture of Rest Splint for Hand and Wrist.

The mould is covered with a single layer of stockinette and a plaster slab is made and placed upon the mould. The slab should overlap slightly around the edges of the aluminium. The patient's hand and forearm are then pressed on the slab (see Fig. 8) and the stockinette pulled tight over them, the thumb being left free. This has the effect of moulding the plaster firmly to the limb. When the plaster has become set, the splint is removed and trimmed and allowed to dry for

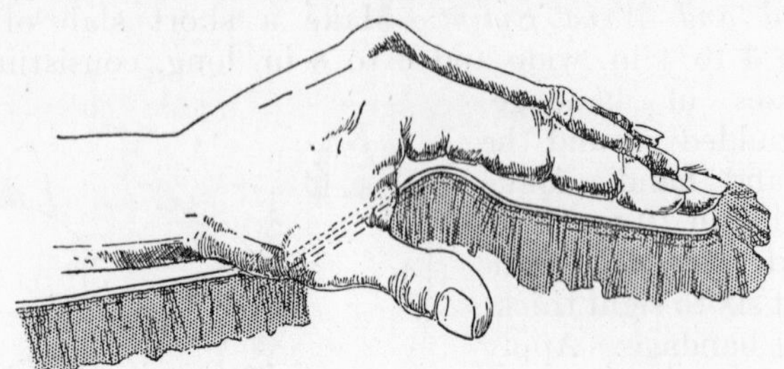

FIG. 8.—The Mould (shown by dotted lines) has been covered with Stockinette. The Hand is resting on the Plaster Slab. The stockinette is used to mould the slab to the hand and wrist as described.

twelve hours. When in use it is kept bandaged firmly to the hand and arm with a crêpe bandage.

The splints described must be adapted and modified to suit each individual case. The measurements given are approximate, and it is essential that the splint should be as light as is compatible with strength.

Serial Plasters for the Correction of Flexion Deformity of the Knees.—The first plaster is applied in the position of deformity to the limb which is encased in stockinette. A plaster slab is made, 4 in. wide and five to six layers of bandage thick, and long enough to extend from the gluteal fold to beyond the toes. It is held in position by an assistant while the first bandage is applied from above downwards. The bandages should be 6 yds. long by 4 in. wide. In order to facilitate the application, the patient's pelvis should be raised on sandbags or a pelvic prop. When two or three bandages are in position the knee should be gently coaxed into the position of maximum extension and the plaster allowed to set. This will allow the limb to be handled more freely without inducing a recurrence of muscular spasm with subsequent loss of extension. A further four or five bandages should be used to complete the plaster, which should extend from the groin to the metatarsophalangeal joints of the toes. The portion of slab extending beyond the toes should be folded back so as to form a sole to the footpiece. Before the last bandage is applied, the stockinette at the upper and lower ends should be folded back on the plaster to cover the edges and prevent chafing of the skin. When the plaster is complete it should be marked with the date and the angle of the knee. On the following day (some workers advise waiting two or three days) the plaster is bivalved (see diagram) so that treatment of the muscles can be resumed. Great care is required in cutting the plaster, as severe pain may be caused by undue pressure over the tender joints and the confidence of the patient may be lost. Considerable experience in the use of plaster shears is required. After the plaster has been cut the splint is kept in position by a bandage or straps, except during treatment to the muscles (see Fig. 9). In five to six days a useful

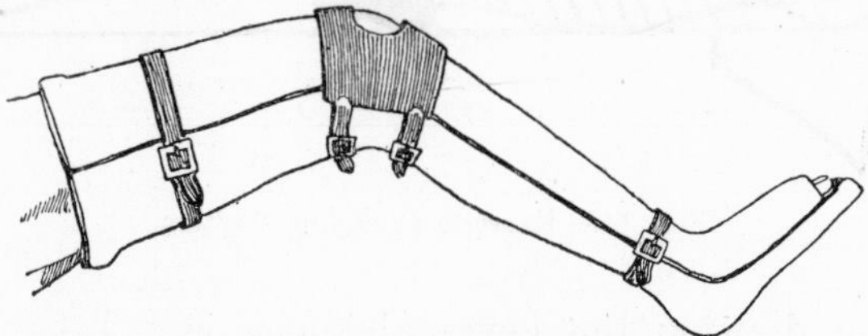

Fig. 9.—Serial Plaster Bivalved and Held in Position by Straps and Kneecap.

gain in extension should have occurred and a new plaster must be applied. The limb should not be removed from the first plaster until everything is ready for the application of the next, as spasm tends to return as soon as the support of the plaster splint is removed, and difficulty may be experienced in consolidating what has been gained. The application of five or six serial plasters may be required for the restoration of full extension of the knee. In more obstinate cases a final manipulation under a general anæsthetic may be required (see p. 920).

Wedge Plasters.—The principles underlying this method have already been explained. The only differences in applying

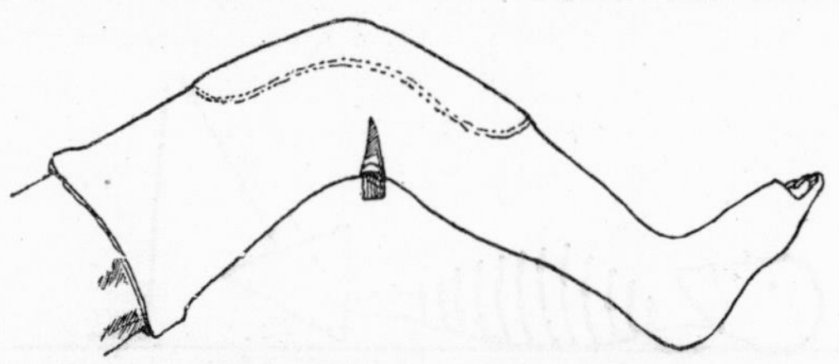

Fig. 10.—Wedge Plaster. Dotted lines show the anterior slab which acts as a hinge.

the plasters are the incorporation of a short anterior slab over the knee to act as a hinge, and, as a whole, the splint is rather heavier than that employed in the serial technique (see Fig. 10).

POSTURAL, BREATHING AND RE-EDUCATIONAL EXERCISES

Exercises for the Abdominal Muscles

Exercise 1.—Lying flat on the back with hands at back of neck or on top of head; if the back is hollow in this position, bend the knees. Breathe deeply, raising the chest; do not allow the lower back to lift. Hold the chest up and

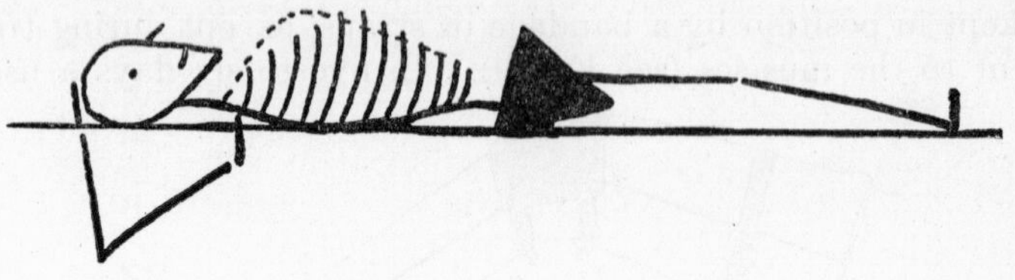

Fig. 11.—Exercise 1: Lying Position.

exhale by drawing the lower abdomen in. Take the next breath against the lifted chest; exhale as before, without allowing the chest to drop. The amount of breath passing is not important; the important points are the constantly lifted chest, which is pushed higher with each breath, and the exhalation by the inward, upward contraction of the lower abdomen.

Exercise 2.—Lying flat on back, hands at back of neck, chin in, knees bent. Contract the lower abdominal muscles with an inward, upward pull; tighten the buttock muscles and so flatten the whole back against the floor; relax and repeat. This is not a breathing exercise, but the chest must be held up and the chin in.

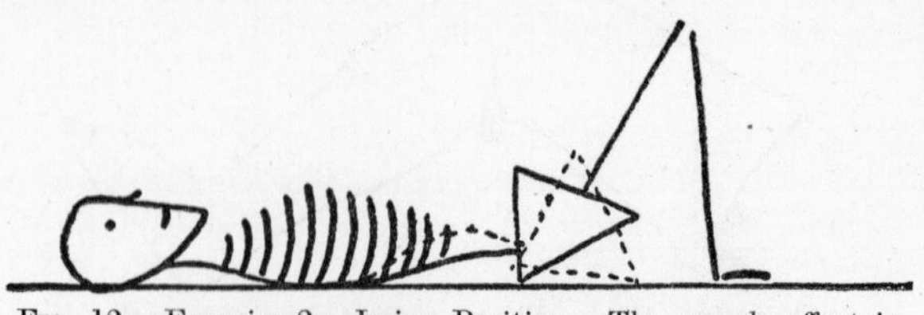

Fig. 12.—Exercise 2: Lying Position. The muscle effort is entirely in the pelvic region and low back.

Exercise 3.—Same position with bent knees. Bend one knee over the chest, straighten leg and lower slowly, holding chest up, chin in, abdomen in, keeping the back flat on the table. Repeat.

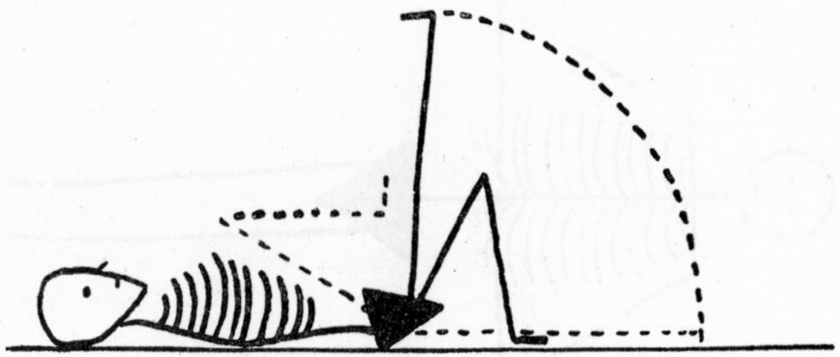

FIG. 13.—Exercise 3: Lying Position.

Exercise 4.—Lying flat with hands clasped on top of head, elbows back, chin in, back flat. Stretch one whole side; feel a lateral upward spread of the ribs; hold the stretch and slightly contract the lateral abdominal muscle on the same side; relax. Repeat, alternate.

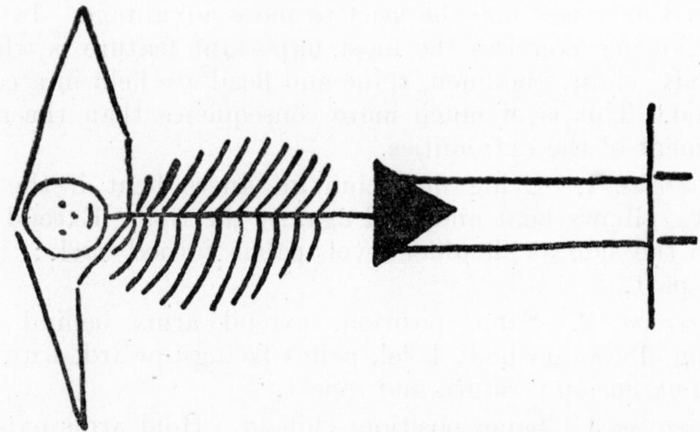

FIG. 14.—Exercise 4: Lying Position. Chest and ribs lifted by lying position. Ribs of one side separated by a muscle pull.

Exercise 5.—Lying flat, chin in, chest up, back flat. Grasp ribs at costal margins firmly with both hands, breathe deeply pulling ribs outwards; hold ribs out and exhale by drawing upper abdomen in. Hold the lateral spread of the ribs and inhale again, spreading the ribs farther. Do not relax until the required number of breaths have been taken. The amount of air passing is not important; the lateral spread of the ribs and the increased motion of the diaphragm are the points worked for.

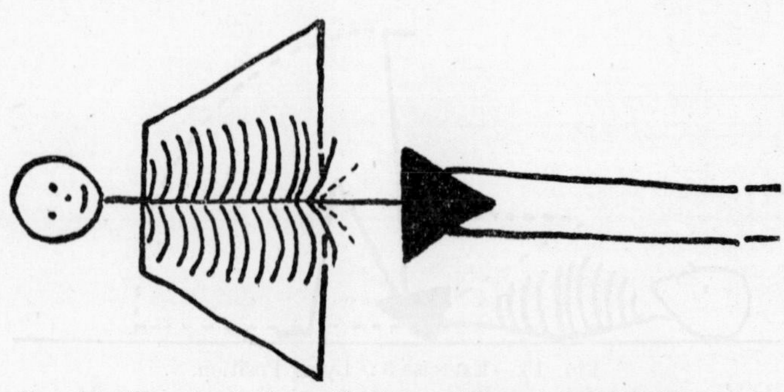

FIG. 15.—Exercise 5: Lying Position. Ribs and chest lifted by lying position. Lateral spread of lower ribs at inhalation.

ARM, NECK AND SHOULDER EXERCISES

Arm, neck and shoulder exercises in the same lying position are of more value than those done while standing, because the body is in good position without muscular effort and localized exercises may be used to more advantage. In all of the following exercises the most important feature is whether the body, chest, abdomen, spine and head are held in a correct position. This is of much more consequence than the actual movement of the extremities.

Exercise 1.—Lying flat, chin in, knees bent if the back hollows, elbows bent and held against the ribs. Extend arms out to the side at shoulder level, palms turned back; return and repeat.

Exercise 2.—Same position, extend arms behind head, keeping elbows on body level, palms facing upward, with arms at full extension; return and repeat.

Exercise 3.—Same position, chin in. Hold arms extended sideways at shoulder level; rotate shoulders and arms backward. Let the shoulders carry the arms in order to allow the rhomboids to contract.

Exercise 4.—Same position, hands at back of neck. Pull chin in, stretching back of neck; relax and repeat. Do not lift the head or shoulders off the table.

Exercise 5.—Same position, hold chin in, turn head to side; alternate.

Exercise 6.—Same position. Hold chin in, bend head to side, toward the shoulders; alternate.

Exercise 7.—Same position, arms straight at sides. Raise arm sideways to back of head, keeping them on body level; stretch whole body upward. Keep chin in and back flat.

Sitting Exercises

Sitting exercises may be undertaken when the lying exercises have been mastered.

The sitting position is preferable to the standing position as the next step in the progression of exercises. The reason is that in the sitting position it is easier to keep the back flat and the abdomen in. The first lateral flexion and rotation should be done in this position because the pelvis and hip joints are locked and the motion is localized in the upper spine.

Exercise 1.—Sit straight and tall, abdomen in, back flat, head up and chin in, hands on hips. Breathe deeply, pushing chest up and forward; hold chest up and exhale by drawing lower abdomen in and up; relax and repeat.

Exercise 2.—Same position, hands clasped on top of head, elbows back, chin in, head up, chest up and forward. Pull lower abdomen in and up; relax and repeat. Do not hunch shoulders. This is not a breathing exercise.

Exercise 3.—Same position. Stretch one whole side, spreading ribs apart, pull abdomen in; alternate. Do not sway or bend the trunk, but simply stretch the whole side.

Exercise 4.—Same position, hands on hips. Bend upper part of trunk to side; alternate.

Exercise 5.—Same position. Turn upper part of trunk to side; alternate.

Exercise 6.—Same position. Tighten buttock muscles; relax and repeat. Hold rest of body in good line.

Exercise 7.—Same position, hands clasped on top of head, elbows back, head up, chin in, back flat. Breathe deeply, pulling chest up; hold chest up and exhale by drawing lower abdomen in.

The progression of exercises is usually from lying, to sitting, to standing work. The progression is made from one to the other as soon as the patient has mastered the fundamentals of good body mechanics. The object of the whole series is a well-poised body with the least amount of muscular effort. If the poise becomes rigid or strained, the aim of the exercises has been missed. The effort should be to teach the use of the whole body in good anatomic and mechanical alignment, which means the least amount of muscle work, and therefore the least amount of strain and fatigue.

A good standing position consists of the following: Feet comfortable, straight ahead, with the weight well forward and on the outside borders; abdomen in, back flat, chest up and forward, head up, chin in, and body relaxed. To relax does not mean to collapse but to balance the weight of the body on the feet like a stick balanced on a finger. With the body in good line, find the balance point and live within. When such a position has been acquired, exercises of any type or theory or "ism" may be done with the greatest amount of benefit as long as they do not force the body into positions of deformity or bad body mechanics.

Exercise 1.—Stand against wall, feet 4 to 6 in. away from wall, head, hips and shoulders against wall, chin in; stretch tall, hands at back of neck. Push elbows back, breathe deeply, hold chest up, exhale by drawing lower abdomen in. Do not let the back arch away from the wall.

Exercise 2.—Same position, hands on hips. Pull lower abdomen in and up, tighten and pull buttocks down to flatten the back against wall; relax and repeat. Keep chest up and

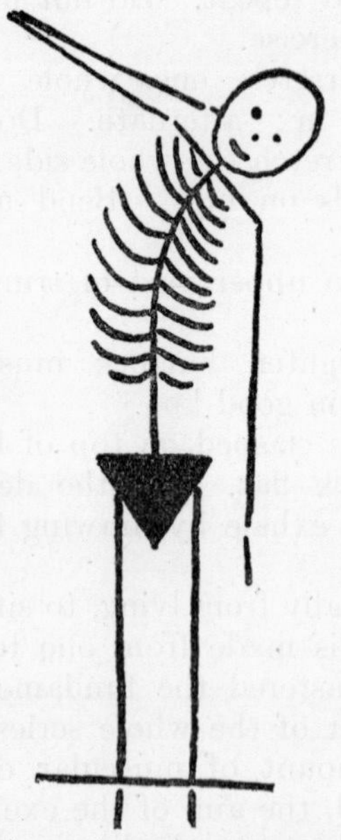

Fig. 16.—Exercise 4: Standing Position. Lateral flexion of dorsal spine. Hips and pelvis fixed. Elbow and head back, chin in.

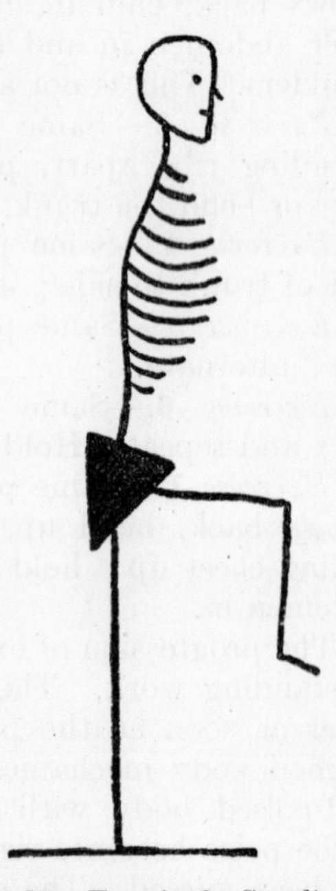

Fig. 17.—Exercise 8: Standing Position. Flexion of the knee and hip. Ribs, chest and head up, back flat.

chin in ; do not bend the knees. This is not a breathing exercise.

Exercise 3.—Same position ; hold abdomen in and chest up. Pull chin in, stretching back of neck ; relax and repeat. Do not lift shoulders or let head leave wall.

Exercise 4.—Good standing position, feet straight, weight well forward and on outer borders, head up, chin in, chest forward, abdomen in, back flat (Fig. 16). One hand at back of neck, elbow back, other hand on thigh. Bend upper part of trunk to side of lower hand, straighten and repeat. Do not let hips sway.

Exercise 5.—Good standing position, feet apart, arms held sideways at shoulder level, palms down, head up, chin in, chest forward, abdomen in, back flat. Bend upper part of trunk to side ; alternate. Do not sway at hips or ankle joints.

Exercise 6.—Same position. Turn upper part of trunk to side ; alternate.

Exercise 7.—Good standing position, hands on hips, weight well forward, head up, chin in. Stretch tall. Walk on straight line, make forward heel meet backward toe, toe in slightly

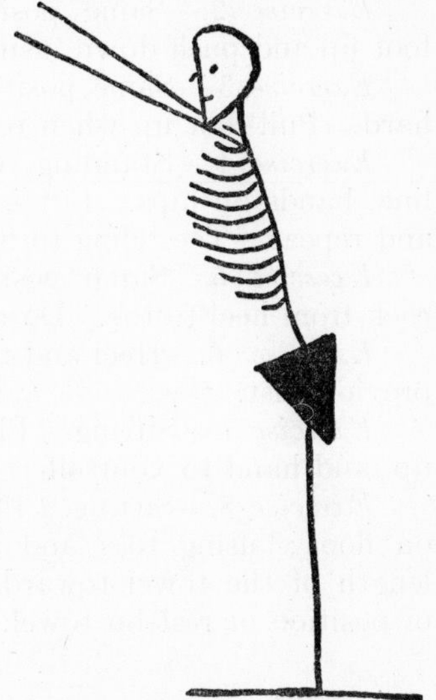

Fig. 18.—Exercise 9 : Standing Position. Forward upward lift of arms, chest and ribs, back flat and head up, weight forward.

Exercise 8.—Good standing position, hands on hips, stretch tall, head up, chin in, chest forward, abdomen in, back flat (Fig. 17). Bend knees up ; alternate. Do not allow the upper part of trunk to sway.

Exercise 9.—Good standing position. Inhale, raising arms forward and upward, rise on toes, stretch tall (Fig. 18). Let arms sink to side as heels sink, exhale by drawing lower abdomen in. Keep chest up and forward and back flat.

Foot Exercises

Exercises to correct faulty body mechanics should always include training in the proper use of the feet. It should be remembered that when a muscle is used in the right way it becomes stronger, and therefore before any foot exercises are given the patient should be shown how to use the feet properly. The correct standing position must begin with the position of the feet in weight bearing. The feet should be comfortably straight ahead with the weight on the outer border, toes on the ground. Use of the feet in this position means correct use of all the foot muscles.

Exercise 1.—Sitting, cross knees. Make half circle with foot, down, in and up. The inward, upward pull is the important result.

Exercise 2.—Same position, turn foot in slightly. Pull foot up and push down, using ankle joint.

Exercise 3.—Same position. Turn foot in, curl toes under hard. Pull foot up when toes are curled.

Exercise 4.—Standing, weight well forward, body in good line, hands on hips. Lift inner borders of feet, relax half-way and repeat. Toes cling to floor.

Exercise 5.—Same position. Lift inner borders of feet, rock from heel to toe. Do not let inner border of feet down.

Exercise 6.—Heel-and-toe walk on line. Described in previous list.

Exercise 7.—Sitting. Pick up marbles with toes, turn foot up, and hand to yourself.

Exercise 8.—Sitting. Place bath towel, folded full length, on floor; using toes and outer border of foot, draw whole length of the towel towards you. Do not let heel move out of position or rest on towel.[1]

Hand Exercises (*Active*)

Starting Position.—Sitting at a table with the forearm at a right angle and supinated to mid-position.

Exercises to Enable Patient to Flex Fingers.—1. Flexion of each joint of the fingers separately into the palm of hand, assisted by other hand or operator.

2. Place a small rubber ball into the palm and tell patient to alternately "squeeze and release." This may be made more difficult by using a soft piece of sponge.

Exercises to Overcome Flexion Deformity.—1. Placing the hand as flat as possible on the table and with the forearm fixed stretch the fingers forward as far as possible.

[1] We are greatly indebted to Drs J. E. Goldthwait, L. T. Brown, L. T. Swaim and J. G. Kuhns, the authors of "Body Mechanics in the Study and Treatment of Disease" (J. B. Lippincott & Coy., Philadelphia), for permission to reproduce the text and diagrams of the postural and breathing exercises quoted above.

2. Stretching fingers and lifting each up off the table separately.

Exercises to Obtain Extension of Wrist.—1.* Forearm supinated, hand over edge of table, wrist extension.

Same exercise may be performed with gravity eliminated, *i.e.*, with forearm in mid-position; or gravity resisting, *i.e.*, forearm pronated.

2. Place forearm on table, palm downwards; raise forearm up, keeping hand fixed.
3. Wringing a duster.
4. Climbing up the wall bars.

Exercises to Obtain Flexion of Wrist.—1. Same as (1*), except the arm is pronated in the first part of exercise and the wrist is moved to the flexed position.

Other Exercises.

1. Stretching the fingers upon the table, separate them as far as possible. If adduction is limited, adduct each finger separately to the middle line of the hand.
2. Forearm supinated, flex the thumb into the palm of the hand.
3. In same position oppose thumb to little finger.
4. With wrists extended and resting on edge of table, perform movements with fingers as if playing piano, taking care not to produce ulnar deviation.
5. Picking up objects (large ones to commence with) such as a reel of cotton with the thumb and each finger separately. This may be progressed by picking up large pins, needles and small pins.
6. Writing with pencil.

DETERMINATION OF THE SEDIMENTATION RATE

The test consists of the measurement of the rate of fall of the blood corpuscles in a perpendicular column of blood maintained at room temperature (65° F.). A standard technique has not yet been universally adopted. Several factors influence the rate of fall, such as anæmia, the bore of the tube employed, the anticoagulant used and the length of time the blood is kept before the test is carried out. To obtain accurate readings an elaborate technique is required, which involves measurements of the cell volume of the sample and adjustment to a standard volume by the addition or removal of plasma. General practitioners have neither the time nor the apparatus for carrying out such a procedure, but a simple method is available (Westergren, 1926) which is sufficiently accurate for practical purposes. Westergren tubes are used, and these can be obtained commercially, mounted on a convenient rack. The tubes are graduated from 0 to 200 mm. The length of the column in millimetres of the supernatant plasma created by the sedimentation of the erythrocytes is noted every half-hour up to two and a half hours. For most purposes the one-hour reading will suffice.

The test is not diagnostic of any particular disease, since an increased sedimentation rate is found in all infections. In a healthy individual the sedimentation rate is 5 mm. or less in an hour. In the acute stage of rheumatoid arthritis the one-hour reading may be 80 to 100 mm. or even more. When the activity abates as a result of treatment, or during a natural remission of the disease, the rate decreases, but any intercurrent infection such as a common cold or influenza will cause a definite rise. If the test is carried out at regular intervals (once weekly) it serves as a useful guide to the progress of the case and the effect of treatment. In addition, it is of value as a diagnostic procedure, particularly in chronic arthritis, as a normal sedimentation rate favours a diagnosis of a degenerative or traumatic condition (osteo-arthritis) rather than a toxic or infective state (rheumatoid arthritis, focal arthritis, etc.).

Method.—Five cubic centimetres of blood are withdrawn from a vein into a dry sterile syringe and immediately ejected into a clean tube containing crystals of potassium oxalate. The amount of anticoagulant required is approximately 2 mg. per cubic centimetre of blood. For 5 c.c. of blood this is roughly the amount which can be conveniently picked up on to the point of a penknife. The blood and anticoagulant must be well mixed by repeatedly inverting the tube. The test should be done as soon as possible after the withdrawal of the blood and certainly within three hours. The Westergren tube is filled by sucking the oxalated blood up to the zero mark and then mounted in the rack provided. Readings are taken at half-hourly intervals, but in most cases the one-hour reading will suffice.

The Organization of a Rheumatism Clinic.—As has already been emphasized, a prolonged stay in hospital is often essential for the treatment of arthritis, especially of the rheumatoid type. On discharge from hospital the patient has to readjust himself to a mode of existence demanding the assumption of a certain degree of independence and responsibility, and too often finds himself unequal to the task. If the best results are to be obtained from institutional treatment, provision must be made for the supervision of such patients on their return to home and occupation. Accordingly an important function of a hospital or clinic for the treatment of chronic rheumatic disease is the provision of a social service department to undertake the care and supervision of patients after their discharge. This service is particularly required for those patients who, for medical or financial reasons, are unable to report at the clinic at regular intervals for medical and orthopædic overhaul. Certain members of the social service department must receive special instruction in the various problems peculiar to the chronic rheumatic diseases. They must visit these patients at regular intervals and report progress to the physician in charge of the case. It is also their duty to improve home conditions where these are unfavourable (see p. 892), and to help the patient find employment which will not predispose to exacerbations of the disease (see p. 893).

It has long been recognized that severe mental shock, profound emotional disturbance and long-continued states of worry and anxiety appear to be of ætiological importance in initiating the onset or precipitating a relapse in patients suffering from rheumatoid arthritis. The psychological aspect is also of importance in patients who, after months or even years in bed, have lost the desire to assume once more the responsibility of independent existence. The correction of this mental attitude is essential, and requires the most careful consideration of the medical and social service. It is only by close co-operation and prolonged supervision that the full benefit of treatment can be ensured.

Occupational Therapy.—One of the most difficult aspects of the treatment of arthritis of the rheumatoid type is the rehabilitation of the patient once the active stage of the disease has passed. Re-educational exercises, physiotherapy, etc. (see p. 915), may do much to improve movement and muscular tone, but restoration of full function in the affected limbs may be very difficult to obtain. In American clinics, occupational therapy has been used with great success for this purpose. Weaving, using a loom driven by hand or foot controls, basket work, metal work, leather work and painting are examples of the types of work employed. The selection of the occupation is determined by the degree of incapacity present and the particular joints involved. In addition to its therapeutic use in restoring function, occupational therapy provides a psychological stimulus of great value. The patient's interest is aroused and his mental outlook improved. Many patients acquire a high degree of skill, and the sale of articles manufactured may provide a source of income where return to a former occupation is impossible.

GOUT

Gout is a disease characterized by recurring attacks of acute pain, swelling and inflammation affecting a joint or joints, and by the deposition of sodium biurate in the form of tophi in and around joints, in bursæ and in the cartilage of the ears. The disease is associated with an inherent abnormality of purine metabolism. The joint most commonly involved is the metatarso-phalangeal joint of the big toe. Gout is extremely rare in women. In the majority of cases a hereditary factor plays some part. A proportion of cases of fibrositis affecting muscles, tendon sheaths and fascial planes are believed to have a gouty basis. As the disease progresses the condition tends to become chronic, and osteo-arthritic changes appear in the joints affected. Acute attacks are usually associated with dietetic indiscretion, but may be precipitated by over-exertion, excessive mental strain, injury, exposure to cold, or a surgical operation. They usually occur in the spring or autumn months. The blood uric acid is elevated at the beginning of an acute attack, but may fall to a normal level between-times. In more chronic cases it tends to remain consistently above normal (normal value in males is 3 to 3·5 mg. per 100 c.c., in females 2·5 to 3 mg. per 100 c.c.). The acute attacks are often preceded by symptoms of dyspepsia or mental depression and irritability.

Treatment of Acute Stage.—Because of the pain, malaise and slight fever, the patient is best confined to bed. The bowels should be opened by the administration of 1 to 2 gr. of calomel or a blue pill at night, followed next morning by a saline purgative. A mixture containing colchicum wine (15 minims), sodium salicylate (20 gr.), potassium bicarbonate (20 gr.) should be administered every two or three hours for the first twelve hours, and thereafter three or four times daily until the acute symptoms have subsided. The alkali is included because it is widely believed that it helps in the excretion of uric, although this is doubtful. Heat should be applied to the inflamed joint in the form of a kaolin poultice, and the pressure of the bedclothes avoided by means of a cradle. A lacto-vegetarian type of diet should be prescribed. Purine-containing foods must be reduced to a minimum. The total calories in the diet should be around 1,500, the reduction being obtained at the expense of protein and fat. Fluids should be taken freely, 3 to 4 pints being drunk daily. A glass of hot water containing 20 to 30 gr. magnesium sulphate or a glass of Vichy water taken first thing in the morning and last thing at night is of particular value. The diet should be constructed from the following foods which are low in purines or purine-free. Milk, cheese, butter, sugar, jam and fruit are purine-free, while bread, cereals, root and green vegetables, tripe and eggs contain less than 0·06 gm. purine nitrogen per 100 gm., and can be considered foods low in purine. Tea, coffee, cocoa and meat extracts must be avoided, since they are beverages rich in purines. Alcohol should be completely forbidden during an acute attack. If the pain is severe, analgesics are necessary. A tablet containing aspirin, phenacetin and codeine (veganin) or one of the barbiturates may be sufficient, but occasionally even morphia may be required. Under this régime the acute symptoms are usually controlled in a few days.

Treatment between Attacks.—When the acute attack has subsided, careful attention must be devoted to the patient's general mode of life.

Diet.—Uric acid in the blood and tissues comes from two sources: endogenous from the breaking down of the body tissues; exogenous from the nucleoproteins contained in the food ingested. Endogenous purine metabolism can be lessened to a limited extent by a reduction in protein intake and of the total caloric value of the diet. Purines from exogenous sources can be curtailed at will by dietetic measures. Therefore the diet in chronic gout is based on three principles: (1) low caloric value; (2) reduced protein and fat intake; (3) low purine intake. While the general principle must be maintained that foods rich in purines should be curtailed, due consideration must be given to the fact that we are dealing with a disease which will persist throughout the patient's life, and a more varied type of diet than that employed in the acute attack must be allowed. The degree of dietetic restriction must be regulated in each individual patient according to the frequency with which the attacks occur and their severity. The following articles should be excluded permanently because of their high purine content: Fish-roe, sweetbreads, whitebait, sprats, sardines, heart, venison, herring, mussels, liver, goose, kidney, bloaters. A small to moderate helping of meat, white or red, should be allowed at one meal during the day, and a small portion of fish at night. It must be noted, however, that the purine content of white fish, sole, haddock and cod is as high as that of chicken or beef. Fish with a high fat content, such as salmon, are generally forbidden, but their purine content is approximately the same as white fish, meat or chicken, while their protein content is lower. Their exclusion can only be justified, therefore, owing to a personal idiosyncrasy or because of their fat content. Plenty of green vegetables and fruit, fresh or stewed, should be taken. If the patient is sensitive to any particular variety, it should be prohibited. Strawberries, spinach and rhubarb are generally prohibited because of their tendency to cause oxaluria. Since some evidence exists that the ability of the serum to dissolve sodium biurate is reduced by sodium salts, it has been suggested that sodium chloride should be used sparingly both in cooking and at the table. It seems unlikely to the authors that the small amount of salt used could affect the level of sodium ions in the blood. In those cases where the gouty tendency is marked, all forms of alcohol should be forbidden. In less severe cases the heavy wines such as burgundy and port should not be indulged in, but a glass of claret or Moselle may be allowed on occasions. A little whisky, well diluted with water, may be taken without harmful results, but beer is best avoided. If the patient is overweight, it is extremely important that the weight should be reduced, due respect being given to the principle of limiting the purine-rich foods in the anti-obesity diet prescribed.

Drugs.—The effect of cinchophen and drugs of a similar type (atophan, agotan) in promoting the excretion of uric acid is well recognized, but their administration is not altogether without danger. In patients sensitive to the drug, toxic reactions may occur, usually in the form of a hepatitis. The danger of toxic reactions has been probably overstressed. If the drug is withheld from elderly patients with cardio-vascular or renal disease and from individuals who give a history of hepatitis or jaundice, cinchophen can safely be employed, provided the measures mentioned below are carried out. It is best reserved for those cases in which the gouty state has become chronic and where the blood uric acid remains consistently high despite dietetic treatment and the general regulation of the patient's life. Such patients may derive considerable benefit from a periodic course of cinchophen. The drug is prescribed in 7½-gr. doses thrice daily for a period of three to four days, then stopped for a week. The simultaneous administration of alkalis (sodium bicarbonate, 30 gr. thrice daily) is said to diminish the irritating effects of the drug on the stomach. Cinchophen should be discontinued when the blood uric acid approaches a normal level. Cinchophen, when given to selected cases on the above lines, is of great value in diminishing the number of acute exacerbations. Some recent work from America suggests that sodium salicylate is equally efficient in promoting the excretion of uric acid. If this is confirmed, there are obvious advantages in using this drug. Doses of 20 gr. three times a day for three days in each week are claimed to be adequate.

General Management.—Exercise in moderation is of undoubted value in the treatment of chronic gout, but over-exertion may precipitate an acute exacerbation. Plenty of fluids should be taken. The daily use of purgatives should be avoided, but an occasional dose of calomel at night followed by a saline laxative the next morning is often of value to the plethoric patient. Clothing must be warm, and the patient should be warned against undue exposure to cold and damp. A daily warm bath followed by a brisk rub down improves the tone of the peripheral circulation and promotes diaphoresis. Sufferers from chronic gout derive great benefit from an annual visit to a spa, where general treatment takes the form of vapour, hot air and immersion baths, while the spa waters, taken internally, have a mild diuretic and laxative effect. Mud packs applied to the liver are said to stimulate its activity. Local treatment to the joints in the form of mud and peat packs, wax baths and the other forms of physiotherapy described on pp. 945 to 947 do much to reduce pain and stiffness. The relief obtained by taking an annual " cure " at a spa is well substantiated in cases of chronic gout, but this form of treatment is best avoided during acute exacerbations. The British spas provide excellent facilities for the treatment of gouty patients, and their waters are as efficacious as those of the more fashionable Continental resorts.

L. S. P. Davidson.
J. J. R. Duthie.

DISEASES OF BONE

HYPERTROPHIC PULMONARY OSTEO-ARTHROPATHY

THIS condition occurs secondarily in chronic diseases of the heart and lungs, and rarely in long-continued toxæmic estates. The terminal phalanges of the fingers and toes become enlarged, giving rise to "clubbing." In the more advanced forms of the disease the bones of the hands, feet, forearms and legs may show thickening. Osteo-arthritic changes may appear in neighbouring joints.

The treatment is that of the primary disease. Should the joints of the hand and feet become painful on account of the osteo-arthritic changes, applications of heat in one or other of its forms may have a palliative effect.

ACHONDROPLASIA

This disease arises during fœtal life and affects bones which develop from cartilage. The long bones, skull and pelvis are commonly involved. Growth is stunted, but although deformed the bones are strongly laid down and there is no impairment of general health.

Apart from the necessity for Cæsarean section in female achondroplasiacs who become pregnant, no treatment is required.

OSTEITIS DEFORMANS

This disease was first described by Sir James Paget in 1877 and is commonly called Paget's disease. Symptoms rarely appear before middle life. The changes in the bones are those of a rarefying osteitis with new bone formation under the periosteum, giving rise to thickening. There is a progressive enlargement of the circumference of the skull, and the long bones become bowed and thickened. The blood phosphatase is raised.

Although calcium, parathyroid extract and vitamin D have

been recommended by various authorities, there is little evidence that any line of treatment exercises an appreciable effect on the course of the disease.

LEONTIASIS OSSEA

This is a descriptive term applied to overgrowth of some or all of the bones of the skull. The cause is unknown and no treatment has been found to have any effect.

OSTEOGENESIS IMPERFECTA

(Fragilitas ossium)

This is a rare condition in which multiple fractures occur during intrauterine life. The fœtus is often born dead. In those which survive the bones are excessively brittle and frequent fractures occur.

Treatment consists of protection from injury and careful surgical treatment of fractures when they occur. Phosphorus internally has been advised.

RICKETS

See section of Deficiency Diseases.

OSTEOMALACIA

(Mollities ossium)

This disease is now believed to be a form of rickets affecting adults. See Deficiency Diseases.

OSTEITIS FIBROSA CYSTICA

(von Recklinghausen's Disease)

This condition is due to tumour or hypertrophy of the parathyroid glands, and is dealt with in the appropriate section (see p. 449).

OXYCEPHALY

In this condition, as a result of premature junction of certain of the cranial sutures, the anteroposterior diameter of the skull is shortened and the height of the vault is greatly increased to provide space for the growing brain. The deformity is usually present at birth. Increased intracranial pressure occurs, giving rise to exophthalmos and eventually to optic atrophy.

Analgesics are required for the relief of headaches. When the signs of intracranial pressure become marked, decompression is advisable.

MULTIPLE MYELOMA

(Myelomatosis ; Kahler's Disease)

In this rare condition there is a diffuse new growth of a sarcomatous nature involving the bone marrow. The bones become softened and spontaneous fractures are common. Anæmia and progressive cachexia occur. The urine of about half the cases contains Bence-Jones protein, which is precipitated on heating the urine to 50° C., dissolves on boiling, and reappears on cooling.

X-ray treatment to bones may alleviate pain, but does nothing to retard the course of the disease. Death usually occurs in about two years.

OSTEOMYELITIS

Up to the present time the treatment of this disease has been a surgical problem, but in view of the success with which other infective diseases and septicæmic states have been treated by the sulphonilamides, it is possible that this form of therapy may prove to be of value in the future.

L. S. P. Davidson.
J. J. R. Duthie.

DISEASES OF THE NERVOUS SYSTEM

Introduction

RECENT advances in our knowledge of diseases of the nervous system have brought forward new methods of treatment. The importance of deficiency diseases and the discovery of the chemical transmission of nerve impulses have provided a new approach to the study of organic nervous disease.

Importance of Early Diagnosis

The neurologist has always laid great emphasis on early and accurate diagnosis; this is now even more important for there are several organic diseases of the nervous system which can be successfully treated only if they are recognised in the early stages of the disease. If, for example, a case of neurosyphilis, of spinal tumour, or of subacute combined degeneration of the cord is not diagnosed in the early stages, gross and permanent damage to the brain or spinal cord will occur, which could have been prevented had the proper treatment been instituted earlier.

Chronic Diseases.—There are still, however, many disorders of the nervous system the ætiology of which is unknown, and for which there is no known specific treatment. The proper management of such cases requires considerable thought and skill. When faced with a case of chronic progressive nervous disease the physician is inclined to picture to himself the plight of the patient in the later stages of the disease, and to adopt an attitude of helplessness and pessimism. This is, of course, unwise, for care should be taken to avoid depressing the patient unnecessarily. What the practitioner says to the patient will depend on the latter's intelligence and curiosity. He may simply point out that the condition is difficult to relieve, that the patient must have considerable patience, and he will see that a course of treatment is arranged. When the patient demands the name of the disease and the exact prognosis in, say, a case of progressive muscular atrophy, the patient may be told frankly that he suffers from a form of muscular atrophy, a disease which sometimes tends to get worse; that it is impossible to restore fully the atrophied muscles, but an attempt will be made to prevent the disease from progressing. Whenever possible, as in disseminated sclerosis, the patient should be told that improvement often occurs, or that the condition may remain stationary for many years. In central diseases, such as paralysis agitans or cerebral thrombosis, reference to disease of *the brain* may with advantage be avoided, as this often suggests insanity to the layman. Reference to degeneration of a *nerve centre* causes less alarm. The practitioner, however, should be careful not to give the impression that he is concealing the truth as to the prognosis. At the same time he must try to avoid making the patient lose all hope of betterment; the mind often adjusts itself to the future as the disease progresses with surprising equanimity. It is obvious that in certain circumstances the physician will be forced to admit to the patient that there is no hope of cure, that the cause of the disease is unknown, or that treatment is experimental; if the patient insists on knowing the truth he is entitled to have his questions truthfully answered. There are, however, many ways of being frank, and it must be remembered that the patient may have years of invalidism before him; it is no kindness to be unnecessarily blunt about the possible developments of the disease. The patient who boasts that the unvarnished truth has no fears for him should be viewed with grave suspicion—his bravado probably conceals a state verging on panic. The precise medical name for the disease is, if possible, kept from the patient, as it is undesirable for his own sake that he should consult medical textbooks. Terms like "muscular atrophy," "degeneration of a nerve centre" or "fibrosis in the spinal cord" will often satisfy even the intelligent layman suffering from bulbar palsy, paralysis agitans or disseminated sclerosis.

In most cases some form of treatment should be given which can be altered from time to time, but when treatment is given merely to let the patient benefit from the feeling that "something is being done," it is unethical to arrange for expensive treatment when something more simple is just as likely to help.

The patient or his relatives may inquire regarding various unorthodox forms of treatment. In such cases the doctor should consider the request patiently, but should point out that, for example, manipulative treatment cannot possibly affect the nerve centres concerned, and, therefore, that the treatment cannot be curative, though the quack will, of course, always claim that he can do good. When the patient is in poor circumstances a considerable responsibility rests on the doctor to protect his patient from being impoverished by unscrupulous persons who claim to be able to help him. When unorthodox treatment is insisted on, the patient may be advised to arrange the cost of treatment in advance. Certain patients suffering from organic disease appear to be incapacitated to a degree which is out of proportion to the severity of the organic disease present. In these cases any form of treatment, if given with confidence, will improve the patient's condition to a surprising extent. The suggestive effect of feeling that " something is being done " is very powerful in many of these cases, so it is not surprising that every form of " healer " at times appears to benefit patients suffering from organic disease. It is difficult and scarcely honest for the physician, knowing as he does the nature of the disease, to prescribe treatment for chronic nervous disease with the confident optimism of the quack.

DISORDERS OF MUSCLE AND OF THE MYONEURAL MECHANISM

Dermatomyositis.—Some muscular diseases fall to be considered here. Rarely the muscles are the site of a progressive replacement by fibrous tissue—a disease called dermatomyositis owing to the associated skin condition which is often present. No treatment is known to help the disease, which is usually fatal within two or three years, but sometimes the condition progresses to a certain stage and becomes stationary. The muscles should be given massage and passive movements to limit the serious contractures which occur. The patient should be carefully protected from catarrhal infections, as these are likely to cause fatal broncho-pneumonia. Active movement should be encouraged while possible. Ten grains of aspirin thrice daily often makes the patient more comfortable. In the later stages morphine may be required.

Volkmann's Ischæmic Contracture usually affects the muscles of the forearm and hand following a severe injury at the elbow. Here again the muscles are replaced by fibrous tissue, and recovery of the affected muscles is impossible. The affected limb should be kept warm, and massage and exercises should be given to help any remaining muscle tissue to contract.

The Muscular Dystrophies form a group of degenerative

diseases in which the muscles atrophy slowly and progressively. The condition is often hereditary. No treatment is known to arrest the condition, but glycine may be helpful. Glycine is a white crystalline substance and can be obtained in $\frac{1}{2}$-lb. tins (price about 15s.). One to two teaspoonfuls of glycine can be given thrice daily and continued indefinitely. Exercises to prevent contractures should be given—massage and electrical treatment are of no value in checking the progress of the disease.

Dystrophia Myotonica (myotonia atrophica) is another hereditary and degenerative disease in which the muscles atrophy along with other organs. No treatment is known to arrest the disease, but the myotonia can often be relieved by giving two 5-gr. tablets of quinine bihydrochloride once daily after breakfast.

Myotonia Congenita is one of the most remarkable of hereditary diseases. The condition does not shorten life, and the myotonia becomes less as the patient becomes older. Myotonia is the only symptom, and can often be relieved temporarily by taking alcohol or quinine. A pint of strong ale may remove the myotonia for three or four hours. Some patients find that they are greatly helped by taking 10 gr. of quinine bihydrochloride by the mouth once daily.

In **myasthenia gravis** the metabolic disturbance at the myoneural junction is the opposite of that seen in myotonia congenita. The disease often shows striking remissions in which complete recovery occurs for a period of perhaps many years, whereas in other cases it is rapidly fatal. The disease behaves to drugs in a manner which is the opposite of that seen in cases of myotonia congenita. Alcohol and quinine make the myasthenia worse, but striking improvement follows the administration of analogues of physostigmine. Prostigmin (Roche)[1] is the most effective of these. Two milligrams may be given hypodermically, preceded by $\frac{1}{150}$ gr. of atropine sulphate (to prevent intestinal colic). A striking improvement in muscular power occurs within fifteen minutes of giving this injection, and the improvement continues for four to eight hours. In some cases good results follow the giving of potassium chloride—a teaspoonful or more taken in milk or water three times daily. It is interesting to note that potassium salts and prostigmin aggravate the myotonia in cases of myotonia congenita. Some patients with severe myasthenia complain that the weakness is worse after the

[1] A concentrated solution of prostigmin, containing 2·5 mgm. per c.cm., is supplied in 5 c.cm. rubber-capped bottles.

effect of the prostigmin has worn off. In many cases, however, prostigmin can be given liberally with great benefit, and remissions often occur while it is being given. There is usually, therefore, no fear of aggravating the disease by temporarily relieving the patient with prostigmin. One of the most dangerous complications of myasthenia gravis is the development of a respiratory infection, for the effort of coughing quickly exhausts the chest muscles. In such cases the free administration of prostigmin—2 mg. every six to eight hours—will usually allow recovery to occur. In one such case a remission with complete recovery of muscular power subsequently occurred. Half-grain ephedrine hydrochloride tablets, three to six daily, and glycine as given to cases of muscular dystrophy (p. 972) are also of considerable value in treating myasthenia gravis.

Familial Periodic Paralysis.—In 1937, Aitken, Allot, Castleden and Walker reported that they could abort the attacks of familial periodic paralysis by giving by the mouth a single dose of 12 gm. potassium chloride in water. A mixture containing the drug should be available, so that it can be given to the patient on the mornings in which he wakens up paralysed.

Sleep Paralysis, in which the individual on waking up is completely paralysed for a period of, perhaps, several minutes, is very alarming to the patient, but is of no pathological significance. The only necessary treatment is to reassure the patient.

Muscular Cramps and Spasms.—The *muscular cramps* of tetany and tetanus are considered elsewhere. When cramp is due to polyneuritis, the latter condition should be treated.

Many normal people suffer occasionally from a painful contraction of a muscle or group of muscles. This may come on while the muscles are at rest and is relieved by exercising the limb and rubbing the muscles. Nocturnal cramp may be very troublesome. In some cases it is brought on by restless movements of the legs in a poor sleeper and may be avoided by the patient simply keeping the limbs quite still. One grain of phenobarbitone or 10 gr. of aspirin taken before retiring is also useful. A light meal only should be taken in the evening, and sometimes cramp is lessened by raising the foot of the bed.

Nocturnal "Jumps."—Some patients complain that, as they are falling asleep, they are suddenly wakened by a sudden jumping of both legs. Sleeping with the head as low as possible or raising the foot of the bed often removes this symptom, which may be due to transient cerebral anæmia.

One grain of phenobarbitone may also be required, especially if the patient is frightened by an associated sensation of faintness which makes him afraid to go to sleep.

Occupational Cramp.—Writer's cramp is the commonest form of occupational cramp (craft palsy), but the condition may develop in all those whose occupation involves the continued use of finely co-ordinated movement. The victim has usually had rather an awkward or stiff style of doing his work, and the cramp appears during a period of strain, particularly when trying to work quicker than usual. The condition is often termed a neurosis, but this is not an entirely satisfactory label, though nervous strain or anxiety will, of course, make it worse.

Treatment is always difficult. Two or more months of complete rest from the exercise which causes the cramp is the first step—a holiday from all work is desirable. The patient should be taught to relax the muscles, and regular exercises of a general type should be practised. Mental relaxation is also important. During the preliminary period of rest the patient may practise doing his work with the other hand or in the case of writer's cramp may use the typewriter—he can do any exercise other than that which causes the cramp. He must be fully warned, however, that all such exercises, and particularly his later attempts to resume his work, must be carried out with the muscles relaxed as far as possible. The conditions at work should be as comfortable as they can be made so that the arm and hand are subjected to the least possible muscle strain. The arm should be kept warm, and a firm bandage sometimes gives confidence. Whenever there is any suspicion of the cramp coming on, the exercise which causes it should be stopped at once, as fighting against the spasm only aggravates it.

DISORDERS OF PERIPHERAL NERVES

Interstitial Neuritis.—The peripheral nerves are frequently the site of a true inflammatory reaction. This type of neuritis may be associated with rheumatic manifestations, the investigation and treatment of which is considered on p. 886. Brachial neuritis and sciatica are common examples of this type of disease. The first principle of the treatment is to put the affected limb at rest in such a way that the inflamed nerves are relaxed. In many instances this rapidly effects a complete cure, especially if strict rest is enforced in the early stages of the disease. The treatment of any possible cause and the use of anti-rheumatic measures should not be neglected (see Rheumatic Diseases, p. 886).

In *brachial neuritis* the arm should be supported under the garments by a sling or bandages as though the clavicle were fractured. The patient will then be unable to put the affected arm in the sleeves of her garments, a movement which stretches the nerves affected. Immobilization should be continued until the pain is relieved. If pain is still present after a week, gentle passive and active movements of the arms should be carried out twice daily to avoid undue stiffness. Heat should be applied over the affected arm, which should never be exposed to cold or draughts. In severe cases rest in bed is advisable until the pain is relieved. Massage is better avoided. Unnecessary exercises which stretch the nerves, such as carrying heavy weights, should be avoided after recovery until all fear of recurrence has passed.

Cervical-occipital Neuritis.—When the upper cervical nerves are also involved with pain up the back of the neck to the occipital region, an attempt should be made to keep the head flexed laterally towards the painful side in order to relax the affected nerves. This may be effected by the patient wearing a cap day and night, the edge of which he can pin or tie with tape to the garment covering the shoulder on the affected side. The resulting relief of pain is often quite dramatic.

Sciatica is the commonest form of interstitial neuritis. Many arthritic and rheumatic conditions affecting the spine and pelvic girdle cause referred pains in the thigh, as also may diseases of the pelvic organs. These conditions should not, however, be confused with true sciatica, which is an interstitial neuritis of the sciatic nerve. Accurate diagnosis with regard to the cause of pain in the sciatic distribution is, therefore, important: the various rheumatic and arthritic conditions which affect the pelvic girdle and spine have been already considered. If they occur along with true sciatica, both conditions can be treated simultaneously. As in the case of brachial neuritis, any condition which impairs health, such as a toxic focus or diabetes, should be corrected (see Rheumatic Diseases, p. 886). Sciatica often follows exposure to wet and cold, and is often preceded by lumbago. Any obvious precipitating circumstance should be noted with a view to advising the patient how to avoid further attacks in the future. Sitting at a football match or driving a draughty car in cold wet weather might, for example, precipitate an attack of sciatica.

The same principles of treatment apply as with brachial

neuritis, and the sooner the condition is thoroughly treated, the easier it is to cure. Relaxation of the affected nerve can only be secured by rest flat in bed, and this should be advised even in slight cases in order to get quick relief. The patient should, if possible, be nursed in bed and not even allowed to sit up in bed to take his food, as this movement, which involves flexion of the thigh, stretches the sciatic nerve. Sitting in a chair is particularly harmful. Local counter-irritation is useful and may be applied by painting the back of the thigh and leg with tinct. iod. or lin. methyl. salicyl. alternately, only one application being used in the day. Massage is better avoided in the acute stage, and the physician should avoid testing to ascertain if stretching the nerve causes pain, as this test is often followed by an increase of pain.

These simple measures, combined with the rest in bed, quickly relieve pain in most cases, and after there has been freedom from pain for a week (or less if the attack is slight), permission may be given to walk a little, but not to sit. A gradual return to usual work is then allowed, but the slightest return of pain should be treated by a day's rest or sometimes simply by not sitting on hard chairs. Motoring commonly aggravates and may, apparently, actually cause sciatica.

Certain cases of sciatic neuritis are very resistant to treatment, and a number of procedures are available for more stubborn cases. If, for example, after a week's rest in bed the pain is still severe, the sciatic nerve or the epidural space may be injected with 50 to 80 c.c. of novocaine solution and normal saline. The technique for carrying out these injections is described on p. 1096. The epidural injection is especially useful when the nerve roots are involved in the neuritic condition—this occurrence may be judged by the state of the cerebrospinal fluid or, more simply, by noting whether a sneeze or cough causes a shooting pain down the line of the nerve. Both forms of injection can be repeated on two or three occasions if necessary. Manipulation of the sacro-iliac and lumbar joints and overstretching of the sciatic nerve under anæsthesia are sometimes useful, especially if there is clinical evidence that these joints are inflamed. Fixation of the thigh with extension applied to the leg or by plaster of Paris may both be successful in relieving severe sciatic neuritis.

Neuritis with Paralysis.—Neuritis is occasionally associated with paralysis of the muscles supplied by the affected nerve. In such cases the muscles usually recover after the neuritis subsides, but the affected muscles should be relaxed with the aid of splinting until the power of voluntary contraction returns. Galvanic stimulation of the paralysed muscles maintains muscular nutrition until the nerves have recovered. Light massage and passive movements are also useful. If the neuritis is so severe that regeneration of the nerve is required, then recovery will not occur for several months.

Neuralgia.—Most cases of "neuralgia" are suffering from the effects of interstitial neuritis of one or more nerve roots. Post-herpetic neuralgia, however, often presents a difficult therapeutic problem. The use of pituitrin in the acute stage is thought to lessen the frequency of neuralgia. The patient should be encouraged by the probability that the pain will gradually become less, but analgesics will be required, especially at night. Ten grains of aspirin with 5 to 10 gr. of veramon is often a useful prescription. X-ray therapy directed at the affected nerve root is sometimes successful. In a few cases division of the affected nerve root by operation is required, but even this operation does not always give complete relief. Opiates must be avoided strictly owing to the great danger in these cases of habit formation.

Trigeminal neuralgia is considered elsewhere (p. 1000). Other forms of neuralgia are best treated by local and general antirheumatic measures (p. 886).

Traumatic Neuritis.—The commonest cause for the sudden onset of paralysis in the distribution of one or more peripheral nerves is pressure on the nerve. Treatment of pressure neuritis consists in tracing the way in which the nerve is injured—often a difficult task—and in taking precautions to avoid any further injury to the nerve involved. Pressure on a nerve during deep sleep is a common cause of traumatic neuritis, and this is the likely explanation if the paralysis is noticed on waking from sleep. Certain occupations may injure a nerve through the muscular contraction of a closely related muscle: the radial nerve and the long thoracic nerve may be injured in this way. The deep palmar branch of the ulnar nerve may be injured in cycling and in many occupations. The external peroneal nerve may be injured during sleep, or by the habit of crossing the legs, and also in occupations involving full flexion at the knee. The treatment is the same as indicated on p. 976 for cases of neuritis with paralysis, but the relaxation of the paralysed muscles should be effected without splints if there is any danger of the splint pressing even lightly on the injured nerve. In most cases of pressure neuritis complete recovery occurs within two or three weeks, but if the nerve is so damaged that regeneration has to occur, prolonged treatment will be necessary.

Pain in Malignant Disease.—The involvement of nerves and nerve roots in cases of malignant disease causes a severe and very painful form of neuritis. In cases of spinal disease, fixation of the spine with plaster of Paris may give great relief. When the disease is likely to cause death within two or three months, the liberal use of opiates is the best treatment, and the dose should be steadily increased as the patient becomes tolerant to the drug used. When the expectation of life is more than two months the question of attempting to "block" the nerves conducting the pain should be considered. The operation of dividing the pain tracts in the spinal cord has occasionally been useful, but the recent discovery that pain can be relieved by the injection of alcohol into the spinal theca offers a better prospect of giving relief by a relatively simple procedure.

Intraspinal Injection of Alcohol.—The technique of this form of treatment requires special study and will not be described in detail here, as it is dangerous to attempt the operation without fully studying the method. The treatment is particularly suitable for the relief of pain in the pelvis and the lower extremities. Alcohol is lighter than cerebrospinal fluid, therefore when a small quantity is introduced into the spinal theca it will at once rise to the highest point of the spinal canal. If, therefore, the patient is placed so that the nerve roots conveying the pain form the highest point of the spinal canal, and if a small quantity (0·5 to 1 c.c.) of alcohol is slowly introduced into the cerebrospinal fluid at this level, the nerve roots conveying the pain become surrounded for a short time by a fairly concentrated solution of alcohol. If the operation is successful the resulting injury to the nerve roots is sufficient to relieve pain without producing anæsthesia or weakness. Unfortunately the margin of safety is small, and an overdose will interfere with sphincter control—a disaster to be avoided at all costs. Another difficulty is that the optimum quantity of alcohol varies greatly from case to case. It is necessary, therefore, to give a small injection of 0·5 c.c. first and repeat the injection if relief is not obtained.

Coccygodynia.—This painful condition of the coccygeal region which occurs in women may often be relieved by the epidural injection of saline (see p. 1096). The sufferers are often highly neurotic, and every effort should be made to allay the unnecessary anxiety which they have regarding the nature of the disease. Local operations are better avoided as they often fail to give relief.

Parenchymatous Neuritis—Polyneuritis.—*Alcoholic Neuritis.*

—This condition is not what its name implies, but is a *degeneration* of the peripheral nerves throughout the body, the longest nerves being most affected. Some of the chronic forms of polyneuritis, including those which occur in chronic alcoholism, pregnancy, beriberi and pernicious anæmia, can be cured by the administration of vitamin B_1. They are, in fact, deficiency diseases. The deficiency may be due either to faulty diet or to a failure in absorption of the vitamin from the alimentary canal.

Arsenical and Lead Poisoning.—Other forms of polyneuritis are associated with poisoning by substances such as arsenic or lead. It is possible, however, that these poisons act partly on the alimentary canal and so interfere with absorption.

All forms of chronic polyneuritis should, therefore, be treated with vitamin B_1, while obviously the patient should be removed from any possible source of poisoning. The vitamin should be given by injection in case there is some interference with absorption. There is no known risk of overdosage. One thousand international units of vitamin B_1 can be given in a 1 c.c. intramuscular injection daily for two weeks. Thereafter an injection can be given every three days until complete recovery occurs. A weekly injection of 5,000 units may be more convenient during the convalescent stage. There are several preparations available at a moderate cost—for example, La Roche market their preparations in 1 c.c. ampoules under the name of Benerva (1,000 units) and Benerva forte (5,000 units) (see also Vitamin B section, p. 404).

Regular passive movements and splinting are required to prevent contractures in severe cases, but massage is better avoided in the acute stage. After improvement has begun, gentle massage, exercises and electricity are useful.

Neuritis in the Aged.—In old people slight polyneuritis may be due to ischæmia of the nerves—a result of vascular disease. Treatment is the same as with general ischæmia of the limbs from arterial disease (p. 731).

Acute Infective Polyneuritis is an alarming disease which is closely related to, if not identical with, Landry's paralysis. The cause of the condition is not known, and vitamin B_1 therapy is probably of no value. No treatment is known to influence the condition, but complete recovery generally occurs if the progressing paralysis does not cause death by involving the respiratory muscles. While paralysis is spreading the patient should be encouraged by the fact that advanced paralysis often develops before the condition becomes stationary, and that, thereafter, gradual but ultimately complete recovery occurs. The patient requires careful nursing. Contractures must be prevented by pillows, sandbags, splints and gentle passive movements. A cradle is required to keep the weight of the bedclothes off the feet. Contractures of the plantar flexors of the feet with drop-foot are very liable to occur. If respiration becomes embarrassed, artificial measures to aid breathing, such as are provided by the Drinker apparatus, may save life. When the cranial nerves are involved, as in polyneuritis cranialis, they also recover completely if the patient survives. After improvement has begun, gentle massage, exercises and electricity will be useful.

Other Forms of Neuritis.—No treatment is known to influence the peroneal type of muscular dystrophy which is probably a form of neuritis. This condition often causes remarkably little incapacity and progresses very slowly. The same can be said of most cases of progressive hypertrophic neuritis. Vitamin B_1 therapy might possibly prove to be beneficial in these diseases.

Neurofibromatosis.—No treatment for this condition is indicated unless one or more of the tumours causes some special disturbance. If a tumour becomes painful or sarcomatous it should be excised. If one of the tumours causes compression on the spinal cord, or increased intracranial pressure, operative removal should be attempted.

DISORDERS OF THE SKULL, VERTEBRÆ AND MENINGES

Osteomyelitis.—The treatment of infections of the skull and of the extradural space is largely a surgical problem. Preventive measures are particularly important, and it should be remembered that serious infection of the skull may be caused by a small wound which perhaps on the surface looks negligible compared with other injuries present. It is dangerous, therefore, to neglect even a small scalp wound. The treatment of spreading infection from the ear and nasal sinuses is also a surgical problem, but when signs of meningitis appear in association with skull infections, treatment of the meningitis should be instituted (see p. 981). Osteomyelitis of the spine is usually fatal, but in some cases the infection is of a low grade and forms an extradural abscess which compresses the spinal cord. Operative relief should always be attempted without, of course, opening the dura mater.

Pott's Disease.—Tuberculous disease of the spine requires prolonged orthopædic treatment which aims at preserving the straightness of the spine until healing occurs. Treatment in hospital with fixation of the spine may be required for a period of one to two years, and general antituberculous measures should not be neglected. Signs, if any, of compression of the cord usually disappear when the spine has been immobilized with extension for a few weeks. If, however, serious signs of progressive pressure on the spinal cord develop, either while the disease is active or in patients suffering from healed spinal disease, an attempt should be made to decompress the cord by laminectomy.

The treatment of syphilitic disease is considered on p. 206.

Meningitis.—Meningitis is always a dangerous disease, but there are certain forms of the disease in which recovery may occur if suitable treatment is instituted at an early stage. Early diagnosis is a matter of vital importance, and this can only be made accurately by examination of the cerebrospinal fluid. Withdrawal of cerebrospinal fluid is also a most valuable therapeutic measure in cases of meningitis, especially if carried out in the early stages of the disease. Lumbar puncture should, therefore, be performed *without any delay* in all cases of suspected meningitis. The technique of lumbar puncture and the method of measuring the pressure of the spinal fluid are described on p. 1090. The operation is more difficult in cases of meningitis owing to spasm of the muscles of the back, but it can usually be performed successfully with the help of only a local anæsthetic; the latter should be allowed five minutes to act before proceeding with the operation, and an injection of morphine given half an hour previously ($\frac{1}{6}$ to $\frac{1}{4}$ gr. for an adult) will help to relax the muscles of the back.

When the pressure of the cerebrospinal fluid is raised and the symptoms and signs point to meningitis, the fluid should be drained off slowly until the flow has almost ceased. Full cytological, bacteriological and chemical examination should be carried out as quickly as possible to establish the diagnosis and to determine the type of infection present. If the tubercle bacillus is isolated, the outlook is hopeless, and further treatment need only be given to relieve symptoms, but in all other forms of meningitis vigorous treatment should be instituted forthwith. In the first place, arrangements should be made for the regular drainage of the cerebrospinal fluid by lumbar puncture at least once in every twelve hours. Operative measures to drain the fluid continuously are of no special value. The secretion of the fluid should be stimulated by giving the patient as much fluid as he can be persuaded to drink. The administration of fluid by the intravenous drip method should be considered if the patient is not too restless. Cisternal or ventricular puncture should be carried out when a block occurs in the free circulation of the cerebrospinal fluid. In those cases which progress favourably the repeated drainage of the spinal fluid should be continued as long as the fluid remains abnormal either as regards its pressure or its cellular content. Persistent headache indicates the need for repeated lumbar puncture in order to avoid the risk of a chronic state of hydrocephalus developing.

The specific treatment of meningococcal meningitis has been considered elsewhere. Antiserum (if used) is best given by the intravenous and intramuscular routes, as intrathecal therapy usually produces a severe meningeal irritation and is of little therapeutic value. Sulphonamide treatment has recently given most encouraging results in meningococcal meningitis.

Sulphonamide treatment now offers some hope of success in cases of streptococcal meningitis. Maximal doses should be given, as the disease is a desperate one (see p. 83). Anti-scarlatinal serum may be given intravenously but, as already stated, should not be given into the theca. No form of specific treatment lessens the urgent need for repeated drainage of the cerebrospinal fluid and for the administration of large quantities of fluid.

Sedatives and analgesics may have to be given freely. Chloral hydrate, veramon or luminal may be useful, but morphia is usually required to relieve severe headache: $\frac{1}{8}$ to $\frac{1}{6}$ gr. of morphine will often be sufficient, larger quantities being given if necessary.

Aseptic Meningitis.—The value of repeated drainage of the spinal fluid is well seen in conditions such as the aseptic meningitis or hydrocephalus associated with middle-ear disease or head injury. The arachnoiditis which sometimes follows spinal anæsthesia also responds well to spinal drainage, as advised above. In these low-grade infective or irritative processes, spinal drainage need only be carried out once daily. Occasionally these measures fail in cases of chronic arachnoiditis with hydrocephalus, and decompressive operations are then required. The thorough treatment of cases of meningeal irritation and inflammation during their acute stages will often prevent those adhesive processes around the brain which may lead to chronic hydrocephalus.

Tumours.—The treatment of tumours arising from the vertebræ, skull or meninges is largely a surgical problem, but certain aspects of these cases are considered on p. 1003. Malignant tumours arising primarily in the spine or skull are sometimes radiosensitive and are best treated by deep X-ray therapy. Secondary deposits of carcinomata in the skull often cause few symptoms. In the spine, however, they often cause severe pain, the relief of which has been considered on p. 978. Simple tumours arising from the meninges, skull and spine can often be removed by operation.

Injury.—Injuries to the skull and spine are considered on p. 1005.

Osteitis Deformans.—No treatment is known to affect the progress of Paget's disease. When compression of the spinal cord occurs, laminectomy should be performed.

DISORDERS OF THE BRAIN AND SPINAL CORD

Infections of the Central Nervous System.—*Pyogenic infection* of the brain may be blood-borne, but it is more commonly due to direct spread from diseased bones of the skull. Abscess formation is preceded by suppurative encephalitis. When the infection is virulent an acute form of meningitis occurs, and treatment is that of meningitis.

When an abscess forms in the brain without any associated meningitis the infecting organism is usually less virulent, and operative drainage of the abscess offers some hope of success. It is unwise, however, to operate hurriedly as soon as local signs of disease of the brain appear, for it is better to allow the abscess to form a wall before attempting to drain it. If operation is performed too soon the natural gliosis around the focus of encephalitis is interfered with. No attempt should be made to search for an abscess unless the neurological localizing signs of the abscess are clearly demonstrable. When in doubt it is better to wait for further evidence than to pass exploring needles through an infected operation field into what may be normal brain tissue ; more brain abscesses have probably been caused by this procedure than have been cured by it.

Chronic Brain Abscess.—In such cases the wall of the abscess becomes thick and tough while the pus contained in it may become sterile : complete surgical removal of the abscess with its wall may then be possible.

The treatment of other infections of the nervous system, including syphilis, is considered elsewhere (see Index).

Disseminated Sclerosis.—The cause of disseminated sclerosis remains a mystery, and the chief difficulty from the point of view of treatment is that periods of improvement constitute the most striking clinical feature of the disease. An important consideration in assessing the effect of any therapy is the fact that a definite course of treatment gives the patient a feeling of confidence which allays anxiety and nervousness. As is well known, any reduction of mental strain such as occurs when the patient has confidence in the treatment, will result in a lessening of the spasticity and tremor which are the common manifestations of disseminated sclerosis. Any form of treatment, therefore, if given with confidence, is likely to be followed by improvement in the clinical condition, and this may be further benefited by the natural remissions which the disease shows.

In the early stages, rest in bed is advisable when the disease is in an active phase and is causing weakness, ataxia or cranial nerve disorders. When the motor and other disturbances subside, the patient may gradually resume his normal activities and can usually return to work. He should, however, be careful to avoid becoming overtired. The physician should not allow his own pessimism regarding the future to alarm his patient, for both the patient and the relatives will become worried about the condition quite soon enough. If pressed for full particulars regarding the condition, he can refer to " small scars " in the spinal cord, and he can usually be confident that improvement will occur. If the physician is forced to admit that the patient has "a form " of disseminated sclerosis, he should point out that the symptoms often disappear for periods of many years. In the more chronic stages of the disease, he should emphasize that, while cure is impossible, an attempt should be made to prevent the condition from becoming worse. The question of the patient marrying has often to be considered. There is no appreciable risk of the disease being transmitted to the next generation, but pregnancy may cause the condition to progress more rapidly. The proposed partner in marriage should know that the disease is likely to cause serious paralysis in the future, and this is sufficient justification to advise against marriage. If, as often happens, such advice is disregarded, the physician may successfully advise postponement of the contract for a year or two, and during this period the progress of the disease may make marriage out of the question.

Specific Treatment.—New methods of treating disseminated sclerosis are reported every year, but, unfortunately, there is no proof that any therapeutic measure has any effect on the condition. The extreme difficulty of assessing the results of treatment in this disease has already been stressed, yet in a disease such as this some form of treatment must be given if only to satisfy the patient.

Arsenic is an old favourite, liq. arsenicalis ♏v thrice daily for periods of six weeks, or a course of six injections of N.A.B. Protein shock therapy (see p. 907) sometimes seems useful in spastic cases. High vitamin diets occasionally seem to give encouraging results, but the writer has also observed great improvement to occur on a diet grossly deficient in vitamins. The regular administration of 5 gr. of quinine sulphate twice daily for an indefinite period has been advocated. Treatment with vitamin B_1, vitamin C and injections of liver extract all have their exponents. There must be some cure for a disease which can cure itself for a period of years, but, unfortunately, it is not yet known.

Exercises.—Regular exercises are of value in re-educating ataxic limbs (see p. 1014). Massage is of no possible value to the underlying pathology, but when combined with passive movements often gives relief.

Later Stages.—When the disease causes severe paresis, every effort should be made to continue daily walking exercises. An advanced case should never be kept in bed, even for a day, if avoidable, as flexion contractures may develop quickly which prevent the patient from ever walking again. While in bed a cradle should be used to remove pressure from bedclothes, and the patient should practice moving the limbs; he should attempt especially to extend the legs by pushing against the end of the bed. Care with regard to these details may delay the painful flexion spasms which are often so troublesome in advanced cases. Regular passive movements three or four times daily are of real value, but great strength is often required to overcome the spasm of the muscles. Splinting to maintain extension at the knees will delay flexion contractures developing. Flexion contractures cannot be relieved even by operation when they become marked, but much can be done to delay their development. Careful nursing is required to prevent bedsores (p. 987).

Allied Diseases.—No treatment is known to benefit diseases such as neuromyelitis optica and encephalitis periaxialis diffusa which seem in some respects to be related to disseminated sclerosis.

Amyotrophic Lateral Sclerosis. — Progressive muscular atrophy, amyotrophic lateral sclerosis and progressive bulbar paralysis are now generally considered to be variations of the one disease. No treatment is known to arrest the progress of the disease, but it is desirable to attempt to improve the patient's general health by the eradication of septic foci should they be present. A slowly developing form of the disease occurs in association with a positive Wassermann reaction in the blood, and antisyphilitic treatment should be instituted in such cases (p. 216). The rate at which the disease progresses varies considerably, and survival for as long as five years occasionally occurs. Some form of treatment should be advised if only for psychological reasons. Electrical treatment is probably harmful, but gentle massage may be given. Injections of 5 c.c. of 5 per cent. calcium gluconate, which may be given twice weekly, have been advocated, but they are of little, if any, value.

DISORDERS OF THE SPINAL CORD

Myelitis is seldom the inflammatory disease that the name implies, for any rapidly developing destruction of a part of the spinal cord is given this designation even when the causal factor is injury or vascular disease.

Myelitis develops so rapidly that a section of the cord is often destroyed before the physician sees the case. When the disease is due to syphilis, antispecific treatment may cautiously be instituted (see p. 216); the prognosis is, however, very bad. When myelitis occurs in the cervical region of the cord it is usually fatal, but it often occurs below this level and causes paralysis of the lower extremities and lower part of the trunk—such a patient is said to be suffering from paraplegia.

Paraplegia.—The proper care of the patient suffering from paraplegia requires considerable nursing skill.

The care of the skin is of particular importance as bedsores are very liable to develop over bony prominences. A bedsore results from: (1) poor nutrition of the anæsthetic skin; (2) prolonged pressure on one area of skin (usually over a bony prominence), which causes interference with the blood circulation in the skin; and (3) chafing of the skin by faulty nursing. Treatment, therefore, consists of:—

1. Distributing the patient's weight over as wide an area of skin as possible and so avoiding much pressure on any one part. This is achieved by using a Dunlop pillow mattress or an air-bed and by taking great care to see that the patient's garments and draw-sheet are free from rucks which cause a local point of pressure on the back. The knees are kept apart by a pillow, and pressure on the heels is avoided by resting the lower part of the leg on a small shallow pillow in such a way that some of the weight of the leg is borne by the back of the calf. Rings of cotton-wool (" crow's nest ") are particularly valuable to protect the heels and other bony prominences.

When flexion spasms prevent this position from being maintained, the same effect may be achieved by bandaging pads of cotton-wool to the limbs in the best position to distribute the weight of the leg and to prevent pressure on bony points.

2. All pressure on the threatened skin is relieved every two to four hours by turning the patient, and the opportunity is then taken to keep the skin clean by washing with soap and water, drying carefully and then rubbing with methylated spirit. Finally the skin is covered with dusting powder, and the bedclothes and patient's clothes having been carefully smoothed, he is returned to his former position. If the skin tends to be dry, omit applying the spirit and powder ; and if necessary apply the following ointment by inunction to soften the skin : ung. zinci, 8 parts ; ol. ricini, 4 parts ; tr. benzoin co., 1 part. Longer periods of relief from pressure, which may sometimes be required, can be obtained by making the patient lie on one or other side.

3. All movements of the patient which cause rubbing of the skin should be avoided, the patient should, therefore, be lifted or turned into a new position, but never pulled across the bed. If, in spite of the above precautions, parts of the skin suffer from rubbing or chafing, a patch of elastoplast (not stretched) may be applied with advantage to the threatened portion of skin and left in position for four or five days, and renewed after an interval of one to two days. Skin over bony prominences around the knees, ankles and pelvic bones can often be protected from friction in this way. Such an application does not, however, lessen the need for relieving pressure on the part concerned.

4. The weight of the bedclothes should be taken by a cradle, and careful precautions must be taken to avoid burning the anæsthetic skin with hot-water bottles.

Bedsores are specially liable to develop over the sacrum, ischial tuberosities, crests of the ilia, greater trochanters of femora and the heels. The treatment consists of redoubling the care with which the skin is protected according to the above principles. In addition a special effort should be made to relieve pressure on the necrotic area. When deep sores develop, dressings should not be introduced into the depths of the wound, as these aggravate pressure on the injured tissues when the patient's weight presses on that part. Treatment with elastic adhesive plaster (elastoplast) has revolutionized the treatment of bedsores. However big the bedsore, and notwithstanding the presence of infection and necrotic tissue, strips of wide elastoplast are applied unstretched across the wound so that the purulent discharges are completely prevented from escaping from the wound. The plaster is left in position for several days, but has to be renewed sooner if the discharges escape from the sore. When the plaster is removed, the wound is washed out with peroxide solution, loose sloughs, if any, are removed, and the skin round the wound is cleansed and rubbed with spirit. After drying the surrounding skin carefully, layers of elastoplast are again applied. This process is repeated until complete healing occurs. The plaster acts not only by preventing friction, but the underlying pus acts as a cushion which prevents excessive pressure on any one spot. This method gives better results than any other form of treatment and relieves the nurse of innumerable dressings, but it does not lessen the need for preventing any avoidable pressure on the sore.

Care of the Bladder.—Retention of urine is a constant accompaniment of paraplegia, though after an interval automatic emptying of the bladder may occur through a low spinal reflex. The chief danger of retention of urine is that infection of the urinary tract is almost certain to occur, *especially if the bladder is allowed to become distended.* Great care must, of course, be taken to catheterize with aseptic precautions, but it is particularly important to avoid distension of the bladder by passing a catheter at least once in every eight hours. The use of an indwelling catheter is to be recommended if there is difficulty in arranging for frequent catheterization. When the spinal lesion is of such severity that recovery of bladder function will, at the best, be slow, suprapubic drainage should be instituted. It should be noted particularly that dangerous distension of the bladder is likely to pass unobserved during the first twenty-four hours following myelitis, secondary to spinal injuries, when attention is more directed to other aspects of the case.

Care of the Bowel.—Severe constipation commonly follows paraplegia. A daily enema should be given and a laxative should be ordered twice weekly. The regular administration of liquid paraffin lessens the danger of hard scybalous masses forming and obstructing the bowel. Abdominal distension may be helped by a subcutaneous injection of 1 c.c. of pituitrin, but rectal examination should first be carried out, and if a mass of hard fæcal matter is found to be distending and obstructing the rectum, removal by the finger may be required. An invalid chair and occupational therapy will help greatly towards alleviating the lot of these unfortunate patients.

Subacute Combined Degeneration of the Spinal Cord.—This

is now a most important disease from the therapeutic standpoint, for, as has already been pointed out, the condition can usually be arrested if properly treated, but if the disease is allowed to progress, paraplegia may be caused by irreparable damage to the spinal cord. The treatment is that of pernicious anæmia (see p. 482), whether or not anæmia is present. Treatment should be continued throughout the remainder of the patient's life, and the blood count should be maintained at the highest possible level with injections of liver extracts. The least suspicion of any neurological involvement necessitates the immediate institution of intensive anti-anæmic treatment (see p. 486). While intensive treatment with liver extracts is by far the most important remedy, the writer has reason to believe that injections of vitamin B_1 (as advised for cases of polyneuritis) have a beneficial effect in some cases of subacute combined degeneration of the cord. Exercises are of value in re-educating the muscles (see p. 1014).

When motor disturbances are already marked before treatment is started, the prognosis depends on the state of the spinal cord. The very spastic cases do not improve greatly, but those cases which show absent tendon reflexes or peripheral sensory loss usually respond dramatically to treatment, for in this type the degenerative changes are largely in the peripheral nerves which have power to regenerate.

Vascular Lesions of the Spinal Cord.—Vascular thrombosis within the spinal cord is a cause of myelitis and has already been considered (p. 986). Hæmatomyelia will be considered on p. 990.

A rare condition closely resembling intermittent claudication of the arteries of the legs, but differing from it in being entirely painless, may be due to impairment of the blood supply to the cord. The condition is liable to proceed to severe myelitis, but the writer has had some success by giving in such cases tab. trinitrin gr. $\frac{1}{100}$—one to be dissolved slowly in the mouth four times daily, and continued indefinitely.

Compression of the Spinal Cord.—In any case showing evidence of a progressive spinal lesion, the possibility that there may be compression of the cord demands careful consideration and expert study of the physical signs. Full examination of the cerebrospinal fluid with pressure readings should be made without delay. Compression will, at a certain stage, quite suddenly cause paralysis and softening of the spinal cord from which there can be no recovery. It is most important, therefore, to relieve the compression by surgical measures as soon as possible. When paraplegia has already developed, operation becomes a matter of great urgency. When spinal compression is due to a simple extradural tumour the results may be very satisfactory.

Syringomyelia.—Deep X-ray therapy often benefits cases of syringomyelia ; it should be applied to the site of disease as indicated by the clinical findings. The treatment may be repeated once a year. When cystic distension of the spinal cord causes obstruction to the subarachnoid circulation, laminectomy with incision of the posterior aspect of the cord may be advisable.

Spina Bifida.—The severe forms of spina bifida are incompatible with life. In cases of spina bifida occulta, a variety of motor, sensory and trophic disturbances may occur. Orthopædic measures to correct paralytic deformities are helpful, but sphincter difficulties, particularly nocturnal enuresis, may be troublesome. In some cases operation on the site of the spinal defect is successful in relieving tension on the nerve roots.

Injury.—Injuries to the spinal cord or cauda equina are usually due to fracture dislocations of the vertebræ, but "concussion" of the spinal cord may occur without bony injury, and may cause temporary interruption of spinal conduction. Fracture dislocations of the vertebræ often cause complete destruction of the spinal cord at the level of the injury, which, of course, results in permanent paralysis below the level of the lesion.

Hæmatomyelia.—Trauma to the spinal cord may bruise or tear the nervous tissues, but in some instances it causes a hæmorrhage into the cord. Hæmatomyelia is, therefore, often traumatic in origin, but may also occur spontaneously or as a complication of syringomyelia.

It is important in all spinal injuries with or without hæmatomyelia to locate the site of injury by clinical examination of the nervous system, and to immobilise the spine at the level of the bony injury in an extended position. First-aid workers should know that in spinal injuries the spine should be kept extended : this can best be done by carrying the patient on a stretcher in the prone position. An X-ray photograph should be taken which centres on the site of the injury, and, if this shows bony displacement, an attempt should be made to reduce the dislocation as soon as the patient's condition will allow. An attempt should be made to nurse the patient in a plaster jacket, but unfortunately the development of bedsores often demands the removal of the plaster of Paris. Operations on the spinal cord after injury are better avoided. The treatment of the resulting paraplegia must be carried out with great care (see p. 986), and particularly the bladder must be drained when the patient is first seen, and subsequently every eight hours, or an indwelling catheter used. Care of the bladder in the early stages will prevent the serious infections of the urinary tract which often cause death in cases of spinal injury.

Prognosis.—If on examination a few hours after the injury the interruption of conduction in the spinal cord is found to be only partial, then an almost complete recovery of function may confidently be anticipated. If in more severe lesions there is any sign of conduction in the cord two or three days after the injury, then a surprising degree of recovery may still occur. When, however, complete interruption of all forms of conduction can be demonstrated a week after the injury, the cord has probably been completely destroyed at the level of the injury. In fracture-dislocation of the lumbar vertebræ, however, a part, or all of the damage, may be to the roots of the cauda equina, and these may regenerate in the course of many months, whereas, no regeneration will occur in the tracts of the spinal cord.

The prognosis depends to some extent on the part of the vertebral column injured. Fracture-dislocations of the thoracic vertebræ usually cause complete severance of the cord, while in the cervical region, where the spinal canal is larger, gross dislocations often occur without the cord suffering severely, and it is owing to this fact that spinal injuries at this level often pass undetected. Injuries to the lower lumbar vertebræ also cause surprisingly little damage to the cauda equina in many instances. When the injury is to the cervical or lumbar region of the spinal cord, atrophic paralysis of groups of muscles in the arms or legs may occur, and the muscles affected in this way should be kept relaxed pending any possible regeneration. Galvanic stimulation and massage are also indicated in such cases.

CONGENITAL DEGENERATIVE DISORDERS

Congenital Diplegia.—*Little's Disease* may be associated with generalized rigidity and mental defect, in which case the prognosis is so bad that surgical and educative measures to improve the usefulness of the limbs are not worth carrying out. In many less severe cases, however, the legs are more affected than the arms, and the mental powers are unimpaired. In the latter type the child can be taught to walk, and operations to relieve spastic deformities of the lower extremities help greatly. Massage, exercises and passive movements are of great value if given with patience and perseverance. The condition tends to improve, and many of the milder cases live to middle age.

Infantile Hemiplegia.—During the acute stage of the disease (which is often a febrile illness) in which infantile hemiplegia develops, the child is unconscious, and removal of cerebrospinal fluid twice daily may be useful in relieving the increased pressure which is commonly present.

Chronic Stage.—After recovery from the acute condition which caused the paralysis, the child should be encouraged to move the paralysed limbs. Massage, passive movements and exercises should be given. It is unwise to give a bad prognosis within a year of the original illness, for in many cases improvement will continue for many months, though in others, permanent paralysis and mental defect result. It is important that contractures should be prevented. The child should not be hampered by splints more than can be avoided, but the parents should be shown how to stretch, at least twice daily, the muscles which are contracting.

OTHER DEGENERATIVE DISEASES

No treatment is known to influence degenerative diseases such as cerebro-macular degeneration, diffuse cerebral sclerosis and tuberose sclerosis. The same can be said of Alzheimer's and Pick's disease which occur in middle life.

Hereditary Ataxias.—The hereditary ataxias, of which Friedreich's ataxia is the most common, run a progressive course which no treatment is known to delay. The ataxia may benefit from exercises of the type given to cases of tabes dorsalis (p. 1014). Operations and appliances to correct deformities of the feet may be useful in the early stages, but when the disease is advanced the patient should be protected from surgical operations which cannot then possibly enable the patient to walk again.

DISORDERS OF THE EXTRA-PYRAMIDAL MOTOR SYSTEM

Encephalitis Lethargica (epidemic encephalitis) is a common cause of extra-pyramidal rigidity and tremor. This Parkinsonian syndrome may develop several years after the acute illness. In some cases the motor disturbances quickly reach a stage at which they become more or less stationary, but in the other examples of the disease the condition is slowly progressive and may ultimately lead to great helplessness. No treatment is known either to prevent the development or to arrest the progress of the condition. In many cases, however, considerable relief is derived from the regular taking of drugs of the belladonna group, which lessen the degree of muscular rigidity and relieve the salivation, which is often a troublesome symptom. They have been taken regularly for several years by many post-encephalitic patients without toxic symptoms occurring. The preparations more commonly used are hyoscine hydrobromide, tincture of belladonna and tincture of stramonium. The dosage is slowly increased until the maximum benefit is obtained without toxic symptoms developing. The latter include mental confusion, dryness of the mouth and gastro-intestinal disturbances. Dimness of vision, which is due to pupillary dilatation and paralysis of accommodation, often occurs. This symptom need give rise to no anxiety, and does not require a reduction of the dose of the drug, for it can be relieved by instilling one drop of $\frac{1}{4}$ per cent. eserine solution into each eye daily or less often as may be required.

℞	Hyoscin. Hydrobrom.		$\frac{1}{150}$ gr.
	Aq. Chlorof.	ad	2 fl. drachms
	Ft. mist. Sig., 2 fl. drachms t.d.s., p.c.		

The dose of this mixture can be increased gradually to 4 or 5 fluid drachms until the maximum effect is obtained.

Tinctura stramonii, B.P. 1932, is only half the strength of the corresponding preparation of the 1914 British Pharmacopœia.

℞	Tinct. Stramon.		30 m.
	Aq. Chlorof.	ad	2 fl. drachms
	Ft. mist. Sig., 2 fl. drachms t.d.s., p.c.		

The dose of this mixture can be increased gradually by increments of 1 drachm up to 8 drachms three times daily.

Oculogyric Crises.—It is usually impossible to arrest completely the oculogyric spasms which are sometimes troublesome. They may be precipitated by emotional factors, and some patients derive benefit from 1 gr. of phenobarbitone taken daily after breakfast and perhaps repeated after the midday meal. Benzedrine sulphate is sometimes of value in relieving these attacks and may be given in doses of 20 to 30 mg. twice daily. Benzedrine tablets (5 mg.) (Menley & James) are obtainable at a price of 3s. 6d. for 50.

Physical Treatment.—Parkinsonian rigidity may cause considerable pain in the affected limbs, which is partly due to the prolonged fixation of the joints in one position. Passive movements of the limbs relieve most of this discomfort, but in severe cases the manipulations have to be carried out every hour or two hours if adequate relief is to be obtained. The relative or nurse in attendance should be instructed in the movements required, and should not hesitate to exert the considerable force needed to overcome the muscular rigidity. The attendance of a skilled masseur is of value, but frequent inexpert manipulations by a relative are of more value than the necessarily less frequent treatment by the expert. The patient suffering from advanced Parkinsonism will often exhaust both the strength and the patience of those in attendance by his requests to be turned into another position. It should be clearly understood, however, that changes of position give great relief to these unfortunate people, and the enforced maintenance of one position causes intolerable discomfort and leads to great mental irritability.

Paralysis Agitans.—The Parkinsonism of paralysis agitans is inevitably progressive. Treatment is the same as is described above. The patient should have walking exercises daily even when the disease is advanced, for every effort should be made to delay the ultimate state of helplessness.

Wilson's Disease.—Other diseases which affect the corpus striatum include progressive hepato-lenticular degeneration (Wilson's disease), while chorea, athetosis and torsion spasm may also develop from diseases affecting this region of the brain. There is little or no prospect of helping these cases, but the treatment of Parkinsonism is worthy of trial.

Chorea.—*Sydenham's Chorea.*—Rheumatic chorea usually affects children. The prognosis is nearly always good as far as the cerebral lesion is concerned, but in a very few cases the disease is so severe that death may result from the exhaustion caused by the extreme violence of the involuntary movements.

Rest in bed with careful nursing in a quiet room is the most important part of the treatment. The child should be isolated from other patients to avoid excitement: screens should be used if the patient is in a hospital ward. If the movements are violent, precautions have to be taken to prevent the child from falling out of bed. If a cot or cot-bed is used the bars should be protected by pillows bandaged in position so that the patient cannot bruise himself. The skin is readily injured by chafing, and the application of elastic adhesive plaster over bony points will often prevent bedsores from developing. Aspirin or calcium aspirin given in doses of 10 gr.

three times daily can be given to a child of ten, and this often has a good effect. The child should remain in bed for at least a month, but associated heart disease may require a longer period of rest. Occasionally stronger sedatives are required, and $\frac{1}{2}$ gr. phenobarbitone may be given three times daily. In chorea gravis sodium bromide and chloral hydrate may be given in sufficient quantity to enable the unfortunate child to get some rest. Nirvanol has been much used in the treatment of chorea, but the reactions are sometimes so severe that it is better avoided. If there is great difficulty in swallowing, sedatives may have to be given subcutaneously, such as a solution of 1 to 3 gr. luminal sodium. Feeding through a stomach tube may then be necessary.

During convalescence the child should be encouraged to use his limbs in order to re-educate the movements. The apparent paralysis which may accompany chorea always recovers completely. A prolonged holiday in healthy surroundings is desirable and should be repeated at intervals of not less than six months for some years in order to lessen the risk of any return of rheumatic disease. Convalescent homes should be used in this way as a form of preventive therapy for children of parents in poor circumstances.

Huntington's Chorea is associated with progressive mental deterioration for which institutional care will ultimately become necessary. No treatment is known to affect the condition. The children of parents affected with the disease should be advised to remain celibate owing to the danger of their transmitting it.

Chorea due to a local lesion (usually vascular) in the nucleus hypothalamicus (corpus luysi) causes violent hemichorea, which may result in death from exhaustion. In other instances the movements gradually subside. The skin of the affected limbs should be protected from the injuries which the violent movements are likely to cause. Full doses of sedatives may be required, as in chorea gravis.

DISORDERS OF THE CEREBRAL CIRCULATION

Cerebral Hæmorrhage.—Cerebro-vascular accidents may be due to hæmorrhage, thrombosis or embolism. The prognosis in cerebral hæmorrhage with high blood pressure is always grave, and if blood is abundant in the cerebrospinal fluid, death is likely to occur within two or three days of the stroke. Treatment should aim at reducing the blood pressure. The patient is kept as quiet as possible with the head slightly raised on two pillows. An ice-bag may be applied to the head, and a pint of blood withdrawn by venesection. Great care is required to prevent bedsores, and regular catheterization will be necessary until consciousness is regained. A purgative should be given, and if the patient is comatose, one drop of croton oil in a little butter will be found suitable. The treatment of the after-effects is considered on p. 998.

Leaking Aneurysm.—When hæmorrhage occurs into the subarachnoid space from a leaking congenital aneurysm, the clinical picture usually indicates clearly that a spontaneous subarachnoid hæmorrhage has occurred. The treatment is as described above, but as the blood pressure is usually normal, the value of venesection is doubtful; the removal, however, of ½ pint of blood may help, and can do no harm. Morphine (⅛ to ¼ gr.) may be required to relieve severe pain in the head and neck. Lumbar puncture should be carried out for diagnostic purposes, and is sometimes of value in subsequent treatment. If, for example, pains in the head continue after hæmorrhage has ceased, the withdrawal of 7 to 8 c.c. of spinal fluid may give relief. Surgical procedures should be avoided in the acute stage unless progressive increase of intracranial pressure threatens to cause death: subtemporal decompression may then be helpful. Even though the aneurysm can sometimes be accurately localised, there is very rarely any prospect of reaching it by operation. In a few cases in which the aneurysm arises near to the upper end of the internal carotid artery, the ligation of this artery has been beneficial: arterial radiography which will locate the diseased vessel accurately is a necessary preliminary before any such operation is attempted. Fortunately most cases of spontaneous subarachnoid hæmorrhage survive the first leakage. The patient should be kept quietly in bed for at least a month and thereafter physical and mental activity should be strictly limited so as to avoid anything which will raise the blood pressure. Straining at stool is particularly dangerous, and can be avoided by prescribing laxatives in adequate quantities.

Cerebral Thrombosis.—When the diagnosis of vascular thrombosis can be made with confidence, stimulants should be given in an attempt to increase the blood supply to the brain. If the patient is seen immediately after the stroke it is reasonable to give a vasodilator as these patients usually have hypertonic arteries. It is possible that spasm of a diseased vessel may simulate thrombosis and in such a case a vasodilator would be of value. A vasodilator will also improve the collateral circulation and so lessen the area of infarction.

Amyl nitrite acts most quickly, but one or two tablets of trinitrin ($\frac{1}{100}$ gr.) dissolved under the tongue is preferable as its effect is less distressing. Alcohol is also useful as it is not only a circulatory stimulant but also dilates the cerebral vessels.

The patient should have the head low and the foot of the bed raised about 9 in. Purgation and venesection should be avoided. Stimulants such as strychnine and coramine may be employed.

Cerebral Arteriosclerosis.—Cerebral thrombosis is usually a complication of disease of the cerebral arteries. Where syphilis or diabetes is associated with the condition, appropriate treatment should be given. In most cases, however, there is little prospect of arresting or even delaying the deterioration of the blood vessels. A prescription such as the following may be tried :—

℞	Pot. Iod.	10 gr.
	Sod. Bicarb.	10 gr.
	Sp. Ammon. Aromat. . . .	30 minims
	Aq. Chlorof. . . . . to	2 fl. drachms

Sig.—2 fl. drachms t.d.s., ex. aq., p.c.

Mild sedative treatment is symptomatically helpful, and phenobarbitone may be used alone or with theocin as in theominal (Bayer) : for the latter preparation one tablet twice daily is an average dose. The mental symptoms which may develop are considered on p. 998.

Cerebral Embolism.—The treatment of cerebral embolism is in most respects the same as that of cerebral thrombosis. A vasodilator may be given in an attempt to dislodge the thrombus into a more distal part of the blocked artery and to open up collateral circulation. Stimulants should not be used as they may dislodge further emboli from the heart. The patient should be kept strictly at rest with the head low for three or four weeks to allow any further potential thrombi to become adherent to the tissue from which they may become liberated. The treatment of the resulting disturbance of function is considered in a following section (p. 998).

Venous Thrombosis.—Thrombosis of the venous sinuses may result from extension of infection from the ear, sinuses or skull. In such cases there is a grave danger of septicæmia. The source of infection should be promptly dealt with surgically, while ligature of the jugular vein may prevent the spread of infective material from the lateral sinus.

Thrombosis of the cavernous sinus is nearly always fatal,

and treatment is symptomatic. Infective thrombosis of the superior longitudinal sinus also ends fatally in most cases. Non-infective thrombosis of the cerebral veins and sinuses may occur, particularly in debilitated children, and may be a cause of infantile hemiplegia or paraplegia, the treatment of which has already been considered.

Treatment of the Effects of Cerebral Lesions

Mental confusion, delirium and aphasia are common effects of cerebral lesions. The patient is often restless, especially at night, and therefore requires considerable supervision. Incontinence may also be troublesome. Patient supervision and nursing attention constitute the main treatment of these cases. A cot-bed is helpful in preventing the patient from falling out of bed. A sleeping draught at night is often necessary, and paraldehyde in doses of 2 drachms is the safest, and can be repeated if necessary. Occasionally the hypodermic administration of $\frac{1}{4}$ gr. morphia with $\frac{1}{100}$ gr. hyoscine hydrobromide (repeated in one hour if necessary) may be required. There is a lack of provision for the proper care of these confused and often aged patients, and it seems to the writer unfortunate that there is a tendency to send such patients to mental hospitals.

Aphasia.—The patient who suffers from aphasia should be encouraged to practice speaking. Simple sentences may often be understood if spoken slowly, and aphasic patients readily know how to convey the negative or affirmative to a question, unless intelligence is greatly impaired. The power of recovery in cases of aphasia varies greatly according to the extent of the lesion and the age of the patient. In young children the prognosis is good and in all those cases in which intelligence is not grossly affected re-education by practising should be attempted.

Hemiplegia.—Recovery after hemiplegia of vascular origin is often surprisingly good owing to the lesion being often smaller than the original disturbance of function suggested. Unless intelligence is grossly impaired, exercises (see p. 1014) to increase the usefulness of the spastic limbs should be regularly carried out. Massage and passive movements are also helpful. When there is loss of positional sense in the limbs the prospects of improvement are not so good, and the patient must use his vision to direct the movements of his limbs.

Hemianopia when homonymous is always a troublesome disturbance of function. When, however, the mental faculties are unimpaired, adjustment to the disability is often surprisingly successful.

Pain referred to a paralysed side is often due to lack of movement of the joints. This can be prevented by frequent passive movements of the limbs: the shoulder joint is especially liable to be affected. Where there are abnormal reactions to pain on the affected side due to thalamic over-reaction, analgesics such as aspirin with phenacetin (10 gr. of each) may be required.

Ataxia due to cerebellar lesions can always be greatly benefited by regular exercises.

DISORDERS OF THE CRANIAL NERVES

Anosmia.—Inability to smell, which has been caused by head injury, chronic meningitis or other intracranial disease, is incurable.

Visual Disturbances.—The treatment of lesions of the optic nerve is that of the underlying condition. Papillœdema due to increased intracranial pressure will lead to irrecoverable loss of vision if operative relief is unduly delayed. When papillœdema of this type begins to interfere appreciably with visual acuity, operation becomes urgently necessary.

Retrobulbar Neuritis may be due to disseminated sclerosis or syphilis. In only a very few cases is the cause referable to the nasal sinuses. Good vision returns in most cases without any operative interference. During an attack of retrobulbar neuritis the eyes should be rested and 10 to 30 gr. potassium iodide three times daily may be given.

Optic Atrophy.—When optic atrophy is discovered, the possibility of direct pressure on the optic nerve by tumour or other pathological process must be carefully considered, as early operation on such a case may be followed by recovery of vision. Other forms of optic atrophy are very resistant to all forms of treatment. Syphilitic optic atrophy usually progresses in spite of treatment (p. 219). The prognosis in cases of tobacco amblyopia is good if smoking is entirely given up.

Oculomotor Disorders which produce symptoms usually cause either diplopia or ptosis. Treatment should be directed to the causal condition, but the discomfort caused by diplopia should be relieved by the wearing of a shade or frosted glass in front of one eye. The use of prisms is usually disappointing. When ptosis interferes with vision a prop can be fitted to a pair of spectacles which will elevate the eyelid.

Trigeminal Nerve.—Neuralgia referred to the distribution of the trigeminal nerve is commonly associated with pathological conditions of the teeth, gums and nasal sinuses. This form of facial neuralgia is relieved by attention to the local pathology.

In paroxysmal trigeminal neuralgia (tic douloureux), however, the pain often becomes progressively more severe notwithstanding the correction of all possible local infective or irritative processes. The milder cases of tic douloureux can be, to some extent, relieved by medicinal treatment. The following may be useful :—

℞		
	Pot. Brom.	10 gr.
	Tinct. Gelsem.	10 minims
	Phenazon.	7 gr.
	Aq.	$\frac{1}{2}$ oz.

Sig.—$\frac{1}{2}$ oz. three times daily.

Butyl chloral hydrate in doses of 10 to 20 gr. may give relief. Occasionally injections of vitamin B_1 as advised for cases of polyneuritis (see p. 979) are beneficial. The inhalation of 15 to 20 drops of trichlorethylene from a piece of gauze relieves the spasm of pain in some cases. The inhalation should not be repeated more than five times daily and the patient should lie down while inhaling the drug. Protein shock therapy has also been used with some success.

In many cases relief can only be obtained by interfering with the conduction of the fifth nerve. When the neuralgia is localized to one small area, the branch to the nerve involved should be injected with alcohol, as this may give relief for a period of years. When, however, injection of the peripheral branch of the nerve has failed, or when the neuralgia involves more than one division of the nerve, a more radical operation is required. In skilled hands resection of the sensory root of the fifth nerve proximal to the Gasserian ganglion is a safe and effective operation : when a neurological surgeon is available, this operation is the treatment of choice. In skilled hands injection of the Gasserian ganglion, according to Dr Wilfred Harris's technique, is also successful in permanently relieving many cases. The patient should be warned of the numbness of one side of the face which will be a permanent result of the operation.

Other Facial Pains.—Pain referred to the face may not have the clinical features of tic douloureux, and in such cases the treatment is difficult. Often there is no evidence of disease of the nasal sinuses or teeth. In some instances antirheumatic measures are helpful, especially if tenderness of the branches of the trigeminal nerve suggests an interstitial inflammation. Rest in a well-heated room free from draughts is helpful and can be combined with the local application of heat or counter-irritation. The administration of 10 gr. each of sodium bromide and sodium salicylate three times daily is also of value (see also section on Fibrositis, p. 931).

In many obscure cases of facial pain there is a large hysterical element, the facial pain being perpetuated by psychological factors (see p. 1016) after the original cause has disappeared.

In some doubtful cases the question of operation on the trigeminal nerve has to be considered. Operation should, however, be avoided if there is any hysterical element in the case, as in such circumstances it will give no relief. In others the effect of the injection of a local anæsthetic into the Gasserian ganglion may be tried in an attempt to judge the probable effect of operation. Such an injection can be accompanied by the suggestion that it will do good, and the beneficial effect of this combination is sometimes surprising. If temporary relief follows the injection of local anæsthetic, and if the pain is severe and of long duration, operation may be advised.

Advanced malignant disease of the mouth, tongue or base of the skull may cause severe pain in the trigeminal distribution, which can be relieved if the trigeminal nerve is interrupted by an alcohol injection of the branch involved, or of the ganglion as in tic douloureux.

The Facial Nerve.—*Bell's Paralysis.*—The most common lesion of the facial nerve is Bell's paralysis. Recovery almost always occurs, but the time taken varies greatly. If, two to three weeks after the onset, there is some return of voluntary movement or some contraction of the muscles to faradism, complete recovery will occur in a few weeks. If, however, there is complete paralysis with reaction of degeneration, recovery may not occur for several months or even for over a year.

During the acute stage the affected side of the face should be kept warm with a pad of cotton-wool. The paralysed muscles of the cheek may be relaxed by means of a piece of wire covered with rubber tubing, one end of which is bent into the angle of the mouth, and the other bent round the ear so as to pull the corner of the mouth into its normal position. Salicylates and iodides are often prescribed, but are probably of no value in this condition. A week after the onset of the paralysis electrical treatment may be commenced, and the muscles should be stimulated every second day with a galvanic current if no response to faradism can be obtained.

There has been a recent tendency in cases of Bell's palsy to decompress the facial nerve in the facial canal. There is no convincing evidence, however, that this hastens recovery. As the prognosis without operation is so good that recovery can almost be promised, there is no obvious justification for operation.

When facial paralysis is caused by disease of, or operation on, the ear, the prognosis is not so good. If after treating the case conservatively for at least a year no regeneration can be demonstrated, operation, such as nerve anastomosis, should be considered.

Chronic Facial Spasm can be ignored when it is slight and causes no inconvenience. As with all involuntary movements it is aggravated by excitement, and is relieved by rest and mental relaxation. When severe and troublesome as, for example, when it causes blepharospasm, relief may be obtained by damaging the facial nerve or some of its branches with an injection of alcohol. This procedure may give relief for as long as a year, but it also causes some paralysis of the muscles of the face.

Facial Hemiatrophy.—No treatment is known to arrest facial hemiatrophy. For cosmetic reasons paraffin preparations may be injected subcutaneously.

The Auditory Nerve.—The treatment of deafness and of inflammation of the middle ear is considered elsewhere (p. 764 *et seq.*).

Tinnitus may be caused by many abnormalities of the hearing mechanism. Some of these can be corrected by the otologist, but many are very resistant to treatment. Sedatives such as 1½ gr. phenobarbitone or 25 gr. sodium bromide taken at night may prevent sleeplessness. In a few severe cases destruction of the eighth nerve or of the cochlea by operation is desirable, but this, of course, causes total and permanent deafness of the ear operated on.

Vertigo.—In cases of recurring aural vertigo (Ménière's syndrome) any detectable abnormality of the ear, Eustachian tube or nasopharynx should be corrected if possible.

In many cases, however, especially when there is an associated tinnitus and progressive deafness, treatment has to be symptomatic. Sufferers from vertigo sometimes receive much benefit from taking regularly for a period of several months either phenobarbitone (½ gr. three times daily), or sodium salicylate and sodium bromide (10 gr. of each three times daily). A salt-poor diet (see p. 671) may also be beneficial. In severe and intractable cases destruction of the labyrinth or division of the eighth nerve by operation will relieve the condition, though these operations also cause permanent deafness on the side operated on.

Seasickness is partly due to stimulation of the labyrinth. For two days prior to embarkation the diet should be light, but with extra sugar added; the bowels should be freely opened. A sedative such as ½ gr. phenobarbitone three times daily or 10 to 15 gr. sodium bromide thrice daily should be taken for two days before embarking. The sedative should be continued after the voyage begins, and if seasickness threatens, two or three extra doses may be taken at intervals of one hour. When on board it may be found helpful to keep the eyes closed, to use coloured glasses and to wear a tight abdominal binder. Only a light diet with glucose drinks should be taken if sickness is threatening.

The Ninth, Tenth, Eleventh and Twelfth Cranial Nerves.—Glossopharyngeal neuralgia may be due to organic disease of the tonsil or pharynx. When there is no obvious local disease, the conservative treatment for trigeminal neuralgia may be tried (p. 1000), but if interruption of the nerve is required, this can only be satisfactorily achieved by operative division of the ninth cranial nerve within the skull.

Dysphagia.—Difficulty in swallowing in organic nervous disease is often associated with weakness of many muscles, including the muscles of respiration. Bulbar paralysis, myasthenia gravis and polyneuritis cranialis may cause marked dysphagia, and consequently a serious danger of the patient choking or of the food passing into the trachea and lungs. Small quantities of semi-solid food can be taken most easily, and the patient should be encouraged to spend a great deal of time attempting to eat, so that he may avoid starvation. Feeding by stomach tube should be instituted when the dysphagia is severe.

HYDROCEPHALUS AND INTRACRANIAL TUMOUR

Operative attempts to relieve congenital hydrocephalus have so far proved to be disappointing.

In cases of acquired hydrocephalus there is a much better prospect of relief. When the condition develops as a result of ear disease, arachnoiditis or meningitis, repeated lumbar puncture will often effect a cure (p. 1090), but decompression is sometimes necessary. Obstructive hydrocephalus will benefit from operation if the obstruction to the circulation of cerebrospinal fluid can be relieved. In all cases of acquired hydrocephalus, operation becomes urgently required if the visual acuity shows evidence of failing.

Intracranial Tumour.—Any mass within the skull, whether or not it is neoplastic in origin, is likely to cause hydrocephalus with increase of intracranial pressure, and damage to the brain or nerves lying within the skull. Certain principles of treatment applicable to such cases require consideration.

A case of possible brain tumour should be investigated fully without delay, for the following reasons :—

1. A small tumour is easier and safer to remove than a large tumour.
2. When intracranial pressure becomes greatly increased, operation becomes much more dangerous, and sudden death may occur.
3. Papillœdema may lead to optic atrophy and loss of vision, which is permanent even if the case is otherwise cured.
4. Irreparable damage may be caused either to the brain or nerves (especially the optic nerve) by the direct growth of a tumour.

The most suitable cases for operation are those in which tumour arises from outside the brain tissue, for it can then often be removed completely. It is occasionally justifiable to delay operation until the position of the tumour can be more accurately localized or when the diagnosis of tumour is not fully established. In such cases a careful watch should be kept on the visual acuity ; if this shows signs of deteriorating, operation, if only to relieve pressure, becomes urgent.

The prognosis in cases of glioma depends on the exact nature of the growth—seldom can it be removed completely. When marked and progressive mental deterioration with aphasia is the first indication of a brain tumour, and if there is little associated increase of intracranial pressure, it is doubtful if operation should be advised. There is no possibility of removing a glioma from the speech hemisphere, and decompressive operations will in such a case only prolong an existence which becomes truly deplorable. X-ray therapy retards the growth of some intracranial tumours, and is often used following decompressive operations when the tumour is not removable. When a gumma of the brain is suspected, antisyphilitic treatment should be given, but operation may also be required to relieve pressure. Intracranial tuberculomata are usually best left alone unless there is increase of intracranial pressure : they tend to become quiescent.

Dehydration.—It is sometimes urgently desirable to relieve intracranial pressure in cases of brain tumour, either to restore consciousness temporarily or to keep the patient alive till operation can be arranged. The injection into the rectum of a warmed solution of 6 to 8 oz. of 25 per cent. magnesium sulphate is usually very effective. The solution should be retained for half an hour. The intravenous injection of hypertonic solutions is more rapidly effective. Fifty cubic centimetres of 50 per cent. solution of sucrose injected very slowly (3 to 4 c.c. per minute) is the best solution to use.

It is important also to restrict the intake of fluids as far as possible, and to keep the patient's head well raised by means of a bed-rest. Should breathing cease, artificial respiration may preserve life until operation is carried out.

INJURY TO THE SKULL AND BRAIN

In the acute stage of head injuries, treatment is directed mainly towards combating shock. When the patient is comatose, blood and nasal secretions may be inhaled into the lungs unless the patient is turned half over on his face. It should be remembered that there may also be other injuries present which are often overlooked owing to the patient's unconscious state. The importance of dealing thoroughly with any scalp injuries has already been stressed (see p. 980).

The possible complications of head injury cannot promptly be recognized and treated unless a neurological examination of the patient is made soon after the injury, and at intervals thereafter. The pulse, respiration rate and temperature should be recorded at hourly intervals. Even more important is the assessment of the degree of unconsciousness and the presence or absence of hemiparesis, neck rigidity or changes in the reflexes. After head injury the patient should become progressively more conscious ; if the reverse process occurs at any stage some complication is developing which may require urgent surgical intervention.

As a general rule, however, surgical treatment of head injuries is better avoided unless a dangerous degree of increase of intracranial pressure develops with progressive loss of consciousness.

After the initial stage of shock has passed, the patient should be allowed a small soft pillow. A quiet room and a special nurse are a great advantage. Retention of urine should be relieved by catheterization as this is a common cause of restlessness. A stage of restlessness and confusion almost always occurs and, indeed, is a step towards recovery. This stage is not necessarily associated with, and is probably seldom due to, cerebral œdema. It is very doubtful whether vigorous measures to prevent cerebral œdema and to reduce intracranial pressure in the early stages after injury are of any real value. The raised intracranial pressure which often follows head injuries is of value in checking hæmorrhage, especially from torn venous sinuses. For the first two or three days, therefore, treatment should be entirely conservative unless there is any complication. Restlessness can be relieved by hypodermic injections of morphine. The effect of a small dose ($\frac{1}{8}$ gr.) should be tried first, as this may be sufficient. The morphine injection may be repeated as required, but the patient should be allowed to recover from the effect of the drug between each dose so that the real degree of unconsciousness can be estimated. A purge should be administered after the stage of shock has passed off.

When it seems desirable to reduce intracranial pressure, the withdrawal of some spinal fluid is the method of choice, and is superior to the use of hypertonic solutions. It may be stated that if loss of consciousness is prolonged for more than two days, if headache is severe, or if the condition is getting worse, withdrawal of a few cubic centimetres of cerebrospinal fluid is of value both for diagnostic and for therapeutic purposes. If necessary, it can be repeated every second day, while if there is any evidence of meningitis developing, the appropriate treatment, including the use of sulphonamide, should be instituted without delay (see p. 981). An injection of morphine prior to lumbar puncture will lessen the patient's restlessness. Two or three strong assistants may be necessary to hold a delirious patient in position during the spinal puncture. A manometer should be used to measure the pressure of the fluid, and the fluid may be withdrawn slowly till the pressure is reduced to about 150 mm. of water. When the intracranial pressure remains high for some days, the patient should be put in the Fowler position to raise the level of the head, and the bowels should be kept freely open.

Rest in bed in quiet surroundings without worry or anxiety constitutes the essential treatment of cases of head injury. The severity of brain injury should be judged not by the presence or absence of fracture of the skull but by the degree and duration of loss of consciousness, the amount of blood in the cerebrospinal fluid and by any other clinical evidence of brain injury.

When there has obviously been severe cerebral contusion a minimum of six weeks in bed should be advised owing to the danger of delayed hæmorrhage. In every case, strict rest in bed without reading or other mental effort should be enforced until pain in the head is relieved. Thereafter a return to active life by very slow stages should be arranged. The duration of post-concussional symptoms cannot be predicted, and the patient should not be unnecessarily alarmed by the persistence of some headache or giddiness for several months. A year or more off work is not an uncommon necessity for the manual worker after a severe head injury. Usually the patient can be assured that complete recovery will occur, and his anxieties with regard to the future should always be relieved as far as possible.

Surgical Complications.—In the absence of a depressed fracture of the skull, surgical treatment is seldom desirable, but large extradural and subdural hæmorrhages cause a dangerous increase of intracranial pressure and require prompt operation. Rarely a large intracerebral hæmorrhage may result from a head injury, and for the relief of the cerebral damage operation is sometimes desirable. In some surgical circles there is a tendency to operate on many cases of head injury, but in the writer's opinion these operations are seldom justifiable: small hæmorrhages below the skull or dura mater require no operative removal, and cerebral œdema can usually be relieved without decompression.

The Post-concussional Syndrome.—Headache, giddiness, loss of mental acuity, nervousness, sleeplessness and irritability are common post-concussional symptoms. A state of anxiety neurosis is commonly associated with the clinical picture, and this aspect of the case should never be ignored for it is often the most important.

The patient should if possible be removed from his domestic environment to a hospital or home. Visitors should be discouraged, preferably excluded, as they often upset the patient by their concern for his health and by reminding him of his home worries. The patient should be surrounded by an atmosphere of kindly understanding combined with confident optimism regarding the future. Rest in bed with no reading or mental effort should be combined with a mild sedative such as 12 gr. of sodium bromide thrice daily and 1 gr. of phenobarbitone at night. Usually the patient will be most comfortable with the head well raised both day and night. If pains in the head fail to respond to rest for two or three weeks along these lines, an encephalogram with the introduction of 25 c.c. of air may be carried out. Though this often causes severe headache for a few days, a remarkable degree of relief is often obtained after the reaction has passed off. Most cases improve greatly with treatment on these lines. The patient's age is an important consideration as regards prognosis, for if he is over forty-five years of age the prospects of recovery are considerably less favourable than they are in younger subjects. Anxieties with regard to matters such as compensation or future employment usually delay recovery, and may, in some instances, lead to permanent disability or mental instability. For these reasons the value of simple psychotherapeutic measures can hardly be overemphasized (see p. 1016). The settlement of a compensation claim by a single payment is sometimes of great therapeutic value.

DISORDERS OF CEREBRAL FUNCTION

Epilepsy.—Epileptic fits are due to abnormal discharges from cells of the brain. These may be stimulated by organic disease of the brain, such as tumour, vascular disease, cysticercosis, syphilis or injury. The investigation of a case of epilepsy involves a search for any possible organic cause, and when such a cause is found the treatment is that of the disease present. Medicinal treatment to control the convulsions is, however, often required in addition.

Traumatic Epilepsy.—Epileptic fits may result from cerebral injury and may begin at any interval up to several years after the initiating trauma. In the great majority of such cases, operation is of no value, but when there is clinical evidence to indicate clearly the exact site at which the cortical discharge originates, operative excision of a portion of brain in this situation is sometimes a successful procedure. The results of operation are, however, so uncertain that conservative medical treatment remains the method of choice in most cases.

Medicinal Treatment.—Apart, therefore, from those cases in which an organic cause for epilepsy can be eradicated, sedative treatment is required to control the number of fits. This applies both to grand mal and to petit mal. In many mild cases of epilepsy the regular administration of a cortical depressant has the striking effect of preventing or greatly reducing the number of fits—the drug apparently makes the brain less sensitive to the irritating factor which causes the cortical discharge. The bromides and phenobarbitone are the chief depressants used in epilepsy. Sodium bromide is usually prescribed with arsenic to lessen the risk of a skin eruption occurring.

℞		
Sod. Brom.	. . . . .	5 to 15 gr.
Liq. Arsen.	. . . . .	3 minims
Aq. Chlorof.	. . . to	2 fl. drachms

Ft. mist. Sig., 2 fl. drachms, t.d.s., p.c.

The addition of sodium biborate (5 to 15 gr.) or tincture of belladonna (5 minims) to each dose is sometimes beneficial. Phenobarbitone is prescribed in tablet form : the dose varies from $\frac{1}{2}$ to $1\frac{1}{2}$ gr. one to three times daily.

Tablets of prominal (Bayer), one (3 gr.) twice daily for an adult, are sometimes effective, and are said to be less depressing than luminal.

Epanutin (P.D. & Co.), which is a derivative of glycolyl urea, has recently been found to be of great value in epilepsy. The dose is one capsule two or three times daily before meals. Each capsule contains 0·1 gm. and bottles of a hundred can be obtained.

It is essential that the depressant should be taken regularly for a period often of many years, for if even a single dose is omitted, a fit will often quickly follow. There is no evidence that the proper administration of sedatives for a long period has a deleterious effect on the patient's mentality : mental deterioration occurs in some cases of epilepsy whether or not sedatives are being given. Even when medicinal treatment controls the fits satisfactorily, treatment should be continued steadily for as long as two years after the last attack : thereafter the amount of the drug should be reduced very gradually. Each case should be considered separately, and the effect of treatment on the number of fits carefully recorded. If, as sometimes happens, sedative treatment has no good effect in reducing the number of fits, the treatment may be discontinued, for it has no known beneficial effect apart from the anticonvulsive action. All the commonly used anticonvulsants should, however, be tried in turn before concluding that medicinal treatment is of no value. The dose of the drug may be gradually increased in order to attempt to obtain the maximum effect without causing drowsiness or other toxic symptoms.

When bromides are used over long periods, the possibility of a cumulative effect producing bromide intoxication should be kept in mind. The initial symptom of bromide intoxication may be excitement or delirium, and this may lead to the disastrous error of increasing the dose of the drug.

Epileptic fits may tend to occur at certain times of the day or night, and when this is the case a larger dose of the sedative used should be given an hour or two before the attack is liable to occur. In nocturnal epilepsy, however, the giving of a sedative before going to sleep may have the unfortunate effect of causing some fits to occur during the day instead of at night. This result should be avoided by stopping treatment if necessary, as the epileptic is fortunate who only has fits while asleep.

In certain cases of epilepsy fits only occur near the time of menstruation: in which case sedatives need not be taken continuously, but only during, and for a few days preceding, menstruation. Operations to stop menstruation are usually of no value in arresting the fits, and should not be advised.

General Management.—The epileptic patient should lead as normal a life as possible even when the fits cannot be fully controlled. Children should, if possible, attend school and be subject to ordinary discipline: intensive study does no harm. Adults should have regular occupation, but obviously must not work in surroundings which would be dangerous should a fit occur. It is impossible to guard the epileptic against all risks, but it is comforting to the patient to know that fits rarely occur during mental concentration: the patient is, for example, very unlikely to have a fit while crossing a busy street, or while faced with a situation requiring careful thought. Fear or excitement, and certain stimuli, such as a sudden sound, may cause a fit in cases of so-called reflex epilepsy.

Fire and Water.—Fire and water provide the main dangers to the epileptic. He may fall on a fire while in a fit or may be drowned in a few inches of water. He must, therefore, be warned about these dangers, and should only take a bath if there is someone at hand who knows the risks to which he is exposed. He is, of course, unfit to drive a car, ride a bicycle or work near machinery. Institutional treatment may be required for severe epileptics, especially if there is associated mental disorder.

Personal Hygiene.—The general health of the epileptic should be kept at the best possible level. Regular physical exercise and study are both beneficial. Constipation should be avoided and the diet should be liberal and nutritious. A ketogenic diet sometimes reduces the number of fits, especially in children, but the results are usually disappointing and the diet is so unpopular with the patients that the results are seldom worth the trouble and inconvenience involved. Such treatment, even when effective in reducing the number of fits, is in no sense curative, for the fits return when the dietetic rules are relaxed.

The Convulsion.—During an epileptic fit the patient should be protected from injuring himself. He is particularly liable to bite his tongue, and something, such as the handle of a spoon, should be placed between the teeth to prevent this injury. The patient should be kept under observation until any possible post-epileptic confusion has passed off.

Status Epilepticus must always be treated vigorously, as the condition may cause death. The administration of paraldehyde by the rectum seldom, if ever, fails to stop the fits. Each dose is dissolved in 6 oz. of normal saline. One ounce of paraldehyde can be given by the rectum in this way for the first dose, and thereafter 2 drachms of paraldehyde in saline by the rectum every half hour until the fits cease. This is a very safe and effective way of treating the condition.

Another method of treating status epilepticus is to give slowly an intravenous injection of a solution of 3 gr. of sodium luminal (convenient ampoules are on the market for this purpose).

Migraine.—Many people who suffer from migraine have attacks at such rare intervals that little treatment is required. Attacks may, in susceptible subjects, be precipitated by indiscretions of diet, overfatigue, eye strain and many other factors. Refractive errors should be corrected, though the part they play in the condition is doubtful. In most cases, however, mere attention to personal hygiene and general health fails to prevent the occurrence of some attacks of migraine, so that treatment has to be given to alleviate or arrest the attack itself. Many sufferers derive great benefit from taking a " headache powder," especially if it is swallowed at the first warning of the developing attack. A powder containing 10 gr. each of phenacetin and aspirin with 5 gr. of caffeine is often effective. If possible the patient should lie down until the attack passes. The powder should be carried by the patient so that it is always available at the first sign of the headache developing.

Treatment with ergotamine tartrate constitutes a distinct advance in the treatment of migraine. The most effective method of administration is by subcutaneous injection : $\frac{1}{4}$ to $\frac{1}{2}$ mg. of ergotamine tartrate should be given as early as possible in the attack, and repeated after one hour if necessary : vomiting sometimes occurs before relief is obtained. The patient should be taught to give the injection to himself. A convenient preparation in ampoules is marketed by Sandoz under the name of femergin. In mild cases two tablets of femergin (each containing 1 mg.) taken by the mouth give relief; the same amount may be repeated one to two hours later if necessary. The drug should not be used during pregnancy, and if any toxic symptoms occur due to ergotism, treatment with the drug should be entirely stopped.

Narcolepsy and Cataplexy.—The regular administration of ephedrine hydrochloride is often of great value in preventing attacks of narcolepsy or cataplexy; ½ gr. taken three times daily is often effective, but the dose should be doubled if necessary. Ephedrine should not be taken late in the evening, as it may then cause sleeplessness.

Spasmodic Torticollis.—It is difficult to determine what part, if any, psychological factors play in the causation of spasmodic torticollis. The more the movement occurs the worse it becomes, so every effort should be made to check the movement in its earliest stages. The patient will often discover that he can arrest the movement by some trick, such as touching his chin with his forefinger. Whatever the apparent cause of the condition in any particular case, it is wise to advise complete mental and physical rest in bed. The patient should go into a nursing home or hospital where he can be removed from home worries, and where visitors can be excluded. A sand-bag placed on each side of the head is often helpful, and some sedative such as 10 gr. of sodium bromide should be given three times daily. It is a good plan to make the patient write down on paper a note of every spasm that occurs. This exercise is particularly useful when there is a hysterical element in the case; the exercise becomes tedious in proportion to the number of spasms, and, therefore, provides a strong stimulus towards betterment. This exercise is beneficial in most cases, and great stress must be laid on its being conscientiously carried out. In intractible cases operation is often attempted in order to divide the nerve supply to the affected muscles. Such operations are, however, often disappointing in their results, and should only be advised as a last resort. Psychotherapeutic treatment may be tried, but it is seldom successful.

Sleeplessness.—*Insomnia* is a common symptom of many diseases. The physiological nature of sleep is not known, but it is obvious that full physical and mental relaxation are required before sleep is possible. In the investigation of the causes of insomnia, therefore, it is necessary to find out exactly why relaxation is not occurring, and then to attempt to correct or remove the disturbing factors which are present. Extraneous factors, such as pain, light, noise, cold or heat are usually obvious to the patient, but the disturbing effect of, say, cold feet is often not fully realized. Attention to detail regarding minor discomforts will often have great success in relieving sleeplessness.

Many patients who are poor sleepers complain that their thoughts become very active as soon as they go to bed, and it is this mental activity which prevents sleep. As this is naturally most troublesome when there are reasons for anxiety or worry, every effort should be made to remove these disturbing factors. The neurotic, however, aggravates the condition by worrying about the consequences of insomnia. The patient will often, for example, fear that insanity may result and it is essential that such a fear should be dogmatically countered, for nobody goes mad from insomnia. The patient should attempt to cultivate an attitude of indifference regarding the amount of sleep obtained and should be reminded that many people do full work with a very few hours of sleep each night. The amount of sleep actually obtained should be investigated; patients may complain bitterly of sleeplessness, whereas on further inquiry there is only a slight reduction in the amount of sleep to which they have been accustomed, and which will therefore do them no harm. Reading in bed is often a most useful and effective method of securing sleep; the light beside the bed should be within easy reach, and the reading matter should not be too stimulating.

Sleep is partly a habit, and when the habit has been disturbed, it is often necessary to give some sedative which will help to re-establish it. Stimulants such as tea and coffee should not be taken within five or six hours of going to bed. Non-stimulating beverages, such as hot milk, are often useful, but should not be taken in large quantities which lead to the patient waking to micturate. Whisky is especially useful in the aged, but should not be advised in the young neurotic patient. When drugs are required, they should be given regularly for a period of, say, two weeks so that the habit of sleep can be regained, and thereafter the amount is gradually reduced until none is required. When the fear of sleeplessness causes insomnia, comfort is often obtained from having at hand a single dose of a mild sedative which the patient knows can be taken if necessary. Large quantities of hypnotics should never be allowed at the bedside, as the patient may forget under the influence of the drug how much she has taken, or may in a fit of depression take an overdose.

Drugs.—In mild cases 10 gr. each of aspirin and sodium bromide may be very effective, but sometimes a single larger dose of sodium bromide (30 gr.) is better. Ten grains of chloral hydrate with 20 gr. of sodium bromide is useful, and in severe cases with restlessness the dose may be doubled and repeated every two hours until sleep occurs. Paraldehyde is a safe and useful hypnotic for old people: 1 to 2 drachms may be given in milk. The barbiturates are much used and are also very valuable: the dangers of giving the patient possession of large quantities of this type of drug have already been stressed. The exact choice of barbituric acid derivative is partly a matter of fashion, for the number of these substances has become very large. One which is quickly excreted is, generally speaking, most suitable as a hypnotic, but the suitability or otherwise of one particular hypnotic is usually a matter for trial in each case.

If the patient can fall asleep readily but wakens early in the morning, a slowly excreted barbiturate such as phenobarbitone (luminal) is most suitable and may be given in doses of 1 to 3 gr.

When there is difficulty in falling asleep a more rapidly excreted preparation is preferable. Medinal (sodium barbitone) is one of the best known of these and may be given in a dose of 5 to 10 gr. Tablets containing 5 and 7½ gr. are supplied. Soneryl tablets (1½ gr.) also act quickly and are rapidly excreted; one or two may be given. As the drug also has analgesic properties it is useful as a post-operative hypnotic.

These quickly acting barbiturates act better if they are absorbed quickly: no food should, therefore, be taken for at least an hour before the tablets are due, as a full stomach delays absorption. Veronal (barbitonum) (dose 5 to 10 gr.) has fallen into disrepute owing to the danger of its cumulative effect when given repeatedly.

Remedial Exercises

Exercises are useful in the treatment of many organic diseases of the nervous system. They should aim at re-training the muscles to carry out movements steadily and accurately. Full use should be made of the patient's own sight, for the visual sense is essential for steadiness of movement if the sense of position in the limbs is impaired. A patient, therefore, who suffers from ataxic paraplegia with impairment of positional sense must *look at his feet* when carrying out walking exercises. Exercises should be as simple as possible.

The Legs.—If the patient is able to stand and to move his legs, he should practice walking along a straight line marked on a floor which is not slippery. He should have a minimum of artificial help, but, if required, he should have support from sticks, crutches or a walking chair, according to the degree of disability. In severe cases he may require to be supported by two people while exercises are attempted. He should be instructed to walk along the marked line with the right foot just to the right of the line and the left foot just to the left. When position sense is greatly impaired, as in tabes dorsalis, a " broader base " for walking will be more successful, and the feet should be placed about 6 in. to right and left of the line. To make the exercise easier, two further lines may be marked on the floor parallel to the first, and 6 in. on either side of it. The patient should aim at making each step approximately the same length : short lines at right angles to the original line and a distance of 1 ft. apart from each other, will help the patient to keep his paces equal. The accuracy with which the feet can be placed depends on the clinical condition : the aim of the exercises is, as has already been stressed, to improve the accuracy of movements : they should, therefore, be made progressively more difficult until the maximum improvement is obtained. If good progress is made, more difficult exercises may be devised, such as walking heel to toe along the centre line.

When the patient is confined to bed, a different form of exercise is required. The patient lies flat in bed with the bed-clothes removed and his head raised on pillows so that he can use his eyes to control the exercises. Precautions must be taken to prevent the patient becoming cold. Three or four small sand-bags or pillows are arranged along the foot of the bed, and the exercise consists of lifting up one leg and moving it slowly and steadily from one sand-bag to the next so that the heel is placed accurately in the centre of each bag. A more difficult exercise consists of sliding one heel up the centre of the opposite shin.

The Upper Extremities.—Exercises to improve co-ordination of the hands and arms should also be simple. The patient may stretch out both arms and slowly and steadily bring the forefingers together so that they all but touch. A box of draughtsmen provides material for a useful exercise, the patient being instructed to pile as many of the pieces, one on top of the other, as he can. This requires both accuracy and steadiness of movement.

The above exercises will be found suitable for most organic diseases of the nervous system. In certain cases, as in poliomyelitis for example, special exercises must be given to develop individual muscles or groups of muscles.

W. R. Russell.

PSYCHOTHERAPY IN GENERAL PRACTICE

EVERYONE in his heart believes that he is a good psychologist even though he may modestly confine outward expression of that belief to the statement that he is a good judge of character. This is natural, for people are endlessly interested in their own personalities, and find their neighbours almost as fascinating a study. But when an attempt is made to dignify this interest by calling it a science, when experts appear who formulate theories which conflict with popular concepts, then we find great divergence of opinion, ranging from slavish acceptance of the formulations of this school or that to aggressive denial that there is anything in psychology at all. A similar reaction has been observed among members of the medical profession towards psychotherapy—a new and importunate branch of healing which has been engaging the attention and disturbing the minds of doctors and patients to an increasing extent during recent years. To the editors of this book of therapeutics, therefore, it seemed fitting that a section should be devoted to the problems in medical psychology which the practitioner encounters in his daily work.

No space need be devoted to emphasizing the importance of good mental health. It is generally accepted that much unhappiness, industrial inefficiency, social unrest and international strife can be traced to individual maladjustment. Neurotic illnesses are much more common than is suspected, and, according to most authorities, there is, in a third of all cases seeking medical aid, a psychogenic factor which must be recognized in planning treatment. The usual procedure is to refer cases in which psychotherapy seems necessary to the nearest clinic or specialist, but this method can deal with only a small proportion of patients who require treatment. Certainly specialists and clinics are at present too few and far between, but even if they were multiplied many times over, there would still be an insufficient number to provide specialist treatment for each patient. Other methods which aim at prevention rather than cure must be found. Provisions already exist in miniature for a broad mental hygiene programme in which child guidance, the inclusion of psychological teaching in the medical curriculum, the training of specialists, the earlier and more active treatment of neuroses and psychoses, and the education of the general public play an important part. Even if these provisions are much more extensive, the burden of treating mild and early cases, the responsibility of eliminating factors which predispose the individual to mental ill-health, must fall on the family physician. No one else has the same opportunity of recognizing and dealing with those intimate environmental and personal conflicts which bring about a disintegration of personality.

That a physician should deem himself capable of undertaking psychotherapy without special training will sound complete heresy to many experts. None the less, it is obvious that the bulk of neurotics will go untreated if they have to depend on the services of specialists, whose exclusive attitude has helped to make the average doctor chary of using even his good common sense in the handling of these patients. Many of the older practitioners were excellent psychotherapists: they gave mental and emotional attitudes their rightful place in the production and cure of illness. To-day the practitioner has little confidence in his ability to deal with psychogenic factors because he has been taught that only the very learned can presume to practice psychotherapy. One hopes that the introduction of psychology into the medical curriculum will serve not only in emphasizing the importance of this branch of medicine but also in helping to produce doctors who have confidence in their ability to use psychotherapy as part of their armamentarium. Much research, it is true, must still be done, not only by specialists but also by general practitioners themselves, on the methods and techniques which can most usefully be employed in general practice. None the less, certain broad principles can be laid down: the purpose of this article is to outline them, to make certain suggestions as to the conduct of treatment and to indicate the scope and limitations which are operative in general practice.

There is little doubt that, even in the last decade, the attitude of the medical profession has changed radically towards patients who suffer from psychogenic illness. To begin with, these disorders have been given a place in reality; patients are no longer told to the same extent that "there is nothing the matter with them except nerves" and, therefore, they no longer leave the doctor's consulting room with a feeling, half of shame and unworthiness and half of fear that their nerves—those mysterious and awesome structures of which they know so little and conjecture so much—are in some way upset or diseased. Even to be told that their trouble is mental rather than physical is a tremendous relief to those frightened and unfortunate people. True, they may protest vigorously against such a diagnosis, but their defence is healthy in comparison with the furtive defiance with which they greet the verdict that they are not ill at all. Their senses, their feelings and thoughts compel them to recognize that something *is* wrong, and naturally they prefer to persuade themselves and their doctors that that something is a physical malfunction. If the liver is out of order, cannot one swallow comforting and magical pills ? If the stomach is upset, are there not well-known powders to be bought ? If anything is wrong with the body it can hardly be one's own fault and there need be no turning over of painful memories, no stirring of the dark and inmost recesses of thought, no facing of unpleasant facts, no thinking that life is too difficult.

Patients thus come to the doctor consciously in misery, consciously eager to get better, but unconsciously determined to do everything in their power to remain ill. Indeed " one may say that they constitute the only condition where the patient comes for help to sustain the disease and resists every effort to cure it." [1] Now when the doctor realizes that the patient, far from wishing to get well, hopes to use him as a means of retaining his symptoms, he is inclined to be filled with righteous indignation and to eject him with harsh words. But no matter how obvious it is that the neurotic wishes to remain ill, the doctor should remember that the patient will be the last to realize it ; that, indeed, his symptoms would be of no use to him did he understand their purpose. Nor must the doctor suddenly blurt out this fact, for if he does, the patient will either frankly disbelieve him and seek a more naïve doctor, or will experience a collapse which may end in suicide. For neurotic symptoms are purposive, in that they defend the patient against something that he dare not face. The patient has come to the doctor for help only because he feels that his protective mechanisms are breaking down and because a corresponding degree of anxiety threatens to overwhelm him. Take away those defences suddenly and disaster will follow. Of course it is a great temptation to make a dramatic cure, but one which the doctor will be more able to resist if he remembers that a neurotic illness is often the result

[1] Jones, Ernest, *Brit. Med. Jour.* (1938), **1**, 1354.

of a lifelong maladjustment, and that one cannot expect to change a man's character, personality and mode of life all in five minutes. The hysteric may seem to be the obvious exception ; for paralyses, anæsthesias and other conversion symptoms may be cured suddenly and with no obvious harm to the patient ; but these dramatic cures, temporarily satisfying though they may be to the physician, the patient and the anxious relatives, are seldom the end of the neurosis. In fact, the sudden cure is only harmless when another symptom appears to make good the patient's defences. Only by a slow process of reintegration can the patient be brought to see what his symptoms mean, and how he may safely discard them for more healthy and permissible mechanisms. It is as if the patient had been treed by a lion and realizes that the tree he has climbed is liable to fall at any minute. A few yards away is a sturdy tree, which would harbour the patient in complete safety, but he is afraid to cross the gap, and comes to the doctor hoping, not that he will help him over the dangerous ground but that he will chase the lion away or tell him that his tree is perfectly safe. Great care is needed in persuading the patient to leave his insecure perch and pass the lion on his way to safety. This analogy is too full of generalizations to bear close scrutiny, but it contains a modicum of truth and is readily understood by patients.

The patient, then, comes to his doctor hoping that he will confirm his dear wish that his symptoms are due to heart disorder, or what you will, and must gently be shown that this is far from the truth. But an even more curious attitude on the part of the doctor must be noted, as Jones points out,[1] which is that the doctor and the patient may both wish to avoid a cure. Both are human beings and both use defensive mechanisms against their unconscious fears. Neither wishes to disturb the dark recesses of the unconscious, for who knows what horrors may emerge if the barricades are torn down. Whether, as Jones implies, this is true of all members of the medical profession or not, it certainly is true in certain cases. Consider the patient who was injured at his work and who later developed vertigo and other very obviously hysterical symptoms. Going to his doctor he asked whether his symptoms were due to head injury. " Well," said the doctor, " you never know with head injuries. Your head is like an orange ; you can squeeze the inside of it into pulp and the outside looks quite undamaged. The outside of your head looks all right." Surely the doctor in this instance was at one with the patient

[1] Jones, Ernest, *Brit. Med. Jour.* (1938), **1**, 1354.

in wishing that there were some organic lesion to account for the symptoms puzzling to him and frightening to the patient. It is much easier to think physiologically rather than psychologically (one has only to read the journals purporting to be devoted to psychiatry to realize this) ; it is difficult to think of man being a psychobiological organism rather than a mind and a body only remotely related. We shrink away from the emotions and their power, encourage the patient to make light of his symptoms, urge him to " pull himself together," to play golf, to get married and, most shamefully of all, to " use his will-power." Would that some prophet would cry from the house-tops, " Will is the organized self in action." How can a neurotic use will-power when his self is disorganized ?

How then can the physician avoid his human tendency to be blind to psychogenic factors in illness ? Jones has suggested that only " real " psycho-analysts (those belonging to the Freudian school) can avoid this pitfall because they have been analysed themselves. It should be pointed out that such an analysis takes about four years, is very expensive and is obviously open only to a minute percentage of medical practitioners. In addition, he would have us believe that psycho-analysis is the only form of psychotherapy of any value. Those of us, however, who are familiar with psycho-analytic thought, are undisturbed by such statements because they are so obviously determined by the lack of insight into their own unconscious processes which so many disciples of Freud show. It is true that the doctor who wishes to practice psychotherapy must be prepared " to face calmly the contents of his own unconscious mind and to have personal experience of resolving the conflicts and anxieties of it." [1] This can be done (one is tempted to add, better) without undergoing an orthodox Freudian analysis.

Now while it is impossible, and indeed inadvisable, in our opinion, for the majority of doctors to be analysed, it is imperative that they should all be alive to the importance of the mental processes in all disease. They must have, as Yellowlees says, " a living interest " in this aspect of medical knowledge. This they should acquire partly from teaching at their medical school, partly by reading, and most of all by experience. The really great physicians are noted chiefly for their deep understanding of human nature and for their sympathy with its frailties. The family doctor has, in particular, an unrivalled opportunity to study not only the individual but his relations to his family, his friends, his work and his

[1] Jones, Ernest, *Brit. Med. Jour.* (1938), **1**, 1354.

recreations. Often he has the privilege of watching him develop from birth to manhood and, unless he be particularly blind, he should be in a unique position to guide him through some, at least, of the difficulties of life. It should be the ambition of every doctor to be the counsellor of his patients both when they are physically ill and when they are in difficulties of a more subtle but perhaps more important character. Of these difficulties there are perhaps three which are most often encountered—parent-child relationships, the adjustment of the sexual instinct and the attitude of the patient to disease. These three subjects are of vast importance in maintaining good mental health, and every physician should have some knowledge of them.

GENERAL PSYCHOGENIC FACTORS

Parent-child Relationships

Precipitating factors are found in most neuroses—the death of a relative, loss of employment, an accident, financial difficulty and misfortunes of many kinds are plain for all to see, but knowledge of them is of little comfort to the patient. The physician must look for more deeply hidden ætiological factors which render the patient potentially neurotic, and which the current difficulty has, by association, stimulated into activity. These latent factors are the conflicts, inevitable in the process of early development, which have remained unresolved. The physician who has a working knowledge of these developmental errors should, through his close association with the family life of his patients, be able to do something to prevent their occurrence or to understand their ætiological significance in later life. Some understanding of the problems of child psychology can be gained by reading such books as "The Inner World of Childhood,"[1] "The Psychoanalytic Study of the Family,"[2] "The Mind in Daily Life,"[3] "Bringing Up Children,"[4] etc., but such study can only be made vital by personal observation of children themselves.

The student of early development will quickly realize that, even in ideal circumstances, the child has many conflicts to resolve during his first few years of life, and that the neuroses of anxiety, aggression, temper-tantrums, feeding and execretory difficulties are common to all children. The infant has to solve conflicts between instinctive reactions and behaviour

[1] Wickes, F., "The Inner World of Childhood." Appleton, 1927.
[2] Flugel, J. C., "The Psychoanalytic Study of the Family." Hogarth, 1921.
[3] Gillespie, R. D., "The Mind in Daily Life." Methuen, 1933.
[4] Rickman, J., "Bringing Up Children."

which is socially acceptable. In those formative years he must pass from a state of primitive savagery to a stage of cultural and social development which mankind has taken untold centuries to attain. Here it is not possible to consider these conflicts in detail, but it is important to note that development takes place smoothly only under ideal circumstances. Either a faulty endowment or a harmful environment, or a combination of the two, will cause a breakdown in childhood or later life. What surprises us is the capacity for adaption to difficulties, the resilience against neuroses and psychoses which the child displays. We understand little of and can do little with a poor hereditary endowment, but we can manipulate the environment so as to relieve undue strain. Study of neuroses in childhood has shown that there are certain conditions for which the child craves in order to make the solving of these inevitable inner conflicts possible, and that the most important is undoubtedly what child psychologists call *security*. By security they mean that the child absorbs from his parents a certain degree of affection, that he should have discipline which can control impulses too strong for himself to deal with, that there should be continuity of home life to compensate for the bewildering changes he experiences within himself, and that the adults around him should demonstrate that they have the power to regulate their own thoughts and feelings. And, lest we become too much absorbed in theory, we should note that these are just the things which wise parents do give their children intuitively.

The child also needs to *play*, for childhood is a period of experiment, trial and preparation. Through play the child is able to dispel his fears. Simple materials are used by the child to create situations of which he is afraid inwardly but over which he feels that he has mastery in a symbolic form. Again and again the child will go through such a performance until his inner fears have found surcease. This phenomenon forms the basis of the most recent technique for dealing with neuroses in childhood.

As an example, we may refer to the case of a child, aged four years, who hated and feared her mother; she had good reason for these feelings, for her mother was most unstable and unwise in the way she treated her. The child, however, knew, perhaps intuitively, perhaps from experience, that it would be unwise to show her antagonism openly, but showed her feelings in the following manner. She was given a family of dolls to play with and at first paid no attention to the mother-doll. After playing with the others for some time, she suddenly picked up the " mother " and, with an expression of ferocity, twisted its head off. On another occasion she made a drawing of a woman and said that this was her mother. When the drawing was completed she regarded it thoughtfully for a time and then asked, " Do people with blue faces die ? " On being told that cyanosis generally heralded death, she seized a blue pencil and carefully coloured her mother's face. Such behaviour is common enough among young children and reminds us of the custom prevalent in primitive civilizations of making a wax or clay image of an enemy and sticking pins into it in the belief that the enemy will thereby suffer harm. It should be added that the child mentioned above seemed relieved by the symbolic expression of her feelings and became more amenable to her real mother thereafter.

Again a child, to develop normally, must have *work* suitable to his intellectual capacity and stage of development. The intellectual faculties are capable of balancing and controlling the emotions, and the child who has no outlet in work becomes a prey to uncontrolled impulses. Work to the infant means the learning of bodily skills, walking, talking and the manipulation of external materials, to the older child it means formal education. Hence Moodie's dictum, "Early and efficient teaching in the fundamental subjects of reading, writing and arithmetic is the corner stone of mental hygiene in children."

Without these fundamental needs of security, play and work, and all that they imply, the child tends to develop a fear of growing up. He is, therefore, potentially vulnerable either during childhood or during adolescence or while facing any of the major life adjustments. Faced with any situation which calls for an integrated and stable personality he will tend to regress to an infantile mode of reaction. And now we see the necessity of uncovering those repressed and unresolved conflicts of childhood when attempting to cure a neurosis in an adult. Unfortunately these conflicts are often deeply buried in the unconscious by the time the individual has reached maturity, and their elucidation may be beyond the skill of anyone but an expert, but the general practitioner can do much to prevent their occurrence by ensuring that the fundamental needs mentioned above are supplied as far as possible, and in certain cases he may be able to deal with them in later life.

The Adjustment of the Sexual Instinct

Probably Freud's discovery of the important part which the sexual instinct plays in the formation of the neurotic's reactions, and of the great influence which this innate force plays in the thoughts, feelings and behaviour of every individual, startled the world more than any other piece of research. His theory lit up the comfortable Victorian world like a flame from the nether regions, and indeed many believed that he was inspired by the dark forces of evil. We are not concerned here with the complexity of Freudian psychology, but there are certain simple facts which have emerged which are of vital importance in the ætiology of the neuroses and which should be known to every medical practitioner. First of all, one must remember that the sexual instinct is a natural force which causes no trouble when given natural outlet. Malinowski [1] has shown that in a primitive tribe where sex is allowed to develop freely there is no such thing as a sexual neurosis. Only in a civilization like our own, where there are so many social and moral taboos, and where there is such an acute feeling of guilt attached to this instinct, does it assume undue significance and power. It is noteworthy that sexual factors are less frequently found to be ætiologically important in centres like London and in the U.S.A., with their less exacting standards, than in certain provincial districts where there are more rigid codes. Significant, also, is the fact that sexual troubles are more often found in the professional classes, where economic factors delay marriage long after the individual has reached maturity, than in the labouring classes, where the individual attains his maximum earning capacity about maturity, or among the rich, where there is no economic bar to marriage. Sex, therefore, is a force, with which the medical profession must reckon only when it is dammed up.

Again one must recognize that the child has a sexual life of its own, but naturally it differs widely from adult sexuality. Much harm is caused by adults who regard the manifestations of sexual activity in children as they would regard similar activity among their coevals. Here the adult is projecting his own knowledge and feelings on to the child and the child suffers feelings of guilt which may colour his attitude to sex all his life. This is illustrated clearly with regard to masturbation. Almost all children masturbate at some time or another, but masturbation in a baby of six months cannot be sexual in the adult sense. In young children and babies autoerotic practices are indulged in mainly for the sake of sensual gratification and are allied to behaviour disorders like thumb-sucking, and should be treated as such. It is practised chiefly

[1] Malinowski, B., "The Sexual Life of Savages in Northwest Melanesia." Routledge, 1929.

by children who are bored, or insecure, or in pain, and appropriate adjustment can be made if steps are taken before a habit is formed. On no account should the child be made to feel guilty. Sexual curiosity is also a very real thing in children, but again it is not dangerous, provided parents are able to satisfy that desire for knowledge in a natural and unemotional manner. If uninstructed, they will gain their knowledge in an undesirable way, or, by brooding over it, conjure up harmful concepts, and either way will spoil their chances of attaining a healthy attitude in later life. Much harm is done because so many parents have themselves feelings of guilt about sex, which are intensified when they try to answer their children's questions. The children sense this and get the impression that there is something shameful about sex, and so the vicious circle is perpetuated. It should be remembered too that children can suffer anxiety or have their sexual feelings prematurely aroused by observation and misinterpretation of sexual behaviour on the part of adults around them.

Masturbation in adolescence must be regarded as something different from autoerotism in children. Our experience shows that it is still necessary to warn doctors that this practice, *per se*, does no physical or mental harm. The harm comes from the feeling of guilt which follows the practice. Masturbation does not weaken the patient, but the emotional disturbance does, especially if the patient has been told so by his doctor, his parents or some would-be counsellor. Most pernicious of all are books like the "Family Physician" or those pseudo-medical, pseudo-religious books [1] which promise to the masturbator as many ills, from tuberculosis of the spine to insanity, as certain proprietary pills claim to cure. What must be realized is that the adolescent masturbator is already over-burdened with guilt and must be relieved of it before he can conquer the habit. "Nor must it be imagined," as Brill says, "that robbing masturbation of its horrors encourages its practice. On the contrary, I have found that as long as patients dread it they masturbate twice as much as when they become convinced that it has none of its former supposed horrors." [2]

We cannot here discuss in any detail the part which sexual maladjustments play in the neuroses of adult life, but mention must be made of the influence which lack of sexual satisfaction

[1] Good examples are "Onania or the Heinous Sin of Self-pollution," an anonymous work published in the eighteenth century, and "Instruction for New Confessors," Salvatori, 1885.

[2] Brill, A. A., "Psychoanalysis," p. 34. Sanders, 1913.

plays in the production of diseases peculiar to women. Gynæcologists are becoming more and more aware that operations performed for the relief of pelvic pain are, in many cases, the wrong treatment. Unfortunately, it is often easier to perform an operation than to discover why the patient is having lower abdominal pain. Such patients are most resistant to a psychogenic interpretation of their condition, partly because they find it difficult to believe that the " real " pain they suffer can have a mental origin, partly because their modesty makes them unwilling to discuss sexual problems. But to the family doctor who knows the patient, the husband and the mode of upbringing, the trouble should be obvious enough.

There are two main types of patients who suffer from pelvic disturbances of a psychological nature. The first is the spinster who, all her life, has been starved emotionally, but whose vague hope, that some day she will marry, maintains fair stability until something makes her realize the poverty of her emotional life. This realization may be activated by the death of a relative, by an unrequited love affair, or merely because advancing age compels her to recognize that soon her hope of romance can no longer be maintained. The pelvic pain expresses, in a symbolic manner, the patient's inability or disinclination to face the bitter fact that she cannot attain her biological end in life. The second, and much more common type, is the married woman who has not obtained sexual satisfaction from her husband. It is true that a high percentage of married women never obtain enjoyment or satisfaction from coitus, yet they do not suffer from psychogenic pain. These women have never had cause to believe that any satisfaction could be obtained from intercourse ; they think of it simply as a somewhat unpleasant duty towards their husbands which they must perform with as good grace as possible. But let them once experience extra-marital satisfaction and trouble soon begins. Here is a typical history. A woman of thirty-seven suffered from such acute pelvic discomfort that a gynæologist performed a hysterectomy. The uterus was successfully removed but the patient complained, during the post-operative period, of headaches, depression, sleeplessness, and weakness, which could not be accounted for on a physical basis. Accordingly a psychiatrist was consulted who elicited the following history : The patient was illegitimate and had married mainly to obtain social status. Her parents-in-law did little to conceal their disapproval of the match and, as they lived in the same town, were able to interfere persistently with her domestic affairs. The husband was inconsiderate and impulsive about intercourse and tended to neglect her in other ways. Her health remained fairly good until she fell so deeply in love with another man that she considered leaving her husband and child. Because her religion forbade this, she decided on the compromise of illicit week-ends, in the course of which she first experienced sexual satisfaction. Then her lover, becoming tired of her, departed to India, and soon the patient began to experience acute pelvic pain, for which the hysterectomy was later performed. Both because no organic disease was found in the uterus and from the psychological history, one can legitimately infer that the pain was defensive, expressing as it did her bitterness at the loss of sexual satisfaction from her lover and acting as a subconscious excuse against intimate relations with her husband. When the operation removed what she consciously believed to be the cause of her pain, she had to develop other symptoms which would subserve the same ends. These symptoms were entirely relieved by psychotherapy, and the patient became much more happy in her marital life.

The Attitude of the Patient to Disease

Disease is perhaps the most dramatic thing which occurs in the life of the average person ; it is little wonder, therefore, that he should take so much interest in it when it does occur. We do not often reflect that physiologically and psychologically our bodies and minds are designed to encounter and deal with considerable dangers in the external world. Our ancestors were constantly meeting danger and reacting to it in an appropriate manner, but now external dangers are rarely encountered. There are occasional wars or threats of war ; there is the danger of traffic but, on the whole, the vast majority of people lead a humdrum existence with no call to feel frightened : but we still have within us a strong instinct of self-preservation which, in the absence of external outlet, tends to be introjected in the form of fears and obsessions about our bodily health. There are, of course, outlets familiar to all ; books on crime and horror have immense sales ; plays and pictures of the gangster type are very popular ; speedway racing and other dangerous sports provide vicarious satisfaction. These things certainly play some part in providing an external outlet for this instinct. The man of to-day will describe his last illness or operation with as much relish and wealth of dramatic detail as the warrior would relate the tale of his latest battle, the explorer his most recent adventure. This is an aspect of disease which has attracted little attention in medical circles, yet surely the doctor's first question on seeing a patient should be, "What attitude does this patient take towards his illness?" His chance of effecting a cure would be much greater if he could allay mental distress, soothe fear and discourage the pleasure and satisfaction which some people get from being ill.

Hysteria.—A good example of a maladjusted attitude is found in the so-called traumatic hysterias. The very name shows that there is much loose thinking in medical as well as legal circles about such cases, for the actual injury does not produce the neurosis; the patient's attitude towards the events after the accident is the real cause. Compensation hysteria would be a more accurate term, for, almost always, the patient is receiving a weekly benefit or attempting to obtain a lump sum. Hysteria does not follow injuries received in sport or when the patient can derive no benefit. Both doctors and lawyers are now beginning to realize that many of these disorders are psychological, but this knowledge does not seem to make them any wiser in their handling of them. Judges and juries are inclined to be either sentimental in their estimate of the mental suffering which the patient has experienced, or mistaken in thinking that hysteria is something like malingering.

Whenever a doctor is called upon to examine a patient suffering from an injury for which compensation may be sought, he should keep in mind the possibility that the symptoms are (1) purely organic in origin; (2) hysterical, *i.e.*, unconsciously determined; (3) the result of malingering, *i.e.*, consciously determined. Certain cases will present a combination of organic and functional elements or organic and malingering, but it is uncommon to find a combination of hysteria and malingering. Such a differential diagnosis is never easy. Physical examination should be as thorough as possible and should be supported by laboratory tests where necessary, the main object being to determine whether the symptoms are of the nature and extent to be expected from the injury. If the symptoms cannot be explained on physical grounds then one must consider whether a functional element is present. Here one must differentiate between an unconsciously determined hysteria and a consciously determined state of malingering. In making a differential diagnosis between those two conditions one should remember that hysteria is a definite disease characterized by certain positive features.[1] These are:—

1. It must prove negative to all clinical and laboratory investigation.

[1] Hall, S. Barton, *The Practitioner* (1938), **141**, 31.

2. There must be found a positive psychogenic basis.
3. The psychogenic factors must bear direct relation to the patient's symptoms.
4. In view of the fact that a psychoneurosis, however suddenly it may appear, has always a background in time, there must be discovered in the life-history of the patient a neurotic trend which, it may be found, has been responsible in the past for the production of subjective states analogous to those under investigation.

Malingering, on the other hand, is characterized by :—

1. A tendency to overact the part. This enables the examiner to devise certain simple pitfalls into which the malingerer readily falls. A simulated anæsthesia, for example, can usually be detected by the response to faradism with a wire brush.
2. The subject is prone to produce any symptom which the examiner appears to expect. This must not be confused with the suggestibility of the hysteric.
3. The malingerer dislikes being examined and is uneasy during the process ; the hysteric, on the other hand, delights in examinations and openly shows his satisfaction in minute investigation of his condition.
4. It is rare for a malingerer to feign new symptoms, rather he pretends that existing symptoms still persist. The hysteric, on the other hand, rarely is content with the *status quo*, and produces a great number of typically hysterical symptoms. Often, indeed, the hysteric will state that his injury has completely healed, but that he has palpitations, vertigo, feelings of pressure in the head, anæsthesias of the glove or stocking type, etc. If the malingerer does produce symptoms *de novo*, they are generally of a dramatic, artificial and exaggerated type.
5. The malingerer plays his rôle only when observed.

So far as treatment of compensation cases is concerned, the mistake is too often made of thinking that a hysterical condition will clear up when a settlement is made. This is by no means true, especially as many cases drag on for months or years : symptoms become fixed reactions and the patient is thus "hoist with his own petard." Therefore, having decided that there is, or may be, a psychogenic element, the doctor should immediately begin psychotherapy. This consists, in the first place, of warning the patient that the worry, disappointment and self-deception, which inevitably occurs, will delay and perhaps prevent recovery. If, in short, the patient goes on with his case, he should do so with full knowledge of what harm may befall him. It may even be necessary to warn a patient, who has got into the hands of an unscrupulous lawyer, that he, the patient, will not benefit as much as his legal adviser if and when compensation is paid. It should be added that even reputable lawyers, who lack medical knowledge, may fail to recognize that human beings are only too eager to exaggerate illness, especially if they are rewarded for doing so. Illness is obviously preferable to work if the former has a maximum of incapacity and a minimum of pain, and if the latter is monotonous and distasteful. Continuing his treatment, the doctor should try to get the patient to realize that his symptoms, real enough to himself, are in the main due to anxiety and not to the original injury. To convince the patient that this is so is by no means easy, and much depends on the physician's own attitude. He must show the patient that he regards functional symptoms as being just as important and worthy of treatment as symptoms arising from organic causes, and must show no sign of despising the patient for having them. Having gained the patient's sympathy, the doctor can then go over the history of the illness chronologically, pointing out which symptoms were directly the result of injury and which arose from the patient's own attitude. This procedure of piecing together the temporal relationships between symptoms and psychological disturbance gives the patient an entirely new attitude towards his illness and is of considerable value in treatment. Further, the patient should be urged to get back to work as soon as possible ; he should, however, be warned that he may have a return of his symptoms when he starts work, but this should only serve to convince him that his symptoms are of mental origin and that they will gradually disappear if he continues with his work. He can be warned that each day he delays will make his symptoms worse, and that no sum of money will compensate for the mental pain he will inevitably suffer.

It should be remembered that the law, as it stands, encourages psychogenic illness because of the delay which takes place before cases are settled, and further, because the patient finds that his right to compensation may be prejudiced by accepting employment before his claim is settled. Therefore, doctor and solicitor should combine in making every effort to settle the compensation case with as little delay as possible.

Before passing from this section dealing with the neurotic reactions which may arise from the patient's attitude towards illness, mention must be made of certain almost traditional fears. A simple example is the fear which many women have of parturition. No doubt this is largely dependent upon the exaggerated accounts of the pain and dangers of child-birth which is passed from mother to daughter, and, of late, the press publicity, which has been given to maternal mortality, has not helped matters. An interesting experiment is being carried out by Miss Margaret Morris who has designed courses of exercises which tell the patient what to expect during child-birth, and what she can do to help. These exercises make the patient interested in the process of parturition and do much to dispel fear. An obstetrician has reported a case whose first two children were delivered by forceps with great pain and difficulty; during the next pregnancy Margaret Morris exercises were practised and the patient became so proud of her skill that she refused all anæsthetics and delivered the child unaided and without difficulty.

Another traditional fear is the dread of cancer. Whole families become hypochondriacal because of a death certificate containing the terrifying words, so much so indeed that some doctors refuse to put malignancy as a cause of death. Doctors should be at pains to point out that there is no evidence to support the common belief that malignant disorder is hereditary. The following history will indicate the insidiousness of this fear: An exceptionally intelligent man, deprived of education by circumstances, developed a duodenal ulcer, as a result of which he experienced a long period of unemployment. He developed toothache and had some teeth extracted but, no doubt, because a dental student did the extraction, his jaw was painful for a day or two afterwards and he asked his doctor for a line to see the dental surgeon at the local hospital. When the doctor made out the line he put, in the space for "conditions for which the patient has already received treatment," carcinoma of the duodenum. The patient, reading this, immediately thought that the pain in his jaw was due to secondary deposits, for, to relieve the boredom of unemployment, he had been reading about cancer in medical textbooks in the public library. It was little wonder that, despite reassurance that there was nothing wrong with his teeth, his pain grew steadily worse and did not disappear until the psychogenic basis of it had been explained to him.

DIFFERENTIAL DIAGNOSIS

Many practitioners find difficulty in making a differential diagnosis between insanity and neurosis. Certainly there are early stages in which even specialists can be baffled, but the vast majority of cases present no difficulty. It is helpful to have in mind a simplified classification of the psychoses for, if one excludes the organic-reaction types such as G.P.I., senile dementia, etc., distinguished by their concomitant physical signs, one is left with only three main types. These are (1) schizophrenia with its delusions, hallucinations, bizarre behaviour and signs that the patient has made a retreat from reality; (2) paranoia, a rare condition in its pure form, with systematized delusions of persecution and otherwise well-preserved personality; and (3) the manic-depressive type where the main symptom is an elation or depression of mood. The neuroses can be classified as neurasthenia, anxiety states, hysteria and obsessional neuroses; the patient suffering from any one of these conditions is commonly called a neurotic. Neurasthenia is much the most difficult to diagnose, for it may be confused with the prodromal stages of G.P.I. Beware of the middle-aged man with no history of previous breakdown, who feels constantly tired, and who complains that he is becoming less efficient. He may have no physical signs, yet his symptoms may be due to the elusive spirochæta, and the true diagnosis may have to be made in the clinical laboratory. Secondly, a diagnostic distinction between neurasthenia and a mild psychotic depression is important, for the former has little risk of suicide whereas in the latter it constitutes the main problem of treatment. The cardinal symptom of neurasthenia is excessive fatigue, but the patient's emotional reactions are most active; a neurasthenic is always tired except when he is talking about himself, and he is loud in his complaint of the handicap from which he suffers. He is eager to work and take an active interest in outside affairs and bewails his inability to do so. The depressed patient, on the other hand, centres his slow thoughts on his own troubles, the outside world means little to him, and he makes no complaint of the limitations which his condition imposes. The risk of suicide is always present with patients showing these symptoms, whether they express a desire to end their lives or not. But it should be remembered that neurotics also may allow themselves to be driven to suicide. This is particularly true of cases of long standing which have their defensive symptoms suddenly removed. If, for instance, a patient has defended himself from some fear by believing that he has a diseased heart and one proves that his heart is sound, he may find his inner adjustment so disorganized, and his distress so great, that he may end his life rather than face it. The sudden cessation of long-standing fears may then be a danger sign. This is understandable enough if one remembers the parable of the man who swept seven devils from his house but neglected to put anything in their place, and seven other devils more terrible than the first entered in and took possession, so that his last state was worse than his first.

PROCEDURES IN TREATMENT

There is a tendency to attach an unnecessary degree of mystery to psychological treatment of the neuroses. Many doctors find themselves baffled and ill at ease when faced with a psychogenic illness ; they have a feeling of helplessness and are constantly asking themselves what they should do. They long for some active procedure and are, of course, encouraged in this by the patient. Here one should remember the very natural unconscious reluctance, mentioned above, of both doctor and patient to uncover the roots of the trouble, no matter how superficial these may be. In a large proportion of cases met with in general practice, there is no need to go deeply into unconscious mechanisms, for the trouble is fairly obvious to an inquiring and unprejudiced mind. Another point is that the physician must not feel that he is doing nothing because he is giving no active physical treatment. The truth is that everything one does with a neurotic is treatment, and the more passive one is, that is, the more one encourages the patient to work out his own problems, the better results one gets. One must have something of the attitude of the angler who is perfectly confident that he is going to catch an enormous fish but is quite happy with his day's sport if he lands nothing. Above all, avoid the temptation of using too much explicit suggestion, do not, for example, use methods of treatment such as tonics which have no effect on the root causes of the trouble. Implicit suggestion is unavoidable and the patient should feel your calm certainty that what you are doing is the correct and only treatment, but you should not encourage that part of him which wants you to say that there is nothing wrong, nothing to fear, and that he, therefore, need not bother himself to face his troubles.

In making a diagnosis of a psychogenic disorder the physician must make quite certain that there is no organic disturbance. This involves a most complete physical examination, supported, if necessary, by laboratory procedures and the advice of specialists. Of course the presence of physical disease does not exclude the possibility that the main trouble is psychological. Autointoxications of various kinds are often present and must receive the appropriate treatment, but the physician should not deceive himself that, in so doing, he is treating the neurosis itself, nor should he allow the patient to think so. Another point is that a neurosis cannot be diagnosed by exclusion. It is not permissible to say that the trouble is psychological just because one has found no organic cause. There are, in fact, some cases in which neither cause can be found, and here one must admit that one has reached the outposts of one's knowledge, and one must await the development of additional signs and symptoms. Having satisfied oneself that no organic disturbance can account for the symptoms, one must tell the patient so, and make sure that there are no doubts left in his mind. Such doubts may, in the course of treatment, recur, but the physician should not re-examine the patient physically unless he is satisfied that there is good cause for doing so. This is one of the reasons why the original examination should be thorough, because certain patients are sure to produce symptoms in any part of the body omitted.

Having assured the patient that there is nothing wrong physically, one must explain that the cause is psychological, illustrating the power of mind over body by simple examples, or, better still, by citing case histories of a similar nature. Examples of the former should be confined to bodily reactions in response to emotional disturbance which are likely to have come within the patient's own experience. Most people have experienced fear or disgust and yet the dramatic bodily changes in response to these emotions are not considered strange or terrifying. The physician should try to show the patient that his symptoms are merely responses of a similar nature which indicate that his body is working normally and not, as he imagines, pathologically. The patient should be asked to think over his own experience from this point of view and an appointment should be made for next day, or soon after, when the physician can conveniently spare at least an hour. Most busy practitioners may feel that they cannot possibly spare so much time on one case, but it is better to allow the patient to talk himself out at one sitting than have him pester you day after day for short periods. If, at this second session, no indication is given as to where the trouble lies, it is probable either that the patient is suffering from an incipient psychosis, or that the case is one for a specialist, or, indeed, that there is no psychological basis at all.

If, however, it is clear to the physician or to the patient (though with the latter this is seldom the case) that the symptoms have a purpose, then subsequent interviews must be arranged. In most cases it is best to see the patient once a week for a month or six weeks and if he is not very much better by that time, or if the physician does not know on what lines to proceed, then a specialist should be consulted. Above all, remember that no rash or hurried interpretation should be given to the patient of the meaning of his symptoms. The physician should interpret mainly mechanisms with which the patient is not familiar, always illustrating from normal reactions or from other cases ; otherwise he should confine himself to criticising or agreeing with the patient's own reading of his case. This can be illustrated by the case of a young man who complained of weakness, palpitation and precordial pain. He explained that he had for many years indulged in masturbation yet enjoyed good health. Immediately prior to the onset of symptoms he had read about the harm which the habit did and, greatly terrified, had stopped it. He attributed his symptoms to the delayed effects of masturbation. Here the physician's function was to point out that his symptoms were due partly to his anxiety and feeling of guilt and partly to the emotional disturbance implicit in the giving up of an act which had served as a relief to the tension of his sexual urges, and not, as he thought, to the harmful effects of masturbation *per se.*

None the less, there are two main lines of inquiry which the physician must keep in mind. The first is simply that a detailed, chronological history of the onset and course of the illness should be gradually built up. This will enable both doctor and patient to see the connection between circumstances and events and the onset of symptoms. The patient will then come to understand the defensive nature of his symptoms and, further, he will realize that there is no longer any need so to protect himself. The history of a patient whose symptoms disappeared in three interviews will illustrate this. He was a man of thirty-seven who, five years previously, had given up an important appointment in the city because he suffered from vehicle sickness and fear of traffic, and had buried himself in a small country town in an unimportant job. When the patient, an only child, was ten, his father died and, by heroic measures, his mother continued his education. He grew up with an intense admiration for his mother and dreamed of the time when he, a successful business man—a captain of industry—would justify her sacrifices and give her a life of ease and luxury. But success of this type is not too easily attained, and, at the age of thirty, he found himself leading a monastic existence in order to send every penny to his mother and still far from being able to marry, or even to live in comfort, far less support his mother. His mother then made a further sacrifice by remarrying, for she saw that her son would miss all the reasonable satisfactions of life in his attempt to pay her back. The patient, suddenly stripped of his former purpose in life, for a time led a life of what to him was riotous living, that is, he moved into comfortable lodgings, no longer stinted his meals, went occasionally to the theatre, and oh, wicked extravagance, took up golf! He even got married himself and, for a time, was quite happy. Then, to his dismay, he found that his step-father, a man whom he disliked and feared, was ill-treating his mother. No doubt because of his anxiety he then made a foolish mistake in his work and was threatened with dismissal. The following morning he became violently sick in the tube going to work and his doctor foolishly sent him away for three months' "complete rest." When he attempted to return to work, he was a confirmed neurotic.

It may be asked why the doctor is considered to have acted foolishly in sending the patient away for a complete rest. The so-called rest cure has been one of the recognized methods of treating nervous disorders from time immemorial and reached its epitome in the Weir Mitchell régime, but very little thought is required to see that rest without active psychological treatment is the worst possible therapy. It is, in fact, an admission that nothing can be done for the patient, and is analogous to immobilizing a patient with an acute abdomen and refusing to operate. The patient is sent away from his habitual occupations, social outlets and work, factors which are of the greatest importance in supporting him against his inner complexes, to a place where he will have nothing to do except struggle with his disturbed emotions and his unresolved mental conflicts. Such a procedure too often results in the symptoms becoming a more habitual reaction than ever. The physician should therefore think very seriously before he takes such an important step as certifying a neurotic as unfit for work. He must evaluate the ætiological factors carefully, for it is only when the environmental influences can be held responsible or mainly responsible for the patient's illness that the cessation of work should be recommended. There are cases, of course, when the patient is ill mainly because of uncongenial work or because of detrimental home conditions, and it may be unfair to expect the patient to adjust under such disadvantageous conditions. Even in those cases, however, the patient should be removed only to an environment which will serve as a stimulus to the patient's recovery, nor should such segregation be regarded as a cure in itself. As a general rule, however, it is best to keep the patient in the environment in which he must live in the future, and to pursue active psychotherapy to enable him to face any environmental difficulty which may exist. Quite early in treatment the patient can be brought to see that his real difficulties lie within himself, and that he cannot run away from inner maladjustments.

The second line of inquiry grows naturally out of the history of the illness, and consists of making a survey of the patient's life. This is necessary if one finds that the current illness was a reaction to some comparatively slight strain or difficulty, and one must ask why this individual was unable to face something which would not distress the average individual unduly. The answer can generally be found in the patient's account of his life, though he himself will be quite unable to see the connection. This second line of inquiry often leads the physician to suspect that there were errors in the patient's early emotional development. If an individual is to face all the "slings and arrows of outrageous fortune," he must have a well-integrated personality, and this is only possible when the foundations of his personality have been well and truly laid. So long as life progresses smoothly and pleasantly the individual remains unaware of his fundamental weakness, nor can this be easily detected by outside observers. Only very small indications are given of this immaturity—a tendency to follow the path of least resistance, an avoidance of responsibilities, an inclination to be overdependent on relatives and friends, or a senseless seeking after frivolous pleasure may be the only clue. Many live and die with their weakness unchallenged, others are vanquished by something which to the onlooker seems trivial. This explains why a national emergency, like the Great War or the economic depression in America, brings to light such large numbers of mental illnesses. In more peaceful times the stress which betrays the individual's poverty of resistance may be a physical illness, the death of a relative, the loss of employment or some business worry.

Now the uncovering and rebuilding of weak foundations is by no means an easy task and generally it lies rather without the scope of the general practitioner's work. It requires great clinical skill and experience to know whether the patient is capable of discarding the props and makeshift buttresses which support his weak personality and of rebuilding his life on a sounder foundation. Such a major operation involves a period of intense dependence on the physician, who must know exactly what is happening and what to do about it. Fortunately, such a proceeding is not always necessary, as most neuroses can be resolved by less drastic means. Every psychological investigation, however, means that the patient must face facts about himself which may be unpleasant, and this may be an entirely novel experience to him. Here the physician must exercise care, for it is almost impossible for an individual to think badly of himself for very long. In the ordinary way his weaknesses and sins are quickly minimized by such mental mechanisms as *projection*, whereby the individual's own thoughts or feelings are attributed to someone else (the motorist is always ready to blame the pedestrian or the other driver for his own lack of skill or judgment), or *rationalization*, whereby we seek to justify our unconsciously determined behaviour as if it was motivated by logical thinking (the deserted wife bewails her lot unaware that her own behaviour has driven her husband away). Should unwelcome self-knowledge become too pressing, some more drastic protection must be sought, and this may take the form of a neurosis, or, in very urgent circumstances, a psychosis. Thus an individual may for years be punishing himself for some sin of which consciously he is unaware, and which he would be unable to face if it intruded itself into consciousness. The physician must therefore be careful of adding to the patient's conscious feeling of inferiority by bringing to light hidden feelings of guilt and unworthiness. Further experience will show that patients who habitually think badly of themselves are difficult to cure. It is useless to assure them that they are suffering from an unwarrantable sense of inferiority, they know that only too well themselves, but it does help them to be assured that there is a perfectly logical reason for their inferiority, and one which can with patience be uncovered and dispelled. This sympathetic, and to them rather surprising, attitude will do much to encourage them to uncover those secret sins which have haunted them probably since childhood, for even in the conscious level they feel guilty and inferior. One must not be misled into thinking that neurotics are people who live private lives of sin ; the opposite, indeed, is true, because they are generally too timid, or have too rigid moral standards, to be sinful. Being shy and reserved they have often built up lurid pictures of themselves, and confession not only relieves their conscious feeling of guilt but helps to release repressed material. This was illustrated in the case of a man who, at the beginning of treatment, could remember nothing before the age of ten. After having written an account of his sex life, which incidentally was really very chaste, he began to remember incidents which occurred at as early an age as three years, and which had an important bearing upon his whole attitude to himself and to the illness from which he was suffering.

One of the first questions which the majority of patients ask is how they should deal with their phobias and obsessions. The patient is, for example, afraid to appear in company or to remain in an enclosed space ; he knows that avoiding his fear only tends to make it more difficult next time, yet panic may overtake him each time he tries. The physician should make it quite clear to the patient that there is some reason for his fear and that he cannot be expected to face it unless he knows that reason. This can be illustrated by case histories or by simple analogies, such as that suggested by Yellowlees.[1] " If a person who is afraid of ghosts becomes aware of what appears to be a ghost standing in the doorway while he is sitting at work, he may adopt either of two methods. On the one hand, he may recall everything he has been told about ghosts, particularly that they do not really exist, and that, even if they did exist, they could not possibly hurt him. Fortified in this way, he may be brave and resolute enough to continue working at his desk, forcing himself to attend to the business in hand and to fight down the uneasy feeling that there is a strange and sinister something standing at the door. If he is of sufficiently heroic mould, he may succeed not only in getting through his work, but in getting through it efficiently. On the other hand, he may determine to deal with the thing once for all. He lays aside his work, and by a supreme effort nerves himself to walk to the door and examine the ghost face to face. He strips it of its white sheet and mask and finds that it turns out to be, let us say, his young brother or his child just dressed up for fun, or, to put it in psychological language, the infantile in himself. If he had dealt faithfully at an earlier stage with his young brother or with his child, or with the infantile in himself, he would not have been troubled thus. Now that he has dealt faithfully with them he can return to

[1] Yellowlees, H., " Clinical Lectures on Psychological Medicine," pp. 221-22. Churchill, 1932.

his work, and he is no longer under the necessity of being heroic. He has no longer got to fight and conquer his fears, for the excellent reason that there are now no fears for him to conquer."

The assurance that a logical explanation for his phobia can be found will both reassure the patient that he is not just a moral weakling or "yellow," and give him hope that he will be cured. He should not, however, be allowed to think that the discovery of the hidden cause of his fear will suddenly dissipate all his fear, as certain psychologists have implied. Rather he should be told that it will give him a new attitude towards his phobia; he will feel as if he had been given an effective weapon with which to fight his adversary, now seen for the first time. His success in fighting his phobia will depend partly on his ability to face and readjust himself to the maladjustment lying behind his fear, and partly on the length of time he has been a prey to it. For habit formation plays an important, though secondary part, in the production of symptoms, and re-education is a vital part of treatment.

The patient should therefore, at the first consultation, be reassured that it is inadvisable for him to try to fight his fears without knowledge, but having discovered what he is really afraid of or why he is afraid he must then begin to make an effort. Comparatively minor or recent acquired fears should be tackled first, the patient keeping in mind all the time, repeating to himself if necessary, why he is afraid. Nor should he expect the procedure to be pleasant, for, to begin with, he will be almost as much afraid as before. The point is that he should credit himself with a victory if he is able to do the thing he fears, whether he is afraid or not; next time he will be less afraid if he has taken the proper attitude at the first attempt, and the emotional tension will gradually lessen. Finally, he will only remember occasionally, with pride and amusement, that he is doing something of which he was formerly afraid. Each fear must be tackled and dealt with in this manner, nor should the patient be satisfied until he is completely able to lead a normal life.

Thus treatment falls into two parts, the first being one of analysis and the second one of re-education. The mistake commonly made is, of course, to miss out the first period altogether, or at least to hurry over it before the true cause has been found. It is our firm belief that no patient can deal successfully with his fears or compulsions until he can use the truth as a weapon. As Yellowlees says: "The aim of all good psychotherapy is to help the patient to face reality." During the second stage also the physician must display considerable skill in knowing just how far the patient has got in the process of re-education, and in being able to forecast what he will or will not be able to do in the immediate future, and how he will feel when doing it. This gives the patient a comforting sense that the physician thoroughly understands his case, and that he is progressing on known and expected lines. Such skill can only be acquired through clinical experience; no textbook can impart the necessary knowledge, but most pitfalls and difficulties can be avoided if the physician has an opportunity of discussing his first cases with an experienced psychotherapist.

Above all, the physician should make himself thoroughly familiar with the patient's environment. It is said that one needs to have a wide general knowledge to be a good psychotherapist, that one must be able to show some understanding of philosophies and religions, of arts and political systems, of trades, professions, and spare-time interests. This may seem a tall order, but the very nature of the work brings one in contact with people of every class, belief and occupation, and one gradually acquires information even about little-known subjects. It is, however, the patient's personal environment which the psychotherapist finds most important. He must know the people who are most important to the patient, and he must have an opportunity of forming a personal judgment of them. To-day psychiatrists think this so important that most clinics have specially trained social workers whose task it is to formulate an accurate picture of the patient's home. In particular, the attitude which the patient has to the several members of his family and, just as important, their attitude to him and to each other, must be investigated. By this means the psychiatrist is able to estimate the stresses and strains to which the patient is continually subjected, and to direct the social worker in that manipulation of the environment which is of so much value in treatment. For example, a wife can be shown that her over-sympathetic attitude only increases her husband's fears. Thus both psychiatrist and relatives will be able to bring the same influence to bear upon the patient.

The general practitioner will have no specially trained assistant of this type, but for obvious reasons he hasn't the same need as the specialist, who only sees the patient at infrequent intervals and his family perhaps not at all. The general practitioner is often in the patient's home and, as a general rule, knows his personal environment intimately. He must make a special point of ensuring that the patient's family understand the nature of the illness and he must outline the best attitude to adopt to the patient. Most neurotics are greatly handicapped by the crude handling, the unsympathetic attitude and lack of understanding which they suffer at the hands of their "nearest and dearest" relatives. The illness may continue unabated unless these handicaps are ameliorated. This is of the utmost importance in the treatment of nervous children, but is also vital in adult cases, as the following history shows. A man of thirty-seven suffered for some ten years from acute anxiety and many fears. The cause of his fears was analysed and treatment had progressed so favourably that he was able to do things which he hadn't been able to attempt for many years. Suddenly and without any warning his wife deserted him and his anxiety and fears returned with all their previous vigour. Now until this happened the patient had spoken little of his wife, except to remark that she was much younger than himself and that she had always been sympathetic and encouraging. Consequently it had not been considered necessary to see her, especially as the patient was poor and lived at a distance from the clinic and there was no social worker to visit the home. After he had been deserted, however, the patient confessed that he had married partly because his doctor advised it and partly because he found his own mother unsympathetic. After marriage he became intensely dependent on his wife. He used her, it seemed, as a mother substitute, for when he was afraid his one thought was to rush home and obtain her sympathy. His fears prevented him from taking her to the pictures and dances, which she craved, and even marital relations were cut down to a minimum. On these grounds her desertion was understandable, but it became more so when she confessed that she was sure he was insane and might attack her at any moment. With these thoughts in her mind her attitude towards the patient could hardly have been helpful; she was sympathetic, perhaps, but that condolence was inspired by fear rather than understanding. Nor could the patient's attitude towards her have been conducive to her happiness, marrying, as he did, to escape his mother and hoping to find in his wife the ideal mother. Cases like this illustrate the futility of attempting psychotherapy without knowledge of the patient's home life.

THE SCOPE AND LIMITATIONS OF PSYCHOTHERAPY IN GENERAL PRACTICE

We can begin this section in no better way than by quoting T. A. Ross,[1] who for many years has advocated psychotherapy in general practice. "There is an idea abroad that no

[1] Ross, T. A., *Brit. Med. Jour.* (1938), 1, 4047.

psychological treatment except psycho-analysis is worth talking about. I have spent my life in trying to show that this is not true. I am saying nothing against psycho-analysis, which is probably the best treatment for certain cases, but there are a great number of patients who do not need it, for whom something quite simple is all that is required. I have no wish that medical students should learn analysis. It would be impossible for them to do so even if it were desirable. Time would make it so. For the same reason, even if psycho-analysis were the only psychotherapy, mental treatment would be impossible for the majority of patients. In my view there are, and have been for a long time, simpler and shorter methods of psychotherapy which are, at least, as old as Freud's system, and of which the greatest exponent was Dejerine of Paris. This depends on the fact that many symptoms are caused by conflicts and anxieties which are not necessarily unconscious in the Freudian sense, but which are not being faced properly." An attempt has been made in the foregoing pages to describe that "something quite simple" in treatment, and now we must try to indicate the type of patient on whom it should be practised.

In contrast to the treatment indicated for neurotic patients, analysis, even of the most mild nature, must never be practised on psychotic patients. The physician can, for his own guidance, allow the patient to pour out his troubles and, for the same reason, can make exhaustive inquiries of the relatives, but no hint of this must be given to the patient. It is, we admit, a great temptation to argue with and exhort a mildly depressed patient, but this only adds to his difficulties. Distinction must, of course, be made between a patient who is depressed and has every reason to be so because of some real trouble and the psychotically depressed patient whose degree of depression bears little or no relation to his circumstances. Treatment should be limited to physical care, guarding the patient from harming himself, and very gentle but oft-repeated reassurance and encouragement. Day after day you may tell the patient that he will, in good time, get better, that one day his depression will lift and he will then be as happy and healthy as ever he was. Meantime he must try to be patient and take what comfort he can from your reassurance. These simple platitudes may seem to have little effect, but the patient will thank you for them when he recovers. With the menopausal depression one may add that the condition is a reaction which commonly results from the physiological changes which are proceeding in the patient.

More difficulty is experienced by the general practitioner in deciding whether to undertake the treatment of a neurosis or not. One must remember that the form of treatment should be suitable to the patient's intellectual capacity and cultural status. The person of average intelligence can hardly understand analytical procedure. This may seem a sweeping statement to make, but few intelligent people have any conception of the limited power of understanding abstract theory displayed by the person of average intelligence, whose abilities are mainly confined to dealing with practical issues. The truth is that the person of average intelligence is just capable of learning to read, write and do simple arithmetic, and could not get further in education than the elementary school. Thus analysis must be limited to those who are capable of going through a high school or university education. Fortunately, those of lesser ability develop less subtle conditions than those who can understand analytical procedures. During the war, officers usually suffered from anxiety or fear states, while other ranks tended to develop crude hysterias. One should therefore be guided by the rule that the less clever a patient is the more one must depend on suggestion, reassurance and simple re-education. Putting it in another way, one might say that the more intelligence a patient displays, the more passive one can become and the more one can allow the patient to analyse his own difficulties.

The non-specialist should be chary of undertaking the treatment of a long-standing condition. If the symptoms have been in evidence for more than a few months the illness will be fixed and difficult to eradicate. If the patient has been, since childhood, a " nervous, highly strung " individual, it is probable that the current illness is but an exaggeration or exacerbation of a habitual tendency to neurotic reaction, and here, again, the non-specialist must not expect success. Another type which presents great difficulty is the patient who shows a marked reaction to comparatively trivial environmental strains, or the patient who can only produce ætiological factors which seem inadequate both to him and to the physician, because experience has shown that his real difficulties will be deeply hidden.

Age, too, is a limiting factor. After a certain age human beings become fixed in their reactions and mode of life ; they resist change so much that they cannot give up defensive symptoms, no matter how inadequate these are. Individuals differ widely, of course, in this respect, but on the whole, patients above the age of fifty are not suitable subjects for psychotherapy. Fortunately it is uncommon to find a neurosis developing so late in life, though an old neurosis may persist to a much later age. When middle age is passed the individual usually reacts to difficulties by developing a psychosis rather than a neurosis.

Of the different neuroses themselves the physician will find greatest success in treating the simple hysterias and the mild anxieties and phobias. Generally speaking, he should avoid obsessional states, for even specialists are chary of undertaking treatment of these cases, despite the fact that they are often eager to be psycho-analysed.

A final limitation applies to the physician himself and is one which he may find difficult to judge. It should be obvious that one cannot expect to obtain results in psychotherapy unless one has a special aptitude for it, just as one cannot paint a picture or play a sonata unless one is gifted in a special way. Psychotherapy, whatever its too-ardent supporters may say, is more of an art than a science, and for its practice one must have, in addition to training and knowledge, an intuitive, inborn capacity. Unfortunately some physicians, who are particularly obtuse about themselves, think that they have this gift and consequently practice what they imagine to be psychological treatment with meagre results. Any success that they do have depends on the powerful suggestive quality of their own belief in their skill. The physician may judge his capacity to practice this difficult art by the degree of his interest in it, by his liking for it, by his capacity to understand how neurotic patients think and feel, and, of course, by the results he obtains, though this last is hardly a criterion for the beginner.

It may be thought that we have imposed so many limitations that the physician will have difficulty in finding suitable cases to treat. This is far from the truth ; in every community there are large numbers of unhappy people who are suffering from some degree of psychological maladjustment. They do not come to the physician complaining that they are neurotic, but that they cannot sleep, or are run-down or have vague pains or strange feelings. Indeed, the general practitioner will find the patient who complains of physical symptoms the most easy to help. Let him keep in mind that emotional disturbance has a physical concomitant in everyone. The patient with a chest will perhaps have asthma, the patient with a tendency to gastric disorder will produce symptoms of ulceration in that region in response to some emotional or mental crises. Others who have no such bodily safety-valve will perhaps produce a more easily recognized neurosis. It behoves every physician to keep this possible ætiology in mind, and if he does so he will not lack material.

In conclusion, the reader may have found less concrete directions for the treatment of psychological conditions in this chapter than he expected. He must remember that this subject is one which can be learned best by practice, and that most attempts to teach or write about it have, as Lewis says, "no reality until given body and meaning in the individual case." He may have found the explanations given here unnecessarily complicated, but must reflect that human nature is unbelievably complex and that simple interpretations are rarely correct. Like most writings on this subject, this chapter may give the impression of irritating vagueness; in this case the lack of sufficient space is partly responsible, but also it must be remembered that there are large gaps in our knowledge which psychologists are constantly trying to fill.

ALCOHOLISM AND DRUG ADDICTION

ALCOHOLISM

Though accurate statistics do not exist, there is undoubtedly less hard drinking in this country to-day than there was, say, at the beginning of this century. Drunken men and women are seldom seen in the streets, Saturday night is no longer the time of carousal it used to be and convictions for drunkenness have decreased. These changes are partly due to the enormous increase in the price of liquor and partly to a change in social and moral codes. None the less, the abuse of alcohol by a certain proportion of the population still constitutes a grave social problem and causes untold suffering to the individual and his relatives. Because of the general decrease in the abuse of alcohol there is much more moral stigma attached to addiction and the addict is more inclined to drink in secret. Doctors, on the other hand, are becoming more conscious that alcoholism is a medical rather than a moral problem. In America the issue is more acute, for with prohibition came a wave of alcoholic excess which beggars description. Hospital wards, psychopathic hospitals and institutions for mental disorders were, and to a lesser extent still are, filled with alcoholic illness of all degrees and varieties. This has led to an intense study of these conditions and to the more recent advances in ætiological and therapeutic knowledge.

Mention should first be made of the part which avitaminosis plays in alcoholic disorders in general. According to recent research alcohol does not have a direct toxic effect on the nerve tissue in alcoholic polyneuritis (*cf.* p. 978) and Wernicke's disease, but the clinical manifestations arise rather from avitaminosis inaugurated by the chronic ingestion of alcohol. According to Alexander (1939) [1] there is much suggestive evidence that Korsakow's psychosis and delirium tremens may also be due essentially to vitamin deficiency. Brodsky (1938) [2] reports that injections of massive doses of crystalline vitamin B (500 to 2,000 units daily) are followed by prompt improvement and complete disappearance of symptoms in cases of chronic alcoholic psychoses. Mainser and Krause (1939) [3] report good results from the treatment of delirium tremens by nicotinic acid. Much of the work on vitamin deficiency in chronic alcoholism is new, but promises to be a field rich in therapeutic results. The deficiency is due to three main factors :—

(*a*) Chronic alcoholics of all classes are notoriously neglectful of their diet.

(*b*) Gastritis and defective liver metabolism cause incomplete absorption and storage of vitamins and minerals.

(*c*) Alcohol has a high calorific value, which necessitates an increased supply of vitamins, especially B. Alexander (*ibid.*) therefore concludes that in order to secure optimum therapeutic results it is best to give very large amounts of vitamins A, B_1, B_2 and C in all types of chronic alcoholic disease.

The excessive use of alcohol gives rise to a variety of disorders, which are classified as *acute* or *chronic*. Here we are concerned with the therapeutic aspect, and for the sake of clarity and simplicity we shall consider the disorder "acute" when the patient may be a danger to himself or others.

Acute Alcoholism.—*Acute or subacute alcoholic poisoning* results from drinking large amounts of alcohol in one or several bouts. Accurate diagnosis is important not only because of treatment but because death from acute or subacute alcoholism must be reported as a case of poisoning. Ideally, specimens of blood (at least 10 c.c.) and urine should be obtained for toxicological analysis. *Dipsomania* is a state of periodic acute

[1] Alexander, L., *Arch. of Neurology and Psychiatry* (July 1939), vol. xli., 179.
[2] Brodsky, M. E., *Jour. Connecticut Med. Soc.* (May 1938), **2**, 228.
[3] Mainser, F., and Krause, M., *Brit. Med. Jour.* (12th August 1939), 331.

intoxication and is usually regarded as being symptomatic of an underlying manic-depressive psychosis or of epilepsy. *Mania à potu* occurs in individuals who are susceptible to alcohol and who become intensely excited and perhaps dangerous after taking comparatively small amounts.

Treatment of these conditions should be directed to detoxication and to obtaining rest. The stomach should be washed out through a soft stomach tube with warm water. Colon lavage with normal saline and, later, saline purgatives also reduce auto-intoxication. Apomorphine hydrochloride (gr. $\frac{1}{10}$ subcutaneously) is strongly recommended [1] for its twofold action of clearing out the stomach and giving restful sleep. Other sedatives are barbitone (gr. x), paraldehyde (at least 3 drachms by mouth), or morphia, gr. $\frac{1}{4}$, and hyoscine, gr. $\frac{1}{100}$, hypodermically. It should be noted that paraldehyde rarely, and hyoscine more commonly, may cause delirium rather than rest.

Delirium Tremens or Acute Alcoholic Delirium.—In this condition it is important to recognize the earliest manifestations, since prompt treatment may avoid the more serious sequelæ. Delirium tremens occurs usually during an excessive bout of drinking when rest and diet have been scanty. Hours or even days before the onset of the psychotic symptoms certain clinical manifestations make their appearance. Tremors, motor restlessness, flightiness of thought and apprehensiveness are danger signals. Other prodromal symptoms are nausea, profuse sweating, headache, rapid pulse and fever. The patient is either sleepless or, if he does sleep, is wakened quickly by nightmares. If treatment is not instituted at this stage the typical delirium appears rapidly with hallucinations and disorientation.

A therapeutic régime somewhat as follows should therefore be adopted :—

(*a*) Alcohol should be stopped immediately and thereafter avoided entirely. To begin with this presents little difficulty, for owing to the confusion of the patient there is little demand for it. If there are symptoms of cardiac collapse, 1 to 2 c.c. of coramine should be given intramuscularly every four hours for six doses.

(*b*) For sedative treatment 3 to 4 drachms of paraldehyde once to thrice daily are recommended. A too liberal use of sedatives should, however, be avoided, and in

[1] Willcox, Sir W., and Carver, A. E., "Encyclopædia of Medical Treatment" (1936), vol. i., p. 289.

preference frequent warm baths should be given. The use of mechanical appliances to restrain the patient forcibly is contraindicated, though this may require an increased nursing staff. If the patient is sleeping he should not be wakened on any account.

(*c*) For elimination 1 oz. of magnesium sulphate should be given, and this may be repeated each morning unless there have been four evacuations on the previous day. Two grammes of sodium chloride should be given in capsules four-hourly in order to encourage the retention of fluids in the tissues (Bowman and Keiser).[1] Although the studies of Cline and Colman (1936) [2] and Piker and Cohn (1937) [3] suggest that fluids should be limited and spinal puncture performed to relieve œdema of the brain, yet later work by Bowman and Keiser (1939) [1] indicates that the reverse type of treatment with salts and forced fluids to relieve systemic acidosis and dehydration is preferable.

(*d*) The diet should be soft or liquid and of a high vitamin content. Daily intramuscular injections of from 500 to 2,000 units of vitamin B_1 (for preparations see pp. 405-7) and nicotinic acid, 0·5 gm. per ounce, twice daily have been recommended.

(*e*) Psychological analysis of the factors underlying the alcoholism should be carried out after the acute phase has passed.

As can be seen there may be difficulty in carrying out the above régime in the patient's house. Sometimes, however, there are no suitable hospitals available and the family doctor has perforce to treat the patient at home. In such cases trained nurses should be engaged and relatives discouraged from taking any part in the routine.

Alcoholic Psychoses.—Psychotic reactions to alcohol require little discussion in this volume, for they necessitate treatment under certificates in a mental hospital. *Alcoholic confusion* is a rare condition which results from sudden and heavy drinking; it is a state allied to other toxic confusional psychoses. The patient is excited, restless, confused in thought and action and may be hallucinated and have fear reactions. There is not

[1] Bowman, K. M., and Keiser, S., *Arch. of Neurology and Psychiatry* (1939), **41,** 702.

[2] Cline, W. B., and Coleman, J. V., *Jour. Amer. Med. Assoc.* (1936), **107**, 404.

[3] Piker, P., and Cohn, J. V., *Jour. Amer. Med. Assoc.* (1937), **108,** 345.

much physical upset. Depression and remorse set in with recovery. *Acute alcoholic hallucinosis* is not uncommon and often accompanies delirium tremens. When threatening auditory hallucinations and delusions of persecution without disorientation occur, hospitalization should be carried out immediately, for such patients are suicidal and unmanageable. Rarer conditions are delusions of jealousy and paranoid reactions. *Korskow's psychosis* is a serious condition in which there are few satisfactory recoveries. The patient should always be sent to a mental hospital and relatives warned that several months' observation will be required to determine whether this will have to be a permanent arrangement. The earliest symptoms are defects of memory, dizziness, headache and mild confusion. It is usually accompanied by signs of neuritis. Rosenbaum and Merritt (1939)[1] have made a valuable study of the factors important in prognosis.

Chronic Alcoholism.—When a patient harms himself or his family by drinking to excess and cannot be made to realize it, or when he no longer has the will or strength to overcome his habit, he should then be regarded as suffering from chronic alcoholism (Diethelm).[2] The development of somatic and personality changes and not the frequency of the bouts of intoxication are the features on which the diagnosis should be based. The only treatment which is flexible enough to be applied to all cases is a combination of personality analysis and re-education under strict supervision.

Ideally every case of chronic alcoholism should be treated in a special institution or hospital where continuous supervision can be given and where there are facilities not only for psychological and medicinal treatment but also for work, games and discipline, which form such an important background to a successful cure. Special institutions for the treatment of alcoholism are a rarity in this country; there are none, for example, in Scotland. They are also comparatively expensive and only a small percentage of patients can afford the fees. There are, however, a number of private hospitals and nursing homes which specialize in the treatment of nervous and mental disorders which are suitable for the treatment of alcoholism. In the writer's opinion too little use is made of the admission blocks of mental hospitals for patients who are unable to afford large fees or who are in the rate-aided classes. By persistent and skilful persuasion many addicts who bring

[1] Rosenbaum, M., and Merritt, H. H., *Arch. of Neurology and Psychiatry* (May 1939), **41,** 978.

[2] Diethelm, O., "Treatment in Psychiatry." (The MacMillan Co., 1936.)

misery to themselves and their families could be induced to become voluntary patients in mental hospitals. But even if full use were made of the existing institutions and hospitals the family physician would find that he was compelled to treat a certain number of patients in their own homes. This presents the greatest difficulty and should only be undertaken in the last resort, for adequate control is uncertain even where nurses are in attendance.

The second major difficulty is to decide whether alcohol should be withdrawn abruptly or "tapered off." The writer has no doubt that abrupt withdrawal is physiologically and psychologically correct in all cases, and this belief is supported without exception by all the recent publications of American authorities who have had a very wide experience in the treatment of alcoholism. Alcohol differs from other drugs like morphia and cocaine in its physiological effects, for the patient does not develop the same physiological need, or the same tolerance, nor does sudden withdrawal lead to the serious symptoms which occur with other drugs. Diethelm [1] states : "There are no serious symptoms of withdrawal and no danger of the development of delirium tremens. Although the average physician claims that he has seen delirium tremens caused by abrupt withdrawal, there are no carefully studied cases in the literature to substantiate this claim." Abrupt withdrawal is also important psychologically, for it shows the patient that there is no medical necessity for alcohol in his case, the realization of which is the beginning of his re-education. In this country there is considerable support given to the theory that abrupt withdrawal *may* be followed by an acute mental state in the nature of a delirium, and it is said that restlessness, excitement and irritability may be so great that unless one deals with the patient sympathetically by allowing some alcohol one loses all contact with him at once. It is true that sympathetic handling must be the keynote of the treatment of alcoholics, but the writer doubts whether the patient will later respect and trust the physician who gives in to his importunities as much as he will the physician who firmly guides him over the first difficult days. The detoxication period is, after all, the shortest and by far the easiest part of the treatment. In the writer's opinion, exception should only be made under two circumstances : first, when the patient is old and feeble and has had a long history of alcoholism ; and, secondly, where the patient is being treated in his own home where nursing and other facilities are inadequate. Information regarding the

[1] Diethelm, O., "Treatment in Psychiatry." (The MacMillan Co., 1936.)

advisability or otherwise of abrupt withdrawal in the latter category is still largely a matter of hearsay, and general practitioners should take every opportunity of carrying out abrupt withdrawal in an attempt to throw some light on what can and what cannot be done. When "tapering" is practised the patient's consumption should be reduced by 25 per cent. each day, so that the whole process takes less than a week. Paraldehyde can be added to the alcohol, for its penetrating odour and taste prevent the patient from knowing how much alcohol he is having, as well as for having a sedative effect.

When possible, then, the patient should spend at least the first two months of treatment in a hospital where absolute supervision and skilled psychotherapy can be given. When the patient is treated at home the first stage should begin where possible with the immediate and absolute withdrawal of alcohol. The patient should be told that he has no need to fear withdrawal symptoms, and certainly not delirium tremens. If required, the use of cardiac stimulants, such as coramine, is permissible. Bloomberg (1938),[1] Reifenstein and Davidoff (1930)[2] advocate the use of benzedrine, in doses of 10 to 30 mg. daily, to relieve depression and to produce a latent interval of sobriety during which psychotherapy may be inaugurated. The patient is usually co-operative for the first month and then begins to be resentful of restraint and unwilling to continue treatment on the grounds that he is completely cured. Unhappily he is often supported in this by his relatives, either because of expense or because they are deceived by the patient's improvement and optimism. The second phase of treatment, which consists of a reorientation of the patient's habits and outlook on life, is, however, most important. Many patients supposed to be cured are still left a prey to the very factors which were originally responsible for their addiction to alcohol. Too little attention is paid to personality analysis and adjustment by skilled psychotherapy, but there is a growing number of special departments attached to general hospitals where adequate domiciliary treatment is available.

The patient should be at work, but his spare time should be well occupied with social activities and physical exercise. Once or twice a week he should see his physician to discuss current difficulties and the management of his life. He must gradually develop fresh interests and group activities and reacquire confidence in his ability to face disappointments,

[1] Bloomberg, W., *Arch. of Neurology and Psychiatry* (1938), **40,** 1051.
[2] Reifenstein, E. C., and Davidoff, E., *Jour. Amer. Med. Assoc.* (1938), **110,** 1811.

failures or depressions without the help of alcohol. When cured he should have a positive feeling that he has no need of alcohol. Nothing less than total abstention should be the object in view and all pleas for moderate drinking should be disallowed.

It is important to carry the co-operation of the relatives throughout the various stages of treatment. They should understand that old associations must be broken, that they must be as abstemious as the patient is trying to be and that they must endeavour to make life new and interesting to him. Relatives are often unable to understand that alcoholism is an illness, preferring to regard it as a moral weakness. Though the majority do their best under exceptionally difficult circumstances, some wives seem to find a perverted satisfaction in sacrificing themselves and their children and are unwilling to co-operate with the physician in enforcing treatment; others, discouraged by broken promises and constant relapses, become indifferent and give the patient no help.

Full discussion of the psychobiological factors underlying alcoholism must be left to works on psychopathology, but some of the commonest can be mentioned briefly. Ætiological factors are seldom on a conscious level and this accounts for the inadequacy of conscious motives and wishes in correcting the desire for alcohol. Smalldon (1938) [1] believes that the underlying psychological factor is best explained on the Freudian hypothesis (*e.g.*, latent homosexuality, repressed sexual forces, partial oral fixations and sadism supply the driving force of desire for alcohol), and that this theory is more acceptable than any other. Knight (1937) [2] calls attention to the fact that the mother of a male patient is usually over-indulgent and protective, quick to satisfy his infantile distresses, vacillating in training and fostering the desire to take something into his mouth for comfort and relief. Such early training stimulates an excessive desire for personal affection which, in later life, is doomed to frustration. Alcohol is used as a solace for the depressing emotions caused by the contrast between early pampering and the frustrations of the adult world. Solitary drinkers are often lonely persons who drink in order to forget their longing for normal social life. Shy, sensitive people seek enough confidence to greet their fellows. An anxiety neurosis or a depression may be the causative factor; nor must we forget that suggestible, inadequate

[1] Smalldon, J. L., *Psychoanalytic Quarterly* (October 1933), **7**, 640.
[2] Knight, R. P., *Jour. of Neurology and Mental Disease* (November 1937), **86**, 538.

personalities, whether or not complicated by low intelligence, are easily persuaded to form drinking habits. There are trades and occupations which encourage alcoholism, and even big business does not despise the aid of alcohol in dealing with customers. Certain games and sports have Bacchus as their patron and the devotees must worship the same god. Considerable controversy exists as to whether people drink primarily for the immediate sensory pleasure of taste ; authorities who themselves are abstainers deny this in a somewhat intolerant manner, but it is generally admitted that taste does not play a major part in the formation of drinking habits.

DRUG ADDICTION

The treatment of drug addiction is based on the same principles as described above for alcoholism, for both conditions point to a personality disorder from which the patient must be freed after the toxic influence of the drug is relieved. There is this difference, however, that in drug addiction the psychological changes following prolonged use are more profound, the symptoms due to withdrawal of the drug more grave and the craving more intense. The development of tolerance is also important, for the addict takes more and more of the drug to satisfy his cravings. His tolerance to the drug still further increases and a vicious circle develops. The general physical deterioration is also greater in drug addicts than in alcoholics.

Morphine Addiction is the most common form of drug habit in this country, the largest group being formed by those who can obtain supplies easily ; thus the highest incidence occurs in doctors, nurses, chemists and their relatives. The craving may have been formed after a long illness in which morphia has been given for the relief of pain. Patients have been known to malinger in order to have another operation and more morphia ; the writer has seen an addict with the scars of thirty-six abdominal operations. It therefore behoves doctors, and especially surgeons, to regard every patient as a potential morphia addict and to exercise corresponding care in prescribing.

Treatment should always be carried out in a hospital where psychological care can be given and where the patient is under discipline. Statutory provisions are of little help, and, in our opinion, a special type of certification should be available. Attempts to treat addiction without restriction ignore the extent of the physiological craving and the complete inability of the patient to co-operate honestly. It is permissible to give morphia to the patient while arrangements are being made for hospitalization, but once this has been accomplished abrupt withdrawal of the drug should take place. The dreaded symptoms of withdrawal have been much exaggerated, and with good medical care and intensive psychotherapy they can be greatly modified and controlled. Subsequent treatment consists of psychotherapy and re-education on the lines suggested for the treatment of chronic alcoholism (see p. 1050).

Cocaine Addiction.—This is fortunately uncommon in this country. It is found especially among criminal and depraved classes. Unhappily every addict is a potential source of danger to the community. The sexual and other urges which follow indulgence make him crave for company and induce him to pervert others. Tolerance, it is important to note, is not acquired, and the increase in consumption is due mainly to a craving for increased sensations. There are no physical symptoms attributable to withdrawal of the drug. Cocaine should, therefore, never be given to a patient who comes for help, no matter what hysterical symptoms he may show or what threats he may make. Treatment should be undertaken in hospital, the drug should be stopped at once and sedative and eliminative treatment instituted. Psychotherapy and re-education play a fundamental part in the management of the case.

D. R. MacCalman.

FEMALE SEX ENDOCRINOLOGY

INTRODUCTION

THE intelligent treatment of menstrual and reproductive abnormalities requires not only some knowledge of the physiological processes involved in normal menstrual function but also an understanding of the actions of the various hormone preparations which are available for clinical use. The following is a brief epitome of the cyclical changes which occur in the ovaries and endometrium during a normal cycle.

1. The activity of the ovaries is regulated by the gonadotropic hormone of the anterior pituitary.

2. The ovaries, stimulated by the pituitary, give rise to several primordial Graafian follicles, and during their development they elaborate a specific hormone, œstradiol. This hormone, in its turn, has a stimulating effect on the growth of the endometrium.

3. One follicle in each cycle reaches full development and ruptures, releasing an ovum. The ruptured follicle, still under the primary pituitary stimulus, becomes luteinized and a corpus luteum is formed. The corpus luteum also elaborates a specific hormone—progesterone—and, in addition, secretes œstradiol. Progesterone changes the character and structure of the endometrium into the so-called secretory or premenstrual stage.

4. If fertilization fails to occur, the endometrium at the end of the secretory phase breaks down and bleeding follows.

Although there are many hypotheses, the actual cause of menstruation itself is not yet explained.

It is difficult to estimate the importance of the rôle played by certain of the endocrine glands, such as the thyroid, adrenal and pancreas, in menstrual and reproductive function. All are essential to a general hormonal balance, and there is evidence to suggest that dysfunction of any one of these glands may adversely affect the reproductive process. Chief interest, however, has been centred round those glands vitally concerned in the menstrual function, namely, the pituitary and ovaries.

GONADOTROPIC HORMONES

It has been conclusively demonstrated that anterior pituitary gland extracts are effective in stimulating gonadal function in the hypophysectomized experimental animal. Such extracts would be of very great value in the treatment of patients exhibiting ovarian hypofunction. Potent extracts, however, are not only very difficult to prepare, but they are so unstable that they readily lose their potency. At the present time there are no reliable anterior pituitary gland extracts procurable. There are, however, substances available which, although not truly hypophyseal in character, have an anterior pituitary-like effect. From the point of view of their therapeutic application it is most important that the action of these two substances should be understood clearly.

The substances are :—

1. Urine or Chorionic Gonadotropic Hormone.
2. Serum or Equine Gonadotropic Hormone.

Urine Gonadotropic Hormone.—This hormone is present in the urine in large amounts during pregnancy and is the basis of the Aschheim-Zondek test for pregnancy. It is also excreted in the urine in cases of chorion epithelioma and certain testicular tumours. The administration of this hormone *does not* stimulate the development of Graafian follicles, but it may produce luteinization in follicles already formed. There are, accordingly, few indications for its clinical use.

Serum Gonadotropic Hormone.—This hormone is found in the blood serum of pregnant mares during the middle third of their pregnancy. It simulates chorionic gonadotropic hormone in that it is probably placental in origin, but differs essentially in action in that it *does* stimulate the growth of primordial follicles. In the latter respect it closely resembles the true anterior pituitary gonadotropic hormone and thus it is a useful therapeutic agent. Experimentally and clinically it has been found that the effect of this preparation can be enhanced by the simultaneous administration of the chorionic gonadotropic hormone. All gonadotropic hormone preparations should be given by intramuscular injection as there is no scientific evidence that they are effective when given by mouth.

Standardization of the Gonadotropic Hormones.—Methods of standardization are based on the minimum amount of the hormone required to induce ovarian changes in immature rats or mice. The unit dosage of the various commercial preparations expressed in rat or mouse units leads to much confusion.

The establishment of a unit in terms of an international standard at an early date will clarify the difficulty in regard to dosage.

Commercial Preparations of Gonadotropic Hormones

Anterior Pituitary Gonadotropic Hormone :—

(*a*) Ambinon (Organon Laboratories). This preparation contains also the thyrotropic factor.
(*b*) Gonadotraphon (Paines & Byrne Ltd.).
(*c*) Preloban (Bayer Ltd.).

Urine Gonadotropic Hormone :—

(*a*) Pregnyl (Organon Laboratories).
(*b*) Gonan (British Drug Houses).
(*c*) Physostab (Boots Ltd.).
(*d*) Antuitrin S (Parke, Davis & Co.).
(*e*) Prolan (Bayer Ltd.).

Serum Gonadotropic Hormone :—

(*a*) Antostab (Boots Ltd.).
(*b*) Serogan (British Drug Houses).
(*c*) Pregnant Mares' Serum (Organon Laboratories).
(*d*) Gonadyl (Roussel Laboratories).

OVARIAN HORMONES

Two hormones are secreted by the ovary: (*a*) œstradiol or œstrogenic hormone, and (*b*) progesterone or corpus luteum hormone.

Œstradiol or Œstrogenic Hormone.—An œstrogenic substance is one which, when injected into the ovariectomized animal, such as the rodent, induces the changes in the reproductive tract characteristic of true œstrus. During œstrus the vaginal epithelium shows cornification and this can readily be demonstrated by the vaginal smear test. Only leucocytes are found in the vaginal smear during diœstrus or resting phase.

The œstrogenic hormone is present in the blood and urine of normal men and women. A very high concentration of the hormone is found in the blood and urine of pregnant women.

Substances with œstrogenic activity have been found widely distributed in the plant and animal kingdom. In the human female three important compounds, each a phenanthrene derivative, have been isolated and purified, viz., œstrone, œstriol and œstradiol. The most powerful of these three compounds is œstradiol, and as it has been recovered from follicular fluid it is believed to be the naturally occurring œstrogenic principle. For clinical use the esterified form of œstradiol—usually œstradiol benzoate—is employed.

Synthetic Œstrogenic Substances.—The identification of the chemical structure of the natural œstrogens has stimulated efforts to synthetize them, but so far with no success. As a result of the research of Dodds and his co-workers, however, several compounds have been isolated which have a high œstrogenic activity. The two principal compounds synthetized —derivatives of stilbene—are diethyl stilbœstrol or stilbœstrol and dihydro-stilbœstrol or hexœstrol. Both substances are very active when given orally, whereas the natural œstrogens are relatively inactive when given by this route. These two synthetic compounds have been tested clinically and experimentally and have been found to simulate all the known functions of the naturally occurring œstrogens. Their high activity by oral administration is important clinically, the only disadvantage being that they have a tendency to cause nausea and vomiting in some cases ; this, however, has been partially eliminated by the use of the propionate ester.

Physiological Actions of the Œstrogenic Hormones

1. They produce œstrus in the castrated or immature experimental animal.

2. They control the development of the secondary sexual characteristics and promote the growth of the reproductive tract in the female.

3. They induce the proliferative or pre-ovulatory change in the uterine endometrium, sensitize the uterine musculature, and stimulate capillary vasodilatation in the uterus.

4. As a result of their action the vaginal epithelium becomes thickened and glycogen is deposited in the cells.

5. They inhibit the anterior pituitary gonadotropic hormone when given in sufficient concentration.

6. It is probable that they promote the development of the duct system of the breasts.

Progesterone or Corpus Luteum Hormone.—The functionally active corpus luteum secretes œstrogenic hormone in addition to its characteristic hormone, progesterone. The latter is essential only for reproductive function. Progesterone does not reproduce its characteristic effect on the endometrium without the prior action of œstrogenic hormone.

There is excreted in the urine in small amounts during the second half of the normal menstrual cycle, and in large amounts during pregnancy, a biologically inactive substance, pregnandiol, which is a metabolic or break-down product of progesterone. Chemical analysis of this product in the urine is proving a fairly reliable index of corpus luteum activity.

Physiological Actions of Progesterone

1. It brings about the secretory phase of the endometrium.

2. It prepares the endometrium for the implantation of the fertilized ovum in that it desensitizes the uterine musculature and maintains pregnancy in the very early stages.

3. The development of the alveolar systems of the breast is probably under the control of progesterone.

Standardization of Ovarian Hormones.—The fixing of an international unit standard in the dosage of œstrogenic hormones brought order out of chaos, but resulted in the dosage being frequently expressed in astronomical figures. The problem has been simplified by expressing the dosage as the actual weight of the hormone in milligrams. One milligram of pure œstrone contains 10,000 international units.

The international unit of progesterone is defined as the progestational activity present in 1 milligram of crystalline corpus luteum hormone. Therapeutically the dosage is expressed in milligrams.

Commercial Preparations of Ovarian Hormones [1]

Œstrogenic Hormones :—

Œstroform (British Drug Houses).
Dimenformon (Organon Laboratories).
Progynon B. Oleosum Forte (Scherings Ltd.)
Theelin (Parke, Davis & Co.).
Benzo-Gynœstryl (Roussel Laboratories).

Synthetic :—

Stilbœstrol Dipropionate.
Hexœstrol.

Progesterone :—

Proluton (Scherings Ltd.).
Progestin (Organon Laboratories).
Progestin (British Drug Houses).

[1] The list of commercial preparations is only representative and is by no means complete.

DISORDERS OF MENSTRUAL FUNCTION

FUNCTIONAL UTERINE BLEEDING

Probably the most common cause of functional uterine bleeding is *metropathia hæmorrhagica*. This condition is characterized pathologically by cystic degeneration of Graafian follicles with absence of recent or active corpora lutea in the ovaries. There is hyperplasia of the uterine muscle with marked hyperplasia of the endometrium and cystic dilatation of the glands. The predominant symptom of the condition is irregular or prolonged uterine bleeding, frequently preceded by a period of amenorrhœa of six to ten weeks' duration. It is more common at puberty and the menopause, but may occur at any time during the period of reproductive life. The clinical and pathological manifestations of the condition are due, undoubtedly, to a dysfunction of the ovaries. It is not clear whether the ovarian dysfunction is due to some change in the structure or reactivity of the ovaries, or if it is associated primarily with an abnormal functioning of the anterior pituitary.

The management of a case of metropathia hæmorrhagica requires the consideration of several specified lines of therapy: (*a*) hormone therapy, (*b*) irradiation, (*c*) surgical treatment.

Hormone Therapy.—This is particularly indicated in the younger woman and in such cases it is, as a rule, successful. Its employment in women towards the end of the period of reproductive life should always be preceded by a very thorough pelvic examination and curettage of the uterus in order to exclude malignant disease. Hormones available for the treatment of metropathia hæmorrhagica are (*a*) progesterone, and (*b*) testosterone.

Progesterone is given intramuscularly in doses of 10 to 20 mgm. daily for four to five days, starting at the onset of the bleeding. If this dosage is not sufficient, then it may be continued for a further two days. The same dosage is again given every third day, starting two weeks after the bleeding has been controlled, giving three doses in all. Relapses do occur with this treatment, but it appears to be rational therapy, and if given a fair trial is usually successful.

Testosterone (male hormone), *e.g.*, Testoviron (Scherings), Sterandyl (Roussel Laboratories), is also effective in metropathia hæmorrhagica. This preparation should be used with caution as it is sometimes associated with unpleasant reactions, such as hirsutism and change of voice. It is given intramuscularly in doses of 100 mgm. daily for eight to ten days. This treatment is frequently followed by a period of amenorrhœa, varying in duration from two to three months, after which there is a return of the normal menstrual cycle.

Thyroid extract (Thyroideum B.P.), 1 gr. once or twice daily, is sometimes useful, especially when the condition occurs in young girls.

It cannot be emphasized too strongly that œstrogenic preparations are contraindicated in metropathia hæmorrhagica.

Irradiation.—The induction of an artificial menopause with radium or X-irradiation of the ovaries is indicated especially in menopausal patients. The employment of a small dosage, however, in *younger* individuals in order to induce a temporary period of amenorrhœa is fraught with danger as there is a marked variation in individual sensitivity to irradiation. The use of this therapeutic agent may in some cases cause permanent ablation of ovarian function.

Surgical Treatment.—Curettage of the uterus is not only diagnostic but is curative in some cases. This being so, it is only reasonable that this simple form of therapy should be employed prior to any more drastic procedure. Hysterectomy is only indicated after all other forms of therapy have failed, and it is probably best reserved as a last resort in patients under the age of thirty-six in whom it is desirable to conserve the ovaries.

MID-MENSTRUAL OR OVULAR BLEEDING

Slight vaginal bleeding midway between the periods is not uncommon. It occurs at the time of ovulation, and it is believed to be associated with a temporary diminution in the concentration of the œstrogenic hormone in the blood just before this is made good by the corpus luteum. It is of no serious significance in the unmarried woman except for the inconvenience, but it may be a cause of sterility in the married woman.

The daily injection of 5 mgm. progesterone for three days at the mid-menstrual interval, given over a period of three months, may control the bleeding effectively.

AMENORRHŒA

Amenorrhœa may represent a physiological condition, may be an expression of a pathological process, or it may be a manifestation of a functional disturbance.

Physiological Amenorrhœa.—Absence of menstruation is physiological before puberty, during pregnancy and lactation, and after the menopause.

Pathological Amenorrhœa.—Pathological lesions situated in the pituitary, ovaries or uterus may cause amenorrhœa. Systemic diseases, such as anæmia, pulmonary tuberculosis, schizophrenia, decompensated mitral stenosis, toxic goitre and diabetes mellitus are also recognized as ætiological factors.

Functional Amenorrhœa.—Any interference with the function of the ovaries and anterior pituitary gland, which normally control the menstrual process, will upset menstrual periodicity. The anterior pituitary gland is under the control of the autonomic nervous system and higher cerebral centres and accordingly in susceptible individuals its function is readily interfered with by extrinsic factors such as psychological trauma. The ovaries and uterus in cases of functional amenorrhœa are capable of being stimulated ; it is the hormonal stimulus to these structures, in the majority of cases, which is deficient or absent.

Management.—A consideration of the ætiological factors involved in amenorrhœa indicates that there is no specific line of treatment, and that only by a review of all the facts accruing from interrogation and examination of the patient can any rational form of therapy be suggested.

In elucidating the patient's history it is important to ascertain if there has been any abnormal psychological stimulus, such as grief, worry, fear, change of surroundings or occupation, etc., within a short time prior to the onset of the amenorrhœa. It is also essential that a careful general examination should be carried out in order that any systemic disease or pathological process, with which amenorrhœa may be associated, may be detected as early as possible. Pregnancy must be excluded in every case. This can be done readily without the patient's knowledge, if there is any doubt, by testing a specimen of urine for the Aschheim-Zondek reaction.

After the exclusion of pathological and physiological causes the amenorrhœa may be considered functional in origin.

The spontaneous onset of menstruation frequently terminates functional amenorrhœa, and this result may be hoped for up to a period of one year. Although it may occur spontaneously after this length of time, it is not advisable to delay the institution of treatment any further. As there is a tendency to obesity in many of these cases, a suitable anti-obesity régime should be instituted if required (see p. 389). Conversely, if the patient is markedly under weight, every effort should be made by rest and an adequate diet to promote nutrition. The initial line of treatment should be directed to the general health of the patient.

A logical scheme of therapy is firstly to give œstrogenic hormone in order to sensitize and induce development of the uterus, which frequently undergoes partial atrophy after a prolonged period of amenorrhœa. This should be followed up by the administration of gonadotropic hormone, since, in the majority of cases, the pituitary stimulus to the ovaries is deficient or in abeyance, and must be supplemented. Five milligrams stilbœstrol dipropionate or hexœstrol are given by mouth thrice daily for a period of ten days. If after a further period of ten days no vaginal bleeding occurs, the same dosage is repeated for another ten days, and so on until bleeding is induced. Except in very resistant patients in whom there may be marked atrophy of the uterus, bleeding occurs six to seven days after the first or second course of therapy. The natural œstrogen, œstradiol benzoate, may be given in place of the synthetic form. It is administered intramuscularly in 5 mgm. doses every third day for five injections, and a similar course is repeated after ten days' interval if no bleeding occurs within that time.

The induction of uterine bleeding may be taken as a rough index of full uterine development. Immediately bleeding occurs serum gonadotropic hormone, 500 rat units, combined with urine gonadotropic hormone, 100 rat units, is given intramuscularly every third day until five injections have been given. After an interval of ten to fourteen days the same course is repeated. It may be necessary to give several courses of these preparations before any effect is produced, and it is advisable to continue their administration during the first half of the cycle for a period of three months after menstruation has been established. Preparations of serum and urine gonadotropic hormone are made up in powder form and are supplied with the necessary solvent. It is important that the powder be completely dissolved and that the site of injection should be thoroughly massaged, as thereby some unpleasant local reactions may be minimized.

MINOR MENSTRUAL DISORDERS

Hypomenorrhœa, or scanty menstrual loss, usually requires no treatment as it is frequently associated with a normal ovarian and uterine cycle. In such cases conception is possible. Although the loss may be normal or scanty, however, many women have incomplete ovarian and uterine cycles due to a failure of ovulation. This type of menstruation is termed anovular and can only be detected by the histological examination of the endometrium immediately prior to the onset of menstruation, or by examination of the urine for its pregnandiol content carried out at the same time.

Oligomenorrhœa or delayed menstruation is common. It is important in that it is frequently associated with lassitude and a feeling of depression and irritability and may be a precursor of amenorrhœa.

Supplementary pituitary therapy is indicated in these disorders as it is probable that they are due to a defective pituitary stimulus to the ovaries. Serum gonadotropic hormone, 500 rat units, combined with 100 rat units chorionic gonadotropic hormone, should be given intramuscularly every third day for five injections, the first injection being given immediately after the cessation of menstrual loss. This treatment should be continued over three menstrual cycles.

RECURRENT ABORTION

General Treatment.—It is essential in the management of a patient who aborts repeatedly that any local pelvic abnormality, such as retroversion of the uterus and cervical lacerations, should be dealt with initially. The Wassermann reaction should be tested and, if positive, specific therapy should be instituted. The patient should be asked to report as soon as conception occurs and given definite instructions. She should be advised to lead as quiet a life as possible, avoiding over-exertion and excitement. The importance of rest must be emphasized and complete rest in bed is desirable during the time when the periods would occur had not pregnancy intervened. Attention should be directed to the careful regulation of the bowel in order to avoid the necessity for any drastic purge which may be disastrous. She should be told that any suspicion of vaginal bleeding is an indication for the immediate cessation of all activities.

Specific Therapy.—The administration intramuscularly of

10 mgm. progesterone twice weekly during the first four months of pregnancy is frequently highly successful. The same dose should be given thrice daily if bleeding occurs and should be continued till it ceases. Vitamin E in the form of Fertilol (Vitamins Ltd.), Viteolin (Glaxo Ltd.) or Ephynal (Hoffman la Roche) is also advocated in the treatment of recurrent abortion. Fertilol and viteolin are extracts of wheat germ oil and are available in capsule form. The dose recommended is one capsule thrice daily throughout pregnancy. Ephynal is a synthetic preparation of vitamin E and is available in tablet form. One tablet is given three times daily throughout pregnancy.

There is some doubtful clinical evidence of the therapeutic effect of urine gonadotropic hormone in this condition. The dose recommended is 100 rat units given intramuscularly twice weekly throughout pregnancy.

THE MENOPAUSE

Some women pass through the climacteric with a minimum of discomfort, while others have a most distressing and hazardous time. These varying effects are possibly determined, in the majority of cases, by the mental status of the individual.

Although the characteristic menopausal symptoms, such as flushes, tachycardia, lassitude, etc., are most frequently associated with the decline of ovarian function, the possibility of systemic disease such as tuberculosis, hyperthyroidism or anæmia being responsible for these symptoms must not be overlooked. Accordingly, a thorough general examination is necessary prior to the institution of treatment directed towards the relief of symptoms. Irregular uterine bleeding at the menopause should not be considered natural and inevitable until the possibility of malignant disease has been excluded.

Many women at the menopause are assailed by doubts and fears regarding the future. It should be explained to them that the change of life is a physiological process and that no ill-effects accrue in the majority of cases. It should be emphasized, however, that it is necessary that they should lead an active and ordered life. Such reassurance, by itself, or given in conjunction with ½ gr. of phenobarbitone twice or thrice daily, is usually effective in women complaining of mild subjective symptoms.

Œstrogenic hormone therapy is usually successful in controlling the more severe symptoms directly associated with the menopausal disturbance. In order to bring the distressing symptoms under control as rapidly as possible large doses of the hormone should be given initially, and thereafter the doses should be gradually reduced. The dosage employed varies according to the severity of the disturbance. In the most severe cases of climacteric disorder the following scheme of treatment is advised. Stilbœstrol dipropionate or hexœstrol in 5 mgm. doses is given thrice daily by mouth until all the subjective phenomena are completely controlled. Thereafter, 5 mgm. of either preparation are given twice daily for one week and once daily for further two weeks. The dose is then reduced to 1 mgm. daily for a further period of two weeks. If the synthetic œstrogen is not well tolerated it is necessary to give œstradiol benzoate intramuscularly. Five milligrams are given daily until the symptoms are controlled, and this is followed by a gradual reduction in the dosage over the ensuing four to six weeks. Uterine bleeding may be induced as a result of this therapy, but it is of no serious significance and requires no treatment.

Patients who have been left untreated over a period of many years or who develop vasomotor and nervous symptoms years after the menopause react favourably to œstrogenic therapy, but a maintenance dose of the hormone may have to be given over a very prolonged period.

POST-MENOPAUSAL DISTURBANCES

Several conditions may develop at varying intervals after the menopause which may directly or indirectly be associated with cessation of ovarian activity. The most important of these are *senile vaginitis*, *kraurosis vulvæ* and *pruritus vulvæ*. Œstrogenic hormone therapy is specific for senile vaginitis and kraurosis vulvæ, while its administration, if not curative, brings about alleviation in many cases of pruritus vulvæ. A large dose of œstrogenic hormone should be administered, either 5 mgm. of stilbœstrol dipropionate thrice daily by mouth or 5 mgm. œstrodial benzoate daily by the intramuscular route. This treatment usually requires to be continued over a period of ten to fourteen days, but varies according to the severity of the condition.

DYSMENORRHŒA

The innumerable therapeutic measures advocated for the relief of primary dysmenorrhœa indicate not only the variety of the ætiological factors concerned, but that several lines of treatment may have to be adopted before success is obtained.

Thus it is evident that there is no single form of therapy suitable for every case. A routine scheme of treatment is recommended, such as the following :—

General Measures.—As there is probably a psychological factor operating in many cases, the initial step should include an investigation of this aspect. It will be found that a brief explanation to the patient of the essentially physiological nature of the menstrual process is often helpful in dispersing the many doubts and superstitions which are founded on a misguided upbringing or unfavourable associations. Every effort should be made to promote a condition of physical fitness, special attention being directed to ensuring sufficient exercise, rest and an adequate diet. As constipation is a very prevalent ætiological factor in the causation of dysmenorrhœa, particularly when present during the pre-menstrual phase, a regular evacuation of the bowels should be ensured by instituting the measures recommended on p. 573. Further, it should be emphasized that if possible menstruation should not be allowed to interfere with the normal daily routine and activities. The adoption of these general measures alone often results in alleviation of the menstrual pain.

Sedative Treatment.—Mild analgesics, such as acetyl salicyl, gr. v, t.i.d., reinforced where necessary by gr. $\frac{1}{4}$ of codein or phenacetin, gr. v, when the pain is severe, are often efficacious.

Hormone Therapy.—If the pain comes on before the onset of the menstrual flow, then it is believed that it is due, in some cases, to an excessive action of the œstrogenic hormone or defective progesterone influence on the uterine musculature. In such cases the administration of 5 mgm. progesterone every second day, starting six days before the expected period, is often beneficial. Conversely, when the pain coincides with the onset of the menstrual flow, it may be due to an excessive action of progesterone on the uterus, and the administration of 5 mgm. stilbœstrol dipropionate t.i.d. for four days before the period is often effective. The treatment in either case should be continued over three menstrual cycles.

Surgical Treatment.—When no pathological pelvic lesion is present dilatation of the cervix should be advised as this is found to be effective in many cases. Severe cases, resistant to the lines of treatment already recommended, should be referred to a specialist, who may consider the injection of alcohol into the cervical ganglia or the division of the presacral nerve.

T. N. MacGregor.

TECHNICAL PROCEDURES AND OXYGEN THERAPY

Introduction

THE procedures to be described in this chapter must be carried out in an aseptic manner. The techniques of hospital or nursing home may have to be modified in general practice, and it will be convenient to begin with an account of the steps common to all.

The hands and forearms of the operator are cleansed by washing for five minutes, preferably in running warm water. A bottle of spirit soap may be carried for this purpose. The use of the nail-brush should be confined to the nails and nail-folds; elsewhere it leads to roughening of the skin. The washing should be done from the elbows downwards, and the final rinsing is of the hands alone. The hands are then immersed in, or swabbed with, a solution of 1 : 1,000 biniodide of mercury in spirit, and the washed area is dried, hands first, on a sterile towel. If this cleansing is, as it should be, scrupulous, it is unnecessary to wear gloves. The *skin of the patient* should be shaved if the part is hairy, and then prepared as are the operator's hands. The spirit solution must not be "slopped" over the area, lest it reach and irritate distant parts—for example, the genitalia, in tapping of the abdomen. To *drape the sterilized area*, it is convenient and economical to employ towels 2 ft. square, with a hole 2 in. square in their middle; a number of these, and a supply of gauze mops, may be sterilized in a drum (in hospital or nursing home, or by a commercial firm), and used as required. The quantity of *local anæsthetic* needed for these minor procedures is best purchased in ampoules; the exterior of these, and the file for opening them, are sterilized by immersion in a mixture of lysol (1 part) and spirit (3 parts) for five minutes. It is safest to boil a *syringe* in distilled water, in the rack in which its component parts lie apart; *hypodermic needles* are wrapped in gauze or lint before they are boiled.

SUBCUTANEOUS ADMINISTRATION OF FLUID

Normal saline (0·9 per cent.) is readily absorbed from subcutaneous areas rich in lymphatic vessels. A " drip " apparatus is used, the delivery tube of which leads to a Y-tube, from which two rubber tubes conduct the fluid to two special " subcutaneous saline " needles. These are of medium bore, and have additional lateral apertures. All the component parts must be sterile. A " head " of about 2 ft. is usual. The system is filled with saline solution, and the delivery tube clamped. The needles are inserted through intradermal wheals of local anæsthetic solution. They may be placed (1) at the outer border of each pectoralis major muscle, directed towards the apex of the axilla ; or (2) on the antero-internal aspect of each thigh, near and directed towards Poupart's ligament. Care must be taken that they do not puncture or rest in a blood vessel. When they are correctly placed the delivery tubes are connected to them by adaptors ; the needles and adaptors are then covered by a piece of sterile gauze, and fixed in position by strapping. The " dripper " is adjusted to deliver 40 to 50 drops a minute. If 10 c.c. of 2 per cent. novocain solution is added to each litre of saline solution, the method does not give rise to pain. The axillæ (or groins) are inspected from time to time, and if the tissues appear tense, or unduly œdematous, the flow is temporarily stopped. In favourable cases fluid may be administered by the subcutaneous route, through the same needle punctures, for two or three days. Occasionally the apertures in a needle become blocked, but this is easily remedied by " stripping " the corresponding delivery tube towards the needle.

RECTAL ADMINISTRATION OF FLUID

Before fluids are administered by the rectum it should be thoroughly emptied by an enema. By this route may be supplied : (1) tap water, which is very well tolerated ; (2) normal (0·9 per cent.) saline solution ; (3) normal (5 per cent.) glucose solution ; and (4) a mixture of (2) and (3). The successful use of the method depends on the avoidance of any distension of the rectum, as this leads to expulsion of its contents.

The apparatus, which need not be sterilized, consists of (1) a " drip " apparatus, which is connected by (2) thick-walled rubber tubing to (3) a wide-bore rectal nozzle of glass or, better, vulcanite (the nozzle used by radiologists for the introduction of a barium enema is a good pattern), and (4) a Y-tube with an additional length of rubber tubing, connected to (5) a glass J-tube. The apparatus is arranged as shown in Fig. 19. The purpose of the thick-walled tubing is to prevent kinking, in order that if necessary flatus may escape by the free limb of the Y-tube, which is hung on the container by the glass J-tube. If the anus is sensitive a little anæsthetic ointment[1] may be smeared on the nozzle. The tubing near the nozzle should be loosely secured to the thigh by a turn of a bandage, rather than by adhesive strapping; the removal of the latter from such a hairy part is painful. A "head" of about 12 in. is all that is necessary, and a suitable rate of flow is 80 drops per minute, or 300 c.c. per hour. The flow may be stopped for one hour in every four, but the nozzle is left in position, unless the bowels are to be moved. Thus about 2 litres of fluid may be given in each twenty-four hours. An alternative method is to run into the rectum through a catheter (size 12) attached to a funnel 300 c.c. of the desired fluid every four hours. The rectum must be washed out daily.

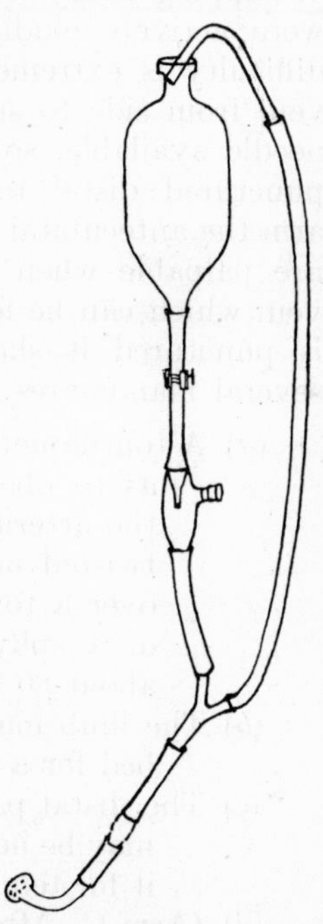

FIG. 19.—Apparatus for Rectal Administration of Fluid.

Occasionally hypertonic solutions are administered by rectum, in order to procure a fluid evacuation and thus to favour the reduction of intracranial pressure. For an adult, 4 to 6 oz. (120-180 c.c.) of a 50 per cent. solution of magnesium sulphate are given slowly by catheter and funnel; the enema must be retained for twenty to thirty minutes to allow time for its hydroscopic action.

VENIPUNCTURE

Puncture of a vein may be necessary (1) for the intravenous introduction of drugs or (2) for the withdrawal of blood, to obtain a sample for analysis, to obtain blood for transfusion, or to deplete the circulation as a therapeutic measure. For any of these purposes, as a rule, a vein in one of the antecubital fossæ is chosen; but sometimes (*e.g.*, in obese patients) an

[1] Such as Anæsthesin or Cycloform.

internal saphenous vein is more accessible. Veins may be visible and prominent, and then they have an irritating habit of slipping easily from side to side under the skin, as if they were actively eluding the point of the needle. When this difficulty is extreme, it may be overcome by transfixing the vein from side to side with the finest hypodermic or cambric needle available, so that it is immobilized ; the vein is then punctured distal to the immobilizing needle. In an obese arm the antecubital veins may not be visible, but as a rule they are palpable when engorged. In practice the least movable vein which can be identified should be utilized. Before a vein is punctured it should be made as prominent as possible ; several manœuvres are available :—

(*a*) A tourniquet may be applied at the root of the limb, so as to obstruct the venous return without stopping the arterial inflow. This may be a turn of bandage twisted on itself ; a piece of rubber tubing applied over a towel and fastened by a forceps, or the cuff of a sphygmomanometer inflated to a pressure of about 80 mm. of mercury.

(*b*) The limb may be allowed to hang over the edge of the bed for a few minutes before the puncture.

(*c*) The distal part of the limb, up to the site of puncture, may be heated by a hot fomentation, or by immersing it for ten minutes in hot (120° F.) water.

(*d*) (Arm.) After the application of the tourniquet the patient may be directed to grasp a roller bandage firmly with his hand at intervals of thirty seconds.

In difficult cases a warm antiseptic solution should be used for cleansing the skin ; cold spirit and ether cause the veins to contract.

1. *Intravenous Medication.*—A fine hypodermic needle should be employed. The fluid to be injected is taken up out of its container, through the needle, into a syringe of appropriate size. The needle should not be passed to the bottom of, *e.g.*, an ampoule, as its point may be turned by this fault ; but the ampoule should be tilted to allow all the fluid to be drawn up with the needle resting on the wall. The syringe and needle are then held vertically, needle uppermost, the barrel is tapped to dislodge any bubbles of air, and the piston pushed onwards until fluid flows from the point of the needle. The needle is pushed through the skin a little to one side of the selected vein, and then brought over it, ready to make the puncture. When the vein is large, the position of the bevel of the point

does not matter, but when the vein is small the bevel should be held downwards, as this minimizes leakage. The needle is then pushed into the vein at an acute angle, and its position verified by slowly [1] withdrawing a little blood into the syringe. When the point is correctly placed, the obstructing cuff or tourniquet is removed and the contents of the syringe slowly injected. *An injection should never be made unless blood has been withdrawn into the syringe, and after this has been done the position of the needle should not be altered until the injection has been completed.* The needle is then quickly withdrawn while the thumb of the left hand makes pressure upon it through a gauze swab or piece of sterile cotton-wool; if the patient flexes his elbow on this pad for a few minutes a dressing is not required.

If the patient moves there is a possibility that the needle may have been dislodged from the vein, and its position within the vein must be verified afresh before the injection is begun or completed. During the injection, if any swelling appears under the skin round the puncture, leakage has occurred, and the injection should be stopped at once, the needle withdrawn, and a new vein in another limb utilized. A hot fomentation, renewed four-hourly over the area of leakage, is the best method of minimizing local irritation.

2. *To Obtain a Sample for Analysis.*—If possible, samples of blood for analysis should be taken from the patient at least eight hours after his last meal (*e.g.*, in the morning before the patient's breakfast); if this is not possible, the interval after the previous meal should be indicated to the laboratory. Samples should be transmitted to the laboratory as soon as possible after their withdrawal. For a single estimation 5 c.c. suffice; for several different estimations 10 to 15 c.c. are necessary. The nature of the samples required for the quantitative estimation of certain constituents of blood, and the normal range of these, is indicated in Tables I and II. When untreated blood is required it is withdrawn into a syringe by venipuncture, and transferred to a sterile test-tube fitted with a *rubber* stopper. When an oxalated sample is necessary, blood withdrawn into a syringe is transferred to a similar test-tube containing crystals of potassium oxalate as an anticoagulant, the test-tube being shaken to ensure solution of the crystals. In practice, it is often very convenient to employ "Venules" [2] for the collection and transmission of

[1] Strong suction may draw the wall of the vein over a correctly placed needle, and so prevent the withdrawal of blood.

[2] "Venules," Behring.

samples of blood. These are small vacuum tubes fitted with a sterile hollow needle ; they may be obtained with or without the addition of, *e.g.*, potassium oxalate crystals.

3. *To Obtain Blood for Transfusion.*—See p. 1082.

4. *To Deplete the Circulation.*—Venipuncture has replaced venesection as a method of depleting the circulation ; in general, the indications for the procedure are cardiac failure, with backward pressure in the systemic veins, hypertension, uræmia and polycythæmia. The technique is similar to that employed in the withdrawal of blood for transfusion : up to 500 c.c. of blood may be withdrawn ; often it must be discarded, but it is a good plan to group such patients, for the blood may occasionally be utilized for transfusion, if direct matching (p. 1079) shows it to be completely suitable.

Table I

Biochemical Estimations, Tests, etc., for which Untreated Blood is required

Constituent.	Normal Range.
Phosphate . . .	3 to 4·5 mg. per cent.
Phosphatase . . .	8 ,, 14 units.
Calcium	9 ,, 11 mg. per cent.
Bilirubin . . .	0·1 ,, 0·5 ,, ,, ,,
Icteric index . . .	3 ,, 6 units.

Van den Bergh's reaction.
Widal and other agglutination reactions.
Wassermann reaction. Kahn reaction.
Serum for grouping or direct testing before transfusions.
Whole blood for culture, transferred direct to flask of medium.

Table II

Biochemical Estimations and Tests for which Oxalated Blood is required

Constituent.	Normal Range.
Sugar	80 to 120 mg. per cent.
Urea	20 ,, 35 ,, ,, ,,
Uric acid . . .	2 ,, 4 ,, ,, ,,
Non-protein nitrogen	20 ,, 40 ,, ,, ,,
Creatinine . . .	1 ,, 2 ,, ,, ,,
Proteins	6 ,, 8·5 gm. per cent.
Cholesterol . . .	140 ,, 200 mg. per cent.
Chlorides . . .	540 ,, 610 ,, ,, ,,
Alkali reserve . . . (CO_2 combining power.)	54 ,, 60 volumes per cent.

Red blood corpuscles, for grouping or direct testing before transfusions.

INTRAVENOUS INFUSION

Fluid may be introduced into a vein either through a needle or through a cannula ; for the latter procedure the vein must be exposed. The chosen fluid may be given in one dose, by allowing it to flow continuously, or its administration may be spread out over a longer period (even for days) by the employment of a " drip " apparatus.

Apparatus for Intravenous Infusion.—In hospital practice, fluids for intravenous infusion are prepared with great care from pure chemicals and distilled water, and thereafter sterilized. Unless every detail in their preparation is scrupulously carried out, reactions may occur during and after their administration. They are transferred for administration to a large funnel or, better, to a container fitted with a rubber stopper through which passes a " thistle tube," the lower end of which does not reach the liquid. In the " thistle " is placed sterile cotton-wool, to act as a filter for the air which displaces the fluid as it flows from the container (Fig. 20). In general practice it is difficult to prepare uniformly satisfactory solutions, and it is highly advisable to procure them ready for administration, from the firms [1] which specialize in their production ; in these circumstances they are delivered to the vein from the container in which they are supplied. The rubber tubing which conveys fluid from container to vein requires special preparation when it is new. It must be boiled in water for an hour, and thereafter its interior washed repeatedly by a stream of water; it is then ready to be sterilized for use. Needles are obtainable in a variety of designs.[2] They should be

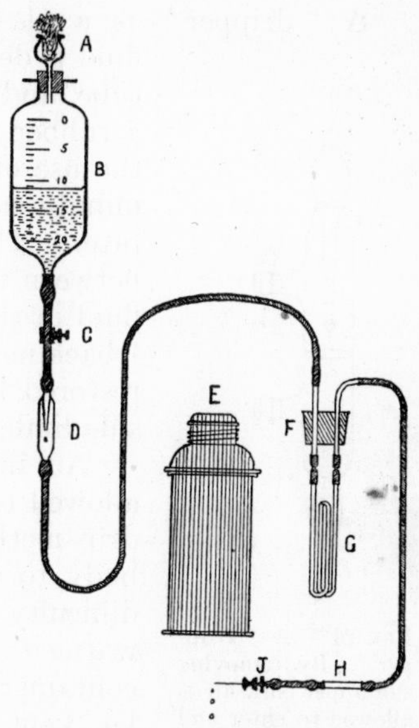

(*By courtesy of Archd. Young & Son Ltd., Edinburgh.*)

FIG. 20.—Diagram of Apparatus. A, Rubber cork and filter funnel, with plug of sterile wool ; B, sterilizable glass flask, 1 pint capacity ; C, screw clip ; D, glass dropping-tube ; E, thermos flask ; F, rubber cork ; G, glass U-tube with double bend ; H, glass connection ; J, " Record " fitting and needle.

[1] The Crookes Laboratories ; Messrs John Bell & Croyden.
[2] Such as those of French, Kaliski or Keynes.

sharp, the bevel should be short, and it is convenient if they are fitted with flanges to facilitate their fixation; they should be made of rustless material. Cannulæ may be of metal or glass; the former should be rustless, and both varieties are best constructed with a slightly bulbous tip, which permits a ligature to be securely tightened upon them. Recently long rubber cannulæ have been introduced for use in "drip" methods; they permit greater freedom of movement of the arm (or leg) after their insertion into the chosen vein.

A "dripper" is a glass tube (Fig. 21) into which the fluid is delivered drop by drop by a narrower tube, and it is connected to the container by a rubber tube on which is a screw clip. By the use of the clip the number of drops per minute can be varied; 40 to 50 is the usual rate. There should be a column of air between the drip-tube and the level of the fluid in the main tube; if this is lost by fluid "backing up" to the drip-tube, it can be restored by removing the rubber cork in the side limb.

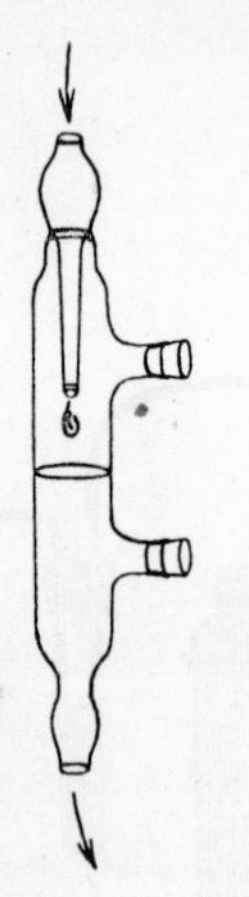

Fig. 21.—A "Dripper." By removing the upper cork air is allowed to enter and displace fluid which may have "backed up" to the inner tube.

An intravenous infusion should not be allowed to chill the patient. If given by the drip method, the fluid can be raised by the body to its own temperature without any difficulty; but if desired, the infusion can be warmed by preliminary immersion of the container in water at 120° F., and it may be kept warm by passing it through a glass coil in a thermos flask containing water at 120° F., or by laying rubber hot-water bottles in the axilla or on the groin. An infusion given continuously (without the intervention of a dripper) should be warmed and kept warm.

A "head" of about 2 ft. is ample. The container may be held in a retort-stand; hung from a hook on the wall; tied to a screen; tied to a pole lashed to the head of the bed; or supported on a regular hospital type of adjustable stand.[1]

Cannula Method.—When the veins are collapsed, as in shock, or after severe hæmorrhage, and when the patient is so fat that they cannot be identified under the skin, a suitable

[1] A convenient and complete set, in a small case for ease of transport, is marketed by Messrs Archibald Young, of Edinburgh. It may be used for intravenous, subcutaneous or rectal administration of fluid.

vein must be exposed for the insertion of a cannula. When a single infusion is to be given, and the matter is urgent, as a rule the most prominent of the veins in both antecubital fossæ is chosen, or an internal saphenous vein in front of one internal malleolus. When the drip method is to be used, the necessary immobilization of the limb is easier and less irksome to the patient, if a vein on the flexor aspect of the forearm is chosen, or a sufficiently large vein on the dorsum of the hand, or an internal saphenous vein.

An intradermal wheal of local anæsthetic is made over the vein at the selected level, about 0·5 c.c. of the solution is deposited in the tissues on each side of the vessel, and the area is compressed for a minute or two in order to distribute the anæsthetic. A tourniquet is applied to make the vein prominent, and an incision about 1 cm. long is made at right angles to the vein, while the skin is steadied by the fingers and thumb of the left hand. The wound is opened up and the vein cleared by inserting a closed small artery forceps on each side of the vessel in turn, and opening the points in a direction parallel to the vein. The closed artery forceps is then passed under the vein, and the tourniquet is released. A double strand of catgut is drawn under the vein by grasping its midpoint with the artery forceps, and the strand is divided so as to provide two ligatures of equal length. The distal of these is drawn to the distal part of the cleared vein, and used to ligate the vessel, the ends of the ligature being left long, and caught by an artery forceps. The proximal ligature is drawn to the proximal end of the cleared vein, and the first loop of a knot is loosely tied with it. Fluid is now allowed to flow through the infusion system and cannula until all air has been displaced, when the flow is stopped by clamping the rubber tubing with an artery forceps, about 15 cm. from the cannula. The cannula is laid on the sterile towel so that it can be picked up conveniently. The vein is now held up and steadied by the distal ligature, and an oblique nick is made into it with fine scissors—a good pair of manicure scissors answers very well. Care must be taken not to divide the vein completely, and yet to make a large enough opening ; about half the circumference of the vein is adequate. Much the best instrument with which to hold the lips of the opening apart is a small sharp hook (" dural hook ") ; it is neater and more efficient than artery forceps or dissecting forceps. While the proximal lip of the opening is retracted with the hook, the cannula is inserted into the lumen of the vein ; care must be taken to elevate the whole thickness of the wall of the vessel so that the glistening intima is displayed, otherwise it is possible for an inexperienced or careless operator to pass the cannula between the coats of the vein instead of into the lumen. The proximal catgut ligature is then tightened upon the cannula, and if the cannula has a " shoulder " the thread must be placed distal to this. The cannula may be fixed more firmly by tying the long ends of the distal ligature round it. As soon as the cannula is in position, the clamp is removed from the rubber tubing, and the flow of fluid started.

When a single infusion is to be given, 500 c.c. may be given in thirty to forty minutes. Before the last of the fluid runs into the vein, the cannula is withdrawn while the proximal ligature, the knot of which has remained half tied, is tightened to occlude the vein. Both ligatures are cut short, and the wound in the skin closed by a single stitch. A sterile pad and bandage are then applied.

Needle Method.—When a vein is readily accessible the infusion can be given through an " intravenous " needle. When the vein is prominent the needle can be inserted directly into it ; or an intradermal wheal of anæsthetic may be made over the vein, the skin divided for a millimetre or two to expose the vein and the needle inserted into the exposed vein. The infusion apparatus (from which all air has been expelled) is connected to the needle by an adaptor, as soon as blood is seen to flow from the needle, and the fluid allowed to flow by unclamping the rubber delivery tube. When the infusion is completed the needle is withdrawn, and a sterile pad and bandage are applied to the site of puncture.

Continuous Infusions.—These are most satisfactorily given by the cannula method. A vein on the flexor aspect of the forearm, the dorsal aspect of the hand, or an internal saphenous vein may be chosen. After the cannula is introduced and fixed in position, the part is bandaged so as to immobilize the terminal 15 cm. of the rubber delivery tube ; if the patient is restless, a splint [1] may be necessary in addition ; and if he is delirious, and an arm is being used for the infusion, the opposite hand must be controlled. The dripper is adjusted to deliver fluid at 50 drops a minute.

In all such cases, and especially when the infusion is to be continued over a number of days, care must be taken that too much fluid is not administered. A record should be kept for each twenty-four hours in which intake is charted against output ; the latter comprising the urine, water lost from the lungs and skin (about 1,500 c.c.), by vomiting and by diarrhœa.

[1] For both arm and leg a moulded plaster of Paris splint is satisfactory.

The appearance of œdema in the legs or about the sacrum is a warning either to discontinue the infusion or to reduce the rate of flow; and the bases of the lungs should be examined daily for signs of œdema. The period during which an infusion into a vein may be continued varies from patient to patient. Sooner or later the vein becomes the site of a non-infective phlebitis, ushered in by a feeling of local soreness; later the tissues in the immediate neighbourhood of the cannula become œdematous, and the skin reddened; and if the infusion is continued the redness and swelling spread proximally along the vein. The appearance of any of these complications is a signal to remove the cannula at once, and, if the infusion must be continued, to introduce the cannula into a vein in another limb.

BLOOD TRANSFUSION

Selection of Donors.—Whenever it is possible the responsibility of matching bloods before transfusion must be delegated to an expert in this procedure. At the present time, in this country, occasions on which this is impossible are rare. In order to illustrate the correct course for a practitioner to follow, certain sets of circumstances will be considered in turn.

A. *A transfusion is urgently required; expert aid is not available; it is not desirable to transfer the patient to a centre where expert aid can be obtained.* In these circumstances, a suitable donor is selected by the *direct test* from those who volunteer. For this test there are required :—

1. A sample of *serum* from the *recipient*. This may be obtained by withdrawing 2 c.c. of blood from a vein by a syringe, and transferring the sample to a small test-tube, or by drawing up in a number—say 6,—of capillary glass tubes blood from a prick of a finger or ear. The serum may be given time to separate, or it may be obtained by centrifuging.[1]
2. A sample of the *corpuscles* of each prospective *donor*. These are obtained either by mixing blood obtained from a prick of a finger or ear in a leucocyte-counting pipette, with normal (0·9 per cent.) saline solution, to a dilution of 1 in 20, or by allowing 2 drops of blood to fall into a small test-tube containing 2 c.c. of normal saline solution, and mixing thoroughly.

[1] A centrifuge may be improvised by fastening the tube(s) by sticking plaster to a blade of the fan of a motor car, or to the "rim end" of a spoke of the back wheel of an upturned bicycle.

Each sample must be labelled carefully with the possible donor's name.

The test is carried out by placing on a microscope slide, or porcelain tile, or plain saucer, a drop of the recipient's serum, and adding to it a drop of the cell suspension from a possible donor; the drops are well mixed with a wooden match, which is at once discarded, and the mixture is gently rocked to and fro. Each test preparation must be labelled carefully with the possible donor's name. If the prospective donor's cells are agglutinated, he is not suitable; at least ten minutes, and in doubtful cases thirty minutes, should be allowed before it is decided that agglutination is not present. If the preparation does not show agglutination, the donor may be used for the transfusion. Minor reactions may occur from agglutination of the recipient's cells by the donor's serum; to avoid these, bloods must be completely compatible. This can be depended upon only if, in addition to the test described above, a similar test between the cells of the recipient and the serum of the donor does not show agglutination.

B. *It is not advisable to move the patient to a centre where expert aid is obtainable; the transfusion is not urgent—or, after a first urgent transfusion, there is a possibility that further transfusions will be required.* In such a case the practitioner must send to the nearest expert :—

1. From the recipient :
   - (*a*) Whole blood (5 c.c.) for serum.
   - (*b*) Red blood corpuscles : 2 drops whole blood received into 2 c.c. of either (and better) 3·8 per cent. sodium citrate solution, or normal (0·9 per cent.) saline solution.

2. From each possible donor :
   - (*a*) Whole blood (5 c.c.) for serum.
   - (*b*) Red blood corpuscles in citrate or saline solution.

In the laboratory, obviously incompatible donors are detected at once by matching the serum of the recipient 1 (*a*) against the cells of the donor 2 (*b*), and discarding any donor whose cells are agglutinated. Each donor not eliminated by this procedure is tested for complete compatibility by testing his serum 2 (*a*) against the cells of the recipient 1 (*b*).

In addition to these direct tests, indirect tests are carried out by the expert, to determine the groups of recipient and donors. This is essential for two reasons :—

1. None of the possible donors may be suitable ; but if the group of the recipient has been determined, a likely donor may be called upon from the local transfusion service ; his cells are then tested directly against the serum of the recipient.
2. The expert has available grouping sera of high titre, the use of which may disclose minimal degrees of incompatibility which would pass undetected by the direct test.

The Indirect (*Grouping*) *Test.*—For this there are required sera of Groups II (A) and III (B), known to be of high titre at the time of the test.

Two clean microscope slides are taken, and marked II and III respectively. On each a drop of the appropriate serum is placed. To each drop is added a drop of the cell-suspension of the person to be grouped, and the drops are thoroughly mixed, a new wooden match being used for each mixing. If agglutination is going to appear, as a rule it does so rapidly ; but an interval of thirty minutes should be allowed before the slides are finally read, during which they are rocked repeatedly. The final appearance may be scrutinized under a low power of a microscope. The group of the tested person is determined thus :—

Table III

Determination of Blood Groups

Agglutination of Unknown Cells by		Unknown belongs to
Group II Serum.	Group III Serum.	
Present (+)	Present (+)	Group I
Absent (−)	Present (+)	Group II
Present (+)	Absent (−)	Group III
Absent (−)	Absent (−)	Group IV

The absence of agglutination from the cells of persons belonging to Group IV explains the use of members of this group as " universal " donors.

C. *Expert assistance is now available.* In such cases the patient is grouped ; and if a compatible donor cannot be found among friends or relatives, a likely prospective donor can be summoned from those on the roster of the transfusion service, *i.e.*, a donor of the same group as the patient, or a Group IV donor. Complete compatibility is finally determined by direct matching.

It must be emphasized that a donor's corpuscles, perfectly compatible at a first transfusion, may at a second transfusion at a later date cause a disastrous accident. Therefore the rule that bloods must be matched directly before a transfusion is absolute.

Donors should be physically healthy and free from any disease transmissible by blood ; for example, syphilis, malaria. If possible a donor should not give blood for transfusion immediately after a meal, especially if the recipient is known to be allergic to any foodstuff.

Collection of Blood for Transfusion.—The donor should be recumbent. A pad is placed behind the elbow, and the skin over and around a suitable antecubital vein is sterilized and isolated. The cuff of the sphygmomanometer, or some other form of tourniquet, is placed round the arm to impede the venous return and make prominent the chosen vein. Two or three drops of local anæsthetic is injected into the skin over the vein at the site to be punctured. After a wait of two or three minutes, a minute nick (about 2 to 3 mm.) is made in the skin with the point of a sharp scalpel. The apparatus for puncturing the vein consists of a needle of uniform bore (*e.g.*, a French's needle) attached to about 12 in. of wide (*e.g.*, $\frac{1}{4}$ in.) rubber tubing, the whole being sterilized by boiling.[1] The blood is received into a sterile graduated jar, which contains sterile isotonic (3·8 per cent.) sodium citrate solution as an anticoagulant. This may be prepared from the pure chemical and freshly distilled water, the solution being sterilized by boiling or in the autoclave ; or a sterile concentrated solution may be purchased,[2] and diluted with sterile distilled water. For each 90 c.c. of blood to be transfused, 10 c.c. of isotonic citrate solution are required. The blood is thoroughly mixed with the citrate solution by rotating the receptacle, or by stirring with a sterile glass rod. Before the needle is inserted into the vein, needle and tubing should be washed through with citrate solution. The vein is punctured through the nick in the skin and the needle is held in position while the blood is flowing ; to avoid clotting in the needle or tube the flow of blood should be maintained at a steady rate by adjustment of the tourniquet, and by directing the donor to clench and

[1] The needle is wrapped in lint or gauze before boiling.

[2] British Drug Houses Ltd. market ampoules containing 1 gm. of sodium citrate in 4 c.c. of distilled water. The contents of two ampoules, made up to 50 c.c. with distilled water, are sufficient for a transfusion of 500 c.c.

unclench his hand at intervals of about thirty seconds. As a rule, about 500 c.c. of blood are obtained from the donor; when the required quantity has been collected, first the tourniquet is released and then the needle is withdrawn. The puncture is covered with a sterile pad of gauze, and the arm is bandaged. The removal of this amount of blood from a healthy donor is not attended by any unpleasant sequel.

The Single Transfusion.—The blood should be given to the recipient as soon as possible after it has been taken from the donor. The technique is that for infusion (p. 1075), and either the needle or the cannula method may be employed. The former is usually possible, but if the veins are collapsed (as in severe shock) they may be difficult to puncture with a needle; in these circumstances, if one attempt with a needle is unsuccessful, the cannula method should be adopted at once. An infusion of saline, or of gum-saline, may be already in progress, and blood may be added to either fluid; in any case a small quantity of saline should be given before and towards the end of the transfusion.

The Continuous Transfusion.—This entails the infusion of quantities of blood up to several litres, over a period of hours or days, by means of a drip apparatus. The method is suitable for hospital practice only. Naturally more than one donor is required; all must belong to the same group, and each must be matched directly with the patient. The technique is the same as that for the continuous administration of other fluids (p. 1078), with the addition that some provision must be made to avoid the settling of the cells in the reservoir. This may be accomplished by gently shaking or stirring its contents from time to time; by adding only small quantities of blood to it at any one time, or by agitating the blood continuously by a stream of oxygen. The oxygen is led from a cylinder through rubber tubing to a sterile glass tube containing a filter of sterile cotton wool; thence through sterile rubber tubing to a second similar filter, and finally through sterile rubber tubing to a glass tube which passes through a rubber stopper nearly to the bottom of the reservoir. A short length of glass tube is inserted through a second hole in the stopper, to provide a vent. To maintain an even suspension the oxygen should be bubbled into the reservoir at double the rate at which the blood is dripping into the delivery tube.

Reactions during Transfusion.—Reactions have resulted from lack of cleanliness or of sterility in the apparatus, from impurity of the citrate solution, and from the use of unwarmed blood; these should not occur. The most important technical cause of reactions is the too rapid administration of blood, and this must be avoided by careful timing, especially in transfusions for any hæmolytic anæmia. Lack of complete compatibility (such as may occur when grouping is used as the only test) may result in a reaction shortly after the transfusion, which may be ushered in by a mild rigor, followed by fever, headache, and perhaps vomiting. This is treated by warmth externally, hot drinks, a powder containing aspirin (10 gr.) and Dover's powder (5 gr.), and in the more serious cases by the subcutaneous injection of 0·5 c.c. (8 minims) of 1 : 1,000 adrenalin hydrochloride solution.

Severe reactions are due to mistakes in matching, resulting in the hæmolysis of the transfused red cells by the plasma of the recipient. After the introduction of a small volume of incompatible blood, the recipient becomes restless and complains of lumbar pain. If the transfusion is continued, respiratory and cardiac collapse occur, and if the patient survives, fever follows, and jaundice and hæmoglobinuria appear. When hæmoglobinuria is excessive and the urine is acid, the pigment may be precipitated in the renal tubules, with suppression of urine and uræmia as possible sequels. At the first sign of any reaction a transfusion must be discontinued, and special vigilance is necessary if the patient is under a general anæsthetic. Adrenalin is given subcutaneously at once, and the measures advised in the preceding paragraph are adopted. As precipitation of hæmoglobin in the kidney is minimal when the urine is alkaline, this should be secured, before the transfusion of large amounts of blood (1 litre or more) and in cases of hæmolytic anæmia, by the administration of potassium citrate (30 gr.) and sodium bicarbonate (30 gr.) at intervals of two hours until the urine is alkaline, and by continuing their administration until the transfusion is completed.

INTRADERMAL INJECTION

Occasionally it is necessary to introduce small amounts of fluid into the skin. This may be needed to test for sensitivity on the part of the patient towards serum, bacterial products or extracts of certain animal and vegetable substances; or the procedure may be a therapeutic one (*e.g.*, sera and egg-albumin in hæmophilia, bee venom in rheumatic disease). The finest of needles should be employed, with a short bevel on its point. A small syringe containing the appropriate quantity of fluid is attached to the needle, and its contents are introduced into the skin where it is hairless, usually on the flexor surface of a forearm. The accurate placement of the fluid is secured by passing the needle into the skin at a very acute angle; if the point of the needle is correctly placed, the injection causes blanching of the skin over a small circular area.

HYPODERMIC INJECTION

By this route are administered (1) certain drugs, (2) vaccines, (3) sera and (4) certain hormones, *e.g.*, insulin.

1. *Drugs.*—These may be already in solution in ampoules. If they are in tablet form, the appropriate dose is dissolved in about 1 c.c. of sterile water. The solution may be made in a china egg-cup, which is boiled in water in a pan from which the required amount of sterile water is removed with a syringe, also boiled in the pan; or if the syringe is already sterile, the necessary amount of water may be boiled in a table-spoon over a spirit lamp or gas jet. The needle should be the finest procurable, and sharp; the ideal is to use a fresh needle for each injection. Areas suitable for hypodermic injections are indicated in Fig. 22. The skin at the selected point is cleansed with spirit, a fold of it is picked up with the finger and thumb of the left hand, and the needle attached to the syringe is plunged rapidly into the *loose subcutaneous tissue* at the extremity of the fold. The piston is then withdrawn slightly, to ensure that the point of the needle is not in a venule; if blood does not enter the syringe, its contents are injected, and the needle withdrawn. Hypodermic injections should never be given into an inflamed area, or into an area which may contain lymphatics draining an inflamed area (*e.g.*, *not* into the arm on the side of a whitlow).

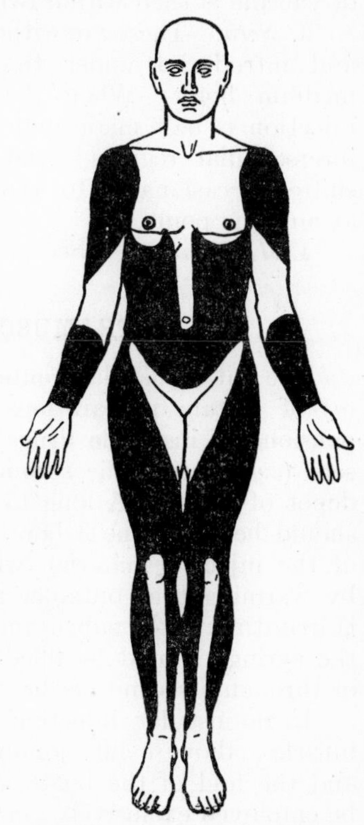

Fig. 22.—The Dark Areas may be used for Hypodermic Injections.

2. *Vaccines.*—These are often supplied in bulk, in bottles with a thin rubber cap. The bottle is well shaken, and the cap is sterilized with spirit ; if the bottle is new, a layer of paraffin wax may have to be removed from the rubber cap. The piston of the syringe is then withdrawn to the level of the dose desired ; the needle is plunged through the rubber cap into the bottle, which is held *inverted* ; air is expelled into the bottle by pushing the piston " home," and the equivalent dose of vaccine is then withdrawn into the syringe.

3. *Sera.*—These are withdrawn from the containing ampoule and introduced under the skin, through a long needle of medium bore. When the amount of serum is large, the injection is best made under the loose skin of the pectoral or interscapular regions ; and the point of the needle may be shifted occasionally, to avoid depositing a " blob " of serum at any one point.

4. *Insulin, etc.*—(See p. 342).

INTRAMUSCULAR INJECTION

The intramuscular route is chosen for the administration (*a*) of certain preparations (*e.g.*, liver extract) ; (*b*) of suspensions of insoluble drugs (*e.g.*, mercury) ; and (*c*) of some sera (*e.g.*, antitetanic serum) when it is desired to provide a depot of serum. A long (5 to 8 cm.) needle is employed ; it should be of as fine a bore as is consistent with the viscosity of the injected material, which may be reduced if necessary by warming the container to about 105° F. If the material is irritating to the subcutaneous tissues (mercurial suspensions) the syringe should be filled either directly, without a needle, or through a second needle.

Intramuscular injections are best made into the gluteal muscles, above a line joining the anterior superior iliac spine and the fold of the buttock (Fig. 24), and this region should be employed exclusively, on alternate sides, when the injections are to be repeated at regular intervals. Single injections of small quantities of sera may be introduced into a pectoralis major muscle. When the gluteal region is chosen, the patient should lie on the opposite side. The skin is sterilized and steadied by the forefinger and thumb of the left hand ; the needle is held in the forefinger and thumb of the right hand, and is plunged through the skin perpendicularly, with a sharp stabbing movement, directly into the muscles. If its point impinges on the ilium, the needle should be withdrawn slightly. It is then held in position with the forefinger and thumb of the left hand, and the charged syringe is attached to it. Gentle suction is applied to ensure that the point of the needle is not in a blood vessel; if it is correctly placed, the injection is slowly and steadily completed. If an irritating substance has been injected, before the needle is removed it is rotated once or twice in its long axis in order to cleanse it. Thereafter the area is massaged firmly for a minute or two, to ensure even dispersion of the injected material.

PARACENTESIS OF THE ABDOMEN

This is indicated when ascites embarrasses movement, respiration or the heart's action.

The point usually chosen for the puncture is in the median line, equidistant from umbilicus and symphysis. The bladder is emptied, if necessary by catheter. If the abdomen is hairy it is shaved. The patient should be in a semi-reclining position, so that the fluid gravitates towards, and the intestines away from, the lower abdomen; and before the abdomen is tapped a broad binder (or roller towel) should be placed round the upper part of the abdomen. This is tightened as the fluid escapes, and thus faintness from the reduction of intra-abdominal pressure is prevented. Either of two methods may be employed.

By Trocar and Cannula.—An instrument of the "piston" type is the most convenient; this has a cannula with a side limb, which opens into the cannula only when the trocar is withdrawn beyond the junction (Fig. 23). To the side limb rubber tubing is attached, long enough to reach a receptacle by the side of the bed. A scalpel with a narrow blade is also necessary. The abdomen is cleansed and the selected point isolated by sterile towels. An intradermal wheal of local anæsthetic is raised here, and the deeper tissues are also infiltrated.

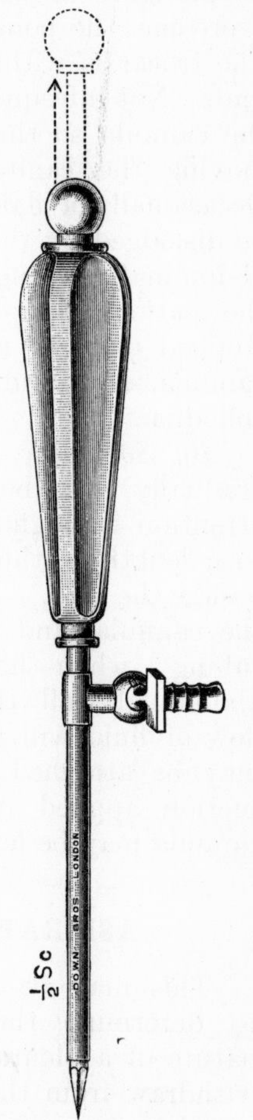

(*By courtesy of Down Bros. Ltd., London.*)

Fig. 23.—Trocar and Cannula for Paracentesis of the Abdomen.

A small cut is made through the skin, of such a size that it will admit the point of the trocar, and stretch to accommodate the cannula. The cannula, with trocar in position, is then pushed slowly through the abdominal wall; the right forefinger is kept firmly upon it to guard against its plunging into the peritoneal cavity. When resistance is overcome, the point of the instrument has reached the cavity. The trocar is withdrawn, and fluid will flow through the side limb. Not infrequently a loop of bowel floats up and obstructs the cannula so that the flow ceases. It can be restarted by moving the cannula up and down, or from side to side. Occasionally a flake of lymph blocks the cannula; this can be dislodged by the cautious reinsertion of the trocar. As the abdominal swelling decreases the binder is tightened; but if the patient complains of faintness the flow is temporarily stopped until he recovers. When the flow finally ceases the cannula is withdrawn, and the tiny wound sealed with collodion.

By Southey's Tube.—This fine tube removes fluid more gradually, and therefore the patient does not require constant attention throughout the drainage. The cannula is connected to a length of thin rubber tubing which reaches a receptacle beside the bed. The tubing is stretched over the mouth of the cannula, and the trocar is inserted *through* the stretched tubing; when the trocar is withdrawn after puncture of the abdominal wall the opening in the tube closes. Often the flow of fluid will begin at once; if it fails to do so a syringe may be attached to the distal end of the tube, and gentle suction applied in order to establish syphon action. The cannula may be left in position for many hours.

ASPIRATION OF THE PLEURAL CAVITY

This may be necessary either as a diagnostic procedure, to determine the physical, cytological and bacteriological nature of a pleural effusion, or as a therapeutic procedure, to withdraw from the cavity a considerable amount of fluid (for example, in metapneumonic empyema, or in cases of cardiac or renal failure).

Although it is occasionally necessary to choose an interspace which lies directly over the site of the effusion, as determined by clinical and especially radiological evidence, as a rule the puncture is made in the eighth intercostal space, in the posterior axillary line, and nearer the ninth than the eighth rib in order to avoid the intercostal nerve and vessels.

The patient may be either in a sitting position or propped up near the edge of the bed in a semi-reclining position, with the arms folded. After the usual preliminary preparation and isolation of the area, an intradermal wheal of local anæsthetic solution is raised at the point selected for the puncture, and 2 c.c. of the solution is then deposited in the deeper tissues ; the needle should be made to impinge on the lower rib. It is well to wait a few minutes in order to give the anæsthetic time to act, and to reach the vicinity of the pleura.

Removal of a Sample.—A rather wide-bore, short-bevelled needle is attached to a 5 c.c. syringe, and the needle is then pushed slowly into the pleural cavity. If a little negative pressure is maintained in the syringe, fluid will flow at once when the cavity is reached, and the needle should not be introduced further. When the syringe is full the needle is withdrawn, and the sample transferred to a sterile test-tube with a closely fitting rubber cork. The puncture is then sealed.

Aspiration as a Part of Treatment.—When it is decided to remove a quantity of fluid, a 50 c.c. syringe is useful. This is connected to the aspirating needle by 6 in. of stout rubber tubing fitted with adaptors. The aspirating needle and small syringe are used as described to ascertain the proper depth ; the large syringe is then coupled to the needle.[1] It is *slowly* filled ; the tubing is then pinched, or clamped with a spring clip, and the syringe is disconnected and emptied. The cycle is repeated until (1) fluid is not obtained, or (2) the patient complains of or shows respiratory embarrassment. The needle is then withdrawn and the puncture sealed. It is a useful plan in cases of empyema to retain from each aspiration a corked test tube almost full of pus ; these are placed in a rack, and the process of " thickening " of the pus can be followed by comparing the levels of cellular sediment in the tubes.

An alternative method is to employ a 20 c.c. syringe to which is coupled a three-way adaptor. One channel of the adaptor leads by way of 6 in. of rubber tubing to the aspirating needle ; to the other channel is attached sufficient rubber tubing to reach a receptacle for the aspirated fluid. The junction of the channels is controlled by a stop-cock, turning of which allows the syringe to be alternately filled from the chest and emptied into the receptacle. This method is

[1] Messrs Down Bros. sell a useful contrivance for maintaining the fixed position of the needle. It consists of a rubber vacuum " sucker " which sticks to the skin. and carries an arm in which the needle rests.

also employed when the aspirated fluid is to be replaced by air; after the syringe is emptied it is filled with a somewhat smaller quantity of air, which is introduced slowly into the pleural cavity. This procedure prevents any sudden disturbance of mediastinal relationships; in favourable cases the lung expands slowly as the air is absorbed. The procedure is repeated as often as clinical and radiological examination indicate the need for it.

Dangers of Pleural Aspiration.—Very rarely puncture of the pleura is immediately followed by *pleural shock*, a condition characterized by extreme cardiac and respiratory failure. If this happens the needle must be withdrawn; the remedial measures include warmth, artificial respiration if necessary, and the subcutaneous injection of 0·5 c.c. (8 minims) of 1 : 1,000 adrenalin hydrochloride, with 2 c.c. of coramine.

LUMBAR PUNCTURE

This consists in the introduction of a hollow needle into the subarachnoid space in the lumbar region, a procedure which is employed for both diagnostic and therapeutic purposes. A lumbar puncture needle must be of fine bore, with a sharp, shortly bevelled point, and a closely fitting stillette; it is so marked that the line of the bevel can be visualized by looking at the base of the needle. Occasionally a needle of large bore is needed to withdraw thick exudate, but even "thick" liquids (such as sera and lipiodol) can be introduced through a fine needle if the ampoule containing the liquid is warmed in a bowl of hot sterile water to a temperature of 110° F., and the barrel of the syringe is kept warm by covering it with relays of gauze swabs soaked in the hot water.

Technique.—In practice most punctures must be performed with the patient in bed, but if his surroundings or size permit, it is more easily carried out as he lies on a firm surface, such as a kitchen table or operating table. He should lie on his left side, and a small pillow is placed under his head in order to keep the cranial and spinal parts of the subarachnoid space at the same level. The patient then bends his head slightly forwards, and clasps his knees with his hands, so as to arch his back and thus open out the spaces between the spinous processes of the lumbar vertebræ (Fig. 24). Only in the most unruly or unco-operative of adults is an anæsthetic needed, and usually a child can be gently but firmly held in the same position. Inhalation anæsthesia interferes with the accurate measurement of cerebrospinal fluid pressure, and if this information is important, omnopon-scopolamine for an adult and chloral hydrate for a child should be tried first.

Usually the needle is inserted between the spines of the third and fourth lumbar vertebræ, a level which corresponds to the point where a line joining the highest points of the iliac crests crosses the spinal column. After the usual preparation, and with a towel in position, this point is identified with the left thumb and an intradermal wheal of local anæsthetic is raised in the median line with a fine hypodermic needle. A larger needle is used to infiltrate the deeper tissues in a forward and slightly cranial direction; the needle should never be sunk to its full extent, for needles break at the junction of shaft and adaptor, and if the patient moves suddenly, a fully inserted needle may snap here, and disappear below the skin. After two or three minutes, to give time for local anæsthesia to develop, the spinal needle is inserted through the same hole in the skin, and with its bevel in the same plane as the spine,[1] and pushed slowly forwards and cranially with the right hand while its direction is maintained by the forefinger of the left, which rests on the skin. At a distance from the surface which varies with age and build (in the average adult, 4 to 5 cm.) the needle is felt to overcome a certain resistance—that of the ligamentum subflavum between the laminæ. If it is pushed onwards for 0·5 cm. it will have pierced the dura and entered the spinal subarachnoid space.

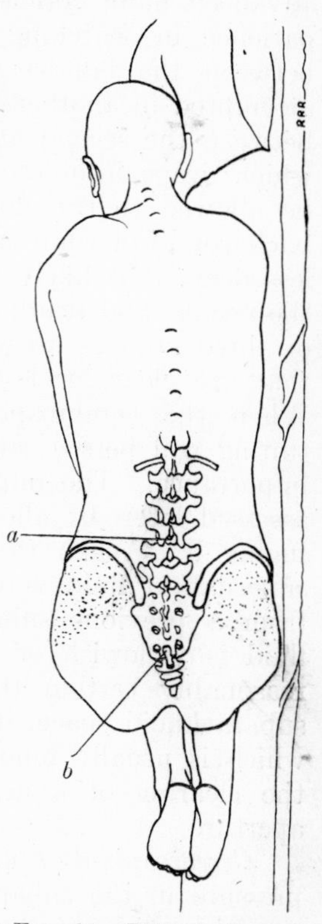

Fig. 24.—Patient in position for Lumbar Puncture. *a*, Site for lumbar puncture; *b*, Site for epidural injection. The stippled areas are suitable for intramuscular injections.

Difficulties in Lumbar Puncture.—Lack of co-operation on the part of the adult patient should be met with only in those who are semiconscious or delirious; in the majority of cases firm holding, careful local anæsthesia and patience will enable the puncture to be completed. The same plan is as a rule successful in children. If the bed is soft, allowance

[1] Held thus it will separate, rather than sever, the longitudinally directed fibres of the dura. On its withdrawal, the small dural slit closes without leaking.

must be made for the tilt of the patient's body, the needle being directed a little downwards as well as forwards and cranially. When the needle impinges on bone before entering the spinal canal, it is usually found to have been pushed in too caudal a direction; it must be withdrawn for 3 cm. before being advanced more cranially. When the spine is arthritic, great patience in searching may be required to find an interval between the laminæ; and the puncture may have to be attempted in another lumbar interspinous space, for example, between the second and third spinous processes. If the fluid which drops from the needle is blood-stained, a little should be allowed to run down the wall of a test tube held on a background of white gauze. If the tint becomes progressively less deep, it is likely that a small vessel has been opened by the needle, and readings of pressure may be taken. Later two or three samples are collected in a series of tubes, and those that are clear (or less deeply tinted) used for investigation. When the cerebrospinal fluid already contains blood, the tinting will persist, and may be assumed to be of diagnostic importance. The importance of admixture of blood may be assessed later, by allowing the sample to settle, or by centrifuging it. When the blood results from local trauma, the supernatant fluid is clear [1]; but when it has been derived from a previous subarachnoid hæmorrhage the supernatant fluid is yellowish or red. If fluid does not flow, and it is reasonably certain that the point of the needle is in the subarachnoid space, it should be slowly rotated, a manœuvre which is usually followed by a flow of fluid as the result of the clearing of a nerve root which previously blocked the aperture.

Cerebrospinal Fluid Pressure.—Investigation of the fluid pressure in the subarachnoid space is usually important and sometimes of essential diagnostic value. It is estimated in terms of millimetres of itself, and the estimation must be made before taking a sample. The needle is connected to a manometer of glass by means of a three-way stopcock and adaptor,[2] and a short length of rubber tubing, to a manometer of glass graduated in centimetres; the whole apparatus must be sterilized by boiling. The stopcock allows the operator (1) to close the lumen of the needle, (2) to allow cerebrospinal fluid into the manometer, and (3) to allow cerebrospinal fluid to flow directly into a single tube. The manometer is held so

[1] Such a mixture may show lysis of red cells if the sample is transmitted to laboratory by post.

[2] Either Greenfield's or Adson's pattern is convenient.

that the zero mark is at the level of the needle. Pressure readings are useless unless the patient is relaxed and breathing quietly, and it may be necessary to wait for this situation, and to secure it by encouragement. Normally the fluid shows oscillations up to 0·5 cm. with each beat of the pulse, and up to 1·0 cm. with each respiration; the mean is taken as the initial pressure.

If the subarachnoid space above the level of the needle is free from obstruction, then variations in its pressure will be at once transmitted to the manometer. The presence of variations of pressure with pulse and respiration is evidence of free communication. The situation may be investigated further by the manœuvre of Queckenstedt. Normally the compression by an assistant of both internal jugular veins for four seconds (the patient having been previously warned) leads to an increase in pressure in the intracranial space of anything up to 30 cm., and if obstruction is absent this is at once reflected by a rise in the manometric reading; and the manometric pressure falls abruptly when the jugular compression is released. If obstruction (*e.g.*, a spinal tumour) is present, then when jugular compression is applied, the manometric pressure may—

1. Remain stationary (complete block).
2. Rise, but remain at a higher level when jugular compression is released (partial block).
3. Rise or fall jerkily ("stair" response) when the jugular pressure is applied or released (partial block).

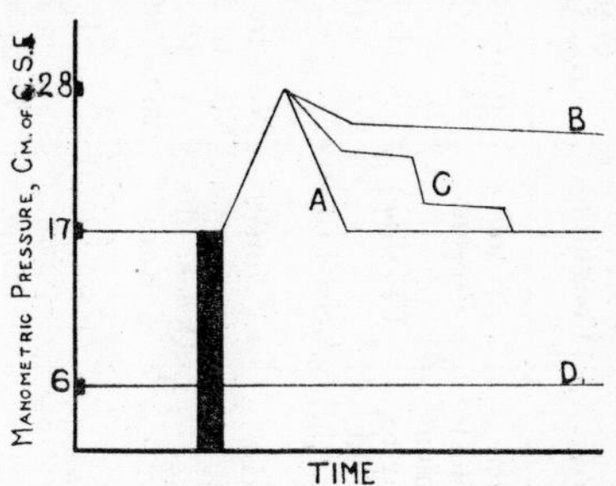

Fig. 25.—Diagrammatic Representation of Manometric Response to Jugular Pressure. The black block represents compression of the internal jugular veins for four seconds. A, normal response; B, new higher level; C, "stairway" fall; and D, lack of response (complete block).

When block is present, the "initial pressure" is low; but manual compression of the abdomen will be followed by a rise in pressure, even when response to jugular compression is absent.

The information that may be obtained from investigation of the pressure of the cerebrospinal fluid is indicated in Fig. 25, and in Table IV.

TABLE IV

Condition.	Pressure. Mm.	Colour.	Coagulum.	Cells. Per Mm.³	Protein. Per Cent.	Glucose. Per Cent.	Chlorides. Per Cent.	Wassermann.
Normal	80 to 175	Clear	None	0 to 3 (S.L.)	0·015 to 0·025	0·04 to 0·08	0·72 to 0·73	Neg.
Acute meningitis	+ + +, to 1,000	Turbid to purulent	Present	+ + + (P.)	0·5 +	Dim. or absent	Nor. to 0·6	,,
Tuberculous meningitis	+ +	Clear to turbid	Us. (fine)	+ + (L.), occas. + (P.)	0·05 to 0·5	,,	Nor. to 0·55	,,
Acute syphilitic meningitis	Us. + to + +	,,	Occas. (fine)	,,	0·04 to 0·4	Us. nor.	V. slt. dim.	Pos., 85 %
Vascular neurosyphilis	Nor. to +	Clear	None	Nor. to + (L.)	0·15 to 0·5	Nor.	Nor.	,, 75 %
Tabes dorsalis	Nor.	,,	,,	Nor. to 200 (L.)	Nor. to 0·1	,,	,,	,, 80 %
Dementia paralytica	Nor. to +	,,	Occas. (fine)	,,	0·25 to 0·5	,,	,,	,, 100 %
Benign lymphocytic meningitis	,,	,,	Rare	25 to 500 + (L.)	0·02 to 0·07	,,	,,	Neg.
Acute anterior poliomyelitis	,,	,,	Occas. (fine)	+ + P., later + L.	0·02 to 0·35	,,	,,	,,
Epidemic encephalitis	Us. nor., rarely +	,,	None	10 to 500 (L.)	Nor. to 0·08	,,	,,	,,
Disseminated sclerosis	Nor.	,,	,,	Us. nor., rarely + (L.)	Nor., or + (0·15)	,,	,,	,,
Polyneuritis (" neuronitis ")	Nor. to +	,,	,,	Nor. to +	Us. +, to 0·75	,,	Nor. to dim.	,,
Aseptic meningeal reactions	Us. + to + +	Clear to turbid	Occas.	To 10,000 (P.)	0·02 to 0·2	,,	,,	,,
Cerebral abscess	,,	Clear to purulent	,,	+ to 800 (P., L.)	+, to 0·2	Nor., occas. dim.	Nor.	,,
Supratentorial cerebral tumour	,,	Clear, occas. yellow	None	Nor. to 150 (L.)	Nor. to 2·0	Nor.	,,	,,
Infratentorial cerebral tumour	,,	,,	,,	,,	Nor. to 0·5	,,	,,	,,
Spinal cord tumour	Low (Block)	Clear to yellow	Occas.	Nor., occas. +	0·04 to 3·5	,,	,,	,,
Spontaneous subarachnoid hæmorrhage	Us. + +	Bloody xanthochromic	None	+ +, R.B.C.	0·02 to 1·0	Nor., occas. dim.	,,	,,

dim. = diminished. L. = Lymphocyte. nor. = normal. P. = Polymorph. us. = usually.

The Collection of Samples.—When manometric readings have been made, fluid is allowed to drip slowly into a tube or series of tubes for further examination. Tubes should be chemically clean and sterile, and should be fitted with stoppers of rubber. Fifteen cubic centimetres of fluid is sufficient for all routine analyses, but when a space-occupying intracranial lesion is present or is suspected, the withdrawal of fluid should be stopped at an amount which does not reduce the manometric pressure by more than one-third of the initial reading. Otherwise the only *contraindication* to lumbar puncture is certainty of diagnosis without the assistance it may afford.

The number of tubes in which the sample is divided depends upon the tests which are desired, and the laboratory or laboratories to which samples are to be sent. Thus information may be desired as to (1) the chemical, (2) the cytological, (3) the bacteriological, and (4) the immunological properties of the fluid (Table IV). Three separate samples should satisfy the most exacting of laboratory colleagues.

After a lumbar puncture the hole in the skin should be sealed with a pledget of cotton wool soaked in collodion or with sterile plaster, and the patient should be kept in the recumbent position for twenty-four hours in order to avoid the unpleasant sequel of " lumbar puncture headache."

NOTE.—If the inexperienced operator be so unfortunate as to have a needle break off under the skin, he should at once mark the puncture by a needle scratch. An incision is made in the median line between the two adjacent spinous processes, the two erector spinæ muscles are separated, and the interspinous tissue (and broken portion of the needle) are grasped between the widely opened jaws of a curved artery forceps applied in the line of the spine. The forceps is then closed and withdrawn.

CISTERNAL PUNCTURE

For diagnostic or therapeutic purposes the *cisterna magna* of the subarachnoid space may be tapped through the atlanto-occipital ligament. This procedure has the advantage over lumbar puncture that it is not attended by the possibility of headache, that the exudate in meningeal infections may be more easily withdrawn and the appropriate sera introduced, and that radio-opaque substances (lipiodol) may be introduced at the cranial end of the spinal canal. It is, however, more potentially dangerous than lumbar puncture because of the proximity of the *medulla oblongata.*

Technique.—The head and neck are shaved below the level of the bases of the mastoid processes and prepared surgically. The patient lies in the left lateral position, the head being raised by a pillow to the level of the cervical spine, and well flexed to open up the interval between occipital bone and atlas. A point is identified in the median line immediately above the spine of the atlas, or, in a thick-necked patient, where a line joining the tips of the mastoid processes crosses the spine. The skin is anæsthetized by intradermal infiltration of local anæsthetic. A spinal puncture needle is then introduced and pushed forwards and cranially, under the control of the left index finger, till it impinges on the occipital bone. It is then withdrawn for 2 cm., the point directed more caudally, and the needle pressed forwards through the atlanto-occipital membrane and dura, which are felt to "give," into the *cisterna magna* ; normally in an adult this lies at a depth of 4 to 6 cm. from the skin. When the needle is disconnected, fluid drops slowly or may be withdrawn by a syringe. Its properties may be investigated as are those of fluid obtained by lumbar puncture. If this route is used to inject fluids into the subarachnoid space, great care must be taken during the injection that pressure on the piston of the syringe does not push the needle onwards, for this mistake may result in injury to the *medulla oblongata*. Throughout an injection the depth to which the needle is allowed to penetrate should be controlled by the thumb and fingers of the left hand. When the needle is withdrawn the puncture is sealed with cotton-wool and collodion.

EPIDURAL INJECTION

By this procedure fluid is forced between the dura and the bony wall of the lower part of the spinal canal. A lumbar puncture needle is used for the injection, and it is introduced between the cornua of the last piece of the sacrum, through the roof of the spinal canal which is here ligamentous.

Technique.—The patient lies face downwards, preferably on a firm surface, with a large pillow under the pelvis. A piece of gauze is placed between the buttocks to prevent the antiseptic from reaching the anus or genitals, and the skin over the sacrum, coccyx and buttocks is cleansed. The position of the sacral cornua is found by palpation, and an intradermal wheal of local anæsthetic is raised between them. The tissues down to the bone are then infiltrated with a somewhat larger hypodermic needle, which can be felt to pierce the ligament bridging the cornua, and two or three minutes are allowed for the anæsthetic to take effect. A lumbar puncture needle is then introduced through the hole already made in the skin, and pushed onwards and cranially at an angle of about 45 degrees with the horizontal, and in the median line, until it is felt to pass through the ligamentous roof of the canal, and come to rest on the posterior surface of the body of the sacrum. The base of the needle is then depressed between the buttocks, to alter its direction, and it is pushed cranially for about 3 cm. along the sacral canal. At this stage its position is verified by making the point impinge on the bony roof of the canal (Fig. 24). A 20 c.c. syringe is then filled with sterile saline, or 0·25 per cent. novocaine solution, and fitted to the needle. The plunger is withdrawn slightly, to make sure the point of the needle is not in a vein; and the contents of the syringe are slowly injected. Very little pressure is needed, and if the plunger has to be forced, the point of the needle is not correctly placed in the sacral canal, but lies between the sacral laminæ and the skin, in the origin of the erector spinæ.[1] When the first 20 c.c. have been injected, it is well to pause for a minute or two; the needle is then slowly pushed onwards in the sacral canal, nearly to its full extent. A second and even a third 20 c.c. of solution are then introduced; as the beneficial effects of the injection may be due partly to its disruptive effect, the writer makes a practice of injecting the final 10 c.c. under pressure. During the injection (which is usually done for sciatica) the patient may complain of exacerbation of pain in the affected leg.

The needle is withdrawn, and the puncture in the skin sealed with a pledget of cotton-wool soaked in collodion. The patient may then turn on his back, but should rest in this position for half to one hour before leaving. When novocaine solution has been used, its correct placement may be verified by the appearance of perianal analgesia within fifteen to twenty minutes.

Difficulties.—Although the injection is usually easy, the sacral cornua may be distorted, and it may take patience and gentle searching with the needle's point to enter the canal. The ease with which fluid may be injected is the best guarantee that the needle has been correctly placed. Occasionally in sensitive patients tachycardia follows the injection of novocaine, and the patient must remain at rest till the pulse-rate returns to normal.

Epidural injection may be utilized to aid in the diagnosis of a tumour compressing the theca below the level of the interval between the third and fourth lumbar vertebræ. Lumbar puncture is performed in the usual way, and manometric readings are taken. A needle is then introduced

[1] If the injection is persisted in when the needle is in the latter position, a palpable and visible lump forms on the back of the sacrum.

into the sacral canal, and fluid is slowly injected. If the canal is unobstructed, the injected fluid displaces a certain volume of cerebrospinal fluid, by compressing the theca, and the pressure in the lumbar manometer rises. If the sacral canal is obstructed by an intradural or extradural tumour, fluid can be introduced only with difficulty, and the pressure does not rise in the lumbar manometer.

J. R. LEARMONTH.

OXYGEN THERAPY

There are few potent therapeutic agents which, both in hospital and in private practice, are in general used to such little effect as oxygen. Considerable misunderstanding exists regarding the indications for its use, and its administration is frequently delayed till the prospects of benefit from its action are negligible. In addition the methods employed are frequently both wasteful and inefficient. Too often it is still administered through a tube and funnel, with totally negative effects, or a nasal catheter (which is quite efficient when properly used) is employed under conditions which cause maximum discomfort to the patient and offer little prospect of effective oxygen administration. The method commonly employed of fixing the catheter to the cheek with adhesive strapping causes considerable discomfort in a man from traction on the growing beard, and irritates an ill patient beyond endurance. The oxygen may be delivered to the catheter from the cylinder through a wash-bottle containing warm water. The succession of bubbles in the fluid indicates the rate of flow of the gas, and unless a considerable turmoil is being caused in the water it may be taken that the oxygen administration is quite inadequate. A flow of 2 litres per minute is the absolute minimum which is found to produce an effect, and when bubbled through such a bottle this flow causes a continuous stream of bubbles at a rate much too fast to count, while the preferable higher rates of 4 or even 6 litres per minute cannot be given by such a method.

It is customary also to give oxygen intermittently, for a definite period of minutes in each hour. This practice is illogical and harmful, and has been likened by Haldane to "dragging a drowning man to the surface once a minute." Oxygen therapy to be fully effective must be continuous, so long as the indications for it persist.

Indications.—The giving of oxygen might be expected to be of value in cases where there is a deficiency of oxygen in the arterial blood, *i.e.*, in anoxæmic states. It should be realized, however, that not all forms of anoxæmia are benefited by oxygen inhalation. In severe uncomplicated anæmias, for example, anoxæmia exists, but such hæmoglobin as remains in circulation is fully saturated with oxygen as it leaves the lungs, and the plasma holds its full complement in solution. The oxygen tension of the blood is therefore normal, and hence additional oxygen in the respired air cannot increase that in the blood to any significant degree. Again, peripheral cyanosis is no certain indication that oxygen therapy will be of value, for the blood leaving the lungs may be fully oxygenated and the cyanosis may be due to slowing of the peripheral blood flow or to admixture of venous with arterial blood as in some cases of congenital heart disease. In those cases, on the other hand, where blood leaves the lungs only partly saturated with oxygen, increase in the oxygen content of the respired air raises its partial pressure in the alveolar air, and improves the oxygen saturation of the arterial blood. Such defective oxygenation, or *anoxic anoxæmia*, arises whenever there is interference with the passage of air to and from the lungs, or with the gaseous interchange in the alveoli. It can arise very readily in the pneumonias, where a number of factors favour its production. If part of the blood in the pulmonary circulation flows through vessels in airless consolidated lung, the blood in the pulmonary veins will not be fully oxygenated. Again, a film of watery or fibrinous exudate over the endothelial surfaces of air-containing alveoli interferes with the gaseous exchange between blood and alveolar air, and the rapid shallow breathing which is common in pneumonia further interferes with the efficiency of pulmonary ventilation. Patchy atelectasis and exudation, as in capillary bronchitis and broncho-pneumonia, lead to a similar state of defective oxygenation of the arterial blood, as does pulmonary congestion and the œdema of cardiac failure. In all these states the timely and efficient administration of oxygen is of great value.

A further important indication for the use of oxygen is in the treatment of carbon monoxide poisoning. The affinity of this gas for hæmoglobin is such that a concentration of 0·05 per cent. of carbon monoxide in the respired air will lead to the conversion of more than half the circulating hæmoglobin to the carbon monoxide compound. A very low concentration of the gas thus leads to a great reduction in the hæmoglobin available for oxygen carriage. The compound of carbon monoxide and hæmoglobin is stable, and will only dissociate to form free carbon monoxide and hæmoglobin in the presence of a high concentration of oxygen. This dissociation may therefore be accelerated in clinical practice by increasing the oxygen content of the respired air, *i.e.*, by oxygen therapy, which comes to be an important part of the resuscitation of patients poisoned by this gas.

Oxygen therapy has been employed in the treatment of cases of heart-failure and of emphysema. In the latter, raising the oxygen in the alveolar air relieves cyanosis to some extent, but from the chronic nature of the disease it is obvious that oxygen therapy is of limited value. It is not feasible to give oxygen by mask or other means for prolonged periods, and in practice oxygen therapy in cases of emphysema is only applicable during periods of excessive oxygen want, as in intercurrent attacks of bronchitis or broncho-pneumonia. In heart failure, likewise, oxygen may be given as a temporary measure, and may be of value to tide the patient over some crisis such as an attack of pulmonary œdema, acute failure following coronary thrombosis, or pulmonary infarction. Under experimental conditions patients have been treated in the oxygen chamber for a long time (*e.g.*, six weeks), but it is not feasible to give oxygen continuously for such periods with ordinary clinical appliances, and its use in cases of chronic heart-failure is therefore of limited value. It is noteworthy that oxygen, even when efficiently given, may yet fail to relieve the dyspnœa of cardiac failure. Cardiac dyspnœa appears to be caused by many factors, of which anoxæmia is not the most important.

The success or failure of oxygen therapy in general cannot be assessed solely by the abolition or persistence of dyspnœa, a point emphasized by Christie,[1] for oxygen lack is a factor of little significance in the production of respiratory embarrassment. Physiologists likewise are agreed that oxygen lack does not cause dyspnœa, a fact well attested by the experiences of those who have subjected themselves to rarefied atmospheres. A patient may stand in desperate need of oxygen without being dyspnœic, and conversely a patient who is both dyspnœic and anoxæmic may derive great benefit from oxygen therapy as regards his anoxæmia and yet may still remain dyspnœic from other causes.

It is sometimes desirable to increase the depth of respiration, as for example in cases of pneumonia with rapid, shallow breathing. As already noted (see p. 1099), this type of breathing aggravates greatly the anoxæmia arising from other causes.

[1] *Lancet*, 1938, **2**, 876.

Again, after anæsthesia with chloroform or ether, deep respiration accelerates the rate at which the drug is excreted by the lungs and shortens the post-operative period of anæsthesia. Deep breathing during the recovery period from such anæsthesia also helps to prevent the plugging of bronchi with sticky mucus, and lessens the risk of post-operative pulmonary collapse. Deep respiration, with efficient ventilation of the bases of the lungs through the action of the diaphragm, also lessens the risk of hypostatic pneumonia in elderly subjects suddenly confined to bed by such accidents as fracture of the femur, etc. In all these conditions the inhalation of a low concentration (5 to 10 per cent.) of carbon dioxide will stimulate respiration considerably, and is therapeutically efficient.

For clinical use oxygen is supplied in cylinders containing the desired percentage (5 or 10 per cent.) of carbon dioxide, and the mixture is given in the same way as simple oxygen (*e.g.*, by simple face mask or nasal tube).

Requirements.—Some idea of the quantity of oxygen required may be gained from consideration of the following points. The tidal air (air inspired and expired at each breath) is about 500 c.c., and with a respiratory rate of 20 per minute this entails a pulmonary ventilation rate of 10 litres per minute. In the case of a patient who is in need of oxygen therapy the total minute ventilation is frequently double this figure, namely, 20 litres per minute. This represents an intake of 4 litres of oxygen every minute, since air contains 20 per cent. of that gas. To raise the oxygen content of the alveolar air to double the normal might be expected, therefore, to require about 4 litres per minute flow of additional oxygen. Since with many methods of administration (nasal catheter, etc.) the gas flows continuously and is wasted during expiration, *i.e.*, during approximately half the respiratory cycle, even higher rates of flow may be required.

Methods.—Many varieties of appliances are available for the clinical administration of oxygen of all degrees of complexity and efficiency. Before reviewing the individual methods it is well to consider the general principles underlying their design. There are four main factors to be studied : efficiency, cost, comfort in use and simplicity in working.

The estimation of efficiency, though possible to some extent by clinical observation, is capable of exact determination only by alveolar air analyses. It is the partial pressure of the oxygen in the alveolar air which determines the amount taken up by the blood, and this pressure depends on the percentage of oxygen in the alveolar air. Normally the alveolar air contains about 14 per cent. of oxygen, which corresponds to a partial pressure of about 100 mm. Hg. An efficient method of oxygen therapy should at least double, or preferably treble, this value, and should raise the alveolar oxygen content to about 40 per cent. The quantity of oxygen per minute required to effect this increase varies considerably with the method of administration. With some methods, *e.g.*, the old tube-and-funnel apparatus, it is frankly impossible to raise the oxygen content of the alveolar air to anything like the essential 40 per cent. level, while with others the required figure can be reached with varying ease. The oxygen flow necessary for various types of apparatus is given by Christie (*loc. cit.*) as follows :—

	Tent.	Face Tent.	Face Mask.	Nasal Mask.	Bifid Nasal Tube.	Nasal Catheter.
Oxygen per cent. in alveolar air.	40 to 50	58	40 to 50	45	45	45
Oxygen flow in litres per min.	4	6	3	3	6	6

There is an extreme range of variation in the cost of different forms of apparatus. At one limit stands the all-steel airtight oxygen chamber, so expensive that only the wealthiest of institutions can afford to install it, and at the other the simple nasal catheter costing a few pence. Between those extremes are those types costing shillings or a few pounds, or like the oxygen tent running up to £50 or £80. As oxygen gas is relatively cheap the actual cost of running varies less. A flow of 1 litre per minute costs only about a penny per hour. The questions of comfort in use and simplicity in running will be considered briefly in the reference to individual methods.

The Oxygen Chamber.—The *oxygen chamber* is an airtight room in which a patient can live for days or weeks in an atmosphere where the oxygen percentage can be raised to any desired level (commonly about 50 per cent.). Such a room must be provided with an air-conditioning plant to cool and dry the enclosed air and to absorb carbon dioxide. Extremely costly to build and to run, such a chamber requires skilled supervision in operation, and is beyond the purse of all but the largest voluntary hospitals in this country. Since only one or two patients can be treated at the same time, it is obviously useless when occasion arises to treat those affected in an epidemic of influenzal broncho-pneumonia, or the victims of gas-warfare. Accordingly, this method needs no further consideration here.

The Tube and Funnel.—At the other extreme stands the "tube-and-funnel" method, formerly popular, and still in use here and there. Here oxygen from a cylinder is delivered through tubing to a glass funnel held near the patient's face. Alveolar air analyses have demonstrated the futility of this procedure; its use represents a waste of time and oxygen. Failure to realize this is a source of potential danger, since a patient in dire need of oxygen may, through such a method, be deprived of the chance of life afforded by efficient treatment. The tube and funnel have no place in oxygen therapy.

The Oxygen Tent.—The oxygen tent was devised in an attempt to surround the patient with an atmosphere rich in oxygen at an economic cost. Here the patient is enclosed in a tent of non-porous material, sealed off from the outside air by tucking the margins of the tent under the mattress, where the apposition of the tent-fabric and a waterproof sheet diminishes loss by leakage. A large window of celluloid material is provided, and oxygen supplied from cylinders to maintain the desired concentration under the tent. Such a tent requires provision for removing water and carbon dioxide from the enclosed air, and for cooling. These ends are achieved by the enclosure of trays of soda-lime and an ice-container. Though very efficient, the tent in use requires skilled supervision, and nursing by trained personnel; the patient is entirely dependent on the oxygen supplied to him from the feed-pipe, and a failure of the oxygen supply will speedily lead to asphyxia unless detected by the attendant; the tent is costly to buy and rather expensive to run; and the confinement is frequently intolerable to a distressed or delirious patient. These points render the tent unsuitable for use in general practice, or even in most nursing-homes or small hospitals; and except in a few large hospitals it is little employed in this country.

Face Tents.—Smaller tents, or box masks (face tents), have been introduced, designed to rest on the shoulders of the patient, and to enclose the head and neck. These are not completely closed boxes, but are open at one end, and are claimed to be less irksome to patients than the complete oxygen tent, the sense of confinement being less marked. With these a high concentration of oxygen may be attained (see table, p. 1102), and with cooling and drying devices they are light and comfortable in use. Restlessness on the part of the patient may, however, dislodge the tent from its optimum position, with consequent loss of efficiency. Relatively cheap to install and economical to run, such face tents can be used efficiently provided nursing supervision is good.

Masks.—One of the most efficient and least costly methods of all is to give oxygen by a *Haldane mask.* Closely applied to the face, however, covering the nose and mouth, it produces a sense of suffocation in many patients, and will rarely be tolerated for any length of time. Despite its efficiency, therefore, the use of the face mask has largely been discontinued. A small *nasal mask,* adapted from a Haldane mask and in current use in anæsthetic practice, has recently been adapted for use in oxygen therapy (see Fig. 26). Designed to

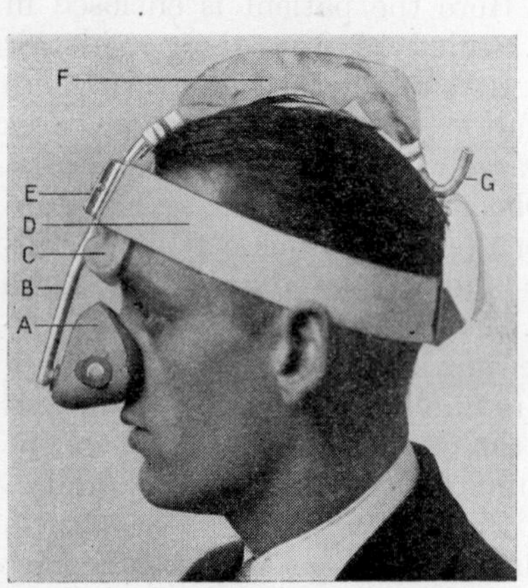

(*By courtesy of "The Lancet" Ltd.*)

Fig. 26.—Nasal Mask and Accessories.

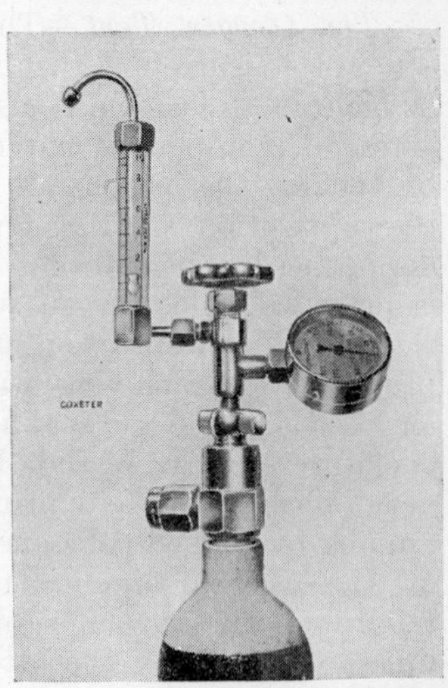

(*By courtesy of Coxeters.*)

Fig. 27.—Valve and Flow-meter for Administration of Oxygen.

fit over the nose only, the mask is for this reason more readily tolerated by the patient, who is less liable to feel suffocated so long as he can breathe through the mouth when he so desires. Analysis of alveolar air samples shows that breathing with the open mouth does not seriously interfere with the efficiency of the apparatus, in which an oxygen flow of 3 litres per minute will raise the alveolar oxygen to 45 per cent. The gas is led to the mask through a thin-walled bag strapped to the crown of the head, from which the tube feeding the mask runs vertically downwards to the nose. Movements of the patient or of his head do not interfere with efficient working of the apparatus. The bag acts as a reservoir, in which the gas accumulates during expiration, like that on the face-piece of an anæsthetic mask. Delivery of the gas through a rigid tube ensures wastage of all the oxygen arriving during the expiratory phase of respiration, *i.e.*, half the total supplied from the cylinder. The introduction of a soft bag which fills during expiration and is emptied by inspiration greatly increases the efficiency of the apparatus. Cheap, efficient and easy to use, this little apparatus is suitable for use in patients' houses or in hospital.

The Nasal Catheter.—Two varieties of intranasal tube are in use, of which the nasal catheter is the more familiar. The catheter should be of soft rubber, size No. 9, and should be lubricated with a bland emollient. A 1 per cent. cocaine ointment is useful for this purpose, combining lubrication with anæsthetic properties. Liquid paraffin or vaseline may be used, but then it will be necessary to apply a local anæsthetic (4 per cent. cocaine spray) to the nostril and nasopharynx before introducing the tube. The tube is usually inserted till the tip touches the back of the nasopharynx, and then withdrawn slightly ($\frac{1}{4}$ to $\frac{1}{2}$ in.). The free end should be carried upwards to the forehead, and fixed there either by adhesive strapping or preferably by a forehead-mirror head band and light clip. The usual practice of affixing the catheter to the cheek with adhesive plaster is undesirable, particularly in men, from the discomfort produced through traction on the growing beard. The other practice so often seen, of fixing the tube to the pillow with a safety-pin, is equally undesirable, since a slight movement of the patient's head may then draw the catheter from the nostril.

A *bifurcated nasal tube* is sometimes substituted for the single rubber catheter, after a method used in 1925 by Davies and Gilchrist,[1] and now in common use. The metal tube, which passes down the front of the face from a forehead band, is divided into two branches which are curved to fit into the nostrils. The metal tips are usually furnished with short pieces of soft rubber tubing for comfort. It is not necessary for these to fit the nostrils closely, but it is essential that the method of fixation to the forehead should not allow of their dislodgment by slight movements. Light and fairly comfortable in use, and cheap to buy, this apparatus is probably slightly more efficient than the nasal catheter. Its main advantage lies probably in the fact that it divides the oxygen stream into two halves, each naturally of less volume than a single undivided stream, and less liable to cause irritation to the nasal passages than a strong single jet.

[1] *Edin. Med. Jour.*, 1925, **32**, 225.

Both these forms of nasal tube require about 6 litres per minute for maximum efficiency, though 4 litres per minute is fairly effective, while a flow of 2 litres per minute represents the minimum with any demonstrable effect. There is considerable discomfort to the patient when 6 litres per minute are delivered through a catheter into the nasopharynx, and this irritation seems to be mainly dependent on the high rate of flow rather than on the temperature or dryness of the gas. These latter irritant qualities can be eliminated by bubbling the gas through a wash-bottle containing warm water. It is to be remembered that even 2 litres per minute passes through the usual wash-bottle in a continuous stream of unbroken bubbles, while higher rates of flow cause splashing of liquid along the delivery tube, or may even blow the stopper out of the bottle. The wash-bottle should not be used as a flow-meter, since, when the bubbles can be counted, the rate of flow is much below the minimum effective level. A simple flow-meter should be considered an essential part of any apparatus for administration of oxygen, together with a fine-adjustment valve for controlling the supply. A simple and compact form of valve and flow-meter is illustrated in Fig. 27, the cost of such an apparatus being between £3 and £4. Without a flow-meter the rate of delivery of the gas is mere guesswork, and efficient working of any apparatus is unlikely.

A final word of warning is necessary regarding the danger of fire, ignorance of which may lead to serious accidents: objects which merely smoulder in air burst into flame in high concentrations of oxygen (*e.g.*, cigarettes); fire may also be caused by lubricating with oil the valves of high-pressure oxygen cylinders. This latter is usually warned against specifically by the manufacturers in printed legends on the cylinder-head.

I. G. W. Hill.

CONVERSION TABLE FOR WEIGHTS AND MEASURES

1 milligram (mg.)	=	0·015	gr.
1 gramme (gm.)	=	15·4	,,
1 gramme	=	0·25	dr.
1 gramme	=	0·03	oz.
1 kilogram (kg.)	=	2·2	lbs.
1 kilogram	=	0·16	st.

1 grain (gr.)	=	64·8	mg.
1 grain	=	0·06	gm.
1 drachm (dr.) = 60 gr.	=	3·9	,,
1 ounce (oz.) = 8 dr.	=	31·1	,,
1 pound (lb.) = 16 oz.	=	0·45	kg.
1 stone (st.) = 14 lbs.	=	6·35	,,

1 cubic centimetre (c.c.)	=	16·9	min.
1 cubic centimetre	=	0·28	fl. dr.
1 cubic centimetre	=	0·035	fl. oz.
1 litre	=	35·2	,,
1 litre	=	1·76	pints.

1 minim (min.)	=	0·058	c.c.
1 fluid drachm (fl. dr.) = 60 min.	=	3·6	,,
1 fluid ounce (fl. oz.) = 8 fl. dr.	=	28·4	,,
1 pint = 20 fl. oz.	=	0·57	litre.
1 pint	=	568·2	c.c.

INDEX

A

Abdomen, paracentesis of (technique), 1087-88
  tapping of, in cirrhosis of liver, 612
Abortion, recurrent, 1065-66
Abortus fever, 241
Abscess, amœbic, 246-47
  cerebral, 983
  complicating sinusitis, 754-55
  lung. *See* LUNG, abscess and gangrene of, 818-20
  peritonsillar, 757
  retro-pharyngeal, 761
  subphrenic, 820
Acacia and the osmotic content of the plasma, 860
Acetabuloplasty, 944
Acetarsone, 207
Acetylarsan, 207
  in cardiovascular syphilis, 657
  in early syphilis, 212
Acetylcholine in paroxysmal tachycardia, 709
  in vascular disease, 738-39
Acetylphenylhydrazine in polycythæmia vera, 505-6
Achalasia of the cardia, 534-35
Achlorhydria in chronic gastritis, 541
  in gastric carcinoma, 561
  in hypochromic anæmia, 467
  in pellagra, 409
  in pernicious anæmia, 483
  in rosacea, 176
  in tuberculosis, 134
Acholuric jaundice, 489
Achondroplasia, 966
Acidosis in chronic interstitial nephritis, 862
  in cyclical vomiting, 297-98
  in diabetes, 351
  in tetany, 425, 426
Acne, 173-75
Acriflavine in drainage of ureter, 881
Acromegaly. *See* ADENOMA OF THE PITUITARY, 457-58
Acute yellow atrophy of the liver, 609
Adams-Stokes attacks in heart-block, 712
Addison's anæmia. *See* PERNICIOUS ANÆMIA, 480-88
  disease, 450-53
Adenitis of cervical glands complicating impetigo of scalp, 164
  tuberculous. *See* GLANDULAR TUBERCULOSIS, 143, 146
Adenoma of the pituitary, 457-58
Adexolin for premature infants, 273
  in acute nephritis, 855
  in anæmia, 487
  in convulsions, 293
  in rheumatoid arthritis, 900, 909
  in rickets, 416
  in vitamin A deficiency, 404
Adherent pericardium, operations for, 714
Adhesions, intrapleural division of, 126-27
Adrenal cortex, 453
Adrenal medulla, 453-54
Adrenalin, and serum therapy in lobar pneumonia, 803, 804, 805
  in Addison's disease, 451
  in asthma, 824-25, 835, 839, 840
  in circulatory collapse in diabetic coma, 353
  in circulatory failure, 644
  in circulatory failure in acute bronchitis, 786-87
  in diarrhœa, 570
  in diphtheria, 24
  in dyspnœic heart failure, 701
  in epistaxis, 747, 748, 751
  in hay fever, 844, 845
  in heat retention, 303
  in purpuras, 513
  in Stokes-Adams seizures, 726-27
  in syncope, 725
  intracardiac injection of, 726
Adrenals, tumours of, 453-54
Agar-agar in constipation, 578
Agarol in constipation, 578
Agotan in gout, 964
Agranulocytic angina, 521-23
  due to sulphonamides, 86
Agranulocytosis. *See* AGRANULOCYTIC ANGINA, 521-23
Air replacement of pleural effusion, 138
Air-swallowers, 563
Albargin in chronic dysentery, 29
Alcohol, causing cirrhosis of liver, 610
  in angina of effort, 697
  in cerebral thrombosis, 997
  in cholera, 243
  in chronic bronchitis, 793
  in circulatory failure in acute bronchitis, 786
  in diet in essential hypertension, 652
  in diet in fibrositis, 937
  in fever diet, 5
  in gastritis, 541
  in gout, 963, 964
  in myotonia congenita, 972
  in peptic ulcer, 546
  in tropical neurasthenia, 256
  injection in facial spasm, 1002
    in neuralgia, 1000
  intraspinal injection of, in malignant disease, 978
Alcoholism, 1046-54
  acute, 1047-50
    alcoholic psychoses, 1049-50
    delirium tremens, 1048-49
    diet in, 1049
    dipsomania, 1047-48
    drugs in, 1048
  and pellagra, 408
  and polyneuritis, 404, 1047
  and scurvy, 410
  avitaminosis and, 1047, 1049
  chronic, 1050-54

Alepol in leprosy, 251
Alfalfa in obstructive jaundice, 517
Alimentary canal, diseases of, 532-601. *See* ŒSOPHAGUS, STOMACH, INTESTINES
Alkalis in gout, 962, 964
  in peptic ulcer, 546-48
  in rheumatoid arthritis, 901
  in urinary infections, 874-76
  tetany due to, 427
Alkalosis following alkali treatment of peptic ulcer, 553-54
Alkalotic tetany, 427
Allen's diets, 355
Allergic factor in asthma, 831-36
  in dermatitis, 180
Allergy, nasal, 751
Aloes in constipation, 577
Alopecia areata, 187
Aluminium acetate in otitis externa, 762
  in syringing ear, 763
Aluminium hydroxide in peptic ulcer, 547
Alum toxoid in diphtheria, 20
Alzheimer's disease, 992
Ambinon, 1058
Amenorrhœa, 455, 1063-64
Amidopyrine causing agranulocytic angina, 521-22
  in rheumatoid arthritis, 900
Ammoket as urinary antiseptic, 878
Ammonium chloride in congestive heart failure, 687-88
  in rickets, 421, 425
  in tetania parathyropriva, 448
  in urinary infections, 874, 877, 878
Amœbic dysentery. *See* DYSENTERY, AMŒBIC, 244-47
  hepatitis, 246
  liver abscess, 246-47
  pulmonary complications, 247
Amyl nitrite in angina of effort, 696
  in cerebral thrombosis, 997
Amyotrophic lateral sclerosis, 985-86
Anabin in amœbic dysentery, 245
Anæmia, achlorhydric, simple, 464
  achrestic, 488
  and menstruation, 465-66
  and pregnancy, 464, 465
  aplastic and hypoplastic, 494-97
  cerebral, 724
  congenital hæmolytic, 489
  due to iron deficiency, 464-79
  following hæmatemesis in peptic ulcer, 552
  hæmolytic, 488-94
    acute, of Lederer, 493-94
    blood transfusion in, 490, 492, 494
    in the newborn, 274-75
    paroxysmal hæmoglobinuria in, 493
  hypochromic, in rheumatoid arthritis, 900
  idiopathic, 494, 497
    hypochromic, 464
  in cancer of the stomach, 562
  in cardiac patient, 648
  in chronic ulcerative colitis, 588
  in cœliac disease, 285
  in myxœdema, 432
  in pregnancy with heart disease, 662
  in scurvy, 412
  in sprue, 247, 248, 250
  iron deficiency in infancy, 284
  megalocytic, 481-88
    classification, 481-82
    in diseases of the liver, 488
    in tropical and non-tropical sprue and pellagra, 487
  microcytic, chronic, 464
  nutritional, prevention of, 272-73
  nutritional hypochromic, chronic, 464-73
    dieto-therapy (Tables I and II), 469-71
    dysphagia in, 468
    gastro-intestinal system in, 467-68
    of infancy and childhood, 473-75
    nervous system in, 468-69
    prophylaxis of, 464-66
    tongue in, 468
Anæmia—*contd.*
  pernicious, Addisonian, 481-86
    blood transfusion in, 482-83
    general measures in, 483
    hog's stomach preparations in, 485
    hydrochloric acid in, 483, 484
    iron in, 483
    liver and liver extract in, 483-84
    maintenance treatment, 485-86
    of pregnancy, 487
  post-hæmorrhagic, acute, 475-79
    chronic, 479
  primary aplastic, 494, 497
  sickle-cell, 494
  splenic, 497-502
    splenectomy in, 498-500
"Anæsthesin" ointment, 737
Anæsthetic in irrigation of urethra, 197
Anæsthetics in diabetic surgery, 383
  in removal of gangrenous digits, 738
  in thyroidectomy, 444
Anahæmin in anæmia, 483, 485
Anal sphincter, spasm of, in infancy, 282-83
Anaphylaxis and serum sickness in lobar pneumonia, 803-4
Androsterone, 454
Aneurin, 405
Aneurysm, congenital leaking, 996
Aneurysms of aorta, 657-58
Angina, agranulocytic, 521-23
Angina decubitus, 699
  operation in, 715-17
Angina innocens, 718
  of effort, 695-99
    in convalescent coronary thrombosis, 697-99
Angina pectoris, operation in, 715-17
Anginal heart failure, 692-99
Angio-neurotic œdema. *See* URTICARIA, 185-86
Aniline dyestuffs, workers with, 320

Ankylostomiasis, 262-64
Anorexia in anæmia, 467
  in digitalis therapy. *See* DIGITALIS, THERAPEUTIC USE OF, 673-84
  in gastritis, 541
  in sulphonamide therapy, 86
  in tuberculosis, 133
  nervosa, 562-63
Anosmia, 999
Anoxæmia and shock, 728-29
Ant-acids, gastric, 546-47
Anthracene series of drugs in constipation, 576
Anthrax, 11-13
Antidysenteric serum in chronic ulcerative colitis, 589-90
  in dysentery, 27
Antileprol, 250
Antimony compounds in kala-azar, 235-36
  in oriental sore, 237
Antiphlogistine in acute bronchitis, 788
Antipyretics, 5-6
Antiseptics in irrigation of urethra, 197-98
  respiratory, 777, 794, 815
  urinary, 876-80
Antostab, 1058
Antuitrin, 455
  G, 458
  S, 175, 1058
Anuria in acute nephritis, 857
Aorta, aneurysms of, 657-58
Aortitis, leutic, 654-58
Aphasia, 998
Apicolysis, 128-29
Apicosan in rheumatoid arthritis, 918
Apomorphine in acute alcoholism, 1048
Appendicostomy in chronic ulcerative colitis, 589
Apple diet, in ulcerative colitis, 597
Argyrol after bladder lavage, 881
  in instillation of urethra, 198, 200
  in ophthalmia neonatorum, 205
  in rhinitis, 749
  in venereal disease, 192, 193
Arsenic in bronchiectasis, 815
  in chronic leukæmia, 527-28
Arsenic—*contd.*
  in disseminated sclerosis, 985
  in Hodgkin's disease, 530
  in leutic aortitis, 655-57
  in lung abscess, 819
  in psoriasis, 191
  in rheumatoid arthritis, 901
  in the senile heart, 660
  poisoning by arseniuretted hydrogen, 309-10
    in polyneuritis, 979
Arsenical compounds in acute necrosis of liver, 609
    in anthrax, 12
    in syphilis, 206-7
      toxic sequels to, 207-10
  drugs and liver function, 213
Arseniuretted hydrogen and arsenic poisoning, 309-10
Arsphenamine "606" in syphilis, 206
Arterectomy, 739
Arteries, obstruction of, gradual, 734-40
    Buerger's exercises in, 739
    induction of intermittent reactive hyperæmia, 739-40
    intermittent claudication, 735
    nutritional changes, 734-35
    operation in, 739
    ulcers in, 737
  intermittent, 740-41
    operative treatment, 741
    Raynaud phenomenon, 740
  sudden, 733-34
    embolus, 733
    thickening of wall of, 732
    treatment of gangrenous area, 734
Arteriosclerosis, cerebral, 997
  in diabetes, 338
Arthritis, ankylosing, 889
  atrophic, 889
  complicating gonorrhœa, 201
  chronic menopausal, 926-27
Arthritis—*contd.*
  chronic villous, 925-27
    climacteric and, 925-27
  degenerative, 890
  gonococcal, 201
  hypertrophic, 890
  in rheumatic fever, 635
  non-ankylosing, 890
  proliferative, 889
  rheumatoid. *See* RHEUMATOID ARTHRITIS, 894-923
Arthrodesing operations, 944
Arthropathies in tabes dorsalis, 220-21
Arthroplasty, 944
Arthrosis, 890
Arthrotomy, 943
Artificial pneumothorax. *See* PNEUMOTHORAX, ARTIFICIAL
Asbestosis, 315-16
Ascariasis, 264
Ascites, 612, 1087-88
Ascorbic acid deficiency. *See* SCURVY, 410-13
  in congestive heart failure, 689
  in dermatitis during syphilis, 208
Aspiration in pericarditis with effusion, 641-42
  of effusion in tuberculous pleurisy, 137
  of the pleural cavity (technique), 1088-90
Aspirin in acute coryza, 780, 782
  in dermatomyositis, 971
  in muscular cramp, 973
  in neuralgia, 977
  in rheumatoid arthritis, 899
  reduction of temperature by, 6
Aspirin, calcium in chorea, 995
Asthma, 823-43
  acute attack, 824-25
  adrenalin hydrochloride in, 824
  and serum sensitivity, 802-3
  management of the asthmatic state, 826-43. *See* ASTHMATIC STATE, MANAGEMENT OF THE, 826-43
  status asthmaticus, 825
Asthma Research Council. "Physical Exercises for Asthma," 843

Asthmatic state, management of the, 826-43
allergic factor, 831-36
climate in, 841-42
desensitization, 834-36
drugs, 838-41
foods causing, 832
gastro-intestinal factor in, 838
infective factor, 836
inhalants causing, 832, 833-34
inhalations, 840-41
nasal factor, 837-38
postural and breathing exercises, 843
psychological factor, 826-31
sensitivity tests, 832-33
spa treatment, 842
Ataxia, 999
in disseminated sclerosis, 984
in tabes dorsalis, 217-18
Ataxias, hereditary, 992
Atebrin (in malaria), 228, 229, 230
Atelectasis, 820-21
Atony, gastric, 565
in infancy, 292
intestinal. *See* CONSTIPATION, 573
Atophan in diseases of the liver, 605, 609
in gout, 964
in rheumatoid arthritis, 901
Atrophy, acute red, 609
acute yellow, 609
optic, 999
progressive muscular, 985
Atropine in achalasia of the ureter, 880
in acute bronchitis, 785
in biliary colic, 619
in cardiac asthma, 700
in cholera, 242
in constipation, 576
in cough in infancy, 288
in gall-bladder disease, 620
in heart-block, 700, 711
in hiccup in cirrhosis of the liver, 614
in muco - membranous colic, 586
in myasthenia gravis, 972
in peptic ulcer, 547
in pulmonary œdema, 790
in pyelitis, 874
in renal colic, 883
in syncope, 725
Auricle, injuries to the, 762
Auricular fibrillation, 703-7
digitalis and, 704-6
quinidine sulphate in, 706-7
Auricular flutter, 707-8
Autohæmotherapy in desensitization in asthma, 836
in plague, 239
Avertin in diseases of the liver, 605
in thyroidectomy, 444
Avitaminosis, 401-23, 1047
Avoleum in vitamin A deficiency, 404
Azotæmia, 861

B

Bacilli, fusiform in sputum in bronchiectasis, 815, 819
Bacilluria, 869
Bacillus acidophilus in diarrhœa, 571
coli in gonorrhœa, 196
in septicæmia, 84
in urinary infections, 871-72, 879
dysenteriæ, 25
paratyphosus B, 30, 31
Pfeiffer in influenza, 40
proteus in urinary infections, 871-72, 879
tuberculosis, in urinary infections, 872
infection with, 93-98
typhosus, 30, 31
Welchii in intestinal obstruction, 594
Bacteriophage, d'Herelle's, 33
in bacillary dysentery, 27
in cholera, 243, 244
in enteric fever, 33
in plague, 239
Balanitis, 226
Banti's disease. *See* ANÆMIA, SPLENIC, 497-502
Barbiturates in acute bronchitis, 784
in auricular fibrillation, 704
in congestive heart failure, 668-69
in extra-systoles, 712
in insomnia, 1035-36
in rheumatoid arthritis, 900
Bargen's serum in chronic ulcerative colitis, 590
Barium chloride in Stokes-Adams seizures, 725
Bartholinian glands in gonorrhœa, 203
Baths in rheumatoid arthritis, 916
Basal narcotics, in hyperthyroidism, 443
Basic ash diets in nephritis, 861
Bayer 205 in African trypanosomiasis, 233
B.C.G. vaccine in tuberculosis, 95
Bednar's ulcers, 279
Bed-sores, in paraplegia, 986-88
Bee venom in rheumatoid arthritis, 902-18
Belladonna in asthma, 839
in chronic ulcerative colitis, 588
in Dietl's crisis, 869
in diseases of the peritoneum, 626
in encephalitis lethargica, 993
in enuresis, 297
in nervous diarrhœa, 571
in renal calculus, 883
Bell's paralysis, 1001
Bemax in anæmia, 469
in deficiency disease, 406
in pink disease, 299
in rheumatoid arthritis, 909
Bence-Jones protein in multiple myeloma, 968
Benerva in beri-beri, 405, 406, 407
in polyneuritis, 979
Bengue's balsam in rheumatoid arthritis, 913
Benzedrine in chronic alcoholism, 1052
in coryza, 780
in encephalitis lethargica, 993
in paroxysmal rhinorrhœa, 847
Benzene poisoning, 313-14
Benzo-Gynœstryl, 1060
Benzol in chronic leukæmia, 528
Berberine sulphate in Oriental sore, 237
Beri-beri, 404-8
Besnier's prurigo, 180-81
Betanaphthol in cestodiasis, 258
Betaxan in beri-beri, 405, 407

Bile, constituents of, 606
Bilharzia. *See* SCHISTOSOMIASIS, 256
Biliary drainage, non-surgical, 617
Biliary tract, diseases of. *See* GALL-BLADDER AND, 614-23
conservative treatment, 620-21
operations in, 621-22
Biliousness, 577
Bilirubin, 606
Bilirubinæmia, 607
Biochemical estimations, tests, etc. (Tables I and II), 1074
Bipalatinoids (in anæmia), 472
Birth injuries, 275-77
Bismarsen in cardiovascular syphilis, 657
Bismostab in yaws, 252, 253
Bismuth arsanilate in yaws, 252
Bismuth arsphenamine sulphonate in yaws, 252
Bismuth in early syphilis, 211
in leutic aortitis, 655-57
in syphilis, 208-10, 214, 216
toxic effects of, 209-10
in tabes dorsalis, 217
Bismuth oxycarbonate, in peptic ulcer, 547
Bismuth-oxychloride in syphilis, 209
Bismuth-salicylate in syphilis, 209
Bismuth subnitrate in amœbic dysentery, 245
Bites, insect, 186
Blackwater fever in malaria, 232-33
Bladder, care of, in paraplegia, 988
lavage of, in drainage of the ureter, 881
Blepharospasm, 1002
Blister, cantharides in pericarditis, 640
Blood, diseases of, 460-531
classification, 461-63
the anæmias, 464-97, *q.v.*
Blood flow, normal peripheral, 731-32
obstruction as a result of trauma, 733
result of local hypersensitivity to cold, 733
Blood flow—*contd.*
pathological processes which reduce, 732-42.
See also ARTERIES
Blood grouping, 1074
Blood groups, determination of (Table III), 1081
Blood, oxalated, tests, etc., 1074
Blood pressure, 396, 650-54, 857, 861
test in serum sensitivity, 802
Blood sedimentation rate in arthritis, 887
in chronic rheumatic diseases, 959-60
in pulmonary tuberculosis, 106
in rheumatic carditis, 638
Blood-sugar curves in pregnancy, 372
in diabetic coma, 352
in diabetes mellitus. *See* HYPOGLYCÆMIA IN DIABETES MELLITUS, 344-47
tests in diabetes mellitus, 349-51
Blood transfusion in anæmia, achrestic, 488
acute hæmolytic, 494
Addisonian pernicious, 482-83
aplastic, 496
secondary hæmolytic, 492
splenic, 502
in benzene poisoning, 314
in carbon monoxide poisoning, 311
in chronic ulcerative colitis, 589
in collapse and shock, 728
in endocarditis, 639
in enterogenous cyanosis, 507
in hæmatemesis of peptic ulcer, 549-50
in hæmophilia, 518, 520
in hæmoptysis, 133
in jaundice, obstructive, 517
of the newborn, 275
in leukæmia, 525, 526
in melæna neonatorum, 274
in purpura and aplastic anæmia in syphilis, 208
Blood transfusion—*contd.*
in purpura hæmorrhagica, 516
in septicæmia, 81-82
technique of, 1079-84
collection of blood for transfusion, 1082
continuous transfusion, 1083
determination of blood groups (Table III), 1081
indirect (grouping) test, 1081
reactions during, 1083-84
selection of donors, 1079
the single transfusion, 1083
Blood vessels of the limbs, diseases of, 731-42. *See* BLOOD FLOW; ARTERIES, OBSTRUCTION OF
Boils. *See* FURUNCULOSIS, 164-65
Bone, diseases of, 966-68
achondroplasia, 966
hypertrophic pulmonary osteo-arthropathy, 966
leontiasis ossea, 967
multiple myeloma, 968
osteitis deformans, 966-67
fibrosa cystica, 967
osteogenesis imperfecta (fragilitas ossium), 967
osteomalacia (mollities ossium), 967
osteomyelitis, 968
oxycephaly, 967-68
Bone-marrow in anæmia. *See* ANÆMIA, APLASTIC, 494-97
Bone-marrow, extracts of, in agranulocytic angina, 523
Boroglycerin as throat paint, 756
Boulay's technique, 141
Bovine bacillus in tuberculosis, 96-97
Brachial neuritis, 975
Brain. *See also* SKULL
Brain abscess, chronic, 983
Brain and spinal cord, disorders of, 983-86
amyotrophic lateral sclerosis, 985-86
disseminated sclerosis, 983-85
infections of the brain and spinal cord, 983

Bran bath in diseases of the skin, 154
Breath-holding attacks in infancy, 294
Breathing exercises in asthma, 843
  in rheumatism, 952
Bright's disease. *See* NEPHRITIS, 851-67
British Health Resorts Association Handbook, 915
Bromide in epilepsy, 1008
Brompton mixture for cough, 691
Bronchial carcinoma, 822-23
Bronchiectasis, 812-18
  artificial pneumothorax in, 818
  bronchoscopic drainage in, 815
  drugs in, 815
  hæmoptysis in, 816
  in infancy, 290-91
  lobectomy, 816-17
  phrenic evulsion in, 817
  postural drainage in, 813-15
  thoracoplasty in, 817
  vaccines in, 816
Bronchitis and pneumonia in infancy, 288-90
Bronchitis, acute, and broncho-pneumonia, 782-92
  circulatory failure in, 785
  convalescence, 791-92
  cough, pain and spit in, 788-90
  cyanosis, 785
  dehydration, 787
  delirium, 785
  diet in, 784
  drugs in, 789
  general measures, 783-84
  insomnia and restlessness, 784-85
  serum therapy, 791
  symptomatic treatment, 784-85
  tympanites, 787-88
Bronchitis, chronic, and emphysema, 792-94
  plastic, 790
Broncho-pneumonia as complication of measles, 46. *See* BRONCHITIS, ACUTE, 782-92
Bronchoscopy in atelectasis, 821
Bubo, climatic, 225
Buerger's exercises, 739
Bulbar paralysis, 985
Bullous eruptions, 186
Burrell's aspirator, 137
Bursitis, subacromial, 40
Butolan in enterobiasis, 264
Butyl chloral hydrate, in neuralgia, 1000

C

Cæcostomy in chronic ulcerative colitis, 589
Cæsarean section in achondroplasia, 966
  in diabetic pregnancy, 373
  in heart disease, 663
  in osteomalacia, 423
Caffein sodium benzoate, 24
Caffeine as diuretic, 688
  group as vasodilators, 699
  in asthma, 841
  in circulatory failure of acute bronchitis, 786-87
Caisson sickness, 304
Calabar swellings, 261
Calamine in diseases of the skin, 159
  lotion in pruritus, 608
Calciferol, 415
Calcium deficiency, 413
  forms of, in rickets, 422
Calcium gluconate in tetania parathyropriva, 447, 448
  in amyotrophic lateral sclerosis, 986
  in chronic interstitial nephritis, 862
  in cœliac disease, 286
  in convulsions, 293
  in rachitic tetany, 425
  in serum sickness, 804
  in tetany of chronic renal disease, 427
Calcium in asthma, 841
  in biliary infection, 615
  in idiopathic steatorrhœa, 592
  in lead poisoning, 307
  in osteitis deformans, 966
  in purpuras, 513
  in rheumatoid arthritis, 890
  in serum sickness, 76, 804
Calcium oxalate in urine, 885
Calcium phosphate, tribasic, in peptic ulcer, 547
Calcium salts in miners' nystagmus, 306
Calcium, serum, and tetany, 424
Calcium therapy in carbon tetrachloride poisoning, 314
Calculi, biliary, 619
  urinary, 882
Calomel in constipation, 577
  in diarrhœa, 569
  in essential hypertension, 654
Calvert's urea concentration range in nephritis, 854
Camphor in diphtheria, 24
  in pruritus, 609
  inhalations, 745
  injection in shock, 729
Campolon in anæmia, 483, 485
  in cœliac disease, 285
  in purpura, 514
  in sprue, 248
Cancer, dread of, in neurotic patients, 1031
  industrial, 319-20
  of the stomach. *See* STOMACH, CANCER OF, 561-63. *See also* TUMOURS
Cannula method of intravenous infusion, 1076-78
Caprokol as urinary antiseptic, 880
Capsulotomy, 944
Carbamic acid ester of p. oxydiphenyl methan, in enterobiasis, 264
Carbarsone in amœbic dysentery, 244, 245
  in yaws, 252, 253
Carbol fuchsin in diseases of the skin, 160
Carbolic acid in pruritus, 609
Carbon dioxide and oxygen in atelectasis, 820, 821
Carbon monoxide poisoning, 311
Carbon tetrachloride in ankylostomiasis, 262, 263
  in ascariasis, 264
  in cestodiasis, 258
  in poisoning of the liver, 605
  in trichuris trichiura, 265
Carbon tetrachloride poisoning, 314
Carbromol (in cancer of the stomach), 562
Carcinoma, bronchial, 822-23. *See* CANCER

Cardia, achalasia of, 534
Cardiac asthma and acute pulmonary œdema, 700
Cardiac disease and diabetes, 378
in obesity, diet for, 396
surgery in, 713-18
Cardiac failure. *See* HEART FAILURE, 665-703
Cardiac failure and beriberi, 408
Cardiac neuroses, 718-22
Cardiac pain, relief of, operations for, 715-17
Cardiac patient, management of the ambulant, 645-50
the senile heart, 658-60
Cardiac therapeutics, principles and limitations of, 627-32
Cardiazol in circulatory failure of acute bronchitis, 786-87
in coronary thrombosis, 693-94
in peripheral vascular dilatation, 644
in shock, 729
Cardiospasm, 534
Cardiovascular syphilis, 214-15, 654-58
Carditis, rheumatic. *See* RHEUMATIC CARDITIS, 633-39
Carriers of acute poliomyelitis, 49
of cerebrospinal fever, 13-15
of diphtheria, 25
of enteric fever, 36-37
of scarlet fever, 59-60
Casbis in yaws, 252
Castor oil in diarrhœa, 569
Cataplasma kaolin in acute bronchitis, 789
Cataplexy, 1012
Cataract in diabetes, 377
Catarrhal jaundice, 607-9
Cauterization in paroxysmal rhinorrhœa, 848
in tuberculosis of the larynx, 140
Cautery in epistaxis, 748
in pharyngitis, 761
Cavernous sinus thrombosis, 997
Celery itch, 318
Central nervous system, syphilis of, 216-24
G.P.I., 221-24
gumma, 217
Central nervous system—*contd.*
meningo-vascular syphilis, 216-17
tabes dorsalis, 217-21
Cephalhæmatoma, 275
Cerebral abscess, 983
Cerebral anæmia, 724
Cerebral birth trauma, 276-77
Cerebral circulation, disorders of, 995-99
arteriosclerosis, 997
embolism, 997
hæmorrhage, 995-96
thrombosis, 996-97
venous thrombosis, 997
Cerebral function, disorders of, 1008-14
epilepsy, 1008-11
migraine, 1011
narcolepsy and cataplexy, 1012
sleeplessness, 1012-13
spasmodic torticollis, 1012
Cerebral thrombosis, 216, 996-97
Cerebral tumours, 1003-5
Cerebro-macular degeneration, 992
Cerebrospinal fever, 13-18
Cerebrospinal fluid in head injuries, 1006
in meningitis, 981-82
in meningo-vascular syphilis, 216
in tabes dorsalis, 217
in vascular syphilis, 217
pressure in lumbar puncture (Table), 1092-94
removal of, in infantile hemiplegia, 992
Certuna in malaria, 228, 230
Cervical glands, tuberculosis of, 144-45
Cervical-occipital neuritis, 975
Cervicitis, chronic, in rheumatoid arthritis, 898
Cervix in gonorrhœa, 202
Cestodiasis, 258-60
Chancroid in syphilis, 224-25
Charcoal in chronic ulcerative colitis, 588
in flatulence, 563
Charcot-Marie-Tooth type of muscular dystrophy. *See* MUSCULAR DYSTROPHY, 972
Charcot's disease of joints in tabes dorsalis, 220
Chaulmoogra oil in leprosy, 250
Chelsea Pensioner in rheumatoid arthritis, 902
Chemical irritation causing dermatitis, 177-78
Chenopodium, oil of, in ankylostomiasis, 262, 263
in ascariasis, 264
in trichuris trichiura, 265
Cheyne-Stokes respiration in dyspnœic heart failure, 699
euphyllin in, 702
Chickenpox, 18-19
Child psychology, 1021-25
Children, diabetes in. *See* DIABETES IN CHILDREN, 363-86
Chloral hydrate for cough in infancy, 288
in acute bronchitis, 784
in birth injuries, 277
in congestive heart failure, 669
in convulsions, 292, 293, 294
in diseases of infancy, 268
in insomnia, 1013
in meningitis, 982
in rachitic tetany, 426
in rheumatoid arthritis, 900
in whooping-cough, 73
Chloramine T in gonorrhœa, 197
Chloranæmia, 464
Chlorine poisoning, 312-13
Chloroform in diseases of the liver, 605
in rabies, 254
Chlorosis, 464
Cholagogues, 616-19
Cholecystectomy, 36
Cholecystitis, 616-21
acute phlegmonous, 616
acute suppurative, 616
and diabetes, 378
and obesity, 618
catarrhal, 616-17
chronic, 619
dietetics, 618
in association with gall-stones, 619-20
in obesity, diet for, 396
spa treatment, 618-19
Cholecystography, 616, 621
Cholelithiasis, 619-21
Cholera, 241-44
Cholera belt, 571
Cholesterol and formation of gall-stones, 606

Choline derivatives. *See* DORYL, 218, 709-10
Chorea, Huntington's, 995
Sydenham's, 994-95
Chromic acid bead in epistaxis, 748
Chrysarobin in diseases of the skin, 159, 161, 162, 190
Chrysops dimidiata, 261
Chrysotherapy. *See* GOLD THERAPY
Chyluria in filariasis, 261
Cicatricine in rheumatoid arthritis, 918
Cignolin in dermatitis with sprue, 250
Cinchona bark, constituents of, 228
Cinchonism, 231, 706-7
Cinchophen and acute necrosis of the liver, 609
in gout, 964
in rheumatoid arthritis, 901
Circulation, cerebral. *See* CEREBRAL CIRCULATION, 995-99
Circulatory failure, acute, 723-30
and beri-beri, 408
cardiac syncope, 725-27
collapse and shock, 727-30
diffusible stimulants, 644
digitalis in, 643
in broncho-pneumonia, 785-86
in diphtheria, 24, 643
in lobar pneumonia, 643
peripheral vascular dilatation, 644
simple syncope, 724-25
Circulatory system and emotional state, 718-19
Cirrhosis, hepatic, in schistosomiasis, 257
of the liver. *See* LIVER, CIRRHOSIS OF, 610-14
Cisternal puncture in meningitis, 982
technique, 1095-96
Citrin in purpura, 514
Claudication, intermittent, 735
Climate in asthma, 841-42
Clostridium tetani, 64
Coagulin ciba in purpura, 514
Cocaine for hiccup in cirrhosis of the liver, 614
Cocaine in asthma, 840
in epistaxis, 747, 748, 751
Cocaine addiction, 1055
Coccygodynia, 978
Codeine in chronic ulcerative colitis, 585
in pulmonary tuberculosis, 131
Codeine phosphate in diarrhœa, 572
in whooping-cough, 73
Codeine, syrup of, for cough in infancy, 288
Cod-liver oil, administration of, 414
in cœliac disease, 285
in congenital heart disease, 664
in feeding of infants, 272-73
in pulmonary fibrosis, 792
in rheumatoid arthritis, 893
prophylactic purposes, 414-15
Cœliac disease, 285-86
Cœliac rickets, 422
Colchicum in fibrositis, 934
in gout, 962
in rheumatoid arthritis, 901
Cold, common, predisposing cause of respiratory disease, 775. *See* CORYZA, ACUTE, 779-82
local hypersensitivity to, and obstruction to blood flow, 733
"Colds" in infancy, 287
Colectomy in chronic ulcerative colitis, 590
Colic, biliary, 619
intestinal, 585-87
lead, 308
renal, 883-84
Colitis, muco-membranous, 585-87
Colitis, ulcerative, 587-91
blood transfusion in, 588-89
dietetics, 588, 597-99
drugs in, 588
treatment, local, 589
Collapse and shock, 727-30
Collapse therapy in pulmonary tuberculosis, 121-30
Colliron, 472
Collosol sulphur in rheumatoid arthritis, 902
Colon, irritable, 585
Colonic irrigations, 578-80
Colsul in rheumatoid arthritis, 902
Coma, cholæmic, 614
diabetic, 351-54
hypoglycæmic, 344-47
uræmic, 862-63
Complement fixation test in gonorrhœa, 199, 204
Compressed air, work in, 304
Compression of the spinal cord, 989-90
Concussion of the brain, 1005-8
Concussion of the spinal cord, 990
Condylomata acuminata, 225
Congenital diplegia, 991-92,
Congenital heart disease, 663-65
Congenital syphilis, 215
Congestive heart failure, 666-92
and paroxysmal tachycardia, 709
complicating coronary thrombosis, 694
convalescent care, 692
cough in, 691
diet in, 669-73
digitalis in, 673-84
diuretics in, 684-89
hydrothorax, ascites, 690
in vitamin deficiency states, 688-89
mechanical procedures, 689-91
oxygen therapy, 691-92
purgatives in, 672-73
rest in, 666-67
sleep and drugs for insomnia, 667-69
thyroidectomy for, 717
treatment, symptomatic, 691-92
venesection in, 689-90
Conjunctivitis and mercury workers, 309
in hay fever, 846
Constipation, 573-80
chronic, diet, specimen, 595-96
classification (Hurst's), 573
diet, 575, 935
drugs, 575-78
dyschezia, 573
enemas and colonic irrigations, 578-80
faulty habits of defæcation, 574
in anæmias, 467-68
in digestive diseases in infancy, 282-83

Constipation—*contd.*
in encephalitis lethargica, 38
in fever, 8
in obesity, 396
in tuberculosis, 134
physical exercise, 574-75
psychic factors in, 574
Contrexeville water in renal calculus, 882
Convulsions due to hypocalcæmia, 293
due to intracranial injury, 293
idiopathic, 293
in epilepsy, 1010-11
in infancy, 292-94
in rachitic tetany, 426
Copper in anæmias, 475
Coramine in alcoholic poisoning, 1048
in anaphylaxis, 803
in circulatory failure of acute bronchitis, 786-87
in coronary thrombosis, 693-94
in septicæmia, 87
in shock, 729
Coreine in constipation, 578
Cornea, perforation of, 206
Corneal ulceration, 206
Coronary thrombosis, 692-95
convalescent, with angina of effort, 697-99
Corsets in visceroptosis, 583
Corticosterone in Addison's disease, 452
Cortin in Addison's disease, 451
in diarrhœa of Graves' disease, 572
Corynebacterium diphtheriæ, 19
Coryza, acute, 779-82
Cough in bronchitis, 784
in bronchitis and pneumonia in infancy, 288-89
in chronic bronchitis, 794
in congestive heart failure, 691
in influenza, 41
in pulmonary tuberculosis, 130-32
mixtures in lobar pneumonia, 796
plates in whooping-cough, 70
recurrent, vaccine for, 779
spit and pain in chest, in acute bronchitis, 788-90
Counter-irritation in fibrositis, 935
in osteo-arthritis, 925
"Crab" yaws, 253
Craft palsy, 974
Cramps and spasms, muscular, 973-74
Cranial nerves, disorders of, 999-1003
anosmia, 999
auditory nerve, 1002-3
facial nerve, 1001-2
ninth, tenth, eleventh and twelfth nerves, 1003
oculomotor disorders, 999
trigeminal nerve, 1000-1
visual disturbances, 999
Creosote for fœtid sputum in bronchiectasis, 815-16
in pulmonary fibrosis and bronchiectasis, 291
Cretinism, mental deficiency in, 295
thyroid in treatment, 430
Crohn's disease, 584-85
Croton oil in cerebral hæmorrhage, 996
Cupping, dry, in asthma, 825
in pulmonary œdema, 791
Curare in rabies, 254
Curd mixture, sweet, 286
Curtis belt, 583
Cushing's syndrome, 458
Cyanogen compounds, poisoning from, 312
Cyanosis, enterogenous, 506-7
in bronchitis and pneumonia in infancy, 289-90
in congenital heart disease, 663-65
in heart disease, 691-92
in sulphonamide poisoning, 86
Cyclical vomiting in infancy, 297-98. *See* VOMITING, CYCLICAL, 297-98
Cyclopropane in thoracoplasty, 129
Cysticercosis, 259
Cystitis associated with phosphaturia, 884
complicating gonorrhœa in the female, 203. *See also* URINARY TRACT, INFECTION OF, 869-82
Cysts in cestodiasis, 259-60

D

Dagenan (M & B 693). *See* SULPHONAMIDE DRUGS
Deaf aids, 770-71
Deafness, nerve in congenital syphilis, 215
progressive middle-ear, 770
Deficiency diseases, 401-23
beri-beri, 404-8
pellagra, 408-10
rickets, 413-23
scurvy, 410-13
tetany, 423-26
vitamin A deficiency, 402-4
Deformities, correction of, in chronic rheumatoid arthritis, 919-23
Delirium in acute bronchitis, 785
in erysipelas, 90-91
in exanthemata, 6-7
Delirium tremens, 1047, 1048-49, 1051
Dental sepsis in rheumatoid arthritis, 898
Depilation, 168-69
Dermatitis, 176-82
due to external causes, 177-79
due to internal causes, 179-81
herpetiformis, 186
in pellagra, 409
in sprue, 250
in syphilis, 208
industrial, 317-19
infantile, 179-80
infective, 178-79
occupational, 182
varicose, 181
X-ray therapy in, 179, 181
Dermatomyositis, 971
Desensitization in asthma, 834-36
in hay fever, 844-46
in urticaria, 186
Desoxycorticosterone-acetate (D.O.C.A.), 452
D'Herelle's bacteriophage, 33
Diabetes insipidus, 456-57
Diabetes mellitus, 323-86
coma in, 351-54
complications of, 376-82
cardiac disease, 378
cataract, 377
cholecystitis, 378
diarrhœa, 379

Diabetes, complications of—*contd.*
fevers, 379
fluid feed in, 379-80
gangrene, 376, 736
light diet in, 381-82
neuritis, 377
pruritus, 377
retinitis, 377
tuberculosis, 376
dietetic treatment, 323-41
bread in, exchanges for, 340
calculation and prescription of diet, 329-32
calories, 324-25
carbohydrate, 325-27
exchange tables, 334-35
fat, 328
fruits, 333
higher carbohydrate, low fat, 338-41
method of adjusting diets, 336
protein, 328
vegetables, 333
furunculosis caused by, 165
hypoglycæmia, with soluble insulin, 344-47
with zinc protamine insulin, 362
in children, 363-72
calories, 364
carbohydrate, 365-66
diet sheets, 368-72
fat, 366
protein, 365-66
vitamins and minerals, 368
insulin treatment. *See* INSULIN IN DIABETES MELLITUS, 341-63
obesity and, 324-36
pregnancy in, 372-76
surgery and, 382-86
Diaphoretics in acute nephritis, 857
Diarrhœa, diet in, 569
drugs in, 569-71
gastrogenous, 571
in Graves' disease, 572
in tuberculosis, 134
infective and toxic, 568-69
intestinal carbohydrate dyspepsia, 571
nervous and lienteric, 571
pancreatic and fatty, 572
Diathermy coagulation in removal of tonsils, 759-60
Diathermy—*contd.*
in furunculosis of ear, 762
in gonorrhœa, 195
in rheumatism, 917
in rosacea, 176
in sinusitis, 753, 754
in tuberculosis of the skin, 148-49
Dick test (in scarlet fever), 54-55
Diet in acute bronchitis, 784
in acute nephritis, 853-55
in alcoholism, 1049
in cholecystitis, 618
in chronic bronchitis, 793
in chronic nephritis, interstitial, 861
nephrotic, 859-60
in chronic pancreatitis, 625
in congestive heart failure, 669-73
in constipation, 575
in cyclical vomiting, 298
in diabetes mellitus. *See* DIABETES MELLITUS, DIETETIC TREATMENT, 323-41
in diarrhœa, 569
in diseases of infancy, 267
in diverticulosis, 599-60
in essential hypertension, 651-52
in fibrositis, 936
in flatulent dyspepsia, 563
in gastro-enteritis of infancy, 283-84
in gonorrhœa, 193-94
in gout, 962-64
in hæmatemesis, 551-52
in infections of urinary tract, 873-74
in Ménière's syndrome, 1002
in nephritis, 863-67
in obesity, 389-96
calories, 389
carbohydrate, 390
diets, sample, with notes, 391-95
fat, 389-90
in complications, 396
protein, 390
salt, 390
in oxaluria, 885
in peptic ulcer, 545
Hurst's, 557-59
Meulengracht's, 560
in phosphaturia, 884
in prevention of respiratory diseases, 777
in pruritus, 184
Diet—*contd.*
in rheumatoid arthritis, 908-10
in sea sickness, 1003
in sprue, 249
in steatorrhœa, 592-93
in ulcerative colitis, 588, 597-99
in urinary infections, 873-74
Dietl's crisis, 584, 868, 869
Dieulafoy's aspirator, 137
Digestion, some common disorders of, 563-64
flatulence, 563
heartburn, 564
hiccup, 564
nausea, 564
water-brash, 563-64
Digifoline in dyspnœic heart failure, 700
Digitaline, Nativelle's, 660
Digitalis in auricular fibrillation, 677-78, 702-4
in auricular flutter, 703-7
in circulatory failure in acute infections, 643
in respiratory diseases, 786
in congestive heart failure, 673-84
dosage and preparations, 675-82
intoxication with, 682-84
in coronary thrombosis, 693
in dyspnœic heart failure, 700
in extra-systoles, 712-13
in heart block, 683, 711
in heart disease in pregnancy, 662
in hyperthyroidism, 443
in paroxysmal fibrillation, 705
in paroxysmal tachycardia, 710
in sino-auricular block, 712
Digoxin, in circulatory failure in acute bronchitis, 786
in congestive heart failure, 678
in dyspnœic heart failure, 700
in the senile heart, 660
intravenous use of, 681-82
Di-iodotyrosine and compounds in thyrotoxicosis, 437

Dimenformon, 1060
Dinitrobenzol poisoning, 315
Dinitrophenol in obesity, 398
Diphtheria, 19-25
antitoxic serum in, 22-23
carriers of, 25
complications in, 23-24
convalescence in, 24-25
immunization against, 20-21
laryngeal, 25
Schick test in, 20
Diplegia, congenital, 991-92
Dipsomania, 1047-48
Disinfection in infectious diseases, 8-11
Disseminated sclerosis, 983-85
Diuretics in acute nephritis, 856
in congestive heart failure, 684-89
ammonium salts, 687
organic mercurials, 684
xanthine, 686-87
in nephrosis, 860
Diuretin, 688
Diverticulitis, 591
Diverticulosis, 591
diet (Spriggs), 599-600
Diverticulum of the œsophagus, 533
of the pharynx, 533
Dmelcos vaccine in chancroid, 224-25
in lympho-granuloma inguinale, 225
Donors in blood transfusion, 1079-80
Doryl in incontinence of urine, 218
in paroxysmal tachycardia, 710
Dover's powder in coryza, 780, 782
Dracunculus Medinensis, 261-62. *See* GUINEA-WORM, 261-62
Drainage, bronchoscopic, 815
"closed" suction, in pyopneumothorax, 812
continuous postural in abscess of the lung, 818
in empyema, 809
postural, in bronchiectasis, 813-15
Dreuw's ointment in diseases of the skin, 162
in psoriasis, 189-90
Drinker apparatus, 980
Drug eruptions, 186
Drugs, addiction to, 1054-55
Drum of the ear, affections, 764
Drunkenness. *See* ALCOHOLISM, 1046-54
Ductless glands, diseases of the, 428-59
gonads, 454-56, 1056-68
parathyroid, 447-50
pituitary, 456-59
suprarenal, 450-54
thyroid, 428-47
Duodenal ileus, chronic, 565
Duodenal ulcer. *See* PEPTIC ULCER, 542-60
Dust diseases, industrial, 315-17. *See* INDUSTRIAL DUST DISEASES, 315-17
Dyschezia, 573, 574
Dysentery, amœbic, 244-47
bacillary, 25-30
chronic, 29
in infancy, 284-85
Dysmenorrhœa, 1067-68
Dyspepsia, flatulent, diet for, 600-1
intestinal carbohydrate, 571
Dysphagia, 533-35, 1003
achalasia of the cardia, 534-35
carcinoma of œsophagus, 534
diverticulum of œsophagus, 533
diverticulum of pharynx, 533-34
Plummer-Vinson syndrome, 534
Dyspnœic heart failure, 699-703
Dystrophia myotonica, 972
Dystrophy, muscular, 972

E

Ear, diseases of the, 762-71
deaf aids, 770-71
external ear, 762-64
affections of the drum, 764
auricle, injuries of, 762
foreign bodies, 764
keratosis obturans, 763
skin affections, 762
wax in, 763
middle ear, 764-70
chronic adhesive process, 770
Ear, diseases of the middle ear—*contd.*
otitis media, acute, 764-68
chronic, 768-70
otosclerosis, 770
Eczema. *See* DERMATITIS, 176-82
Effleurage in rheumatoid arthritis, 913, 917
Effort syndrome, 718, 722
Egg white in hæmophilia, 520
Ektomak in pernicious anæmia, 485
Elastoplast in arthritis, 927
in bed-sores during paraplegia, 987
in furunculosis, 165
in impetigo, 163
Electrical treatment in Bell's paralysis, 1001-2
in herpes simplex, 187
in rheumatoid arthritis, 816
Electrocardiographic control in auricular fibrillation, 708
Elephantiasis in filariasis, 260
Embolism, air, in artificial pneumothorax, 125
and the blood flow, 732, 733
cerebral, 997
complicating coronary thrombosis, 694
pulmonary and infarction, 821-22
Emetine, and preparations in amœbic dysentery, 244
in schistomiasis, 256, 257
Emetine injections in chronic ulcerative colitis, 590
Emotional state and the circulatory system, 718-19
Emphysema, 794
and dyspnœic failure, 702-3
interstitial in artificial pneumothorax, 125
Empyema, acute, 808-10
in infancy, 290
Encephalitis lethargica, 37-38, 92-94
Encephalitis periaxialis diffusa, 985
Encephalitis, suppurative, 983
Encephalogram in post-concussional syndrome, 1007

Endocarditis, non-rheumatic, 639-40
simple rheumatic, 633-39
subacute bacterial, 639-40
ulcerative, 640
Endrine in coryza, 780
in paroxysmal rhinorrhœa, 847
Enemas and colonic irrigations, 578-80
Enesol in lichen planus, 189
Entamœba histolytica in amœbic dysentery, 246
Enteric fever, 30-37
bacteriophage in, 33
carriers of, 36-37
complications in, 36
constipation in, 34
diarrhœa in, 34
diet in, 33-34
hæmorrhage and perforation in, 35
meteorism in, 34
phlebitis in, 35
toxæmia in, 34-35
Enteritis, 584-93
tuberculous, 134
Enterobiasis, 264
Enterogenous cyanosis, 506-7
Enuresis in infancy, 296-97
Eosinophil adenoma. *See* PITUITARY ADENOMATA, 457-58
Epanutin in epilepsy, 1009
Ephedrine for cough in congestive heart failure, 691
for cough in infancy, 289
in asthma, 825, 839, 840
in diseases of the nose, 745
in hay fever, 844
in myasthenia gravis, 973
in narcolepsy, 1012
in nasal allergy, 751
in paroxysmal rhinorrhœa, 847
in serum sickness, 804
in sinusitis, 752, 754
in Stokes-Adams seizures, 725
in syncope, 724
Ephregel in paroxysmal rhinorrhœa, 847
Ephynal, 1066
Epidermophytosis. *See* RINGWORM OF BODY FOLDS, 170-71
Epididymis, tuberculosis of, 143
Epididymitis complicating gonorrhœa, 199
Epidural injection (technique), 1096-98
in coccygodynia, 978
in sciatica, 976
Epilepsy, 1008-11
Epistaxis, 746-49
Ergosterol in deficiency disease, 421
irradiated, in idiopathic steatorrhœa, 592
Ergotamine tartrate in migraine, 1011
Eruptions, bullous, 186
drug, 186
iodide, 186
pemphigoid, 186
Erysipelas, 88-91
Erythræmia, 502
Erythrocyanosis, 741-42
Erythrocytosis, 503
Erythrœdema polyneuritis. *See* PINK DISEASE, 299
Erythrol tetranitrate in essential hypertension, 653
Eschatin in Addison's disease, 451
in diarrhœa of Graves' disease, 572
Eserine for dimness of vision in encephalitis lethargica, 993
in enuresis, 297
Essential hypertension. *See* HYPERTENSION, ESSENTIAL, 650-54
Esthiomene, 225
Ether and olive oil per rectum in asthma, 825
Ethyl hydnocarpate injection for tuberculosis of the skin, 149
Eucalyptus in acute coryza, 782
inhalations, 745
Eucortone in shock, 728
Eumydrine in hypertrophic pyloric stenosis, 282
in pylorospasm, 280
Euparatone in tetania parathyropriva, 447
Euphyllin as diuretic in congestive heart failure, 688
as vasodilator, 699
for dyspnœa in coronary thrombosis, 694
in dyspnœic heart failure, 701, 702
to check Cheyne-Stokes breathing, 702
Eusol in post-operative empyema, 810
Eustachian tube, inflation of, in otitis media, 767
Exercise and obesity, 388-89
and rheumatic carditis, 637
Exercises, deep-breathing, in pulmonary fibrosis and bronchiectasis, 291
for cardiac patient, 647-48
in asthma, 843
in chronic rheumatic arthritis, 923, 952-59
in rheumatoid arthritis, 896-917
physical, benefiting constipation, 574-75
remedial, in diseases of the nervous system, 1014-15
Exophthalmic goitre. *See* HYPERTHYROIDISM, 432-47
Expectorants, in adult respiratory diseases, 789-90
in children, 288
Extra-pyramidal motor system, diseases of, 992-95
encephalitis lethargica, 992-94
paralysis agitans, 994
Extra-systoles, 712-13
Eye, gonococcal infection of, 205-6

F

Face tents in oxygen therapy, 1103
Facial hemiatrophy, 1002
nerve, Bell's paralysis, 1001-2
pains, 1000-1
spasm, chronic, 1002
Factories Act (1937), 301
Fairley's operation for removal of worm in guinea-worm, 262
Feeding in infancy, methods of, 268
of premature infants, 272-73
Fehling's blood-sugar test, 349
Fehling's urine test in diabetes mellitus, 336
Female sex endocrinology, 1056-68
Femergin in migraine, 1011
Femur, drilling of the head of, 944

Ferronyl, 472
Ferrous sulphate in anæmia, 471-73
Fersolate in iron deficiency, 472, 475
Fertilol, 1066
Festan in pancreatic disease, 624
Fever, 1-77
  cerebrospinal. *See* Cerebrospinal Fever, 13-18
  definition of, 1
  diet in, 4
  discharges from body during, 9
  disinfection after, 8-11
  drugs in, 5-6
  enteric. *See* Enteric Fever, 30-37
  fresh air in, 4
  glandular. *See* Glandular Fever, 38-39
  hay. *See* Hay Fever, 843-46
  inanition. *See* Inanition Fever, 273
  in pulmonary tuberculosis, 136
  nursing in, 2-4
  relief of symptoms, 5-8
  rest in, 1-2
  scarlet. *See* Scarlet Fever, 54-60
  therapy in G.P.I., 221-24
  undulant. *See* Undulant Fever, 240-41
Fibrolysin in rheumatoid arthritis, 918
Fibrosis, pulmonary, 791-92
Fibrositis, 931-42
  acute, 933-35
  ætiology, 931-32
  cervical spine and occipital region, 939
  diet, 936-37
  drugs, 937
  hydrotherapy, 936
  intercostal, 934
  local infiltration, 937-38
  lumbago, 940-41
  manipulation, 938-39
  massage, 935
  shoulder, 939
  subacromial bursitis, 940
  subacute and chronic, 935
Filaria bancrofti, 260
Filaria loa, 260, 261
Filaria Malayi, 260
Filarial abscess, 260
Filariasis, 260-62
Filix mas in cestodiasis, 258
Finsen-Lomholt lamp irradiation in tuberculosis of the skin, 148
Fits, epileptic, 1008-11
  in acute uræmia, 857
  in hypoglycæmia, 345
  in infancy, 292-94
Flat-foot in rheumatoid arthritis, 922
Flatulence, 563
Flavine in septicæmia, 83
Flexner and Sonne infections, 27, 29
Flexner organisms in dysentery of infancy, 284
Fluid, methods of giving, in diseases of infancy, 269
  "continuous drip," 271, 1075-76
  intraperitoneal route, 269
  intravenous route, 270, 1075-79
  rectal administration of, 269, 1070-71
  subcutaneous route, 269, 1070
Foot, perforating ulcer of, in tabes dorsalis, 220
Forapin in rheumatoid arthritis, 918
Foreign bodies, in the ear, 764
  in the nose, 751-52
  in the œsophagus, 532
Formalin spray in disinfection, 11
Formol toxoid, 20
Fouadin in kala-azar, 235, 236
  in schistosomiasis, 256, 257
Fowler's solution in leukæmia, 528
  in rheumatoid arthritis, 901
Fractures in the newborn, 276
  of the nose, 746
  pathological in tabes dorsalis, 220
Fragilitas ossium, 967
Frei's test, in lymphogranuloma inguinale, 225
French equivalent, Fourneau 309 and 270, in African trypanosomiasis, 233
Friars' balsam inhalation in acute coryza, 782
  in pharyngitis, 760
Friedreich's ataxia, 992
Funiculitis in filariasis, 260
Furunculosis, 164-65
  of the ear, 760

G

Gall-bladder and biliary tract, diseases of, 614-23
  biliary stasis, 615
  carcinoma of, 622
  cholecystitis, 616-21
  conservative treatment of diseases of the biliary tract, 620-21
  gall-bladder, 616
  gall-stones, 619-20
  microbic infection, 614-15
  surgery, 616
  typhoid fever and, 615
Gall-bladder disease in relation to heart disease, 644
Gall-stones, 619-20
Galvanism in lead paralysis, 308
Galvano-cautery in diseases of the nose, 745
Gangrene, dry, 737
  amputation in, 738
  in diabetes, 376-77, 738
  of extremities following embolism, 733
  of lung. *See* Lung Abscess and Gangrene of, 818-20
Gargles in tonsillitis, 756
Gas gangrene causing secondary hæmolytic anæmia, 492
Gases, poisonous, 310-15
  ammonia refrigerating plant, 310
  benzene, 313-14
    nitro derivatives of, 315
  carbon monoxide, 311-12
  carbon tetrachloride, 314
  chlorine, 312-13
  classification of, 310-11
  cyanogen compounds, 312
  nitrous fumes, 312
  sulphuretted hydrogen, 313-14
  tetrachlorethane, 314
Gasserian ganglion, injection of, in neuralgia, 998, 1000, 1001
Gastrectomy in peptic ulcer, 554-56
  partial, in cancer of the stomach, 561
Gastric and duodenal ulcer. *See* Ulcer, Peptic, 542-60

Gastric lavage in gastric carcinoma, 561
in gastritis, 541
in pyloric stenosis, 553
of infancy, 280-81
Gastritis, 540-42
Gastro-enteritis in infancy, 283-84
Gastro-enterostomy in gastric carcinoma, 561
in peptic ulcer, 554-56
Gaucher's disease, 508, 524
Gavage method of feeding infants, 272
Gee-Thaysen's disease. *See* IDIOPATHIC STEATORRHŒA, 591-93
General paralysis of the insane (G.P.I.), 221-24
Gentian, in gastritis, 542
Gentian violet, in diseases of the skin, 160
in furunculosis, 164
in otitis externa, 762
German measles. *See* RUBELLA, 53-54
Germanin in African trypanosomiasis, 233
Gerson-Sauerbruch diet in pulmonary tuberculosis, 111
Glandular fever, 38-39
Glandular tuberculosis, 143-46
Globulin, immune, in measles, 43-44
Glossina swynnertoni in African trypanosomiasis, 235
Glosso-pharyngeal tic, 761
Glucose, and acute necrosis of the liver, 609
for coma in cirrhosis of the liver, 614
in acute bronchitis, 787
in anuria, 857
in asthma, 840
in cyclical vomiting, 297-98
in diphtheria, 22-23
in fever diet, 5
in liver treatment, 604
in tonsillitis, 756
intravenous administration of, 622
intravenous hypertonic in peripheral vascular dilatation, 644
lemonade constituents, 622-23
in catarrhal jaundice, 608
Glucose, lemonade constituents—*contd.*
in pre-cirrhotic hepatitis, 611
Glyceryltrinitrate in essential hypertension, 653
Glycine in muscular dystrophies, 972
in myasthenia gravis, 973
Goggles in ultra-violet radiation, 321-22
Goitre, simple, 428-30
toxic. *See* HYPERTHYROIDISM, 432-47
Gold therapy in pulmonary tuberculosis, 119-21
in rheumatoid arthritis, 903-5
prevention of gold salt reactions, 903
sedimentation rate in, 905
in tuberculosis of the larynx, 139
Gomenol in bronchiectasis, 815
Gonadotraphon, 1058
Gonadotropic hormones, 454-55, 1057-58
in amenorrhœa, 1064
in recurrent abortion, 1066
Gonadyl, 1058
Gonorrhœa, 193-206
antiseptic irrigations and instillations in, 196-98
arthritis in, 200-1
bartholinian glands in, 203
conjunctivitis in, 206
cystitis, 202-3
Dagenan (M & B 693) in, 195-96
diathermy in, 195
diet in, 193-94
dysuria in, 194-95
epididymitis in, 199
in the female, 201-5
in the male, 198-201
iridocyclitis in, 201
iritis in, 201
nursing and isolation in, 194
ophthalmia neonatorum in, 205-6
prostatis in, 199-200
salpingitis in, 203
sexual intercourse in, 193
sulphapyridine treatment in, 195-96
synovitis in, 200-1
trichomonas vaginalis in, 204
Gonorrhœa—*contd.*
vaccines in, 196
vulvovaginitis in, 194, 204-5
vesiculitis in, 199-200
Gout, acute stage, 962-65
treatment between attacks, 963-65
"Grain itch," 319
Grancher system, 95
Granulocytopenia. *See* AGRANULOCYTIC ANGINA, 521-23
Graves' disease. *See* HYPERTHYROIDISM, 432-47
Gregory's powder in catarrhal jaundice, 608
in constipation, 576
Grey powder in gastro-enteritis of infancy, 284
Guinea-worm, 261-62
Gumma, cerebral, 217

H

Hæmatemesis and melæna in peptic ulcer, 548-52
blood transfusion in, 549-50
treatment, immediate, 548-49
subsequent, 549
Hæmatoma of the nose, 746
Hæmatomyelia, 90-91
Hæmoglobinuria, paroxysmal, 493
Hæmolytic anæmia and jaundice, 274
Hæmophilia, 518-20
Hæmophilus influenzæ, 84
Hæmophilus pertussis, 70
Hæmoplastin in purpura, 514
Hæmoptysis in bronchiectasis, 816
in pulmonary tuberculosis, 132
Hæmorrhage, cerebral, 995-96
gastro-duodenal, dietetic treatment (Meulengracht), 560
in enteric fever, 35
in thyroidectomy, 446-47
Hæmorrhagic diseases of the newborn, 274
Hæmostatic preparations in purpura, 514
Haffkine prophylactic vaccine, 240
Halarsol in yaws, 252

Haldane mask, in oxygen therapy, 790, 1104
Halibut-liver oil, 404, 415
Hand and wrist splint, 949
Hand - Schüller - Christian disease, 524
Hay fever, 843-46
Head injuries, 1005-8
surgical complications, 1007
Headache and malaise in fever, 6
Heart and circulation, diseases of, 627-730
acute circulatory failure, 723-30
cardiac therapeutics, principles and limitations of, 627-32
neuroses, 718-22
circulatory failure in acute infections, 643-44
endocarditis, non-rheumatic, 639-40
essential hypertension, 650-54
focal sepsis in relation to heart disease, 644-45
heart and circulation in infections, 633-45
management of the ambulant cardiac patient, 645-50
pericarditis, 640-43
rheumatic carditis, 633-39
rhythm disorders and indications for treatment, 703-13
treatment of types of heart failure, 665-703
surgery in, 713-18
Heart disease, congenital. *See* Congenital Heart Disease, 663-65
in relation to pregnancy, 660-63
Heart failure, types of, 665-703
anginal, 692-99
congestive, 666-92
dyspnœic, 699-703
Heart, "strained," 720
the senile, 658-60
Heart-block, 711-12
and Adams-Stokes attacks, 712
in digitalis treatment, 683
Heartburn, 564
Heat, cramps, 302
exhaustion, 303
in fibrositis, 933
Heat—*contd.*
in rheumatic arthritis, 912-13, 916
methods of applying in chronic rheumatic disease, 945-47
retention, 303
Heliotherapy, 416-17
in prophylaxis of rickets, 417
in pulmonary tuberculosis, 110
in tuberculosis of the cervical glands, 145
of the skin, 148
Helminthic infections, 256-65
Hemianopia, 998-99
Hemiparesis, 216
Hemiplegia, 216, 998
infantile, 992
Henoch's purpura, 508
Hepastab in anæmia, 483
Hepatex in anæmia, 483
Hepatitis, amœbic, 246
chronic interstitial. *See* Liver, Cirrhosis of, 610-14
Hereditary ataxias, 992
Hering-Breuer reflexes, 790
Heroin in bronchial carcinoma, 823
in lobar pneumonia, 797
in thyroidectomy, 444
Herpes genitalis, 225-26
of the ear drum, 764
simplex, 186-87
zoster, 187
Hexamine as urinary antiseptic, 879-80
in cholecystitis, 617
Hexœstrol, 1059, 1060
Hexyl-resorcinol as urinary antiseptic, 880
Hiccup, 564
in cirrhosis of the liver, 614
Hippocrates' diet in fever, 4
Hirschsprung's disease, 594-95
Histamine in rheumatoid arthritis, 902, 918
Histidin in peptic ulcer, 548
Hodgkin's disease, 530-31
affecting the mediastinal glands, 823
Hog's stomach preparations in anæmia, 485
Honsaker apparatus for fever therapy, 223-24
Hook-worm. *See* Ankylostomiasis, 262-64
Hormone preparations, follicular in essential hypertension, 653
Hormones, gonadotropic, 454-55, 1057-58
corpus luteum, 456, 1059-60
male, 456, 1061-62
œstrogenic, 455-56, 1058-59
Hour-glass stomach in peptic ulcer, 553
Huntington's chorea, 995
Hurst diet in peptic ulcer, 545
Hurst's régime of treatment in peptic ulcer, 557-59
Hutchinson's pill in cardiovascular syphilis, 656
Hydatid disease, 259-60
Hydnocarpus wightiana, 250
Hydræmic syndrome, 858
Hydramnios in babies of diabetics, 373
Hydrocele in filariasis, 260
Hydrocephalus and intracranial tumour, 1003-5
as complication of cerebrospinal fever, 17
Hydrochloric acid in anæmia, 483
in diseases of the stomach, 538, 541
causing ulcer, 542-43
in gastrogenous diarrhœa, 571
in phosphaturia, 884
in tetania parathyropriva, 448
Hydrocyanic acid poisoning, 312
Hydrogen peroxide, in epistaxis, 747
in otitis media, 766, 769
Hydrology in osteo-arthritis 925
in rheumatoid arthritis, 915-18
Hydronephrosis, 865-67
Hydropneumothorax, 126
Hydrotherapy in fibrositis, 936
Hydrothorax in congestive heart failure, 690
Hyoscine in acute alcoholism, 1048
in cerebral lesions, 998
in encephalitis lethargica, 993
in erysipelas, 91
in labour with heart disease, 663
in thyroidectomy, 444

Hyperæmia, intermittent reactive, induction of, 739
Hyperchlorhydria. *See* Ulcer, Peptic, 542-68
Hyperparathyroidism, 449-50
Hyperpyrexia, 6
Hypertension, essential, 650-54
  and the climacteric, 653
  blood-letting, 653
  diet in, 651-52
  drugs in, 652-53
  giddiness, headache and tinnitus in, 653
  in obesity, 396
  surgical measures in, 653-54
Hyperthyroidism, 432-47
  causes, 433-34
  diet, 434-36
  general management of, 432-34
  iodine in, 436-38
  radiation in, 439-40
  sedatives in, 434
  thyroidectomy, 441-42
Hypertonic saline solution in cholera, 242-43
Hypervitaminosis D, 421
Hypochlorhydria in tuberculosis, 134
Hypodermic injection, technique, 1085-86
Hypoglycæmia in diabetes mellitus, 344-47
Hypoparathyroidism, idiopathic, 449
Hypophosphorus acid in iron therapy, 474
Hypovitaminosis, 401-2
Hysteria, 1028

I

Ice-bag in pericarditis, 641
Ichthyol and glycerin, in diseases of the ear, 762
  in rhinitis, 750
Ichthyol in diseases of the skin, 159, 161
Icterus, hæmolytic, 489
  neonatorum, 274-75
Ileocolitis, 26
  acute, in infancy, 284-85
Iliostomy in chronic ulcerative colitis, 589
Immunization against diphtheria, 20-21
  against measles, 43
  against scarlet fever, 55
  against tetanus, 65
Immunization—*contd.*
  against whooping-cough, 71
Impetigo contagiosa, 162-64
Inanition fever, 273
Inductotherm, 223
Industrial diseases, 300-22
  cancer, 319-20
  compressed air, workers in, 304
  dermatitis, 317-19
  dust diseases, 315-17
  heat disease, 302-3
  high temperature effects, 302-3
  Medical Boards in, 315-16
  miners' nystagmus, 305-6
  pneumatic drills, work with, 304-5
  poisoning by metals, 306-10
  poisonous gases, 310-15
  prevention of, 300-2
  radio-active substances, injury from, 320-22
Industrial dust diseases, 315-17
Infancy, anæmia in. *See* Anæmia
Infancy and early childhood, disorders in, 266-99
  diet in, 267
  digestive system in, 278-87
    cœliac disease. 285-86
    constipation, 282-83
    feeding, 278
    gastro-enteritis, 283-84
    hypertrophic pyloric stenosis, 280-82
    ileocolitis, acute, 284-85
    milk modifications, 286-87
    seasonal disturbances, 278
    stomatitis, 278-79
    vomiting, 279-82
  drugs, 267-68
    dosage formula, 267
  feeding, methods of, 268-69
  medicine, method of giving, 268
  neonatal conditions. *See* Neonatal Conditions, 271-77
  nervous system in, 292-99
    convulsions, 292-94
    cyclical vomiting, 297-98
    enuresis, 296-97
    mental deficiency, 295
    pink disease, 299
    nursing in, 266-68
Infancy and early childhood—*contd.*
  respiratory system in, 287-92
    atelectasis, 292
    infections, 287-91
    thymic enlargement, 292
  scratching in, 266
Infantile dermatitis, 179-80
  hemiplegia, 992
Infantilism, pituitary, 458-59
Infarction. *See* Coronary Thrombosis, 692-95; Pulmonary Embolism, 821-22
Infection, "droplet," in disease of respiratory system, 287
  in glandular fever, 38
  in mumps, 47
Infections in respiratory diseases in infancy, 287-91
Inferiority sense, 1038-39
Infiltration in fibrositis, 938-39
Influenza, 40-42
  predisposing cause of respiratory diseases, 775
Infra-red rays in nasal allergy, 751
Infusion, intravenous, technique, 1075-79
Inhalants causing asthma, 832
Inhalations in acute coryza, 782
  in asthma, 840-41
  in bronchiectasis, 815
  in diseases of the nose, 745
  in tonsillitis, 757
Injury and compensation in psychotherapy, 1028-30
  of the spinal cord, 990-91
Insane, general paralysis of the. *See* General Paralysis of the Insane, 221-24
Insanity and neurosis, differential diagnosis, 1032-33
Insect bites, 186
Insomnia, 1012-14
  and delirium, in fever, relief of, 6-7
  in acute bronchitis, 784-85
  in congestive heart failure, 667-69
  in erysipelas, 90
  in heart disease in pregnancy, 662
  in the senile heart, 658-59

Insulin in anorexia nervosa, 563
Insulin in diabetes mellitus, 341-63
blood-sugar tests in, 349-51
dosage, 347-49
hypoglycæmia with, 344-47
in diabetic coma, 351-53
injection of, pain with, 343-44
technique of, 342-44
Insulin, zinc protamine, in diabetes mellitus, 354-63
age and, 361
and diabetic coma (charts), 362-63
and soluble, 355-63
technique, 359
diet in conversion from soluble to Z.P., 361
hypoglycæmic reactions with, 362
exercise and, 362
in new case, 359-60
strengths of, 355
transition period, from soluble to Z.P. insulin, 356-57
Intestinal obstruction, 593-94
Intestines, diseases of, 565-601
chronic regional ileitis, 584-85
chronic ulcerative colitis, 587-91
constipation, 573-80
diarrhœa, 567-73
diets, 595-601
diverticulosis and diverticulitis, 591
enteritis, 584
idiopathic steatorrhœa, 591-93
megacolon, 594-95
muco-membranous colic, 585-87
obstruction, 593-94
visceroptosis, 580-84
Intermittent claudication, 735
sympathectomy in, 739
Interstitial keratitis in congenital syphilis, 215
Intracardiac injection, 726
Intracranial tumour, 1004-5
dehydration in, 1005
Intradermal injection, 1084-85
Intradermal test for serum sensitivity, 801-2
Intramuscular injection, 1086-87
Intrapleural division of adhesions, 126-27
Intrathoracic new growths, 822-23
Intravenous infusion (technique), 1075-79
apparatus, 1075-76
cannula method, 1076-78
continuous infusions, 1078-79
needle method, 1078
Iodide eruptions, 186
Iodides in cardiovascular syphilis, 656, 657
in syphilis, 210, 213, 214, 216, 217
Iodine in chronic leukæmia, 528
in hyperthyroidism, 436-38
post-operative, 445
in pharyngitis, 761
in rheumatoid arthritis, 901
in sciatica, 976
in simple goitre, 428-29
in spontaneous pneumothorax, 811
Iodine-Basedow, 429
Iodoform and eucalyptus inhalation, 291
Iodolysin in rheumatoid arthritis, 918
Ionization in chronic otitis media, 769
Iridocyclitis in gonorrhœa, 201
Iritis in gonorrhœa, 201
Iron content of cheaper foodstuffs, 470
deficiency. *See* ANÆMIA
preparations, 472-73, 474-75
Irradiated milk, 416
Irradiation in polycythæmia, 503-4
Ischæmic contracture (Volkmann's), 971

J

Jaundice, 606-9
acholuric, 489-90
catarrhal, 607-9
and yellow atrophy of liver, 607
hæmolytic, 607
in arsenical therapy, 208
Jaundice—*contd.*
in gold therapy, 904
in the newborn, 274-75
in syphilis, 208
in Weil's disease, 238
infectious, 238
obstructive, 607
bleeding tendency in, 517
toxic and infective, 607
Jejunal or gastro-jejunal ulcer, 555-56

K

Kahler's disease, 968
Kahn reaction, 193, 1074
in early syphilis, 212
Kala-azar, 235-37
Kaolin in chronic ulcerative colitis, 588
in diarrhœa, 570
poultice in asthma, 825
Karell diet in congestive heart failure, 670-71
Kellogg's all-bran in obesity, 396
Keratitis in congenital syphilis, 215
Ketosis, 297-98
in the surgical diabetic, 383
induction of, in pyelitis, 877
Kharsulphan, in cardiovascular syphilis, 656
in syphilis, 207
Kidneys. *See* RENAL DISEASES, 851-85
in late syphilis, 213
tuberculosis of, 141-43
Klebs-Löffler bacillus, 749
Knees, serial plasters for the correction of flexion deformity, 950-51
Koch's old tuberculin, 835
Kondoleon's operation in elephantiasis, 260
Koplik's spots, 43
Korsakow's syndrome, 1047, 1050
Kraurosis vulvæ, 1067
Kurchi bark in amœbic dysentery, 245

L

Lactic acid milk, 287
Lactose in diarrhœa, 571
in urine during pregnancy, 372
Lævulinate, 447

Laminectomy in Paget's disease, 983
Landry's paralysis, 979-80
Lanolin in dermatitis, 318
Larostidin in peptic ulcer, 548
Laryngitis, 771-73
  acute, 771-72
  chronic, 772-73
Larynx, diseases of the, 771-74
  tuberculosis of, 138-41
Lasegue's sign, 941
Lead in diseases of the skin, 160
Lead poisoning, 306-8
  in polyneuritis, 979
Leather-bottle stomach, 562
Lederle laboratories, sera of, in pneumonia, 290
Lederer, acute hæmolytic anæmia of, 493-94
Leduc's insufflator, 141
Leishmaniasis, 235-38. *See* KALA-AZAR, 235-37; ORIENTAL SORE, 237-38
Lenhartz diet in peptic ulcer, 545
Leontiasis ossea, 967
Leprosy, 250-52
Leptospira icterohæmorrhagica, 238
Leucopenia in gold therapy, 904
Leukæmias, 524-31
  acute, 529
  aleukæmic, 529-30
  chronic, 525-29
  drug treatment, 527-29
  Hodgkin's disease in, 530-31
  X-ray treatment of, 526-27
Lichen planus, 188-89
Linseed poultice in asthma, 824
Lipiodol examination in bronchiectasis, 816-18
Little's area in epistaxis, 746
Little's disease, 991
Liver abscess, amœbic, 246
Liver, acute necrosis of, 609
  and arsenical drugs, 213
  carcinoma of, 614
  cirrhosis of, 610-14
    advanced, 611-14
    alcohol as cause of, 610
    anæmia in, 613
    coma in, 614
    hæmorrhage in, 613
    hiccup in, 614
    in splenic anæmia, 497-502
Liver, cirrhosis of—*contd.*
    œdema of legs and scrotum, 613
    pre-cirrhotic hepatitis, 611
    prophylactic treatment, 610-11
    Talma-Morison operation in, 613
    tapping of abdomen, 612-13
  damaged, 603-5
  diseases of, 602-26
  extract in chronic leukæmia, 529
  in late syphilis, 213, 214
  in pellagra, 409
  in pernicious anæmia, 483, 484, 486
  in purpuras, 514
  in subacute combined degeneration of the spinal cord, 989
  specific infections of, 614
  therapy in benzene poisoning, 314
    in tetrachlorethane poisoning, 315
Loa loa, 260, 261
Lobar pneumonia. *See* PNEUMONIA, LOBAR, 795-808
Lobelia in asthma, 839
Lobelin Ingelheim in carbon monoxide poisoning, 311
  in poisoning from cyanogen compounds, 312
Lotio phenolis in Hodgkin's disease, 530
Lotio picis carbonis alkalina in Hodgkin's disease, 530
Lugol's solution in chronic leukæmia, 529
  in rheumatoid arthritis, 901
  in simple goitre, 429
  in thyroidectomy, 443, 445, 446
  in thyrotoxicos, 436
Lumbago, 934, 940
Lumbar puncture, cerebrospinal fluid pressure (Table) in, 1092-94
  in convulsions, 293
  in leaking aneurysm, 996
  in meningitis, 981
  in uræmia of acute nephritis, 857-58
  in uræmia of chronic interstitial nephritis, 862
  technique, 1090-95
Luminal. *See* PHENOBARBITONE
Lung, abscess and gangrene of, 818-20
  specific non-tuberculous infection of, 823
Lupus vulgaris, 148-49
Lymph scrotum in filariasis, 260
Lymphadenitis filarial, 260
Lymphangitis in filariasis, 260
Lympho-granuloma inguinale, 225
Lymphosarcoma affecting the mediastinal glands, 823

M

M'Mahon's inspiratory exercises, 810
Magnesium phosphate, tribasic, in peptic ulcer, 547
Magnesium sulphate, in anuria, 857
  in cholecystitis, 617
  in chronic interstitial nephritis, 862
  in uræmia, 858
  pre-rectum, in intracranial tumour, 1005
Magnesium trisilicate, in peptic ulcer, 547
Magsorbent in peptic ulcer, 559
Malaria, 228-33
  acute primary attack of 228-30
  blackwater fever in, 232
  cerebral, 231
  drugs, 228-31
    toxic effects of, 231
  general management of, 232
  in pregnancy, 231
  malignant tertian, 229
  prophylaxis of, 232-33
  relapses in, 230-31
  therapy in G.P.I., 221-23
  treatment, non-specific, 231-32
Male fern in cestodiasis. *See* FELIX MAS, 258
Malignant disease, pain in, 978
Malingering, 1028-29
Mandecal, urinary antiseptic, 872

Mandelic acid as urinary antiseptic, 877-79
Mandelix, urinary antiseptic, 878
Mandl's throat pain, 758, 760, 774
Manganese in anæmias, 475
Mania à potu, 1048
Manipulation in chronic rheumatoid arthritis, 920-21
Mantoux test in tuberculosis, 118
Marchiafava-Micheli syndrome, 493
Marie-Strumpell syndrome, 890
Marmite, in anæmia, 469, 487
in bacillary dysentery, 28
in cœliac disease, 286
in deficiency diseases, 405, 406, 407
in diabetes mellitus, 328, 331
in idiopathic steatorrhœa, 592
in pink disease, 299
in rheumatoid arthritis, 900, 909
Masks in oxygen therapy, 1104
Massage in osteo-arthritis, 925
in rheumatoid arthritis, 896-917
in subacute fibrositis, 935
Masturbation, 1024-25, 1035
M & B 693. *See* SULPHONAMIDE DRUGS
Mayer-Tanret reagent, in malaria, 229-30
Measles, 42-47
complications of, 46-47
general management in, 44-45
German. *See* RUBELLA, 53-54
preventive treatment, 43-44
prophylactic preparations, 43-44
Mechanical supports in visceroptosis, 582-83
Mecholin in paroxysmal tachycardia, 708
Mediastinal glands, tuberculosis of, 145-46
Mediastinum, displacement of, in artificial pneumothorax, 125-26
Medical Boards for prevention of silicosis and asbestosis, 315-16
Medinal. *See* BARBITURATES
Megacolon, 594-95
Melæna in peptic ulcer. *See* ULCER, PEPTIC, HÆMATEMESIS AND MELÆNA IN, 548-52
Melæna neonatorum, 274
Mellin's food in cœliac, disease, 285
Ménière's syndrome, 1002
Meningitis, 981-82
complicating sinusitis, 754-55
following septicæmia, 85
meningococcal. *See* CEREBROSPINAL FEVER, 13-18
Menopause, disturbances of, 1066-67
Menstruation and anæmias, 465-66
and epileptic fits, 1010
disorders of function, 1061-68
Mental deficiency in infancy, 295
Mental disorder and pruritus, 184
Menthol and zinc oxide in pruritus, 609
Menthol inhalations in acute coryza, 782
in bronchiectasis, 815
in nasal affections, 745
in rhinitis, 749
Mercurials, organic, in congestive heart failure, 684-88
Mercurochrome in plague, 239
in undulant fever, 241
Mercury in leutic aortitis, 656, 657
in syphilis, 210, 214
poisoning, 308-9
preparations in constipation, 577
Mercury-vapour lamp, 418
Mersalyl in congestive heart failure, 685-88
Mesenteric lymph-glands, tuberculosis of, 146
Metabolic diseases, 323-427
deficiency diseases, 401-23
diabetes mellitus, 323-86
obesity, 387-400
Metals, poisoning by, 306-10
Meteorism. *See* TYMPANITES, 787
Methæmoglobinæmia. *See* ENTEROGENOUS CYANOSIS, 506
Methyl salicylate, in rheumatism, 635
in sciatica, 976
Methylene blue, 86
Metropathia hæmorrhagica, 1061-62
Meulengracht diet in peptic ulcer, 545, 551
Mid-menstrual bleeding, 1062
Migraine, 1011
Milk and undulant fever, 241
and vitamin D content, 418
certified, 97
citrated, in peptic ulcer, 551
of œsophagus, 536
desensitizing agent in asthma, 836
in acute nephritis, 853-54
irradiated, 416
modifications in digestive diseases in infancy, 286-87
pasteurized, 97
tuberculin-tested, 97
with low percentage of fat, 286
Miners' nystagmus, 305-6
Mitalin, protection against mosquito bites, 233
Mitral stenosis, operation for, 714
Moccasin snake venom, 514
Mollities ossium, 967
Mongolian idiocy, 295
Moogral in leprosy, 250, 251
Morphia, addiction to, 1054
cause of drug eruptions, 186
in acute bronchitis, 785, 786
in acute leukæmias, 529
in asthma, 825, 840
in atelectasis, 821
in auricular fibrillation, 704
in biliary colic, 619, 620
in bronchial carcinoma, 823
in cancer of the stomach, 562
in cerebral lesions, 998
in cholera, 243
in chronic kidney disease, 863
in congestive heart failure, 668

Morphia—*contd.*
in coronary thrombosis, 691
and embolism, 693
in dyspnœic heart failure, 700, 702
in epistaxis, 748
in erysipelas, 91
in gangrene, 738
in hæmatemesis, 548
in hæmoptysis, 132
in labour with heart disease, 663
in meningitis, 978, 979
in paroxysmal tachycardia, 709
in pericarditis, 640
in pneumonia, 796-97
in post-hæmorrhagic anæmia, 476
in pulmonary embolism, 691, 822
in pulmonary œdema, 790
in pyelitis, 874
in renal colic, 883
in shock, 729
in spontaneous pneumothorax, 811
in thyroidectomy, 444
in whooping-cough, 74
Morphine addiction, 1054-55
Morris, Margaret, exercises in pregnancy, 1031
Mosquitoes, protection against bites of, 233
Mouth, care of, in fevers, 3. *See* Stomatitis, 278-79
Mucous colitis and bodily habitus, 581. *See* Colic, Muco-membranous, 585-87
Mucous membranes in diseases of the nose, 743-45
in coryza, 780
Mud-pack in chronic rheumatic diseases, 946
Mulberry stone, 885
Multiple myeloma, 968
Mumps, 47-49
Muscle and the myoneural mechanism, disorders of, 971-74
dermatomyositis, 971
dystrophia myotonica, 972
familial periodic paralysis, 973
muscular dystrophies, 971-73
myasthenia gravis, 972-73
Muscle—*contd.*
myotonia congenita, 972
sleep paralysis, 973
Volkmann's ischæmic contracture, 971
Muscular atrophy, progressive, 985-86
cramps and spasms, 973-74
dystrophies, 972
dystrophy, peroneal type of, 980
Mustard plaster in acute bronchitis, 789
Mustard poultice in asthma, 825
Myasthenia gravis, 972-73
Myelitis, 986
Myeloma, multiple, 968
Myocrisin in rheumatoid arthritis, 904
Myoneural mechanism. *See* Muscle and the, Disorders of, 971-74
Myotonia atrophica, 972
Myotonia congenita, 972
Myringitis bullosa, 764
Myxœdema, 431-32
after thyroidectomy, 447

N

N. meningitidis, 13, 16
N.A.B. in bronchiectasis, 815
in lung abscess, 819
in syphilis, 206
Nails, ringworm of. *See* Ringworm of Nails
Narcolepsy, 1012
Nasal accessory sinuses, physiology of, 743-45
allergy, 751
catheter in oxygen therapy, 1105-6
polypi, 750-51
remedies, common, 744-45
tube, bifurcated, in oxygen therapy, 1105-6
Nativelle's digitaline-granules, 680
in auricular fibrillation, 705
Nausea, 564
and vomiting in fever, relief of, 7-8
Nembutal in thyroidectomy, 444
Neoantimosan in kala-azar, 235, 236
Neoarsphenamine "914," 206
Neoarsphenanime in cardiovascular syphilis, 657
in early syphilis, 211
in rat-bite fever, 239
Neocardyl in syphilis, 209
Neo-hepatex in pernicious anæmia, 483
Neoket, urinary antiseptic, 878
Neokharsivan in syphilis, 206
Neonatal conditions, 271-77
birth injuries, 275-77
hæmolytic anæmia and jaundice, 274-75
hæmorrhagic diseases of the newborn, 274
inanition fever, 273
prematurity, 271-73
sepsis neonatorum, 273
Neoprotosil in instillation of urethra, 198
in venereal diseases, 192, 193
Neosalvarsan in syphilis, 206
in yaws, 252, 253
Neostibosan in kala-azar, 235, 236, 237
Neotropin, urinary antiseptic, 880
Nephritis, 851-67
acute, 852-58
after-care, 858
as complication of erysipelas, 91
diet, 853-55
drugs, 856-57
focal sepsis, 855-56
rest, 853
schemes of treatment, 863-67
symptomatic treatment, 857-58
urea concentration range, 854
and mercury workers, 309
chronic interstitial, 861
and tetany, 425
diet in, 861
diets, 864-67
chronic parenchymatous, 858
chronic, with œdema, 858
Diet V, 866-67
glomerulonephritis (second stage), 858-60
(third stage), 861-63
uræmia, 862-63
Nephrosis, chronic, 858-60
high protein diet, 859
Diet V, 866-67

Neptal in congestive heart failure, 685
Nerve, seventh cranial, in the newborn, 277
Nervous system, congenital degenerative disorders, 991-92
  diseases of the, 969-1015
    of the brain and spinal cord, 983-86
    of the cerebral circulation, 995-99
    of cerebral function, 1008-14
    of the cranial nerves, 999-1003
    of the extra-pyramidal motor system, 992-95
    of the peripheral nerves, 974-80
    of the skull, vertebræ and meninges, 980-83
    of the spinal cord, 986-91
  hydrocephalus and intracranial tumour, 1003-5
  in infancy, 292-99
    convulsions, 292-94
    cyclical vomiting, 297-98
    enuresis, 296-97
    mental deficiency, 295
    pink disease, 299
  injury to the skull and brain, 1003-8
  remedial exercises, 1014-15
Nervous system in anæmia, 468-69
Neufeld method of serum administration, 802
Neuralgia, 977
  glossopharyngeal, 1003
  paroxysmal trigeminal, 1000
Neurasthenia, 1032
  tropical. *See* TRYPANOSOMIASIS, AFRICAN, 233-35
Neuritis, alcoholic, 978-79
  arsenical, 979
  brachial, 975
  cervical-occipital, 975
  in diabetes, 377
  in diphtheria, 24
  in the aged, 979
  interstitial, 974-77
  lead, 979
  neuralgia, 977
  parenchymatous, 978-79
  progressive hypertrophic, 980
Neuritis—*contd.*
  retrobulbar, 999
  sciatica, 975-76
  traumatic, 977
  vitamin B_1 deficiency and, 404-8
  with paralysis, 976-77
Neurofibromatosis, 980
Neuromyelitis optica, 985
Neuroses, cardiac. *See* CARDIAC NEUROSES, 716-21
Neurosis and insanity, differential diagnosis, 1032-33
Neurosis, sensory, 761
Neurosyphilis, 216-24
Neurotic reactions of patients to illness, 1027-31
  treatment of the, 1033-42
Neutropenia, malignant and primary, 521. *See* AGRANULOCYTIC ANGINA, 521-23
Nickel, test for skin sensitiveness, 318
Nicotinic acid in alcoholism, 1047, 1049
  in pellagra, 409-10
Niemann-Pick disease, 524
Nirvanol in chorea, 995
Nitrites in angina, 696-99
  in essential hypertension, 653
Nitro derivatives of benzene, poisoning from, 315
Nitroglycerin in angina of effort, 696-97, 699
Nitrous fumes, poisoning from, 312
Nocturnal jumps, 973
Normacol in constipation, 578
Nose, affections of, 743-55
    common nasal remedies, 744-45
    foreign bodies in, 749-50
    nasal allergy, 751
    nasal polypi, 750-51
    rhinitis, 749-50
    sinusitis, 752-55
  epistaxis, 746-49
  fractures, 746
  hæmatoma, 746
  injuries of the, 745-49
Nose, throat and ear, diseases of, 743-74
  ear, 762-71
  larynx, 771-73
  nose, 743-55
Nose, throat and ear, diseases of—*contd.*
  pharynx, 755-61
  prescriptions (Appendix), 773-74
Novarsenobillon in oral sepsis, 513
  in syphilis, 206
Novocain in chronic rheumatoid arthritis, 922
  in sciatica, 976
  infiltration in fibrositis, 937-38, 939
Novurit in congestive heart failure, 685
Nutrition and visceroptosis, 581-82
Nux vomica in gastritis, 542
Nyctalopia in vitamin A deficiency, 403
Nystagmus, miner's, 305-6

O

Obesity, 387-400
  and amenorrhœa, 1064
  and angina, 697
  and cholecystitis, 618
  and gall-stones, 620
  and hypertension, 651-52
  arthritis and, 926
  associated complaints, 387
  complications, diet in, 396
  dietetics, 389-96. *See* DIETETICS IN OBESITY, 389-96
  exercise and, 388-89
  thyroid in, 396-98
  types of, exogenous and endogenous, 388
Obsessions, 1039
Occupational cramp, 974
  dermatitis, 182
  factor in fibrositis, 932
  therapy in rheumatism, 961-62
Oculogyric crises in encephalitis lethargica, 993
Oculomotor disorders, 999
Œdema in acute nephritis, 857
  in congestive heart failure, 666-92
  in hepatic cirrhosis, 612-13
  in nephrosis, 858-60
  pulmonary, 790-91
Œsophageal atresia and cardiospasm in infancy, 280
Œsophagitis, 532-33
Œsophagus, carcinoma of, 534
  diverticulum of, 533
  peptic ulcer of, 535-36

Œstradiol, 1056, 1058-59
Œstrin, 455-56
Œstroform, 455, 456, 1060
Ointments in skin diseases, 156-57
Oleothorax in spontaneous pneumothorax, 811
Oleum chenopodium in cestodiasis, 258
Olive oil enemata, 579
 in cholecystitis, 618
 in gall-stones, 619
 in peptic ulcer, 547
Omnopon in congestive heart failure, 668
 in diarrhœa, 572
 in septicæmia, 87
 in thyroidectomy, 444
Onchocerca cæcutiens, 262
Onchocerca volvulus, in filariasis, 262
Oöphorectomy in osteomalacia, 423
Ophthalmia neonatorum, 194, 205-6
 sulphonamides in, 206
Ophthalmic test for serum sensitivity, 801
Ophthalmic zoster, 187
Opium in acute bronchitis, 785
 in cancer of the stomach, 562
 in congestive heart failure, 668
 in coronary thrombosis, 693
 in diarrhœa, 569
 in digitalis therapy, 680
 in dyspnœic heart failure, 702
 in rheumatoid arthritis, 900
Optic atrophy, 999
 in G.P.I., 221
 in tabes dorsalis, 219-20
Optochin in lobar pneumonia, 798
Oral sepsis in rheumatoid arthritis, 898
Orange juice in scurvy, 410-11
Orarsan in syphilis, 207
Orchitis as complication of mumps, 48
 in filariasis, 260
Oriental sore, 237-38
Orisol in oriental sore, 237
Orris root sensitivity in asthma, 834
Orthoform, 140-41
Ortho-iodoxy benzoic acid in rheumatoid arthritis, 901
Orthopædic procedures in osteo-arthritis, 925
Osler's disease. *See* POLYCYTHÆMIA VERA, 502-6
Osteitis deformans, 966-67, 983
Osteitis, fibro-cystic, 449, 967
Ostelin in cœliac disease, 285
 in convulsions, 293
 in deficiency diseases, 416
 in neonatal conditions, 273
 in rheumatoid arthritis, 900
Osteo-arthritis, 890, 893-94, 923-26
 drugs in, 924
 obesity in, 923
 occupational factor, 893, 923
 orthopædic procedures, 925-26
 prophylaxis, 893-94
 trauma causing, 893
 treatment, general, 923-24
  local, 924-25
Osteo-arthropathy, hypertrophic pulmonary, 966
Osteogenesis imperfecta, 967
Osteomalacia and rickets, 422-23
Osteomyelitis, 968, 980-81
 Pott's disease, 980-81
 sinusitis and, 754-55
Osteotomy, 944
Otitis externa, 762-63
Otitis media, acute, 764-68
  complications, 768
  paracentesis, 767-68
  prevention of deafness, 767
  suction, 766-67
  treatment after discharge appears, 765-66
   before discharge appears, 765
 chronic, 768-70
 in infancy, 287-88
Otosclerosis, 770
Ovarian hormones, 1058-60
Oxaluria, 885
Oxo in diabetes mellitus, 328, 331
Oxycephaly, 967-68
Oxygen and carbon dioxide inhalation in carbon monoxide poisoning, 311
Oxygen chamber in oxygen therapy, 1102
Oxygen in acute bronchitis, 785, 787
 in anoxæmia, 728-29
 in congestive heart failure, 691-92
 in dyspnœic heart failure, 702
 in pulmonary œdema, 790
 in thyroidectomy, 446
 inhalation in poisoning from nitrous fumes, 312
  in poisoning from sulphuretted hydrogen, 313
 tent in cyanosis, 289
  in oxygen therapy, 1103
 therapy (technique), 1098-1106
  indications, 1098
  methods, 1101-6
   bifurcated nasal tube, 1105-6
   face tents, 1103-4
   masks, 1104-5
   nasal catheter, 1105-6
   oxygen chamber, 1102-3
   oxygen tent, 1103
   tube and funnel, 1103
  requirements, 1101
Ozæna, 750

P

Paget's disease, 983, 966
Panacoids in pancreatic disease, 624
Pancreas, diseases of the, 623-25. *See also* DIABETES MELLITUS, 523-63
 chronic, 624-25
 cyst of the pancreas, 624
 pancreatic stone, 624
Papaverin in muco-membranous colic, 586
Paracentesis in pericarditis with effusion, 641-42
 indications for, in otitis media, 767-68
 of the abdomen (technique), 1087-88
 of the pleural cavity (technique), 1088-89

Paraffin and agar emulsion in congestive heart failure, 672
enemata, 579
in constipation, 577-78
in pediculosis, 172
wax baths in rheumatoid arthritis, 913, 946-47
Paraldehyde in acute bronchitis, 784
in alcoholism, 1048, 1052
in cerebral lesions, 998
in epilepsy, 1011
in insomnia, 1013
in status epilepticus, 292
in the senile heart, 659
in thyroidectomy, 444
Paralysis agitans, 994
and beri-beri, 407
Bell's, 1001
brachial, in the newborn, 277
diphtheritic, 24
familial periodic, 973
general, of the insane. *See* G.P.I.
Landry's, 979
neuritis with, 976-77
progressive bulbar, 985
sleep, 973
Paraplegia, 986-88
Parathormone in lead poisoning, 308
in tetania parathyropriva, 447
Parathyroid extract, in osteitis deformans, 966
in tetany, 424
Parathyroid glands, 447-50
hyperparathyroidism, 449-50
tetania parathyropriva, 447-49
Paratyphoid. *See* ENTERIC FEVER, 30-37
Parkinsonian syndrome, 992
Paroidin in tetania parathyropriva, 447
Paroxysmal fibrillation and digitalis, 705
hæmoglobinuria, 493
tachycardia *See* TACHYCARDIA, PAROXYSMAL, 708-11
Patch tests in industrial dermatitis, 317, 318-19
Paterson-Kelly syndrome, 761
Pediculosis, 172-73
Pellagra, 408-10
Pelvic pain, psychotherapy of, 1026
Pemphigoid eruptions, 186
Pemphigus in sepsis neonatorum, 273
Pentnucleotide in agranulocytic angina, 523
Pepsac in pernicious anæmia, 485
Pepsin in diseases of the stomach, 538
Peptic ulcer. *See* ULCER, PEPTIC, 542-60
in diabetes, 378
Peptone, as desensitizing agent in asthma, 835
injections in dermatitis, 177
in rheumatoid arthritis, 908
Peptonized milk, 286
Perandren, 456
Perforation in enteric fever, 35
Perforation of peptic ulcer, 552
Pericardial disease, operation for, 714
Pericarditis, 640-43
Perichondritis, 762
Peripheral blood flow, normal, 731-42
Peripheral nerves, disorders of, 974-80
coccygodynia, 978
interstitial neuritis, 974-77
neurofibromatosis, 980
other forms of neuritis, 980
pain in malignant disease, 978
parenchymatous neuritis, 978-79
polyneuritis, 978-80
traumatic neuritis, 977
Peripheral vascular dilatation, 644
Peritoneal tuberculosis, 147-48
Peritoneum, diseases of the, 625-26
Peri-urethral abscess, complicating gonorrhœa, 199, 200
Pernicious anæmia. *See* ANÆMIA, PERNICIOUS, ADDISONIAN, 481-86
Pertussis. *See* WHOOPING-COUGH, 70-74
Pessaries, carbasone, 204
Petrolagar in constipation, 578
in infancy, 283
Pharyngitis, 760-61
Pharynx, anæsthesia of, 761
diseases of, 755-61
neuroses of, 761
pharyngitis, 760-61
tonsillitis, 755-61
diverticulum of, 533-34
Phenacetin in agranulocytic angina, 522
Phenazone in rheumatoid arthritis, 900
Phenobarbitone in asthma, 838
in chorea, 995
in encephalitis lethargica, 993
in epilepsy, 1008
in essential hypertension, 652-53
in hyperthyroidism, 434
in insomnia, 1013
in muscular cramp, 973, 974
in peptic ulcer, 547
in sea-sickness, 1003
in thyroidectomy, 442
in tinnitus, 1002
in vertigo, 1002
in X-ray sickness, 527
Phenolphthalein in constipation, 577, 578
Phenylhydrazine hydrochloride in polycythæmia, 504-5
Phlebitis as complication of enteric fever, 35
Phobias and obsessions, 1039
Phosphaturia, 884
Phosphorus in diseases of the liver, 605
Phrenic avulsion in bronchiectasis, 291, 818
Phrenicectomy in pulmonary tuberculosis, 127-28
Phthisis. *See* PULMONARY TUBERCULOSIS
Physostab, 1058
Pick's disease, 992
Piles in cirrhosis of the liver, 611
Pine oil inhalations, 745
Pink disease in infancy, 299
Pistany mud in applying heat, 946
Pitressin in diabetes insipidus, 457
Pituitary, 456-59
adenomata, 457-58
diabetes insipidus, 456-57
extract, 457
in reticulo-endotheliosis, 524

Pituitary—*contd.*
infantilism, 458-59
Simmond's disease, 459
Pituitrin in asthma, 825
in circulatory failure of acute bronchitis, 786-87
in constipation in paraplegia, 988
in herpes zoster, 187
in neuralgia, 977
in peripheral vascular dilatation, 644
in post-hæmorrhagic anæmia, 477
in tympanites, 788
Pityriasis rosea, 188
Placental extract in hæmophilia, 520
Plague, 239-40
Plasma albumin concentration in chronic nephrosis, 859
Plasmoquine, in malaria, 228, 230
Plasters, serial, in chronic rheumatoid arthritis, 919-20
wedge, in rheumatoid arthritis, 920, 951
Plastules, in anæmia, 472
Pleural cavity, aspiration of (technique), 1088-90
Pleural effusion in artificial pneumothorax, 126
shock in artificial pneumothorax treatment, 125
Pleurisy, dry, in pneumonia, 796-97
Pleurisy, tuberculous, with effusion, 136-38
Pleurodynia, 934
Plummer-Vinson syndrome, 462, 534, 761
Pneumatic drills, work with, 304-5
Pneumokoniosis. *See* Dust Diseases, Industrial, 315-17
Pneumolysis, internal, 126-27
Pneumonia, lobar, 795-808
artificial pneumothorax in, 797-98
chemotherapy, 806-8
cough mixtures, 796
feeding, 795-96
M & B 693 in, 807-8
morphia in, 796-97
pain and restlessness in, 796-97
quinine 798

Pneumonia, lobar—*contd.*
serum therapy, 798-806
sleep and, 796
strapping, 797
types, 799
Pneumothorax, artificial, in bronchiectasis, 818
in lobar pneumonia, 797-98
in pulmonary fibrosis, 291
in pulmonary tuberculosis, 123-26
air embolism in, 125
bilateral, 124
displacement of mediastinum in, 125-26
extra-pleural, 129-30
induction and management of, 124-25
interstitial emphysema in, 125
pleural effusion in, 126
pleural shock in, 125
termination of treatment, 125
spontaneous, 810-12
Poisoning by gases, 310-15
by metals, 306-10. *See* Lead Poisoning, Mercury Poisoning, etc.
Poisons, corrosive, causing œsophagitis, 532
Poliomyelitis, acute, 49-52
Pollen extract in hay fever, desensitization, 844-45
Polycythæmia vera, 502-6
acetylphenylhydrazine in, 505-6
diet in, 503
irradiation, 504
phenylhydrazine hydrochloride, 504-5
symptomatic treatment, 506
venesection, 503-4
Polymorph-lymphocyte-monocyte ratio in pulmonary tuberculosis, 107
Polyneuritis, 978-80
acute infective, 979-80
arsenical and lead poisoning in, 979
vitamin B_1 deficiency causing, 404-5
Polypi, nasal, 750-51
Ponndorf's vaccine, 929
Poro-adenitis, 225
Postural drainage in pulmonary fibrosis and bronchitis, 291

Posture and breathing in prevention of respiratory disease, 778
Potain's aspirator, 137
Potassium bicarbonate in acute nephritis, 856
Potassium bromide in acute bronchitis, 784
in asthma, 838
in congestive heart failure, 668-69
in epilepsy, 1008-9
in rheumatoid arthritis, 900
in whooping-cough, 73
Potassium chloride in familial periodic paralysis, 973
in myasthenia gravis, 972
Potassium citrate in acute nephritis, 856
in polycythæmia vera, 506
in renal calculus, 882
in rheumatoid arthritis, 901
Potassium iodide in gastric syphilis, 565
in heart-block, 711
in thyrotoxicosis, 436. *See also* Iodides
Potassium permanganate bath in diseases of the skin, 154
in gonorrhœa, 197
Pott's disease, 980-81
Poultices in skin diseases, 155-56
Powders in skin diseases, 154-55
Pregnancy and acute yellow atrophy, 609
and anæmia, 464, 465
and biliary stasis, 615
and cholera, 243
and diabetes. *See* Diabetes and Pregnancy, 372-76
and gonorrhœa, 203
and intra-abdominal pressure, 580
and lactation in vitamin B_1 deficiency, 405
and pyelitis, 870, 880
and syphilis, 214
and tuberculosis, 115
in relation to heart disease, 660-63
malaria in, 231
Pregnandiol, 1060
Pregnyl, 455
Preloban, 455

Prematurity, 271-73
Prepalin in vitamin A deficiency, 404
Progesterone, 456
in metropathia hæmorrhagica, 1061
in mid-menstrual bleeding, 1062
in recurrent abortion, 1066
Progestin, 456
Progressive muscular atrophy, 985-86
Progynon, 455-56
Prolac in cœliac rickets, 422
Prolan, 454-55
Proluton, 456
Prominal in convulsions, 294
in epilepsy, 1009
Prontosil. *See* SULPHONAMIDE DRUGS
Proof-puncture in sinusitis, 753-54
Proseptasine as urinary antiseptic, 876
in septicæmia, 84
Prostatitis and seminal vesiculitis complicating gonorrhœa, 199-200
Prostigmin in myasthenia gravis, 972, 973
Protamine zinc insulin, 354-63. *See* INSULIN Z.P.
Protargol in dysentery, 29
in rhinitis, 749
Protein in acute nephritis, 853-55
in chronic interstitial nephritis, 861
in diabetes mellitus, 328-29
Protein milk, 286
Protein, sensitizing agent in asthma, 831
Protein shock therapy in disseminated sclerosis, 983
in gonorrhœa, 196
in leprosy, 251
in lympho-granuloma inguinale, 225
in neuralgia, 1000
in rheumatoid arthritis, 907-8
in undulant fever, 241
Prurigo, Besnier's, 180-81
Pruritus, 182-84
in catarrhal jaundice, 608
in diabetes, 377
in serum sickness, 76
vulvæ, 1067
Psittacosis, 52-53
Psoriasis, 189-91
Psycho-analysis in psychotherapy, 1043
Psychological factor in asthma, 826-31
Psychology, child. *See* CHILD PSYCHOLOGY, 1021-25
Psychotherapy in general practice, 1016-46
adjustment of the sexual instinct, 1023-27
attitude of the patient to disease, 1027-31
differential diagnosis, 1032-33
parent-child relationships, 1021-23
pelvic pain, 1026
procedures in treatment, 1033-42
scope and limitations, 1042-46
Pulmonary abscess, 818-20
Pulmonary complications, post-operative, 820-22
Pulmonary disease in relation to dyspnœic failure, 702-3
Pulmonary embolism and infarction, 821-22
thrombophlebitis causing, 822
Pulmonary embolism in congestive heart failure, 689
Pulmonary fibrosis, 791-92
and bronchiectasis in infancy, 290-91
Pulmonary œdema, acute, 699, 790-91
Pulmonary stenosis with septal defect, 663
Pulmonary tuberculosis. *See* TUBERCULOSIS, PULMONARY, 100-136
Pulse-deficit in digitalis administration, 676-77
Pulses in vascular insufficiency, 735
Pulsus bigeminus, 711
Purgatives in constipation, 576-77
Purpura and aplastic anæmia in syphilis, 208
Purpuras, 507-17
adrenalin and calcium in, 513
bleeding from gums, 510
from nose, 511-12
from tooth-sockets, 510-11
Purpuras—*contd.*
classification, 507-8
hæmorrhage, severe, 516-17
hæmorrhagic lesions, 510-17
hæmostatic preparations, 514
Henoch's, 508
idiopathic, thrombocytopenic, 508
liver extracts in, 514
local measures, 509
protein, foreign, therapy, 515-16
Schönlein's, 508
simplex, 509
snake venom in, 514
splenectomy in, 509
X-rays to the spleen, 515
Pus in urine in urinary infections, 871
Pyelitis, 869-82
acute, 870-71
diet in, 873
drainage of ureter, 880
in pregnancy, 870, 880
Pylephlebitis, suppurative, 614
Pyloric stenosis, hypertrophic, in infancy, 280-82
organic, in peptic ulcer, 553
Pylorospasm, 280
in peptic ulcer, 552-53
Pyogenic infection of the brain, 983
Pyonephrosis, 867
Pyopneumothorax, 126, 811-12
Pyramidon in fever, 6
in rheumatoid arthritis, 900
Pyrexia, 1
relief of, 5-6
Pyrexial treatment in G.P.I., 223
Pyridine as urinary antiseptic, 880
Pyrolactin D in fibrositis 937
in rheumatoid arthritis, 902, 908
Pyuria, 871, 876

Q

Quassia in enterobiasis, 264
Queckenstedt's manœuvre, 1093

Quinidine sulphate, in auricular fibrillation, 706-7
in auricular flutter, 708
in coronary thrombosis, 693
in extra-systoles, 713
in paroxysmal tachycardia, 709, 710, 711
in Stokes-Adams seizures, 727
in thyrotoxicosis, post-operative, 707
Quinine in lobar pneumonia, 798
in malaria, 228-30
in myotonia, 972
Mayer-Tanret reagent for, 229-30
Quinolor in sycosis, 167
Quinoxyl in amœbic dysentery, 244
Quinsy, 757

R

Rabies, 254-55
Rachitic tetany, 425-26
Radiant-heat baths in sinusitis, 753
Radiation in hyperthyroidism, 439
in nasal allergy, 751
in tonsillitis, 758-59
Radio-active compounds in rheumatoid arthritis, 903
Radio-active substances, injury from, 320-22
Radiostol in cœliac disease, 285
in idiopathic steatorrhœa, 592
in premature infancy, 273
in vitamin D deficiency, 416
Radiostoleum in anæmia, 487
in rheumatoid arthritis, 909
in vitamin A deficiency, 404
in vitamin D deficiency, 416
Radium for removal of warts, 320
for thymic enlargement, 292
in nasal allergy, 751
in paroxysmal rhinorrhœa, 848
Radium—*contd.*
needles in bronchial carcinoma, 822
over-exposure to. *See* RADIO-ACTIVE SUBSTANCES, INJURY FROM, 320-22
Radon seeds in bronchial carcinoma, 822
Ramstedt operation, 281
Rat-bite fever, 239
Raynaud's disease, 740
Reaction, Kahn. *See* KAHN REACTION
Van den Bergh. *See* VAN DEN BERGH REACTION
Wassermann. *See* WASSERMANN REACTION
Widal. *See* WIDAL REACTION
Rectal administration of fluid in diseases of infancy, 269
technique, 1070-71
Redoxon in the purpuras, 513
in scurvy, 411
Reenstierna's test for chancroid, 224
Refrigerating plant, ammonia, 310
Renal calcinosis, 421
Renal calculus, 882-84
Renal diseases, 851-85
calculus, 882-84
chronic, tetany of, 426-27
hydronephrosis, 867-69
infections of the urinary tract, 869-82
nephritis, 851-67
oxaluria, 885
phosphaturia, 884-85
Renal dwarfs, 296
rickets, 422
tuberculosis, 141-43
Renal function tests, 854
Respirators in industrial dust diseases, 315
in oxygen therapy, 1101-6
Respiratory system, diseases of the, 775-850
abscess and gangrene of the lung, 818-20
acute bronchitis and broncho-pneumonia, 782-92
acute coryza, 779-82
acute empyema, 808-10
acute œdema of the lungs, 823
asthma, 823-43
bronchiectasis, 812-18
Respiratory system—*contd.*
hay fever, 843-46
in infancy. *See* INFANCY, RESPIRATORY SYSTEM IN, 287-92
intrathoracic new growths, 822-23
lobar pneumonia, 795-808
paroxysmal rhinorrhœa, 846-48
post-operative pulmonary complications, 820-22
prescriptions (Appendix), 848-50
prevention of acute respiratory disease, 775-79
diet and tonics, 777-78
faulty posture and breathing, 778
predisposing causes, 775-76
vaccine therapy, 778-79
specific non-tuberculous infection of the lung, 823
spontaneous pneumothorax, 810-12
Reticulo-endothelial system, diseases of, 524
Retinitis in diabetes, 377
Rheumatic carditis, 633-39
after-care in, 638-39
antistreptococcal serum in, 636-37
blood sedimentation rate in, 638
convalescence in, 638
focal sepsis, 635-36
future occupation, 639
joint changes, 635
joint involvement, 637
local treatment, 635
rest in, 633
salicylate administration, 633-35
sinus arrhythmia in, 637
tonsillectomy, 636
Rheumatic diseases, chronic, 886-965
ætiology, 888
age incidence, 891-92
blood sedimentation rate, 887
determination of, 959-60
classification, 889-91
chronic menopausal arthritis, 926-27
exercises, 952-59
fibrositis, 931-42
gout, 962-65

Rheumatic diseases—*contd.*
osteo-arthritis, 923-26
prophylaxis, 891-94
rheumatoid arthritis, 894-923
splints, manufacture of, 947-51
spondylitis, 927-30
Still's disease, 931
surgery in. *See* SURGERY IN RHEUMATIC DISEASES, 942-45
Rheumatic fever. *See* RHEUMATIC CARDITIS, 633-39
Rheumatism clinic, organisation of, 960-61
Rheumatoid arthritis, 894-923
acute, 895-913
clinical features, 895
diet in, 908-10
drugs in, 899-907
gastro-intestinal tract in, 910
non-specific protein therapy, 907-8
removal of septic foci, 897-99
rest in, 895-96
splints in, 911-12
treatment, general, 895-99
local, 910-13
vaccines in, 905-7
chronic, 918-23
correction of deformities, 919-23
diet, 892
prophylaxis, 892-93
spa treatment, 892
subacute, 913-18
drugs in, 918
physiotherapy, 914-18
Rheumogen in rheumatoid arthritis, 913
Rhinitis, acute. *See* CORYZA, 779-82
chronic, 749-50
Rhinorrhœa, paroxysmal, 846-48
Rhythm, disorders of, 703-13
auricular fibrillation, 703-7
auricular flutter, 707-8
coupled, 683
extra-systoles, 712-13
heart-block, 711-12
paroxysmal tachycardia, 708-11
sino-auricular block, nodal rhythm, etc., 713
Rice in beri-beri, 406
Rickets, 413-23
ætiology, 413
cœliac, 422
diet in, 419-20
hypervitaminosis D, 421
maternal treatment in, 419
osteomalacia, 422-23
prevention of, 272-73, 418-19
renal, 422
sun-burn and, 417
vitamin D, forms of, 414-18
Ringworm, 167-71
of body folds, 170-71
of nails, 171
of scalp, 168-70
Rosacea, 175-76
Round-worm. *See* ASCARIASIS, 264
Rubella, 53-54
Rubiazol in septicæmia, 84
Rumination in infancy, 279-80
Rupture of the drum, 764
Russell's viper venom in purpura, 510
in hæmophilia, 518

S

Salicin and salicylates in psoriasis, 191
Salicylates in fibrositis, 934
in rheumatic fever, 633-35
in rheumatoid arthritis, 899
Saline infusions, technique of, 1075-79
Salines in constipation, 577
Salpingitis in gonorrhœa, 203
Salt in acute alcoholism, 1049
in acute nephritis, 855
in chronic nephrosis, 859
in congestive heart failure, 670-72
Salvarsan and derivatives in rat-bite fever, 239
Salvarsan in anthrax, 12
in yaws, 252
Salyrgan in cirrhosis of the liver, 613
in chronic nephrosis, 860
in congestive heart failure, 685, 686
Sanatorium treatment in tuberculosis, 101-2
Sand-fly in onchocerca volvulus, 262
Sanitary pad, tampon type of, in gonorrhœa, 193
Sanocrysin in tuberculosis, 120
Santonin in ascariasis, 264
in diseases of the liver, 605
Saxin or saccharine in obesity diets, 392, 395
Scabies, 171-72
Scalp, impetigo of, 163
lotions and ointment, 161
ringworm of. *See* RINGWORM OF SCALP, 168-70
Scarlet fever, 54-60
carriers in, 59-60
complications in, 58
Dick test in, 54-55
quarantine in, 56
sulphonamide in, 56
toxic and septic attacks, 58-59
treatment, curative, 56-59
general, 57-58
preventive, 54-56
Schick test in diphtheria, 20
Schistosoma hæmatobium, 257
Schistosoma japonica, 257
Schistosoma mansoni, 257
Schistosomiasis, acute attack of, 256-57
Schmidt's test intestinal diet, 597
Schönlein's purpura, 508
Sciatica, 934, 938, 941-42, 975-76
Sclavo's anti-anthrax serum, 12
Sclerosis, diffuse cerebral, 992
tuberose, 992
Scopolamine-morphine in thyroidectomy, 444
Scott's dressing in rheumatoid arthritis, 913
Scratching, to prevent, in diseases of infancy, 266
Scurvy, 410-13
Seasickness, 1003
Seborrhœa. *See* DERMATITIS, 176-82
Sedatives in peptic ulcer, 547
Sedimentation rate, determination of, in chronic rheumatic disease, 959-60
in tuberculosis, 106-7

Seloram in acute nephritis, 855
Semb, apicolysis of, 129
Senile heart disease, 658-60
vaginitis, 1067
Senna in constipation, 576
Sensitivity, serum, reactions, 800-1
tests for, 801-3
Sepsis causing secondary hæmolytic anæmia, 491
Sepsis neonatorum, 273
Septicæmia, 78-88
agranulocytosis complicating, 86
blood cultures in, 80
blood transfusion in, 81-82
causes of, 78
chemotherapy in, 83-87
diet in, 86, 87
focal lesion in, 81
general measures in, 87
in sinusitis, 755
management of, 80
of septic abortion, 80
prophylaxis in, 88
seras and vaccines in, 82-83
sulphonamide preparations in, 83-87, 88
toxic effects of drugs in, 86-87
types of, 79-80
Sera in hæmophilia, 518-20
in septicæmia, 82, 83
Serogan, 1058
Serum, antiscarlatinal in meningitis, 982
antitoxic, in diphtheria, 22
in tetanus, 66
gonadotropic hormone, 1057
horse, 74-75
skin test after injection of, 76
Serum sickness, 74-77
in lobar pneumonia, 803-4
Serum therapy in acute poliomyelitis, 50-51
in anthrax, 12
in bacillary dysentery, 27
in broncho-pneumonia, 781
in cerebrospinal fever, 15
in enteric fever, 32
in lobar pneumonia, 798-806
administration, 805-6
anaphylaxis and serum sickness, 803-4
Serum therapy in lobar pneumonia—*contd.*
dosage, 805-6
pneumococcal serum (Felton process), 800
reactions, 800
serum sensitivity, 800-3
sulphonamide and, 800
thermal reactions, 804-5
vasovagal attacks, 804
in scarlet fever, 56-57
Sexual instinct, adjustment of, 1023-27
intercourse in gonorrhœa, 193, 199
in syphilis, 211
Ship-breaking by use of oxyacetylene, 307
Shock, 727-30
Shock therapy, non-specific in elephantiasis, 260
Shoulder, fibrositis, 939
Sickle-cell anæmia, 494
Silicosis, 315-16
Silver nitrate in diseases of the skin, 161
in drainage of ureter, 881
in laryngitis, 772
in pharyngitis, 761
Simmond's disease, 459
Sino-auricular block, 713
Sinus arrhythmia, 703
and carditis, 637
Sinuses, accessory air, in rheumatoid arthritis, 898
Sinusitis, 752-55
Sippy diet in peptic ulcer, 545
Skin, bacterial infections of, 162-67
care of, in rheumatoid arthritis, 896
common diseases of, 150-91
baths in, 154
formulæ for common local applications, 159-62
lotions in treatment of, 156, 159-61
ointments and pastes in, 156, 160-61
paints in, 158, 159-61
pastes in, 155, 160-61
permanent fixed dressings in, 158
poultices in, 155
powders in, 154
tar applications in, 160-61
Skin—*contd.*
erythema of, in gold therapy, 904
parasitic infections of, 167-73
purpura of, in gold therapy, 904
tuberculosis of, 148-49
Skull and brain, injury to, 1005-8
post-concussional syndrome, 1007-8
surgical complications, 1007
Skull, vertebræ and meninges, disorders of, 980-83
meningitis, 981-82
osteomyelitis, 980-81
tumours, 982
Sleep paralysis, 973
Sleeping sickness. *See* TRYPANOSOMIASIS, 233-35
Sleeplessness, 1012-14. *See also* INSOMNIA
Smallpox, 60-64
vaccination against, 61
Smoking and atelectasis, 820
and chronic bronchitis, 793
and peptic ulcer, 544, 546
and pulmonary tuberculosis, 110
and thrombo-angiitis obliterans, 736
Snake venom in purpuras, 514-15
Sodium and potassium tartrate in yaws, 252
Sodium biborate in epilepsy, 1009
in pyelitis, 874-75
Sodium-bismuth tartrate in yaws, 252
Sodium bromide in epilepsy, 1009
in insomnia, 1013
in post-concussional syndrome, 1007
in spasmodic torticollis, 1012
Sodium chloride and tetany, 427. *See also* SALT
Sodium citrate as anticoagulant in blood transfusion, 1082
in pyelitis, 874-76
Sodium luminal in epilepsy, 1011
Sodium mandelate mixture, 878
Sodium phenobarbitone in the senile heart, 659

Sodium salicylate in cholecystitis, 617
in gout, 962-65
in rheumatic fever, 633-35
in seasickness, 1003
in vertigo, 1002
Sodium salts in Addison's disease, 451-53
Sodium sulphate in anuria, 857
Sodium thiosulphate in syphilis, 208, 209
Solganol in tuberculosis, 120
Solustibosan, 561
in kala-azar, 235, 236, 237
Soneryl in insomnia, 1014
Sonne organisms in dysentery of infancy, 284
Southey's tubes in congestive heart failure, 690-91
paracentesis by, 1098
Spa treatment, British Health Resorts Assoc. Handbook, 915
in cholecystitis, 618-19
in gastritis, 542
in gout, 965
in menopausal arthritis, 927
in rheumatoid arthritis, 892, 914
Spastic colon. *See* Colic, Muco-membranous, 585-87
diet for, 596
Spes phthisica, 113
Sphagnum moss in enuresis, 297
Spina bifida, 990
Spinal cord, compression of, 989-90
disorders of, 986-91
injury, 990-91
myelitis, 986
paraplegia, 986-88
spina bifida, 990
subacute combined degeneration of, 988-89
in anæmia, 486-87
syringomyelia, 990
vascular lesions of, 989
Spine, arthritis affecting the. *See* Spondylitis, 927-30
cervical, fibrositis, 939
tuberculous disease of the, 980-81
Spirochæta pallida, 206
Spirochætes in lung abscess, 819
in sputum in bronchiectasis, 815
Spirochætosis icterohæmorrhagiæ, 238
Spirocid in syphilis, 207
Splenectomy and purpura, 509
contraindicated in polycythæmia vera, 503
in severe purpura hæmorrhagica, 516-17
in acholuric jaundice, 489-90
in splenic anæmia, 498-500
in thrombosis of splenic vein, 500
Splenic anæmia, 497-502
Splenic vein, thrombosis of, 500
Splenomegaly in schistosomiasis, 257
Splints, aeroplane, 921
in neuritis with paralysis, 976
in rheumatoid arthritis, 911-12
plaster, manufacture of, 947-51
Spondylitis, 927-30
ankylosing, 928-29
Spondylose rhizomélique, 890
Spontaneous pneumothorax, 810-12
Sprays, oily, in diseases of the nose, 745
Sprue, 247-50
non-tropical. *See* Idiopathic Steatorrhœa, 591-93
Sprulac in idiopathic steatorrhœa, 592
Stabilarsan in syphilis, 206
Stabismol in syphilis, 209
Starch and opium enema in chronic ulcerative colitis, 589
bath in diseases of the skin, 154
in pruritus, 609
poultice in impetigo contagiosa, 162
in ringworm, 169
in sycosis, 166
Status asthmaticus, 825
Status epilepticus, 292, 1011
Steatorrhœa, idiopathic, 572, 591-93
anæmia in, 592
diet in, 592
Sterilization in heart disease, 663
Stibosan in Leishmaniasis, 235
Stilbœstrol, 1059-60
in amenorrhœa, 1064
in menopausal disturbances, 1067
in post-menopausal disturbances, 1067
Still's disease, 931
Stokes-Adams seizures, 725-27
intracardiac injection in, 726
Stomach, diseases of the, 536-65
anorexia nervosa, 562-63
cancer of, 561-62
common disorders of digestion, 563-64
gastric and duodenal ulcer, 542-60
gastritis, 540-42
uncommon disorders of the stomach and duodenum, 565-66
acute dilatation, 565
chronic duodenal ileus (stasis), 565
syphilis, 564-65
Stomach, hour-glass, in peptic ulcer, 553
Stomach preparations in anæmia, 485
Stomatitis in infancy, 278-79
in pellagra, 409
Stoneworkers, 316
Stovarsol in amœbic dysentery, 244
in syphilis, 207
in yaws, 252
Stramonium in asthma, 839
in encephalitis lethargica, 993
Strapping in lobar pneumonia, 797
Streptococcal septicæmia causing secondary hæmolytic anæmia, 491
S. hæmolyticus, 59-60, 640
S. pyogenes, 44
S. viridans, 644
in endocarditis, 639
Stricture, simple in œsophagitis, 532-33
Strophanthin in chlorine poisoning, 313
in treatment of congestive heart failure, 682
intravenous use, 81
Strychnine in cerebral thrombosis, 997

Strychnine—*contd.*
in circulatory failure, 644
in circulatory failure in acute bronchitis, 786-87
in diphtheria, 24
in post-hæmorrhagic anæmia, 477
in septicæmia, 87
in shock, 729
iron and arsenic combined in rheumatoid arthritis, 900
Stypven in control of hæmorrhage, 510
Subcutaneous administration of fluid (technique), 1070
Sulphæmoglobinæmia. *See* ENTEROGENOUS CYANOSIS, 506-7
Sulphanilamide. *See* SULPHONAMIDE DRUGS
Sulphapyridine. *See* SULPHONAMIDE DRUGS
Sulpharsenol in syphilis, 207
Sulpharsphenamine in bronchiectasis, 815
in lung abscess, 819
in syphilis, 207
Sulphonamide drugs causing acute hæmolytic anæmia, 492
agranulocytosis, 86
enterogenous cyanosis, 86, 506
nausea and vomiting, 86
sulphæmoglobinæmia, 86
in acute bronchitis and broncho-pneumonia, 791
in acute nephritis, 856
in cerebrospinal fever, 15
in chancroid, 224
in endocarditis, 638, 640
in erysipelas, 89-91
in gonorrhœa, 195-96, 198-99, 201-2, 203
in infections of the urinary tract, 876
in lobar pneumonia, 800, 806-8
in meningitis, 15, 982
in ophthalmia neonatorum, 205
in osteomyelitis, 968
in otitis media, 765
in pneumonia in infancy, 290
in rheumatoid arthritis, 903
in scarlet fever, 56, 57
in septicæmia, 83-87
Sulphonamide—*contd.*
in tonsillitis, 758
in vulvovaginitis of children, 204-5
in undulant fever, 241
toxic effects of, 86-87
Sulphostab in cardiovascular syphilis, 657
in syphilis, 207
Sulphur bath in diseases of the skin, 154
desensitizing agent in asthma, 836
in rheumatoid arthritis, 902
Sulphuretted hydrogen poisoning, 313
Sulphuric acid orangeade, 307
Sunlight, artificial, in asthma, 841
in pulmonary tuberculosis, 110
in rickets, 416-18
in tuberculosis of the skin, 148
in tuberculous adenitis, 145
cause of dermatitis, 177. *See also* ULTRA-VIOLET RADIATION
Suprarenal glands, 450-54
Addison's disease, 450-53
tumours of the adrenals, 453-54
Surgery in rheumatic diseases, 942-45
Surgery in treatment of cardiac disease. *See* CARDIAC DISEASES, SURGERY IN, 713-18
Sweating in pulmonary tuberculosis, 135-36
Sycosis, 165-67
Sydenham's chorea, 994-95
Sympathectomy for relief of cardiac pain, 716
in rheumatic diseases, 945
to improve blood supply, 739
Syncope, cardiac, 725-27
simple, 724
Stokes-Adams seizures, 725-27
Syndrome, hydræmic, 858
Marchiafava-Micheli, 493
Ménière's, 1002
nephrotic, 858
Parkinsonian, 992
Paterson-Kelly, 761
Plummer-Vinson, 761
post-concussional, 1007-8
Synovectomy, 943
Synovitis complicating gonorrhœa, 200-1
in filariasis, 260-61
Syphilis, 206-26
alopecia in, 187
and cardiovascular system, 214-15
and cold hæmoglobinuria, 493
and myelitis, 986
arsenic in, 206-7
toxic effects of, 207-8
bismuth in, 208-10
toxic effects of, 209-10
cardiovascular. *See* CARDIOVASCULAR SYPHILIS, 654-58
chancroid in, 224-25
coitus during, 211
congenital, 215
interstitial keratitis in, 215
nerve deafness in, 215
drug treatment of, 206-10
during pregnancy, 214
early, 210-12
gumma in, 217
in diseases of the stomach, 564-65
iodides in, 210
jaundice in, 208
late, 212-14
meningo-vascular, 216
cerebrospinal fluid in, 216
mercury in, 210
ulcus molle of, 224-25
vascular, 216-17
Syringing of the ear, 763
in otitis media, 766, 769
Syringomyelia, 990

T

T.A.B. vaccine, desensitizing agent in asthma, 836
in elephantiasis, 260
in leprosy, 251
in lympho-granuloma inguinale, 225
in rheumatoid arthritis, 907
in undulant fever, 241
T. rhodesiense, 235
Tabes dorsalis, 217-21
arthropathies in, 220-21
ataxia in, 217-18
incontinence of urine in, 218

Tabes dorsalis—*contd.*
lightning pains and crises in, 218-19
optic atrophy in, 219-20
Tabes mesenterica. *See* TUBERCULOSIS OF MESENTERIC LYMPH GLANDS, 146
Tachycardia, paroxysmal, 708-11
Tœnia echinococcus granulosis, 259-60
Tœnia saginata, 258
Tœnia solium, 259
Taka-diastase in diarrhœa, 572
Talma-Morison operation, in cirrhosis of the liver, 613
in splenic anæmia, 500
Tampax in gonorrhœa, 193
Tannic acid enema in chronic ulcerative colitis, 589
Tape worm. *See* TÆNIA SAGINATA, 258
Tar in diseases of the skin, 160
in sycosis, 166
Tartar emetic in schistosomiasis, 256
Technical procedures and oxygen therapy, 1069-1106
aseptic precautions, 1069
aspiration of the pleural cavity, 1088-90
blood transfusion, 1079-84
cisternal puncture, 1095-96
epidural injection, 1096-98
hypodermic injection, 1085-86
intradermal injection, 1084-85
intramuscular injection, 1086-87
intravenous infusion, 1075-79
lumbar puncture, 1090-95
oxygen therapy, 1098-1106
paracentesis of the abdomen, 1087-88
rectal administration of fluid, 1070-71
subcutaneous administration of fluid, 1070
venipuncture, 1071-74
Teeth and peptic ulcer, 544
influence of vitamin deficiency on, 419
Teeth and peptic ulcer—*contd.*
in mercury poisoning, 308-9
in rheumatism, 898
Temperatures, effects of high, 302-3
Test, blood-sugar. *See* BLOOD-SUGAR TEST
Dick. *See* DICK TEST
Fehling, in diabetes, 336
for blood sedimentation rate in arthritis, 887
Frei's. *See* FREI'S TEST
indirect grouping, 1081
Kahn. *See* KAHN TEST
Mantoux. *See* MANTOUX TEST
Mayer-Tanret. *See* MAYER-TANRET REAGENT
Reenstierna's. *See* REENSTIERNA'S TEST
Schick. *See* SCHICK TEST
tuberculin, 118
Van den Bergh. *See* VAN DEN BERGH REACTION
Wassermann. *See* WASSERMANN REACTION
Testicular extracts, in metropathia hæmorrhagica, 1061-62
Testoviron for retarded puberty, 456
Tests, cutaneous scratch, with foreign proteins in urticaria, 185
desensitization, in hay fever, 845
patch, in industrial dermatitis, 317, 318-19
sensitivity, in asthma, 832-33
for serum sensitivity, 801-3
Tetania parathyropriva, 447-49
Tetanus, 64-67
Tetany, alkalotic, 427
and rickets, 420
and uræmia, 862
associated with cœliac disease, 286, 426
associated with vitamin D deficiency, 425-26
clinical varieties: hypocalæmic and eucalcæmic, 423
following removal of parathyroid tumour, 448
gastric, in pyloric stenosis during peptic ulcer, 553
Tetany—*contd.*
of chronic renal disease, 426-27
parathyroid. *See* PARATHYROID GLANDS, 447-50
rachitic, 425-26
serum calcium level in, 424
acid-producing substances, 424-25
parathyroid extract, 424
parenteral administration of calcium, 424
vitamin D supply, 424
Tetrachlorethane in diseases of the liver, 605
poisoning, 314-15
Thallium for epilation in ringworm of the scalp, 168-69
Theelin, 1060
Theelol, in sterility, etc., 455
Theobromine and phenobarbitone as coronary vasodilator, 699
Theobromine as diuretic, 688
in essential hypertension, 653
Theocine as diuretic in congestive heart failure, 688
Theominal in cerebral arteriosclerosis, 997
in essential hypertension, 652-53
Theophylline as diuretic in congestive heart failure, 685, 688
Thiamin in beri-beri, 405
Thiosianamine group of drugs in rheumatoid arthritis, 902, 918
Thiosulphate, sodium, 208
Thoracoplasty, 128-29
in bronchiectasis, 817
Thoracoscope, 127
Thoracotomy in lung abscess, 819
Thread-worm. *See* ENTEROBIASIS, 264
Thrombo-angiitis obliterans, induction of intermittent reactive hyperæmia, 739
local removal of a digit, 738
Thrombocytopenia, 508
Thrombophlebitis causing pulmonary embolism, 822

Thrombosis and the blood flow, 732
Thrombosis, cerebral, 996-97
in typhoid fever, 35
Thrush, 279
Thymic enlargement in infancy, 292
Thymol in ankylostomiasis, 262, 263
in pruritus, 609
in trichuris trichiura, 265
Thyroid extract in cretinism, 295, 430
in essential hypertension, 653
in metropathia hæmorrhagica, 1062
in myxœdema, 431
in nephrosis, 860
in obesity, 396-98
in psoriasis, 191
in rheumatoid arthritis, 900
in simple goitre, 429
Thyroid gland, diseases of, 428-47
cretinism, 430
goitre, simple, 428-30
hyperthyroidism, 432-47
myxœdema, 431-32
Thyroidectomy, 441-42
hæmorrhage in, 446
hyperthyroid crisis in, 445-46
in congestive heart failure, 666, 717
in relief of cardiac pain, 715
myxœdema after, 447
post-operative treatment, 444-47
complications, 445-47
pre-operative, treatment, 442-44
pulmonary infections in, 445
subtotal, in cases of cardiac decompensation, 717-18
in cases of thyrotoxicosis, 717-18
Thyrotoxicosis. *See* HYPERTHYROIDISM, 432-47
Thyroxine in myxœdema, 431
in obesity, 398
Tic douloureux, 1000
Tinnitus, 1002
Tobacco, in angina pectoris, 697
Tobacco—*contd.*
in bronchitis, 793
in pulmonary tuberculosis, 110
in retrobulbar neuritis, 999
in thrombo-angiitis, 736
Tongue in anæmia, 468
Tonic water and pre-cirrhotic hepatitis, 611
constituents, 623
Tonsillar sepsis in rheumatoid arthritis, 898
Tonsillectomy during acute nephritis, 856
Tonsillitis, 755-60
acute, 755-58
chronic, 758-60
complications, 757-58
diet, 756
removal of tonsils, 759
sulphonamide in, 758
Tophi in gout, 962
Torticollis, spasmodic, 1012
Totaquina in malaria, 228
Toxæmia in enteric fever, 34-35
Toxic adenoma, 441
Toxoid-antitoxin floccules in immunization against diphtheria, 20
Tracheotomy in diphtheria, 25
Transfusion, blood, 1079-84
Tribrom-ethyl-alcohol. *See* AVERTIN
Trichloracetic acid in tuberculosis of the skin, 149
Trichlorethylene in ankylostomiasis, 262
in neuralgia, 1000
Trichomonas vaginalis in gonorrhœa, 204
Trichuris trichiura, 265
Trigeminal nerve disorders, 1000-1
Trinitrin in cerebral thrombosis, 997
in vascular lesions of the spinal cord, 989
Trinitrotoluene in diseases of the liver, 605
poisoning, 315
Trocar and cannula, paracentesis by, 1087-88
Tropical diseases, common, 227-65
Tropical neurasthenia, 255-56
Trypan blue in leprosy, 251
Trypanosomiasis, African, 233-35
Tryparsamide in African trypanosomiasis, 233
in G.P.I., 221
in optic atrophy, 219
in syphilis, 207, 216
in tabes dorsalis, 217
Trypflavine in undulant fever, 241
Tube and funnel in oxygen therapy, 1103
Tuberculin as desensitizing agent in asthma, 835
Tuberculin test, 118
Tuberculin treatment of tuberculosis, 116-19
Tuberculomata, 1004-5
Tuberculosis, 92-149
and diabetes, 376
and environmental conditions in, 98
and marriage, 114
and mercury workers, 309
and overcrowding, 98
and pregnancy, 115
diseases predisposing to, 99
"droplet infection" in, 96
due to bovine bacillus, 96-97
early diagnosis in, 99
glandular, 143-46
heliotherapy in, 110
immunity to reinfection, 94
infection, 93-97
prevention of, in children, 95-97
resistance to, 97-99
milk supply in, 97
morbidity due to professional contact, 94
mortality, cause of decline in, 92-93
of cervical glands, 144-45
of epididymis, 143
heliotherapy in, 145
surgical treatment of, 144
of larynx, cauterization in, 140
complicating pulmonary tuberculosis, 138-41
gold treatment of, 139
palliative treatment, 140-41
silence in, 139-40
of mediastinal glands, 145-46
of mesenteric glands, 146

Tuberculosis—*contd.*
of the skin, 148-49
of the spine, 980-81
of urinary tract, 141-43
peritoneal, 147-48
prevention of, 92-99
nutrition in, 98-99
pulmonary, 100-36
after-care in, 113
apicolysis in, 128-29
artificial pneumothorax in, 123-26
blood sedimentation rate, 106
chronic fibroid, 115-16
climate in, 102-3
clothing in, 110
collapse therapy, 121-30
constipation in, 134
cough in, 130-32
diarrhœa in, 134
diet in, 110-12
employment after, 114
exercise in, 104
extrapleural pneumothorax in, 129-30
fever in, 136
fresh air in, 108-10
gastro-intestinal symptoms in, 133-35
general management of, 100-1
gold treatment in, 119-21
hæmoptysis in, 132
intrapleural division of adhesions in, 126-27
pain in, 135
phrenicectomy in, 127-28
polymorph - lymphocyte-monocyte ratio in, 107
pulse-rate in, 105
radiography in, 106
rest in, 103-8
sanatorium treatment in, 101
smoking in, 110
sweating in, 135-36
temperature in, 104
thoracoplasty in, 128-29
tuberculin in, 116-19
tuberculosis of larynx and, 138-41
tuberculous enteritis in, 134
weight in, 107
renal, 141-43

Tuberculosis—*contd.*
segregation of young children, 95-96
Tuberculous epididymitis, 199
meningitis, 981
pleurisy with effusion, 136-38
"Tulip fingers," 319
Tumour, intracranial, 1004-5
Tumours, malignant, 822-23
bronchial carcinoma, 822-23
Hodgkin's disease, 823
lymphosarcoma, 823
of the adrenals, 453-54
of the skull, vertebræ or meninges, 981-83
Turkish baths and obesity, 389
Turpentine enemata, 579
in enteric fever, 34
stupes in asthma, 825
in diarrhœa, 570
"Twilight sleep" in thyroidectomy, 444
Tympanites in acute bronchitis, 787-88
Typhoid fever. *See* ENTERIC FEVER, 30-37
Typhoid fever and the biliary tract, 615
Typhus fever, 67-70

U

Ulcer, gastric and duodenal. *See* ULCER, PEPTIC, 542-60
jejunal or gastrojejunal, 555-56
peptic, 542-60
ætiology, 542
alkalosis following alkali treatment, 553-54
chronic, 542
complications of, 548-54
diabetes and, 378
diet (Meulengracht) in gastro-duodenal hæmorrhage, 560
dietetic treatment, 544-46
Hurst's régime, 557-59
drugs in, 546-48

Ulcer, peptic—*contd.*
gastro - enterostomy and gastrectomy, 555
hæmatemesis and melæna in, 548-52
anæmia following, 552
dietetics following, 551-52
hæmostatics in, 550
operation in, 550-51
hour-glass stomach, 553
hydrochloric acid and, 542-43
initial management of, 543-44
medical treatment before and after operation, 556
of the œsophagus, 535-36
organic pyloric stenosis, 553
perforation, 552
pylorospasm, 552-53
surgery, medical aspects of, 554-56
Ulcerative colitis, 587-91
endocarditis, 640
Ulcers, intestinal, dysenteric. *See* DYSENTERY, 25-27
tuberculous, 134-35
typhoid. *See* ENTERIC FEVER, 30-37
lingual, in anæmia, 468
perforating, in tabes, 220
Ulcus molle of syphilis, 224-25
Uleron in septicæmia, 84, 85
Ultra-violet radiation, and congenital heart disease, 664
and fat tolerance, 418
in alopecia, 187
in cœliac disease, 285
in furunculosis, 762
in industrial dermatitis, 319
in rheumatoid arthritis, 896
in rickets, 418
in tuberculosis of the larynx, 141
in tuberculosis of the skin, 148
in tuberculous adenitis, 145
in tuberculous enteritis, 134

Ultra-violet radiation—*contd.*
protective measures, 321-22
special glass permeable to rays, 417
vitamin D and, 416-18
Undulant fever, 240-41
Unguentum capsici in rheumatoid arthritis, 913
Unna's ichthyol zinc gelatin, in diseases of the skin, 158, 181
Uræmia, in carbon tetrachloride poisoning, 314
in nephritis, acute, 857
chronic, 862-63
Urea as a diuretic in nephrosis, 860
Urea concentration range in nephritis, 854
Urea hydrochloride and quinine in lobar pneumonia, 798
Urea stibamine in Leishmaniasis, 235, 237
Ureter, achalasia of, 880
drainage of, in urinary infections, 880-81
Urethra, instillation of, in gonorrhœa, 196-98, 202-3
Urethra, irrigation of, in gonorrhœa, 196-97
in prostatitis, 199-200
Urethritis. *See* GONORRHŒA, 193-205
Uric acid, in gout, 962-65
Urinary antiseptics, 876-80
hexamine, 879-80
hexyl-resorcinol, 880
mandelic acid, 877-79
pyridine, 880
sulphonamide, 876
Urinary tract, infections of, 869-82
alkalis in, 874-76
antiseptics in, 876-80
bowels, regulation of, 873
control of pain in pyrexia, 874
diet in, 873-74
drainage of the ureter, 880-81
general management of, 872-73
organisms, 871-72
predisposing causes, 870
Urinary tract—*contd.*
pyelitis, 869-71
tuberculosis of, 141-43
Urine, calcium oxalate in, 885
gonadotropic hormone, 1057
in infections of the urinary tract, 871
in multiple myeloma, 968
incontinence of, in tabes dorsalis, 218
microscopic examination, 871
phosphate in, 884
reaction in pyelitis, 874-75
specific gravity of, in nephritis, 854
Urogenital tract, sepsis of, in rheumatoid arthritis, 898
Urotropine in infections of the urinary tract, 879
in enteric fever, 36
Urticaria, 185-86
Uterine bleeding, functional, 1061-62

V

Vaccination for enteric fever, 31
for herpes simplex, 187
for smallpox, 61-62
Vaccine, Haffkine prophylactic, in plague, 240
(T.A.B.) in elephantiasis, 260
in rabies, 254-55
(Ponndorf's) in spondylitis, 929
(B.C.G.) in tuberculosis, 95
Vaccine therapy contraindicated in rosacea, 176
contraindicated in sycosis, 167
in acne, 175
in asthma, 836
in bacillary dysentery, 26
in bronchiectasis, 816
in bronchitis, 793
in enteric fever, 33
in furunculosis, 165
in gonorrhœa, 196
Vaccine therapy—*contd.*
in prevention of respiratory disease, 778-79
in rheumatoid arthritis, 905-7
in septicæmia, 82, 83
in whooping-cough, 70, 71
Vagina, in gonorrhœa, 202
Vaginitis, senile, 1067
Valvulotome, in mitral stenosis, 714
Van den Bergh reaction, 1074
in sprue, 247
Vaquez's disease. *See* POLYCYTHÆMIA VERA, 502-6
Varicose dermatitis, 181
Variola. *See* SMALLPOX, 60-64
Varix in filariasis, 260
Vascular syphilis, 216-17
Vasodilators, coronary, 699
Vasopressin in reticulo-endotheliosis, 524
Vaso-vagal attacks. *See* SIMPLE SYNCOPE, 724-25
Venereal diseases, 192-226. *See also* GONORRHŒA, SYPHILIS, ETC.
Venereal warts, 225
Venesection in cardiac asthma and acute pulmonary œdema, 700
in cerebral hæmorrhage, 996
in congestive heart failure, 689-90
in cyanosis in bronchopneumonia, 785
in hypertension, 653
in polycythæmia, 503-4
in pulmonary œdema, 790
in uræmia, 857, 862
Venipuncture, technique of, 1071-74
intravenous medication, 1072-73
to deplete the circulation, 1074
to obtain a sample for analysis, 1073
Venom, bee, in rheumatism, 918
snake, in purpuras, 514
Ventricular fibrillation, 727
puncture in meningitis, 982